BNF
for children
2010–2011

Royal
Pharmaceutical
Society
of Great Britain

Royal College of
Paediatrics and
Child Health

Published by
BMJ Group
Tavistock Square, London WC1H 9JP, UK

Pharmaceutical Press
Pharmaceutical Press is the publishing division
of the Royal Pharmaceutical Society of Great
Britain
1 Lambeth High Street, London, SE1 7JN, UK

RCPCH Publications Ltd
5–11 Theobalds Road, London WC1X 8SH, UK

Copyright © BMJ Group, Pharmaceutical
Press, and RCPCH Publications Ltd 2010

ISBN: 978 0 85369 927 9

ISSN: 1747–5503

Printed by CPI Clausen & Bosse, Leck, Germany

A catalogue record for this book is available
from the British Library.

Paper copies may be obtained through any
bookseller or direct from:

Pharmaceutical Press
c/o Macmillan Distribution (MDL)
Brunel Rd
Houndmills
Basingstoke
RG21 6XS
UK
Tel: +44 (0) 1256 302 692
Fax: +44 (0) 1256 812 521
E-mail: direct@macmillan.co.uk
www.pharmpress.com

Pharmaceutical Press also supplies *BNF for
Children* in digital formats suitable for standalone use and for use on a personal digital
assistant (PDA).

Distribution of BNFCs
The UK health departments distribute BNFCs to
NHS hospitals, doctors, dental surgeons, and
community pharmacies.
In **England**, BNFCs are mailed individually to
NHS general practitioners and community
pharmacies; contact the DH Publication
Orderline for extra copies or changes relating to
mailed BNFCs
Tel: 0300 123 1002
In **Wales**, telephone the Business Services
Centre
Tel: 01495 332 000
For further information on the supply of copies
of the BNFC to NHS organisations, see
www.library.nhs.uk/orderingbnf

The *BNF for Children* is for use by health
professionals engaged in prescribing, dispensing, and administering medicines to
children. It has been prepared under the
guidance of the Paediatric Formulary Committee.

BNF for Children has been constructed using
robust procedures for gathering, assessing
and assimilating information on paediatric
drug treatment. It is, however, expected that
the reader will be relying on appropriate
professional knowledge and expertise to
interpret the contents in the context of the
circumstances of the individual child. *BNF for
Children* should be used in conjunction with
other appropriate and up-to-date literature
and, where necessary, supplemented by
expert advice. *Special care is required in
managing childhood conditions with unlicensed
medicines or with licensed medicines for unlicensed uses.*

Responsibility for the appropriate use of
medicines lies solely with the individual
health professional.

Contents

Preface

BNF for Children aims to provide prescribers, pharmacists and other healthcare professionals with sound up-to-date information on the use of medicines for treating children.

A joint publication of the British Medical Association, the Royal Pharmaceutical Society of Great Britain, the Royal College of Paediatrics and Child Health, and the Neonatal and Paediatric Pharmacists Group, *BNF for Children* ('BNFC') is published under the authority of a Paediatric Formulary Committee.

Many areas of paediatric practice have suffered from inadequate information on effective medicines. BNFC addresses this significant knowledge gap by providing practical information on the use of medicines in children of all ages from birth to adolescence. *Medicines for Children* (RCPCH Publications Ltd) and the *British National Formulary* itself form the basis for BNFC. Information in BNFC has been validated against emerging evidence, best-practice guidelines, and crucially, advice from a network of clinical experts.

Drawing information from manufacturers' literature where appropriate, BNFC also includes a great deal of advice that goes beyond marketing authorisations (product licences). This is necessary because licensed indications frequently do not cover the clinical needs of children; in some cases, products for use in children need to be specially manufactured or imported. Careful consideration has been given to establishing the clinical need for unlicensed interventions with respect to the evidence and experience of their safety and efficacy; local paediatric formularies, clinical literature and national information resources have been invaluable in this process.

BNFC has been designed for rapid reference and the information presented has been carefully selected to aid decisions on prescribing, dispensing and administration of medicines. Less detail is given on areas such as malignant disease and the very specialist use of medicines generally undertaken in tertiary centres. BNFC should be interpreted in the light of professional knowledge and it should be supplemented as necessary by specialised publications. Information is also available from medicines information services (see inside front cover).

The website (bnfc.org) includes additional information of relevance to healthcare professionals. BNFC is also available on other digital platforms.

BNFC aims to provide information suited to the needs of the clinician and recognises that, although this edition represents a considerable advance in the content and presentation of information on the paediatric use of medicines, further changes will be necessary. Comments from healthcare professionals are therefore very welcome and should be sent to:

British National Formulary Publications, Royal Pharmaceutical Society of Great Britain, 1 Lambeth High Street, London SE1 7JN. bnfc@bnf.org

Acknowledgements

The Paediatric Formulary Committee is grateful to individuals and organisations that have provided advice and information to the *BNF for Children*.

The principal contributors for this edition were: I.H. Ahmed-Jushuf, M.N. Badminton, S. Bailey, T.G. Barrett, D.N. Bateman, G.D.L. Bates, H. Bedford, M.W. Beresford, R.M. Bingham, I.W. Booth, L. Brook, K.G. Brownlee, R.J. Buckley, M. Burch, I.F. Burgess, A. Cant, L.J. Carr, R. Carr, E.A. Chalmers, T.D. Cheetham, A.J. Cotgrove, J.B.S. Coulter, B.G. Craig, S.M. Creighton, J.H. Cross, A. Dhawan, P.N. Durrington, A. Durward, A.B. Edgar, J.A. Edge, D.A.C. Elliman, N.D. Embleton, P.J. Goadsby, J. Gray, J.W. Gregory, P. Gringras, J.P. Harcourt, P.J. Helms, C. Hendriksz, R.F. Howard, R.G. Hull, H.R. Jenkins, S. Jones, B.A. Judd, C.J.H. Kelnar, P.T. Khaw, J.M.W. Kirk, P.J. Lee, T.H. Lee, S. Lewis-Jones, E.G.H. Lyall, A. MacDonald, D.J. Macrae, P.S. Malone, A.Y. Manzur, S.D. Marks, A.G. Marson, P.J. McKiernan, L.M. Melvin, E. Miller, C. Moss, P. Mulholland, J.M. Neuberger, K.K. Nischal, C.Y. Ng, L.P. Omerod, J.Y. Paton, G.A. Pearson, M.M. Ramsay, J.M. Rennie, I.A.G. Roberts, J. Rogers, K.E. Rogstad, P.C. Rubin, J.W. Sander, N.J. Scolding, M.R. Sharland, N.J. Shaw, G.J. Shortland, O.F.W. Stumper, A.G. Sutcliffe, A. Sutherland, A.M. Szarewski, E.A. Taylor, A.H. Thomson, M.A. Thomson, J.A. Vale, J.O. Warner, D.A. Warrell, N.J.A. Webb, A.D. Weeks, R. Welbury, W.P. Whitehouse, C.E. Willoughby, C. Wren, A. Wright, M.M. Yaqoob, Z. Zaiwalla, and S.M. Zuberi.

Members of the British Association of Dermatologists Therapy Guidelines Subcommittee, L.C. Fuller, J. Hughes, S. Hulley, J. Lear, N.J. Levell, A.J. McDonagh, N. Morar, S. Punjabi, M.J. Tidman, P.D. Yesudian, and M.F.M. Mustapa (Secretariat) have provided valuable advice.

Members of the Advisory Committee on Malaria Prevention, B.A. Bannister, R.H. Behrens, P.L. Chiodini, F. Genasi, L. Goodyer, A. Green, D. Hill, G. Kassianos, D.G. Lalloo, G. Lea, G. Pasvol, M. Powell, D.V. Shingadia, D.A. Warrell, C.J.M. Whitty, and C. Lucas (Secretariat) have also provided valuable advice.

R. Suvarna and colleagues at the MHRA have provided valuable assistance.

Correspondents in the pharmaceutical industry have provided information on new products and commented on products in the *BNF for Children*. NHS Prescription Services has supplied the prices of products in the *BNF for Children*.

Numerous doctors, pharmacists, nurses and others have sent comments and suggestions.

The *BNF for Children* has valuable access to the *Martindale* data banks by courtesy of S. Sweetman and staff.

J. E. Macintyre and staff provided valuable technical assistance

C. Adetola, O. Akporobaro-Iwudibia, K.L. d'Almeida, N. Bansal, A. Breewood, J.J. Coleman, M. Davis, J.A. Dickin, C. Fischetti, S. Foad, E.H. Glover, D.T.H. Griffiths, T. Hamp, A. Holmes, J. Humphreys, J.M. James, E. Laughton, H.M.N. Neill, O. Ojeleye, J.L. Palmer, R.M. Patel, S.J. Qureshi, J. Reynolds, and E.J. Tong provided considerable assistance during the production of this edition of *BNF for Children*.

Xpage have provided technical assistance with the editorial database and typesetting software.

BNF Staff

Managing Editor: Knowledge Creation
John Martin *BPharm, PhD, MRPharmS*

Assistant Editors
Leigh-Anne Claase *BSc, PhD, MRPharmS*
Bryony Jordan *BSc, DipPharmPract, MRPharmS*
Colin R. Macfarlane *BPharm, MSc, MRPharmS*
Paul S. Maycock *MPharm, DipPharmPract, MRPharmS*
Allison F. Patterson *BPharm, MRPharmS*
Rachel S. M. Ryan *BPharm, MRPharmS*
Shama M. S. Wagle *BPharm, DipPharmPract, MRPharmS*

Staff Editors
Sejal Amin *BPharm, MSc, MRPharmS*
Angela K. Bennett *MPharm, DipPharmPract, MRPharmS*
Shena S. Chauhan *BPharm, MRPharmS*
Susan E. Clarke *BPharm, DipClinPharm, MRPharmS*
Belén Granell Villen *BSc, PGDipClinPharm, MRPharmS*
Manjula Halai *BScChem, MPharm, MRPharmS*
Emma E. Harris *MPharm, DipPharmPract, MRPharmS*
Amy E. Harvey *MPharm, PGDipCommPharm, MRPharmS*
Amber F. Lauder *BPharm, PGCertPharm, MRPharmS*
Angela M. G. McFarlane *BSc, DipClinPharm, MRPharmS*
Jaime M. Miks *MPharm, DipClinPharm, MRPharmS*
Elizabeth Nix *DipPharm(NZ), MRPharmS*
Sanjay Patel *BPharm, MRPharmS*
Claire L. Preston *BPharm, MRPharmS*
Nirvashi Ramgoolam *BPharm, MRPharmS*
Vinaya K. Sharma *BPharm, MSc, PGDipPIM, MRPharmS*

Editorial Assistants
Rebecca S. Bastable *BA, BTEC*
Cristina Lopez-Bueno *BA*

Senior BNF Administrator
Heidi Homar *BA*

Administrative Assistant
Zoe Daniel

Managing Editor: Digital Development and Delivery
Cornelia Schnelle *MPhil*

Digital Development Editor
Philip D. Lee *BSc, PhD*

Digital Development Assistants
Robert C. Buckingham *BSc*
Michelle Cartwright
Zephyr M. Wastell *BTEC*

Terminologist
Sarah Peck *BSc*

Head of Publishing Services
John Wilson

BNF Publishing Director
Duncan S.T. Enright *MA, PGCE, MInstP, FIDM*

Managing Director, Pharmaceutical Press
Robert Bolick *BA, MA*

Senior Medical Adviser
Martin J. Kendall *OBE, MB, ChB, MD, FRCP, FFPM*

Paediatric Formulary Committee 2009–2010

Chair
Warren Lenny
MD, FRCP, FRCPCH, DCH

Committee Members
Jeffrey K. Aronson
MA, MBChB, DPhil, FRCP, FBPharmacolS, FFPM

Judith H. Cope
BPharm, MSc, MRPharmS

Ian Costello
BPharm, MSc, MRPharmS

Simon Keady
BSc, MRPharmS, SP

Martin J. Kendall
OBE, MB, ChB, MD, FRCP, FFPM (Chair, Content Strategy Committee)

James H. Larcombe
MB, ChB, FRCGP, DipAdvGP

Neena Modi
MB, ChB, MD, FRCP, FRCPCH

Matthew J. Thatcher
MBBS, FRCS, DRCOG, DMRD

William G. van't Hoff
BSc, MB, MD, FRCPCH, FRCP

Edward R. Wozniak
BSc, MB, BS, FRCP, FRCPCH, DCH

Observer
Jane Houghton
RGN, RSCN, DNCert, MSc

Executive Secretary
Heidi Homar
BA

Dental Advisory Group 2009–2010

Chair
David Wray
MD, BDS, MB ChB, FDSRCPS, FDSRCS Ed, F MedSci

Committee Members
Christine Arnold
BDS, DDPHRCS, MCDH

Barry Cockcroft
BDS, FFDS (Eng)

Duncan S.T. Enright *MA, PGCE, MInstP, FIDM*

Amy E. Harvey *MPharm, PGDipCommPharm, MRPharmS*

Martin J. Kendall
OBE, MB, ChB, MD, FRCP, FFPM

Lesley P. Longman
BSc, BDS, FDSRCS Ed, PhD

John Martin
BPharm, PhD, MRPharmS

Michelle Moffat
BDS, MFDS RCS Ed, M Paed Dent RPCS, FDS (Paed Dent) RSC Ed

Richard J. Oliver
BDS, BSc, PhD, FDSRCPS, FDS (OS) RCPS

Rachel S.M. Ryan
BPharm, MRPharmS

Secretary
Arianne J. Matlin
MA, MSc, PhD

Executive Secretary
Heidi Homar
BA

> **Advice on dental practice**
> The **British Dental Association** has contributed to the advice on medicines for dental practice through its representatives on the Dental Advisory Group.

Nurse Prescribers' Advisory Group 2009–2010

Chair
Nicky A. Cullum
PhD, RGN

Committee Members
Shena S. Chauhan
BPharm, MRPharmS

Rebecca F. Cheatle
BSc, RGN

Michele L. Cossey
BPharm, MSc, MRPharmS

Molly Courtenay
PhD, MSc, Cert Ed, BSc, RGN

Duncan S.T. Enright
MA, PGCE, MInstP, FIDM

Penny M. Franklin
RN, RCN, RSCPHN(HV), MA, PGCE

Margaret F. Helliwell
MB, BS, BSc, MFPHM

Bryony Jordan
BSc, DipPharmPract, MRPharmS

Martin J. Kendall
OBE, MB, ChB, MD, FRCP, FFPM

Fiona Lynch
BSc, MSc, RGN, RSCN

John Martin
BPharm, PhD, MRPharmS

Maureen P. Morgan
RN, RHV, MBA

Elizabeth J. Plastow
RMN, RGN, RSCPHN(HV), MSc, PGDipEd

Paul G.H. Robinson

Gul Root
BSc, MRPharmS, DMS

Jill M. Shearer
BSc, RGN, RM

Rabina Tindale
RN, RSCN, BSc, DipAEN, PGCE

Vicky Vidler
MA, RGN, RSCN

Executive Secretary
Heidi Homar
BA

How *BNF for Children* is constructed

BNF for Children (BNFC) is unique in bringing together authoritative, independent guidance on best practice with clinically validated drug information, enabling healthcare professionals to select safe and effective medicines for individual children.

Information in BNFC has been validated against emerging evidence, best-practice guidelines, and advice from a network of clinical experts. BNFC includes a great deal of advice that goes beyond marketing authorisations (product licences or summaries of product characteristics). This is necessary because licensed indications frequently do not cover the clinical needs of children; in some cases, products for use in children need to be specially manufactured or imported. Careful consideration has been given to establishing the clinical need for unlicensed interventions with respect to the evidence and experience of their safety and efficacy.

Hundreds of changes are made between editions, and the most clinically significant changes are listed at the front of each edition.

Paediatric Formulary Committee

The Paediatric Formulary Committee (PFC) is responsible for the content of BNFC. The PFC includes a neonatologist and paediatricians appointed by the Royal College of Paediatrics and Child Health, paediatric pharmacists appointed by the Royal Pharmaceutical Society of Great Britain and the Neonatal and Paediatric Pharmacists Group, doctors appointed by the BMJ Publishing Group, a GP appointed by the Royal College of General Practitioners, and representatives from the Medicines and Healthcare products Regulatory Agency (MHRA) and the UK health departments. The PFC decides on matters of policy and reviews amendments to BNFC in the light of new evidence and expert advice. The Committee meets every 6 months and each member also receives proofs of all BNFC chapters for review before publication.

Dental Advisory Group

The Dental Advisory Group oversees the preparation of advice on the drug management of dental and oral conditions; the group includes representatives from the British Dental Association.

Editorial team

BNFC staff editors are pharmacists with a sound understanding of how drugs are used in clinical practice, including paediatrics. Each staff editor is responsible for editing, maintaining, and updating specific chapters of BNFC. During the publication cycle the staff editors review information in BNFC against a variety of sources (see below).

Amendments to the text are drafted when the editors are satisfied that any new information is reliable and relevant. The draft amendments are passed to expert advisers for comment and then presented to the Paediatric Formulary Committee for consideration. Additionally, for each edition, sections are chosen from every chapter for thorough review. These planned reviews aim to verify all the information in the selected sections and to draft any amendments to reflect current best practice.

Staff editors prepare the text for publication and undertake a number of checks on the knowledge at various stages of the production.

Expert advisers

BNFC uses about 80 expert clinical advisers (including doctors, pharmacists, nurses, and dentists) throughout the UK to help with the production of each edition. The role of these expert advisers is to review existing text and to comment on amendments drafted by the staff editors. These clinical experts help to ensure that BNFC remains reliable by:

- commenting on the relevance of the text in the context of best clinical practice in the UK;

- checking draft amendments for appropriate interpretation of any new evidence;
- providing expert opinion in areas of controversy or when reliable evidence is lacking;
- advising on areas where BNFC diverges from summaries of product characteristics;
- advising on the use of unlicensed medicines or of licensed medicines for unlicensed uses ('off-label' use);
- providing independent advice on drug interactions, prescribing in hepatic impairment, renal impairment, pregnancy, breast-feeding, neonatal care, palliative care, and the emergency treatment of poisoning.

In addition to consulting with regular advisers, BNFC calls on other clinical specialists for specific developments when particular expertise is required.

BNFC also works closely with a number of expert bodies that produce clinical guidelines. Drafts or pre-publication copies of guidelines are routinely received for comment and for assimilation into BNFC.

Sources of BNFC information

BNFC uses a variety of sources for its information; the main ones are shown below.

Summaries of product characteristics   BNFC receives summaries of product characteristics (SPCs) of all new products as well as revised SPCs for existing products. The SPCs are a key source of product information and are carefully processed, despite the ever-increasing volume of information being issued by the pharmaceutical industry. Such processing involves:

- verifying the approved names of all relevant ingredients including 'non-active' ingredients (BNFC is committed to using approved names and descriptions as laid down by the Medicines Act);
- comparing the indications, cautions, contra-indications, and side-effects with similar existing drugs. Where these are different from the expected pattern, justification is sought for their inclusion or exclusion;
- seeking independent data on the use of drugs in pregnancy and breast-feeding;
- incorporating the information into BNFC using established criteria for the presentation and inclusion of the data;
- checking interpretation of the information by two staff editors before submitting to a senior editor; changes relating to doses receive an extra check;
- identifying potential clinical problems or omissions and seeking further information from manufacturers or from expert advisers;
- careful validation of any areas of divergence of BNFC from the SPC before discussion by the Committee (in the light of supporting evidence);
- constructing, with the help of expert advisers, a comment on the role of the drug in the context of similar drugs.

Much of this processing is applicable to the following sources as well.

Expert advisers   The role of expert clinical advisers in providing the appropriate clinical context for all BNFC information is discussed above.

Literature   Staff editors monitor core medical, paediatric, and pharmaceutical journals. Research papers and reviews relating to drug therapy are carefully processed. When a difference between the advice in BNFC and the paper is noted, the new information is assessed for reliability and relevance to UK clinical practice. If necessary, new text is drafted and discussed with expert advisers and the Paediatric Formulary Committee. BNFC enjoys a close working relationship with a number of national information providers.

Systematic reviews   BNFC has access to various databases of systematic reviews (including the Cochrane Library and various web-based resources). These are used for answering specific queries, for reviewing existing text and for constructing new text. Staff editors receive training in critical appraisal, literature evaluation, and search strategies. Reviews published in Clinical Evidence are used to validate BNFC advice.

Consensus guidelines   The advice in BNFC is checked against consensus guidelines produced by expert bodies. A number of bodies make drafts or pre-publication copies of the guidelines available to BNFC; it is therefore possible to ensure that a consistent message is disseminated. BNFC routinely processes guidelines from the National Institute for Health and Clinical Excellence (NICE), the Scottish Medicines Consortium (SMC), and the Scottish Intercollegiate Guidelines Network (SIGN).

Reference sources   Paediatric formularies and reference sources are used to provide background information for the review of existing text or for the construction of new text. The BNFC team works closely with the editorial team that produces *Martindale: The Complete Drug Reference*. BNFC has access to *Martindale* information resources and each team keeps the other informed of significant developments and shifts in the trends of drug usage.

Statutory information   BNFC routinely processes relevant information from various Government bodies including Statutory Instruments and regulations affecting the Prescription only Medicines Order. Official compendia such as the British Pharmacopoeia and its addenda are processed routinely to ensure that BNFC complies with the relevant sections of the Medicines Act.

BNFC maintains close links with the Home Office (in relation to controlled drug regulations) and the Medicines and Healthcare products Regulatory Agency (including the British Pharmacopoeia Commission). Safety warnings issued by the Commission on Human Medicines (CHM) and guidelines on drug use issued by the UK health departments are processed as a matter of routine.

Relevant professional statements issued by the Royal Pharmaceutical Society of Great Britain are included in BNFC as are guidelines from bodies such as the Royal College of Paediatrics and Child Health.

BNFC reflects information from the Drug Tariff, the Scottish Drug Tariff, and the Northern Ireland Drug Tariff.

Pricing information   NHS Prescription Services provide information on prices of medicinal products and appliances in BNFC. BNFC also receives and processes price lists from product suppliers.

Comments from readers   Readers of BNFC are invited to send in comments. Numerous letters and emails are received during the preparation of each edition. Such feedback helps to ensure that BNFC provides practical and clinically relevant information. Many changes in the presentation and scope of BNFC have resulted from comments sent in by users.

Comments from industry   Close scrutiny of BNFC by the manufacturers provides an additional check and allows them an opportunity to raise issues about BNFC's presentation of the role of various drugs; this is yet another check on the balance of BNFC advice. All comments are looked at with care and, where necessary, additional information and expert advice are sought.

Virtual user groups   BNFC has set up virtual user groups across various healthcare professions (e.g. doctors, pharmacists, nurses). The aim of these groups will be to provide feedback to the editors and publishers to ensure that BNF publications continue to serve the needs of its users.

Market research   Market research is conducted at regular intervals to gather feedback on specific areas of development, such as drug interactions or changes to the way information is presented in digital formats.

> BNFC is an independent professional publication that is kept up-to-date and addresses the day-to-day prescribing information needs of healthcare professionals treating children. Use of this resource throughout the health service helps to ensure that medicines are used safely, effectively, and appropriately in children.

How to use *BNF for Children*

> The *BNF for Children* provides information on the use of medicines in children ranging from neonates (including preterm neonates) to adolescents. The terms infant, child, and adolescent are not used consistently in the literature; to avoid ambiguity actual ages are used in the dose statements in *BNF for Children*. The term neonate is used to describe a newborn infant aged 0–28 days. The terms child or children are used generically to describe the entire range from infant to adolescent in *BNF for Children*.

BNF for Children is divided into the following broad areas.

General Guidance

The section on general guidance includes general advice on the use of medicines for managing childhood conditions. It also includes information on prescribing controlled drugs and the management of palliative care. Advice is given on the reporting of adverse reactions. General principles on the use of medicines in hepatic impairment, renal impairment, pregnancy, and breast-feeding are also included in this section.

Notes on conditions, drugs and preparations

The main text consists of classified notes on clinical conditions, drugs and preparations. These notes are divided into 15 chapters, each of which is related to a particular system of the body or to an aspect of neonatal and paediatric medical care. Each chapter is then divided into sections which begin with *notes* on the selection and use of medicines. Guidance on dental and oral conditions is identified by means of a relevant heading (e.g. Dental and Orofacial pain) in the appropriate sections. The notes are followed by details of relevant drugs and preparations.

Drug entries

Drugs appear under pharmacopoeial or other non-proprietary titles. When there is an *appropriate current monograph* (Medicines Act 1968, Section 65) preference is given to a name at the head of that monograph; otherwise a British Approved Name (BAN), if available, is used. Information on the properties of each drug is organised as shown in the illustration below; the information on cautions, contra-indications, side-effects, dose and indications reflects, as far as possible, the manufacturer's summary of product characteristics.

Side-effects are generally listed in order of frequency and arranged broadly by body systems. Occasionally a rare side-effect might be listed first if it is considered to be particularly important because of its seriousness.

For the majority of drugs, *doses* are expressed in terms of body-weight (i.e. standardised by weight). To calculate the dose for a given child the weight-standardised dose is multiplied by the child's weight (or occasionally by the child's ideal body-weight). The calculated dose should not normally exceed the maximum recommended dose for an adult. For example if the dose is 8 mg/kg (max. 300 mg) a child of 10 kg body-weight should receive 80 mg but a child of 40 kg body-weight should receive 300 mg (rather than 320 mg).

> Doses are expressed for specific age ranges; neonatal doses are preceded by the word Neonate, all other doses are preceded by the word Child. Age ranges in the BNF for Children are described as follows:
>
> Child 1 month–4 years refers to a child from 1 month old up to their 4th birthday;
>
> Child 4–10 years refers to a child from the day of their 4th birthday up to their 10th birthday.
>
> However, a pragmatic approach should be applied to these cut-off points depending on the child's physiological development, condition, and if weight is appropriate for the child's age.

DRUG NAME ◢◀

Cautions details of precautions required and also any monitoring required
Counselling Verbal explanation to the patient of specific details of the drug treatment (e.g. posture when taking a medicine)

Contra-indications details of any contra-indications to use of drug

Hepatic impairment advice on the use of a drug in hepatic impairment

Renal impairment advice on the use of a drug in renal impairment

Pregnancy advice on the use of a drug during pregnancy

Breast-feeding advice on the use of a drug during breast-feeding

Side-effects details of common and more serious side-effects

Licensed use licensing status where this is of clinical relevance

Indication and dose
Details of uses and indications
● By route
　Child dose and frequency of administration (max. dose) for specific age group

● By alternative route
　Child dose and frequency

[1]**Approved Name** (Non-proprietary) [PoM] ◀
Pharmaceutical form colour, coating, active ingredient and amount in dosage form, net price, pack size = basic NHS price. Label: (as in Appendix 3)
1. Exceptions to the prescribing status are indicated by a note or footnote.

Proprietary Name (Manufacturer) [PoM] [NHS] ◀
Pharmaceutical form sugar-free, active ingredient mg/mL, net price, pack size = basic NHS price. Label: (as in Appendix 3)
Excipients include clinically important excipients or electrolytes
Note Specific notes about the product e.g. handling

Preparations

Preparations usually follow immediately after the drug which is their main ingredient.

Preparations are included under a non-proprietary title, if they are marketed under such a title, if they are not otherwise prescribable under the NHS, or if they may be prepared extemporaneously.

If proprietary preparations are of a distinctive colour this is stated.

In the case of compound preparations the indications, cautions, contra-indications, side-effects, and interactions of all constituents should be taken into account for prescribing.

When no suitable licensed preparation is available details of preparations that may be imported or formulations available as manufactured specials or extemporaneous preparations are included.

Drugs

The symbol ◢ is used to denote those preparations considered to be less suitable for prescribing. Although such preparations may not be considered as drugs of first choice, their use may be justifiable in certain circumstances.

Prescription-only medicines

This symbol [PoM] has been placed against preparations that are available only on a prescription from an appropriate practitioner.

The symbol [CD] indicates that the preparation is subject to the prescription requirements of the Misuse of Drugs Act. For advice on prescribing such preparations see Prescribing Controlled Drugs.

Preparations not available for NHS prescription

This symbol [NHS] has been placed against preparations that are not prescribable under the NHS. Those prescribable only for specific disorders have a footnote specifying the condition(s) for which the preparation remains available. Some preparations which are not *prescribable* by brand name under the NHS may nevertheless be *dispensed* using the brand name provided that the prescription shows an appropriate non-proprietary name.

Prices

Prices have been calculated from the basic cost used in pricing NHS prescriptions. The price for an extemporaneously prepared preparation has been omitted where the net cost of the ingredients used to make it would give a misleadingly low impression of the final price. Since the prices shown in the *BNF for Children* do not include professional fees and overhead allowances, they are not suitable for quoting to patients seeking private prescriptions or contemplating over-the-counter purchase.

How to use BNFC

Emergency treatment of poisoning

This chapter provides information on the management of acute poisoning when first seen, although aspects of hospital-based treatment are mentioned.

Appendices and indices

The appendices include information on interactions, borderline substances, and cautionary and advisory labels for dispensed medicines. They are designed for use in association with the main body of the text.

The Dental Practitioners' List and the Nurse Prescribers' List are also included in this section. The indices consist of the Index of Manufacturers and the Main Index.

Patient Packs

Directive 92/27/EEC specifies the requirements for the labelling of medicines and outlines the format and content of patient information leaflets to be supplied with every medicine; the directive also requires the use of Recommended International Non-proprietary Names for drugs.

All medicines have approved labelling and patient information leaflets; anyone who supplies a medicine is responsible for providing the relevant information to the patient (see also Appendix 3).

Many medicines are available in manufacturers' original packs complete with patient information leaflets. Where patient packs are available, the *BNF for Children* shows the number of dose units in the packs. In particular clinical circumstances, where patient packs need to be split or medicines are provided in bulk dispensing packs, manufacturers will provide additional supplies of patient information leaflets on request.

During the revision of each edition of this publication careful note is taken of the information that appears on the patient information leaflets. Where it is considered appropriate to alert a prescriber to some specific limitation appearing on the patient information leaflet (for example, in relation to pregnancy) this advice now appears in the *BNF for Children*, see also General guidance, patient information leaflets.

The patient information leaflet also includes details of all inactive ingredients in the medicine. A list of common E numbers and the inactive ingredients to which they correspond is now therefore included in the *BNF for Children* (see inside back cover).

PACT and SPA

PACT (Prescribing Analyses and Cost) and SPA (Scottish Prescribing Analysis) provide prescribers with information about their prescribing.

The *PACT Standard Report*, or in Scotland SPA *Level 1 Report*, is sent to all general practitioners on a quarterly basis. The PACT Standard Report contains an analysis of the practitioner's prescribing and the practice prescribing over the last 3 months, and gives comparisons with the local Primary Care Trust equivalent practice and with a national equivalent. The report also contains details of the practice prescribing for a specific topic; a different topic is chosen each quarter.

The *PACT Catalogue*, or in Scotland SPA *Level 2 Report*, provides a full inventory of the prescriptions issued by a prescriber. The PACT catalogue is available on request for periods between 1 and 24 months. To allow the prescriber to target specific areas of prescribing, a Catalogue may be requested to cover individual preparations, BNF sections, or combinations of BNF chapters.

PACT is also available electronically (www.nhsbsa.nhs.uk). This system gives users on-line access through NHSnet to the 3 years' prescribing data held on the NHS Prescription Services' database; tools for analysing the data are also provided.

Prices in the *BNF for Children*

Basic **net prices** are given in the *BNF for Children* to provide an indication of relative cost. Where there is a choice of suitable preparations for a particular disease or condition the relative cost may be used in making a selection. Cost-effective prescribing must, however, take into account other factors (such as dose frequency and duration of treatment) that affect the total cost. The use of more expensive drugs is justified if it will result in better treatment of the patient or a reduction of the length of an illness or the time spent in hospital.

Prices have generally been calculated from the net cost used in pricing NHS prescriptions dispensed in November 2009; unless an original pack is available these prices are based on the largest pack size of the preparation in use in community pharmacies. The price for an extemporaneously prepared preparation has been omitted where the net cost of the ingredients used to make it would give a misleadingly low impression of the final price.

The unit of 20 is still sometimes used as a basis for comparison, but where suitable original packs or patient packs are available these are priced instead.

Gross prices vary as follows:

1. Costs to the NHS are greater than the net prices quoted and include professional fees and overhead allowances;
2. Private prescription charges are calculated on a separate basis;
3. Over-the-counter sales are at retail price, as opposed to basic net price, and include VAT.

> *BNF for Children* prices are not, therefore, suitable for quoting to patients seeking private prescriptions or contemplating over-the-counter purchases.

A fuller explanation of costs to the NHS may be obtained from the Drug Tariff.

It should be noted that separate Drug Tariffs are applicable to England and Wales, Scotland, and Northern Ireland. Prices in the different tariffs may vary.

Changes for this edition

Significant changes

The *BNF for Children* is revised yearly and numerous changes are made between issues. All copies of *BNF for Children 2009* should therefore be withdrawn and replaced by *BNF for Children 2010–2011*. Significant changes have been made in the following sections for *BNF for Children 2010–2011*:

Equivalent doses of morphine sulphate and diamorphine hydrochloride [table amended], Prescribing in palliative care

Benzodiazepine poisoning, Emergency treatment of poisoning

Paracetamol poisoning, Emergency treatment of poisoning

Constipation, section 1.6

Oral anticoagulants: Haemorrhage [management of elevated values in adults], section 2.8.2

Blood products [new section], section 2.11

Lipid-regulating drugs [management of hypercholesterolaemia], section 2.12

Symbicort® [maintenance and reliever therapy for children 12–18 years], section 3.2

Treatment of schizophrenia, section 4.2.1

Aripiprazole [monograph added], section 4.2.1

Treatment of bipolar disorder, section 4.2.3

Treatment of depression, section 4.3

Tricyclic antidepressant drugs [section updated and reorganised], section 4.3.1

Zolmitriptan [monograph added], section 4.7.4.1

Clostridium difficile infection and peritonitis, section 5.1, Table 1

Pneumonia possibly caused by atypical pathogens, section 5.1, Table 1

Syphilis and pelvic inflammatory disease, section 5.1, Table 1

Osteomyelitis and septic arthritis, section 5.1, Table 1

Congenital gonococcal conjunctivitis, section 5.1, Table 1

Staphylococcal scalded skin syndrome, section 5.1, Table 1

Prevention of *Staphylococcus aureus* lung infection in cystic fibrosis, section 5.1, Table 2

Prevention of infection in gastro-intestinal procedures, section 5.1, Table 2

Ceftriaxone [contra-indications and administration], section 5.1.2

Minocycline [application of 'less suitable for prescribing' symbol], section 5.1.3

Treatment of fungal infections: deep and disseminated candidiasis, section 5.2

Treatment of fungal infections: Immunocompromised children, section 5.2

Ketoconazole [addition of 'less suitable for prescribing' symbol], section 5.2

Prophylaxis and treatment of influenza in pregnancy and breast-feeding, section 5.3.4

Intravenous quinine for benign malaria in children unable to take oral therapy, section 5.4.1

Prophylaxis against malaria, recommendations for Cambodia and Jamaica, section 5.4.1

Measurement of HbA$_{1c}$ [update on units], section 6.1

Examples of insulin regimens, section 6.1.1

Diabetes and surgery, section 6.1.1

Insulin detemir and insulin glargine for type 2 diabetes [NICE guidance updated], section 6.1.1.2

Oral hypoglycaemic drugs for type 2 diabetes during pregnancy and breast-feeding, section 6.1.2

Diabetic ketoacidosis, section 6.1.3

Monitoring devices for diabetes mellitus [meters and test strips], section 6.1.6

Bisphosphonates and osteonecrosis of the jaw [MHRA/CHM advice], section 6.6.2

Information on safe systems for cytotoxic medicines, extra information on dosing and National Patient Safety Agency advice on prescribing and use of oral cytotoxic medicines, section 8.1

Rationalisation of folinic acid monograph, section 8.1

Rationalisation of levofolinic acid monograph, section 8.1

Azathioprine and thiopurine methyltransferase (TPMT) testing, section 8.2.1

Prescribing of oral ciclosporin by brand and formulation and switching between formulations [updated advice], section 8.2.2

Tacrolimus [correct use of formulations], section 8.2.2

Drugs unsafe for use in acute porphyrias, section 9.8.2

Piroxicam [application of 'less suitable for prescribing' symbol], section 10.1.1

Removal of ear wax, section 12.1.3

Topical nasal decongestants, section 12.2.2

Isotretinoin [pregnancy prevention], section 13.6.2

Vaccinations in babies born preterm, section 14.1

Immunoglobulins [section reorganised and updated], section 14.5

Foods for special diets [gluten-free and low-protein foods—sections reorganised], section A2.6

Dose changes

Changes in dose statements introduced into *BNF for Children 2010–2011*:

Aciclovir [neonatal prophy-laxis of chickenpox], p. 392

Adcortyl® Intra-articular/Intra-dermal [intra-articular dose], p. 617

Adenosine, p. 111

Alprostadil, p. 168

AmBisome®, p. 371

Aminophylline [severe acute asthma], p. 183

Amoxicillin [community-acquired pneumonia, sal-monellosis, and Lyme dis-ease], p. 320

Ampicillin [community-aquired pneumonia and sal-monellosis], p. 321

Anapen®, p. 204

Atracurium besilate [neuro-muscular blockade during intensive care], p. 790

Atropine [control of muscari-nic side-effects of neo-stigmine in reversal of com-petitive neuromuscular block], p. 780

Avamys®, p. 659

Baclofen [by mouth], p. 626

Bisacodyl, p. 79

Carnitine [primary deficiency and organic acidaemias], p. 597

Caspofungin, p. 371

Ceftriaxone [uncomplicated gonorrhoea], p. 330

Cefuroxime [Lyme disease], p. 331

Chloral hydrate [neonatal dose deleted], p. 216

Ciprofloxacin, p. 365

Deferasirox, p. 549

Dexamfetamine, p. 241

Diamorphine [intranasal], p. 259

Diazepam [rectal dose for status epilepticus], p. 291

Dinoprostone, p. 169

Docusate sodium, p. 80

Ephedrine hydrochloride [nasal drops], p. 661

Epipen®, p. 205

Fentanyl [peri-operative and intensive care, all doses], p. 788

Fluconazole [tinea capitis caused by *Trichophyton* spp.], p. 372

Furosemide [intravenous injection dose for oedema in 1 month–12 years], p. 104

Hydrocortisone [intravenous injection for acute asthma], p. 171

Imiglucerase, p. 598

Isoniazid [tuberculosis, stan-dard unsupervised treatment regimen], p. 355

Kenalog® Intra-articular/Intra-muscular [intra-articular dose], p. 617

Lactulose, p. 82

Levetiracetam [monotherapy on partial seizures], p. 280

Lisinopril, p. 134

Loratadine, p. 197

Losartan, p. 134

Manevac® granules, p. 81

Mebendazole [roundworms], p. 420

Metoprolol [hypertension], p. 119

Metronidazole [intestinal amoebiasis], p. 413

Miconazole [oral local lesions], p. 666

Mirena®, p. 495

Morphine [pain], p. 262

Movicol® *Paediatric Plain*, p. 84

Naloxone [reversal of respir-atory depression caused by medicinal use of opioids], p. 796

NeoRecormon®, p. 547

Neostigmine [reversal of non-depolarising muscle block], p. 794

Omalizumab, p. 202

Ondansetron, p. 250

Oseltamivir, p. 397

Otrivine-Antistin®, p. 637

Paracetamol, p. 254

Paraldehyde, p. 293

Pentamidine [*Pneumocystis jir-ovecii*], p. 418

Pentasa® tablets, p. 69

Pethidine, p. 265

Prednisolone [acute asthma], p. 171

Propofol [induction of anaes-thesia], p. 775

Pyridostigmine, p. 625

Risperidone [short-term treat-ment of severe aggression in autism], p. 229

Salbutamol [aerosol inhalation for acute asthma], p. 171

Salbutamol [nebulised solution for severe acute asthma], p. 171

Sapropterin dihydrochloride [Tetrahydrobiopterin defi-ciency], p. 571

Senna tablets, p. 81

Senokot® syrup, p. 81

Simvastatin, p. 164

Sodium picosulfate, p. 81

Suxamethonium [by intra-venous injection, and neo-natal dose by intramuscular injection], p. 793

T-Gel®, p. 714

Triamcinolone acetonide [nasal spray], p. 660

Trihexyphenidyl, p. 297

Vancomycin [*Clostridium diffi-cile* infection], p. 349

Vecuronium bromide [in neo-nates], p. 792

Xylometazoline [paediatric nasal drops], p. 661

New Names

Budelin Novolizer® [formerly *Novolizer*®], p. 190

Classification changes

Classification changes have been made in the following sections of *BNF for Children 2010–2011*:

Section 1.6.5 Bowel Cleansing Preparations [title change]

Section 10.1.4 Gout and cytotoxic-induced hyperuricaemia [title change]

Section 13.11 Skin cleansers, antiseptics, and preparations for the promotion of wound healing [title change]

Section 14.5.1 Normal immunoglobulin [new sub-section]

Section 14.5.2 Disease-specific immunoglobulins [new sub-section]

Section 14.5.3 Anti-D (Rh$_0$) immunoglobulin [new sub-section]

Deleted preparations

Preparations listed below have been discontinued during the compilation of *BNF for Children 2010–2011*, or are still available but are not considered suitable for inclusion by the Paediatric Formulary Committee (see footnote):

Adcortyl in Orabase®
Alpha Keri Bath®
Amphocil®
Angettes 75®
Augmentin® dispersible tablets
Beclazone Easi-Breathe®
Betadine® ointment
Calcium gluconate tablets
Canesten® powder
Carace®
Clinitar® preparations
Dromadol® SR
Econacort®
Ecostatin® preparations
E45® Sun

Fucidin H® ointment
Full Marks®
Fungilin®
Haemaccel®
Imuderm® Bath Oil
Isopto Atropine®
Konakion® tablets
Luborant®
Lubri-Tears®
Maxolon® syrup and paediatric liquid
Methydopa[1]
NeoRecormon® Reco-Pen
Nicotinamide tablets
Nystan® tablets
Paraplatin®

Phenothrin
Polytrim®
Prioderm®
Propine®
Prosulf® injection
Quellada M®
Rennie® Duo suspension
Robinul® injection
Robinul-Neostigmine®
Sustanon 100®
Synercid®
Tinaderm-M®
Vallergan®
Velosef®
Vistamethasone N®

New preparations included in this edition

Preparations included in the relevant sections of *BNF for Children 2010–2011*:

Acrivastine, p. 196
Albunorm® [albumin], p. 566
Aptivus® oral solution [tipranavir], p. 388
Balneum® cream, p. 676
Berinert® [C1-esterase inhibitor], p. 206
Carnitor® [L-carnitine] tablets, p. 597
Cozaar® oral suspension [losartan], p. 135
Denzapine® suspension [clozapine], p. 228
Dermovate NN®, p. 686
Deximune® [ciclosporin], p. 530
EllaOne® [ulipristal], p. 499
Epaderm® cream, p. 675
Glucophage® oral powder [metformin], p. 438
Glypressin® solution for injection [terlipressin], p. 474

Hydromol® Intensive, p. 676
Hylo-Forte® [sodium hyaluronate], p. 648
Hylo-Tear® [sodium hyaluronate], p. 648
Ilaris® [canakinumab], p. 536
Lescol® [fluvastatin], p. 163
Levest® [ethinylestradiol with levonorgestrel], p. 489
Menveo® [meningococcal A, C, W135, and Y conjugate vaccine], p. 753
Mepact® [mifamurtide], p. 536
Modigraf® [tacrolimus], p. 531
Nexium® [esomeprazole], p. 62
Novgos® [goserelin], p. 465
Orencia® [abatacept], p. 621
Panadol OA® [paracetamol], p. 255
Periogard® [chlorhexidine gluconate], p. 668

Prevenar 13® [pneumococcal polysaccharide conjugate vaccine (adsorbed)], p. 755
Qlaira® [estradiol valerate with dienogest], p. 491
Rupafin® [rupatadine], p. 198
Savene® [dexrazoxane], p. 508
Synflorix® [pneumococcal polysaccharide conjugate vaccine (adsorbed)], p. 755
Systane® [hydroxypropyl guar], p. 647
Tramacet® effervescent tablets [tramadol with paracetamol], p. 267
Vedrop® [alpha tocopherol], p. 592
Xamiol® [betametasone with calcipotriol], p. 694
Xerotin® oral spray, p. 670
Xomolix® [droperidol], p. 248
Zarzio® [filgrastim], p. 554

1. Not considered suitable for inclusion by the Paediatric Formulary Committee

General guidance

Medicines should be given to children only when they are necessary, and in all cases the potential benefit of administering the medicine should be considered in relation to the risk involved. This is particularly important during pregnancy, when the risk to both mother and fetus must be considered (for further details see Prescribing in Pregnancy, p. 22).

It is important to discuss treatment options carefully with the child and the child's carer (see also Taking Medicines to Best Effect, below). In particular, the child and the child's carer should be helped to distinguish the adverse effects of prescribed drugs from the effects of the medical disorder. When the beneficial effects of the medicine are likely to be delayed, this should be highlighted.

Taking medicines to best effect   Difficulties in adherence to drug treatment occur regardless of age. Factors that contribute to poor compliance with prescribed medicines include:

- difficulty in taking the medicine (e.g. inability to swallow the medicine);
- unattractive formulation (e.g. unpleasant taste);
- prescription not collected or not dispensed;
- purpose of medicine not clear;
- perceived lack of efficacy;
- real or perceived adverse effects;
- carers' or child's perception of the risk and severity of side-effects may differ from that of the prescriber;
- instructions for administration not clear.

The prescriber, the child's carer, and the child (if appropriate) should agree on the health outcomes desired and on the strategy for achieving them ('concordance'). The prescriber should be sensitive to religious, cultural, and personal beliefs of the child's family that can affect acceptance of medicines.

Taking the time to explain to the child (and carers) the rationale and the potential adverse effects of treatment may improve adherence. Reinforcement and elaboration of the physician's instructions by the pharmacist and other members of the healthcare team can be important. Giving advice on the management of adverse effects and the possibility of alternative treatments may encourage carers and children to seek advice rather than merely abandon unacceptable treatment.

Simplifying the drug regimen may help; the need for frequent administration may reduce adherence, although there appears to be little difference in adherence between once-daily and twice-daily administration. Combination products reduce the number of drugs taken but at the expense of the ability to titrate individual doses.

Administration of medicines to children   Children should be involved in decisions about taking medicines and encouraged to take responsibility for using them correctly. The degree of such involvement will depend on the child's age, understanding, and personal circumstances.

Occasionally a medicine or its taste has to be disguised or masked with small quantities of food. However, unless specifically permitted (e.g. some formulations of pancreatin), a medicine should **not** be mixed with large quantities of food because the full dose might not be taken and the child might develop an aversion to food if the medicine imparts an unpleasant taste. Medicines should **not** be mixed or administered in a baby's feeding bottle.

Children under 5 years (and some older children) find a liquid formulation more acceptable than tablets or capsules. However, for long-term treatment it may be possible for a child to be taught to take tablets or capsules.

An oral syringe (see below) should be used for accurate measurement and controlled administration of an oral liquid medicine. The unpleasant taste of an oral liquid can be disguised by flavouring it or by giving a favourite food or drink immediately afterwards, but the potential for food-drug interactions should be considered.

Advice should be given on dental hygiene to those receiving medicines containing cariogenic sugars for long-term treatment; sugar-free medicines should be provided whenever possible.

Children with nasal feeding tubes in place for prolonged periods should be encouraged to take medicines by mouth if possible; enteral feeding should generally be interrupted before the medicine is given (particularly if enteral feeds reduce the absorption of a particular drug). Oral liquids can be given through the tube provided that precautions are taken to guard against blockage; the dose should be washed down with warm water. When a medicine is given through a nasogastric tube to a neonate, **sterile water** must be used to accompany the medicine or to wash it down.

The intravenous route is generally chosen when a medicine cannot be given by mouth; reliable access, often a central vein, should be used for children whose treatment involves irritant or inotropic drugs or who need to receive the medicine over a long period or for home therapy. The subcutaneous route is used most commonly for insulin administration. Intramuscular injections should preferably be **avoided** in children, particularly neonates, infants, and young children. However, the intramuscular route may be advantageous for administration of single doses of medicines when intravenous cannulation would be more problematic or painful to the child. Certain drugs, e.g. some vaccines, are only administered intramuscularly.

The intrathecal, epidural and intraosseous routes should be used **only** by staff specially trained to administer medicines by these routes. Local protocols for the management of intrathecal injections must be in place (section 8.1).

Managing medicines in school   Administration of a medicine during schooltime should be avoided if possible; medicines should be prescribed for once or twice-daily administration whenever practicable. If the medicine needs to be taken in school, this should be discussed with parents or carers and the necessary arrangements made in advance; where appropriate, involvement of a school nurse should be sought. *Managing Medicines in Schools and Early Years Settings* produced by the Department of Health provides guidance on using medicines in schools (www.dh.gov.uk).

Patient information leaflets   Manufacturers' patient information leaflets that accompany a medicine, cover only the licensed use of the medicine (see *BNF for Children* and Marketing Authorisation, below). Therefore, when a medicine is used outside its licence, it may be appropriate to advise the child and the child's parent or carer that some of the information in the leaflet might not apply to the child's treatment. Where necessary, inappropriate advice in the patient information leaflet should be identified and reassurance provided about the correct use in the context of the child's condition.

Biosimilar medicines   A biosimilar medicine is a new biological product that is similar to a medicine that has already been authorised to be marketed (the biological reference medicine) in the European Union. The active substance of a biosimilar medicine is similar, but not identical, to the biological reference medicine. Biological products are different from standard chemical products in terms of their complexity and although theoretically there should be no important differences between the biosimilar and biological reference medicine in terms of safety or efficacy, when prescribing biological products, it is good practice to use the brand name. This will ensure that substitution of a biosimilar medicine does not occur when the medicine is dispensed.

Biosimilar medicines have black triangle status (▼, see p. 16) at the time of initial marketing. It is important to report suspected adverse reactions to biosimilar medicines using the Yellow Card Scheme (p. 15). For biosimilar medicines, adverse reaction reports should clearly state the brand name of the suspected medicine.

Complementary and alternative medicine   An increasing amount of information on complementary and alternative medicine is becoming available. Where appropriate, the child and the child's carers should be asked about the use of their medicines, including dietary supplements and topical products. The scope of *BNF for Children* is restricted to the discussion of conventional medicines but reference is made to complementary treatments if they affect conventional therapy (e.g. interactions with St John's wort—see Appendix 1). Further information on herbal medicines is available at www.mhra.gov.uk.

BNF for Children and marketing authorisation   Where appropriate the *doses, indications, cautions, contra-indications,* and *side-effects* in *BNF for Children* reflect those in the manufacturers' Summaries of Product Characteristics (SPCs) which, in turn, reflect those in the corresponding marketing authorisations (formerly known as Product Licences). *BNF for Children* does not generally include proprietary medicines that are not supported by a valid Summary of Product Characteristics or when the marketing authorisation holder has not been able to supply essential information. When a preparation is available from more than one manufacturer, *BNF for Children* reflects advice that is the most clinically relevant regardless of any variation in the marketing authorisation. Unlicensed products can be obtained from 'special-order' manufacturers or specialist importing companies, see p. 957.

As far as possible, medicines should be prescribed within the terms of the marketing authorisation. However, many children require medicines not specifically licensed for paediatric use. Although medicines cannot be promoted outside the limits of the licence, the Medicines Act does not prohibit the use of unlicensed medicines.

BNF for Children includes advice involving the use of unlicensed medicines or of licensed medicines for unlicensed uses ('off-label' use). Such advice reflects careful consideration of the options available to manage a given condition and the weight of evidence and experience of the unlicensed intervention (see also Unlicensed Medicines, p. 7). Where the advice falls outside a drug's marketing authorisation, *BNF for Children* shows the licensing status in the drug monograph. However, limitations of the marketing authorisation should not preclude unlicensed use where clinically appropriate.

> Prescribing unlicensed medicines or medicines outside the recommendations of their marketing authorisation alters (and probably increases) the prescriber's professional responsibility and potential liability. The prescriber should be able to justify and feel competent in using such medicines.

Drugs and skilled tasks   Prescribers and other healthcare professionals should advise children and their carers if treatment is likely to affect their ability to perform skilled tasks (e.g. driving). This applies especially to drugs with sedative effects; patients should be warned that these effects are increased by alcohol. General information about a patient's fitness to drive is available from the Driver and Vehicle Licensing Agency at www.dvla.gov.uk.

Oral syringes   An **oral syringe** is supplied when oral liquid medicines are prescribed in doses other than multiples of 5 mL. The oral syringe is marked in 0.5-mL divisions from 1 to 5 mL to measure doses of less than 5 mL (other sizes of oral syringe may also be available). It is provided with an adaptor and an instruction leaflet. The *5-mL spoon* is used for doses of 5 mL (or multiples thereof).

Excipients   Branded oral liquid preparations that do not contain *fructose, glucose,* or *sucrose* are described as 'sugar-free' in *BNF for Children*. Preparations containing hydrogenated glucose syrup, mannitol, maltitol, sorbitol, or xylitol are also marked 'sugar-free' since they do not cause dental caries. Children receiving medicines containing cariogenic sugars, or their carers, should be advised of dental hygiene measures to prevent caries. Sugar-free preparations should be used whenever possible, particularly if treatment is required for a long period.

Where information on the presence of *alcohol, aspartame, gluten, sulphites, tartrazine, arachis (peanut) oil* or *sesame oil* is available, this is indicated in *BNF for Children* against the relevant preparation.

Information is provided on *selected excipients* in skin preparations (section 13.1.3), in vaccines (section 14.1), and on *selected preservatives* and *excipients* in eye drops and injections. Pressurised metered aerosols containing *chlorofluorocarbon* (CFC) or *hydrofluoroalkane* (HFA) propellants have also been identified throughout Chapter 3 of *BNF for Children*.

General guidance

The presence of *benzyl alcohol* and *polyoxyl castor oil* (polyethoxylated castor oil) in injections is indicated in *BNF for Children*. Benzyl alcohol has been associated with a fatal toxic syndrome in preterm neonates, and therefore, parenteral preparations containing the preservative should not be used in neonates. Polyoxyl castor oils, used as vehicles in intravenous injections, have been associated with severe anaphylactoid reactions.

The presence of *propylene glycol* in oral or parenteral medicines is indicated in *BNF for Children*; it can cause adverse effects if its elimination is impaired, e.g. in renal failure, in neonates and young children, and in slow metabolisers of the substance. It may interact with metronidazole.

The *lactose* content in most medicines is too small to cause problems in most lactose-intolerant children. However in severe lactose intolerance, the lactose content should be determined before prescribing. The amount of lactose varies according to manufacturer, product, formulation, and strength.

In the absence of information on excipients in *BNF for Children* and in the product literature (available at www.emc.medicines.org.uk), contact the manufacturer (see Index of Manufacturers) if it is essential to check details.

Health and safety   When handling chemical or biological materials particular attention should be given to the possibility of allergy, fire, explosion, radiation, or poisoning. Care is required to avoid sources of heat (including hair dryers) when flammable substances are used on the skin or hair. Substances, such as corticosteroids, some antimicrobials, phenothiazines, and many cytotoxics, are irritant or very potent and should be handled with caution; contact with the skin and inhalation of dust should be avoided. Healthcare professionals and carers should guard against exposure to sensitising, toxic or irritant substances if it is necessary to crush tablets or open capsules.

Security of prescriptions   The Councils of the British Medical Association and the Royal Pharmaceutical Society have issued a joint statement on the security and validity of prescriptions.

In particular, prescription forms should:

- not be left unattended at reception desks;
- not be left in a car where they may be visible; and
- when not in use, be kept in a locked drawer within the surgery and at home.

Patient group direction (PGD)   In most cases, the most appropriate clinical care will be provided on an individual basis by a prescriber to a specific child. However, a Patient Group Direction for supply and administration of medicines by other healthcare professionals can be used where it would benefit the child's care without compromising safety.

A Patient Group Direction is a written direction relating to the supply and administration (or administration only) of a licensed prescription-only medicine by certain classes of healthcare professionals; the Direction is signed by a doctor (or dentist) and by a pharmacist. Further information on Patient Group Directions is available in Health Service Circular HSC 2000/026 (England), HDL (2001) 7 (Scotland), and WHC (2000) 116 (Wales) and at www.portal.nelm.nhs.uk/pgd.

NICE and Scottish Medicines Consortium   Advice issued by the National Institute for Health and Clinical Excellence (NICE) and by the Scottish Medicines Consortium (SMC) is included in *BNF for Children* when relevant. If advice within a NICE Single Technology Appraisal differs from SMC advice, the Scottish Executive expects NHS Boards within NHS Scotland to comply with the SMC advice. Details of the advice together with updates can be obtained from www.nice.org.uk and from www.scottishmedicines.org.

Prescription writing

> **Shared care**
> In its guidelines on responsibility for prescribing (circular EL (91) 127)
> between hospitals and general practitioners, the Department of Health has
> advised that legal responsibility for prescribing lies with the doctor who signs
> the prescription.

Prescriptions[1] should be written legibly in ink or otherwise so as to be indelible[2], should be dated, should state the full name and address of the patient, and should be signed in ink by the prescriber[3]. The age and the date of birth of the child should preferably be stated, and it is a legal requirement in the case of prescription-only medicines to state the age for children under 12 years.

Wherever appropriate the prescriber should state the current weight of the child to enable the dose prescribed to be checked. Consideration should also be given to including the dose per unit mass e.g. mg/kg or the dose per m² body-surface area e.g. mg/m² where this would reduce error.

The following should be noted:

(a) The unnecessary use of decimal points should be avoided, e.g. 3 mg, not 3.0 mg.

Quantities of 1 gram or more should be written as 1 g, etc.

Quantities less than 1 gram should be written in milligrams, e.g. 500 mg, not 0.5 g.

Quantities less than 1 mg should be written in micrograms, e.g. 100 micrograms, not 0.1 mg.

When decimals are unavoidable a zero should be written in front of the decimal point where there is no other figure, e.g. 0.5 mL, not .5 mL.

Use of the decimal point is acceptable to express a range, e.g. 0.5 to 1 g.

(b) 'Microgrms' and 'nanograms' should **not** be abbreviated. Similarly 'units' should **not** be abbreviated.

(c) The term 'millilitre' (ml or mL)[4] is used in medicine and pharmacy, and cubic centimetre, c.c., or cm³ should not be used.

(d) Dose and dose frequency should be stated; in the case of preparations to be taken 'as required' a **minimum dose interval** should be specified.

Care should be taken to ensure the child receives the correct dose of the active drug. Therefore, the dose should normally be stated in terms of the mass of the active drug (e.g. '125 mg 3 times daily'); terms such as '5 mL' or '1 tablet' should be avoided except for compound preparations.

When doses other than multiples of 5 mL are prescribed for *oral liquid preparations* the dose-volume will be provided by means of an **oral syringe**, see p. 3 (except for preparations intended to be measured with a pipette).

(e) For suitable quantities of dermatological preparations, see section 13.1.2.

(f) The names of drugs and preparations should be written clearly and **not** abbreviated, using approved titles **only** (see also advice in box on p. 6 to **avoid** creating generic titles for modified-release preparations).

(g) The quantity to be supplied may be stated by indicating the number of days of treatment required in the box provided on NHS forms. In most cases the exact amount will be supplied. This does not apply to items directed to be used as required—if the dose and frequency are not given then the quantity to be supplied needs to be stated.

When several items are ordered on one form the box can be marked with the number of days of treatment provided the quantity is added for any item for which the amount cannot be calculated.

(h) Although directions should preferably be in **English without abbreviation**, it is recognised that some Latin abbreviations are used (for details see Inside Back Cover).

General guidance

---

1. These recommendations are acceptable for **prescription-only medicines** (POM). For items marked CD see also Prescribing Controlled Drugs, p. 11.
2. It is permissible to issue carbon copies of NHS prescriptions as long as they are signed in ink.
3. Computer-generated facsimile signatures do not meet the legal requirement.
4. The use of capital 'L' in mL is a printing convention throughout *BNF for Children*; both 'mL' and 'ml' are recognised SI abbreviations.

For a sample prescription, see below.

Abbreviation of titles   In general, titles of drugs and preparations should be written *in full*. Unofficial abbreviations should **not** be used as they may be misinterpreted.

Non-proprietary titles   Where non-proprietary ('generic') titles are given, they should be used for prescribing. This will enable any suitable product to be dispensed, thereby saving delay to the patient and sometimes expense to the health service. The only exception is where there is a demonstrable difference in clinical effect between each manufacturer's version of the formulation, making it important that the child should always receive the same brand; in such cases, the brand name or the manufacturer should be stated.

> Non-proprietary names of **compound preparations** e.g. co-codamol that appear in *BNF for Children* are those that have been introduced by the British Pharmacopoeia Commission or another recognised body; whenever possible they reflect the names of the active ingredients.
>
> Prescribers should avoid creating their own compound names for the purposes of generic prescribing; such names do not have an approved definition and can be misinterpreted.
>
> Special care should be taken to avoid errors when prescribing compound preparations; in particular the hyphen in the prefix 'co-' should be retained.
>
> Special care should also be taken to avoid creating generic names for **modified-release** preparations where the use of these names could lead to confusion between formulations with different duration of action.

Strengths and quantities   The strength or quantity to be contained in capsules, lozenges, tablets, etc. should be stated by the prescriber. In particular, strengths of liquid preparations should be clearly stated (e.g. 125 mg/ 5 mL).

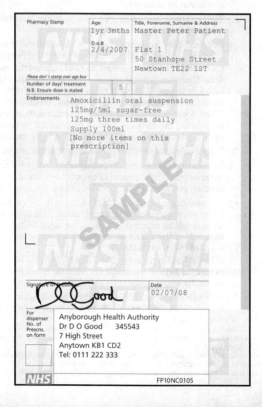

Supply of medicines

When supplying a medicine for a child, the pharmacist should ensure that the child and the child's carer understand the nature and identity of the medicine and how it should be used. The child and the carer should be provided with appropriate information (e.g. how long the medicine should be taken for and what to do if a dose is missed or the child vomits soon after the dose is given).

Safety in the home   Carers and relatives of children must be warned to keep all medicines out of the reach and sight of children. Tablets, capsules and oral and external liquid preparations must be dispensed in a reclosable *child-resistant container* unless:

- the medicine is in an original pack or patient pack such as to make this inadvisable;
- the child's carer will have difficulty in opening a child-resistant container;
- a specific request is made that the product shall not be dispensed in a child-resistant container;
- no suitable child-resistant container exists for a particular liquid preparation.

All patients should be advised to dispose of *unwanted medicines* by returning them to a pharmacy for destruction.

Validity of prescriptions   Where there is any doubt about the authenticity of a prescription, the pharmacist should contact the prescriber. If this is done by telephone, the number should be obtained from the directory rather than relying on the information on the prescription form, which may be false.

Strength and quantities   If a pharmacist receives an incomplete prescription for a systemically administered preparation[1] and considers it would not be appropriate for the patient to return to the prescriber, the following procedures will apply:

(a) an attempt must always be made to contact the prescriber to ascertain the intention;

(b) if the attempt is successful the pharmacist must, where practicable, subsequently arrange for details of quantity, strength where applicable, and dosage to be inserted by the prescriber on the incomplete form;

(c) where, although the prescriber has been contacted, it has not proved possible to obtain the written intention regarding an incomplete prescription, the pharmacist may endorse the form 'p.c.' (prescriber contacted) and add details of the quantity and strength where applicable of the preparation supplied, and of the dose indicated. The endorsement should be initialled and dated by the pharmacist;

(d) where the prescriber cannot be contacted and the pharmacist has sufficient information to make a professional judgement the preparation may be dispensed. If the quantity is missing the pharmacist may supply sufficient to complete up to 5 days' treatment; except that where a combination pack (i.e. a proprietary pack containing more than one medicinal product) or oral contraceptive is prescribed by name only, the smallest pack shall be dispensed. In all cases the prescription must be endorsed 'p.n.c.' (prescriber not contacted), the quantity, the dose, and the strength (where applicable) of the preparation supplied must be indicated, and the endorsement must be initialled and dated;

(e) if the pharmacist has any doubt about exercising discretion, an incomplete prescription must be referred back to the prescriber.

Unlicensed medicines   A drug or formulation that is not covered by a marketing authorisation (see also *BNF for Children* and Marketing Authorisation) may be obtained from a pharmaceutical company, imported by a specialist importer, manufactured by a commercial or hospital licensed manufacturing unit (see Special-order Manufacturers, p. 957), or prepared extemporaneously (see below) against a prescription.

The safeguards that apply to products with marketing authorisation should be extended, as far as possible, to the use of unlicensed medicines. The safety,

General guidance

---

1. With the exception of temazepam, an incomplete prescription is **not** acceptable for controlled drugs in schedules 2 and 3 of the Misuse of Drugs Regulations 2001.

General guidance

efficacy, and quality (including labelling) of unlicensed medicines should be assured by means of clear policies on their prescribing, purchase, supply, and administration. Extra care is required with unlicensed medicines because less information may be available on the drug and any formulation of the drug.

The following should be agreed with the supplier when ordering an unlicensed or extemporaneously prepared medicine:

- the specification of the formulation;
- documentation confirming the specification and quality of the product supplied (e.g. a certificate of conformity or of analysis);
- for imported preparations product and licensing information should be supplied in English.

Extemporaneous preparations   A product should be dispensed extemporaneously only when no product with a marketing authorisation is available. Every effort should be made to ensure that an extemporaneously prepared product is stable and that it delivers the requisite dose reliably; the child should be provided with a consistent formulation regardless of where the medicine is supplied to minimise variations in quality. Where there is doubt about the formulation, advice should be sought from a medicines information centre, the pharmacy at a children's hospital, a hospital production unit, a hospital quality control department, or the manufacturer.

In many cases it is preferable to give a licensed product by an unlicensed route (e.g. an injection solution given by mouth) than to prepare a special formulation. When tablets or capsules are cut, dispersed, or used for preparing liquids immediately before administration, it is important to confirm uniform dispersal of the active ingredient, especially if only a portion of the solid content (e.g. a tablet segment) is used or if only an aliquot of the liquid is to be administered.

In some cases the child's clinical condition may require a dose to be administered in the absence of full information on the method of administration. It is important to ensure that the appropriate supporting information is available at the earliest opportunity.

Preparation of products that produce harmful dust (e.g. cytotoxic drugs, hormones, or potentially sensitising drugs such as neomycin) should be **avoided** or undertaken with appropriate precautions to protect staff and carers (see also Safety in the Home, above).

The BP direction that a preparation must be *freshly prepared* indicates that it must be made not more than 24 hours before it is issued for use. The direction that a preparation should be *recently prepared* indicates that deterioration is likely if the preparation is stored for longer than about 4 weeks at 15–25° C.

The term **water** used without qualification means either potable water freshly drawn direct from the public supply and suitable for drinking or freshly boiled and cooled purified water. The latter should be used if the public supply is from a local storage tank or if the potable water is unsuitable for a particular preparation. See also Water for Injections, section 9.2.2.

Labelling medicines   The *name* of the medicine should appear on the label unless the prescriber indicates otherwise; the name shown on the label should be that written on the prescription. The *strength* should also be stated on the label in the case of preparations that are available in different strengths.

Labels should indicate the *total quantity* of the product dispensed in the container to which the label refers. This requirement applies equally to solid, liquid, internal, and external preparations. If a product is dispensed in more than one container, the reference should be to the amount in each container.

Emergency supply of medicines

Emergency supply requested by member of the public

Pharmacists are sometimes called upon by members of the public to make an emergency supply of medicines. The Prescription Only Medicines (Human Use) Order 1997 allows exemptions from the Prescription Only requirements for emergency supply to be made by a person lawfully conducting a retail pharmacy business provided:

(a) that the pharmacist has interviewed the person requesting the prescription-only medicine and is satisfied:

    (i) that there is immediate need for the prescription-only medicine and that it is impracticable in the circumstances to obtain a prescription without undue delay;

    (ii) that treatment with the prescription-only medicine has on a previous occasion been prescribed for the person requesting it;

    (iii) as to the dose that it would be appropriate for the person to take;

(b) that no greater quantity shall be supplied than will provide 5 days' treatment of phenobarbital, phenobarbital sodium, or Controlled Drugs in Schedules 4 or 5,[1] or 30 days' treatment for other prescription-only medicines, except when the prescription-only medicine is:

    (i) insulin, an ointment or cream, or a preparation for the relief of asthma in an aerosol dispenser when the smallest pack can be supplied;

    (ii) an oral contraceptive when a full cycle may be supplied;

    (iii) an antibiotic in liquid form for oral administration when the smallest quantity that will provide a full course of treatment can be supplied;

(c) that an entry shall be made by the pharmacist in the prescription book stating:

    (i) the date of supply;

    (ii) the name, quantity, and, where appropriate, the pharmaceutical form and strength;

    (iii) the name and address of the patient;

    (iv) the nature of the emergency;

(d) that the container or package must be labelled to show:

    (i) the date of supply;

    (ii) the name, quantity, and, where appropriate, the pharmaceutical form and strength;

    (iii) the name of the patient;

    (iv) the name and address of the pharmacy;

    (v) the words 'Emergency supply';

    (vi) the words 'Keep out of the reach of children' (or similar warning);

(e) that the prescription-only medicine is not a substance specifically excluded from the emergency supply provision, and does not contain a Controlled Drug specified in Schedules 1, 2, or 3 to the Misuse of Drugs Regulations 2001 except for phenobarbital or phenobarbital sodium for the treatment of epilepsy: for details see *Medicines, Ethics and Practice*, No. 33, London, Pharmaceutical Press, 2009 (and subsequent editions as available).[1]

General guidance

---

1. Doctors or dentists from the European Economic Area and Switzerland, or their patients, cannot request an emergency supply of Controlled Drugs, or drugs that do not have a UK marketing authorisation.

Emergency supply requested by prescriber

Emergency supply of a prescription-only medicine may also be made at the request of a doctor, a dentist, a supplementary prescriber, a community practitioner nurse prescriber, a nurse, pharmacist or optometrist independent prescriber, or a doctor or dentist from the European Economic Area or Switzerland, provided:

(a) that the pharmacist is satisfied that the prescriber by reason of some emergency is unable to furnish a prescription immediately;

(b) that the prescriber has undertaken to furnish a prescription within 72 hours;

(c) that the medicine is supplied in accordance with the directions of the prescriber requesting it;

(d) that the medicine is not a Controlled Drug specified in Schedules 1, 2, or 3 to the Misuse of Drugs Regulations 2001 except for phenobarbital or phenobarbital sodium for the treatment of epilepsy: for details see *Medicines, Ethics and Practice*, No. 33, London, Pharmaceutical Press, 2009 (and subsequent editions as available);[1]

(e) that an entry shall be made in the prescription book stating:

　(i) the date of supply;

　(ii) the name, quantity, and, where appropriate, the pharmaceutical form and strength;

　(iii) the name and address of the practitioner requesting the emergency supply;

　(iv) the name and address of the patient;

　(v) the date on the prescription;

　(vi) when the prescription is received the entry should be amended to include the date on which it is received.

Royal Pharmaceutical Society's guidelines

1. The pharmacist should consider the medical consequences of *not* supplying a medicine in an emergency.

2. If the pharmacist is unable to make an emergency supply of a medicine the pharmacist should advise the patient how to obtain essential medical care.

For conditions that apply to supplies made at the request of a patient, see *Medicines, Ethics and Practice*, No. 33, London Pharmaceutical Press, 2009 (and subsequent editions).

General guidance

1. Doctors or dentists from the European Economic Area and Switzerland, or their patients, cannot request an emergency supply of Controlled Drugs, or drugs that do not have a UK marketing authorisation.

Prescribing Controlled Drugs

The Misuse of Drugs Act, 1971 prohibits certain activities in relation to 'Controlled Drugs', in particular their manufacture, supply, and possession. The penalties applicable to offences involving the different drugs are graded broadly according to the *harmfulness attributable to a drug when it is misused* and for this purpose the drugs are defined in the following three classes:

Class A includes: alfentanil, cocaine, diamorphine (heroin), dipipanone, lysergide (LSD), methadone, methylenedioxymethamfetamine (MDMA, 'ecstasy'), morphine, opium, pethidine, phencyclidine, remifentanil, and class B substances when prepared for injection

Class B includes: oral amphetamines, barbiturates, cannabis, cannabis resin, codeine, ethylmorphine, glutethimide, nabilone, pentazocine, phenmetrazine, and pholcodine

Class C includes: certain drugs related to the amphetamines such as benzfetamine and chlorphentermine, buprenorphine, diethylpropion, mazindol, meprobamate, pemoline, pipradrol, most benzodiazepines, zolpidem, androgenic and anabolic steroids, clenbuterol, chorionic gonadotrophin (HCG), non-human chorionic gonadotrophin, somatotropin, somatrem, and somatropin

The Misuse of Drugs Regulations 2001 define the classes of person who are authorised to supply and possess controlled drugs while acting in their professional capacities and lay down the conditions under which these activities may be carried out. In the regulations drugs are divided into five schedules each specifying the requirements governing such activities as import, export, production, supply, possession, prescribing, and record keeping which apply to them.

Schedule 1 includes drugs such as cannabis and lysergide which are not used medicinally. Possession and supply are prohibited except in accordance with Home Office authority.

Schedule 2 includes drugs such as diamorphine (heroin), morphine, nabilone, remifentanil, pethidine, secobarbital, glutethimide, amfetamine, and cocaine and are subject to the full controlled drug requirements relating to prescriptions, safe custody (except for secobarbital), the need to keep registers, etc. (unless exempted in Schedule 5).

Schedule 3 includes the barbiturates (except secobarbital, now Schedule 2), buprenorphine, diethylpropion, mazindol, meprobamate, midazolam, pentazocine, phentermine, and temazepam. They are subject to the special prescription requirements (except for temazepam) and to the safe custody requirements (except for any 5,5 disubstituted barbituric acid (e.g. phenobarbital), mazindol, meprobamate, midazolam, pentazocine, phentermine, or any stereoisomeric form or salts of the above). Records in registers do not need to be kept (although there are requirements for the retention of invoices for 2 years).

Schedule 4 includes in Part I benzodiazepines (except temazepam and midazolam which are in Schedule 3) and zolpidem, which are subject to minimal control. Part II includes androgenic and anabolic steroids, clenbuterol, chorionic gonadotrophin (HCG), non-human chorionic gonadotrophin, somatotropin, somatrem, and somatropin. Controlled Drug prescription requirements do not apply (but see Department of Health Guidance, p. 12) and Schedule 4 Controlled Drugs are not subject to safe custody requirements.

Schedule 5 includes those preparations which, because of their strength, are exempt from virtually all Controlled Drug requirements other than retention of invoices for two years.

Prescriptions Preparations in Schedules 2 and 3 of the Misuse of Drugs Regulations 2001 (and subsequent amendments) are identified throughout *BNF for Children* by the symbol ⸤CD⸥ (Controlled Drug). The principal legal requirements relating to medical prescriptions are listed below (see also Department of Health Guidance, p. 12).

General guidance

General guidance

> **Prescription requirements**
> Prescriptions for Controlled Drugs that are subject to prescription requirements[1] must be indelible[2] and must be *signed* by the prescriber, *be dated*, and specify the prescriber's *address*. The prescription must always state:
> - The name and address of the patient;
> - In the case of a preparation, the form[3] and where appropriate the strength[4] of the preparation;
> - either the total quantity (in both words and figures) of the preparation,[5] or the number (in both words and figures) of dosage units, as appropriate, to be supplied; in any other case, the total quantity (in both words and figures) of the Controlled Drug to be supplied;
> - The dose;[6]
> - The words 'for dental treatment only' if issued by a dentist.

A pharmacist is **not** allowed to dispense a Controlled Drug unless all the information required by law is given on the prescription. In the case of a prescription for a Controlled Drug in Schedule 2 or 3, a pharmacist can amend the prescription if it specifies the total quantity only in words or in figures or if it contains minor typographical errors, provided that such amendments are indelible and clearly attributable to the pharmacist.[7] Failure to comply with the regulations concerning the writing of prescriptions will result in inconvenience to patients and carers and delay in supply of the necessary medicine. A prescription for a Controlled Drug in Schedules 2, 3, or 4 is valid for 28 days from the date stated thereon.[8]

Instalments and 'repeats'   A prescription may order a Controlled Drug to be dispensed by instalments; the amount of instalments and the intervals to be observed must be specified.[9] Prescriptions ordering 'repeats' on the same form are **not** permitted for Controlled Drugs in Schedules 2 or 3.

Private prescriptions   Private prescriptions for Controlled Drugs in Schedules 2 and 3 must be written on specially designated forms provided by Primary Care Trusts in England, Health Boards in Scotland, Local Health Boards in Wales or the Northern Ireland Central Services Agency; in addition, prescriptions must specify the *prescriber's identification number*. Prescriptions to be supplied by a pharmacist in hospital are exempt from the requirement for private prescriptions.

Department of Health guidance   Guidance (June 2006) issued by the Department of Health in England on prescribing and dispensing of Controlled Drugs requires:

- in general, prescriptions for Controlled Drugs in Schedules 2, 3, and 4 to be limited to a supply of up to 30 days' treatment; exceptionally, to cover a justifiable clinical need and after consideration of any risk, a prescription can be issued for a longer period, but the reasons for the decision should be recorded on the patient's notes;
- the patient's identifier to be shown on NHS and private prescriptions for Controlled Drugs in Schedules 2 and 3.

Further information is available at www.dh.gov.uk.

For a sample prescription, see p. 13.

Dependence and misuse   The most serious drugs of addiction are **cocaine**, **diamorphine** (heroin), **morphine**, and the **synthetic opioids**.

---

1. All preparations in Schedules 2 and 3, except temazepam.
2. A machine-written prescription is acceptable. The prescriber's signature must be handwritten.
3. The dosage form (e.g. tablets) must be included on a Controlled Drug prescription irrespective of whether it is implicit in the proprietary name (e.g. *MST Continus*) or whether only one form is available.
4. When more than one strength of a preparation exists the strength required must be specified.
5. The Home Office has advised that quantities of liquid preparations such as methadone mixture should be written in millilitres.
6. The instruction 'one as directed' constitutes a dose but 'as directed' does not.
7. Implementation date for *N. Ireland* not confirmed.
8. The prescriber may forward-date the prescription; the start date may also be specified in the body of the prescription.
9. A total of 14 days' treatment by instalment of any drug listed in Schedule 2 of the Misuse of Drugs Regulations, buprenorphine and diazepam may be prescribed in England. In *England*, forms FP10(MDA) (blue) and FP10H(MDA) (blue) should be used. In *Scotland*, forms GP10 (peach), HBP (blue), or HBPA (pink) should be used. In *Wales* a total of 14 days' treatment by instalment of any drug listed in Schedules 2–5 of the Misuse of Drugs Regulations may be prescribed. In Wales, form WP10(MDA) or form WP10HP(AD) should be used.

Despite marked reduction in the prescribing of **amphetamines** there is concern that abuse of illicit amfetamine and related compounds is widespread.

Benzodiazepines are commonly misused. However, the misuse of **barbiturates** is now uncommon because of their declining medicinal use and consequent availability.

Cannabis (Indian hemp) has no approved medicinal use and cannot be prescribed by doctors. Its use is illegal but widespread. Cannabis is a mild hallucinogen seldom accompanied by a desire to increase the dose; withdrawal symptoms are unusual. **Lysergide** (lysergic acid diethylamide, LSD) is a much more potent hallucinogen; its use can lead to severe psychotic states which can be life-threatening.

There are concerns over increases in the availability and the misuse of other drugs with variously combined hallucinogenic, anaesthetic, or sedative properties. These include ketamine and gamma-hydroxybutyrate (sodium oxybate, GHB).

Prescribing drugs likely to cause dependence or misuse   The prescriber has three main responsibilities:

- to avoid creating dependence by introducing drugs to patients without sufficient reason. In this context, the proper use of the morphine-like drugs is well understood. The dangers of other Controlled Drugs are less clear because recognition of dependence is not easy and its effects, and those of withdrawal, are less obvious;

- to see that the patient does not gradually increase the dose of a drug, given for good medical reasons, to the point where dependence becomes more likely. The prescriber should keep a close eye on the amount prescribed to prevent patients or their carers from accumulating stocks. A minimal amount should be prescribed in the first instance, or when seeing a new patient for the first time;

- to avoid being used as an unwitting source of supply for addicts and being vigilant to methods for obtaining medicines which include visiting more than one doctor, fabricating stories, and forging prescriptions.

General guidance

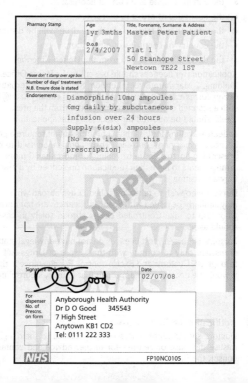

Patients under temporary care should be given only small supplies of drugs unless they present an unequivocal letter from their own doctor. It is sensible to reduce dosages steadily or to issue weekly or even daily prescriptions for small amounts if dependence is suspected.

The stealing and misuse of prescription forms could be minimised by the following precautions:

(a) do not leave unattended if called away from the consulting room or at reception desks; do not leave in a car where they may be visible; when not in use, keep in a locked drawer within the surgery and at home;

(b) draw a diagonal line across the blank part of the form under the prescription;

(c) the quantity should be shown in words and figures when prescribing drugs prone to abuse; this is obligatory for controlled drugs (see Prescriptions, above);

(d) alterations are best avoided but if any are made they should be clear and unambiguous; add initials against altered items;

(e) if prescriptions are left for collection they should be left in a safe place in a sealed envelope.

Travelling abroad   Prescribed drugs listed in Schedule 4 Part II (CD Anab) and Schedule 5 of the Misuse of Drugs Regulations 2001 are not subject to export or import licensing. However, patients intending to travel abroad for more than 3 months carrying any amount of drugs listed in Schedules 2, 3, or 4 Part I (CD Benz) will require a personal export/import licence. Further details can be obtained at www.drugs.homeoffice.gov.uk/drugs-laws/licensing/personal, or from the Home Office by contacting licensing_enquiry.aadu@homeoffice.gsi.gov.uk (in cases of emergency, telephone (020) 7035 0484).

Applications must be supported by a covering letter from the prescriber and should give details of:

• the patient's name and current address;

• the quantities of drugs to be carried;

• the strength and form in which the drugs will be dispensed;

• the country or countries of destination;

• the dates of travel to and from the United Kingdom.

Applications for licences should be sent to the Home Office, Drugs Licensing, Peel Building, 2 Marsham Street, London, SW1P 4DF. Alternatively, completed application forms can be emailed to licensing_enquiry.aadu@homeoffice.gsi.gov.uk with a scanned copy of the covering letter from the prescriber. A minimum of two weeks should be allowed for processing the application.

Patients travelling for less than 3 months do not require a personal export/import licence for carrying Controlled Drugs, but are advised to carry a letter from the prescribing doctor. Those travelling for more than 3 months are advised to make arrangements to have their medication prescribed by a practitioner in the country they are visiting.

Doctors who wish to take Controlled Drugs abroad while accompanying patients may similarly be issued with licences. Licences are not normally issued to doctors who wish to take Controlled Drugs abroad solely in case a family emergency should arise.

Personal export/import licences do not have any legal status outside the UK and are issued only to comply with the Misuse of Drugs Act and facilitate passage through UK Customs and Excise control. For clearance in the country to be visited it would be necessary to approach that country's consulate in the UK.

Notification of drug misusers

Doctors should report cases of drug misuse to their regional or national drug misuse database or centre—for further advice and contact telephone numbers consult the BNF.

Adverse reactions to drugs

Any drug may produce unwanted or unexpected adverse reactions. Rapid detection and recording of adverse drug reactions is of vital importance so that unrecognised hazards are identified promptly and appropriate regulatory action is taken to ensure that medicines are used safely. Healthcare professionals and coroners (see also Self-reporting, below) are urged to report suspected adverse drug reactions directly to the Medicines and Healthcare products Regulatory Agency (MHRA) through the Yellow Card Scheme using the electronic form at www.yellowcard.gov.uk. Alternatively, prepaid Yellow Cards for reporting are available from the address below and are also bound in this book (inside back cover).

Medicines and Healthcare products Regulatory Agency
CHM
Freepost SW2991
London, SW8 5BR.
Tel: 0800 731 6789

Suspected adverse drug reactions to *any* therapeutic agent should be reported, including drugs *(self-medication* as well as those *prescribed)*, blood products, vaccines, radiographic contrast media, complementary and herbal products.

The reporting of **all** suspected adverse drug reactions, no matter how minor, in children under 18 years, including those relating to unlicensed or off-label use of medicines, is **strongly encouraged** through the Yellow Card Scheme even if the intensive monitoring symbol (▼, see below) has been removed. This is because experience in children may still be limited.

The identification and reporting of adverse reactions to drugs in children is particularly important because:

- the action of the drug and its pharmacokinetics in children (especially in the very young) may be different from that in adults;

- drugs may not be extensively tested in children;

- children may be more susceptible to developmental disorders or they may have delayed adverse reactions which do not occur in adults;

- many drugs are not specifically licensed for use in children and are used 'off-label';

- suitable formulations may not be available to allow precise dosing in children;

- the nature and course of illnesses and adverse drug reactions may differ between adults and children.

Spontaneous reporting is particularly valuable for recognising possible new hazards rapidly. An adverse reaction should be reported even if it is not certain that the drug has caused it, or if the reaction is well recognised, or if other drugs have been given at the same time. Reports of overdoses (deliberate or accidental) can complicate the assessment of adverse drug reactions, but provide important information on the potential toxicity of drugs.

A 24-hour Freefone service is available to all parts of the UK for advice and information on suspected adverse drug reactions; contact the National Yellow Card Information Service at the MHRA on 0800 731 6789. Outside office hours a telephone-answering machine will take messages.

The following Yellow Card Centres can be contacted for further information:

Yellow Card Centre, North West
Freepost SW2991
70 Pembroke Place
Liverpool, L69 3GF.
Tel: (0151) 794 8122

Yellow Card Centre, West Midlands
Freepost SW2991
City Hospital
Birmingham, B18 7QH.
Tel: (0121) 507 5672

Yellow Card Centre, Wales
Freepost SW2991
University Hospital of Wales
Cardiff, CF4 1ZZ.
Tel: (029) 2074 4181

Yellow Card Centre, Scotland
Freepost NAT3271
CARDS, Royal Infirmary of Edinburgh
Edinburgh, EH16 4SA.
Tel: (0131) 242 2919

General guidance

Yellow Card Centre, Northern & Yorkshire
Freepost SW2991
Wolfson Unit
Claremont Place
Newcastle upon Tyne, NE2 4HH.
Tel: (0191) 260 6181

The MHRA's database facilitates the monitoring of adverse drug reactions.

More detailed information on reporting and a list of products currently under intensive monitoring can be found on the MHRA website: www.mhra.gov.uk

> Drug Safety Update is a monthly newsletter from the MHRA and the Commission on Human Medicines (CHM); it is available at www.mhra.gov.uk/mhra/drugsafetyupdate

Self-reporting   Patients and their carers can also report suspected adverse drug reactions to the MHRA. Reports can be submitted directly to the MHRA through the Yellow Card Scheme using the electronic form at www.yellowcard.gov.uk or by telephone on 0808 100 3352. Alternatively, patient Yellow Cards are available from pharmacies and GP surgeries, or can be downloaded from www.mhra.gov.uk where more detailed information on patient reporting is available.

Prescription-event monitoring   In addition to the MHRA's Yellow Card Scheme, an independent scheme monitors the safety of new medicines using a different approach. The Drug Safety Research Unit identifies patients who have been prescribed selected new medicines and collects data on clinical events in these patients. The data are submitted on a voluntary basis by general practitioners on green forms. More information about the scheme and the Unit's educational material is available from www.dsru.org

Newer drugs and vaccines   Only limited information is available from clinical trials on the safety of new medicines. Further understanding about the safety of medicines depends on the availability of information from routine clinical practice.

The black triangle symbol (▼) identifies newly licensed medicines that are monitored intensively by the MHRA. Such medicines include new active substances, biosimilar medicines, medicines that have been licensed for administration by a new route or drug delivery system, or for significant new indications which may alter the established risks and benefits of that drug, or that contain a new combination of active substances. There is no standard time for which products retain a black triangle; safety data are usually reviewed after 2 years.

Adverse reactions to medical devices   Suspected adverse reactions to medical devices including dental or surgical materials, intra-uterine devices, and contact lens fluids should be reported. Information on reporting these can be found at: www.mhra.gov.uk

Side-effects in the *BNF for Children*   The *BNF for Children* includes clinically relevant side-effects for most drugs; an exhaustive list is not included for drugs that are used by specialists (e.g. cytotoxic drugs and drugs used in anaesthesia). Where causality has not been established, side-effects in the manufacturers' literature may be omitted from the *BNF for Children*.

In the product literature the frequency of side-effects is generally described as follows:

Very common	greater than 1 in 10
Common	1 in 100 to 1 in 10
Uncommon ['less commonly' in *BNF for Children*]	1 in 1000 to 1 in 100
Rare	1 in 10 000 to 1 in 1000
Very rare	less than 1 in 10 000

Special problems

Symptoms   Children may be poor at expressing the symptoms of an adverse drug reaction and parental opinion may be required.

Delayed drug effects   Some reactions (e.g. cancers and effects on development) may become manifest months or years after exposure. Any suspicion of such an association should be reported directly to the MHRA through the Yellow Card Scheme.

Congenital abnormalities   When an infant is born with a congenital abnormality or there is a malformed aborted fetus doctors are asked to consider whether this might be an adverse reaction to a drug and to report all drugs (including self-medication) taken during pregnancy.

Prevention of adverse reactions

Adverse reactions may be prevented as follows:

- never use any drug unless there is a good indication. If the patient is pregnant do not use a drug unless the need for it is imperative;

- allergy and idiosyncrasy are important causes of adverse drug reactions. Ask if the child has had previous reactions to the drug or formulation;

- prescribe as few drugs as possible and give very clear instructions to the child, parent, or carer;

- whenever possible use a familiar drug; with a new drug be particularly alert for adverse reactions or unexpected events;

- consider if excipients (e.g. colouring agents) may be contributing to the adverse reaction. If the reaction is minor, a trial of an alternative formulation of the same drug may be considered before abandoning the drug;

- obtain a full drug history including asking if the child is already taking other drugs *including over-the-counter medicines*; interactions may occur;

- age and hepatic or renal disease may alter the metabolism or excretion of drugs, particularly in neonates, which can affect the potential for adverse effects. Genetic factors may also be responsible for variations in metabolism, and therefore for the adverse effects of the drug;

- warn the child, parent, or carer if serious adverse reactions are liable to occur.

Defective medicines

During the manufacture or distribution of a medicine an error or accident may occur whereby the finished product does not conform to its specification. While such a defect may impair the therapeutic effect of the product and could adversely affect the health of a patient, it should **not** be confused with an Adverse Drug Reaction where the product conforms to its specification.

The Defective Medicines Report Centre assists with the investigation of problems arising from licensed medicinal products thought to be defective and co-ordinates any necessary protective action. Reports on suspect defective medicinal products should include the brand or the non-proprietary name, the name of the manufacturer or supplier, the strength and dosage form of the product, the product licence number, the batch number or numbers of the product, the nature of the defect, and an account of any action already taken in consequence. The Centre can be contacted at:

The Defective Medicines Report Centre

Medicines and Healthcare products Regulatory Agency

17–157 Market Towers

1 Nine Elms Lane

London SW8 5NQ

(020) 7084 2574 (weekdays 9.00 am–5.00 pm)

or (020) 7210 3000 (urgent calls any other time)

info@mhra.gsi.gov.uk

General guidance

Drug treatment in children

Children, and particularly neonates, differ from adults in their response to drugs. Special care is needed in the neonatal period (first 28 days of life) and doses should always be calculated with care; the risk of toxicity is increased by a reduced rate of drug clearance and differing target organ sensitivity.

Many children's doses in *BNF for Children* are standardised by **weight** (and therefore require multiplying by the body-weight in kilograms to determine the child's dose); occasionally, the doses have been standardised by **body surface area** (in m²) (see also How to Use *BNF for Children*, p. xii). Body surface area can be estimated from weight; see inside back cover. These methods should be used rather than attempting to calculate a child's dose on the basis of doses used in adults. If a dose is not stated, prescribers should seek advice from a medicines information centre.

For some drugs the neonatal dose varies according to the **postmenstrual age** of the neonate. Postmenstrual age is the neonate's total age expressed in weeks from the start of the mother's last menstrual period. For example, a 3 week old baby born at 27 weeks gestation is treated as having a postmenstrual age of 30 weeks. A term baby has a postmenstrual age of 37–42 weeks when born. For most other drugs, the dose can be based on the child's actual date of birth irrespective of postmenstrual age. However, the degree of prematurity, the maturity of renal and hepatic function, and the clinical properties of the drug need to be considered on an individual basis.

For most drugs the adult maximum dose should not be exceeded. For example if the dose is 8 mg/kg (max. 300 mg) a child of 10 kg body-weight should receive 80 mg but a child of 40 kg body-weight should receive 300 mg (rather than 320 mg). For certain drugs, young children may require a higher dose per kilogram than adults because of their higher metabolic rates. Calculation by body-weight in the overweight child may result in much higher doses being administered than necessary; in such cases, the dose should be calculated from an ideal weight, related to height and age.

Body surface area (BSA) estimates are sometimes preferable to body-weight for calculating paediatric doses since many physiological phenomena correlate better with body surface area.

Where the dose for children is not stated, prescribers should seek advice from a medicines information centre.

Dose frequency   Most drugs can be administered at slightly irregular intervals during the day. Some drugs, e.g. antimicrobials, are best given at regular intervals. Some flexibility should be allowed in children to avoid waking them during the night. For example, the night-time dose may be given at the child's bedtime.

Prescribing in hepatic impairment

Children have a large reserve of hepatic metabolic capacity and modification of the choice and dosage of drugs is usually unnecessary even in apparently severe liver disease. However, special consideration is required in the following situations:

- liver failure characterised by severe derangement of liver enzymes and profound jaundice; the use of sedative drugs, opioids, and drugs such as diuretics and amphotericin which produce hypokalaemia may precipitate hepatic encephalopathy;

- impaired coagulation, which can affect response to oral anticoagulants;

- in cholestatic jaundice elimination may be impaired of drugs such as fusidic acid and rifampicin which are excreted in the bile;

- in hypoproteinaemia, the effect of highly protein-bound drugs such as phenytoin, prednisolone, warfarin, and benzodiazepines may be increased;

- use of hepatotoxic drugs is more likely to cause toxicity in children with liver disease; such drugs should be avoided if possible;

- in neonates, particularly preterm neonates, and also in infants metabolic pathways may differ from older children and adults because liver enzyme pathways may be immature.

Where care is needed when prescribing in hepatic impairment, this is indicated under the relevant drug in *BNF for Children*.

General guidance

Prescribing in renal impairment

The use of drugs in children with reduced renal function can give rise to problems for several reasons:

- reduced renal excretion of a drug or its metabolites may produce toxicity;
- sensitivity to some drugs is increased even if elimination is unimpaired;
- many side-effects are tolerated poorly by children with renal impairment;
- some drugs are not effective when renal function is reduced;
- neonates, particularly preterm, may have immature renal function.

Many of these problems can be avoided by reducing the dose or by using alternative drugs.

Principles of dose adjustment in renal impairment

The level of renal function below which the dose of a drug must be reduced depends on the proportion of the drug eliminated by renal excretion and its toxicity.

For many drugs with only minor or no dose-related side-effects, very precise modification of the dose regimen is unnecessary and a simple scheme for dose reduction is sufficient

For more toxic drugs with a small safety margin dose regimens based on glomerular filtration rate should be used. When both efficacy and toxicity are closely related to plasma-drug concentration, recommended regimens should be regarded only as a guide to initial treatment; subsequent doses must be adjusted according to clinical response and plasma-drug concentration.

The total daily maintenance dose of a drug can be reduced either by reducing the size of the individual doses or by increasing the interval between doses. For some drugs, although the size of the maintenance dose is reduced it is important to give a loading dose if an immediate effect is required. This is because it takes about five times the half-life of the drug to achieve steady-state plasma concentration. Because the plasma half-life of drugs excreted by the kidney is prolonged in renal impairment, it can take many doses at the reduced dosage to achieve a therapeutic plasma concentration. The loading dose should usually be the same as the initial dose for a child with normal renal function.

Nephrotoxic drugs should, if possible, be avoided in children with renal disease because the consequences of nephrotoxicity are likely to be more serious when the renal reserve is already reduced.

Glomerular filtration rate is low at birth and increases rapidly during the first 6 months. Thereafter, glomerular filtration rate increases gradually to reach adult levels by 1–2 years of age, when standardised to a typical adult body surface area ($1.73\,\mathrm{m}^2$). In the first weeks after birth, serum creatinine falls; a single measure of serum creatinine provides only a crude estimate of renal function and observing the change over days is of more use. In the neonate, a sustained rise in serum creatinine or a lack of the expected postnatal decline, is indicative of a reduced glomerular filtration rate.

Dose recommendations are based on the severity of renal impairment. This is expressed in terms of **glomerular filtration rate** ($\mathrm{mL/minute/1.73\,m^2}$).

The following equations provide a guide to glomerular filtration rate.

Child over 1 year:
Estimated glomerular filtration rate ($\mathrm{mL/minute/1.73\,m^2}$)$= 40^{1} \times$ height (cm)/ serum creatinine (micromol/litre)

Neonate:
Estimated glomerular filtration rate ($\mathrm{mL/minute/1.73\,m^2}$)$= 30^{1} \times$ height (cm)/ serum creatinine (micromol/litre)

The serum-creatinine concentration is sometimes used as a measure of renal function but is only a **rough guide** even when corrected for age, weight, and sex.

1. The values used in these formulas may differ according to locality or laboratory.

General guidance

> **Important**
>
> The information on dose adjustment in *BNF for Children* is expressed in terms of estimated glomerular filtration rate.
>
> Renal function in adults is increasingly being reported as estimated glomerular filtration rate (eGFR) normalised to a body surface area of $1.73\,m^2$; however, eGFR is derived from the MDRD (Modification of Diet in Renal Disease) formula which is not validated for use in children. eGFR derived from the MDRD formula should **not** be used to adjust drug doses in children with renal impairment.

In *BNF for Children*, values for measures of renal function are included where possible. However, where such values are not available, the *BNF for Children* reflects the terms used in the published information.

*Chronic kidney disease in **adults**: UK guidelines for identification, management and referral* (March 2006) defines renal function as follows:

Degree of impairment	eGFR[1] mL/minute/$1.73\,m^2$
Normal: Stage 1	More than 90 (with other evidence of kidney damage)
Mild: Stage 2	60–89 (with other evidence of kidney damage)
Moderate[2]: Stage 3	30–59
Severe: Stage 4	15–29
Established renal failure: Stage 5	Less than 15

1. Estimated glomerular filtration rate (eGFR) derived from the Modification of Diet in Renal Disease (MDRD) formula for use in patients over 18 years
2. NICE clinical guideline 73 (September 2008)—Chronic kidney disease: Stage 3A eGFR = 45–59, Stage 3B eGFR = 30–44

> **Dialysis**
>
> For prescribing in children on renal replacement therapy consult specialist literature.

Drug prescribing should be kept to the minimum in all children with severe renal disease.

If even mild renal impairment is considered likely on clinical grounds, renal function should be checked before prescribing **any** drug which requires dose modification.

Where care is needed when prescribing in renal impairment, this is indicated under the relevant drug in *BNF for Children*.

General guidance

Prescribing in pregnancy

Drugs can have harmful effects on the fetus at any time during pregnancy. It is important to bear this in mind when prescribing for a female of *childbearing age* or for men *trying to father* a child.

During the *first trimester* drugs may produce congenital malformations (teratogenesis), and the period of greatest risk is from the third to the eleventh week of pregnancy.

During the *second* and *third trimesters* drugs may affect the growth and functional development of the fetus or have toxic effects on fetal tissues; and drugs given shortly before term or during labour may have adverse effects on labour or on the neonate after delivery.

BNF for Children identifies drugs which:

- may have harmful effects in pregnancy and indicates the trimester of risk;
- are not known to be harmful in pregnancy.

The information is based on human data but information on *animal* studies has been included for some drugs when its omission might be misleading. Maternal drug doses may require adjustment during pregnancy due to changes in maternal physiology but this is beyond the scope of *BNF for Children*.

Where care is needed when prescribing in pregnancy, this is indicated under the relevant drug in *BNF for Children*.

Drugs should be prescribed in pregnancy only if the expected benefit to the mother is thought to be greater than the risk to the fetus, and all drugs should be avoided if possible during the first trimester. Drugs which have been extensively used in pregnancy and appear to be usually safe should be prescribed in preference to new or untried drugs; and the smallest effective dose should be used.

Few drugs have been shown conclusively to be teratogenic in humans but no drug is safe beyond all doubt in early pregnancy. Screening procedures are available where there is a known risk of certain defects.

Absence of information does not imply safety.

It should be noted that *BNF for Children* provides independent advice and may not always agree with the product literature.

Information on drugs and pregnancy is also available from the UK Teratology Information Service.

Tel: (0844) 892 0909 (08:30–17:00 Monday to Friday)
Fax: (0191) 260 6193
Outside of these hours, urgent enquiries only
www.uktis.org

General guidance

Prescribing in breast-feeding

Breast-feeding is beneficial; the immunological and nutritional value of breast milk to the infant is greater than that of formula feeds.

Although there is concern that drugs taken by the mother might affect the infant, there is very little information on this. In the absence of evidence of an effect, the potential for harm to the infant can be inferred from:

- the amount of drug or active metabolite of the drug delivered to the infant (dependent on the pharmacokinetic characteristics of the drug in the mother);
- the efficiency of absorption, distribution and elimination of the drug by the infant (infant pharmacokinetics);
- the nature of the effect of the drug on the infant (pharmacodynamic properties of the drug in the infant).

Most medicines given to a mother cause no harm to breast-fed infants and there are few contra-indications to breast-feeding when maternal medicines are necessary. However, administration of some drugs to nursing mothers can harm the infant. In the first week of life, some such as preterm or jaundiced infants are at a slightly higher risk of toxicity.

Toxicity to the infant can occur if the drug enters the milk in pharmacologically significant quantities. The concentration in milk of some drugs (e.g. fluvastatin) may exceed the concentration in maternal plasma so that therapeutic doses in the mother can cause toxicity to the infant. Some drugs inhibit the infant's sucking reflex (e.g. phenobarbital) while others can affect lactation (e.g. bromocriptine). Drugs in breast milk may, at least theoretically, cause hypersensitivity in the infant even when concentration is too low for a pharmacological effect. *BNF for Children* identifies drugs:

- which should be used with caution or which are contra-indicated in breast-feeding for the reasons given above;
- which, on present evidence, may be given to the mother during breast-feeding, because they appear in milk in amounts which are too small to be harmful to the infant;
- which are not known to be harmful to the infant although they are present in milk in significant amounts.

Where care is needed when prescribing in breast-feeding, this is indicated under the relevant drug in *BNF for Children*.

> For many drugs insufficient evidence is available to provide guidance and it is advisable to administer only essential drugs to a mother during breast-feeding. Because of the inadequacy of information on drugs in breast milk information in *BNF for Children* should be used only as a guide; absence of information does not imply safety.

General guidance

Prescribing in palliative care

Palliative care is the active total care of children and young adults who have incurable, life-limiting conditions and are not expected to survive beyond young adulthood.

The child may be cared for in a hospice or at home according to the needs of the child and the child's family. In all cases, children should receive total care of their physical, emotional, social, and spiritual needs, and their families should be supported throughout. In particular, specialist palliative care is essential for end-of-life care of the child and for supporting the family through death and bereavement.

Drug treatment   The number of drugs should be as few as possible. Oral medication is usually appropriate unless there is severe nausea and vomiting, dysphagia, weakness, or coma, when parenteral medication may be necessary.

Pain

Analgesics are more effective in preventing pain than in the relief of established pain; it is important that they are given regularly.

Paracetamol (p. 254) or a **NSAID** (section 10.1.1) given regularly will often make the use of opioid analgesics unnecessary. A NSAID may also control the pain of *bone secondaries*. Radiotherapy and bisphosphonates (section 6.6.2) may also be useful for pain due to bone metastases.

An opioid analgesic (section 4.7.2) such as **codeine** (p. 259), alone or in combination with a non-opioid analgesic at adequate dosage, may be helpful in the control of moderate pain if non-opioid analgesics alone are not sufficient. If these preparations do not control the pain, **morphine** (p. 262) is the most useful opioid analgesic. Alternatives to morphine, including transdermal **fentanyl** (see below and p. 260), are best initiated by those with experience in palliative care. Initiation of an opioid analgesic should not be delayed by concern over a theoretical likelihood of psychological or physical dependence (addiction).

Equivalent single doses of opioid analgesics	
These equivalences are intended **only** as an approximate guide; patients should be carefully monitored after **any** change in medication and dose titration may be required	
Analgesic	Dose
Morphine salts (oral)	10 mg
Diamorphine hydrochloride (subcutaneous)	3 mg
Hydromorphone hydrochloride	1.3 mg
Oxycodone (oral)	5 mg

Oral route   Morphine (p. 262) is given *by mouth* as an oral solution or as standard ('immediate release') tablets regularly every 4 hours, the initial dose depending largely on the patient's previous treatment. If the first dose of morphine is no more effective than the previous analgesic, the next dose should be increased by 30–50%, the aim being to choose the lowest dose that prevents pain. The dose should be adjusted with careful assessment of the pain, and the use of adjuvant analgesics (such as NSAIDs) should also be considered. Although low doses of morphine are usually adequate there should be no hesitation in increasing the dose stepwise according to response if necessary.

When the pain is controlled and the patient's 24-hour morphine requirement is established, the daily dose can be given as a single dose or in 2 divided doses as a *modified-release preparation*. The first dose of the modified-release preparation is given with, or within 4 hours of, the last dose of the oral solution. The child should be reviewed regularly for treatment efficacy and side-effects.

MST Continus® tablets or suspension (p. 263) are designed for twice daily administration; *MXL*® capsules (p. 263) allow administration of the total daily morphine requirement as a single dose.

Alternatively, a *modified-release preparation* may be commenced immediately and the dose adjusted according to pain control. The starting dose of modified-release preparations designed for twice daily administration is usually 200–800 micrograms/kg every 12 hours if no other analgesic (or only paracetamol) has been taken previously, but to replace a weaker opioid analgesic (such as codeine) the starting dose is usually higher. Increments should be made to the dose, not to the frequency of administration, which should remain at every 12 hours.

If pain occurs between regular doses of morphine ('breakthrough pain'), an additional dose ('rescue dose') should be given. An additional dose should also be given 30 minutes before an activity that causes pain (e.g. wound dressing). Morphine, as oral solution or standard formulation tablets, should be prescribed for breakthrough pain. The standard dose of a strong opioid for breakthrough pain is usually 10% of the regular 24 hour total daily dose, but may vary from 5–20%, repeated every 4 hours if necessary (review pain management if analgesic required more frequently). Each child should be assessed on an individual basis.

Children often require a higher dose of morphine in proportion to their body-weight compared to adults. Children are more susceptible to certain adverse effects of opioids such as urinary retention (which can be eased by carbachol or bethanechol), and opioid-induced pruritus.

Oxycodone (p. 264) is used in a child who requires an opioid but cannot tolerate morphine. If the child is already receiving an opioid, oxycodone should be started at a dose equivalent to the current analgesic (see p. 24).

Parenteral route   Diamorphine (p. 259) is preferred for injection because, being more soluble, it can be given in a smaller volume. The equivalent subcutaneous dose is approximately a third of the oral dose of morphine. *Subcutaneous infusion* of diamorphine via a continuous infusion device can be useful (for details, see p. 28).

If the child can resume taking medicines by mouth, then oral morphine may be substituted for subcutaneous infusion of diamorphine. See table of approximate equivalent doses of morphine and diamorphine, p. 29.

Rectal route   Morphine (p. 263) is also available for *rectal administration* as suppositories.

Transdermal route   Transdermal preparations of fentanyl (p. 261) are available; they are not suitable for acute pain or in those children whose analgesic requirements are changing rapidly because the long time to steady state prevents rapid titration of the dose. Prescribers should ensure that they are familiar with the correct use of transdermal preparations (see under fentanyl, p. 260) because inappropriate use has caused fatalities.

The following 24-hour doses of morphine **by mouth** are considered to be approximately equivalent to the fentanyl patches shown:

> Morphine salt 45 mg daily ≡ fentanyl '12' patch
>
> Morphine salt 90 mg daily ≡ fentanyl '25' patch
>
> Morphine salt 180 mg daily ≡ fentanyl '50' patch
>
> Morphine salt 270 mg daily ≡ fentanyl '75' patch
>
> Morphine salt 360 mg daily ≡ fentanyl '100' patch

Morphine (as oral solution or standard formulation tablets) is given for breakthrough pain.

Gastro-intestinal pain   The pain of *bowel colic* may be reduced by loperamide (p. 65). Hyoscine hydrobromide (p. 252) may also be helpful in reducing the frequency of spasms; it is given sublingually at a dose of 10 micrograms/kg (max. 300 micrograms) 3 times daily as *Kwells®* tablets. For the dose by subcutaneous infusion, see p. 28.

Gastric distension pain due to pressure on the stomach may be helped by a preparation incorporating an antacid with an antiflatulent (p. 51) and a prokinetic such as domperidone (p. 57) before meals.

Muscle spasm   The pain of muscle spasm can be helped by a muscle relaxant such as diazepam (p. 628) or baclofen (p. 626).

Neuropathic pain   Patients with neuropathic pain (p. 267) may benefit from a trial of a tricyclic antidepressant, most commonly amitriptyline (p. 236), for several weeks. An anticonvulsant, most commonly carbamazepine (p. 274), may be added or substituted if pain persists; gabapentin is licensed for neuropathic

General guidance

pain in adults. Ketamine is sometimes used under specialist supervision as an adjuvant for neuropathic pain that responds poorly to opioid analgesics.

Pain due to nerve compression may be reduced by a corticosteroid such as dexamethasone, which reduces oedema around the tumour, thus reducing compression.

Nerve blocks can be considered when pain is localised to a specific area. **Transcutaneous electrical nerve stimulation** (TENS) may also help.

Miscellaneous conditions

> Unlicensed indications or routes
> Several recommendations in this section involve unlicensed indications or routes.

Anorexia   Anorexia may be helped by prednisolone or dexamethasone.

Anxiety   Anxiety can be treated with a long-acting benzodiazepine such as diazepam, or by continuous infusion of the short-acting benzodiazepine midazolam. Interventions for more acute episodes of anxiety (such as panic attacks) include short-acting benzodiazepines such as lorazepam given sublingually or midazolam given subcutaneously. Temazepam provides useful night-time sedation in some children.

Capillary bleeding   Capillary bleeding can be treated with tranexamic acid (p. 158) by mouth; treatment is usually continued for one week after the bleeding has stopped but it can be continued at a reduced dose if bleeding persists. Alternatively, gauze soaked in tranexamic acid 100 mg/mL or adrenaline (epinephrine) solution 1 mg/mL (1 in 1000) can be applied to the affected area.

Vitamin K may be useful for the treatment and prevention of bleeding associated with prolonged clotting in liver disease. In severe chronic cholestasis, absorption of vitamin K may be impaired; either parenteral or water-soluble oral vitamin K should be considered (section 9.6.6).

Constipation   Constipation is a very common cause of distress and is almost invariable after administration of an opioid analgesic. It should be prevented if possible by the regular administration of laxatives. Suitable laxatives include osmotic laxatives (p. 82) (such as lactulose or macrogols), stimulant laxatives (p. 79) (such as co-danthramer and senna) or the combination of lactulose and a senna preparation. Naloxone given by mouth may help relieve opioid-induced constipation; it is poorly absorbed but opioid withdrawal reactions have been reported.

Convulsions   Intractable seizures are relatively common in children dying from non-malignant conditions. Phenobarbital by mouth or as a continuous subcutaneous infusion may be beneficial; continuous infusion of midazolam is an alternative. Both cause drowsiness, but this is rarely a concern in the context of intractable seizures. For breakthrough convulsions diazepam (p. 291) given rectally (as a solution), buccal midazolam (p. 293), or paraldehyde (p. 293) as an enema may be appropriate.

For the use of midazolam by subcutaneous infusion using a continuous infusion device, see p. 28.

Dry mouth   Dry mouth may be caused by certain medications including opioid analgesics, antimuscarinic drugs (e.g. hyoscine), antidepressants and some antiemetics; if possible, an alternative preparation should be considered. Dry mouth may be relieved by good mouth care and measures such as chewing sugar-free gum, sucking ice or pineapple chunks, or the use of artificial saliva (p. 669); dry mouth associated with candidiasis can be treated by oral preparations of nystatin (p. 667) or miconazole (p. 666); alternatively, fluconazole (p. 372) can be given by mouth.

Dysphagia   A corticosteroid such as dexamethasone may help, temporarily, if there is an obstruction due to tumour. See also Dry Mouth, above.

Dyspnoea   Breathlessness at rest may be relieved by regular oral morphine in carefully titrated doses. Diazepam may be helpful for dyspnoea associated with anxiety. Sublingual lorazepam or subcutaneous or buccal midazolam are alternatives. A nebulised short-acting beta$_2$ agonist (section 3.1.1.1) or a corticosteroid (section 3.2), such as dexamethasone or prednisolone, may also be helpful for bronchospasm or partial obstruction.

Excessive respiratory secretion   Excessive respiratory secretion (death rattle) may be reduced by hyoscine hydrobromide patches (p. 252) or by subcutaneous or intravenous injection of hyoscine hydrobromide 10 micrograms/kg (max. 600 micrograms) every 4 to 8 hours; however, care must be taken to avoid the discomfort of dry mouth. Alternatively, glycopyrronium (p. 780) may be given.

For the administration of hyoscine hydrobromide by subcutaneous or intravenous infusion using a continuous infusion device, see p. 28.

Fungating tumours   Fungating tumours can be treated by regular dressing and antibacterial drugs; systemic treatment with metronidazole (p. 362) is often required to reduce malodour, but topical metronidazole (p. 718) is also used.

Hiccup   Hiccup due to gastric distension may be helped by a preparation incorporating an antacid with an antiflatulent (p. 52).

Hypercalcaemia   See section 9.5.1.2.

Insomnia   Children with advanced cancer may not sleep because of discomfort, cramps, night sweats, joint stiffness, or fear. There should be appropriate treatment of these problems before hypnotics (p. 216) are used. Benzodiazepines, such as temazepam, may be useful.

Intractable cough   Intractable cough may be relieved by moist inhalations or by regular administration of oral morphine every 4 hours. Methadone linctus should be avoided because it has a long duration of action and tends to accumulate.

Mucosal bleeding   Mucosal bleeding from the mouth and nose occurs commonly in the terminal phase, particularly in a child suffering from haemopoeitic malignancy. Bleeding from the nose caused by a single bleeding point can be arrested by cauterisation or by dressing it. Tranexamic acid (p. 158) may be effective applied topically or given systemically.

Nausea and vomiting   Nausea and vomiting are common in children with advanced cancer. Ideally, the cause should be determined before treatment with an antiemetic (section 4.6) is started.

Nausea and vomiting with opioid therapy are less common in children than in adults but may occur particularly in the initial stages and can be prevented by giving an antiemetic. An antiemetic is usually necessary only for the first 4 or 5 days and therefore combined preparations containing an opioid with an antiemetic are not recommended because they lead to unnecessary antiemetic therapy (and associated side-effects when used long-term).

Metoclopramide has a prokinetic action and is used by mouth for nausea and vomiting associated with gastritis, gastric stasis, and functional bowel obstruction. Drugs with antimuscarinic effects antagonise prokinetic drugs and, if possible, should not therefore be used concurrently.

Haloperidol (p. 223) is used by mouth or by continuous intravenous or subcutaneous infusion for most metabolic causes of vomiting (e.g. hypercalcaemia, renal failure).

Cyclizine (p. 246) is used for nausea and vomiting due to mechanical bowel obstruction, raised intracranial pressure, and motion sickness.

Ondansetron (p. 250) is most effective when the vomiting is due to damaged or irritated gut mucosa (e.g. after chemotherapy or radiotherapy).

Antiemetic therapy should be reviewed every 24 hours; it may be necessary to substitute the antiemetic or to add another one.

Levomepromazine (methotrimeprazine) (p. 224) can be used if first-line antiemetics are inadequate. Dexamethasone by mouth can be used as an adjunct.

For the administration of antiemetics by subcutaneous infusion using a continuous infusion device, see below.

For the treatment of nausea and vomiting associated with cancer chemotherapy, see section 8.1.

Pruritus   Pruritus, even when associated with obstructive jaundice, often responds to simple measures such as application of emollients (p. 674). Ondansetron may be effective in some children. Where opioid analgesics cause pruritus it may be appropriate to review the dose or to switch to an alternative opioid analgesic. In the case of obstructive jaundice, further measures include adminis-tration of colestyramine (p. 93).

Raised intracranial pressure   Headache due to raised intracranial pressure often responds to a high dose of a corticosteroid, such as dexamethasone, for 4 to 5 days, subsequently reduced if possible; dexamethasone should be given before 6 p.m. to reduce the risk of insomnia. Treatment of headache and of associated nausea and vomiting should also be considered.

Restlessness and confusion   Restlessness and confusion may require treatment with haloperidol (p. 223) 10–20 micrograms/kg by mouth every 8–12 hours. Levomepromazine (methotrimeprazine) (p. 224) is also used occasionally for restlessness. See also below.

Continuous infusion devices

Although drugs can usually be administered *by mouth* to control symptoms in palliative care, the parenteral route may sometimes be necessary. Repeated administration of *intramuscular injections* should be avoided in children, particu-larly if cachectic. This has led to the use of portable continuous infusion devices such as syringe drivers to give a *continuous subcutaneous infusion*, which can provide good control of symptoms with little discomfort or inconvenience to the patient.

> **Syringe driver rate settings**
> Staff using syringe drivers should be **adequately trained** and different rate settings should be **clearly identified** and **differentiated**; incorrect use of syringe drivers is a common cause of medication errors.

Indications for the **parenteral route** are:

- inability to take medicines by mouth owing to *nausea and vomiting, dysphagia, severe weakness,* or *coma;*
- *malignant bowel obstruction* for which surgery is inappropriate (avoiding the need for an intravenous infusion or for insertion of a nasogastric tube);
- refusal by the child to take regular medication by mouth.

Bowel colic and excessive respiratory secretions   Hyoscine hydrobromide (p. 252) effectively reduces respiratory secretions and is sedative (but occasionally causes paradoxical agitation); it is given in a *subcutaneous* or *intravenous infusion dose* of 40–60 micrograms/kg/24 hours. Glycopyrronium (p. 780) may also be used.

Hyoscine butylbromide (p. 55) is effective in bowel colic, is less sedative than hyoscine hydrobromide, but is not always adequate for the control of respiratory secretions; it is given by *subcutaneous infusion* (**important:** *hyoscine butylbromide* must not be confused with *hyoscine hydrobromide,* above).

Convulsions   If a child has previously been receiving an antiepileptic drug *or* has a primary or secondary cerebral tumour *or* is at risk of convulsion (e.g. owing to uraemia) antiepileptic medication should not be stopped. Midazolam (p. 293) is the benzodiazepine antiepileptic of choice for *continuous subcutaneous infusion.*

Nausea and vomiting   Levomepromazine (methotrimeprazine) (p. 224) causes sedation in about 50% of patients. Haloperidol (p. 223) has little sedative effect.

Cyclizine (p. 246) is particularly likely to precipitate if mixed with diamorphine or other drugs (see under Mixing and Compatibility); it is given by *subcutaneous infusion.*

Pain control   Diamorphine (p. 259) is the preferred opioid since its high solubility permits a large dose to be given in a small volume (see under Mixing and Compatibility). The table on p. 29 shows approximate equivalent doses of mor-phine and diamorphine.

Restlessness and confusion   Haloperidol has little sedative effect. Levomepro-mazine (methotrimeprazine) (p. 224) has a sedative effect. Midazolam is a seda-tive and an antiepileptic that may be suitable for a very restless patient.

Mixing and compatibility   The general principle that injections should be given into separate sites (and should not be mixed) does not apply to the use of syringe drivers in palliative care. Provided that there is evidence of compatibility, selected injections can be mixed in syringe drivers. Not all types of medication can be used in a subcutaneous infusion. In particular, chlorpromazine, prochlorperazine, and diazepam are **contra-indicated** as they cause skin reactions at the injection site; to a lesser extent cyclizine and levomepromazine (methotrimeprazine) also sometimes cause local irritation.

In theory injections dissolved in water for injections are more likely to be associated with pain (possibly owing to their hypotonicity). The use of physiological saline (sodium chloride 0.9%) however increases the likelihood of precipitation when more than one drug is used; moreover subcutaneous infusion rates are so slow (0.1–0.3 mL/hour) that pain is not usually a problem when water is used as a diluent.

Diamorphine can be given by subcutaneous infusion in a strength of up to 250 mg/mL; up to a strength of 40 mg/mL either *water for injections* or *physiological saline* (sodium chloride 0.9%) is a suitable diluent—above that strength only *water for injections* is used (to avoid precipitation).

The following can be mixed with *diamorphine*:

Cyclizine[1]	Hyoscine hydrobromide
Dexamethasone[2]	Levomepromazine
Haloperidol[3]	Metoclopramide[4]
Hyoscine butylbromide	Midazolam

Subcutaneous infusion solution should be monitored regularly both to check for precipitation (and discoloration) and to ensure that the infusion is running at the correct rate.

Equivalent doses of morphine sulphate and diamorphine hydrochloride given over 24 hours

These equivalences are *approximate only* and may need to be adjusted according to response

MORPHINE		PARENTERAL DIAMORPHINE
Oral morphine sulphate	Subcutaneous infusion of morphine sulphate	Subcutaneous infusion of diamorphine hydrochloride
over 24 hours	**over 24 hours**	**over 24 hours**
30 mg	15 mg	10 mg
60 mg	30 mg	20 mg
90 mg	45 mg	30 mg
120 mg	60 mg	40 mg
180 mg	90 mg	60 mg
240 mg	120 mg	80 mg
360 mg	180 mg	120 mg
480 mg	240 mg	160 mg
600 mg	300 mg	200 mg
780 mg	390 mg	260 mg
960 mg	480 mg	320 mg
1200 mg	600 mg	400 mg

If breakthrough pain occurs give a subcutaneous injection equivalent to 10% (but may vary from 5–20%) of the total 24-hour subcutaneous infusion dose. With an intermittent subcutaneous injection absorption is smoother so that the risk of adverse effects at peak absorption is avoided (an even better method is to use a subcutaneous butterfly needle).

To minimise the risk of infection no subcutaneous infusion solution should be used for longer than 24 hours.

1. Cyclizine may precipitate at concentrations above 10 mg/mL *or* in the presence of sodium chloride 0.9% *or* as the concentration of diamorphine relative to cyclizine increases; mixtures of diamorphine and cyclizine are also likely to precipitate after 24 hours.
2. Special care is needed to avoid precipitation of dexamethasone when preparing it.
3. Mixtures of haloperidol and diamorphine are likely to precipitate after 24 hours if haloperidol concentration is above 2 mg/mL.
4. Under some conditions, infusions containing metoclopramide become discoloured; such solutions should be discarded.

Problems encountered with syringe drivers   The following are problems that may be encountered with syringe drivers and the action that should be taken:

- if the subcutaneous infusion runs *too quickly* check the rate setting and the calculation;

- if the subcutaneous infusion runs *too slowly* check the start button, the battery, the syringe driver, the cannula, and make sure that the injection site is not inflamed;

- if there is an *injection site reaction* make sure that the site does not need to be changed—firmness or swelling at the site of injection is not in itself an indication for change, but pain or obvious inflammation is.

Prescribing in dental practice

> Advice on the drug management of dental and oral conditions is covered in the main text. For ease of access, guidance on such conditions is usually identified by means of a relevant heading (e.g. Dental and Orofacial Pain) in the appropriate sections.

The following is a list of topics of particular relevance to dental surgeons.

General guidance

Drugs and sport

UK Anti-Doping advises that athletes are personally responsible should a prohibited substance be detected in their body. An advice card listing examples of permitted and prohibited substances is available from:

UK Anti-Doping
Oceanic House
1a Cockspur Street
London, SW1Y 5BG.
Tel: (020) 7766 7350
information@ukad.org.uk
www.ukad.org.uk

A similar card detailing classes of drugs and doping methods prohibited in football is available from the Football Association. This contains information specific to the Football Association Doping Control Regulations including the Football Association's policy on social drugs. Further information is available at www.thefa.com.

> **General Medical Council's advice**
> Doctors who prescribe or collude in the provision of drugs or treatment with the intention of improperly enhancing an individual's performance in sport contravene the GMC's guidance, and such actions would usually raise a question of a doctor's continued registration. This does not preclude the provision of any care or treatment where the doctor's intention is to protect or improve the patient's health.

Emergency treatment of poisoning

These notes provide only an overview of the treatment of poisoning and it is strongly recommended that either **TOXBASE** or the **UK National Poisons Information Service** (see below) be consulted when there is doubt about the degree of risk or about appropriate management.

Most childhood poisoning is accidental. Other causes include intentional overdose, drug abuse, iatrogenic and deliberate poisoning. The drugs most commonly involved in childhood poisoning are paracetamol, ibuprofen, orally ingested creams, aspirin, iron preparations, cough medicines, and the contraceptive pill.

Hospital admission   Children who have features of poisoning should generally be admitted to hospital. Children who have taken poisons with delayed actions should also be admitted, even if they appear well. Delayed-action poisons include aspirin, iron, paracetamol, tricyclic antidepressants, and co-phenotrope (diphenoxylate with atropine, *Lomotil*®); the effects of modified-release preparations are also delayed. A note of all relevant information, including what treatment has been given, should accompany the patient to hospital.

Further information and advice

TOXBASE, the primary clinical toxicology database of the National Poisons Information Service, is available on the Internet to registered users at www.toxbase.org (a backup site is available at www.toxbasebackup.org if the main site cannot be accessed). It provides information about routine diagnosis, treatment, and management of patients exposed to drugs, household products, and industrial and agricultural chemicals.

Specialist information and advice on the treatment of poisoning is available day and night from the **UK National Poisons Information Service** on the following number:
Tel: 0844 892 0111

Advice on laboratory analytical services can be obtained from TOXBASE or from the National Poisons Information Service.

Help with identifying capsules or tablets may be available from a regional medicines information centre (see inside front cover) or (out of hours) from the National Poisons Information Service.

General care

It is often impossible to establish with certainty the identity of the poison and the size of the dose. This is not usually important because only a few poisons (such as opioids, paracetamol, and iron) have specific antidotes; few children require active removal of the poison. In most children, treatment is directed at managing symptoms as they arise. Nevertheless, knowledge of the type and timing of poisoning can help in anticipating the course of events. All relevant information should be sought from the poisoned child and from their carers. However, such information should be interpreted with care because it may not be complete or entirely reliable. Sometimes symptoms arise from other illnesses, and children should be assessed carefully. Accidents may involve a number of domestic and industrial products (the contents of which are not generally known). The **National Poisons Information Service** should be consulted when there is doubt about any aspect of suspected poisoning.

Respiration

Respiration is often impaired in unconscious children. An obstructed airway requires immediate attention. In the absence of trauma, the airway should be opened with simple measures such as chin lift or jaw thrust. An oropharyngeal or nasopharyngeal airway may be useful in children with reduced consciousness to prevent obstruction, provided ventilation is adequate. Intubation and ventilation should be considered in children whose airway cannot be protected or who have respiratory acidosis because of inadequate ventilation; such children should be monitored in a critical care area.

Most poisons that impair consciousness also depress respiration. Assisted ventilation (either mouth-to-mouth or using a bag-valve-mask device) may be needed. Oxygen is not a substitute for adequate ventilation, although it should be given in the highest concentration possible in poisoning with carbon monoxide and irritant gases.

The potential for pulmonary aspiration of gastric contents should be considered.

> The **National Poisons Information Service** (Tel: 0844 892 0111) will provide specialist advice on all aspects of poisoning day and night

Blood pressure

Hypotension is common in severe poisoning with central nervous system depressants; if severe this may lead to irreversible brain damage or renal tubular necrosis. Hypotension should be corrected initially by tilting down the head of the bed and administration of either sodium chloride intravenous infusion or a colloidal infusion. Vasoconstrictor sympathomimetics (section 2.7.2) are rarely required and their use may be discussed with the National Poisons Information Service.

Fluid depletion without hypotension is common after prolonged coma and after aspirin poisoning due to vomiting, sweating, and hyperpnoea.

Hypertension, often transient, occurs less frequently than hypotension in poisoning; it may be associated with sympathomimetic drugs such as amphetamines, phencyclidine, and cocaine.

Heart

Cardiac conduction defects and arrhythmias can occur in acute poisoning, notably with tricyclic antidepressants, some antipsychotics, and some antihistamines. Arrhythmias often respond to correction of underlying hypoxia, acidosis, or other biochemical abnormalities, but ventricular arrhythmias that cause serious hypotension may require treatment (section 2.3.1). If the QT interval is prolonged, specialist advice should be sought because the use of some anti-arrhythmic drugs may be inappropriate. Supraventricular arrhythmias are seldom life-threatening and drug treatment is best withheld until the child reaches hospital.

Body temperature

Hypothermia may develop in patients of any age who have been deeply unconscious for some hours, particularly following overdose with barbiturates or phenothiazines. It may be missed unless core temperature is measured using a low-reading rectal thermometer or by some other means. Hypothermia is best treated by wrapping the patient (e.g. in a 'space blanket') to conserve body heat.

Hyperthermia can develop in children taking CNS stimulants; children are also at risk when taking therapeutic doses of drugs with antimuscarinic properties. Hyperthermia is initially managed by removing all unnecessary clothing and using a fan. Sponging with **tepid** water will promote evaporation. Advice should be sought from the National Poisons Information Service on the management of severe hyperthermia resulting from conditions such as the serotonin syndrome.

Both hypothermia and hyperthermia require **urgent** hospitalisation for assessment and supportive treatment.

Convulsions

Single short-lived convulsions do not require treatment. If convulsions are protracted or recur frequently, lorazepam 100 micrograms/kg (max. 4 mg) or diazepam (preferably as emulsion) 300–400 micrograms/kg (max. 20 mg) should be given by slow intravenous injection into a large vein. Benzodiazepines should not be given by the intramuscular route for convulsions. If the intravenous route is not readily available, diazepam can be administered as a rectal solution or midazolam [unlicensed use] can be given by the buccal route (section 4.8.2).

Removal and elimination

Prevention of absorption   Given by mouth, **activated charcoal** can adsorb many poisons in the gastro-intestinal system, thereby *reducing their absorption*. The **sooner** it is given the **more effective** it is, but it may still be effective up to 1 hour after ingestion of the poison—longer in the case of modified-release preparations or of drugs with antimuscarinic (anticholinergic) properties. It is particularly useful for the prevention of absorption of poisons that are toxic in small amounts such as antidepressants.

A second dose may occasionally be required when blood-drug concentration continues to rise suggesting delayed drug release or delayed gastric emptying.

For the use of charcoal in active elimination techniques, see below.

Active elimination techniques   Repeated doses of **activated charcoal** by mouth may *enhance the elimination* of some drugs after they have been absorbed; repeated doses are given after overdosage with:

Carbamazepine	Quinine
Dapsone	Theophylline
Phenobarbital	

Vomiting should be treated (e.g. with an antiemetic drug) since it may reduce the efficacy of charcoal treatment. In cases of intolerance, the dose may be reduced and the frequency increased but this may compromise efficacy.

Other techniques intended to enhance the elimination of poisons after absorption are only practicable in hospital and are only suitable for a small number of severely poisoned patients. Moreover, they only apply to a limited number of poisons. Examples include:

- haemodialysis for ethylene glycol, lithium, methanol, phenobarbital, salicylates, and sodium valproate
- alkalinisation of the urine for salicylates.

Removal from the gastro-intestinal tract   Gastric lavage is rarely required as benefit rarely outweighs risk; advice should be sought from the National Poisons Information Service if a significant quantity of iron or lithium has been ingested within the previous hour.

Whole bowel irrigation (by means of a bowel cleansing preparation) has been used in poisoning with certain modified-release or enteric-coated formulations, in severe poisoning with lithium salts, and if illicit drugs are carried in the gastro-intestinal tract ('body-packing'). However, it is not clear that the procedure improves outcome and advice should be sought from a poisons information centre.

The administration of **laxatives** alone has no role in the management of the poisoned child and is not a recommended method of gut decontamination. The routine use of a laxative in combination with activated charcoal has mostly been abandoned. Laxatives should not be administered to young children because of the likelihood of fluid and electrolyte imbalance.

CHARCOAL, ACTIVATED

Cautions drowsy or comatose child (risk of aspiration); reduced gastro-intestinal motility (risk of obstruction); **not** for poisoning with petroleum distillates, corrosive substances, alcohols, malathion, and metal salts including iron and lithium salts

Contra-indications unprotected airway; gastro-intestinal tract not intact

Side-effects black stools

Indication and dose

Reduction of absorption of poisons
- By mouth

Neonate 1 g/kg

Child 1 month–12 years 1 g/kg (max. 50 g)

Child 12–18 years 50 g

Active elimination of poisons
- By mouth

Neonate 1 g/kg every 4 hours

Child 1 month–12 years 1 g/kg (max. 50 g) every 4 hours

Child 12–18 years 50 g every 4 hours

Administration suspension or reconstituted powder may be mixed with soft drinks (e.g. caffeine-free diet cola) or fruit juices to mask the taste

◻ **CHARCOAL, ACTIVATED** (*continued*)

Actidose-Aqua® Advance (Alliance)
Oral suspension, activated charcoal 1.04 g/5 mL,
net price 50-g pack (240 mL) = £8.69

Charcodote® (TEVA UK)
Oral suspension, activated charcoal 1 g/5 mL, net
price 50-g pack = £11.88

Carbomix® (Beacon)
Powder, activated charcoal, net price 25-g pack =
£8.50, 50-g pack = £11.90

Specific drugs

Alcohol

Acute intoxication with alcohol (ethanol) is common in adults but also occurs in
children. The features include ataxia, dysarthria, nystagmus, and drowsiness,
which may progress to coma, with hypotension and acidosis. Aspiration of
vomit is a special hazard and hypoglycaemia may occur in children and some
adults. Patients are managed supportively, with particular attention to maintaining
a clear airway and measures to reduce the risk of aspiration of gastric contents.
The blood glucose is measured and glucose given if indicated.

Analgesics (non-opioid)

Aspirin   The main features of salicylate poisoning are hyperventilation, tinnitus,
deafness, vasodilatation, and sweating. Coma is uncommon but indicates very
severe poisoning. The associated acid-base disturbances are complex.

Treatment must be in hospital, where plasma salicylate, pH, and electrolytes
(particularly potassium) can be measured; absorption of aspirin may be slow and
the plasma-salicylate concentration may continue to rise for several hours,
requiring repeated measurement. Plasma-salicylate concentration may not correlate with clinical severity in children, and clinical and biochemical assessment is
necessary. Generally, the clinical severity of poisoning is less below a plasma-
salicylate concentration of 500 mg/litre (3.6 mmol/litre) unless there is evidence
of metabolic acidosis. Activated charcoal should be given within 1 hour of
ingesting more than 125 mg/kg aspirin. Fluid losses should be replaced and
intravenous sodium bicarbonate may be given (ensuring plasma-potassium concentration is maintained within the reference range) to enhance urinary salicylate
excretion (optimum urinary pH 7.5–8.5); treatment should be given in a high
dependency unit.

Plasma-potassium concentration should be corrected before giving sodium
bicarbonate as hypokalaemia may complicate alkalinisation of the urine.

Haemodialysis is the treatment of choice for severe salicylate poisoning and
should be considered when the plasma-salicylate concentration exceeds 700 mg/
litre (5.1 mmol/litre) or in the presence of severe metabolic acidosis, convulsions,
renal failure, pulmonary oedema or persistently high plasma-salicylate concentrations unresponsive to urinary alkalinisation.

NSAIDs   Mefenamic acid has important consequences in overdosage because it
can cause convulsions, which if prolonged or recurrent, require treatment with
intravenous lorazepam or diazepam.

Overdosage with ibuprofen may cause nausea, vomiting, epigastric pain, and
tinnitus, but more serious toxicity is very uncommon. Activated charcoal followed
by symptomatic measures are indicated if more than 400 mg/kg has been
ingested within the preceding hour.

Paracetamol   Single or repeated doses totalling as little as 150 mg/kg of paracetamol taken within 24 hours may cause severe hepatocellular necrosis and,
much less frequently, renal tubular necrosis. Children at *high-risk* of liver damage,
including those taking enzyme-inducing drugs or who are malnourished (see

below), may develop liver toxicity with as little as 75 mg/kg of paracetamol taken within 24 hours. Nausea and vomiting, the only early features of poisoning, usually settle within 24 hours. Persistence beyond this time, often associated with the onset of right subcostal pain and tenderness, usually indicates development of hepatic necrosis. Liver damage is maximal 3–4 days after ingestion and may lead to encephalopathy, haemorrhage, hypoglycaemia, cerebral oedema, and death.

Therefore, despite a lack of significant early symptoms, patients who have taken an overdose of paracetamol should be transferred to hospital **urgently**.

Administration of activated charcoal should be considered if paracetamol in excess of 150 mg/kg (or in excess of 75 mg/kg for those considered to be at *high-risk*, see below) is thought to have been ingested within the previous hour.

Acetylcysteine protects the liver if infused within 24 hours of ingesting para-cetamol. It is most effective if given within 8 hours of ingestion, after which effectiveness declines; in children who present 8–36 hours after a potentially toxic ingestion, acetylcysteine treatment should commence immediately even if plasma-paracetamol concentrations are not yet available. If more than 24 hours have elapsed advice should be sought from the National Poisons Information Service. Giving acetylcysteine by mouth [unlicensed route] is an alternative if intravenous access is not possible—contact the National Poisons Information Service for advice. In remote areas, **methionine** by mouth is an alternative only if acetylcysteine cannot be given promptly. Once the child reaches hospital the need to continue treatment with the antidote will be assessed from the plasma-para-cetamol concentration (related to the time from ingestion).

Children at risk of liver damage and therefore requiring treatment can be identified from a single measurement of the plasma-paracetamol concentration, related to the time from ingestion, provided this time interval is not less than 4 hours; earlier samples may be misleading. The concentration is plotted on a paracetamol treatment graph, with a reference line ('normal treatment line') joining plots of 200 mg/litre (1.32 mmol/litre) at 4 hours and 6.25 mg/litre (0.04 mmol/litre) at 24 hours (see p. 38). Those whose plasma-paracetamol concentration is above the *normal treatment line* are treated with acetylcysteine by intravenous infusion (or, if acetylcysteine is not available, with methionine by mouth, provided the overdose has been taken **within 10–12 hours** *and* the child is not vomiting).

Children at *high-risk* of liver damage include those:

- taking liver enzyme-inducing drugs (e.g. carbamazepine, phenobarbital, phenytoin, primidone, rifampicin, rifabutin, efavirenz, nevirapine, alcohol, St John's wort);
- who are malnourished (e.g. in anorexia or bulimia, cystic fibrosis, hepatitis C, in underweight children with 'failure to thrive', in alcoholism, or those who are HIV-positive);
- who have a febrile illness;
- who have not eaten for a few days.

These children may develop toxicity at **lower** plasma-paracetamol concentra-tions and should be treated if the concentration is above the *high-risk treatment line* (which joins plots that are at 50% of the plasma-paracetamol concentrations of the normal treatment line). The prognostic accuracy of plasma-paracetamol concentration taken after 15 hours is uncertain, but a concentration above the relevant treatment line should be regarded as carrying a serious risk of liver damage.

The plasma-paracetamol concentration may be difficult to interpret when para-cetamol has been ingested over several hours (staggered overdose). If there is doubt about timing or the need for treatment then the child should be treated with acetylcysteine.

The **National Poisons Information Service** (Tel: 0844 892 0111) will provide specialist advice on all aspects of poisoning day and night

Emergency treatment of poisoning

Time (hours)

Patients whose plasma-paracetamol concentrations are above the **normal treatment line** should be treated with acetylcysteine by intravenous infusion (or, if acetylcysteine cannot be used, with methionine by mouth, provided the overdose has been taken **within 10–12 hours** and the patient is not vomiting).

Children at *high-risk* of liver damage include those:
- taking liver enzyme-inducing drugs (e.g. carbamazepine, phenobarbital, phenytoin, primidone, rifampicin, rifabutin, efavirenz, nevirapine, alcohol, St John's wort);
- who are malnourished (e.g. in anorexia or bulimia, cystic fibrosis, hepatitis C, in underweight children with failure to thrive, in alcoholism, or those who are HIV-positive);
- who have a febrile illness;
- who have not eaten for a few days.

These children should be treated if their plasma-paracetamol concentration is above the **high-risk treatment line.**

The prognostic accuracy after 15 hours is uncertain but a plasma-paracetamol concentration above the relevant treatment line should be regarded as carrying a serious risk of liver damage.

Graph reproduced courtesy of University of Wales College of Medicine Therapeutics and Toxicology Centre

ACETYLCYSTEINE

Cautions asthma (see side-effects below, but do not delay acetylcysteine treatment)

Side-effects hypersensitivity-like reactions managed by reducing infusion rate or suspending until reaction settled (rash also managed by giving antihistamine; acute asthma managed by giving nebulised short-acting beta$_2$ agonist)—contact the National Poisons Information Service if reaction severe

◁ **ACETYLCYSTEINE** (*continued*)

Indication and dose

Paracetamol overdosage see notes above
• **By intravenous infusion**

Neonate initially 150 mg/kg in 3 mL/kg Glucose 5% and given over 15 minutes, followed by 50 mg/kg in 7 mL/kg Glucose 5% and given over 4 hours, then 100 mg/kg in 14 mL/kg Glucose 5% and given over 16 hours

Child 1 month–5 years (or body-weight under 20 kg) initially 150 mg/kg in 3 mL/kg Glucose 5% and given over 15 minutes, followed by 50 mg/kg in 7 mL/kg Glucose 5% and given over 4 hours, then 100 mg/kg in 14 mL/kg Glucose 5% and given over 16 hours

Child 5–12 years (or body-weight over 20 kg) initially 150 mg/kg in 100 mL Glucose 5% and given over 15 minutes, followed by 50 mg/kg in 250 mL Glucose 5% and given over 4 hours, then 100 mg/kg in 500 mL Glucose 5% and given over 16 hours

Child 12–18 years initially 150 mg/kg (max. 16.5 g) in 200 mL Glucose 5% and given over 15 minutes, followed by 50 mg/kg (max. 5.5 g) in 500 mL Glucose 5% and given over 4 hours, then 100 mg/kg (max.11 g) in 1 litre Glucose 5% and given over 16 hours

Note Manufacturer also recommends other infusion fluids, but Glucose 5% is preferable

Acetylcysteine (Non-proprietary) ℗ｏＭ
Injection, acetylcysteine 200 mg/mL, net price 10-mL amp = £2.50

Parvolex® (UCB Pharma) ℗ｏＭ
Injection, acetylcysteine 200 mg/mL, net price 10-mL amp = £2.25

▊ METHIONINE

Hepatic impairment may precipitate coma

Side-effects nausea, vomiting, drowsiness, irritability

Indication and dose

Paracetamol overdosage see notes above
• **By mouth**

Child under 6 years 1 g every 4 hours for a total of 4 doses

Child 6–18 years 2.5 g every 4 hours for a total of 4 doses

Methionine (Pharma Nord)
Tablets, f/c, methionine 500 mg, net price 20-tab pack = £9.95

▊ Analgesics (opioid)

Opioids (narcotic analgesics) cause varying degrees of coma, respiratory depression, and pinpoint pupils. The specific antidote **naloxone** is indicated if there is coma or bradypnoea. Since naloxone has a shorter duration of action than many opioids, close monitoring and repeated injections are necessary according to the respiratory rate and depth of coma. When repeated administration of naloxone is required, it can be given by continuous intravenous infusion instead and the rate of infusion adjusted according to vital signs. All children should be observed for at least 6 hours after the last dose of naloxone. The effects of some opioids, such as buprenorphine, are only partially reversed by naloxone. Dextropropoxyphene and methadone have very long durations of action; patients may need to be monitored for long periods following large overdoses.

Naloxone reverses the opioid effects of dextropropoxyphene; the long duration of action of dextropropoxyphene calls for prolonged monitoring and further doses of naloxone may be required. Norpropoxyphene, a metabolite of dextropropoxyphene, also has cardiotoxic effects which may require treatment with **sodium bicarbonate**, or **magnesium sulphate**, or both; arrhythmias may occur for up to 12 hours.

The **National Poisons Information Service** (Tel: 0844 892 0111) will provide specialist advice on all aspects of poisoning day and night

▊ NALOXONE HYDROCHLORIDE

Cautions physical dependence on opioids; cardiac irritability; naloxone is short-acting, see notes above

Pregnancy section 15.1.7
Breast-feeding section 15.1.7

Emergency treatment of poisoning

◻ **NALOXONE HYDROCHLORIDE** (*continued*)

Indication and dose

> Safe Practice Doses used in acute opioid overdosage may not be appropriate for the management of opioid-induced respiratory depression and sedation in those receiving palliative care and in chronic opioid use; see also section 15.1.7 for management of postoperative respiratory depression

Overdosage with opioids
• **By intravenous injection**

Neonate 10 micrograms/kg; if no response give subsequent dose of 100 micrograms/kg (then review diagnosis); further doses may be required if respiratory function deteriorates

Child 1 month–12 years 10 micrograms/kg; if no response give subsequent dose of 100 micrograms/kg (then review diagnosis); further doses may be required if respiratory function deteriorates

Child 12–18 years 0.4–2 mg; if no response repeat at intervals of 2–3 minutes to a max. of 10 mg (then review diagnosis); further doses may be required if respiratory function deteriorates

• **By subcutaneous or intramuscular injection**
As intravenous injection but only if intravenous route not feasible (onset of action slower)

• **By continuous intravenous infusion using an infusion pump**

Neonate 5–20 micrograms/kg/hour, adjusted according to response

Child 1 month–12 years 5–20 micrograms/kg/hour, adjusted according to response

Child 12–18 years initially 0.24–1.2 mg infused over 1 hour, then using a solution of 4 micrograms/mL infuse at a rate adjusted according to response

Reversal of postoperative respiratory depression, reversal of respiratory and CNS depression in neonate following maternal opioid use during labour section 15.1.7

Administration for *continuous intravenous infusion*, dilute to a concentration of 4 micrograms/mL with Glucose 5% *or* Sodium Chloride 0.9% infusion

Naloxone (Non-proprietary) ᴘᴏᴹ
Injection, naloxone hydrochloride 400 micrograms/mL, net price 1-mL amp = £4.50; 1 mg/mL, 2-mL prefilled syringe = £8.36

Minijet® Naloxone (UCB Pharma) ᴘᴏᴹ
Injection, naloxone hydrochloride 400 micrograms/mL, net price 1-mL disposable syringe = £19.90, 2-mL disposable syringe = £12.96, 5-mL disposable syringe = £12.68

Antidepressants

Tricyclic and related antidepressants   Tricyclic and related antidepressants cause dry mouth, coma of varying degree, hypotension, hypothermia, hyperreflexia, extensor plantar responses, convulsions, respiratory failure, cardiac conduction defects, and arrhythmias. Dilated pupils and urinary retention also occur. Metabolic acidosis may complicate severe poisoning; delirium with confusion, agitation, and visual and auditory hallucinations, are common during recovery.

Assessment in hospital is strongly advised in case of poisoning by *tricyclic and related antidepressants* but symptomatic treatment can be given before transfer. Supportive measures to ensure a clear airway and adequate ventilation during transfer are mandatory. Intravenous lorazepam or diazepam (preferably in emulsion form) may be required to treat convulsions. Activated charcoal given within 1 hour of the overdose reduces absorption of the drug. Although arrhythmias are worrying, some will respond to correction of hypoxia and acidosis. The use of anti-arrhythmic drugs is best avoided, but intravenous infusion of sodium bicarbonate can arrest arrhythmias or prevent them in those with an extended QRS duration. Diazepam given by mouth is usually adequate to sedate delirious children but large doses may be required.

Selective serotonin re-uptake inhibitors (SSRIs)   Symptoms of poisoning by selective serotonin re-uptake inhibitors include nausea, vomiting, agitation, tremor, nystagmus, drowsiness, and sinus tachycardia; convulsions may occur. Rarely, severe poisoning results in the serotonin syndrome, with marked neuropsychiatric effects, neuromuscular hyperactivity, and autonomic instability; hyperthermia, rhabdomyolysis, renal failure, and coagulopathies may develop.

Management of SSRI poisoning is supportive. Activated charcoal given within 1 hour of the overdose reduces absorption of the drug. Convulsions can be treated with lorazepam, diazepam, or buccal midazolam [unlicensed use] (see p. 34). Contact the National Poisons Information Service for the management of hyperthermia or the serotonin syndrome.

Antimalarials

Overdosage with quinine, chloroquine, or hydroxychloroquine is extremely hazardous and difficult to treat. Urgent advice from the National Poisons Information Service is essential. Life-threatening features include arrhythmias (which can have a very rapid onset) and convulsions (which can be intractable).

Beta-blockers

Therapeutic overdosages with beta-blockers may cause lightheadedness, dizziness, and possibly syncope as a result of bradycardia and hypotension; heart failure may be precipitated or exacerbated. These complications are most likely in children with conduction system disorders or impaired myocardial function. Bradycardia is the most common arrhythmia caused by beta-blockers, but sotalol may induce ventricular tachyarrhythmias (sometimes of the torsade de pointes type). The effects of massive overdosage can vary from one beta-blocker to another; propranolol overdosage in particular may cause coma and convulsions.

Acute massive overdosage must be managed in hospital and expert advice should be obtained. Maintenance of a clear airway and adequate ventilation is mandatory. An intravenous injection of atropine is required to treat bradycardia (40 micrograms/kg, max. 3 mg). Cardiogenic shock unresponsive to atropine is probably best treated with an intravenous injection of glucagon (50–150 micrograms/kg, max. 10 mg) [unlicensed indication and dose] in glucose 5% (with precautions to protect the airway in case of vomiting) followed by an intravenous infusion of 50 micrograms/kg/hour. If glucagon is not available, intravenous isoprenaline (available from 'special-order' manufacturers or specialist importing companies, see p. 957) is an alternative. A cardiac pacemaker can be used to increase the heart rate.

Calcium-channel blockers

Features of calcium-channel blocker poisoning include nausea, vomiting, dizziness, agitation, confusion, and coma in severe poisoning. Metabolic acidosis and hyperglycaemia may occur. Verapamil and diltiazem have a profound cardiac depressant effect causing hypotension and arrhythmias, including complete heart block and asystole. The dihydropyridine calcium-channel blockers cause severe hypotension secondary to profound peripheral vasodilatation.

Activated charcoal should be considered if the child presents within 1 hour of overdosage with a calcium-channel blocker; repeated doses of activated charcoal are considered if a modified-release preparation is involved (although activated charcoal may be effective beyond 1 hour with modified-release preparations). In children with significant features of poisoning, calcium chloride or calcium gluconate (section 9.5.1.1) is given by injection; atropine is given to correct symptomatic bradycardia. In severe cases, an insulin and glucose infusion may be required in the management of hypotension and myocardial failure. For the management of hypotension, the choice of inotropic sympathomimetic depends on whether hypotension is secondary to vasodilatation or to myocardial depression—advice should be sought from the National Poisons Information Service.

> The **National Poisons Information Service** (Tel: 0844 892 0111) will provide specialist advice on all aspects of poisoning day and night

Hypnotics and anxiolytics

Benzodiazepines   Benzodiazepines taken alone cause drowsiness, ataxia, dysarthria, nystagmus, and occasionally respiratory depression, and coma. They potentiate the effects of other central nervous system depressants taken concomitantly. Activated charcoal can be given within 1 hour of ingesting a significant quantity of benzodiazepine, provided the child is awake and the airway is protected. Use of the benzodiazepine antagonist flumazenil [unlicensed indication] can be hazardous, particularly in mixed overdoses involving tricyclic antidepressants or in benzodiazepine-dependent patients. Flumazenil may prevent the need for ventilation, particularly in children with severe respiratory disorders; it should be used on expert advice and not as a diagnostic test in children with a reduced level of consciousness.

Iron salts

Iron poisoning in childhood is usually accidental. The symptoms are nausea, vomiting, abdominal pain, diarrhoea, haematemesis, and rectal bleeding. Hypotension and hepatocellular necrosis can occur later. Coma, shock and metabolic acidosis indicate severe poisoning.

Advice should be sought from the National Poisons Information Service if a significant quantity of iron has been ingested within the previous hour.

Mortality is reduced by intensive and specific therapy with **desferrioxamine**, which chelates iron. The serum-iron concentration is measured as an emergency and intravenous desferrioxamine given to chelate absorbed iron in excess of the expected iron binding capacity. In **severe toxicity** intravenous desferrioxamine should be given *immediately* without waiting for the result of the serum-iron measurement.

DESFERRIOXAMINE MESILATE

(Deferoxamine Mesilate)

Cautions section 9.1.3

Renal impairment section 9.1.3

Pregnancy section 9.1.3

Breast-feeding section 9.1.3

Side-effects section 9.1.3

Licensed use licensed for use in children (age range not specified by manufacturer)

Indication and dose

Iron poisoning
- **By continuous intravenous infusion**

  Neonate up to 15 mg/kg/hour, reduced after 4–6 hours; max. 80 mg/kg in 24 hours (in severe cases, higher doses on advice from the National Poisons Information Service)

  Child 1 month–18 years up to 15 mg/kg/hour, reduced after 4–6 hours; max. 80 mg/kg in 24 hours (in severe cases, higher doses on advice from the National Poisons Information Service)

Chronic iron overload section 9.1.3

◀Preparations
Section 9.1.3

Lithium

Lithium intoxication can occur as a complication of long-term therapy and is caused by reduced excretion of the drug due to a variety of factors including dehydration, deterioration of renal function, infections, and co-administration of diuretics or NSAIDs (or other drugs that interact). Acute deliberate overdoses may also occur with delayed onset of symptoms (12 hours or more) due to slow entry of lithium into the tissues and continuing absorption from modified-release formulations.

The early clinical features are non-specific and may include apathy and restlessness which could be confused with mental changes due to the child's depressive illness. Vomiting, diarrhoea, ataxia, weakness, dysarthria, muscle twitching, and tremor may follow. Severe poisoning is associated with convulsions, coma, renal failure, electrolyte imbalance, dehydration, and hypotension.

Therapeutic lithium concentrations are within the range of 0.6–1 mmol/litre; concentrations in excess of 2 mmol/litre are usually associated with serious toxicity and such cases may need treatment with haemodialysis if neurological symptoms or renal failure are present. In acute overdosage, much higher serum-litium concentrations may be present without features of toxicity and all that is usually necessary is to take measures to increase urine output (e.g. by increasing fluid intake, but avoiding diuretics). Otherwise, treatment is supportive with special regard to electrolyte balance, renal function, and control of convulsions. Whole-bowel irrigation should be considered for significant ingestion, but advice should be sought from the National Poisons Information Service, p. 33.

The **National Poisons Information Service** (Tel: 0844 892 0111) will provide specialist advice on all aspects of poisoning day and night

Phenothiazines and related drugs

Phenothiazines cause less depression of consciousness and respiration than other sedatives. Hypotension, hypothermia, sinus tachycardia, and arrhythmias may complicate poisoning. Dystonic reactions can occur with therapeutic doses (particularly with prochlorperazine and trifluoperazine), and convulsions may occur in severe cases. Arrhythmias may respond to correction of hypoxia, acidosis, and other biochemical abnormalities, but specialist advice should be sought if arrhythmias result from a prolonged QT interval; the use of some anti-arrhythmic drugs can worsen such arrhythmias. Dystonic reactions are rapidly abolished by injection of drugs such as procyclidine (section 4.9.2) or diazepam (section 4.8.2, emulsion preferred).

Atypical antipsychotic drugs

Features of poisoning by atypical antipsychotic drugs (section 4.2.1) include drowsiness, convulsions, extrapyramidal symptoms, hypotension, and ECG abnormalities (including prolongation of the QT interval). Management is supportive. Activated charcoal can be given within 1 hour of ingesting a significant quantity of an atypical antipsychotic drug.

Stimulants

Amphetamines These cause wakefulness, excessive activity, paranoia, hallucinations, and hypertension followed by exhaustion, convulsions, hyperthermia, and coma. The early stages can be controlled by diazepam or lorazepam; advice should be sought from the National Poisons Information Service (p. 33) on the management of hypertension. Later, tepid sponging, anticonvulsants, and artificial respiration may be needed.

Cocaine Cocaine stimulates the central nervous system, causing agitation, dilated pupils, tachycardia, hypertension, hallucinations, hyperthermia, hypertonia, and hyperreflexia; cardiac effects include chest pain, myocardial infarction, and arrhythmias.

Initial treatment of cocaine poisoning involves intravenous administration of diazepam to control agitation and cooling measures for hyperthermia (see p. 34); hypertension and cardiac effects require specific treatment and expert advice should be sought.

Ecstasy Ecstasy (methylenedioxymethamfetamine, MDMA) may cause severe reactions, even at doses that were previously tolerated. The most serious effects are delirium, coma, convulsions, ventricular arrhythmias, hyperthermia, rhabdomyolysis, acute renal failure, acute hepatitis, disseminated intravascular coagulation, adult respiratory distress syndrome, hyperreflexia, hypotension and intracerebral haemorrhage; hyponatraemia has also been associated with ecstasy use and syndrome of inappropriate antidiuretic hormone secretion (SIADH) can occur.

Treatment of methylenedioxymethamfetamine poisoning is supportive, with diazepam to control severe agitation or persistent convulsions and close monitoring including ECG. Self-induced water intoxication should be considered in patients with ecstasy poisoning.

'Liquid ecstasy' is a term used for sodium oxybate (gamma-hydroxybutyrate, GHB), which is a sedative.

Theophylline

Theophylline and related drugs are often prescribed as modified-release formulations and toxicity can therefore be delayed. They cause vomiting (which may be severe and intractable), agitation, restlessness, dilated pupils, sinus tachycardia, and hyperglycaemia. More serious effects are haematemesis, convulsions, and supraventricular and ventricular arrhythmias. Severe hypokalaemia may develop rapidly.

Repeated doses of activated charcoal can be used to eliminate theophylline even if more than 1 hour has elapsed after ingestion and especially if a modified-release preparation has been taken (see also under Active Elimination Techniques). Ondansetron (section 4.6) may be effective for severe vomiting that is resistant to other antiemetics. Hypokalaemia is corrected by intravenous infusion of potassium chloride in 0.9% sodium chloride and may be so severe as to require high doses under ECG monitoring. Convulsions should be controlled by intravenous administration of lorazepam or diazepam (see Convulsions, p. 34). Sedation with diazepam (emulsion preferred) may be necessary in agitated children.

Provided the child does **not** suffer from asthma, a short-acting beta-blocker (section 2.4) can be administered intravenously to reverse severe tachycardia, hypokalaemia, and hyperglycaemia.

Emergency treatment of poisoning

Other poisons

Consult either the National Poisons Information Service day and night or TOX-BASE, see p. 33.

> The **National Poisons Information Service** (Tel: 0844 892 0111) will provide specialist advice on all aspects of poisoning day and night

Cyanides

Oxygen should be administered to children with cyanide poisoning. The choice of antidote depends on the severity of poisoning, certainty of diagnosis, and the cause. Dicobalt edetate is the antidote of choice when there is a strong clinical suspicion of severe cyanide poisoning. Dicobalt edetate itself is toxic, associated with anaphylactoid reactions, and is potentially fatal if administered in the absence of cyanide poisoning. A regimen of sodium nitrite followed by sodium thiosulphate is an alternative if dicobalt edetate is not available.

Hydroxocobalamin can be considered for victims of smoke inhalation who show signs of significant cyanide poisoning. The usual dose is 70 mg/kg (max. 5 g) by intravenous infusion (given once or twice according to severity). *Cyanokit®* provides hydroxocobalamin 2.5 g/bottle (no other preparation of hydroxocobalamin is suitable)—contact the National Poisons Information Service for advice.

DICOBALT EDETATE

Cautions owing to toxicity to be used only for definite cyanide poisoning when patient tending to lose, or has lost, consciousness; **not** to be used as a precautionary measure

Side-effects hypotension, tachycardia, and vomiting; anaphylactoid reactions including facial and laryngeal oedema and cardiac abnormalities

Indication and dose

Severe poisoning with cyanides
- By intravenous injection
  Consult the National Poisons Information Service

[1]**Dicobalt Edetate** (Non-proprietary) PoM
  Injection, dicobalt edetate 15 mg/mL, net price 20-mL (300-mg) amp = £13.75
  1. PoM restriction does not apply where administration is for saving life in emergency

SODIUM NITRITE

Side-effects flushing and headache due to vasodilatation

Indication and dose

Poisoning with cyanides (used in conjunction with sodium thiosulphate)
  See under preparation

[1]**Sodium Nitrite** PoM
  Injection, sodium nitrite 3% (30 mg/mL) in water for injections
Dose
- By intravenous injection over 5–20 minutes
  Child 1 month–18 years 4–10 mg/kg max. 300 mg (0.13–0.33 mL/kg, max. 10 mL, of 3% solution) followed by sodium thiosulphate injection 400 mg/kg, max. 12.5 g (0.8 mL/kg, max. 25 mL, of 50% solution) over 10 minutes

  Available from 'special-order' manufacturers or specialist importing companies, see p. 957
  1. PoM restriction does not apply where administration is for saving life in emergency

SODIUM THIOSULPHATE

Indication and dose

Poisoning with cyanides (used in conjunction with sodium nitrite)

  See above under Sodium Nitrite

[1]**Sodium Thiosulphate** PoM
  Injection, sodium thiosulphate 50% (500 mg/mL) in water for injections
  Available from 'special-order' manufacturers or specialist importing companies, see p. 957
  1. PoM restriction does not apply where administration is for saving life in emergency

Ethylene glycol and methanol

Fomepizole (available from 'special-order' manufacturers or specialist importing companies, see p. 957) is the treatment of choice for ethylene glycol and methanol (methyl alcohol) poisoning. If necessary, **ethanol** (by mouth or by intravenous infusion) can be used, but with caution. Advice on the treatment of ethylene glycol and methanol poisoning should be obtained from the National Poisons Information Service. It is important to start antidote treatment promptly in cases of suspected poisoning with these agents.

Heavy metals

Heavy metal antidotes include succimer (DMSA) [unlicensed], unithiol (DMPS) [unlicensed], sodium calcium edetate, and dimercaprol. Dimercaprol in the management of heavy metal poisoning has been superseded by other chelating agents. In all cases of heavy metal poisoning, the advice of the National Poisons Information Service should be sought.

DIMERCAPROL
(BAL)

Cautions hypertension; **interactions**: Appendix 1 (dimercaprol)

Contra-indications not indicated for iron, cadmium, or selenium poisoning

Hepatic impairment avoid in severe impairment (unless due to arsenic poisoning)

Renal impairment discontinue or use with extreme caution if impairment develops during treatment

Pregnancy manufacturer advises use with caution, but benefits outweigh potential risks

Breast-feeding manufacturer advises use with caution—no information available

Side-effects hypertension, tachycardia, malaise, nausea, vomiting, salivation, lacrimation, sweating, burning sensation (mouth, throat, and eyes), feeling of constriction of throat and chest, headache, muscle spasm, abdominal pain, tingling of extremities; pyrexia; local pain and abscess at injection site

Licensed use licensed for use in children (age range not specified by manufacturer)

Indication and dose

Poisoning by antimony, arsenic, bismuth, gold see also notes above

• By intramuscular injection

Child 1 month–18 years 2.5–3 mg/kg every 4 hours for 2 days, 2–4 times on the third day, then 1–2 times daily for 10 days or until recovery

Dimercaprol (Sovereign) ℗ℴℳ
Injection, dimercaprol 50 mg/mL. Net price 2-mL amp = £42.73

Note Contains arachis (peanut) oil as solvent

SODIUM CALCIUM EDETATE
(Sodium Calciumedetate)

Renal impairment use with caution in mild impairment; avoid in moderate to severe impairment—contact the National Poisons Information Service for advice

Side-effects nausea, diarrhoea, abdominal pain, pain at site of injection, thrombophlebitis if given too rapidly, renal damage particularly in overdosage; hypotension, lacrimation, myalgia, nasal congestion, sneezing, malaise, thirst, fever, chills, headache and zinc depletion also reported

Licensed use licensed for use in children (age range not specified by manufacturer)

Indication and dose

Lead poisoning

• By intravenous infusion

Child 1 month–18 years 40 mg/kg twice daily for up to 5 days; if necessary a second course can be given at least 7 days after the first course, and a third course can be given at least 7 days after the second course

Administration for *intravenous infusion*, dilute to a concentration of not more 30 mg/mL with Glucose 5% *or* Sodium Chloride 0.9%; give over at least 1 hour

Ledclair® (Durbin) ℗ℴℳ
Injection, sodium calcium edetate 200 mg/mL, net price 5-mL amp = £7.29

Noxious gases

Carbon monoxide Carbon monoxide poisoning is usually due to inhalation of smoke, car exhaust, or fumes caused by blocked flues or incomplete combustion of fuel gases in confined spaces.

Immediate treatment of carbon monoxide poisoning is essential. The child should be moved to fresh air, the airway cleared, and high-flow **oxygen** 100% administered as soon as available. Artificial respiration should be given as necessary and continued until adequate spontaneous breathing starts, or stopped only after persistent and efficient treatment of cardiac arrest has failed. The child should be admitted to hospital because complications may arise after a delay of hours or days. Cerebral oedema may occur in severe poisoning and is treated with an intravenous infusion of mannitol (section 2.2.5). Referral for hyperbaric oxygen treatment should be discussed with the National Poisons Information Service if the patient is pregnant or in cases of severe poisoning such as if the child is or has been unconscious, or has psychiatric or neurological features other than a headache or has myocardial ischaemia or an arrhythmia, or has a blood carboxyhaemoglobin concentration of more than 20%.

Sulphur dioxide, chlorine, phosgene, ammonia   All of these gases can cause upper respiratory tract and conjunctival irritation. Pulmonary oedema, with severe breathlessness and cyanosis may develop suddenly up to 36 hours after exposure. Death may occur. Children are kept under observation and those who develop pulmonary oedema are given oxygen. Assisted ventilation may be necessary in the most serious cases.

CS Spray

CS spray, which is used for riot control, irritates the eyes (hence 'tear gas') and the respiratory tract; symptoms normally settle spontaneously within 15 minutes. If symptoms persist, the patient should be removed to a well-ventilated area, and the exposed skin washed with soap and water after removal of contaminated clothing. Contact lenses should be removed and rigid ones washed (soft ones should be discarded). Eye symptoms should be treated by irrigating the eyes with physiological saline (or water if saline is not available) and advice sought from an ophthalmologist. Patients with features of severe poisoning, particularly respiratory complications, should be admitted to hospital for symptomatic treatment.

Nerve agents

Treatment of nerve agent poisoning is similar to organophosphorus insecticide poisoning (see below), but advice must be sought from the National Poisons Information Service. The risk of cross-contamination is significant; adequate decontamination and protective clothing for healthcare personnel are essential. In emergencies involving the release of nerve agents, kits ('NAAS pods') containing **pralidoxime** can be obtained through the Ambulance Service from the National Blood Service (or the Welsh Blood Service in South Wales or designated hospital pharmacies in Northern Ireland and Scotland—see TOXBASE for list of designated centres).

> The **National Poisons Information Service** (Tel: 0844 892 0111) will provide specialist advice on all aspects of poisoning day and night

Pesticides

Organophosphorus insecticides   Organophosphorus insecticides are usually supplied as powders or dissolved in organic solvents. All are absorbed through the bronchi and intact skin as well as through the gut and inhibit cholinesterase activity, thereby prolonging and intensifying the effects of acetylcholine. Toxicity between different compounds varies considerably, and onset may be delayed after skin exposure.

Anxiety, restlessness, dizziness, headache, miosis, nausea, hypersalivation, vomiting, abdominal colic, diarrhoea, bradycardia, and sweating are common features of organophosphorus poisoning. Muscle weakness and fasciculation may develop and progress to generalised flaccid paralysis, including the ocular and respiratory muscles. Convulsions, coma, pulmonary oedema with copious bronchial secretions, hypoxia, and arrhythmias occur in severe cases. Hyperglycaemia and glycosuria without ketonuria may also be present.

Further absorption of the organophosphorus insecticide should be prevented by moving the child to fresh air, removing soiled clothing, and washing contaminated skin. In severe poisoning it is vital to ensure a clear airway, frequent removal of bronchial secretions, and adequate ventilation and oxygenation; gastric lavage may be considered provided that the airway is protected. **Atropine** will reverse the muscarinic effects of acetylcholine and is given by intravenous injection in a dose of 20 micrograms/kg (max. 2 mg) as atropine sulphate every 5 to 10 minutes (according to the severity of poisoning) until the skin becomes flushed and dry, the pupils dilate, and bradycardia is abolished.

Pralidoxime chloride, a cholinesterase reactivator, is used as an adjunct to atropine in moderate or severe poisoning. It improves muscle tone within 30 minutes of administration. Pralidoxime chloride is continued until the patient has not required atropine for 12 hours. Pralidoxime chloride can be obtained from designated centres, the names of which are held by the National Poisons Information Service (see p. 33).

PRALIDOXIME CHLORIDE

Cautions myasthenia gravis

Contra-indications poisoning with carbamates or organophosphorus compounds without anticholinesterase activity

Renal impairment use with caution

Side-effects drowsiness, dizziness, disturbances of vision, nausea, tachycardia, headache, hyperventilation, and muscular weakness

Licensed use licensed for use in children (age range not specified by manufacturer)

Indication and dose

Adjunct to atropine in the treatment of poisoning by organophosphorus insecticide or nerve agent

• **By intravenous infusion** over 20 minutes

Child under 18 years initially 30 mg/kg, followed by 8 mg/kg/hour; usual max. 12 g in 24 hours

Note The loading dose may be administered **by intravenous injection** (diluted to a concentration of 50 mg/mL with water for injections) over at least 5 minutes if pulmonary oedema is present or if it is not practical to administer an intravenous infusion; pralidoxime chloride doses may differ from those in product literature

[1]**Pralidoxime chloride** (PoM)

Injection, powder for reconstitution pralidoxime chloride 1 g/vial

Available as *Protopam*® (from designated centres for organophosphorus insecticide poisoning or from the National Blood Service (or Welsh Ambulance Services for Mid West and South East Wales) — see TOXBASE for list of designated centres)

1. (PoM) restriction does not apply where administration is for saving life in emergency

Snake bites and animal stings

Snake bites Envenoming from snake bite is uncommon in the UK. Many exotic snakes are kept, some illegally, but the only indigenous venomous snake is the adder (*Vipera berus*). The bite may cause local and systemic effects. Local effects include pain, swelling, bruising, and tender enlargement of regional lymph nodes. Systemic effects include early anaphylactic symptoms (transient hypotension with syncope, angioedema, urticaria, abdominal colic, diarrhoea, and vomiting), with later persistent or recurrent hypotension, ECG abnormalities, spontaneous systemic bleeding, coagulopathy, adult respiratory distress syndrome, and acute renal failure. Fatal envenoming is rare but the potential for severe envenoming must not be underestimated.

Early anaphylactic symptoms should be treated with **adrenaline (epinephrine)** (section 3.4.3). Indications for antivenom treatment include *systemic envenoming*, especially hypotension (see above), ECG abnormalities, vomiting, haemostatic abnormalities, and marked local envenoming such that after bites on the hand or foot, swelling extends beyond the wrist or ankle within 4 hours of the bite. The contents of one vial (10 mL) of **European viper venom antiserum** (available from Movianto) is given *by intravenous injection* over 10–15 minutes or *by intravenous infusion* over 30 minutes after diluting in sodium chloride intravenous infusion 0.9% (use 5 mL diluent/kg body-weight). The **same dose** should be used for **adults** and **children**. The dose can be repeated in 1–2 hours if symptoms of *systemic envenoming* persist. However, for those children who present with clinical features of *severe envenoming* (e.g. shock, ECG abnormalities, or local swelling that has advanced from the foot to above the knee or from the hand to above the elbow within 2 hours of the bite), an initial dose of 2 vials (20 mL) of the antiserum is recommended; if symptoms of *systemic envenoming* persist contact the National Poisons Information Service. Adrenaline (epinephrine) injection must be immediately to hand for treatment of anaphylactic reactions to the antivenom (for the management of anaphylaxis see section 3.4.3).

Antivenom is available for bites by certain foreign snakes and spiders, stings by scorpions and fish. For information on identification, management, and for supply in an emergency, telephone the National Poisons Information Service. Whenever possible the TOXBASE entry should be read, and relevant information collected, before telephoning the National Poisons Information Service (see p. 33).

Insect stings   Stings from ants, wasps, hornets, and bees cause local pain and swelling but seldom cause severe direct toxicity unless many stings are inflicted at the same time. If the sting is in the mouth or on the tongue local swelling may threaten the upper airway. The stings from these insects are usually treated by cleaning the area with a topical antiseptic. Bee stings should be removed as quickly as possible. Anaphylactic reactions require immediate treatment with intramuscular **adrenaline (epinephrine)**; self-administered (or administered by a carer) intramuscular adrenaline (e.g. *EpiPen®*) is the best first-aid treatment for children with severe hypersensitivity. An inhaled bronchodilator should be used for asthmatic reactions. For the management of anaphylaxis, see section 3.4.3. A short course of an **oral antihistamine** or a **topical corticosteroid** may help to reduce inflammation and relieve itching. A vaccine containing extracts of bee and wasp venom can be used to reduce the risk of severe anaphylaxis and systemic reactions in children with systemic hypersensitivity to bee or wasp stings (section 3.4.2).

Marine stings   The severe pain of weeverfish (*Trachinus vipera*) and Portuguese man-o'-war stings can be relieved by immersing the stung area immediately in uncomfortably hot, but not scalding, water (not more than 45° C). Children stung by jellyfish and Portuguese man-o'-war around the UK coast should be removed from the sea as soon as possible. Adherent tentacles should be lifted off carefully (wearing gloves or using tweezers) or washed off with seawater. Alcoholic solutions, including suntan lotions, should **not** be applied because they can cause further discharge of stinging hairs. Ice packs will reduce pain and a slurry of baking soda (sodium bicarbonate), but not vinegar, may be useful for treating stings from UK species.

> The **National Poisons Information Service** (Tel: 0844 892 0111) will provide specialist advice on all aspects of poisoning day and night

1 Gastro-intestinal system

1

Gastro-intestinal system

This chapter includes advice on the drug management of the following:
- *Clostridium difficile* infection, p. 67
- constipation, p. 76
- Crohn's disease, p. 66
- food allergy, p. 76
- *Helicobacter pylori* infection, p. 58
- irritable bowel syndrome, p. 67
- malabsorption syndromes, p. 68
- NSAID-associated ulcers, p. 59
- ulcerative colitis, p. 66

1.1 Dyspepsia and gastro-oesophageal reflux disease

1.1.1 Antacids and simeticone
1.1.2 Compound alginate preparations

Dyspepsia

Dyspepsia covers pain, fullness, early satiety, bloating, and nausea. It can occur with gastric and duodenal ulceration (section 1.3), gastro-oesophageal reflux disease, gastritis, and upper gastro-intestinal motility disorders, but most commonly it is of uncertain origin.

Children with dyspepsia should be advised about lifestyle changes (see Gastro-oesophageal reflux disease, below). Some medications may cause dyspepsia—these should be stopped, if possible.

A compound alginate preparation (section 1.1.2) may provide relief from dyspepsia; persistent dyspepsia requires investigation. Treatment with a H$_2$-receptor antagonist (section 1.3.1) or a proton pump inhibitor (section 1.3.5) should be initiated only on the advice of a hospital specialist.

Helicobacter pylori may be present in children with dyspepsia. *H. pylori* eradication therapy (section 1.3) should be considered for persistent dyspepsia if it is ulcer-like. However, most children with functional (investigated, non-ulcer) dyspepsia do not benefit symptomatically from *H. pylori* eradication.

Gastro-oesophageal reflux disease

Gastro-oesophageal reflux disease includes non-erosive gastro-oesophageal reflux and erosive oesophagitis. Uncomplicated gastro-oesophageal reflux is common in infancy and most symptoms, such as intermittent vomiting or repeated, effortless regurgitation, resolve without treatment between 12 and 18 months of age. Older children with gastro-oesophageal reflux disease may have heartburn, acid regurgitation and dysphagia. Oesophageal inflammation (oesophagitis), ulceration or stricture formation may develop in early childhood; gastro-oesophageal reflux disease may also be associated with chronic respiratory disorders including asthma.

Parents and carers of *neonates* and *infants* should be reassured that most symptoms of uncomplicated gastro-oesophageal reflux resolve without treatment. An increase in the frequency and a decrease in the volume of feeds may reduce symptoms. A feed thickener or pre-thickened formula feed (Appendix 2) can be used on the advice of a dietician. If necessary, a suitable alginate-containing preparation (section 1.1.2) can be used instead of thickened feeds.

Older children should be advised about life-style changes such as weight reduction if overweight, and the avoidance of alcohol and smoking. An alginate-containing antacid (section 1.1.2) can be used to relieve symptoms.

Children who do not respond to these measures or who have problems such as respiratory disorders or suspected oesophagitis need to be referred to hospital. On the advice of a paediatrician, a **histamine H$_2$-receptor antagonist** (section 1.3.1) can be used to relieve symptoms of gastro-oesophageal reflux disease, promote mucosal healing and permit reduction in antacid consumption. A **proton pump inhibitor** (section 1.3.5) can be used for the treatment of moderate, non-erosive oesophagitis that is unresponsive to an H$_2$-receptor antagonist. Endoscopically confirmed *erosive*, *ulcerative*, or *stricturing* disease in children is usually treated with a proton pump inhibitor. Reassessment is necessary if symptoms persist despite 4–6 weeks of treatment; long-term use of an H$_2$-receptor antagonist or proton pump inhibitor should not be undertaken without full assessment of the underlying condition. For endoscopically confirmed *erosive*, *ulcerative*, or *stricturing* disease, the proton pump inhibitor usually needs to be maintained at the minimum effective dose.

Motility stimulants (section 1.2), such as domperidone or erythromycin may improve gastro-oesophageal sphincter contraction and accelerate gastric emptying. Evidence for the long-term efficacy of motility stimulants in the management of gastro-oesophageal reflux in children is unconvincing.

For advice on specialised formula feeds, see section 9.4.2.

1.1.1 Antacids and simeticone

Antacids (usually containing aluminium or magnesium compounds) can be used for short-term relief of intermittent symptoms of *ulcer dyspepsia* and *non-erosive gastro-oesophageal reflux* (see section 1.1) in children; they are also used in functional (non-ulcer) dyspepsia, but the evidence of benefit is uncertain.

Aluminium- and **magnesium-containing** antacids, being relatively insoluble in water, are long-acting if retained in the stomach. Magnesium-containing antacids tend to be laxative whereas aluminium-containing antacids may be constipating; antacids containing both magnesium and aluminium may reduce these colonic side-effects. Aluminium-containing antacids should not be used in children with renal impairment, or in neonates and infants because accumulation may lead to increased plasma-aluminium concentrations.

Complexes such as **hydrotalcite** confer no special advantage.

Calcium-containing antacids can induce rebound acid secretion; with modest doses the clinical significance of this is doubtful, but prolonged high doses also cause hypercalcaemia and alkalosis.

Simeticone (activated dimeticone) is used to treat infantile colic, but the evidence of benefit is uncertain. Simeticone is added to an antacid as an antifoaming agent to relieve flatulence; such preparations may also be useful for the relief of hiccup in palliative care (see Prescribing in Palliative Care, p. 27).

Alginates act as mucosal protectants in gastro-oesophageal reflux disease (section 1.1.2). The amount of additional ingredient or antacid in individual preparations varies widely, as does their sodium content, so that preparations may not be freely interchangeable.

Hepatic impairment   In children with fluid retention, avoid antacids containing large amounts of sodium. Avoid antacids that cause constipation because this can precipitate coma. Avoid antacids containing magnesium salts in hepatic coma if there is a risk of renal failure.

Renal impairment   There is a risk of accumulation and aluminium toxicity with antacids containing aluminium salts. Absorption of aluminium from aluminium salts is increased by citrates, which are contained in many effervescent preparations (such as effervescent analgesics). Antacids containing magnesium salts should be avoided or used at a reduced dose because there is an increased risk of toxicity.

Interactions   Antacids should preferably not be taken at the same time as other drugs since they may impair absorption. Antacids may also damage enteric coatings designed to prevent dissolution in the stomach. See also **Appendix 1** (antacids, calcium salts).

> **Low Na$^+$**
> The words 'low Na$^+$' added after some preparations indicate a sodium content of less than 1 mmol per tablet or 10-mL dose.

1 Gastro-intestinal system

Aluminium- and magnesium-containing antacids

ALUMINIUM HYDROXIDE

Cautions see notes above; **interactions:** Appendix 1 (antacids)

Contra-indications hypophosphataemia; neonates and infants

Hepatic impairment see notes above

Renal impairment see notes above

Side-effects see notes above

Indication and dose

Dyspepsia for dose see preparations

Hyperphosphataemia section 9.5.2.2

◢**Co-magaldrox**
Co-magaldrox is a mixture of aluminium hydroxide and magnesium hydroxide; the proportions are expressed in the form *x*/*y* where *x* and *y* are the strengths in milligrams per unit dose of magnesium hydroxide and aluminium hydroxide respectively

Maalox® (Sanofi-Aventis)
Suspension, sugar-free, co-magaldrox 195/220 (magnesium hydroxide 195 mg, dried aluminium hydroxide 220 mg/5 mL (low Na$^+$)). Net price 500 mL = £2.79

Dose
- **By mouth**
  Child 14–18 years 10–20 mL 20–60 minutes after meals and at bedtime, or when required

◻ **ALUMINIUM HYDROXIDE** (*continued*)

Mucogel® (Chemidex)
Suspension, sugar-free, co-magaldrox 195/220
(magnesium hydroxide 195 mg, dried aluminium
hydroxide 220 mg/5 mL (low Na⁺)). Net price
500 mL = £1.71

Dose
• **By mouth**
  Child 12–18 years 10–20 mL 3 times daily, 20–60
  minutes after meals and at bedtime, or when required

MAGNESIUM TRISILICATE

Cautions heart failure, hypertension; metabolic or
respiratory alkalosis, hypermagnesaemia; **interactions**: Appendix 1 (antacids)

Contra-indications severe renal failure; hypophosphataemia

Hepatic impairment see notes above

Renal impairment see notes above; magnesium
trisilicate mixture has a high sodium content

Side-effects see notes above; silica-based renal
stones reported on long-term treatment

Indication and dose

Dyspepsia for dose see under preparation

Magnesium Trisilicate Mixture, BP
(Magnesium Trisilicate Oral Suspension)
Oral suspension, 5% each of magnesium trisilicate,
light magnesium carbonate, and sodium bicarbonate in a suitable vehicle with a peppermint flavour. Contains about 6 mmol Na⁺/10 mL

Dose
• **By mouth**
  Child 5–12 years 5–10 mL with water 3 times daily or
  as required
  Child 12–18 years 10–20 mL with water 3 times daily
  or as required

Aluminium-magnesium complexes

HYDROTALCITE

Aluminium magnesium carbonate hydroxide
hydrate

Cautions see notes above; **interactions**: Appendix 1 (antacids)

Hepatic impairment see notes above

Renal impairment see notes above

Side-effects see notes above

Indication and dose

Dyspepsia for dose see under preparation

◢With simeticone
Altacite Plus® (Non-proprietary)
see below

Antacid preparations containing simeticone

Altacite Plus® (Peckforton)
Suspension, sugar-free, co-simalcite 125/500
(simeticone 125 mg, hydrotalcite 500 mg)/5 mL
(low Na⁺). Net price 500 mL = £1.96

Dose
• **By mouth**
  Child 8–12 years 5 mL 4 times daily (between meals
  and at bedtime) when required
  Child 12–18 years 10 mL 4 times daily (between
  meals and at bedtime) when required

Asilone® (Thornton & Ross)
Suspension, sugar-free, dried aluminium hydroxide
420 mg, simeticone 135 mg, light magnesium oxide
70 mg/5 mL (low Na⁺). Net price 500 mL = £1.95

Dose
• **By mouth**
  Child 12–18 years 5–10 mL after meals and at bed-
  time or when required up to 4 times daily

Maalox Plus® (Sanofi-Aventis)
Suspension, sugar-free, dried aluminium hydroxide
220 mg, simeticone 25 mg, magnesium hydroxide
195 mg/5 mL (low Na⁺). Net price 500 mL = £2.79

Dose
• **By mouth**
  Child 2–5 years 5 mL 3 times daily
  Child 5–12 years 5–10 mL 3–4 times daily
  Child 12–18 years 5–10 mL 4 times daily (after meals
  and at bedtime) or when required

Simeticone alone

SIMETICONE

Activated dimeticone

Indication and dose

Colic or wind pain for dose see under individual
preparations

Dentinox® (DDD) ◢
Colic drops (= emulsion), simeticone 21 mg/2.5-
mL dose. Net price 100 mL = £1.73

Dose
• **By mouth**
  Neonate 2.5 mL with or after each feed (max. 6 doses
  in 24 hours); may be added to bottle feed

⌐ SIMETICONE (*continued*)

Child 1 month–2 years 2.5 mL with or after each feed (max. 6 doses in 24 hours); may be added to bottle feed

Note The brand name *Dentinox®* is also used for other preparations including teething gel

Infacol® (Forest) ⌐
Liquid, sugar-free, simeticone 40 mg/mL (low Na$^+$). Net price 50 mL = £2.26. Counselling, use of dropper

Dose
- **By mouth**

  Neonate 0.5–1 mL before feeds

  Child 1 month–2 years 0.5–1 mL before feeds

1.1.2 Compound alginate preparations

Alginate taken in combination with an antacid increases the viscosity of stomach contents and can protect the oesophageal mucosa from acid reflux. Some alginate-containing preparations form a viscous gel ('raft') that floats on the surface of the stomach contents, thereby reducing symptoms of reflux. Alginate-containing preparations are used in the management of mild symptoms of dyspepsia and gastro-oesophageal reflux disease (see section 1.1). Antacids may damage enteric coatings designed to prevent dissolution in the stomach. For **interactions**, see Appendix 1 (antacids, calcium salts).

Preparations containing aluminium should not be used in children with renal impairment, or in neonates and infants.

Alginate raft-forming oral suspensions

The following preparations contain sodium alginate, sodium bicarbonate, and calcium carbonate in a suitable flavoured vehicle, and conform to the specification for Alginate Raft-forming Oral Suspension, BP.

Acidex® (Pinewood)
Liquid, sugar-free, sodium alginate 250 mg, sodium bicarbonate 133.5 mg, calcium carbonate 80 mg/5 mL. Contains about 3 mmol Na$^+$/5 mL, net price 500 mL (aniseed- or peppermint-flavour) = £2.30

Dose
- **By mouth**

  Child 6–12 years 5–10 mL after meals and at bedtime

  Child 12–18 years 10–20 mL after meals and at bedtime

Peptac® (IVAX)
Suspension, sugar-free, sodium bicarbonate 133.5 mg, sodium alginate 250 mg, calcium carbonate 80 mg/5 mL. Contains 3.1 mmol Na$^+$/5 mL. Net price 500 mL (aniseed- or peppermint-flavoured) = £2.16

Dose
- **By mouth**

  Child 6–12 years 5–10 mL after meals and at bedtime

  Child 12–18 years 10–20 mL after meals and at bedtime

Other compound alginate preparations

Gastrocote® (Actavis)
Tablets, alginic acid 200 mg, dried aluminium hydroxide 80 mg, magnesium trisilicate 40 mg, sodium bicarbonate 70 mg. Contains about 1 mmol Na$^+$/tablet. Net price 100-tab pack = £3.51
Cautions diabetes mellitus (high sugar content)

Dose
- **By mouth**

  Child 6–18 years 1–2 tablets chewed 4 times daily (after meals and at bedtime)

Liquid, sugar-free, peach-coloured, dried aluminium hydroxide 80 mg, magnesium trisilicate 40 mg, sodium alginate 220 mg, sodium bicarbonate 70 mg/5 mL. Contains 2.13 mmol Na$^+$/5 mL. Net price 500 mL = £2.67

Dose
- **By mouth**

  Child 6–12 years 5–10 mL 4 times daily (after meals and at bedtime)

  Child 12–18 years 5–15 mL 4 times daily (after meals and at bedtime)

Gaviscon® Advance (Reckitt Benckiser)
Tablets, sugar-free, sodium alginate 500 mg, potassium bicarbonate 100 mg. Contains 2.25 mmol Na$^+$, 1 mmol K$^+$/tablet. Net price 60-tab pack (peppermint-flavour) = £3.13
Excipients include aspartame (section 9.4.1)

Dose
- **By mouth**

  Child 6–12 years 1 tablet to be chewed after meals and at bedtime (under medical advice only)

  Child 12–18 years 1–2 tablets to be chewed after meals and at bedtime

Suspension, sugar-free, aniseed- or peppermint-flavour, sodium alginate 500 mg, potassium bicarbonate 100 mg/5 mL. Contains 2.3 mmol Na$^+$, 1 mmol K$^+$/5 mL, net price 250 mL = £2.61, 500 mL = £5.21

Dose
- **By mouth**

  Child 2–12 years 2.5–5 mL after meals and at bedtime (under medical advice only)

  Child 12–18 years 5–10 mL after meals and at bedtime

1 Gastro-intestinal system

Gaviscon® Infant (Reckitt Benckiser)
Oral powder, sugar-free, sodium alginate 225 mg, magnesium alginate 87.5 mg, with colloidal silica and mannitol/dose. Contains 0.92 mmol Na$^+$/dose. Net price 30 doses = £2.46

Dose

- **By mouth**

  Neonate body-weight under 4.5 kg 1 'dose' mixed with feeds (or water, for breast-fed infants) when required (max. 6 times in 24 hours)

  Neonate body-weight over 4.5 kg 2 'doses' mixed with feeds (or water, for breast-fed infants) when required (max. 6 times in 24 hours)

  Child 1 month–2 years

  Body-weight under 4.5 kg dose as for neonate

  Body-weight over 4.5 kg 2 'doses' mixed with feeds (or water, for breast-fed infants) when required (max. 6 times in 24 hours)

Note Not to be used in preterm neonates, or where excessive water loss likely (e.g. fever, diarrhoea, vomiting, high room temperature), or if intestinal obstruction. Not to be used with other preparations containing thickening agents

> Safe Practice Each half of the dual sachet is identified as 'one dose'. To avoid errors prescribe with directions in terms of 'dose'

Topal® (Fabre)
Tablets, alginic acid 200 mg, dried aluminium hydroxide 30 mg, light magnesium carbonate 40 mg with lactose 220 mg, sucrose 880 mg, sodium bicarbonate 40 mg (low Na$^+$). Net price 42-tab pack = £1.67

  Cautions diabetes mellitus (high sugar content)

Dose

- **By mouth**

  Child 12–18 years 1–3 tablets chewed 4 times daily (after meals and at bedtime)

1.2 Antispasmodics and other drugs altering gut motility

Drugs in this section include antimuscarinic compounds and drugs believed to be direct relaxants of intestinal smooth muscle. The smooth muscle relaxant properties of antimuscarinic and other antispasmodic drugs may be useful in *irritable bowel syndrome*.

The dopamine-receptor antagonist **domperidone** stimulates transit in the gut.

Antimuscarinics

Antimuscarinics (formerly termed 'anticholinergics') reduce intestinal motility. They are occasionally used for the management of *irritable bowel syndrome* but the evidence of their value has not been established and response varies. Other indications for antimuscarinic drugs include asthma and airways disease (section 3.1.2), motion sickness (section 4.6), urinary frequency and enuresis (section 7.4.2), mydriasis and cycloplegia (section 11.5), premedication (section 15.1.3), palliative care (p. 27), and as an antidote to organophosphorus poisoning (p. 46).

Antimuscarinics that are used for gastro-intestinal smooth muscle spasm include the tertiary amine **dicycloverine hydrochloride** (dicyclomine hydrochloride) and the quaternary ammonium compounds **propantheline bromide** and **hyoscine butylbromide**. The quaternary ammonium compounds are less lipid soluble than atropine and so are less likely to cross the blood-brain barrier; they are also less well absorbed from the gastro-intestinal tract.

Dicycloverine hydrochloride may also have some direct action on smooth muscle. Hyoscine butylbromide is advocated as a gastro-intestinal antispasmodic, but it is poorly absorbed; the injection may be useful in endoscopy and radiology.

Cautions   Antimuscarinics should be used with caution in children (especially children with Down's syndrome) due to increased risk of side-effects; they should also be used with caution in hypertension, conditions characterised by tachycardia (including hyperthyroidism, cardiac insufficiency, cardiac surgery), pyrexia, and in children susceptible to angle-closure glaucoma. Antimuscarinics are not used in children with gastro-oesophageal reflux disease, diarrhoea or ulcerative colitis. **Interactions:** Appendix 1 (antimuscarinics).

Contra-indications   Antimuscarinics are contra-indicated in myasthenia gravis (but may be used to decrease muscarinic side-effects of anticholinesterases—section 10.2.1), paralytic ileus, and pyloric stenosis.

Side-effects   Side-effects of antimuscarinics include constipation, transient bradycardia (followed by tachycardia, palpitation and arrhythmias), reduced bronchial secretions, urinary urgency and retention, dilatation of the pupils with loss of accommodation, photophobia, dry mouth, flushing and dryness of the skin. Side-effects that occur occasionally include nausea, vomiting, and giddiness; very rarely, angle closure glaucoma may occur.

DICYCLOVERINE HYDROCHLORIDE
(Dicyclomine hydrochloride)

Cautions see notes above

Contra-indications see notes above; child under 6 months

Pregnancy use with caution

Breast-feeding avoid—present in milk; apnoea reported in infant

Side-effects see notes above

Indication and dose

Symptomatic relief of gastro-intestinal disorders characterised by smooth muscle spasm
- **By mouth**

  Child 6 months–2 years 5–10 mg 3–4 times daily 15 minutes before feeds

  Child 2–12 years 10 mg 3 times daily

  Child 12–18 years 10–20 mg 3 times daily

Merbentyl® (Sanofi-Aventis) PoM

Tablets, dicycloverine hydrochloride 10 mg, net price 100-tab pack = £4.84; 20 mg (*Merbentyl 20®*), 84-tab pack = £8.14

Syrup, dicycloverine hydrochloride 10 mg/5 mL, net price 120 mL = £1.77

Note Dicycloverine hydrochloride can be sold to the public provided that max. single dose is 10 mg and max. daily dose is 60 mg

◢Compound preparations
Kolanticon® (Peckforton)

Gel, sugar-free, dicycloverine hydrochloride 2.5 mg, dried aluminium hydroxide 200 mg, light magnesium oxide 100 mg, simeticone 20 mg/5 mL, net price 200 mL = £2.21, 500 mL = £2.79

Dose

  Child 12–18 years 10–20 mL every 4 hours when required

HYOSCINE BUTYLBROMIDE

Cautions see notes above; also intestinal and urinary outlet obstruction

Contra-indications see notes above

Pregnancy manufacturer advises use only if potential benefit outweighs risk

Breast-feeding amount too small to be harmful

Side-effects see notes above

Licensed use *tablets* not licensed for use in children under 6 years; *injection* not licensed for use in children (age range not specified by manufacturer)

Indication and dose

Symptomatic relief of gastro-intestinal or genito-urinary disorders characterised by smooth muscle spasm
- **By mouth**

  Child 6–12 years 10 mg 3 times daily

  Child 12–18 years 20 mg 4 times daily

Excessive respiratory secretions and bowel colic in palliative care (see also p. 28)
- **By mouth**

  Child 1 month–2 years 300–500 micrograms/kg (max. 5 mg) 3–4 times daily

  Child 2–5 years 5 mg 3–4 times daily

  Child 5–12 years 10 mg 3–4 times daily

  Child 12–18 years 10–20 mg 3–4 times daily

- **By intramuscular or intravenous injection**

  Child 1 month–4 years 300–500 micrograms/kg (max. 5 mg) 3–4 times daily

  Child 5–12 years 5–10 mg 3–4 times daily

  Child 12–18 years 10–20 mg 3–4 times daily

Acute spasm, spasm in diagnostic procedures
- **By intramuscular or intravenous injection**

  Child 2–6 years 5 mg repeated after 30 minutes if necessary (may be repeated more frequently in endoscopy), max. 15 mg daily

  Child 6–12 years 5–10 mg repeated after 30 minutes if necessary (may be repeated more frequently in endoscopy), max. 30 mg daily

  Child 12–18 years 20 mg repeated after 30 minutes if necessary (may be repeated more frequently in endoscopy), max. 80 mg daily

Administration for *intravenous injection*, may be diluted with Glucose 5% *or* Sodium Chloride 0.9%; give over at least 1 minute.

For administration *by mouth*, injection solution may be used; content of ampoule may be stored in a refrigerator for up to 24 hours after opening

Buscopan® (Boehringer Ingelheim) PoM

Tablets, coated, hyoscine butylbromide 10 mg, net price 56-tab pack = £2.25

Note Hyoscine butylbromide tablets can be sold to the public for medically confirmed irritable bowel syndrome, provided single dose does not exceed 20 mg, daily dose does not exceed 80 mg, and pack does not contain a total of more than 240 mg

Injection, hyoscine butylbromide 20 mg/mL. Net price 1-mL amp = 22p

PROPANTHELINE BROMIDE

Cautions see notes above

Contra-indications see notes above

Hepatic impairment manufacturer advises caution

Renal impairment manufacturer advises caution

Pregnancy manufacturer advises avoid

Breast-feeding may suppress lactation

Side-effects see notes above

Licensed use *tablets* not licensed for use in children under 12 years

Gastro-intestinal system

1

◻ **PROPANTHELINE BROMIDE** (*continued*)

Indication and dose

Symptomatic relief of gastro-intestinal disorders characterised by smooth muscle spasm

• **By mouth**

Child 1 month–12 years 300 micrograms/kg (max. 15 mg) 3–4 times daily at least one hour before food

Child 12–18 years 15 mg 3 times daily at least one hour before meals and 30 mg at night (max. 120 mg daily)

Pro-Banthine® (Archimedes) ⟨PoM⟩
Tablets, pink, s/c, propantheline bromide 15 mg, net price 112-tab pack = £18.38. Label: 23

▲Extemporaneous formulations available see Extemporaneous Preparations, p. 8

Other antispasmodics

Alverine, **mebeverine**, and **peppermint oil** are believed to be direct relaxants of intestinal smooth muscle and may relieve pain in *irritable bowel syndrome* and primary dysmenorrhoea. They have no serious adverse effects; peppermint oil occasionally causes heartburn.

ALVERINE CITRATE

Contra-indications paralytic ileus
Pregnancy use with caution
Breast-feeding manufacturer advises avoid—limited information available
Side-effects nausea; headache, dizziness; pruritus, rash; hepatitis also reported

Indication and dose

Adjunct in gastro-intestinal disorders characterised by smooth muscle spasm, dysmenorrhoea

• **By mouth**

Child 12–18 years 60–120 mg 1–3 times daily

Spasmonal® (Norgine)
Capsules, alverine citrate 60 mg (blue/grey), net price 100-cap pack = £11.48; 120 mg (*Spasmonal® Forte*, blue/grey), 60-cap pack = £13.26

MEBEVERINE HYDROCHLORIDE

Cautions avoid in acute porphyria (section 9.8.2)
Contra-indications paralytic ileus
Pregnancy not known to be harmful—manufacturers advise caution
Side-effects allergic reactions (including rash, urticaria, angioedema) reported
Licensed use *tablets and liquid* not licensed for use in children under 10 years; *granules* not licensed for use in children under 12 years; *modified-release capsules* not licensed for use in children under 18 years

Indication and dose

Adjunct in gastro-intestinal disorders characterised by smooth muscle spasm

• **By mouth**

Child 3–4 years 25 mg 3 times daily, preferably 20 minutes before meals

Child 4–8 years 50 mg 3 times daily, preferably 20 minutes before meals

Child 8–10 years 100 mg 3 times daily, preferably 20 minutes before meals

Child 10–18 years 135–150 mg 3 times daily, preferably 20 minutes before meals

Mebeverine Hydrochloride (Non-proprietary) ⟨PoM⟩
Tablets, mebeverine hydrochloride 135 mg, net price 100-tab pack = £6.24

Oral suspension, mebeverine hydrochloride (as mebeverine embonate) 50 mg/5 mL, net price 300 mL = £107.00

Colofac® (Solvay) ⟨PoM⟩
Tablets, s/c, mebeverine hydrochloride 135 mg, net price 100-tab pack = £7.52

▲Modified release
Colofac® MR (Solvay) ⟨PoM⟩
Capsules, m/r, mebeverine hydrochloride 200 mg, net price 60-cap pack = £6.67. Label: 25

Dose

Irritable bowel syndrome
• **By mouth**
Child 12–18 years 1 capsule twice daily preferably 20 minutes before food

▲Compound preparations
[1]**Fybogel® Mebeverine** (Reckitt Benckiser) ⟨PoM⟩
Granules, buff, effervescent, ispaghula husk 3.5 g, mebeverine hydrochloride 135 mg/sachet, net price 10 sachets = £2.50. Label: 13, 22, counselling, see below
Excipients include aspartame (section 9.4.1)
Electrolytes K⁺ 2.5 mmol/sachet

Dose

Irritable bowel syndrome
• **By mouth**
Child 12–18 years 1 sachet in water, morning and evening 30 minutes before food; an additional sachet may also be taken before the midday meal if necessary

Counselling Preparations that swell in contact with liquid should always be carefully swallowed with water and should not be taken immediately before going to bed
1. 10-sachet pack can be sold to the public for use in children over 12 years

◢ PEPPERMINT OIL

Cautions sensitivity to menthol

Breast-feeding significant levels of menthol in breast milk unlikely

Side-effects heartburn, perianal irritation; *rarely*, allergic reactions (including rash, headache, bradycardia, muscle tremor, ataxia)

Local irritation Capsules should not be broken or chewed because peppermint oil may irritate mouth or oesophagus

Indication and dose

Relief of abdominal colic and distension, particularly in irritable bowel syndrome
• **By mouth**

  Child 15–18 years 1–2 capsules, swallowed whole with water, 3 times daily for up to 3 months if necessary

Colpermin® (McNeil)

Capsules, e/c, light blue/dark blue, blue band, peppermint oil 0.2 mL. Net price 100-cap pack = £12.05. Label: 5, 25
Excipients include arachis (peanut) oil

Motility stimulants

Domperidone and **metoclopramide** (section 4.6) are dopamine receptor antagonists which stimulate gastric emptying and small intestinal transit, and enhance the strength of oesophageal sphincter contraction. Metoclopramide and occasionally domperidone can cause acute dystonic reactions—for further details of this and other side-effects, see section 4.6.

A low dose of **erythromycin** stimulates gastro-intestinal motility and may be used on the advice of a paediatric gastroenterologist to promote tolerance of enteral feeds; erythromycin may be less effective as a prokinetic drug in preterm neonates than in older children.

◢ DOMPERIDONE

Cautions see under Domperidone (section 4.6)

Side-effects see under Domperidone (section 4.6); also QT-interval prolongation reported

Licensed use not licensed for use in gastro-intestinal stasis; not licensed for use in children for gastro-oesophageal reflux disease

Indication and dose

Gastro-oesophageal reflux disease (but efficacy not proven, see section 1.1), gastro-intestinal stasis
• **By mouth**

  Neonate 100–300 micrograms/kg 4–6 times daily before feeds

  Child 1 month–12 years 200–400 micrograms/kg (max. 20 mg) 3–4 times daily before food

  Child 12–18 years 10–20 mg, 3–4 times daily before food

  Nausea and vomiting section 4.6

◢Preparations
Section 4.6

◢ ERYTHROMYCIN

Cautions see section 5.1.5; **interactions:** Appendix 1 (macrolides)

Side-effects see section 5.1.5

Licensed use not licensed for use in gastro-intestinal stasis

Indication and dose

Gastro-intestinal stasis
• **By mouth**

  Neonate 3 mg/kg 4 times daily

  Child 1 month–18 years 3 mg/kg 4 times daily
• **By intravenous infusion**

  Neonate 3 mg/kg 4 times daily

  Child 1 month–1 year 3 mg/kg 4 times daily

◢Preparations
Section 5.1.5

Gastro-intestinal system

1.3 **Antisecretory drugs and mucosal protectants**

1.3.1 H₂-receptor antagonists
1.3.2 Selective antimuscarinics
1.3.3 Chelates and complexes
1.3.4 Prostaglandin analogues
1.3.5 Proton pump inhibitors

Peptic ulceration commonly involves the stomach, duodenum, and lower oeso-phagus; after gastric surgery it involves the gastro-enterostomy stoma.

Healing can be promoted by general measures, stopping smoking and taking antacids and by antisecretory drug treatment, but relapse is common when treatment ceases. Nearly all duodenal ulcers and most gastric ulcers not asso-ciated with NSAIDs are caused by *Helicobacter pylori*.

The management of *H. pylori* infection and of NSAID-associated ulcers is dis-cussed below.

Helicobacter pylori infection

Eradication of *Helicobacter pylori* reduces the recurrence of gastric and duodenal ulcers and the risk of rebleeding. The presence of *H. pylori* should be confirmed before starting eradication treatment. If possible, the antibacterial sensitivity of the organism should be established at the time of endoscopy and biopsy. Acid inhibition combined with antibacterial treatment is highly effective in the eradica-tion of *H. pylori*; reinfection is rare. Antibiotic-associated colitis is an uncommon risk.

Treatment to eradicate *H. pylori* infection in children should be initiated under specialist supervision. One-week triple-therapy regimens that comprise ome-prazole, amoxicillin, and either clarithromycin or metronidazole are recom-mended. Resistance to clarithromycin or to metronidazole is much more common than to amoxicillin and can develop during treatment. A regimen containing amoxicillin and clarithromycin is therefore recommended for initial therapy and one containing amoxicillin and metronidazole for eradication failure. There is usually no need to continue antisecretory treatment (with a proton pump inhibitor or H₂-receptor antagonist); however, if the ulcer is large, or complicated by haemorrhage or perforation then antisecretory treatment is continued for a further 3 weeks. Lansoprazole may be considered if omeprazole is unsuitable. Treatment failure usually indicates antibacterial resistance or poor compliance.

Two-week triple-therapy regimens offer the possibility of higher eradication rates compared to one-week regimens, but adverse effects are common and poor compliance is likely to offset any possible gain.

Recommended regimens for *Helicobacter pylori* eradication

Eradication therapy	Age range	Oral dose (to be used in combination with omeprazole, section 1.3.5)
Amoxicillin	1–6 years	250 mg twice daily (with clarithromycin)
		125 mg 3 times daily (with metronidazole)
	6–12 years	500 mg twice daily (with clarithromycin)
		250 mg 3 times daily (with metronidazole)
	12–18 years	1 g twice daily (with clarithromycin)
		500 mg 3 times daily (with metronidazole)
Clarithromycin	1–12 years	7.5 mg/kg (max. 500 mg) twice daily (with metronidazole or amoxicillin)
	12–18 years	500 mg twice daily (with metronidazole or amoxicillin)
Metronidazole	1–6 years	100 mg twice daily (with clarithromycin)
		100 mg 3 times daily (with amoxicillin)
	6–12 years	200 mg twice daily (with clarithromycin)
		200 mg 3 times daily (with amoxicillin)
	12–18 years	400 mg twice daily (with clarithromycin)
		400 mg 3 times daily (with amoxicillin)

1 Gastro-intestinal system

Two-week dual-therapy regimens using a proton pump inhibitor and a single antibacterial produce low rates of *H. pylori* eradication and are **not** recommended.

For the role of *H. pylori* eradication therapy in children starting or taking NSAIDs, see NSAID-associated ulcers, below.

Test for *Helicobacter pylori*

^{13}C-Urea breath test kits are available for confirming the presence of gastro-duodenal infection with *Helicobacter pylori*. The test involves collection of breath samples before and after ingestion of an oral solution of ^{13}C-urea; the samples are sent for analysis by an appropriate laboratory. The test should not be performed within 4 weeks of treatment with an antibacterial or within 2 weeks of treatment with an antisecretory drug. A specific ^{13}C-Urea breath test kit for children is available (*Helicobacter Test INFAI for children of the age 3–11*®). However the appropriateness of testing for *H. pylori* infection in children has not been established. Breath, saliva, faecal, and urine tests for *H. pylori* are frequently unreliable in children; the most accurate method of diagnosis is endoscopy with biopsy.

Helicobacter Test INFAI for children of the age 3–11® (Infai) [PoM]
Oral powder, ^{13}C-urea 45 mg, net price 1 kit (including 4 breath sample containers, straws) = £19.20 (spectrometric analysis included)

Helicobacter Test INFAI® (Infai) [PoM]
Oral powder, ^{13}C-urea 75 mg, net price 1 kit (including 4 breath-sample containers, straws) = £19.20 (spectrometric analysis included); 1 kit (including 2 breath bags) = £14.20 (spectroscopic analysis not included); 50-test set = £855.00 (spectrometric analysis included)

NSAID-associated ulcers

Gastro-intestinal bleeding and ulceration can occur with NSAID use (section 10.1.1). In adults, the risk of serious upper gastro-intestinal side-effects varies between individual NSAIDs (see Gastro-intestinal side-effects, p. 611). Whenever possible, NSAIDs should be **withdrawn** if an ulcer occurs.

Children at high risk of developing gastro-intestinal complications include those with a history of peptic ulcer disease or serious upper gastro-intestinal complication, those taking other medicines that increase the risk of upper gastro-intestinal side-effects, or those with serious co-morbidity. In children at risk of ulceration, a proton pump inhibitor (section 1.3.5) or an H₂-receptor antagonist, such as ranitidine, may be considered for protection against gastric and duodenal ulcers associated with non-selective NSAIDs.

NSAID use and *H. pylori* infection are independent risk factors for gastro-intestinal bleeding and ulceration. In children already taking a NSAID, eradication of *H. pylori* is unlikely to reduce the risk of NSAID-induced bleeding or ulceration. However, in children about to start long-term NSAID treatment who are *H. pylori* positive and have dyspepsia or a history of gastric or duodenal ulcer, eradication of *H. pylori* may reduce the overall risk of ulceration.

If the *NSAID can be discontinued* in a child who has developed an ulcer, a proton pump inhibitor usually produces the most rapid healing, alternatively the ulcer can be treated with an H₂-receptor antagonist.

If *NSAID treatment needs to continue*, the ulcer is treated with a proton pump inhibitor (section 1.3.5).

1.3.1 H₂-receptor antagonists

Histamine H₂-receptor antagonists heal *gastric* and *duodenal ulcers* by reducing gastric acid output as a result of histamine H₂-receptor blockade; they are also used to relieve symptoms of *dyspepsia* and *gastro-oesophageal reflux disease* (section 1.1). H₂-receptor antagonists should not normally be used for *Zollinger–Ellison syndrome* because proton pump inhibitors (section 1.3.5) are more effective.

Maintenance treatment with low doses has largely been replaced in *Helicobacter pylori* positive children by eradication regimens (section 1.3).

H₂-receptor antagonist therapy can promote healing of *NSAID-associated ulcers* (section 1.3).

1

Gastro-intestinal system

Treatment with a H$_2$-receptor antagonist has not been shown to be beneficial in haematemesis and melaena, but prophylactic use reduces the frequency of bleeding from *gastroduodenal erosions in hepatic coma*, and possibly in other conditions requiring intensive care. Treatment also reduces the risk of *acid aspiration* in obstetric patients at delivery (Mendelson's syndrome).

H$_2$-receptor antagonists are also used to reduce the degradation of pancreatic enzyme supplements (section 1.9.4) in children with cystic fibrosis.

Side-effects   Side-effects of the H$_2$-receptor antagonists include diarrhoea and other gastro-intestinal disturbances, altered liver function tests (rarely liver damage), headache, dizziness, rash, and tiredness. Rare side-effects include acute pancreatitis, bradycardia, AV block, confusion, depression, and hallucinations particularly in the very ill, hypersensitivity reactions (including fever, arthralgia, myalgia, anaphylaxis), blood disorders (including agranulocytosis, leucopenia, pancytopenia, thrombocytopenia), and skin reactions (including erythema multiforme and toxic epidermal necrolysis). There have been occasional reports of gynaecomastia and impotence.

RANITIDINE

Cautions acute porphyria; **interactions:** Appendix 1 (histamine H$_2$-antagonists)

Renal impairment use half normal dose if estimated glomerular filtration rate less than 50 mL/minute/1.73 m^2

Pregnancy manufacturer advises avoid unless essential, but not known to be harmful

Breast-feeding significant amount present in milk, but not known to be harmful

Side-effects see notes above; also *rarely* tachycardia, agitation, visual disturbances, alopecia; *very rarely* interstitial nephritis

Licensed use *oral* preparations not licensed for use in children under 3 years; *injection* not licensed for use in children under 6 months

Indication and dose

Reflux oesophagitis, benign gastric and duodenal ulceration, prophylaxis of stress ulceration, other conditions where gastric acid reduction is beneficial (see notes above and section 1.9.4)

• By mouth

Neonate 2 mg/kg 3 times daily but absorption unreliable; max. 3 mg/kg 3 times daily

Child 1–6 months 1 mg/kg 3 times daily; max. 3 mg/kg 3 times daily

Child 6 months–3 years 2–4 mg/kg twice daily

Child 3–12 years 2–4 mg/kg (max. 150 mg) twice daily; increased up to 5 mg/kg (max. 300 mg) twice daily in severe gastro-oesophageal reflux disease

Child 12–18 years 150 mg twice daily *or* 300 mg at night; increased if necessary, to 300 mg twice daily *or* 150 mg 4 times daily for up to 12 weeks in moderate to severe gastro-oesophageal reflux disease

Note In fat malabsorption syndrome, give 1–2 hours before food to enhance effects of pancreatic enzyme replacement

• By slow intravenous injection

Neonate 0.5–1 mg/kg every 6–8 hours

Child 1 month–18 years 1 mg/kg (max. 50 mg) every 6–8 hours (may be given as an intermittent infusion at a rate of 25 mg/hour)

Zollinger–Ellison syndrome (but see notes above)

• By mouth

Child 12–18 years 150 mg 3 times daily (doses up to 6 g daily in divided doses have been used)

Administration For *slow intravenous injection* dilute to a concentration of 2.5 mg/mL with Glucose 5%, Sodium Chloride 0.9%, *or* Compound Sodium Lactate. Give over at least 3 minutes

[1]**Ranitidine** (Non-proprietary) ⓅⓄⓂ
Tablets, ranitidine (as hydrochloride) 150 mg, net price 60-tab pack = £1.37; 300 mg, 30-tab pack = £1.45
Brands include *Ranitic*®

Effervescent tablets, ranitidine (as hydrochloride) 150 mg, net price 60-tab pack = £10.51; 300 mg, 30-tab pack = £11.22. Label: 13
Excipients may include sodium (check with supplier)

Oral solution, ranitidine (as hydrochloride) 75 mg/5 mL, 100 mL = £7.44, 300 mL = £19.70
Excipients may include alcohol (check with supplier)

1. Ranitidine can be sold to the public for children over 16 years (provided packs do not contain more than 2 weeks' supply) for the short-term symptomatic relief of heartburn, dyspepsia, and hyperacidity, and for the prevention of these symptoms when associated with consumption of food or drink (max. single dose 75 mg, max. daily dose 300 mg)

Zantac® (GSK) ⓅⓄⓂ
Tablets, f/c, ranitidine (as hydrochloride) 150 mg, net price 60-tab pack = £1.30; 300 mg, 30-tab pack = £1.30

Effervescent tablets, pale yellow, ranitidine (as hydrochloride) 150 mg (contains 14.3 mmol Na$^+$/tablet), net price 60-tab pack = £24.93; 300 mg (contains 20.8 mmol Na$^+$/tablet), 30-tab pack = £24.52. Label: 13
Excipients include aspartame (section 9.4.1)

Syrup, sugar-free, ranitidine (as hydrochloride) 75 mg/5 mL. Net price 300 mL = £20.76
Excipients include alcohol 8%

Injection, ranitidine (as hydrochloride) 25 mg/mL. Net price 2-mL amp = 57p

1.3.2 Selective antimuscarinics

Classification not used in *BNF for Children*.

1.3.3 Chelates and complexes

Sucralfate is a complex of aluminium hydroxide and sulphated sucrose that appears to act by protecting the mucosa from acid-pepsin attack; it has minimal antacid properties. Sucralfate can be used to prevent stress ulceration in children receiving intensive care. It should be used with caution in this situation (**important**: reports of bezoar formation, see CSM advice below).

SUCRALFATE

Cautions administration of sucralfate and enteral feeds should be separated by 1 hour; **interactions**: Appendix 1 (sucralfate)

Bezoar formation Following reports of bezoar formation associated with sucralfate, the **CSM** has advised caution in seriously ill patients, especially those receiving concomitant enteral feeds or those with predisposing conditions such as delayed gastric emptying

Renal impairment use with caution; aluminium is absorbed and may accumulate

Pregnancy use with caution

Breast-feeding amount probably too small to be harmful

Side-effects constipation; *less frequently* diarrhoea, nausea, indigestion, flatulence, gastric discomfort, back pain, dizziness, headache, drowsiness, bezoar formation (see above), dry mouth, and rash

Licensed use not licensed for use in children under 15 years; tablets not licensed for prophylaxis of stress ulceration

Indication and dose

Prophylaxis of stress ulceration in child under intensive care
- **By mouth**
  Child 1 month–2 years 250 mg 4–6 times daily
  Child 2–12 years 500 mg 4–6 times daily
  Child 12–15 years 1 g 4–6 times daily
  Child 15–18 years 1 g 6 times daily; max. 8 g daily

Benign gastric and duodenal ulceration
- **By mouth**
  Child 1 month–2 years 250 mg 4–6 times daily
  Child 2–12 years 500 mg 4–6 times daily
  Child 12–15 years 1 g 4–6 times daily
  Child 15–18 years 2 g twice daily (on rising and at bedtime) *or* 1 g 4 times daily (1 hour before meals and at bedtime) taken for 4–6 weeks, or in resistant cases up to 12 weeks; max. 8 g daily

Administration for administration *by mouth*, sucralfate should be given 1 hour before meals, see also Cautions, above; *oral suspension* blocks fine-bore feeding tubes; crushed *tablets* may be dispersed in water.

Antepsin® (Chugai) (PoM)
Tablets, scored, sucralfate 1 g, net price 50-tab pack = £5.53. Label: 5

Suspension, sucralfate, 1 g/5 mL, net price 250 mL (aniseed- and caramel-flavoured) = £5.53. Label: 5

1.3.4 Prostaglandin analogues

Classification not used in *BNF for Children*.

1.3.5 Proton pump inhibitors

Proton pump inhibitors inhibit gastric acid secretion by blocking the hydrogen-potassium adenosine triphosphatase enzyme system (the 'proton pump') of the gastric parietal cell. **Omeprazole** is currently only licensed in children for the treatment of *gastro-oesophageal reflux disease* with severe symptoms. **Lansoprazole** is not licensed for use in children, but may be considered when the available formulations of omeprazole are unsuitable. Proton pump inhibitors are effective short-term treatments for *gastric* and *duodenal ulcers*; they are also used in combination with antibacterials for the eradication of *Helicobacter pylori* (see p. 58 for specific regimens). An initial short course of a proton pump inhibitor is the treatment of choice in *gastro-oesophageal reflux disease* with severe symptoms; children with endoscopically confirmed *erosive*, *ulcerative*, or *stricturing oesophagitis* usually need to be maintained on a proton pump inhibitor.

Proton pump inhibitors are also used for the prevention and treatment of NSAID-associated ulcers (see p. 59). In children who need to continue NSAID treatment after an ulcer has healed, the dose of proton pump inhibitor should not normally be reduced because asymptomatic ulcer deterioration may occur.

1 Gastro-intestinal system

Proton pump inhibitors are effective in the treatment of the *Zollinger-Ellison syndrome* (including cases resistant to other treatment). They are also used to reduce the degradation of pancreatic enzyme supplements (section 1.9.4) in children with cystic fibrosis.

Side-effects   Side-effects of the proton pump inhibitors include gastro-intestinal disturbances (including nausea, vomiting, abdominal pain, flatulence, diarrhoea, constipation), and headache. Less frequent side-effects include dry mouth, peripheral oedema, dizziness, sleep disturbances, fatigue, paraesthesia, arthralgia, myalgia, rash, and pruritus. Other side-effects reported *rarely* or *very rarely* include taste disturbance, stomatitis, hepatitis, jaundice, hypersensitivity reactions (including anaphylaxis, bronchospasm), fever, depression, hallucinations, confusion, gynaecomastia, interstitial nephritis, hyponatraemia, blood disorders (including leucopenia, leucocytosis, pancytopenia, thrombocytopenia), visual disturbances, sweating, photosensitivity, alopecia, Stevens-Johnson syndrome, and toxic epidermal necrolysis. By decreasing gastric acidity, proton pump inhibitors may increase the risk of gastro-intestinal infections (including *Clostridium difficile* infection).

ESOMEPRAZOLE

Cautions interactions: Appendix 1 (proton pump inhibitors)

Hepatic impairment child 1–12 years max. 10 mg daily in severe impairment; child 12–18 years max. 20 mg daily in severe impairment

Renal impairment manufacturer advises caution in severe renal insufficiency

Pregnancy manufacturer advises caution—no information available

Breast-feeding manufacturer advises avoid—no information available

Side-effects see notes above

Licensed use tablets not licensed for use in children 1–12 years

Indication and dose

> Gastro-oesophageal reflux disease (in the presence of erosive reflux oesophagitis)
> * By mouth
>
> **Child 1–12 years**
>
> **Body-weight 10–20 kg** 10 mg once daily for 8 weeks
>
> **Body-weight over 20 kg** 10–20 mg once daily for 8 weeks
>
> **Child 12–18 years** 40 mg once daily for 4 weeks, continued for further 4 weeks if not fully healed or symptoms persist; maintenance 20 mg daily

> Symptomatic treatment of gastro-oesophageal reflux disease (in the absence of oesophagitis)
> * By mouth
>
> **Child 1–12 years, body-weight over 10 kg** 10 mg once daily for up to 8 weeks
>
> **Child 12–18 years** 20 mg once daily for up to 4 weeks

Nexium® (AstraZeneca) PoM
Tablets, f/c, esomeprazole (as magnesium trihydrate) 20 mg (light pink), net price 28-tab pack = £18.50; 40 mg (pink), 28-tab pack = £25.19. Counselling, administration

Administration Swallow whole or disperse in water; do not chew or crush tablets

Granules, yellow, e/c, esomeprazole (as magnesium trihydrate) 10 mg/sachet, net price 28-sachet pack = £25.19. Label: 25, counselling, administration

Administration Disperse the contents of each sachet in approx. 15 mL water. Stir and leave to thicken for a few minutes; stir again before administration and use within 30 minutes; rinse container with 15 mL water to obtain full dose; can be administered through nasogastric or gastric tube

LANSOPRAZOLE

Cautions interactions: Appendix 1 (proton pump inhibitors)

Hepatic impairment may accumulate in severe impairment

Pregnancy manufacturer advises avoid

Breast-feeding avoid unless essential—present in milk in *animal* studies

Side-effects see notes above; also glossitis, pancreatitis, anorexia, restlessness, tremor, impotence, petechiae, and purpura; *very rarely* colitis, raised serum cholesterol or triglycerides

Licensed use not licensed for use in children

Indication and dose

> Gastro-oesophageal reflux disease, acid-related dyspepsia, treatment of duodenal and benign gastric ulcer including those complicating NSAID therapy, fat malabsorption despite pancreatic enzyme replacement therapy in cystic fibrosis
> * By mouth
>
> **Child body-weight under 30 kg** 0.5–1 mg/kg (max. 15 mg) once daily in the morning
>
> **Child body-weight over 30 kg** 15–30 mg once daily in the morning

◻ **LANSOPRAZOLE** (*continued*)

Administration for administration by a *nasogastric tube* or an *oral syringe*, *Zoton FasTab®* can be dispersed in a small amount of water

Zoton® (Wyeth) ⒫ⓄⓂ
FasTab® (= orodispersible tablet), lansoprazole 15 mg, net price 28-tab pack = £2.99; 30 mg, 28-tab pack = £5.50. Label: 5, 22, counselling, administration
Excipients include aspartame (section 9.4.1)

Counselling Tablets should be placed on the tongue, allowed to disperse and swallowed, or may be swallowed whole with a glass of water.

■ OMEPRAZOLE

Cautions interactions: Appendix 1 (proton pump inhibitors)

Hepatic impairment no more than 700 micrograms/kg (max. 20 mg) once daily

Pregnancy not known to be harmful

Breast-feeding present in milk but not known to be harmful

Side-effects see notes above; also agitation and impotence

Licensed use *capsules* and *tablets* not licensed for use in children except for severe ulcerating reflux oesophagitis in children over 1 year; *injection* not licensed for use in children under 12 years

Indication and dose

> Gastro-oesophageal reflux disease, acid-related dyspepsia, treatment of duodenal and benign gastric ulcers including those complicating NSAID therapy, prophylaxis of acid aspiration, Zollinger-Ellison syndrome, fat malabsorption despite pancreatic enzyme replacement therapy in cystic fibrosis
>
> • **By mouth**
>
> **Neonate** 700 micrograms/kg once daily, increased if necessary after 7–14 days to 1.4 mg/kg; some neonates may require up to 2.8 mg/kg once daily
>
> **Child 1 month–2 years** 700 micrograms/kg once daily, increased if necessary to 3 mg/kg (max. 20 mg) once daily
>
> **Child body-weight 10–20 kg** 10 mg once daily increased if necessary to 20 mg once daily (in severe ulcerating reflux oesophagitis, max. 12 weeks at higher dose)
>
> **Child body-weight over 20 kg** 20 mg once daily increased if necessary to 40 mg once daily (in severe ulcerating reflux oesophagitis, max. 12 weeks at higher dose)
>
> • **By intravenous injection over 5 minutes** *or* **by intravenous infusion**
>
> **Child 1 month–12 years** initially 500 micrograms/kg (max. 20 mg) once daily, increased to 2 mg/kg (max. 40 mg) once daily if necessary
>
> **Child 12–18 years** 40 mg once daily

Helicobacter pylori eradication (in combination with antibacterials see p. 58)

> • **By mouth**
>
> **Child 1–12 years** 1–2 mg/kg (max. 40 mg) once daily
>
> **Child 12–18 years** 40 mg once daily

Administration for administration *by mouth*, swallow whole, *or* disperse *Losec MUPS®* tablets in water, *or* mix capsule contents or *Losec MUPS®* tablets with fruit juice or yoghurt. Preparations consisting of an e/c tablet within a capsule should **not** be opened.

For administration through an *enteral feeding tube*, use *Losec MUPS®* or the contents of a capsule containing omeprazole dispersed in a large volume of water, or in 10 mL Sodium Bicarbonate 8.4% (1 mmol Na^+/mL) (allow to stand for 10 minutes before administration).

For *intermittent intravenous infusion*, dilute reconstituted solution to a concentration of 400 micrograms/mL with Glucose 5% *or* Sodium Chloride 0.9%; give over 20–30 minutes

Omeprazole (Non-proprietary) ⒫ⓄⓂ
Capsules, enclosing e/c granules, omeprazole 10 mg, net price 28-cap pack = £1.77; 20 mg, 28-cap pack = £1.77; 40 mg, 7-cap pack = £2.12; 28-cap pack = £21.65. Counselling, administration
Note Some preparations consist of an e/c tablet within a capsule
Brands include *Mepradec®*
Dental prescribing on NHS Gastro-resistant omeprazole capsules may be prescribed

Tablets, e/c, omeprazole 10 mg, net price 28-tab pack = £4.59; 20 mg, 28-tab pack = £5.91; 40 mg, 7-tab pack = £5.68. Label: 25

Intravenous infusion, powder for reconstitution, omeprazole (as sodium salt), net price 40-mg vial = £5.18

Losec® (AstraZeneca) ⒫ⓄⓂ
MUPS® (multiple-unit pellet system = dispersible tablets), f/c, omeprazole 10 mg (light pink), net price 28-tab pack = £7.75; 20 mg (pink), 28-tab pack = £11.60; 40 mg (red-brown), 7-tab pack = £5.80. Counselling, administration

Capsules, enclosing e/c granules, omeprazole 10 mg (pink), net price 28-cap pack = £7.75; 20 mg (pink/brown), 28-cap pack = £11.60; 40 mg (brown), 7-cap pack = £5.80. Counselling, administration

Intravenous infusion, powder for reconstitution, omeprazole (as sodium salt), net price 40-mg vial = £5.41

Injection, powder for reconstitution, omeprazole (as sodium salt), net price 40-mg vial (with solvent) = £5.41

1.4 Acute diarrhoea

1.4.1 Adsorbents and bulk-forming drugs
1.4.2 Antimotility drugs

The priority in acute diarrhoea, as in gastro-enteritis, is the prevention or reversal of fluid and electrolyte depletion—this is particularly important in infants. For details of **oral rehydration preparations**, see section 9.2.1.2. Severe dehydration requires immediate admission to hospital and urgent replacement of fluid and electrolytes.

Antimotility drugs (section 1.4.2) relieve symptoms of diarrhoea. They are used in the management of uncomplicated acute diarrhoea in adults, but are **not** recommended for use in children under 12 years. Fluid and electrolyte replacement (section 9.2.1.2) are of prime importance in the treatment of acute diarrhoea.

Antispasmodics (section 1.2) are occasionally of value in treating abdominal cramp associated with diarrhoea but they should **not** be used for primary treatment. Antispasmodics and antiemetics should be **avoided** in young children with gastro-enteritis since they are rarely effective and have troublesome side-effects.

Antibacterial drugs are generally unnecessary in simple gastro-enteritis because the complaint usually resolves quickly without such treatment, and infective diarrhoeas in the UK often have a viral cause. Systemic bacterial infection does, however, need appropriate systemic treatment; for drugs used in campylobacter enteritis, shigellosis, and salmonellosis, see p. 305

Colestyramine (cholestyramine, section 1.9.2) binds unabsorbed bile salts and provides symptomatic relief of diarrhoea following ileal disease or resection.

1.4.1 Adsorbents and bulk-forming drugs

Adsorbents such as kaolin are **not** recommended for *acute diarrhoeas*. Bulk-forming drugs, such as ispaghula, methylcellulose, and sterculia (section 1.6.1) are rarely effective in controlling faecal consistency in ileostomy and colostomy.

1.4.2 Antimotility drugs

Antimotility drugs have a role in the management of uncomplicated *acute diarrhoea* in adults but not in children under 12 years; see also section 1.4. However, in the case of dehydration, fluid and electrolyte replacement (section 9.2.1.2) are of primary importance.

For comments on their role in *chronic bowel disorders* see section 1.5. Antimotility drugs are also used in children with *stoma* (section 1.8).

CODEINE PHOSPHATE

Cautions see section 4.7.2; tolerance and dependence may occur with prolonged use; **interactions:** Appendix 1 (opioid analgesics)

Contra-indications see section 4.7.2; also conditions where inhibition of peristalsis should be avoided, where abdominal distension develops, or in acute diarrhoeal conditions such as acute ulcerative colitis or antibiotic-associated colitis

Hepatic impairment section 4.7.2
Renal impairment section 4.7.2
Pregnancy section 4.7.2
Breast-feeding section 4.7.2
Side-effects section 4.7.2

Indication and dose

Diarrhoea (but see notes above)
● **By mouth**
Child **12–18 years** 30 mg (range 15–60 mg) 3–4 times daily

Pain section 4.7.2

Codeine Phosphate (Non-proprietary) ⓅⓄⓂ
Tablets, codeine phosphate 15 mg, net price 28 = £1.08; 30 mg, 28 = £1.24; 60 mg, 28 = £1.73. Label: 2

Note As for schedule 2 controlled drugs, travellers needing to take codeine phosphate tablets abroad may require a doctor's letter explaining why codeine is necessary.

▲ CO-PHENOTROPE

A mixture of diphenoxylate hydrochloride and atropine sulphate in the mass proportions 100 parts to 1 part respectively

Cautions see under Codeine Phosphate (section 4.7.2); also young children are particularly susceptible to **overdosage** and symptoms may be delayed and observation is needed for at least 48 hours after ingestion; presence of subclinical doses of atropine may give rise to atropine side-effects in susceptible individuals or in overdosage (section 1.2); **interactions:** Appendix 1 (antimuscarinics, opioid analgesics)

Contra-indications see under Antimuscarinics (section 1.2) and Codeine Phosphate (section 4.7.2); also jaundice

Hepatic impairment section 4.7.2

Renal impairment section 4.7.2

Pregnancy section 4.7.2

Breast-feeding may be present in milk

Side-effects see under Antimuscarinics (section 1.2) and Codeine Phosphate (section 4.7.2); also fever

Licensed use not licensed for use in children under 4 years

Indication and dose
> See preparations

Administration for administration *by mouth* tablets may be crushed

Co-phenotrope (Non-proprietary) ⒫ₒₘ
> Tablets, co-phenotrope 2.5/0.025 (diphenoxylate hydrochloride 2.5 mg, atropine sulphate 25 micrograms), net price 100 = £8.95
> Brands include *Lomotil®*

Dose
> Control of faecal consistency after colostomy or ileostomy, adjunct to rehydration in acute diarrhoea (but see notes above)
> • By mouth
>> Child 2–4 years half tablet 3 times daily
>> Child 4–9 years 1 tablet 3 times daily
>> Child 9–12 years 1 tablet 4 times daily
>> Child 12–16 years 2 tablets 3 times daily
>> Child 16–18 years initially 4 tablets then 2 tablets 4 times daily
>
> Note Co-phenotrope 2.5/0.025 can be sold to the public for children over 16 years (provided packs do not contain more than 20 tablets) as an adjunct to rehydration in acute diarrhoea (max. daily dose 10 tablets)

▲ LOPERAMIDE HYDROCHLORIDE

Cautions see notes above; **interactions:** Appendix 1 (loperamide)

Contra-indications conditions where inhibition of peristalsis should be avoided, where abdominal distension develops, or in conditions such as active ulcerative colitis or antibiotic-associated colitis

Hepatic impairment risk of accumulation—manufacturer advises caution

Pregnancy manufacturer advises avoid—no information available

Breast-feeding amount probably too small to be harmful

Side-effects abdominal cramps, dizziness, drowsiness, and skin reactions including urticaria; paralytic ileus and abdominal bloating also reported

Licensed use *capsules* not licensed for use in children under 8 years; *syrup* not licensed for use in children under 4 years; not licensed for use in children for chronic diarrhoea

Indication and dose
> Chronic diarrhoea
> • By mouth
>> Child 1 month–1 year 100–200 micrograms/kg twice daily, 30 minutes before feeds; up to 2 mg/kg daily in divided doses occasionally required
>> Child 1–12 years 100–200 micrograms/kg (max. 2 mg) 3–4 times daily; up to 1.25 mg/kg daily in divided doses may be required (max. 16 mg daily)
>> Child 12–18 years 2–4 mg 2–4 times daily (max. 16 mg daily)

> Acute diarrhoea (but see notes above)
> • By mouth
>> Child 4–8 years 1 mg 3–4 times daily for *up to 3 days only*
>> Child 8–12 years 2 mg 4 times daily for up to 5 days
>> Child 12–18 years initially 4 mg, then 2 mg after each loose stool for up to 5 days (usual dose 6–8 mg daily; max. 16 mg daily)

Loperamide (Non-proprietary) ⒫ₒₘ
> Capsules, loperamide hydrochloride 2 mg, net price 30-cap pack = £1.07
> Tablets, loperamide hydrochloride 2 mg, net price 30-tab pack = £2.15
> Brands include *Norimode®*

Note Loperamide can be sold to the public, for use in children over 12 years, provided it is licensed and labelled for the treatment of acute diarrhoea

Imodium® (Janssen-Cilag) ⒫ₒₘ
> Capsules, green/grey, loperamide hydrochloride 2 mg. Net price 30-cap pack = £1.09
> Syrup, sugar-free, red, loperamide hydrochloride 1 mg/5 mL. Net price 100 mL = 94p

◢ Compound preparations

Imodium® Plus (McNeil)
> Caplets (= tablets), loperamide hydrochloride 2 mg, simeticone 125 mg, net price 6-tab pack = £2.27, 12-tab pack = £3.58

Dose
> Acute diarrhoea with abdominal colic
>> Child 12–18 years initially 1 caplet, then 1 caplet after each loose stool; max. 4 caplets daily for up to 2 days

1 Gastro-intestinal system

1.5 Chronic bowel disorders

Individual symptoms of chronic bowel disorders need specific treatment including dietary manipulation as well as drug treatment and the maintenance of a liberal fluid intake.

Gastro-intestinal system   **1**

Inflammatory bowel disease

Chronic inflammatory bowel diseases include *ulcerative colitis* and *Crohn's disease*. The treatment of inflammatory bowel disease in children should be initiated and supervised by a paediatric gastroenterologist. Effective management requires drug therapy, attention to nutrition, and in severe or chronic active disease, surgery.

Aminosalicylates (balsalazide, mesalazine, olsalazine, and sulfasalazine), **corticosteroids** (hydrocortisone, budesonide, and prednisolone), and **drugs that affect the immune response** are used in the treatment of inflammatory bowel disease.

Treatment of acute ulcerative colitis and Crohn's disease Acute mild to moderate disease affecting the rectum (proctitis) or the recto-sigmoid (distal colitis) is treated initially with local application of an aminosalicylate (section 1.5.1); alternatively a local corticosteroid (section 1.5.2) can be used but it is less effective. Foam preparations and suppositories are useful for children who have difficulty retaining liquid enemas.

Diffuse inflammatory bowel disease or disease that does not respond to local therapy requires oral treatment. Mild disease affecting the proximal colon can be treated with an oral aminosalicylate alone; a combination of a local and an oral aminosalicylate can be used in proctitis or distal colitis. Refractory or moderate inflammatory bowel disease usually requires adjunctive use of an oral corticosteroid such as **prednisolone** (section 1.5.2) for 4–8 weeks. Modified-release **budesonide** is used for children with Crohn's disease affecting the ileum and the ascending colon; it causes fewer systemic side-effects than oral prednisolone but may be less effective. As an alternative to an oral corticosteroid, **enteral nutrition** (Appendix 2) may be used for 6–8 weeks in children with active Crohn's disease.

Severe inflammatory bowel disease calls for hospital admission and treatment with an intravenous corticosteroid such as **hydrocortisone** (p. 458) or **methylprednisolone** (p. 459); other therapy may include intravenous fluid and electrolyte replacement, and possibly parenteral nutrition. Children with ulcerative colitis that fails to respond adequately to these measures may benefit from a short course of ciclosporin. Children with unresponsive or chronically active Crohn's disease may benefit from azathioprine, mercaptopurine, or once-weekly methotrexate; these drugs have a slow onset of action.

Infliximab (section 1.5.3) is used in specialist centres for children with severe active Crohn's disease whose condition has not responded adequately to treatment with a corticosteroid and a conventional immunosuppressant or who are intolerant of them. Infliximab has also been used for the treatment of severe, refractory ulcerative colitis. There are concerns about the long-term safety of infliximab in children; hepatosplenic T-cell lymphoma has been reported.

Crohn's disease of the mouth or of the perineum is more common in children than in adults and it is difficult to treat; elimination diets and the use of a topical corticosteroid (section 13.4) may be beneficial, but a systemic corticosteroid (section 6.3.2) and occasionally azathioprine may be required in severe cases.

NICE guidance

Infliximab for Crohn's disease (April 2002)

Infliximab is recommended for the treatment of severe active Crohn's disease (with or without fistulae) when treatment with immunomodulating drugs and corticosteroids has failed or is not tolerated and when surgery is inappropriate. Treatment may be repeated if the condition responded to the initial course but relapsed subsequently. Infliximab should be prescribed only by a gastroenterologist.

> **NICE guidance**
>
> Infliximab for subacute manifestations of ulcerative colitis (April 2008)
> Infliximab is **not** recommended for the treatment of subacute manifestations
> of moderate to severe active ulcerative colitis that would normally be man-
> aged in an outpatient setting.

Maintenance of remission of acute ulcerative colitis and Crohn's disease
Smoking cessation (section 4.10) reduces the risk of relapse in Crohn's disease
and should be encouraged. **Aminosalicylates** are of great value in the maintenance of remission of ulcerative colitis. They are of less value in the maintenance of remission of Crohn's disease; an oral formulation of mesalazine is
available for the long-term management of ileal disease. Corticosteroids are **not**
suitable for maintenance treatment because of their side-effects. In resistant or
frequently relapsing cases either **azathioprine** (section 1.5.3) or **mercaptopurine**
(section 1.5.3) may be helpful. **Methotrexate** (section 1.5.3) is used in Crohn's
disease when azathioprine or mercaptopurine are ineffective or not tolerated.
Infliximab (p. 75) can be used for maintenance therapy in Crohn's disease or
ulcerative colitis in children who respond to the initial induction course of this
drug. There are concerns about the long-term safety of infliximab in children.

Fistulating Crohn's disease   Treatment may not be necessary for simple,
asymptomatic perianal fistulas. **Metronidazole** (section 5.1.11) or **ciprofloxacin**
(section 5.1.12) may be beneficial for the treatment of fistulating Crohn's disease
[both unlicensed for this indication]. Metronidazole by mouth is used at a dose of
7.5 mg/kg 3 times daily, usually for 1 month; it should not be used for longer than
3 months because of concerns about peripheral neuropathy. Ciprofloxacin by
mouth is given at a dose of 5 mg/kg twice daily. Other antibacterials should be
given if specifically indicated (e.g. sepsis associated with fistulas and perianal
disease) and for managing bacterial overgrowth in the small bowel. Fistulas may
also require surgical exploration and local drainage.

Either **azathioprine** or **mercaptopurine** is used as a second-line treatment for
fistulating Crohn's disease and continued for maintenance. **Infliximab** is used for
fistulating Crohn's disease refractory to conventional treatments and it can be
continued as maintenance therapy.

Adjunctive treatment of inflammatory bowel disease   Due attention should be
paid to diet; high-fibre or low-residue diets should be used as appropriate.

Antimotility drugs such as codeine phosphate and loperamide, and antispasmodic
drugs may precipitate paralytic ileus and megacolon in active ulcerative colitis;
treatment of the inflammation is more logical. Laxatives may be required in
proctitis. Diarrhoea resulting from the loss of bile-salt absorption (e.g. in terminal
ileal disease or bowel resection) may improve with **colestyramine** (section 1.9.2),
which binds bile salts.

Irritable bowel syndrome

Irritable bowel syndrome can present with pain, constipation, or diarrhoea. Some
children have important psychological aggravating factors which respond to
reassurance. The **fibre** intake of children with irritable bowel syndrome should
be reviewed. If an increase in dietary fibre is required, soluble fibre (e.g. oats,
ispaghula husk, or sterculia) is recommended; insoluble fibre (e.g. bran) should be
avoided. A **laxative** (section 1.6) can be used to treat constipation. An osmotic
laxative, such as a macrogol, is preferred; lactulose may cause bloating. **Loperamide** (section 1.4.2) may relieve diarrhoea and antispasmodic drugs (section
1.2) may relieve pain. Opioids with a central action, such as codeine, are better
avoided because of the risk of dependence.

Clostridium difficile infection

Clostridium difficile infection is caused by colonisation of the colon with *Clostridium
difficile* and production of toxin. It often follows antibiotic therapy and is usually of
acute onset, but may become chronic. It is a particular hazard of ampicillin,
amoxicillin, co-amoxiclav, second- and third-generation cephalosporins, clindamycin, and quinolones, but few antibacterials are free of this side-effect. Oral
metronidazole (section 5.1.11) or oral **vancomycin** (section 5.1.7) are used as
specific treatment; vancomycin may be preferred for very sick patients. Metronidazole can be given by intravenous infusion if oral treatment is inappropriate.

Malabsorption syndromes

Individual conditions need specific management and also general nutritional consideration. Coeliac disease (gluten enteropathy) usually needs a gluten-free diet (Appendix 2) and pancreatic insufficiency needs pancreatin supplements (section 1.9.4).

For further information on foods for special diets (ACBS), see Appendix 2.

1.5.1   Aminosalicylates

Sulfasalazine is a combination of 5-aminosalicylic acid ('5-ASA') and sulfapyridine; sulfapyridine acts only as a carrier to the colonic site of action but still causes side-effects. In the newer aminosalicylates, **mesalazine** (5-aminosalicylic acid), **balsalazide** (a prodrug of 5-aminosalicylic acid) and **olsalazine** (a dimer of 5-aminosalicylic acid which cleaves in the lower bowel), the sulphonamide-related side-effects of sulfasalazine are avoided, but 5-aminosalicylic acid alone can still cause side-effects including blood disorders (see recommendation below) and lupus-like syndrome also seen with sulfasalazine.

Cautions   Renal function should be monitored before starting an oral aminosalicylate, at 3 months of treatment, and then annually during treatment (more frequently in renal impairment). Blood disorders can occur with aminosalicylates (see recommendation below).

> **Blood disorders**
>
> Children receiving aminosalicylates and their carers should be advised to report any unexplained bleeding, bruising, purpura, sore throat, fever or malaise that occurs during treatment. A blood count should be performed and the drug stopped immediately if there is suspicion of a blood dyscrasia.

Contra-indications   Aminosalicylates should be avoided in salicylate hypersensitivity.

Side-effects   Side-effects of the aminosalicylates include diarrhoea, nausea, vomiting, abdominal pain, exacerbation of symptoms of colitis, headache, hypersensitivity reactions (including rash and urticaria); side-effects that occur rarely include acute pancreatitis, hepatitis, myocarditis, pericarditis, lung disorders (including eosinophilia and fibrosing alveolitis), peripheral neuropathy, blood disorders (including agranulocytosis, aplastic anaemia, leucopenia, methaemoglobinaemia, neutropenia, and thrombocytopenia—see also recommendation above), renal dysfunction (interstitial nephritis, nephrotic syndrome), myalgia, arthralgia, skin reactions (including lupus erythematosus-like syndrome, Stevens-Johnson syndrome), alopecia.

BALSALAZIDE SODIUM

Cautions see notes above; also history of asthma; **interactions:** Appendix 1 (aminosalicylates)
Blood disorders see recommendation above

Contra-indications see notes above

Hepatic impairment avoid in severe impairment

Renal impairment manufacturer advises avoid in moderate to severe impairment

Pregnancy manufacturer advises avoid

Breast-feeding monitor infant for diarrhoea

Side-effects see notes above; also cholelithiasis

Licensed use not licensed for use in children under 18 years

Indication and dose

Treatment of mild to moderate ulcerative colitis and maintenance of remission

• By mouth

   Child 12–18 years acute attack, 2.25 g 3 times daily until remission occurs or for up to max. 12 weeks; maintenance, 1.5 g twice daily, adjusted according to response (max. 3 g twice daily)

Colazide® (Almirall) ▣PoM
Capsules, beige, balsalazide sodium 750 mg, net price 130-cap pack = £30.42. Label: 21, 25, counselling, blood disorder symptoms (see recommendation above)

MESALAZINE

Cautions see notes above; **interactions:** Appendix 1 (aminosalicylates)
Blood disorders see recommendation above

Contra-indications see notes above; blood clotting abnormalities

Hepatic impairment avoid in severe impairment

◹ **MESALAZINE** *(continued)*

Renal impairment use with caution; avoid if estimated glomerular filtration rate less than 20 mL/minute/1.73 m²

Pregnancy negligible quantity crosses placenta

Breast-feeding diarrhoea reported but negligible amounts detected in breast milk; monitor infant for diarrhoea

Side-effects see notes above

Licensed use *Asacol®* (all preparations), *Ipocol®*, *Salofalk® rectal enema*, not licensed for use in children under 18 years; *Pentasa® tablets* and *suppositories*, *Salofalk® tablets* and *suppositories*, not licensed for use in children under 15 years; *Mesren MR®*, *Pentasa® granules*, *Salofalk® rectal foam*, not licensed for use in children under 12 years; *Salofalk® granules* not licensed for use in children under 6 years; *Pentasa® retention enema*, no dose recommendation for children (age range not specified by manufacturer)

Indication and dose

Treatment of mild to moderate ulcerative colitis and maintenance of remission for dose see under preparations below

Note The delivery characteristics of oral mesalazine preparations may vary; these preparations should not be considered interchangeable

Asacol® (Procter & Gamble Pharm.) PoM
Foam enema, mesalazine 1 g/metered application, net price 14-application canister with disposable applicators and plastic bags = £27.26. Counselling, blood disorder symptoms (see recommendation above)
Excipients include disodium edetate, hydroxybenzoates (parabens), polysorbate 20, sodium metabisulphite

Dose

Acute attack affecting the rectosigmoid region
• By rectum
   Child 12–18 years 1 metered application (mesalazine 1 g) into the rectum daily for 4–6 weeks

Acute attack affecting the descending colon
• By rectum
   Child 12–18 years 2 metered applications (mesalazine 2 g) once daily for 4–6 weeks

Suppositories, mesalazine 250 mg, net price 20-suppos pack = £4.92; 500 mg, 10-suppos pack = £4.92. Counselling, blood disorder symptoms (see recommendation above)

Dose

Treatment and maintenance of remission of ulcerative colitis affecting the rectosigmoid region
• By rectum
   Child 12–18 years 250–500 mg 3 times daily, with last dose at bedtime

Asacol® MR (Procter & Gamble Pharm.) PoM
Tablets, red, e/c, mesalazine 400 mg, net price 90-tab pack = £30.00, 120-tab pack = £40.00. Label: 5, 25, counselling, blood disorder symptoms (see recommendation above)

Dose

Acute attack
• By mouth
   Child 12–18 years 800 mg 3 times daily

Maintenance of remission of ulcerative colitis and Crohn's ileo-colitis
• By mouth
   Child 12–18 years 400–800 mg 2–3 times daily

Note Preparations that lower stool pH (e.g. lactulose) may prevent release of mesalazine

Ipocol® (Sandoz) PoM
Tablets, e/c, mesalazine 400 mg, net price 120-tab pack = £41.62. Label: 5, 25, counselling, blood disorder symptoms (see recommendation above)

Dose

Acute attack
• By mouth
   Child 12–18 years 800 mg 3 times daily

Maintenance of remission
• By mouth
   Child 12–18 years 400–800 mg 3 times daily

Mesren MR® (IVAX) PoM
Tablets, red-brown, e/c, mesalazine 400 mg, net price 90-tab pack = £19.50, 120-tab pack = £26.00. Label: 5, 25, counselling, blood disorder symptoms (see recommendation above)

Dose

Acute attack
• By mouth
   Child 12–18 years 800 mg 3 times daily

Maintenance of remission
• By mouth
   Child 12–18 years 400–800 mg 3 times daily

Pentasa® (Ferring) PoM
Tablets, m/r, scored, mesalazine 500 mg (grey), net price 100-tab pack = £24.21. Counselling, administration (see dose), blood disorder symptoms (see recommendation above)

Dose

Acute attack
• By mouth
   Child 5–15 years 15–20 mg/kg (max. 1 g) 3 times daily
   Child 15–18 years 1–2 g twice daily; total daily dose may alternatively be given in 3 divided doses

Maintenance of remission
• By mouth
   Child 5–15 years 10 mg/kg (max. 500 mg) 2–3 times daily
   Child 15–18 years 2 g once daily

Administration tablets may be halved, quartered, or dispersed in water, but should not be chewed

Granules, m/r, pale brown, mesalazine 1 g/sachet, net price 50-sachet pack = £28.82; 2 g/sachet, 60-sachet pack = £72.05. Counselling, administration (see dose), blood disorder symptoms (see recommendation above)

Dose

Acute attack
• By mouth
   Child 5–12 years 15–20 mg/kg (max. 1 g) 3 times daily
   Child 12–18 years 1–2 g twice daily; total daily dose may alternatively be given in 3–4 divided doses

1

Gastro-intestinal system

◻ **MESALAZINE (continued)**

Maintenance of remission
• **By mouth**
  Child 5–12 years 10 mg/kg (max. 500 mg) 2–3 times daily
  Child 12–18 years 2 g once daily

Administration contents of one sachet should be weighed and divided immediately before use; discard any remaining granules. Granules should be placed on tongue and washed down with water or orange juice without chewing

Retention enema, mesalazine 1 g in 100-mL pack, net price 7 enemas = £17.73. Counselling, blood disorder symptoms (see recommendation above)

Dose
Acute attack affecting the rectosigmoid region
• **By rectum**
  Child 12–18 years 1 g at bedtime

Suppositories, mesalazine 1 g, net price 28-suppos pack = £40.01. Counselling, blood disorder symptoms (see recommendation above)

Dose
Acute attack, ulcerative proctitis
• **By rectum**
  Child 12–18 years 1 g daily for 2–4 weeks

Maintenance, ulcerative proctitis
• **By rectum**
  Child 12–18 years 1 g daily

Salofalk® (Dr Falk) PoM
Tablets, e/c, yellow, mesalazine 250 mg. Net price 100-tab pack = £16.50. Label: 5, 25, counselling, blood disorder symptoms (see recommendation above)

Dose
Acute attack
• **By mouth**
  Child 12–18 years 500 mg 3 times daily

Maintenance of remission
• **By mouth**
  Child 12–18 years 250–500 mg 2–3 times daily

Granules, m/r, grey, e/c, vanilla-flavoured, mesalazine 500 mg/sachet, net price 100-sachet pack = £29.30; 1 g/sachet, 50-sachet pack = £29.30; 1.5 g/sachet, 60-sachet pack = £49.80. Counselling, administration (see dose), blood disorder symptoms (see recommendation above)
Excipients include aspartame (section 9.4.1)

Dose
Acute attack
• **By mouth**
  Child 6–15 years and body-weight under 40 kg 10–15 mg/kg 3 times daily

Child 6–15 years and body-weight over 40 kg 1.5–3 g once daily (preferably in the morning) or 0.5–1 g 3 times daily

Child 15–18 years 1.5–3 g once daily (preferably in the morning) or 0.5–1 g 3 times daily

Maintenance of remission
• **By mouth**
  Child 6–15 years and body-weight under 40 kg 7.5–15 mg/kg twice daily or 250 mg 3 times daily
  Child 6–15 years and body-weight over 40 kg 500 mg 3 times daily
  Child 15–18 years 500 mg 3 times daily

Administration Granules should be placed on tongue and washed down with water without chewing
Note Preparations that lower stool pH (e.g. lactulose) may prevent release of mesalazine

Suppositories, mesalazine 500 mg. Net price 30-suppos pack = £15.10. Counselling, blood disorder symptoms (see recommendation above)

Dose
Acute attack
• **By rectum**
  Child 12–18 years 0.5–1 g 2–3 times daily adjusted according to response

Enema, mesalazine 2 g in 59-mL pack. Net price 7 enemas = £30.50. Counselling, blood disorder symptoms (see recommendation above)

Dose
Acute attack or maintenance
• **By mouth**
  Child 12–18 years 2 g once daily at bedtime

Rectal foam, mesalazine 1 g/metered application, net price 14-application canister with disposable applicators and plastic bags = £30.75. Counselling, blood disorder symptoms (see recommendation above)
Excipients include cetostearyl alcohol, disodium edetate, polysorbate 60, propylene glycol, sodium metabisulphite

Dose
Mild ulcerative colitis affecting sigmoid colon and rectum
• **By rectum**
  Child 12–18 years 2 metered applications (mesalazine 2 g) into the rectum at bedtime increased if necessary to 2 metered applications (mesalazine 2 g) twice daily

▰ **OLSALAZINE SODIUM**

Cautions see notes above; **interactions:** Appendix 1 (aminosalicylates)
Blood disorders see recommendation above

Contra-indications see notes above

Renal impairment use with caution; manufacturer advises avoid in significant impairment

Pregnancy manufacturer advises avoid unless potential benefit outweighs risk

Breast-feeding monitor infant for diarrhoea

Side-effects see notes above; watery diarrhoea common; also reported, tachycardia, palpitation, pyrexia, blurred vision, and photosensitivity

Licensed use not licensed for use in children under 12 years

◁ **OLSALAZINE SODIUM** (*continued*)

Indication and dose

Treatment of acute attack of mild ulcerative colitis

• **By mouth**

  Child 2–18 years 500 mg twice daily after food increased if necessary over 1 week to max. 1 g 3 times daily

Maintenance of remission of mild ulcerative colitis

• **By mouth**

  Child 2–18 years 250–500 mg twice daily after food

Administration Capsules can be opened and contents sprinkled on food

Dipentum® (UCB Pharma) ℗ℴ𝕄

Capsules, brown, olsalazine sodium 250 mg. Net price 112-cap pack = £19.77. Label: 21, counselling, blood disorder symptoms (see recommendation above)

Tablets, yellow, scored, olsalazine sodium 500 mg. Net price 60-tab pack = £21.18. Label: 21, counselling, blood disorder symptoms (see recommendation above)

▲ SULFASALAZINE
(Sulphasalazine)

Cautions see notes above; also history of allergy or asthma; G6PD deficiency (section 9.1.5); slow acetylator status; risk of haematological and hepatic toxicity (differential white cell, red cell, and platelet counts initially and at monthly intervals for first 3 months; liver function tests at monthly intervals for first 3 months); maintain adequate fluid intake; upper gastro-intestinal side-effects common with doses over 4 g daily; acute porphyria (section 9.8.2); **interactions:** Appendix 1 (aminosalicylates)

Blood disorders see recommendation above

Contra-indications see notes above; also sulphonamide hypersensitivity; child under 2 years of age

Hepatic impairment use with caution

Renal impairment risk of toxicity, including crystalluria, in moderate impairment—ensure high fluid intake; avoid in severe impairment

Pregnancy theoretical risk of neonatal haemolysis in third trimester; adequate folate supplements should be given to mother

Breast-feeding small amount in milk (1 report of bloody diarrhoea and rashes); theoretical risk of neonatal haemolysis especially in G6PD-deficient infants

Side-effects see notes above; also cough, insomnia, dizziness, fever, blood disorders (including Heinz body anaemia, megaloblastic anaemia), proteinuria, tinnitus, stomatitis, taste disturbances, and pruritus; *less commonly* dyspnoea, depression, convulsions, vasculitis, and alopecia; also reported loss of appetite, hypersensitivity reactions (including exfoliative dermatitis, epidermal necrolysis, photosensitivity, anaphylaxis, serum sickness), ataxia, hallucinations, aseptic meningitis, oligospermia, crystalluria, disturbances of smell, and parotitis; yellow-orange discoloration of skin, urine, and other body fluids; some soft contact lenses may be stained

Indication and dose

Treatment of acute attack of mild to moderate and severe ulcerative colitis, active Crohn's disease

• **By mouth**

  Child 2–12 years 10–15 mg/kg (max. 1 g) 4–6 times daily until remission occurs; increased to max. 60 mg/kg daily in divided doses, if necessary

  Child 12–18 years 1–2 g 4 times daily until remission occurs

Maintenance of remission of mild to moderate and severe ulcerative colitis

• **By mouth**

  Child 2–12 years 5–7.5 mg/kg (max. 500 mg) 4 times daily

  Child 12–18 years 500 mg 4 times daily

Treatment of mild to moderate or severe ulcerative colitis and maintenance of remission, active Crohn's disease

• **By rectum as suppositories**

  Child 5–8 years 500 mg twice daily

  Child 8–12 years 500 mg in the morning and 1 g at night

  Child 12–18 years 0.5–1 g twice daily

Juvenile idiopathic arthritis section 10.1.3

Sulfasalazine (Non-proprietary) ℗ℴ𝕄

Tablets, sulfasalazine 500 mg, net price 112 = £8.46. Label: 14, counselling, blood disorder symptoms (see recommendation above), contact lenses may be stained

Tablets, e/c, sulfasalazine 500 mg. Net price 112-tab pack = £14.92. Label: 5, 14, 25, counselling, blood disorder symptoms (see recommendation above), contact lenses may be stained
Brands include *Sulazine EC®*

Suspension, sulfasalazine 250 mg/5 mL, net price 500 mL = £28.00. Label: 14, counselling, blood disorder symptoms (see recommendation above), contact lenses may be stained
Excipients may include alcohol

Salazopyrin® (Pharmacia) ℗ℴ𝕄

Tablets, yellow, scored, sulfasalazine 500 mg. Net price 112-tab pack = £6.97. Label: 14, counselling, blood disorder symptoms (see recommendation above), contact lenses may be stained

EN-Tabs® (= tablets e/c), yellow, f/c, sulfasalazine 500 mg. Net price 112-tab pack = £8.43. Label: 5, 14, 25, counselling, blood disorder symptoms (see

1 Gastro-intestinal system

◁ **SULFASALAZINE (continued)**

recommendation above), contact lenses may be stained

Suppositories, yellow, sulfasalazine 500 mg. Net price 10 = £3.30. Label: 14, counselling, blood

disorder symptoms (see recommendation above), contact lenses may be stained

1.5.2 Corticosteroids

For the role of corticosteroids in acute ulcerative colitis and Crohn's disease, see Inflammatory Bowel Disease, p. 66.

BUDESONIDE

Cautions section 6.3.2; **interactions:** Appendix 1 (corticosteroids)

Contra-indications section 6.3.2

Hepatic impairment section 6.3.2

Pregnancy section 6.3.2

Breast-feeding section 6.3.2

Side-effects section 6.3.2

Licensed use not licensed for use in children

Indication and dose

See preparations

Administration Capsules can be opened and the contents mixed with apple or orange juice

Budenofalk® (Dr Falk) [PoM]

Capsules, pink, enclosing e/c granules, budesonide 3 mg, net price 100-cap pack = £76.70. Label: 5, 10, steroid card, 22, 25

Dose

> Mild to moderate Crohn's disease affecting ileum or ascending colon, chronic diarrhoea due to collagenous colitis
> • By mouth
> Child 12–18 years 3 mg 3 times daily for up to 8 weeks; reduce dose for the last 2 weeks of treatment. See also section 6.3.2

Entocort® (AstraZeneca) [PoM]

CR Capsules, grey/pink, enclosing e/c, m/r granules, budesonide 3 mg, net price 100-cap pack = £99.00. Label: 5, 10, steroid card, 22, 25

Note Dispense in original container (contains desiccant)

Dose

> Mild to moderate Crohn's disease affecting the ileum or ascending colon
> • By mouth
> Child 12–18 years 9 mg once daily in the morning before breakfast for up to 8 weeks; reduce dose for the last 2–4 weeks of treatment. See also section 6.3.2

Enema, budesonide 2 mg/100 mL when dispersible tablet reconstituted in isotonic saline vehicle, net price pack of 7 dispersible tablets and bottles of vehicle = £33.00

Dose

> Ulcerative colitis involving rectal and recto-sigmoid disease
> • By rectum
> Child 12–18 years 1 enema at bedtime for 4 weeks

HYDROCORTISONE

Cautions section 6.3.2; systemic absorption may occur; prolonged use should be avoided

Contra-indications intestinal obstruction, bowel perforation, recent intestinal anastomoses, extensive fistulas; untreated infection

Side-effects section 6.3.2; also local irritation

Indication and dose

Inflammatory bowel disease
• By intravenous administration
See p. 458

• By rectum
See preparations

Colifoam® (Meda) [PoM]

Foam in aerosol pack, hydrocortisone acetate 10%, net price 14-application cannister with applicator = £8.21

Excipients include cetyl alcohol, hydroxybenzoates (parabens), propylene glycol

Dose

> Ulcerative colitis, proctitis, proctosigmoiditis
> • By rectum
> Child 2–18 years initially 1 metered application (125 mg hydrocortisone acetate) inserted into the rectum once or twice daily for 2–3 weeks, then once on alternate days

PREDNISOLONE

Cautions section 6.3.2; systemic absorption may occur; prolonged use should be avoided

Contra-indications section 6.3.2; intestinal obstruction, bowel perforation, recent intestinal anastomoses, extensive fistulas; untreated infection

Hepatic impairment section 6.3.2

Renal impairment section 6.3.2

Pregnancy section 6.3.2

Breast-feeding section 6.3.2

Side-effects section 6.3.2

Licensed use *Predfoam®*, *Predsol®* retention enema not licensed for use in children (age range not specified by manufacturer)

▱ PREDNISOLONE (continued)

Indication and dose

Ulcerative colitis, Crohn's disease see also
under preparations, below
- **By mouth**
  Child 2–18 years 2 mg/kg (max. 60 mg) once
  daily until remission occurs, followed by redu-
  cing doses
- **By rectum**
  See under preparations

Other indications section 6.3.2

◢ Oral preparations
Section 6.3.2

◢ Rectal preparations
Predenema® (Forest) [PoM]
Retention enema, prednisolone 20 mg (as sodium
metasulphobenzoate) in 100-mL single-dose disposable pack. Net price 1 (standard tube) = 71p, 1
(long tube) = £1.21

Dose
Ulcerative colitis
- **By rectum**
  Child 12–18 years initially 20 mg at bedtime for 2–4
  weeks, continued if good response

Predfoam® (Forest) [PoM]
Foam in aerosol pack, prednisolone 20 mg (as
metasulphobenzoate sodium)/metered application, net price 14-application cannister with disposable applicators = £6.32
Excipients include cetostearyl alcohol, disodium edetate,
polysorbate 20, sorbic acid

Dose
Proctitis and distal ulcerative colitis
- **By rectum**
  Child 12–18 years 1 metered application (20 mg
  prednisolone) inserted into the rectum once or twice
  daily for 2 weeks, continued for further 2 weeks if good
  response

Predsol® (UCB Pharma) [PoM]
Suppositories, prednisolone 5 mg (as sodium
phosphate). Net price 10 = £1.35

Dose
Proctitis and rectal complications of Crohn's disease
- **By rectum**
  Child 2–18 years 5 mg inserted night and morning
  after a bowel movement

1.5.3 Drugs affecting the immune response

Azathioprine, **mercaptopurine**, or once weekly **methotrexate** are used to
induce remission in unresponsive or chronically active Crohn's disease. Azathioprine or mercaptopurine may also be helpful for retaining remission in frequently
relapsing inflammatory bowel disease; once weekly methotrexate is used in
Crohn's disease when azathioprine or mercaptopurine are ineffective or not
tolerated. Response to azathioprine or mercaptopurine may not become apparent
for several months. Folic acid (section 9.1.2) should be given to reduce the
possibility of methotrexate toxicity. Folic acid can be given at a dose of 5 mg
weekly; alternative regimens may be used in some settings.

Ciclosporin (cyclosporin) is a potent immunosuppressant and is markedly
nephrotoxic. In children with severe ulcerative colitis unresponsive to other
treatment, ciclosporin may reduce the need for urgent colorectal surgery.

◤ AZATHIOPRINE

Cautions section 8.2.1; **interactions:** Appendix 1
  (azathioprine)
Contra-indications section 8.2.1
Hepatic impairment section 8.2.1
Renal impairment section 8.2.1
Pregnancy section 8.2.1
Breast-feeding section 8.2.1
Side-effects section 8.2.1
Licensed use not licensed for use in ulcerative
  colitis or Crohn's disease

Indication and dose

Severe ulcerative colitis and Crohn's disease
- **By mouth**
  Child 2–18 years initially 2 mg/kg (if necessary
  up to 3 mg/kg) once daily, then reduced

according to response to lowest effective dose;
total daily dose may alternatively be given in 2
divided doses

Transplantation rejection section 8.2.1

Rheumatic diseases section 10.1.3

◢ Preparations
Section 8.2.1

1

Gastro-intestinal system

CICLOSPORIN

Cautions section 8.2.2; **interactions**: Appendix 1 (ciclosporin)

Hepatic impairment section 8.2.2

Renal impairment section 8.2.2

Pregnancy section 8.2.2

Breast-feeding section 8.2.2

Side-effects section 8.2.2

Licensed use not licensed for use in ulcerative colitis

Indication and dose

Refractory ulcerative colitis
- By mouth

  Child 2–18 years initially 2 mg/kg twice daily, dose adjusted according to blood-ciclosporin concentration and response; max. 5 mg/kg twice daily

  Important For advice on counselling and conversion between preparations, see section 8.2.2

- By intravenous infusion

  Child 3–18 years initially 0.5–1 mg/kg twice daily, dose adjusted according to blood-ciclosporin concentration and response

Nephrotic syndrome section 8.2.2

Transplantation rejection and auto-immune conditions section 8.2.2

Atopic dermatitis and psoriasis section 13.5.3

Administration for *intermittent intravenous infusion*, dilute to a concentration of 0.5–2.5 mg/mL with Glucose 5% *or* Sodium Chloride 0.9% and give over 2–6 hours; not to be used with PVC equipment; observe patient for signs of anaphylaxis for at least 30 minutes after starting infusion and at frequent intervals thereafter

◢Preparations
Section 8.2.2

MERCAPTOPURINE

Cautions section 8.1.3; see also Azathioprine, section 8.2.1

Contra-indications section 8.1.3

Hepatic impairment section 8.1.3

Renal impairment section 8.1.3

Pregnancy section 8.1.3

Breast-feeding section 8.1.3

Side-effects section 8.1.3

Licensed use not licensed for use in severe ulcerative colitis and Crohn's disease; for other indications, see section 8.1.3

Indication and dose

Severe ulcerative colitis and Crohn's disease
- By mouth

  Child 2–18 years 1–1.5 mg/kg once daily (initial max. 50 mg; may be increased to 75 mg once daily)

Acute leukaemias section 8.1.3

◢Preparations
Section 8.1.3

METHOTREXATE

Cautions section 10.1.3

Contra-indications section 10.1.3

Hepatic impairment section 10.1.3

Renal impairment section 8.1.3

Pregnancy section 8.1.3

Breast-feeding section 8.1.3

Side-effects section 10.1.3

Licensed use not licensed for use in children for non-malignant conditions

Indication and dose

Severe acute Crohn's disease
- By subcutaneous or intramuscular injection

  Child 7–18 years 15 mg/m^2 (max. 25 mg) once weekly

Maintenance of remission of severe Crohn's disease
- By mouth or by subcutaneous or intramuscular injection

  Child 7–18 years 15 mg/m^2 (max. 25 mg) once weekly; dose reduced according to response to lowest effective dose

Safe Practice Note that the above dose is a **weekly** dose. To avoid error with low-dose methotrexate, it is recommended that:

- the child or their carer is carefully advised of the **dose** and **frequency** and the reason for taking methotrexate and any other prescribed medicine (e.g. folic acid);
- only one strength of methotrexate tablet (usually 2.5 mg) is prescribed and dispensed;
- the prescription and the dispensing label clearly show the dose and frequency of methotrexate administration;
- the child or their carer is warned to report immediately the onset of any feature of blood disorders (e.g. sore throat, bruising, and mouth ulcers), liver toxicity (e.g. nausea, vomiting, abdominal discomfort, and dark urine), and respiratory effects (e.g. shortness of breath).

Malignant disease section 8.1.3

Rheumatic disease section 10.1.3

Psoriasis section 13.5.3

◢Preparations
Section 10.1.3

> **Cytokine modulators**
>
> **Infliximab** is a monoclonal antibody which inhibits the pro-inflammatory cytokine, tumour necrosis factor alpha. It should be administered under specialist supervision where adequate resuscitation facilities are available and is used in the treatment of severe refractory or fistulating Crohn's disease in children. Infliximab should be used only when treatment with other immunomodulating drugs has failed or is not tolerated and for children in whom surgery is inappropriate.

INFLIXIMAB

Cautions monitor for infections before, during, and for 6 months after treatment (see also Tuberculosis below); predisposition to infection; chronic hepatitis B—monitor for active infection; heart failure (discontinue if symptoms develop or worsen; avoid in moderate or severe heart failure); demyelinating CNS disorders (risk of exacerbation); history of malignancy (consider discontinuing treatment if malignancy develops); history of prolonged immunosuppressant or PUVA treatment in patients with psoriasis; **interactions:** Appendix 1 (infliximab)

Tuberculosis Children should be evaluated for tuberculosis before treatment. Active tuberculosis should be treated with standard treatment (section 5.1.9) for at least 2 months before starting infliximab. Children who have previously received adequate treatment for tuberculosis can start infliximab but should be monitored every 3 months for possible recurrence. In those without active tuberculosis but who were previously not treated adequately, chemoprophylaxis should ideally be completed before starting infliximab. In children at high risk of tuberculosis who cannot be assessed by tuberculin skin test, chemoprophylaxis can be given concurrently with infliximab. Children and their carers should be advised to seek medical attention if symptoms suggestive of tuberculosis (e.g. persistent cough, weight loss, and fever) develop

Hypersensitivity reactions Hypersensitivity reactions (including fever, chest pain, hypotension, hypertension, dyspnoea, pruritus, urticaria, serum sickness-like reactions, angioedema, anaphylaxis) reported during or within 1–2 hours after infusion (risk greatest during first or second infusion or in children who discontinue other immunosuppressants). All children should be observed carefully for 1–2 hours after infusion and resuscitation equipment should be available for immediate use. Prophylactic antipyretics, antihistamines, or hydrocortisone may be administered. Readministration not recommended after infliximab-free interval of more than 16 weeks—risk of delayed hypersensitivity reactions. Children and carers should be advised to keep Alert card with them at all times and seek medical advice if symptoms of delayed hypersensitivity develop

Contra-indications severe infections (see also under cautions)

Pregnancy use only if essential; manufacturer advises adequate contraception during and for at least 6 months after last dose

Breast-feeding amount probably too small to be harmful

Side-effects see under Cytokine Modulators (section 10.1.3) and Cautions above; also diarrhoea, dyspepsia; flushing, chest pain; dyspnoea; dizziness, fatigue; sinusitis; rash, increased sweating, dry skin; *less commonly* constipation, gastro-oesophageal reflux, cholecystitis, palpitation, arrhythmia, hypertension, hypotension, vasospasm, cyanosis, bradycardia, syncope, oedema, thrombophlebitis, epistaxis, pleurisy, confusion, agitation, nervousness, amnesia, sleep disturbances, vaginitis, demyelinating disorders, antibody formation, pyelonephritis, myalgia, arthralgia, eye disorders, abnormal skin pigmentation, ecchymosis, cheilitis, and alopecia; *rarely* hepatitis, intestinal stenosis, intestinal perforation, gastro-intestinal haemorrhage, pancreatitis, lymphoma (including hepatosplenic T-cell lymphoma), circulatory failure, meningitis, and seizure; *very rarely* pericardial effusion, and skin reactions (including Stevens-Johnson syndrome and toxic epidermal necrolysis); also reported interstitial lung disease, transverse myelitis, neuropathy, and paraesthesia

Licensed use not licensed for fistulating Crohn's disease in children

Indication and dose

> **Severe active Crohn's disease**
> - **By intravenous infusion**
>
>   **Child 6–18 years** initially 5 mg/kg, then 5 mg/kg 2 weeks and 6 weeks after initial dose, then 5 mg/kg every 8 weeks; interval between maintenance doses adjusted according to response; discontinue if no response within 10 weeks of initial dose

> **Fistulating Crohn's disease**
> - **By intravenous infusion**
>
>   **Child 6–18 years** initially 5 mg/kg, then 5 mg/kg 2 weeks and 6 weeks after initial dose, then if condition has responded, consult literature for guidance on further doses

Administration for *intravenous infusion* reconstitute each 100-mg vial of powder with 10 mL Water for Injections; to dissolve, gently swirl vial without shaking; allow to stand for 5 minutes; dilute required dose with Sodium Chloride 0.9% to a final volume of 250 mL and give through a low protein-binding filter (1.2 micron or less) over at least 2 hours; start infusion within 3 hours of reconstitution

Remicade® (Schering-Plough) ℗ₒₘ
Intravenous infusion, powder for reconstitution, infliximab, net price 100-mg vial = £419.62.
Label: 10, alert card, counselling, tuberculosis and hypersensitivity reactions

1

Gastro-intestinal system

1.5.4 Food allergy

Allergy with classical symptoms of vomiting, colic and diarrhoea caused by specific foods such as cow's milk should be managed by strict avoidance. The condition should be distinguished from symptoms of occasional food intolerance in children with irritable bowel syndrome. **Sodium cromoglicate** (sodium cromoglycate) may be helpful as an adjunct to dietary avoidance.

SODIUM CROMOGLICATE

(Sodium cromoglycate)

Pregnancy not known to be harmful

Breast-feeding unlikely to be present in milk

Side-effects occasional nausea, rashes, and joint pain

Indication and dose

Food allergy (in conjunction with dietary restriction)

- By mouth

  Child 2–14 years 100 mg 4 times daily before meals, dose may be increased after 2–3 weeks to a max. 40 mg/kg daily and then reduced according to response

  Child 14–18 years 200 mg 4 times daily before meals, dose may be increased after 2–3 weeks to max. 40 mg/kg daily and then reduced according to response

Asthma section 3.3

Allergic conjunctivitis section 11.4.2

Allergic rhinitis section 12.2.1

Administration capsules may be swallowed whole or the contents dissolved in hot water and diluted with cold water before taking

Nalcrom® (Sanofi-Aventis) [PoM]

Capsules, sodium cromoglicate 100 mg. Net price 100-cap pack = £59.75. Label: 22, counselling, administration

1.6 Laxatives

1.6.1 Bulk-forming laxatives
1.6.2 Stimulant laxatives
1.6.3 Faecal softeners
1.6.4 Osmotic laxatives
1.6.5 Bowel cleansing preparations
1.6.6 Peripheral opioid-receptor antagonists

Before prescribing laxatives it is important to be sure that the child *is* constipated and that the constipation is *not* secondary to an underlying undiagnosed complaint.

Laxatives should be prescribed by a healthcare professional experienced in the management of constipation in children. Delays of greater than 3 days between stools may increase the likelihood of pain on passing hard stools leading to anal fissure, anal spasm and eventually to a learned response to avoid defaecation.

In *infants*, increased intake of fluids, particularly fruit juice containing sorbitol (e.g. prune, pear, or apple), may be sufficient to soften the stool. In infants under 1 year of age with mild constipation, **lactulose** (section 1.6.4) can be used to soften the stool; either an oral preparation containing **macrogols** or, rarely, **glycerol** suppositories can be used to clear faecal impaction. The infant should be referred to a hospital paediatric specialist if these measures fail.

The diet of *children over 1 year of age* should be reviewed to ensure that it includes an adequate intake of fibre and fluid. An osmotic laxative containing **macrogols** (section 1.6.4) can also be used, particularly in children with chronic constipation; **lactulose** is an alternative in children who cannot tolerate a macrogol. If there is an inadequate response to the osmotic laxative, a **stimulant laxative** (section 1.6.2) can be added.

Treatment of faecal impaction may initially increase symptoms of soiling and abdominal pain. In children over 1 year of age with faecal impaction, an oral preparation containing **macrogols** (section 1.6.4) is used to clear faecal mass and to establish and maintain soft well-formed stools. If disimpaction does not occur after 2 weeks, a **stimulant laxative** (section 1.6.2) can be added. If the impacted mass is not expelled following treatment with macrogols and a stimulant laxative, a **sodium citrate** enema can be administered. Although rectal administration of laxatives may be effective, this route is frequently distressing for the child and may lead to persistence of withholding. A **phosphate enema** may be administered under specialist supervision if disimpaction does not occur after a sodium citrate enema; a **bowel cleansing preparation** (section 1.6.5) is an alternative. Manual evacuation under anaesthetic may be necessary if disimpaction does not occur after oral and rectal treatment, or if the child is afraid.

Long-term regular use of laxatives is essential to maintain well-formed stools and prevent recurrence in children with chronic constipation or a history of faecal impaction; intermittent use may provoke relapses.

> For children with chronic constipation, it may be necessary to exceed the licensed doses of some laxatives. Parents and carers of children should be advised to adjust the dose of laxative in order to establish a regular pattern of bowel movements in which stools are soft, well-formed, and passed without discomfort.
>
> Laxatives should be administered at a time that produces an effect that is likely to fit in with the child's toilet routine.

For the role of laxatives in the treatment of irritable bowel syndrome, see p. 67.

Pregnancy If dietary and lifestyle changes fail to control constipation in pregnancy, moderate doses of poorly absorbed laxatives may be used. A bulk-forming laxative should be tried first. An osmotic laxative, such as lactulose, can also be used. Bisacodyl or senna may be suitable, if a stimulant effect is necessary.

Laxatives are also of value in *drug-induced constipation* (see Prescribing in Palliative Care, p. 26), in *distal intestinal obstruction syndrome* in children with cystic fibrosis, for the expulsion of *parasites* after anthelmintic treatment, and to clear the alimentary tract before *surgery and radiological procedures* (section 1.6.5).

> The laxatives that follow have been divided into 5 main groups (sections 1.6.1–1.6.5). This simple classification disguises the fact that some laxatives have a complex action.

1.6.1 Bulk-forming laxatives

Bulk-forming laxatives are of value if the diet is deficient in fibre. They relieve constipation by increasing faecal mass which stimulates peristalsis; children and their carers should be advised that the full effect may take some days to develop.

During treatment with bulk-forming laxatives, adequate fluid intake must be maintained to avoid intestinal obstruction. Proprietary preparations containing a bulking agent such as ispaghula husk are often difficult to administer to children. Finely ground bran, though more palatable, has poorer water-retaining properties, but can be taken as bran bread or biscuits in appropriately increased quantities. Oat bran is also used.

Bulk-forming laxatives may be used in the management of children with *haemorrhoids*, *anal fissure*, and *irritable bowel syndrome*.

ISPAGHULA HUSK

Cautions adequate fluid intake should be maintained to avoid intestinal obstruction

Contra-indications difficulty in swallowing, intestinal obstruction, colonic atony, faecal impaction

Side-effects flatulence and abdominal distension (especially during the first few days of treatment), gastro-intestinal obstruction or impaction; hypersensitivity reported

Licensed use *Regulan*® not licensed for use in children under 6 years; *Fybogel*® and *Ispagel Orange*® not licensed for use in children under 6 years (unless on specialist practitioner's advice);

Isogel® licensed for use in children (age range not specified by manufacturer)

Indication and dose

See under preparations

Counselling Preparations that swell in contact with liquid should always be carefully swallowed with water and should not be taken immediately before going to bed

Fibrelief® (Manx)

Granules, sugar- and gluten-free, ispaghula husk 3.5 g/sachet (natural or orange flavour), net price

Gastro-intestinal system

1

◁ **ISPAGHULA HUSK** *(continued)*

10 sachets = £1.23, 30 sachets = £2.07. Label: 13, counselling, see above
Excipients include aspartame (section 9.4.1)

Dose

> Constipation
> • By mouth
> > **Child 12–18 years** 1–6 sachets daily in water in 1–3 divided doses

Fybogel® (Reckitt Benckiser)

Granules, buff, effervescent, sugar- and gluten-free, ispaghula husk 3.5 g/sachet (low Na⁺), net price 30 sachets (plain, lemon, or orange flavour) = £1.84. Label: 13, counselling, see above
Excipients include aspartame 16 mg/sachet (see section 9.4.1)

Dose

> Constipation
> • By mouth
> > **Child 2–12 years** ½–1 level 5-mL spoonful in water twice daily preferably after meals
> > **Child 12–18 years** 1 sachet (or 2 level 5-mL spoonfuls) in water twice daily preferably after meals

Isogel® (Potters)

Granules, brown, sugar- and gluten-free, ispaghula husk 90%. Net price 200 g = £2.67. Label: 13, counselling, see above

Dose

> Constipation
> • By mouth
> > **Child 2–12 years** 1 level 5-mL spoonful in water once or twice daily, preferably at mealtimes

> **Child 12–18 years** 2 level 5-mL spoonfuls in water once or twice daily, preferably at mealtimes

Note May be difficult to obtain

Ispagel Orange® (LPC)

Granules, beige, effervescent, sugar- and gluten-free, ispaghula husk 3.5 g/sachet, net price 30 sachets = £2.10. Label: 13, counselling, see above
Excipients include aspartame (section 9.4.1)

Dose

> Constipation
> • By mouth
> > **Child 2–12 years** ½–1 level 5-mL spoonful in water twice daily preferably after meals
> > **Child 12–18 years** 1 sachet (or 2 level 5-mL spoonfuls) in water 1–3 times daily preferably after meals

Regulan® (Procter & Gamble)

Powder, beige, sugar- and gluten-free, ispaghula husk 3.4 g/5.85-g sachet (orange or lemon/lime flavour). Net price 30 sachets = £2.44. Label: 13, counselling, see above
Excipients include aspartame (section 9.4.1)

Dose

> Constipation
> • By mouth
> > **Child 2–12 years** ½–1 level 5-mL spoonful in water 1–3 times daily
> > **Child 12–18 years** 1 sachet in 150 mL water 1–3 times daily

METHYLCELLULOSE

Cautions see under Ispaghula Husk
Contra-indications see under Ispaghula Husk; also infective bowel disease
Side-effects see under Ispaghula Husk
Licensed use no age limit specified by manufacturer

Indication and dose

> See under preparation below

> Counselling Preparations that swell in contact with liquid should always be carefully swallowed with water and should not be taken immediately before going to bed

Celevac® (Amdipharm)

Tablets, pink, scored, methylcellulose '450' 500 mg, net price 112-tab pack = £3.22.Counselling, see above and dose

Dose

> Constipation, diarrhoea (see notes above)
> • By mouth
> > **Child 7–12 years** 2 tablets twice daily
> > **Child 12–18 years** 3–6 tablets twice daily

Administration In constipation the dose should be taken with at least 300 mL liquid. In diarrhoea, ileostomy, and colostomy control, avoid liquid intake for 30 minutes before and after dose

◢ Extemporaneous formulations available see Extemporaneous Preparations, p. 8

STERCULIA

Cautions see under Ispaghula Husk
Contra-indications see under Ispaghula Husk
Side-effects see under Ispaghula Husk

Indication and dose

> Constipation for dose see under preparation

> Counselling Preparations that swell in contact with liquid should always be carefully swallowed with water and should not be taken immediately before going to bed

Normacol® (Norgine)

Granules, coated, gluten-free, sterculia 62%. Net price 500 g = £5.94; 60 × 7-g sachets = £4.99. Label: 25, 27, counselling, see above

Dose

> • By mouth
> > **Child 6–12 years** ½–1 heaped 5-mL spoonful *or* the contents of ½–1 sachet, washed down without chewing with plenty of liquid once or twice daily after meals

◻ **STERCULIA (continued)**

Child 12–18 years 1–2 heaped 5-mL spoonfuls *or the* contents of 1–2 sachets, washed down without chewing with plenty of liquid once or twice daily after meals

Administration May be mixed with soft food (e.g. yoghurt) before swallowing, followed by plenty of liquid.

Normacol Plus® (Norgine)
Granules, brown, coated, gluten-free, sterculia 62%, frangula (standardised) 8%. Net price 500 g = £6.34; 60 × 7 g sachets = £5.34. Label: 25, 27, Counselling, see above

Dose
• **By mouth**
Child 6–12 years ½–1 heaped 5-mL spoonful *or the* contents of ½–1 sachet, washed down without chewing with plenty of liquid, once or twice daily after meals

Child 12–18 years 1–2 heaped 5-mL spoonfuls *or the* contents of 1–2 sachets, washed down without chewing with plenty of liquid, once or twice daily after meals

1.6.2 Stimulant laxatives

Stimulant laxatives include **bisacodyl**, **sodium picosulfate**, and members of the **anthraquinone** group, **senna** and **dantron** (danthron). The indications for dantron are limited (see below) by its potential carcinogenicity (based on *rodent* carcinogenicity studies) and evidence of genotoxicity. Powerful stimulants such as **cascara** (an anthraquinone) and **castor oil** are obsolete. **Docusate sodium** probably acts both as a stimulant and as a softening agent.

Stimulant laxatives increase intestinal motility and often cause abdominal cramp; they should be avoided in intestinal obstruction. Stools should be softened by increasing dietary fibre and liquid or with an osmotic laxative (section 1.6.4) before giving a stimulant laxative. In chronic constipation, especially where withholding of stool occurs, additional doses of a stimulant laxative may be required. Long-term use of stimulant laxatives is sometimes necessary (see section 1.6), but excessive use can cause diarrhoea and related effects such as hypokalaemia.

Glycerol suppositories act as a lubricant and as a rectal stimulant by virtue of the mildly irritant action of glycerol.

◢ BISACODYL

Cautions prolonged use (risk of electrolyte imbalance)

Contra-indications intestinal obstruction, acute abdominal conditions, acute inflammatory bowel disease, severe dehydration

Pregnancy see Pregnancy, p. 77

Side-effects see notes above; nausea and vomiting; colitis also reported; *suppositories* local irritation

Indication and dose

Constipation (tablets act in 10–12 hours; suppositories act in 20–60 minutes)

• **By mouth**
Child 4–18 years 5–20 mg once daily, adjusted according to response

• **By rectum (suppositories)**
Child 2–18 years 5–10 mg once daily, adjusted according to response

Bowel clearance before radiological procedures and surgery

• **By mouth and by rectum**
Child 4–10 years *by mouth*, 5 mg at bedtime for 2 days before procedure and, if necessary, *by rectum*, 5 mg suppository 1 hour before procedure

Child 10–18 years *by mouth*, 10 mg at bedtime for 2 days before procedure and, if necessary, *by rectum*, 10 mg suppository 1 hour before procedure

Bisacodyl (Non-proprietary)
Tablets, e/c, bisacodyl 5 mg, net price 100 = £3.27. Label: 5, 25

Suppositories, bisacodyl 10 mg, net price 12 = 99p

Paediatric suppositories, bisacodyl 5 mg, net price 5 = 94p

Note The brand name *Dulcolax®* (ℕℍ𝕊) (Boehringer Ingelheim) is used for bisacodyl tablets, net price 10-tab pack = 74p; suppositories (10 mg), 10 = £1.57; paediatric suppositories (5 mg), 5 = 94p
The brand names *Dulcolax® Liquid* and *Dulcolax® Perles* are used for sodium picosulfate preparations

◢ DANTRON
(Danthron)

Cautions avoid prolonged contact with skin (as in incontinent patients or infants wearing nappies)—risk of irritation and excoriation; *rodent* studies indicate potential carcinogenic risk

Contra-indications see Bisacodyl above

Pregnancy manufacturers of co-danthramer and co-danthrusate advise avoid—no information available

Breast-feeding manufacturers of co-danthramer and co-danthrusate advise avoid—limited information available

1 · Gastro-intestinal system

◁ **DANTRON (***continued***)**

Side-effects see notes above; also urine may be coloured red

Indication and dose

Constipation in terminally ill children for dose see under preparations

▰**With poloxamer '188' (as co-danthramer)**

Note Co-danthramer suspension 5 mL = one co-danthramer capsule, **but** strong co-danthramer suspension 5 mL = two strong co-danthramer capsules

Co-danthramer (Non-proprietary) PoM

Capsules, co-danthramer 25/200 (dantron 25 mg, poloxamer '188' 200 mg). Net price 60-cap pack = £12.86. Label: 14, (urine red)

Dose

• By mouth

Child 6–12 years 1 capsule at night (restricted indications, see notes above)

Child 12–18 years 1–2 capsules at night (restricted indications, see notes above)

Strong capsules, co-danthramer 37.5/500 (dantron 37.5 mg, poloxamer '188' 500 mg). Net price 60-cap pack = £15.55. Label: 14, (urine red)

Dose

• By mouth

Child 12–18 years 1–2 capsules at night (restricted indications, see notes above)

Suspension, co-danthramer 25/200 in 5 mL (dantron 25 mg, poloxamer '188' 200 mg/5 mL). Net price 300 mL = £11.27, 1 litre = £37.57. Label: 14, (urine red)

Brands include *Codalax*® JHS, *Danlax*®

Dose

• By mouth

Child 2–12 years 2.5–5 mL at night (restricted indications, see notes above)

Child 12–18 years 5–10 mL at night (restricted indications, see notes above)

Strong suspension, co-danthramer 75/1000 in 5 mL (dantron 75 mg, poloxamer '188' 1 g/5 mL). Net price 300 mL = £30.13. Label: 14, (urine red)

Brands include *Codalax Forte*® JHS

Dose

• By mouth

Child 12–18 years 5 mL at night (restricted indications, see notes above)

▰**With docusate sodium (as co-danthrusate)**

Co-danthrusate (Non-proprietary) PoM

Capsules, co-danthrusate 50/60 (dantron 50 mg, docusate sodium 60 mg). Net price 63-cap pack = £14.50. Label: 14, (urine red)

Brands include *Normax*® JHS

Dose

• By mouth

Child 6–12 years 1 capsule at night (restricted indications, see notes above)

Child 12–18 years 1–3 capsules at night (restricted indications, see notes above)

Suspension, yellow, co-danthrusate 50/60 (dantron 50 mg, docusate sodium 60 mg/5 mL). Net price 200 mL = £8.75. Label: 14, (urine red)

Brands include *Normax*®

Dose

• By mouth

Child 6–12 years 5 mL at night (restricted indications, see notes above)

Child 12–18 years 5–15 mL at night (restricted indications, see notes above)

▰ **DOCUSATE SODIUM**

(Dioctyl sodium sulphosuccinate)

Cautions see notes above; do not give with liquid paraffin

Contra-indications see notes above; also for *rectal preparations*, haemorrhoids or anal fissure

Pregnancy not known to be harmful—manufacturer advises caution

Breast-feeding present in milk following oral administration—manufacturer advises caution; rectal administration not known to be harmful

Side-effects see notes above

Licensed use *adult oral solution and capsules* not licensed for use in children under 12 years

Indication and dose

Constipation

• By mouth

Child 6 months–2 years 12.5 mg 3 times daily, adjusted according to response (use paediatric oral solution)

Child 2–12 years 12.5–25 mg 3 times daily, adjusted according to response (use paediatric oral solution)

Child 12–18 years up to 500 mg daily in divided doses, adjusted according to response

Note Oral preparations act within 1–2 days; response to rectal administration usually occurs within 20 minutes

Adjunct in abdominal radiological procedures

• By mouth

Child 12–18 years 400 mg with barium meal

Administration for administration *by mouth*, solution may be mixed with milk or squash

Dioctyl® (UCB Pharma)

Capsules, yellow/white, docusate sodium 100 mg, net price 30-cap pack = £1.92, 100-cap pack = £6.40

Docusol® (Typharm)

Adult oral solution, sugar-free, docusate sodium 50 mg/5 mL, net price 300 mL = £5.49

Paediatric oral solution, sugar-free, docusate sodium 12.5 mg/5 mL, net price 300 mL = £5.29

◁ **DOCUSATE SODIUM** (*continued*)

◢ **Rectal preparations**

Norgalax Micro-enema® (Norgine)
Enema, docusate sodium 120 mg in 10-g single-dose disposable packs. Net price 10-g unit = 57p

Dose
• **By rectum**
    Child 12–18 years 1 enema as a single dose

◢ **GLYCEROL**

(Glycerin)

Indication and dose

Constipation
• **By rectum**
    Child 1 month–1 year 1-g suppository as required
    Child 1–12 years 2-g suppository as required
    Child 12–18 years 4-g suppository as required

Glycerol Suppositories, BP
(Glycerin Suppositories)
Suppositories, gelatin 140 mg, glycerol 700 mg, purified water to 1 g, net price 12 = £1.02 (1 g), £1.02 (2 g), £1.58 (4 g)

Administration Moisten with water before insertion

◢ **SENNA**

Cautions see notes above

Contra-indications see notes above

Pregnancy see Pregnancy, p. 77

Breast-feeding not known to be harmful

Side-effects see notes above

Licensed use *tablets* not licensed for use in children under 6 years; *syrup* not licensed for use in children under 2 years

Indication and dose

Constipation for dose see under preparations
    Note Onset of action 8–12 hours; initial dose should be low

Senna (Non-proprietary)
Tablets, total sennosides (calculated as sennoside B) 7.5 mg. Net price 60 = £2.13
Brands include *Senokot®* ᴺᴴˢ

Dose
• **By mouth**
    Child 2–4 years ½–2 tablets once daily, adjusted according to response
    Child 4–6 years ½–4 tablets once daily, adjusted according to response
    Child 6–18 years 1–4 tablets once daily, adjusted according to response

Manevac® (HFA Healthcare)
Granules, coated, senna fruit 12.4%, ispaghula 54.2%, net price 400 g = £7.45. Label: 25, counselling, administration
Excipients include sucrose 800 mg per level 5-mL spoonful of granules

Dose
• **By mouth**
    Child 12–18 years 1–2 level 5-mL spoonfuls at night with at least 150 mL water, fruit juice, milk, or warm drink

Counselling Preparations that swell in contact with liquid should always be carefully swallowed with water or appropriate fluid and should not be taken immediately before going to bed

Senokot® (Reckitt Benckiser)
Tablets ᴺᴴˢ, see above

Syrup, sugar-free, brown, total sennosides (calculated as sennoside B) 7.5 mg/5 mL. Net price 500 mL = £2.69

Dose
• **By mouth**
    Child 1 month–4 years 2.5–10 mL once daily, adjusted according to response
    Child 4–18 years 2.5–20 mL once daily, adjusted according to response

---

◢ **SODIUM PICOSULFATE**

(Sodium picosulphate)

Cautions see notes above; active inflammatory bowel disease (avoid if fulminant)

Contra-indications see notes above; severe dehydration

Pregnancy see Pregnancy, p. 77

Breast-feeding not known to be present in milk but manufacturer advises avoid unless potential benefit outweighs risk

Side-effects see notes above

Licensed use *elixir*, licensed for use in children (age range not specified by manufacturer); *Perles®* not licensed for use in children under 4 years

Indication and dose

Constipation
• **By mouth**
    Child 1 month–4 years 2.5–10 mg once daily, adjusted according to response
    Child 4–18 years 2.5–20 mg once daily, adjusted according to response
    Note onset of action 6–12 hours

Bowel evacuation before abdominal radiological and endoscopic procedures on the colon, and surgery section 1.6.5

1

Gastro-intestinal system

1 Gastro-intestinal system

◻ **SODIUM PICOSULFATE** (*continued*)

Sodium Picosulfate (Non-proprietary)
Elixir, sodium picosulfate 5 mg/5 mL, net price
100 mL = £1.85

Note The brand name *Dulcolax*® *Liquid* (Boehringer
Ingelheim) is used for sodium picosulfate elixir 5 mg/
5 mL

Dulcolax® (Boehringer Ingelheim)
Perles® (= capsules), sodium picosulfate 2.5 mg,
net price 20-cap pack = £1.93, 50-cap pack = £2.73

Note The brand name *Dulcolax*® is also used for bisacodyl
tablets and suppositories

◢Bowel cleansing preparations
Section 1.6.5

1.6.3 Faecal softeners

Enemas containing **arachis oil** (ground-nut oil, peanut oil) lubricate and soften
impacted faeces and promote a bowel movement.

Bulk laxatives (section 1.6.1) and non-ionic surfactant 'wetting' agents e.g. docusate sodium (section 1.6.2) also have softening properties. Such drugs are useful
for oral administration in the management of anal fissure; glycerol suppositories
(section 1.6.2) are useful for rectal use.

◢ ARACHIS OIL

Cautions intestinal obstruction; hypersensitivity
to soya

Contra-indications inflammatory bowel disease,
hypersensitivity to arachis oil or peanuts

Licensed use licensed for use in children (age
range not specified by manufacturer

Indication and dose

Impacted faeces
• By rectum
Child 3–7 years 45–65 mL as required

Child 7–12 years 65–100 mL as required

Child 12–18 years 100–130 mL as required

Administration warm enema in warm water
before use

Arachis Oil Enema (Non-proprietary)
Enema, arachis (peanut) oil in 130-mL single-dose
disposable packs. Net price 130 mL = £7.98

1.6.4 Osmotic laxatives

Osmotic laxatives increase the amount of water in the large bowel, either by
drawing fluid from the body into the bowel or by retaining the fluid they were
administered with.

Lactulose is a semi-synthetic disaccharide which is not absorbed from the gastro-
intestinal tract. It produces an osmotic diarrhoea of low faecal pH, and dis-
courages the proliferation of ammonia-producing organisms. It is therefore useful
in the treatment of *hepatic encephalopathy*.

Macrogols are inert polymers of ethylene glycol which sequester fluid in the
bowel; giving fluid with macrogols may reduce the dehydrating effect sometimes
seen with osmotic laxatives. Macrogols are an effective non-traumatic means of
evacuation in children with faecal impaction and can be used in the long-term
management of chronic constipation.

Saline purgatives such as **magnesium hydroxide** are commonly abused but are
satisfactory for occasional use; adequate fluid intake should be maintained.
Magnesium salts are useful where rapid bowel evacuation is required. **Sodium
salts** should be avoided as they may give rise to sodium and water retention in
susceptible individuals. **Phosphate enemas** are useful in bowel clearance before
radiology, endoscopy, and surgery. Enemas containing **phosphate** or **sodium
citrate**, and oral **bowel cleansing preparations** (section 1.6.5) should only be
used on the advice of a specialist practitioner.

◢ LACTULOSE

Cautions lactose intolerance; **interactions:**
Appendix 1 (lactulose)

Contra-indications galactosaemia, intestinal
obstruction

Pregnancy not known to be harmful; see also
Pregnancy, p. 77

Side-effects nausea (can be reduced by administration with water, fruit juice or with meals),
vomiting, flatulence, cramps, and abdominal
discomfort

Licensed use not licensed for use in children for
hepatic encephalopathy

◁ **LACTULOSE** *(continued)*

Indication and dose

Constipation (may take up to 48 hours to act)
- **By mouth**

    Child 1 month–1 year 2.5 mL twice daily, adjusted according to response

    Child 1–5 years 2.5–10 mL twice daily, adjusted according to response

    Child 5–18 years 5–20 mL twice daily, adjusted according to response

Hepatic encephalopathy
- **By mouth**

    Child 12–18 years 30–50 mL 3 times daily; adjust dose to produce 2–3 soft stools per day

Lactulose (Non-proprietary)
Solution, lactulose 3.1–3.7 g/5 mL with other ketoses. Net price 300-mL pack = £2.24, 500-mL pack = £2.96
Brands include *Duphalac®* ⒹⒽⓈ, *Lactugal®*, *Regulose®*

▰ MACROGOLS
(Polyethylene glycols)

Cautions discontinue if symptoms of fluid and electrolyte disturbance; see also preparations below

Contra-indications intestinal perforation or obstruction, paralytic ileus, severe inflammatory conditions of the intestinal tract (such as Crohn's disease, ulcerative colitis, and toxic megacolon); see also preparations below

Pregnancy manufacturers advise use only if essential—no information available

Breast-feeding manufacturers advise use only if essential—no information available

Side-effects abdominal distension and pain, nausea, flatulence

Licensed use *Movicol® Paediatric Plain* not licensed for use in faecal impaction in children under 5 years, or for chronic constipation in children under 2 years

Indication and dose

See under preparations below

Macrogol Oral Powder, Compound (Non-proprietary)
Oral powder, macrogol '3350' (polyethylene glycol '3350') 13.125 g, sodium bicarbonate 178.5 mg, sodium chloride 350.7 mg, potassium chloride 46.6 mg/sachet, net price 20-sachet pack = £4.45, 30-sachet pack = £6.68. Label: 13
Brands include *Laxido®*, *Molaxole®*

Cautions patients with cardiovascular impairment should not take more than 2 sachets in any 1 hour

Dose

Chronic constipation
- **By mouth**

    Child 12–18 years 1–3 sachets daily in divided doses usually for up to 2 weeks; maintenance, 1–2 sachets daily

    Administration Mix contents of each sachet in half a glass (approx. 125 mL) of water

Faecal impaction
- **By mouth**

    Child 12–18 years 8 sachets daily, usually for max. 3 days

    Administration Mix contents of 8 sachets in 1 litre of water, and drink within 6 hours. After reconstitution the solution should be kept in a refrigerator and discarded if unused after 6 hours

Movicol® (Norgine)
Oral powder, macrogol '3350' (polyethylene glycol '3350') 13.125 g, sodium bicarbonate 178.5 mg, sodium chloride 350.7 mg, potassium chloride 46.6 mg/sachet, net price 20-sachet pack (lime-

and lemon- flavoured) = £4.45, 30-sachet pack (lime- and lemon- or chocolate- or plain- flavoured) = £6.68, 50-sachet pack (lime- and lemon- or plain-flavoured) = £11.13. Label: 13

Note Amount of potassium chloride varies according to flavour of *Movicol®* as follows: plain-flavour (sugar-free) = 50.2 mg/sachet; lime and lemon flavour = 46.6 mg/sachet; chocolate flavour = 31.7 mg/sachet. 1 sachet when reconstituted with 125 mL water provides K^+ 5.4 mmol/litre

Cautions patients with cardiovascular impairment should not take more than 2 sachets in any 1 hour

Dose

Chronic constipation
- **By mouth**

    Child 12–18 years 1–3 sachets daily in divided doses usually for up to 2 weeks; maintenance, 1–2 sachets daily

    Administration Mix contents of each sachet in half a glass (approx. 125 mL) of water

Faecal impaction
- **By mouth**

    Child 12–18 years 8 sachets daily, usually for max. 3 days

    Administration Mix contents of 8 sachets in 1 litre of water and drink within 6 hours. After reconstitution the solution should be kept in a refrigerator and discarded if unused after 6 hours

Movicol®-Half (Norgine)
Oral powder, sugar-free, macrogol '3350' (polyethylene glycol '3350') 6.563 g, sodium bicarbonate 89.3 mg, sodium chloride 175.4 mg, potassium chloride 23.3 mg/sachet, net price 20-sachet pack (lime and lemon flavour) = £2.67, 30-sachet pack = £4.01. Label: 13

Cautions patients with impaired cardiovascular function should not take more than 4 sachets in any 1 hour

Dose

Chronic constipation
- **By mouth**

    Child 12–18 years 2–6 sachets daily in divided doses usually for up to 2 weeks; maintenance, 2–4 sachets daily

    Administration Mix contents of each sachet in quarter of a glass (approx. 60–65 mL) of water

Faecal impaction
- **By mouth**

    Child 12–18 years 16 sachets daily, usually for max. 3 days

    Administration Mix contents of 16 sachets in 1 litre of water and drink within 6 hours. After reconstitution the solution should be kept in a refrigerator and discarded if unused after 6 hours

◻ **MACROGOLS** (*continued*)

Movicol® Paediatric Plain (Norgine) ⟨PoM⟩
Oral powder, sugar-free, macrogol '3350' (poly-ethylene glycol '3350') 6.563 g, sodium bicarbonate 89.3 mg, sodium chloride 175.4 mg, potassium chloride 25.1 mg/sachet, net price 30-sachet pack = £4.45. Label: 13

Cautions *with high doses*, impaired gag reflex, reflux oesophagitis, impaired consciousness
Contra-indications cardiovascular impairment, renal impairment——no information available

Dose

> Chronic constipation, prevention of faecal impaction
> • By mouth
>   **Child under 1 year** ½–1 sachet daily
>
>   **Child 1–6 years** 1 sachet daily; adjust dose to produce regular soft stools (max. 4 sachets daily)

> **Child 6–12 years** 2 sachets daily; adjust dose to produce regular soft stools (max. 4 sachets daily)
> Administration Mix content of each sachet in quarter of a glass (approx. 60–65 mL) of water

> Faecal impaction
> • By mouth
>   **Child under 1 year** ½–1 sachet daily
>
>   **Child 1–5 years** (treat until impaction resolves) 2 sachets on first day, then 4 sachets daily for 2 days, then 6 sachets daily for 2 days, then 8 sachets daily
>
>   **Child 5–12 years** (treat until impaction resolves) 4 sachets on first day, then increased in steps of 2 sachets daily to max. 12 sachets daily
>   Administration Mix each sachet in quarter of a glass (approx. 60–65 mL) of water; total daily dose to be taken over a 12-hour period

---

◼ **MAGNESIUM SALTS**

Cautions see also notes above; **interactions:** Appendix 1 (antacids)
Contra-indications acute gastro-intestinal conditions
Hepatic impairment avoid in hepatic coma if risk of renal failure
Renal impairment avoid or reduce dose; increased risk of toxicity
Side-effects colic

Indication and dose

> Constipation see under preparations below

◢ Magnesium hydroxide
Magnesium Hydroxide Mixture, BP
Aqueous suspension containing about 8% hydrated magnesium oxide. Do not store in cold place

Dose
> • By mouth
>   **Child 3–12 years** 5–10 mL with water at bedtime when required
>
>   **Child 12–18 years** 30–45 mL with water at bedtime when required

◢ Bowel cleansing preparations
Section 1.6.5

◼ **PHOSPHATES (RECTAL)**

Cautions see also notes above; *with enema*, electrolyte disturbances, congestive heart failure, ascites, uncontrolled hypertension, maintain adequate hydration
Contra-indications acute gastro-intestinal conditions (including gastro-intestinal obstruction, inflammatory bowel disease, and conditions associated with increased colonic absorption)
Renal impairment use enema with caution
Side-effects local irritation; *with enema*, electrolyte disturbances

Indication and dose

> Constipation, bowel evacuation before abdominal radiological procedures, endoscopy, and surgery
>   For dose see preparations

Carbalax® (Forest)
Suppositories, sodium acid phosphate (anhydrous) 1.3 g, sodium bicarbonate 1.08 g, net price 12 = £2.01

Dose
> • By rectum
>   **Child 12–18 years** 1 suppository, inserted 30 minutes before evacuation required; moisten with water before use

Fleet® Ready-to-use Enema (De Witt)
Enema, sodium acid phosphate 21.4 g, sodium phosphate 9.4 g/118 mL, net price 133-mL pack (delivers 118 mL dose) with standard tube = 57p

Dose
> • By rectum
>   **Child 3–7 years** 40–60 mL once daily
>
>   **Child 7–12 years** 60–90 mL once daily
>
>   **Child 12–18 years** 90–118 mL once daily

Phosphates Enema BP Formula B
Enema, sodium dihydrogen phosphate dihydrate 12.8 g, disodium phosphate dodecahydrate 10.24 g, purified water, freshly boiled and cooled, to 128 mL. Net price 128 mL with standard tube = £2.98, with long rectal tube = £3.98

Dose
> • By rectum
>   **Child 3–7 years** 45–65 mL once daily
>
>   **Child 7–12 years** 65–100 mL once daily
>
>   **Child 12–18 years** 100–128 mL once daily

◾ SODIUM CITRATE (RECTAL)

Cautions see notes above

Contra-indications acute gastro-intestinal conditions

Indication and dose

Constipation for dose see under preparations

Micolette Micro-enema® (Pinewood)

Enema, sodium citrate 450 mg, sodium lauryl sulphoacetate 45 mg, glycerol 625 mg, together with citric acid, potassium sorbate, and sorbitol in a viscous solution, in 5-mL single-dose disposable packs with nozzle. Net price 5 mL = 38p

Dose
- **By rectum**
  Child 3–18 years 5–10 mL as a single dose

Micralax Micro-enema® (UCB Pharma)

Enema, sodium citrate 450 mg, sodium alkylsulphoacetate 45 mg, sorbic acid 5 mg, together with

glycerol and sorbitol in a viscous solution in 5-mL single-dose disposable packs with nozzle. Net price 5 mL = 41p

Dose
- **By rectum**
  Child 3–18 years 5 mL as a single dose

Relaxit Micro-enema® (Crawford)

Enema, sodium citrate 450 mg, sodium lauryl sulphate 75 mg, sorbic acid 5 mg, together with glycerol and sorbitol in a viscous solution in 5-mL single-dose disposable packs with nozzle. Net price 5 mL = 32p

Dose
- **By rectum**
  Child 1 month–18 years 5 mL as a single dose (insert only half nozzle length in child under 3 years)

1.6.5 Bowel cleansing preparations

Bowel cleansing preparations are used before colonic surgery, colonoscopy, or radiological examination to ensure the bowel is free of solid contents. They are **not** treatments for constipation.

Cautions   Bowel cleansing preparations should be used with caution in children, particularly those with fluid and electrolyte disturbances. Adequate hydration should be maintained during treatment. Bowel cleansing preparations should also be used with caution in colitis (avoid if severe), or in those who are debilitated.

Contra-indications   Bowel cleansing preparations are contra-indicated in patients with gastro-intestinal obstruction or perforation, gastric retention, acute severe colitis, or toxic megacolon.

Side-effects   Side-effects of bowel cleansing preparations include nausea, vomiting, abdominal pain (usually transient—reduced by taking more slowly), and abdominal distention. Less frequent side-effects include headache, dizziness, dehydration, and electrolyte disturbances.

◾ MACROGOLS

Cautions see notes above; also heart failure; impaired gag reflex, impaired consciousness or possibility of regurgitation or aspiration

Contra-indications see notes above; also gastro-intestinal ulceration

Pregnancy manufacturers advise use only if essential—no information available

Breast-feeding manufacturers advise use only if essential—no information available

Side-effects see notes above; also anal discomfort

Licensed use *Klean-Prep®* not licensed for use in children

Indication and dose

See preparations

Klean-Prep® (Norgine)

Oral powder, sugar-free, macrogol '3350' (polyethylene glycol '3350') 59 g, anhydrous sodium sulphate 5.685 g, sodium bicarbonate 1.685 g, sodium chloride 1.465 g, potassium chloride 743 mg/

sachet, net price 4 sachets = £8.23. Label: 10, patient information leaflet, counselling

Excipients include aspartame (section 9.4.1)

Electrolytes 1 sachet when reconstituted with 1 litre water provides Na^+ 125 mmol, K^+ 10 mmol, Cl^- 35 mmol, HCO_3^- 20 mmol

Dose

Bowel cleansing before radiological examination, colonoscopy or surgery
- **By mouth**
  Child 12–18 years a glass (approx. 250 mL) of reconstituted solution every 10–15 minutes, or by nasogastric tube 20–30 mL/minute, until 4 litres have been consumed or watery stools are free of solid matter. The solution from all 4 sachets should be drunk within 4–6 hours (250 mL drunk rapidly every 10–15 minutes)

  Alternatively total volume for administration given in 2 divided doses, first dose taken on the evening before examination and second dose on the morning of the examination

Distal intestinal obstruction syndrome
- **By mouth, nasogastric or gastrostomy tube**
  Child 1–18 years 10 mL/kg/hour for 30 minutes, then 20 mL/kg/hour for 30 minutes, then increase to 25 mL/kg/hour if tolerated; max. 100 mL/kg (or 4

1

Gastro-intestinal system

◻ **MACROGOLS** (*continued*)

litres) over 4 hours; repeat 4-hour treatment if necessary.

Administration Each sachet should be made up to 1 litre with water; flavouring such as clear fruit cordials may be added if required; to facilitate gastric emptying domperidone (section 1.2) may be given 30 minutes before starting. After reconstitution the solution should be kept in a refrigerator and discarded if unused after 24 hours.

▰ MAGNESIUM CITRATE

Reconstitution of a sachet containing 11.57 g magnesium carbonate and 17.79 g anhydrous citric acid produces a solution containing magnesium citrate

Cautions see notes above

Contra-indications see notes above

Hepatic impairment avoid in hepatic coma if risk of renal failure

Renal impairment avoid if estimated glomerular filtration rate less than 30 mL/minute/1.73 m²—risk of hypermagnesaemia

Pregnancy caution

Breast-feeding caution

Side-effects see notes above

Indication and dose

See preparations

Citramag® (Sanochemia)
Oral powder, sugar-free, effervescent, magnesium carbonate 11.57 g, anhydrous citric acid 17.79 g/ sachet, net price 10-sachet pack (lemon and lime flavour) = £17.20. Label: 10, patient information leaflet, 13, counselling, see below

Dose

> Bowel evacuation on day before radiological examination, colonoscopy, or surgery
> • By mouth
>   **Child 5–10 years** on day before procedure, one-third of a sachet at 8 a.m. and one-third of a sachet between 2 and 4 p.m.
>
>   **Child 10–18 years** on day before procedure, ½–1 sachet at 8 a.m. and ½–1 sachet between 2 and 4 p.m.

Counselling The patient information leaflet advises that hot water (200 mL) is needed to make the solution and provides guidance on the timing and procedure for reconstitution; it also mentions need for high fluid, low residue diet beforehand (according to hospital advice), and explains that only clear fluids can be taken after *Citramag®* until procedure completed

▰ PHOSPHATES (ORAL)

Cautions see notes above; also cardiac disease (avoid in congestive cardiac failure)

Contra-indications see notes above; also ascites; congestive cardiac failure

Renal impairment manufacturer of *Fleet Phospho-soda®* advises avoid in significant impairment

Pregnancy caution

Breast-feeding caution

Side-effects see notes above; also chest pain and asthenia

Licensed use *Fleet Phospho-soda®* not licensed for use in children

Indication and dose

See preparations

Fleet Phospho-soda® (De Witt)
Oral solution, sugar-free, sodium dihydrogen phosphate dihydrate 24.4 g, disodium phosphate dodecahydrate 10.8 g/45 mL. Net price 2 × 45-mL bottles = £4.79. Label: 10, patient information leaflet, counselling

Electrolytes Na⁺ 217 mmol, phosphate 186 mmol/45 mL

Dose

> Bowel evacuation before colonic surgery, colonoscopy, or radiological examination
> • By mouth
>   **Child 15–18 years** 45 mL diluted with half a glass (120 mL) of cold water, followed by one full glass (240 mL) of cold water
>
>   Timing of doses is dependent on the time of the procedure
>
>   For morning procedure, first dose should be taken at 7 a.m. and second at 7 p.m. on day before the procedure
>
>   For afternoon procedure, first dose should be taken at 7 p.m. on day before and second dose at 7 a.m. on day of the procedure
>
>   Solid food must not be taken during dosing period; clear liquids or water should be substituted for meals
>
>   Acts within half to 6 hours of first dose

▰ SODIUM PICOSULFATE WITH MAGNESIUM CITRATE

Cautions see notes above; also recent gastrointestinal surgery; cardiac disease (avoid in congestive cardiac failure)

Contra-indications see notes above; also gastrointestinal ulceration; ascites; congestive cardiac failure

Hepatic impairment avoid in hepatic coma if risk of renal failure

Renal impairment avoid if estimated glomerular filtration rate less than 30 mL/minute/1.73 m²—risk of hypermagnesaemia

Pregnancy caution

Breast-feeding caution

Side-effects see notes above; also anal discomfort, sleep disturbances, fatigue, and rash

Indication and dose

See preparations

Picolax® (Ferring)
Oral powder, sugar-free, sodium picosulfate 10 mg/ sachet, with magnesium citrate. Contains 87 mmol Mg²⁺ and 5 mmol K⁺/sachet. Net price 20-sachet

Gastro-intestinal system — 1

△ **SODIUM PICOSULFATE WITH MAGNESIUM CITRATE** (*continued*)

pack = £33.90. Label: 10, patient information leaflet, 13, counselling, see below

Dose

> **Bowel evacuation on day before radiological procedure, endoscopy, or surgery**
>
> • **By mouth**
>
> **Child 1–2 years** ¼ sachet before 8 a.m. then ¼ sachet 6–8 hours later
>
> **Child 2–4 years** ½ sachet before 8 a.m. then ½ sachet 6–8 hours later
>
> **Child 4–9 years** 1 sachet before 8 a.m. then ½ sachet 6–8 hours later

> **Child 9–18 years** 1 sachet before 8 a.m. then 1 sachet 6–8 hours later

Note Acts within 3 hours of first dose. Low residue diet recommended on the day before procedure and copious intake of water or other clear fluids recommended during treatment

Counselling One sachet should be reconstituted with 150 mL (approx. half a glass) of cold water; children and carers should be warned that heat is generated during reconstitution and that the solution should be allowed to cool before drinking

---

Amidotrizoates

Gastrografin® is an **amidotrizoate** radiological contrast medium with high osmolality; it is used in the treatment of meconium ileus in neonates and in the management of distal intestinal obstruction syndrome in children with cystic fibrosis.

◼ AMIDOTRIZOATES

Diatrizoates

Cautions asthma or history of allergy, latent hyperthyroidism, dehydration and electrolyte disturbance (correct first); in children with oesophageal fistulae (aspiration may lead to pulmonary oedema); benign nodular goitre; enteritis; risk of anaphylactoid reactions increased by concomitant administration of beta-blockers

Contra-indications hypersensitivity to iodine, hyperthyroidism

Pregnancy manufacturer advises caution

Side-effects diarrhoea, nausea, vomiting; also reported, abdominal pain, intestinal perforation, bowel necrosis, oral mucosal blistering, hypersensitivity reactions, pyrexia, headache, dizziness, disturbances in consciousness, hyperthyroidism, electrolyte disturbances, and skin reactions (including toxic epidermal necrolysis)

Licensed use not licensed for use in distal intestinal obstruction syndrome

Indication and dose

> **Uncomplicated meconium ileus**
>
> • **By rectum**
>
> **Neonate** 15–30 mL as a single dose

> **Distal intestinal obstruction syndrome**
>
> • **By mouth or by rectum**
>
> **Child 1 month–2 years** 15–30 mL as a single dose

> **Child body-weight 15–25 kg** 50 mL as a single dose
>
> **Child body-weight over 25 kg** 100 mL as a single dose

Administration Intravenous prehydration is essential in neonates and infants. Fluid intake should be encouraged for 3 hours after administration. *By mouth*, for child bodyweight under 25 kg, dilute *Gastrografin*® with 3 times its volume of water or fruit juice; for child bodyweight over 25 kg, dilute *Gastrografin*® with twice its volume of water or fruit juice. *By rectum*, administration must be carried out slowly under radiological supervision to ensure required site is reached. For child under 5 years, dilute *Gastrografin*® with 5 times its volume of water; for child over 5 years dilute *Gastrografin*® with 4 times its volume of water.

Radiological investigations dose to be recommended by radiologist

Gastrografin® (Bayer Schering)
Solution, sodium amidotrizoate 100 mg, meglumine amidotrizoate 660 mg/mL, net price 100-mL bottle = £14.97
Excipients include disodium edetate

1.6.6 Peripheral opioid-receptor antagonists

Classification not used in *BNF for Children*.

1.7 Local preparations for anal and rectal disorders

1.7.1 Soothing anal and rectal preparations
1.7.2 Compound anal and rectal preparations with corticosteroids
1.7.3 Rectal sclerosants
1.7.4 Management of anal fissures

In children with perianal soreness or pruritus ani, good toilet hygiene is essential; the use of alcohol-free 'wet-wipes' after each bowel motion, regular bathing and the avoidance of local irritants such as bath additives is recommended.

Gastro-intestinal system

Excoriated skin is best treated with a protective barrier emollient (section 13.2.2); in children over 1 month, **hydrocortisone** ointment or cream (section 13.4) or a compound rectal preparation (section 1.7.2) may be used for a short period of time, up to a maximum of 7 days.

Pruritus ani caused by threadworm infection requires treatment with an anthelmintic (section 5.5.1). Topical application of **white soft paraffin** or other bland emollient (section 13.2.1) may reduce anal irritation caused by threadworms.

Perianal erythema caused by streptococcal infection should be treated initially with an oral antibacterial such as **phenoxymethylpenicillin** (section 5.1.1.1) or **erythromycin** (section 5.1.5), while awaiting results of culture and sensitivity testing.

Perianal candidiasis (thrush) requires treatment with a topical antifungal preparation (section 13.10.2). For treatment of vulvovaginal candidiasis, see section 7.2.2.

Proctitis associated with inflammatory bowel disease in children is treated with corticosteroids and aminosalicylates (section 1.5).

For the management of anal fissures, see section 1.7.4.

1.7.1 Soothing anal and rectal preparations

Haemorrhoids in children are rare, but may occur in infants with portal hypertension. Soothing rectal preparations containing mild astringents such as bismuth subgallate, zinc oxide, and hammamelis may provide symptomatic relief, but proprietary preparations which also contain lubricants, vasoconstrictors, or mild antiseptics may cause further perianal irritation.

Local anaesthetics may be used to relieve pain in children with anal fissures or pruritus ani, but local anaesthetics are absorbed through the rectal mucosa and may cause sensitisation of the anal skin. Excessive use of local anaesthetics may result in systemic effects, see section 15.2. Preparations containing local anaesthetics should be used for no longer than 2–3 days.

Lidocaine (lignocaine) ointment (section 15.2) may be applied before defaecation to relieve pain associated with anal fissure, but local anaesthetics can cause stinging initially and this may aggravate the child's fear of pain.

Other local anaesthetics such as tetracaine (amethocaine), cinchocaine (dibucaine), and pramocaine (pramoxine) may be included in rectal preparations, but these are more irritant than lidocaine.

Corticosteroids are often combined with local anaesthetics and soothing agents in topical preparations for haemorrhoids and proctitis. Topical preparations containing corticosteroids (section 1.7.2) should not be used long-term or if infection (such as herpes simplex) is present. For further information on the use of topical corticosteroids, see section 13.4.

1.7.2 Compound anal and rectal preparations with corticosteroids

Anugesic-HC® (Pfizer) (PoM)
Cream, benzyl benzoate 1.2%, bismuth oxide 0.875%, hydrocortisone acetate 0.5%, Peru balsam 1.85%, pramocaine hydrochloride 1%, zinc oxide 12.35%. Net price 30 g (with rectal nozzle) = £3.71

Dose

Haemorrhoids, pruritus ani
• By rectum
Child 12–18 years apply night and morning and after a bowel movement; do not use for longer than 7 days

Suppositories, buff, benzyl benzoate 33 mg, bismuth oxide 24 mg, bismuth subgallate 59 mg, hydrocortisone acetate 5 mg, Peru balsam 49 mg,

pramocaine hydrochloride 27 mg, zinc oxide 296 mg, net price 12 = £2.69

Dose

Haemorrhoids, pruritus ani
• By rectum
Child 12–18 years insert 1 suppository night and morning and after a bowel movement; do not use for longer than 7 days

Anusol-HC® (McNeil) (PoM)
Ointment, benzyl benzoate 1.25%, bismuth oxide 0.875%, bismuth subgallate 2.25%, hydrocortisone acetate 0.25%, Peru balsam 1.875%, zinc oxide 10.75%. Net price 30 g (with rectal nozzle) = £3.50

Dose

Haemorrhoids, pruritus ani
• By rectum
Child 12–18 years apply night and morning and after a bowel movement; do not use for longer than 7 days

Suppositories, benzyl benzoate 33 mg, bismuth oxide 24 mg, bismuth subgallate 59 mg, hydrocortisone acetate 10 mg, Peru balsam 49 mg, zinc oxide 296 mg. Net price 12 = £2.46

Dose

> Haemorrhoids, pruritus ani
> • **By rectum**
> **Child 12–18 years** insert 1 suppository night and morning and after a bowel movement; do not use for longer than 7 days

Perinal® (Dermal)

Spray application, hydrocortisone 0.2%, lidocaine hydrochloride 1%. Net price 30-mL pack = £6.21

Dose

> Haemorrhoids, pruritus ani
> • **By rectum**
> **Child 2–18 years** spray once over the affected area up to 3 times daily; do not use for longer than 7 days without medical advice (child under 14 years, on medical advice only)

Proctofoam HC® (Meda) [PoM]

Foam in aerosol pack, hydrocortisone acetate 1%, pramocaine hydrochloride 1%. Net price 21.2-g pack (approx. 40 applications) with applicator = £5.06

Dose

> Pain and irritation associated with local, non-infected anal or perianal conditions
> • **By rectum**
> **Child 12–18 years** 1 applicatorful (4–6 mg hydrocortisone acetate, 4–6 mg pramocaine hydrochloride) by rectum 2–3 times daily and after a bowel movement (max. 4 times daily); do not use for longer than 7 days

Proctosedyl® (Sanofi-Aventis) [PoM]

Ointment, cinchocaine (dibucaine) hydrochloride 0.5%, hydrocortisone 0.5%, net price 30 g = £10.34 (with cannula)

Dose

> Haemorrhoids, pruritus ani
> • **By rectum**
> **Child 1 month–18 years** apply morning and night and after a bowel movement, externally or by rectum; do not use for longer than 7 days

Suppositories, cinchocaine (dibucaine) hydrochloride 5 mg, hydrocortisone 5 mg, net price 12 = £4.66

Dose

> Haemorrhoids, pruritus ani
> • **By rectum**
> **Child 12–18 years** insert 1 suppository night and morning and after a bowel movement; do not use for longer than 7 days

Scheriproct® (Valeant) [PoM]

Ointment, cinchocaine (dibucaine) hydrochloride 0.5%, prednisolone hexanoate 0.19%, net price 30 g = £3.00

Dose

> Haemorrhoids, pruritus ani
> • **By rectum**
> **Child 1 month–18 years** apply twice daily for 5–7 days (3–4 times daily on 1st day if necessary), then once daily for a few days after symptoms have cleared

Suppositories, cinchocaine (dibucaine) hydrochloride 1 mg, prednisolone hexanoate 1.3 mg, net price 12 = £1.41

Dose

> Haemorrhoids, pruritus ani
> • **By rectum**
> **Child 12–18 years** insert 1 suppository daily after a bowel movement, for 5–7 days (in severe cases initially 2–3 times daily)

Ultraproct® (Meadow) [PoM]

Ointment, cinchocaine (dibucaine) hydrochloride 0.5%, fluocortolone caproate 0.095%, fluocortolone pivalate 0.092%, net price 30 g (with rectal nozzle) = £4.57

Dose

> Haemorrhoids, pruritus ani
> • **By rectum**
> **Child 1 month–18 years** apply twice daily for 5–7 days (3–4 times daily on 1st day if necessary), then once daily for a few days after symptoms have cleared

Suppositories, cinchocaine (dibucaine) hydrochloride 1 mg, fluocortolone caproate 630 micrograms, fluocortolone pivalate 610 micrograms, net price 12 = £2.15

Dose

> Haemorrhoids, pruritus ani
> • **By rectum**
> **Child 12–18 years** insert 1 suppository daily after a bowel movement, for 5–7 days (in severe cases initially 2–3 times daily) then 1 suppository every other day for 1 week

Uniroid-HC® (Chemidex) [PoM]

Ointment, cinchocaine (dibucaine) hydrochloride 0.5%, hydrocortisone 0.5%, net price 30 g (with applicator) = £4.23

Dose

> Haemorrhoids, pruritus ani
> • **By rectum**
> **Child 1 month–18 years** apply twice daily and after a bowel movement, externally or by rectum; do not use for longer than 7 days (child under 12 years, on medical advice only)

Suppositories, cinchocaine (dibucaine) hydrochloride 5 mg, hydrocortisone 5 mg, net price 12 = £1.91

Dose

> Haemorrhoids, pruritus ani
> • **By rectum**
> **Child 12–18 years** insert 1 suppository twice daily and after a bowel movement; do not use for longer than 7 days

Xyloproct® (AstraZeneca) [PoM]

Ointment (water-miscible), aluminium acetate 3.5%, hydrocortisone acetate 0.275%, lidocaine 5%, zinc oxide 18%, net price 20 g (with applicator) = £2.26

Dose

> Haemorrhoids, pruritus ani
> • **By rectum**
> **Child 1 month–18 years** apply several times daily; short-term use only

1

Gastro-intestinal system

1 Gastro-intestinal system

1.7.3 Rectal sclerosants

Classification not used in *BNF for Children*.

1.7.4 Management of anal fissures

The management of anal fissures includes stool softening (section 1.6) and the short-term use of a topical preparation containing a local anaesthetic (section 1.7.1). If these measures are inadequate, children with chronic anal fissures should be referred for specialist treatment in hospital. Topical **glyceryl trinitrate**, 0.05% or 0.1% ointment, may be used in children to relax the anal sphincter, relieve pain and aid healing of anal fissures. Excessive application of topical nitrates causes side-effects such as headache, flushing, dizziness, and postural hypotension.

Before considering surgery, **diltiazem** 2% ointment may be used in children with chronic anal fissures resistant to topical nitrates.

Ointments containing glyceryl trinitrate in a range of strengths or diltiazem 2% are available as manufactured specials (see Special-order Manufacturers, p. 957).

1.8 Stoma and enteral feeding tubes

Stoma

Prescribing for children with stoma calls for special care. The following is a brief account of some of the main points to be borne in mind.

When a solid-dose formulation such as a capsule or a tablet is given the contents of the ostomy bag should be checked for any remnants; response to treatment should be carefully monitored because of the possibility of incomplete absorption. *Enteric-coated* and *modified-release* preparations are **unsuitable**, particularly in children with an ileostomy, as there may not be sufficient release of the active ingredient.

Laxatives   Enemas and washouts should be used in children with stoma only under specialist supervision; they should **not** be prescribed for those with an ileostomy as they may cause rapid and severe loss of water and electrolytes.

Children with colostomy may suffer from constipation and whenever possible it should be treated by increasing fluid intake or dietary fibre. If a laxative (section 1.6) is required, it should generally be used for short periods only.

Antidiarrhoeals   Loperamide, **codeine phosphate,** and **co-phenotrope** (section 1.4.2) are effective for controlling excessive stool losses. Bulk-forming drugs (section 1.6.1) may be tried but it is often difficult to adjust the dose appropriately.

Antibacterials should **not** be given for an episode of acute diarrhoea.

Antacids   The tendency to diarrhoea from magnesium salts or constipation from aluminium salts may be increased in children with stoma.

Diuretics   Diuretics should be used with caution in children with an ileostomy because they may become excessively dehydrated and potassium depletion may easily occur. It is usually advisable to use a **potassium-sparing** diuretic (section 2.2.3).

Digoxin   Children with stoma are particularly susceptible to hypokalaemia. This predisposes children on digoxin to digoxin toxicity; potassium supplements (section 9.2.1.1) or a potassium-sparing diuretic (section 2.2.3) may be advisable.

Analgesics   Opioid analgesics (section 4.7.2) may cause troublesome constipation in children with colostomy. When a non-opioid analgesic is required **paracetamol** is usually suitable; anti-inflammatory analgesics may cause gastric irritation and bleeding.

Iron preparations   Iron supplements may cause loose stools and sore skin at the stoma site. If this is troublesome and if iron is definitely indicated a parenteral iron preparation (section 9.1.1.2) should be used. Modified-release iron preparations should be **avoided**.

Care of stoma   Children and carers are usually given advice about the use of *cleansing agents*, *protective creams*, *lotions*, *deodorants*, or *sealants* whilst in hospital, either by the surgeon or by a stoma-care nurse. Voluntary organisations offer help and support to patients with stoma.

Enteral feeding tubes

Care is required in choosing an appropriate formulation of a drug for administration through a nasogastric narrow-bore feeding tube or through a percutaneous endoscopic gastrostomy (PEG) or jejunostomy tube. Liquid preparations (or soluble tablets) are preferred; injection solutions may also be suitable for administration through an enteral tube.

If a solid formulation of a medicine needs to be given, it should be given as a suspension of particles fine enough to pass through the tube. It is possible to crush many immediate-release tablets but enteric-coated or modified-release preparations should **not** be crushed.

Enteral feeds may affect the absorption of drugs and it is therefore important to consider the timing of drug administration in relation to feeds. If more than one drug needs to be given, they should be given separately and the tube should be flushed with water after each drug has been given.

Clearing blockages   Carbonated (sugar-free) drinks may be marginally more effective than water in unblocking feeding tubes, but mildly acidic liquids (such as pineapple juice or cola-based drinks) can coagulate protein in feeds, causing further blockage. If these measures fail to clear the enteral feeding tube, an alkaline solution containing pancreatic enzymes may be introduced into the tube (followed after at least 5 minutes by water). Specific products designed to break up blockages caused by formula feeds are also available.

1.9   Drugs affecting intestinal secretions

1.9.1 Drugs affecting biliary composition and flow
1.9.2 Bile acid sequestrants
1.9.3 Aprotinin
1.9.4 Pancreatin

1.9.1   Drugs affecting biliary composition and flow

Bile acids (**ursodeoxycholic** and **chenodeoxycholic acid**) may be used as dietary supplements in children with inborn errors of bile acid synthesis. Ursodeoxycholic acid is used to improve the flow of bile in children with cholestatic conditions such as familial intrahepatic cholestasis, biliary atresia in infants, cystic-fibrosis-related liver disease, and cholestasis caused by total parenteral nutrition or following liver transplantation. Ursodeoxycholic acid may also relieve the severe itching associated with cholestasis.

In sclerosing cholangitis, ursodeoxycholic acid is used to lower liver enzyme and serum-bilirubin concentrations.

Ursodeoxycholic acid is also used in the treatment of intrahepatic cholestasis in pregnancy.

Smith-Lemli-Opitz syndrome   Chenodeoxycholic and ursodeoxycholic acid have been used with cholesterol in children with Smith-Lemli-Opitz syndrome. Chenodeoxycholic acid is also used in combination with cholic acid to treat bile acid synthesis defects but cholic acid is difficult to obtain. Chenodeoxycholic acid and cholesterol are available from 'special-order' manufacturers or specialist importing companies, see p. 957.

URSODEOXYCHOLIC ACID

Cautions interactions: Appendix 1 (ursodeoxycholic acid)

Contra-indications radio-opaque stones; non-functioning gall bladder (in patients with radiolucent gallstones)

1   Gastro-intestinal system

Gastro-intestinal system

1

◁ URSODEOXYCHOLIC ACID (*continued*)

Hepatic impairment avoid in chronic liver disease (but used in primary biliary cirrhosis)

Pregnancy no evidence of harm but manufacturer advises avoid

Breast-feeding not known to be harmful but manufacturer advises avoid

Side-effects *rarely*, diarrhoea

Licensed use not licensed for use in children for indications shown below

Indication and dose

Cholestasis
- **By mouth**

  Neonate 5 mg/kg 3 times daily, adjust dose and frequency according to response, max. 10 mg/kg 3 times daily

  Child 1 month–2 years 5 mg/kg 3 times daily, adjust dose and frequency according to response, max. 10 mg/kg 3 times daily

Improvement of hepatic metabolism of essential fatty acids and bile flow, in children with cystic fibrosis
- **By mouth**

  Child 1 month–18 years 10–15 mg/kg twice daily; total daily dose may alternatively be given in 3 divided doses

Cholestasis associated with total parenteral nutrition
- **By mouth**

  Neonate 10 mg/kg 3 times daily

  Child 1 month–18 years 10 mg/kg 3 times daily

Sclerosing cholangitis
- **By mouth**

  Child 1 month–18 years 5–10 mg/kg 2–3 times daily, adjusted according to response, max. 15 mg/kg 3 times daily

Ursodeoxycholic Acid (Non-proprietary) (PoM)
Tablets, ursodeoxycholic acid 150 mg, net price 60-tab pack = £18.51. Label: 21

Capsules, ursodeoxycholic acid 250 mg, net price 60-cap pack = £35.11. Label: 21

Destolit® (Norgine) (PoM)
Tablets, scored, ursodeoxycholic acid 150 mg, net price 60-tab pack = £17.67. Label: 21

Urdox® (CP) (PoM)
Tablets, f/c, ursodeoxycholic acid 300 mg, net price 60-tab pack = £26.50. Label: 21

Ursofalk® (Dr Falk) (PoM)
Capsules, ursodeoxycholic acid 250 mg, net price 60-cap pack = £30.75, 100-cap pack = £32.50. Label: 21

Suspension, sugar-free, ursodeoxycholic acid 250 mg/5 mL, net price 250 mL = £27.50. Label: 21

Ursogal® (Galen) (PoM)
Tablets, scored, ursodeoxycholic acid 150 mg, net price 60-tab pack = £17.05. Label: 21

Capsules, ursodeoxycholic acid 250 mg, net price 60-cap pack = £30.50. Label: 21

Other preparations for bile synthesis defects

CHENODEOXYCHOLIC ACID

Cautions see under Ursodeoxycholic Acid

Contra-indications see under Ursodeoxycholic Acid

Pregnancy avoid—fetotoxicity reported in *animal* studies

Side-effects see under Ursodeoxycholic Acid

Licensed use not licensed

Indication and dose

Cerebrotendinous xanthomatosis
- **By mouth**

  Neonate 5 mg/kg 3 times daily

  Child 1 month–18 years 5 mg/kg 3 times daily

Defective synthesis of bile acid
- **By mouth**

  Neonate initially 5 mg/kg 3 times daily, reduced to 2.5 mg/kg 3 times daily

  Child 1 month–18 years initially 5 mg/kg 3 times daily, reduced to 2.5 mg/kg 3 times daily

Smith-Lemli-Opitz syndrome see notes above
- **By mouth**

  Neonate 7 mg/kg once daily or in divided doses

  Child 1 month–18 years 7 mg/kg once daily or in divided doses

Administration for administration *by mouth*, add the contents of a 250-mg capsule to 25 mL of sodium bicarbonate solution 8.4% (1 mmol/mL) to produce a suspension containing chenodeoxycholic acid 10 mg/mL; use immediately after preparation, discard any remaining suspension

Chenofalk® (Non-proprietary) (PoM)
Capsules, chenodeoxycholic acid 250 mg
Available from 'special-order' manufacturers or specialist importing companies, see p. 957

CHOLESTEROL

Cautions consult product literature
Contra-indications consult product literature
Licensed use not licensed

Indication and dose

> Smith-Lemli-Opitz syndrome
>
> • By mouth
>
> > Neonate 5–10 mg/kg 3–4 times daily

> Child 1 month–18 years 5–10 mg/kg 3–4 times daily (doses up to 15 mg/kg 4 times daily have been used)

Administration cholesterol powder can be mixed with a vegetable oil before administration

Cholesterol Powder (Non-proprietary)
Available from 'special-order' manufacturers or specialist importing companies, see p. 957

1.9.2   Bile acid sequestrants

Colestyramine (cholestyramine) is an anion-exchange resin that forms an insoluble complex with bile acids in the gastro-intestinal tract; it is used to relieve diarrhoea associated with surgical procedures such as ileal resection, or following radiation therapy. Colestyramine is also used in the treatment of familial hypercholesterolaemia (see section 2.12), and to relieve pruritus in children with partial biliary obstruction, (for treatment of pruritus, see section 3.4.1). Colestyramine is not absorbed from the gastro-intestinal tract, but will interfere with the absorption of a number of drugs, so timing of administration is important.

COLESTYRAMINE
(Cholestyramine)

Cautions section 2.12
Contra-indications section 2.12
Pregnancy section 2.12
Breast-feeding section 2.12
Side-effects section 2.12
Licensed use not licensed for use in children under 6 years

Indication and dose

> Pruritus associated with partial biliary obstruction and primary biliary cirrhosis, diarrhoea associated with Crohn's disease, ileal resection, vagotomy, diabetic vagal neuropathy, and radiation
>
> • By mouth
>
> > Child 1 month–1 year 1 g once daily in a suitable liquid, adjusted according to response; total daily dose may alternatively be given in 2–4 divided doses (max. 9 g daily)
> >
> > Child 1–6 years 2 g once daily in a suitable liquid, adjusted according to response; total daily dose may alternatively be given in 2–4 divided doses (max. 18 g daily)

> > Child 6–12 years 4 g once daily in a suitable liquid, adjusted according to response; total daily dose may alternatively be given in 2–4 divided doses (max. 24 g daily)
> >
> > Child 12–18 years 4–8 g once daily in a suitable liquid, adjusted according to response; total daily dose may alternatively be given in 2–4 divided doses (max. 36 g daily)
> > Counselling Other drugs should be taken at least 1 hour before or 4–6 hours after colestyramine to reduce possible interference with absorption
> > Note For treatment of diarrhoea induced by bile acid malabsorption, if no response within 3 days an alternative therapy should be initiated

> Hypercholesterolaemia section 2.12

Administration The contents of one sachet should be mixed with at least 150 mL of water or other suitable liquid such as fruit juice, skimmed milk, thin soups, or pulpy fruits with a high moisture content

◢Preparations
Section 2.12

1.9.3   Aprotinin

Classification not used in *BNF for Children*.

1.9.4   Pancreatin

Pancreatin, containing a mixture of protease, lipase and amylase in varying proportions, aids the digestion of starch, fat, and protein. Supplements of pancreatin are given by mouth to compensate for reduced or absent exocrine secretion in cystic fibrosis, and following pancreatectomy, total gastrectomy, or chronic pancreatitis.

The dose of pancreatin is adjusted according to size, number, and consistency of stools, and the nutritional status of the child; extra allowance will be needed if snacks are taken between meals. Daily dose should not exceed 10 000 lipase units per kg body-weight per day, (**important**: see CSM advice on Higher-strength preparations below).

1   Gastro-intestinal system

Pancreatin preparations

Preparation	Protease units	Amylase units	Lipase units
Creon® 10 000 capsule, e/c granules	600	8000	10 000
Creon® Micro e/c granules (per 100 mg)	200	3600	5000
Nutrizym 10® capsule, e/c minitablets	500	9000	10 000
Pancrex® granules (per gram)	300	4000	5000
Pancrex V® capsule, powder	430	9000	8000
Pancrex V '125'® capsule, powder	160	3300	2950
Pancrex V® e/c tablet	110	1700	1900
Pancrex V® Forte e/c tablet	330	5000	5600
Pancrex V® powder (per gram)	1400	30 000	25 000

Higher-strength pancreatin preparations *Pancrease HL®* and *Nutrizym 22®* have been associated with the development of large bowel strictures (fibrosing colonopathy) in children with cystic fibrosis aged between 2 and 13 years. The CSM (1995) has recommended the following:

- *Pancrease HL®*, *Nutrizym 22®* should not be used in children under 16 years with cystic fibrosis;

- the total dose of pancreatic enzyme supplements used in patients with cystic fibrosis should not usually exceed 10 000 units of lipase per kg body-weight daily;

- if a patient on any pancreatin preparation develops new abdominal symptoms (or any change in existing abdominal symptoms) the patient should be reviewed to exclude the possibility of colonic damage.

Possible risk factors are gender (boys at greater risk than girls), more severe cystic fibrosis, and concomitant use of laxatives. The peak age for developing fibrosing colonopathy is between 2 and 8 years.

Higher-strength pancreatin preparations

Preparation	Protease units	Amylase units	Lipase units
Creon® 25 000 capsule, e/c pellets	1000	18 000	25 000
Creon® 40 000 capsule, e/c granules	1600	25 000	40 000
Nutrizym 22® capsule, e/c minitablets	1100	19 800	22 000
Pancrease HL® capsule, e/c minitablets	1250	22 500	25 000

Pancreatin is inactivated by gastric acid therefore pancreatin preparations are best taken with food (or immediately before or after food). In children with cystic fibrosis with persistent fat malabsorption despite optimal use of enzyme replacement, an H_2-receptor antagonist (section 1.3.1), or a **proton pump inhibitor** (section 1.3.5) may improve fat digestion and absorption. Enteric-coated preparations are designed to deliver a higher enzyme concentration in the duodenum (provided the capsule contents are swallowed whole without chewing). If the capsules are opened the enteric-coated granules should be mixed with milk, slightly acidic soft food or liquid such as apple juice, and then swallowed immediately without chewing. Any left-over food or liquid containing pancreatin should be discarded. Since pancreatin is also inactivated by heat, excessive heat should be avoided if preparations are mixed with liquids or food.

Pancreatin can irritate the perioral skin and buccal mucosa if retained in the mouth, and excessive doses can cause perianal irritation. Hypersensitivity reactions may occur particularly if the powder is handled.

PANCREATIN

Cautions see CSM advice above; hyperuricaemia and hyperuricosuria have been associated with very high doses; **interactions:** Appendix 1 (pancreatin)

Pregnancy not known to be harmful

Side-effects nausea, vomiting, abdominal discomfort; skin and mucosal irritation (see notes above)

Indication and dose

Pancreatic insufficiency for dose see individual preparations, below

☐ PANCREATIN (continued)

Creon® 10 000 (Solvay)

Capsules, brown/clear, enclosing buff-coloured e/c granules of pancreatin (pork), providing: protease 600 units, lipase 10 000 units, amylase 8000 units, net price 100-cap pack = £14.00. Counselling, see dose

Dose

- **By mouth**

  Child 1 month–18 years initially 1–2 capsules with each meal either taken whole or contents mixed with fluid or soft food (then swallowed immediately without chewing), see notes above

Creon® Micro (Solvay)

Gastro-resistant granules, brown, pancreatin (pork): protease 200 units, lipase 5000 units, amylase 3600 units per 100 mg, net price 20 g = £31.50. Counselling, see dose

Dose

- **By mouth**

  Neonate initially 100 mg before each feed; granules can be mixed with a small amount of breast milk or formula feed and administered immediately (manufacturer recommends mixing with a small amount of apple juice before administration)

  Child 1 month–18 years initially 100 mg before each feed or meal; granules can be mixed with a small amount of milk or soft food and administered immediately (manufacturer recommends mixing with acidic liquid or pureed fruit before administration); see notes above

  Note 100 mg granules = one measured scoopful (scoop supplied with product). Granules should not be chewed before swallowing.

Nutrizym 10® (Merck Serono)

Capsules, red/yellow, enclosing e/c minitablets of pancreatin (pork) providing minimum of: protease 500 units, lipase 10 000 units, amylase 9000 units. Net price 100 = £14.47. Counselling, see dose

Dose

- **By mouth**

  Child 1 month–18 years 1–2 capsules with meals and 1 capsule with snacks, swallowed whole or contents taken with water or mixed with soft food (then swallowed immediately without chewing, see notes above); higher doses may be required according to response

Pancrex® (Paines & Byrne)

Granules, pancreatin (pork), providing minimum of: protease 300 units, lipase 5000 units, amylase 4000 units/g. Net price 300 g = £20.39. Label: 25, counselling, see dose

Excipients include lactose (7 g per 10 g dose)

Dose

- **By mouth**

  Child 2–18 years 5–10 g just before meals washed down or mixed with milk or water

Pancrex V® (Paines & Byrne)

Capsules, pancreatin (pork), providing minimum of: protease 430 units, lipase 8000 units, amylase 9000 units, net price 300-cap pack = £15.80. Counselling, see dose

Dose

- **By mouth**

  Child 1 month–1 year contents of 1–2 capsules mixed with feeds

---

Child 1–18 years 2–6 capsules with meals, swallowed whole or sprinkled on food

Capsules '125', pancreatin (pork), providing minimum of: protease 160 units, lipase 2950 units, amylase 3300 units, net price 300-cap pack = £9.72. Counselling, see dose

Dose

- **By mouth**

  Neonate contents of 1–2 capsules in each feed (or mix with feed and give by spoon)

Tablets, e/c, pancreatin (pork), providing minimum of: protease 110 units, lipase 1900 units, amylase 1700 units, net price 300-tab pack = £4.51. Label: 5, 25, counselling, see dose

Dose

- **By mouth**

  Child 2–18 years 5–15 tablets before meals

Tablets forte, e/c, pancreatin (pork), providing minimum of: protease 330 units, lipase 5600 units, amylase 5000 units, net price 300-tab pack = £13.74. Label: 5, 25, counselling, see dose

Dose

- **By mouth**

  Child 2–18 years 6–10 tablets before meals

Powder, pancreatin (pork), providing minimum of: protease 1400 units, lipase 25 000 units, amylase 30 000 units/g, net price 300 g = £24.28. Counselling, see dose

Dose

- **By mouth**

  Neonate 250–500 mg with each feed

  Child 1 month–18 years 0.5–2 g with meals, washed down or mixed with milk or water

◢ Higher-strength preparations

See **CSM** warning above

Counselling It is important to ensure adequate hydration at all times in children receiving higher-strength pancreatin preparations.

Creon® 25 000 (Solvay) PoM

Capsules, orange/clear, enclosing brown-coloured e/c pellets of pancreatin (pork), providing: protease (total) 1000 units, lipase 25 000 units, amylase 18 000 units, net price 100-cap pack = £28.25. Counselling, see above and under dose

Dose

- **By mouth**

  Child 2–18 years initially 1 capsule with meals either taken whole or contents mixed with fluid or soft food (then swallowed immediately without chewing), see notes above

Creon® 40 000 (Solvay) PoM

Capsules, brown/clear, enclosing brown-coloured e/c granules of pancreatin (pork), providing: protease (total) 1600 units, lipase 40 000 units, amylase 25 000 units, net price 100-cap pack = £60.00. Counselling, see above and under dose

Dose

- **By mouth**

  Child 2–18 years initially 1–2 capsules with meals either taken whole or contents mixed with fluid or soft

◻ **PANCREATIN (*continued*)**

food (then swallowed immediately without chewing), see notes above

Nutrizym 22® (Merck Serono) PoM

Capsules, red/yellow, enclosing e/c minitablets of pancreatin (pork), providing minimum of: protease 1100 units, lipase 22 000 units, amylase 19 800 units, net price 100-cap pack = £33.33. Counselling, see above and under dose

Dose

• **By mouth**

Child 15–18 years 1–2 capsules with meals and 1 capsule with snacks, swallowed whole or contents taken with water or mixed with soft food (then swallowed immediately without chewing), see notes above

Pancrease HL® (Janssen-Cilag) PoM

Capsules, enclosing light brown e/c minitablets of pancreatin (pork), providing minimum of: protease 1250 units, lipase 25 000 units, amylase 22 500 units. Net price 100 = £32.34. Counselling, see above and under dose

Dose

• **By mouth**

Child 15–18 years 1–2 capsules during each meal and 1 capsule with snacks swallowed whole or contents mixed with slightly acidic liquid or soft food (then swallowed immediately without chewing), see notes above

2 Cardiovascular system

2 Cardiovascular system

> This chapter also includes advice on the drug management of the following:
> arrhythmias, p. 108
> heart failure, p. 101
> hypertension, p. 120
> pulmonary hypertension, p. 124

arrhythmias, p. 108
heart failure, p. 101
hypertension, p. 120
pulmonary hypertension, p. 124

2.1 Positive inotropic drugs

2.1.1 Cardiac glycosides
2.1.2 Phosphodiesterase inhibitors

Positive inotropic drugs increase the force of contraction of the myocardium. Drugs which produce inotropic effects include cardiac glycosides, phosphodiesterase inhibitors, and some sympathomimetics (section 2.7.1).

2.1.1 Cardiac glycosides

The cardiac glycoside digoxin increases the force of myocardial contraction and reduces conductivity within the atrioventricular (AV) node.

Digoxin is most useful in the treatment of supraventricular tachycardias, especially for controlling ventricular response in persistent atrial fibrillation (section 2.3.1). Digoxin has a limited role in children with chronic heart failure; for reference to the role of digoxin in heart failure, see section 2.2.

For the management of atrial fibrillation, the maintenance dose of digoxin is determined on the basis of the ventricular rate at rest, which should not be allowed to fall below an acceptable level for the child.

Digoxin is now rarely used for rapid control of heart rate (see section 2.3.2), even with intravenous administration, response may take many hours; persistence of tachycardia is therefore not an indication for exceeding the recommended dose. The intramuscular route is **not** recommended.

In children with heart failure who are in sinus rhythm, a loading dose may not be required.

Unwanted effects depend both on the concentration of digoxin in the plasma and on the sensitivity of the conducting system or of the myocardium, which is often increased in heart disease. It can sometimes be difficult to distinguish between toxic effects and clinical deterioration because the symptoms of both are similar. The plasma-digoxin concentration alone cannot indicate toxicity reliably, but the likelihood of toxicity increases progressively through the range 1.5 to 3 micrograms/litre for digoxin. Renal function is very important in determining digoxin dosage.

Hypokalaemia predisposes the child to digitalis toxicity and should be avoided; it is managed by giving a potassium-sparing diuretic or, if necessary, potassium supplements.

If toxicity occurs, digoxin should be withdrawn; serious manifestations require urgent specialist management. **Digoxin-specific antibody fragments** are available for reversal of life-threatening overdosage (see below).

DIGOXIN

Cautions sick sinus syndrome; thyroid disease; hypoxia; severe respiratory disease; avoid hypokalaemia, hypomagnesaemia, hypercalcaemia, and hypoxia (risk of digitalis toxicity); monitor serum electrolytes and renal function; avoid rapid intravenous administration (risk of hypertension and reduced coronary flow); **interactions:** Appendix 1 (cardiac glycosides)

Contra-indications intermittent complete heart block, second degree AV block; supraventricular arrhythmias associated with accessory conducting pathways e.g. Wolff-Parkinson-White syndrome (although can be used in infancy); ventricular tachycardia or fibrillation; hypertrophic cardiomyopathy (unless concomitant atrial fibrillation and heart failure—but use with caution); myocarditis; constrictive pericarditis (unless for atrial fibrillation or improve systolic dysfunction—but use with caution)

Renal impairment reduce dose; toxicity increased by electrolyte disturbances, adjust dose according to plasma-digoxin concentration

◻ **DIGOXIN** *(continued)*

Pregnancy may need dosage adjustment

Breast-feeding amount too small to be harmful

Side-effects see notes above; also nausea, vomiting, diarrhoea; arrhythmias, conduction disturbances; dizziness; blurred or yellow vision; rash, eosinophilia; *less commonly* depression; *very rarely* anorexia, intestinal ischaemia and necrosis, psychosis, apathy, confusion, headache, fatigue, weakness, gynaecomastia on long-term use, and thrombocytopenia

Pharmacokinetics For plasma-digoxin concentration assay, blood should ideally be taken at least 6 hours after a dose; plasma-digoxin concentration should be maintained in the range 0.8–2 micrograms/litre (see also notes above)

Licensed use heart failure, supraventricular arrhythmias

Indication and dose

Supraventricular arrhythmias and chronic heart failure (see also notes above) consult product literature for details

• By mouth

Neonate under 1.5 kg initially 25 micrograms/kg in 3 divided doses for 24 hours then 4–6 micrograms/kg daily in 1–2 divided doses

Neonate 1.5–2.5 kg initially 30 micrograms/kg in 3 divided doses for 24 hours then 4–6 micrograms/kg daily in 1–2 divided doses

Neonate over 2.5 kg initially 45 micrograms/kg in 3 divided doses for 24 hours then 10 micrograms/kg daily in 1–2 divided doses

Child 1 month–2 years initially 45 micrograms/kg in 3 divided doses for 24 hours then 10 micrograms/kg daily in 1–2 divided doses

Child 2–5 years initially 35 micrograms/kg in 3 divided doses for 24 hours then 10 micrograms/kg daily in 1–2 divided doses

Child 5–10 years initially 25 micrograms/kg (max. 750 micrograms) in 3 divided doses for 24 hours then 6 micrograms/kg daily (max. 250 micrograms daily) in 1–2 divided doses

Child 10–18 years initially 0.75–1.5 mg in 3 divided doses for 24 hours then 62.5–250 micrograms daily in 1–2 divided doses (higher doses may be necessary)

• By intravenous infusion (but rarely necessary)

Neonate under 1.5 kg initially 20 micrograms/kg in 3 divided doses for 24 hours then 4–6 micrograms/kg daily in 1–2 divided doses

Neonate 1.5–2.5 kg initially 30 micrograms/kg in 3 divided doses for 24 hours then 4–6 micrograms/kg daily in 1–2 divided doses

Neonate over 2.5 kg initially 35 micrograms/kg in 3 divided doses for 24 hours then 10 micrograms/kg daily in 1–2 divided doses

Child 1 month–2 years initially 35 micrograms/kg in 3 divided doses for 24 hours then 10 micrograms/kg daily in 1–2 divided doses

Child 2–5 years initially 35 micrograms/kg in 3 divided doses for 24 hours then 10 micrograms/kg daily in 1–2 divided doses

Child 5–10 years initially 25 micrograms/kg (max. 500 micrograms) in 3 divided doses for 24 hours then 6 micrograms/kg daily (max. 250 micrograms daily) in 1–2 divided doses

Child 10–18 years initially 0.5–1 mg in 3 divided doses for 24 hours then 62.5–250 micrograms daily in 1–2 divided doses (higher doses may be necessary)

Note The above doses may need to be reduced if digoxin (or another cardiac glycoside) has been given in the preceding 2 weeks. When switching from intravenous to oral route may need to increase dose by 20–30% to maintain the same plasma-digoxin concentration. Plasma monitoring may be required when changing formulation to take account of varying bioavailabilities. For plasma concentration monitoring, blood should ideally be taken at least 6 hours after a dose

Administration for *intravenous infusion*, dilute with Sodium Chloride 0.9% or Glucose 5% to a max. concentration of 62.5 micrograms/mL; loading doses should be given over 30–60 minutes and maintenance dose over 10–20 minutes. Protect infusion from light.

For *oral* administration, oral solution must **not** be diluted

Digoxin (Non-proprietary) ℗ℴ𝕄

Tablets, digoxin 62.5 micrograms, net price 28-tab pack = £1.64; 125 micrograms, 28-tab pack = £1.18; 250 micrograms, 28-tab pack = £1.19

Injection, digoxin 250 micrograms/mL, net price 2-mL amp = 70p

Excipients include alcohol, propylene glycol (see Excipients, p. 3)

Paediatric injection, digoxin 100 micrograms/mL

Available from 'special-order' manufacturers or specialist importing companies, see p. 957

Lanoxin® (Aspen) ℗ℴ𝕄

Tablets, digoxin 125 micrograms, net price 500-tab pack = £8.09; 250 micrograms (scored), 500-tab pack = £8.09

Injection, digoxin 250 micrograms/mL, net price 2-mL amp = 66p

Lanoxin-PG® (Aspen) ℗ℴ𝕄

Tablets, blue, digoxin 62.5 micrograms, net price 500-tab pack = £8.09

Elixir, yellow, digoxin 50 micrograms/mL. Do not dilute, measure with pipette. Net price 60 mL = £5.35. Counselling, use of pipette

2

Cardiovascular system

Digoxin-specific antibody

Digoxin-specific antibody fragments are indicated for the treatment of known or strongly suspected digoxin or digitoxin overdosage when measures beyond the withdrawal of the cardiac glycoside and correction of any electrolyte abnormalities are felt to be necessary (see also notes above).

Digibind® (GSK) [PoM]
Injection, powder for preparation of infusion, digoxin-specific antibody fragments (F(ab)) 38 mg. Net price per vial = £93.97 (hosp. and poisons centres only)

Dose
Consult product literature or Poisons Information Centre

2.1.2 Phosphodiesterase inhibitors

Enoximone and **milrinone** are selective phosphodiesterase inhibitors that exert most of their effect on the myocardium. They possess positive inotropic and vasodilator activity and are useful in infants and children with low cardiac output especially after cardiac surgery. Phosphodiesterase inhibitors should be limited to short-term use because long-term oral administration has been associated with increased mortality in adults with congestive heart failure.

ENOXIMONE

Cautions heart failure associated with hypertrophic cardiomyopathy, stenotic or obstructive valvular disease or other outlet obstruction; monitor blood pressure, heart rate, ECG, central venous pressure, fluid and electrolyte status, renal function, platelet count, hepatic enzymes; avoid extravasation; **interactions:** Appendix 1 (phosphodiesterase inhibitors)

Hepatic impairment dose reduction may be required

Renal impairment consider dose reduction

Pregnancy manufacturer advises use only if potential benefit outweighs risk

Breast-feeding manufacturer advises caution—no information available

Side-effects ectopic beats; less frequently ventricular tachycardia or supraventricular arrhythmias (more likely in children with pre-existing arrhythmias); hypotension; also headache, insomnia, nausea and vomiting, diarrhoea; occasionally, chills, oliguria, fever, urinary retention; upper and lower limb pain

Licensed use not licensed for use in children

Indication and dose

Congestive heart failure, low cardiac output following cardiac surgery
- By intravenous injection and continuous intravenous infusion

  Neonate initial loading dose of 500 micrograms/kg *by slow intravenous injection*, followed by 5–20 micrograms/kg/minute *by continuous intravenous infusion* over 24 hours adjusted according to response; max 24 mg/kg over 24 hours

  Child 1 month–18 years initial loading dose of 500 micrograms/kg *by slow intravenous injection*, followed by 5–20 micrograms/kg/minute *by continuous intravenous infusion* over 24 hours adjusted according to response; max. 24 mg/kg over 24 hours

Administration for *intravenous administration*, dilute to concentration of 2.5 mg/mL with Sodium Chloride 0.9% *or* Water for Injections; the initial loading dose should be given by slow intravenous injection over at least 15 minutes. Use plastic apparatus—crystal formation if glass used

Perfan® (INCA-Pharm) [PoM]
Injection, enoximone 5 mg/mL. For dilution before use. Net price 20-mL amp = £15.02
Excipients include alcohol, propylene glycol (see Excipients, p. 3)

MILRINONE

Cautions see under Enoximone; also correct hypokalaemia; monitor renal function; **interactions:** Appendix 1 (phosphodiesterase inhibitors)

Renal impairment reduce dose and monitor response if estimated glomerular filtration rate less than $50 \, mL/minute/1.73 \, m^2$

Pregnancy manufacturer advises use only if potential benefit outweighs risk

Breast-feeding manufacturer advises caution—no information available

Side-effects ectopic beats, ventricular tachycardia, supraventricular arrhythmias (more likely in children with pre-existing arrhythmias), hypotension; headache; *less commonly* ventricular fibrillation, chest pain, tremor, hypokalaemia, thrombocytopenia; *very rarely* bronchospasm, anaphylaxis, and rash

Licensed use not licensed for use in children under 18 years

Indication and dose

Congestive heart failure, low cardiac output following cardiac surgery, shock
- By intravenous infusion

  Neonate initially 50–75 micrograms/kg over 30–60 minutes (reduce or omit initial dose if at risk of hypotension) then 30–45 micrograms/kg/hour by *continuous intravenous infusion* for 2–3 days (usually for 12 hours after cardiac surgery)

  Child 1 month–18 years initially 50–75 micrograms/kg over 30–60 minutes (reduce or omit initial dose if at risk of hypotension) then 30–45 micrograms/kg/hour by *continuous intra-*

2 Cardiovascular system

◻ **MILRINONE (continued)**

venous infusion for 2–3 days (usually for 12 hours after cardiac surgery)

Administration for *intravenous infusion* dilute with Glucose 5% *or* Sodium Chloride 0.9% *or* Sodium Chloride and Glucose intravenous infusion to a concentration of 200 micrograms/mL (higher concentrations of 400 micrograms/mL have

been used); loading dose may be given undiluted if fluid-restricted

Primacor® (Sanofi-Aventis) [PoM]
Injection, milrinone (as lactate) 1 mg/mL, net price 10-mL amp = £16.61

2.2 Diuretics

Diuretics are used for a variety of conditions in children including pulmonary oedema (caused by conditions such as respiratory distress syndrome and bronchopulmonary dysplasia), congestive heart failure, and hypertension. Hypertension in children is often resistant to therapy and may require the use of several drugs in combination (see section 2.5). Maintenance of fluid and electrolyte balance can be difficult in children on diuretics, particularly neonates whose renal function may be immature.

Loop diuretics (section 2.2.2) are used for pulmonary oedema, congestive heart failure, and in renal disease.

Thiazides (section 2.2.1) are used less commonly than loop diuretics but are often used in combination with loop diuretics or spironolactone in the management of pulmonary oedema and, in lower doses, for hypertension associated with cardiac disease.

Aminophylline infusion has been used with intravenous furosemide to relieve fluid overload in critically ill children.

Heart failure Heart failure is less common in children than in adults; it can occur as a result of congenital heart disease (e.g. septal defects), dilated cardiomyopathy, myocarditis, or cardiac surgery. Drug treatment of heart failure due to left ventricular systolic dysfunction is covered below; optimal management of heart failure with preserved left ventricular function has not been established.

Acute heart failure can occur after cardiac surgery or as a complication in severe acute infections with or without myocarditis. Therapy consists of volume loading, vasodilator or inotropic drugs.

Chronic heart failure is initially treated with a **loop diuretic** (section 2.2.2), usually furosemide supplemented with spironolactone, amiloride, or potassium. If diuresis with furosemide is insufficient, the addition of metolazone or a thiazide diuretic (section 2.2.1) can be considered. With metolazone, the resulting diuresis can be profound and care is needed to avoid potentially dangerous electrolyte disturbance.

If diuretics are insufficient an ACE inhibitor, titrated to the maximum tolerated dose, can be used. **ACE inhibitors** (section 2.5.5.1) are used for the treatment of all grades of heart failure in adults and can also be useful for children with heart failure. Addition of **digoxin** (section 2.1.1) can be considered in children who remain symptomatic despite treatment with a diuretic and an ACE inhibitor.

Some beta-blockers improve outcome in adults with heart failure, but data on beta-blockers in children are limited. **Carvedilol** (section 2.4) has vasodilatory properties and therefore (like ACE inhibitors) also lowers afterload.

In children receiving specialist cardiology care, the selective phosphodiesterase inhibitor **enoximone** is sometimes used by mouth for its inotropic and vasodilator effects. **Spironolactone** (section 2.2.3) is usually used as a potassium-sparing drug with a loop diuretic; in adults low doses of spironolactone are effective in the treatment of heart failure. Careful monitoring of serum potassium is necessary if spironolactone is used in combination with an ACE inhibitor.

Potassium loss Hypokalaemia can occur with both thiazide and loop diuretics. The risk of hypokalaemia depends on the duration of action as well as the potency and is thus greater with thiazides than with an equipotent dose of a loop diuretic.

2

Cardiovascular system

Hypokalaemia is particularly dangerous in children being treated with cardiac glycosides. In hepatic failure hypokalaemia caused by diuretics can precipitate encephalopathy.

The use of potassium-sparing diuretics (section 2.2.3) avoids the need to take potassium supplements.

2.2.1 Thiazides and related diuretics

Thiazides and related compounds are moderately potent diuretics; they inhibit sodium reabsorption at the beginning of the distal convoluted tubule. They are usually administered early in the day so that the diuresis does not interfere with sleep.

In the management of *hypertension* a low dose of a thiazide produces a maximal or near-maximal blood pressure lowering effect, with very little biochemical disturbance. Higher doses cause more marked changes in plasma potassium, sodium, uric acid, glucose, and lipids, with little advantage in blood pressure control. For reference to the use of thiazides in chronic heart failure see section 2.2.

Bendroflumethiazide is licensed for use in children; **chlorothiazide** is also used.

Chlortalidone (chlorthalidone), a thiazide-related compound, has a longer duration of action than the thiazides and may be given on alternate days in younger children.

Metolazone is particularly effective when combined with a loop diuretic (even in renal failure) and is most effective when given 30–60 minutes before furosemide; profound diuresis can occur and the child should therefore be monitored carefully.

Cautions See also section 2.2. Thiazides and related diuretics can exacerbate diabetes, gout, and systemic lupus erythematosus. Electrolytes should be monitored particularly with high doses, long-term use, or in renal impairment. Thiazides and related diuretics should also be used with caution in nephrotic syndrome, hyperaldosteronism, and malnourishment; **interactions:** Appendix 1 (diuretics).

Contra-indications Thiazides and related diuretics should be avoided in refractory hypokalaemia, hyponatraemia, and hypercalcaemia, symptomatic hyperuricaemia, and Addison's disease.

Hepatic impairment Thiazides and related diuretics should be used with caution in mild to moderate impairment and avoided in severe impairment. Hypokalaemia may precipitate coma, although hypokalaemia can be prevented by using a potassium-sparing diuretic.

Renal impairment Thiazides and related diuretics should be used with caution because they can further reduce renal function. They are ineffective if estimated glomerular filtration rate is less than $30\,mL/minute/1.73\,m^2$ and should be avoided; metolazone remains effective but with a risk of excessive diuresis.

Pregnancy Thiazides and related diuretics should not be used to treat gestational hypertension. They may cause neonatal thrombocytopenia, bone marrow suppression, jaundice, electrolyte disturbances, and hypoglycaemia; placental perfusion may also be reduced. Stimulation of labour, uterine inertia, and meconium staining have also been reported.

Breast-feeding The amount of bendroflumethiazide, chlorothiazide, chlortalidone, and metolazone present in milk is too small to be harmful; large doses may suppress lactation.

Side-effects Side-effects of thiazides and related diuretics include mild gastrointestinal disturbances, postural hypotension, altered plasma-lipid concentrations, metabolic and electrolyte disturbances including hypokalaemia (see also notes above), hyponatraemia, hypomagnesaemia, hypercalcaemia, hyperglycaemia, hypochloraemic alkalosis, and hyperuricaemia, and gout. Less common side-effects include blood disorders including agranulocytosis, leucopenia and thrombocytopenia, and impotence. Pancreatitis, intrahepatic cholestasis, cardiac arrhythmias, headache, dizziness, paraesthesia, visual disturbances, and hypersensitivity reactions (including pneumonitis, pulmonary oedema, photosensitivity, and severe skin reactions) have also been reported.

BENDROFLUMETHIAZIDE
(Bendrofluazide)

Cautions see notes above
Contra-indications see notes above
Hepatic impairment see notes above
Renal impairment see notes above
Pregnancy see notes above
Breast-feeding see notes above
Side-effects see notes above

Indication and dose

Oedema and hypertension
• By mouth
  Child 1 month–2 years 50–100 micrograms/kg daily adjusted according to response

Child 2–12 years initially 50–400 micrograms/kg daily (max. 10 mg daily) then 50–100 micrograms/kg daily adjusted according to response

Child 12–18 years initially 5–10 mg daily or on alternate days (2.5 mg daily in hypertension) as a single morning dose, adjusted according to response

Bendroflumethiazide (Non-proprietary) ℗
Tablets, bendroflumethiazide 2.5 mg, net price 28 = 85p; 5 mg, 28 = 94p
Brands include *Aprinox®, Neo-NaClex®*

◢Extemporaneous formulations available see Extemporaneous Preparations, p. 8

CHLOROTHIAZIDE

Cautions see notes above; also neonate (theoretical risk of kernicterus if very jaundiced)
Contra-indications see notes above
Hepatic impairment see notes above
Renal impairment see notes above
Pregnancy see notes above
Breast-feeding see notes above
Side-effects see notes above
Licensed use not licensed

Indication and dose

Heart failure, hypertension, ascites
• By mouth
  Neonate 10–20 mg/kg twice daily

  Child 1–6 months 10–20 mg/kg twice daily

Child 6 months–12 years 10 mg/kg twice daily (max. 1 g daily)

Child 12–18 years 0.25–1 g once daily *or* 125–500 mg twice daily

Chronic hypoglycaemia section 6.1.4

Diabetes insipidus section 6.5.2

◢Preparations
Chlorothiazide oral suspension 250 mg/5 mL is available from 'special-order' manufacturers or specialist importing companies, see p. 957

CHLORTALIDONE
(Chlorthalidone)

Cautions see notes above
Contra-indications see notes above
Hepatic impairment see notes above
Renal impairment see notes above
Pregnancy see notes above
Breast-feeding see notes above
Side-effects see notes above; also *rarely* jaundice

Indication and dose

Hypertension
• By mouth
  Child 5–12 years 0.5–1 mg/kg in the morning every 48 hours; max. 1.7 mg/kg every 48 hours

  Child 12–18 years 25 mg daily in the morning, increased to 50 mg daily if necessary (but see notes above)

Stable heart failure
• By mouth
  Child 5–12 years 0.5–1 mg/kg in the morning every 48 hours; max. 1.7 mg/kg every 48 hours

  Child 12–18 years 25–50 mg daily in the morning, increased if necessary to 100–200 mg daily (reduce to lowest effective dose for maintenance)

Ascites, oedema in nephrotic syndrome
• By mouth
  Child 5–12 years 0.5–1 mg/kg in the morning every 48 hours; max. 1.7 mg/kg every 48 hours
  Child 12–18 years up to 50 mg daily

Hygroton® (Alliance) ℗
Tablets, yellow, scored, chlortalidone 50 mg, net price 28-tab pack = £1.52

METOLAZONE

Cautions see notes above; also acute porphyria (section 9.8.2)
Contra-indications see notes above
Hepatic impairment see notes above
Renal impairment see notes above
Pregnancy see notes above
Breast-feeding see notes above
Side-effects see notes above; also chills, chest pain
Licensed use not licensed for use in children

◻ **METOLAZONE** (*continued*)

Indication and dose

Oedema resistant to loop diuretics; adjunct to loop diuretics to induce diuresis

• **By mouth**

Child 1 month–12 years 100–200 micrograms/kg once or twice daily

Child 12–18 years 5–10 mg once daily in the morning, increased to 5–10 mg twice daily in resistant oedema

Administration Tablets may be crushed and mixed with water immediately before use

Metenix 5® (Sanofi-Aventis) [PoM]
Tablets, blue, metolazone 5 mg, net price 100-tab pack = £18.20

◢ Extemporaneous formulations available see Extemporaneous Preparations, p. 8

2.2.2 Loop diuretics

Loop diuretics inhibit reabsorption of sodium, potassium, and chloride from the ascending limb of the loop of Henlé in the renal tubule and are powerful diuretics.

Furosemide (frusemide) and **bumetanide** are similar in activity; they produce dose-related diuresis. Furosemide is used extensively in children. It can be used for pulmonary oedema (e.g. in respiratory distress syndrome and bronchopulmonary dysplasia), congestive heart failure, and in renal disease.

Cautions Hypovolaemia and hypotension should be corrected before initiation of treatment with loop diuretics; electrolytes should be monitored during treatment (see also Potassium Loss, section 2.2). Loop diuretics should be used with caution in comatose and precomatose states associated with liver cirrhosis. Loop diuretics can exacerbate diabetes (but hyperglycaemia less likely than with thiazides) and gout; they can also cause acute urinary retention in children with obstruction of urinary outflow, therefore adequate urinary output should be established before initiating treatment.

Contra-indications Loop diuretics should be avoided in severe hypokalaemia, severe hyponatraemia, anuria, and in renal failure due to nephrotoxic or hepatotoxic drugs.

Hepatic impairment Hypokalaemia induced by loop diuretics may precipitate hepatic encephalopathy and coma—potassium-sparing diuretics can be used to prevent this.

Renal impairment High doses of loop diuretics may occasionally be needed; high doses or rapid intravenous administration can cause tinnitus and deafness; high doses of bumetanide can also cause musculoskeletal pain.

Pregnancy Furosemide and bumetanide should not be used to treat gestational hypertension because of the maternal hypovolaemia associated with this condition.

Side-effects Side-effects of loop diuretics include mild gastro-intestinal disturbances, pancreatitis, hepatic encephalopathy, postural hypotension, temporary increase in serum-cholesterol and triglyceride concentration, hyperglycaemia (less common than with thiazides), acute urinary retention, electrolyte disturbances (including hyponatraemia, hypokalaemia (see section 2.2), increased calcium excretion (nephrocalcinosis and nephrolithiasis reported with long-term use of furosemide in preterm infants), hypochloraemia, and hypomagnesaemia), metabolic alkalosis, blood disorders (including bone marrow depression, thrombocytopenia, and leucopenia), hyperuricaemia, visual disturbances, tinnitus and deafness (usually with high doses and rapid intravenous administration, and in renal impairment), rash, and photosensitivity.

◢ FUROSEMIDE

(Frusemide)

Cautions see notes above; also hypoproteinaemia may reduce effect and increase risk of side-effects; hepatorenal syndrome; risk of ototoxicity may be reduced by giving high oral doses in 2 or more divided doses; effect may be prolonged in neonates; some liquid preparations contain alcohol, caution especially in neonates; **interactions:** Appendix 1 (diuretics)

Contra-indications see notes above

Hepatic impairment see notes above

Renal impairment see notes above; also lower rate of infusion may be necessary

Pregnancy see notes above

Breast-feeding amount too small to be harmful; may inhibit lactation

◁ **FUROSEMIDE** (*continued*)

Side-effects see notes above; also intrahepatic cholestasis and gout

Indication and dose

Oedema

• **By mouth**

Neonate 0.5–2 mg/kg every 12–24 hours (every 24 hours if postmenstrual age under 31 weeks)

Child 1 month–12 years 0.5–2 mg/kg 2–3 times daily (every 24 hours if postmenstrual age under 31 weeks); higher doses may be required in resistant oedema; max. 12 mg/kg daily, not to exceed 80 mg daily

Child 12–18 years 20–40 mg daily, increased in resistant oedema to 80–120 mg daily

• **By slow intravenous injection**

Neonate 0.5–1 mg/kg every 12–24 hours (every 24 hours if post-menstrual age under 31 weeks)

Child 1 month–12 years 0.5–1 mg/kg repeated every 8 hours as necessary; max. 2 mg/kg (max. 40 mg) every 8 hours

Child 12–18 years 20–40 mg repeated every 8 hours as necessary; higher doses may be required in resistant cases

• **By continuous intravenous infusion**

Child 1 month–18 years 0.1–2 mg/kg/hour (following cardiac surgery, initially 100 micrograms/kg/hour, doubled every 2 hours until urine output exceeds 1 mL/kg/hour)

Oliguria

• **By mouth**

Child 12–18 years initially 250 mg daily; if necessary, dose increased in steps of 250 mg given every 4–6 hours; max. single dose 2 g (rarely used)

• **By intravenous infusion**

Child 1 month–12 years 2–5 mg/kg up to 4 times daily (max. 1 g daily)

Child 12–18 years initially 250 mg over 1 hour (rate not exceeding 4 mg/minute), increase to 500 mg over 2 hours if satisfactory urine output not obtained, then give a further 1 g over 4 hours if no satisfactory response within subsequent hour, if no response obtained dialysis probably required; effective dose (up to 1 g) can be repeated every 24 hours

Administration for administration *by mouth* tablets can be crushed and mixed with water *or* injection solution diluted and given by mouth.

For *intravenous injection*, give over 5–10 minutes at a usual rate of 100 micrograms/kg/minute (not exceeding 500 micrograms/kg/minute), max. 4 mg/minute.

For *intravenous infusion* dilute with Sodium Chloride 0.9% to a concentration of 1–2 mg/mL—glucose solutions unsuitable (infusion pH must be above 5.5)

Furosemide (Non-proprietary) ⓅⓄⓂ

Tablets, furosemide 20 mg, net price 28 = 85p; 40 mg, 28-tab pack = 90p; 500 mg, 28 = £3.73
Brands include *Froop®, Rusyde®*

Oral solution, sugar-free, furosemide, net price 20 mg/5 mL, 150 mL = £12.41; 40 mg/5 mL, 150 mL = £15.92; 50 mg/5 mL, 150 mL = £17.32
Brands include *Frusol®* (contains alcohol 10%)

Injection, furosemide 10 mg/mL, net price 2-mL amp = 30p; 5-mL amp = 38p; 25-mL amp = £2.50

Lasix® (Sanofi-Aventis) ⓅⓄⓂ

Injection, furosemide 10 mg/mL, net price 2-mL amp = 75p

Note Large-volume furosemide injections also available; brands include *Minijet®*

▰ **BUMETANIDE**

Cautions see notes above
Contra-indications see notes above
Hepatic impairment see notes above
Renal impairment see notes above
Pregnancy see notes above
Breast-feeding no information available; may inhibit lactation
Side-effects see notes above; also gynaecomastia, breast pain, musculoskeletal pain (associated with high doses in renal failure)
Licensed use not licensed for use in children under 12 years

Indication and dose

Oedema

• **By mouth**

Child 1 month–12 years 15–50 micrograms/kg 1–4 times daily (max. single dose 2 mg); do not exceed 5 mg daily

Child 12–18 years 1 mg in the morning, repeated after 6–8 hours if necessary; severe cases up to 5 mg daily

• **By intravenous injection**

Child 12–18 years 1–2 mg, repeated after 20 minutes if necessary

• **By intravenous infusion over 30–60 minutes**

Child 1 month–12 years 25–50 micrograms/kg

Child 12–18 years 1–5 mg

Administration for *intravenous infusion*, dilute with Glucose 5% *or* Sodium Chloride 0.9%; concentrations above 25 micrograms/mL may cause precipitation

Bumetanide (Non-proprietary) ⓅⓄⓂ

Tablets, bumetanide 1 mg, net price 28-tab pack = £1.12; 5 mg, 28-tab pack = £3.89

Oral liquid, bumetanide 1 mg/5 mL, net price 150 mL = £128.00

Injection, bumetanide 500 micrograms/mL, net price 4-mL amp = £1.79

Burinex® (LEO) ⓅⓄⓂ

Tablets, scored, bumetanide 1 mg, net price 28-tab pack = £1.52; 5 mg, 28-tab pack = £9.67

◂ Extemporaneous formulations available see Extemporaneous Preparations, p. 8

2.2.3 Potassium-sparing diuretics and aldosterone antagonists

Spironolactone is the most commonly used potassium-sparing diuretic in children; it is an aldosterone antagonist and enhances potassium retention and sodium excretion in the distal tubule. Spironolactone is combined with other diuretics to reduce urinary potassium loss. It is also used in nephrotic syndrome, the long-term management of Bartter's syndrome, and high doses can help to control ascites in babies with chronic neonatal hepatitis. The clinical value of spironolactone in the management of pulmonary oedema in preterm neonates with chronic lung disease is uncertain.

Potassium canrenoate, given intravenously, is an alternative aldosterone antagonist that may be useful if a potassium-sparing diuretic is required and the child is unable to take oral medication. It is metabolised to canrenone, which is also a metabolite of spironolactone.

Amiloride on its own is a weak diuretic. It causes retention of potassium and is therefore given with thiazide or loop diuretics as an alternative to giving potassium supplements (see section 2.2.4 for compound preparations with thiazides or loop diuretics).

A potassium-sparing diuretic such as spironolactone or amiloride may also be used in the management of amphotericin-induced hypokalaemia.

Potassium supplements must **not** be given with potassium-sparing diuretics. Administration of a potassium-sparing diuretic to a child receiving an ACE inhibitor or an angiotensin-II receptor antagonist (section 2.5.5) can also cause severe hyperkalaemia.

AMILORIDE HYDROCHLORIDE

Cautions monitor electrolytes; diabetes mellitus; interactions: Appendix 1 (diuretics)

Contra-indications hyperkalaemia; anuria; Addison's disease

Renal impairment monitor plasma-potassium concentration (high risk of hyperkalaemia in renal impairment); manufacturers advise avoid in severe impairment

Pregnancy not to be used for treating hypertension in pregnancy

Breast-feeding manufacturer advises avoid—no information available

Side-effects include gastro-intestinal disturbances, dry mouth, rashes, confusion, postural hypotension, hyperkalaemia, hyponatraemia

Licensed use Not licensed for use in children

Indication and dose

Adjunct to thiazide or loop diuretics in oedema or congestive heart failure (where potassium conservation desirable)
* **By mouth**
  Neonate 100–200 micrograms/kg twice daily
  Child 1 month–12 years 100–200 micrograms/kg twice daily; max. 20 mg daily
  Child 12–18 years 5–10 mg twice daily

Amiloride (Non-proprietary) [PoM]
Tablets, amiloride hydrochloride 5 mg, net price 28-tab pack = £1.00
Oral solution, sugar-free, amiloride hydrochloride 5 mg/5 mL, net price 150 mL = £39.73
Brands include *Amilamont*® (*excipients include* propylene glycol, see Excipients p. 3)

◢Compound preparations with thiazide or loop diuretics
See section 2.2.4

Aldosterone antagonists

SPIRONOLACTONE

Cautions potential metabolic products carcinogenic in *rodents*; monitor electrolytes (discontinue if hyperkalaemia); acute porphyria (section 9.8.2); interactions: Appendix 1 (diuretics)

Contra-indications hyperkalaemia, hyponatraemia; anuria; Addison's disease

Renal impairment monitor plasma-potassium concentration (high risk of hyperkalaemia in renal impairment); avoid if rapidly deteriorating or severe impairment

Pregnancy feminisation of male fetus in *animal* studies

Breast-feeding metabolites present in milk but unlikely to be harmful

Side-effects gastro-intestinal disturbances, hepatotoxicity; malaise, headache, confusion, drowsiness, dizziness; gynaecomastia, benign breast tumour, breast pain, menstrual disturbances, changes in libido; hyperkalaemia (discontinue), hyponatraemia, acute renal failure, hyperuricaemia, leucopenia, agranulocytosis, thrombocytopenia; leg cramps; alopecia, hirsutism, rash, and Stevens-Johnson syndrome

◁ **SPIRONOLACTONE** *(continued)*

Licensed use not licensed for reduction of hypo-kalaemia induced by diuretics or amphotericin

Indication and dose

> Diuresis in congestive heart failure, ascites and oedema, nephrotic syndrome, reduction of hypokalaemia induced by diuretics or amphotericin
>
> • **By mouth**
>
> > **Neonate** 1–2 mg/kg daily in 1–2 divided doses; up to 7 mg/kg daily in resistant ascites
> >
> > **Child 1 month–12 years** 1–3 mg/kg daily in 1–2 divided doses; up to 9 mg/kg daily in resistant ascites
> >
> > **Child 12–18 years** 50–100 mg daily in 1–2 divided doses; up to 9 mg/kg daily (max. 400 mg daily) in resistant ascites

Spironolactone (Non-proprietary) ⒫ₒ̄ₘ̄
Tablets, spironolactone 25 mg, net price 28 = £1.82; 50 mg, 28 = £2.44; 100 mg, 28 = £3.19. Label: 21

Oral suspensions, spironolactone 5 mg/5 mL, 10 mg/5 mL, 25 mg/5 mL, 50 mg/5 mL, and 100 mg/5 mL
Available from 'special-order' manufacturers or specialist importing companies, see p. 957

Aldactone® (Pharmacia) ⒫ₒ̄ₘ̄
Tablets, f/c, spironolactone 25 mg (buff), net price 100-tab pack = £8.89; 50 mg (white), 100-tab pack = £17.78; 100 mg (buff), 28-tab pack = £9.96. Label: 21

■ **POTASSIUM CANRENOATE**

Cautions potential metabolic products carcinogenic in *rodents*; monitor electrolytes (discontinue if hyperkalaemia); hypotension; acute porphyria (section 9.8.2); **interactions:** Appendix 1 (diuretics)

Contra-indications hyperkalaemia; hyponatraemia

Renal impairment use with caution and monitor plasma-potassium concentration if estimated glomerular filtration rate 30–60 mL/minute/1.73 m²; avoid if estimated glomerular filtration rate less than 30 mL/minute/1.73 m²

Pregnancy crosses placenta; feminisation and undescended testes in male fetus in *animal* studies—manufacturer advises avoid

Breast-feeding present in breast milk—manufacturer advises avoid

Side-effects drowsiness, headache, ataxia; menstrual irregularities; hyperuricaemia; pain at injection site on rapid administration; *less commonly* thrombocytopenia, eosinophilia, and hyperkalaemia; *rarely* hepatotoxicity, agranulocytosis, osteomalacia, hoarseness and deepening of voice, hypersensitivity reactions (including urticaria and erythema), and alopecia; also gastro-intestinal disturbances, hypotension, transient confusion with high doses, hyponatraemia, hypochloraemic acidosis, mastalgia, gynaecomastia, and hirsutism

Licensed use not licensed for use in the UK

Indication and dose

> Short-term diuresis in congestive heart failure, oedema, and ascites
>
> • **By intravenous injection over at least 3 minutes or intravenous infusion**
>
> > **Neonate** 1–2 mg/kg twice daily
> >
> > **Child 1 month–12 years** 1–2 mg/kg twice daily
> >
> > **Child 12–18 years** 1–2 mg/kg (max. 200 mg) twice daily

Note To convert to equivalent oral spironolactone dose, multiply potassium canrenoate dose by 0.7

Administration consult product literature

◢**Preparations**

Potassium canrenoate injection is available from 'special-order' manufacturers or specialist importing companies, see p. 957

2.2.4 Potassium-sparing diuretics with other diuretics

Although it is preferable to prescribe diuretics separately in children, the use of fixed combinations may be justified in older children if compliance is a problem. The most commonly used preparations are listed below (but they may not be licensed for use in children—consult product literature), for other preparations see the BNF. For **interactions**, see Appendix 1 (diuretics).

◢**Amiloride with thiazides**

Co-amilozide (Non-proprietary) ⒫ₒ̄ₘ̄
Tablets, co-amilozide 2.5/25 (amiloride hydrochloride 2.5 mg, hydrochlorothiazide 25 mg), net price 28-tab pack = £2.41
Brands include *Moduret 25*®

◢**Amiloride with loop diuretics**

Co-amilofruse (Non-proprietary) ⒫ₒ̄ₘ̄
Tablets, co-amilofruse 2.5/20 (amiloride hydrochloride 2.5 mg, furosemide 20 mg). Net price 28-tab pack = £1.24, 56-tab pack = £1.61
Brands include *Frumil LS*®

Tablets, co-amilofruse 5/40 (amiloride hydrochloride 5 mg, furosemide 40 mg). Net price 28-tab pack = £1.30, 56-tab pack = £1.64
Brands include *Frumil*®

Tablets, co-amilofruse 10/80 (amiloride hydrochloride 10 mg, furosemide 80 mg), net price 28-tab pack = £9.33

2

Cardiovascular system

2.2.5 Osmotic diuretics

Mannitol is used to treat cerebral oedema, raised intra-ocular pressure, periph-eral oedema, and ascites.

MANNITOL

Cautions extravasation causes inflammation and thrombophlebitis; monitor fluid and electrolyte balance, serum osmolality, and pulmonary and renal function; assess cardiac function before and during treatment; **interactions:** Appendix 1 (mannitol)

Contra-indications severe heart failure; severe pulmonary oedema; intracranial bleeding (except during craniotomy); anuria; severe dehydration

Renal impairment use with caution in severe impairment

Pregnancy manufacturer advises avoid unless essential—no information available

Breast-feeding manufacturer advises avoid unless essential—no information available

Side-effects *less commonly* hypotension, throm-bophlebitis, fluid and electrolyte imbalance; *rarely* dry mouth, thirst, nausea, vomiting, oedema, raised intracranial pressure, arrhythmia, hypertension, pulmonary oedema, chest pain, headache, convulsions, dizziness, chills, fever, urinary retention, focal osmotic nephrosis, dehy-dration, cramp, blurred vision, rhinitis, skin necrosis, and hypersensitivity reactions (includ-ing urticaria and anaphylaxis); *very rarely* con-gestive heart failure and acute renal failure

Licensed use not licensed for use in children under 12 years

Indication and dose

Cerebral oedema, raised intra-ocular pressure
- By intravenous infusion over 30–60 minutes
  Child 1 month–12 years 0.25–1.5 g/kg repeated if necessary 1–2 times after 4–8 hours
  Child 12–18 years 0.25–2 g/kg repeated if necessary 1–2 times after 4–8 hours

Peripheral oedema and ascites
- By intravenous infusion over 2–6 hours
  Child 1 month–18 years 1–2 g/kg

Administration examine infusion for crystals; if crystals present, dissolve by warming infusion fluid (allow to cool to body temperature before administration); for mannitol 20%, an in-line filter is recommended (15-micron filters have been used)

Mannitol (Baxter) [PoM]
Intravenous infusion, mannitol 10%, net price 500-mL *Viaflex*® bag = £1.87, 500-mL *Viaflo*® bag = £2.15; 20%, 250-mL *Viaflex*® bag = £2.70, 250-mL *Viaflo*® bag = £3.10, 500-mL *Viaflex*® bag = £2.72, 500-mL *Viaflo*® bag = £3.12

2.2.6 Mercurial diuretics

Classification not used in *BNF for Children*.

2.2.7 Carbonic anhydrase inhibitors

The carbonic anhydrase inhibitor **acetazolamide** is a weak diuretic although it is little used for its diuretic effect. Acetazolamide and eye drops of dorzolamide and brinzolamide inhibit the formation of aqueous humour and are used in glaucoma (section 11.6). In children, acetazolamide is also used in the treatment of epilepsy (section 4.8.1), and raised intracranial pressure (section 11.6).

2.2.8 Diuretics with potassium

Diuretics and potassium supplements should be prescribed separately for chil-dren.

2.3 Anti-arrhythmic drugs

2.3.1 Management of arrhythmias
2.3.2 Drugs for arrhythmias

2.3.1 Management of arrhythmias

Management of an arrhythmia requires precise diagnosis of the type of arrhyth-mia; electrocardiography and referral to a paediatric cardiologist is essential; underlying causes such as heart failure require appropriate treatment.

Arrhythmias may be broadly divided into bradycardias, supraventricular tachy-cardias, and ventricular arrhythmias.

Bradycardia Adrenaline (epinephrine) is useful in the treatment of symptomatic bradycardia in an infant or child.

Supraventricular tachycardias

In supraventricular tachycardia adenosine is given by rapid intravenous injection. If adenosine is ineffective, intravenous amiodarone, flecainide, or a beta-blocker (such as esmolol, see section 2.4) can be tried; verapamil can also be considered in children over 1 year. Atenolol, sotalol (section 2.4), and flecainide are used for the prophylaxis of paroxysmal supraventricular tachycardias.

The use of d.c. shock and vagal stimulation also have a role in the treatment of supraventricular tachycardia.

Syndromes associated with accessory conducting pathways   Amiodarone, flecainide, or a beta-blocker is used to prevent recurrence of supraventricular tachycardia in infants and young children with these syndromes (e.g. Wolff-Parkinson-White syndrome).

Atrial flutter   In atrial flutter without structural heart defects, sinus rhythm is restored with d.c. shock or cardiac pacing; drug treatment is usually not necessary. Amiodarone is used in atrial flutter when structural heart defects are present or after heart surgery. Sotalol (section 2.4) may also be considered.

Atrial fibrillation   Atrial fibrillation is very rare in children. To restore sinus rhythm d.c. shock is used; beta-blockers, alone or together with digoxin, may be useful for ventricular rate control.

Ectopic tachycardia   Intravenous amiodarone is used in conjunction with body cooling and synchronised pacing in *postoperative* junctional ectopic tachycardia. Oral amiodarone or flecainide are used in *congenital* junctional ectopic tachycardia.

Amiodarone, flecainide, or a beta-blocker are used in atrial ectopic tachycardia; amiodarone is preferred in those with poor ventricular function.

Ventricular tachycardia and ventricular fibrillation

Pulseless ventricular tachycardia or ventricular fibrillation require resuscitation, see Paediatric Advanced Life Support algorithm (inside back cover). Amiodarone is used in resuscitation for pulseless ventricular tachycardia or ventricular fibrillation unresponsive to d.c. shock; lidocaine can be used as an alternative only if amiodarone is not available.

Amiodarone is also used in a haemodynamically stable child when drug treatment is required; lidocaine can be used as an alternative only if amiodarone is not available.

Torsade de pointes   Torsade de pointes is a form of ventricular tachycardia associated with long QT syndrome, which may be congenital or drug induced. Episodes may be self-limiting, but are frequently recurrent and can cause impairment or loss of consciousness. If not controlled, the arrhythmia can progress to ventricular fibrillation and sometimes death. Intravenous magnesium sulphate (section 9.5.1.3) can be used to treat torsade de pointes (dose recommendations vary—consult local guidelines). Anti-arrhythmics can further prolong the QT interval, thus worsening the condition.

2.3.2 Drugs for arrhythmias

Anti-arrhythmic drugs can be classified clinically as those acting on supraventricular arrhythmias (adenosine, digoxin, and verapamil), those acting on both supraventricular and ventricular arrhythmias (amiodarone, beta-blockers, flecainide, and procainamide), and those acting on ventricular arrhythmias (lidocaine (lignocaine)). For the treatment of bradycardia, see section 2.3.1.

Anti-arrhythmic drugs can also be classified according to their effects on the electrical behaviour of myocardial cells during activity (the Vaughan Williams classification) although this classification is of less clinical significance:

Class I: membrane stabilising drugs (e.g. lidocaine, flecainide)

Class II: beta-blockers

Class III: amiodarone; sotalol (also Class II)

Class IV: calcium-channel blockers (includes verapamil but not dihydropyridines)

2

Cardiovascular system

Cautions The negative inotropic effects of anti-arrhythmic drugs tend to be additive. Therefore special care should be taken if two or more are used, especially if myocardial function is impaired. Most drugs that are effective in countering arrhythmias can also provoke them in some circumstances; moreover, hypokalaemia enhances the arrhythmogenic (pro-arrhythmic) effect of many drugs.

Adenosine is the treatment of choice for terminating supraventricular tachycardias, including those associated with accessory conducting pathways (e.g. Wolff-Parkinson-White syndrome). It is also used in the diagnosis of supraventricular arrhythmias. It is not negatively inotropic and does not cause significant hypotension; it can be used safely in children with impaired cardiac function or postoperative arrhythmias. The injection should be administered by rapid intravenous injection into a central or large peripheral vein.

Amiodarone is useful in the management of both supraventricular and ventricular tachyarrhythmias. It can be given by intravenous infusion and by mouth, and causes little or no myocardial depression. Unlike oral amiodarone, intravenous amiodarone acts relatively rapidly. Intravenous amiodarone is also used in cardiopulmonary resuscitation for ventricular fibrillation or pulseless ventricular tachycardia unresponsive to d.c. shock (see algorithm, inside back cover).

Amiodarone has a very long half-life (extending to several weeks) and only needs to be given once daily (but high doses may cause nausea unless divided). Many weeks or months may be required to achieve steady-state plasma-amiodarone concentration; this is particularly important when drug interactions are likely (see also Appendix 1).

Most patients taking amiodarone develop corneal microdeposits (reversible on withdrawal of treatment); these rarely interfere with vision, but drivers may be dazzled by headlights at night. However, if vision is impaired or if optic neuritis or optic neuropathy occur, amiodarone must be stopped to prevent blindness and expert advice sought. Because of the possibility of phototoxic reactions, children and carers should be advised to shield the child's skin from light during treatment and for several months after discontinuing amiodarone; a wide-spectrum sunscreen (section 13.8.1) should be used to protect against both long-wave ultraviolet and visible light.

Amiodarone contains iodine and can cause disorders of thyroid function; both hypothyroidism and hyperthyroidism can occur. Clinical assessment alone is unreliable, and laboratory tests should be performed before treatment and every 6 months. Thyroxine (T4) may be raised in the absence of hyperthyroidism; therefore tri-iodothyronine (T3), T4, and thyroid-stimulating hormone (thyrotrophin, TSH) should all be measured. A raised T3 and T4 with a very low or undetectable TSH concentration suggests the development of thyrotoxicosis. The thyrotoxicosis may be very refractory, and amiodarone should usually be withdrawn at least temporarily to help achieve control; treatment with carbimazole may be required. Hypothyroidism can be treated with replacement therapy without withdrawing amiodarone if it is essential; careful supervision is required.

Pneumonitis should always be suspected if new or progressive shortness of breath or cough develops in a patient taking amiodarone. Fresh neurological symptoms should raise the possibility of peripheral neuropathy. Amiodarone is also associated with hepatotoxicity (see under amiodarone, below).

Beta-blockers act as anti-arrhythmic drugs principally by attenuating the effects of the sympathetic system on automaticity and conductivity within the heart, for details see section 2.4. For special reference to the role of **sotalol** in ventricular arrhythmias, see section 2.4.

Oral administration of **digoxin** (section 2.1.1) slows the ventricular rate in atrial fibrillation and in atrial flutter. However, intravenous infusion of digoxin is rarely effective for rapid control of ventricular rate.

Flecainide is useful for the treatment of resistant re-entry supraventricular tachycardia, ventricular tachycardia, ventricular ectopic beats, arrhythmias associated with accessory conducting pathways (e.g. Wolff-Parkinson-White syndrome), and paroxysmal atrial fibrillation. Flecainide crosses the placenta and can be used to control fetal supraventricular arrhythmias.

Lidocaine (lignocaine) can be used in cardiopulmonary resuscitation in children with ventricular fibrillation or pulseless ventricular tachycardia unresponsive to d.c. shock, but only if amiodarone is not available. Doses may need to be reduced in children with persistently poor cardiac output and hepatic or renal failure (see under lidocaine, below).

Verapamil (section 2.6.2) can cause severe haemodynamic compromise (refractory hypotension and cardiac arrest) when used for the acute treatment of arrhythmias in neonates and infants; it is contra-indicated in children under 1 year. It is also contra-indicated in those with congestive heart failure, syndromes associated with accessory conducting pathways (e.g. Wolff-Parkinson-White syndrome) and in most receiving concomitant beta-blockers. It can be useful in older children with supraventricular tachycardia.

ADENOSINE

Cautions monitor ECG and have resuscitation facilities available; atrial fibrillation or flutter with accessory pathway (conduction down anomalous pathway may increase); first degree AV block; bundle branch block; left main coronary artery stenosis; uncorrected hypovolaemia; stenotic valvular heart disease; left to right shunt; pericarditis; pericardial effusion; autonomic dysfunction; stenotic carotid artery disease with cerebrovascular insufficiency; recent myocardial infarction; heart failure; heart transplant (see dose); **interactions:** Appendix 1 (adenosine)

Contra-indications second- or third-degree AV block and sick sinus syndrome (unless pacemaker fitted); long QT syndrome; severe hypotension; decompensated heart failure; asthma

Pregnancy large doses may produce fetal toxicity; manufacturer advises use only if essential

Breast-feeding no information available—unlikely to be present in milk owing to short half-life

Side-effects nausea; arrhythmia (discontinue if asystole or severe bradycardia occur), sinus pause, AV block, flushing, angina (discontinue), dizziness; dyspnoea; headache; *less commonly* metallic taste, palpitation, hyperventilation, weakness, blurred vision, sweating; *very rarely* transient worsening of intracranial hypertension, bronchospasm, injection-site reactions; *also reported* vomiting, syncope, hypotension (discontinue if severe), cardiac arrest, respiratory failure (discontinue), and convulsions

Licensed use not licensed for use in children

Indication and dose

Arrhythmias (see also section 2.3.1), diagnosis of arrhythmias
• **By rapid intravenous injection**

Neonates 150 micrograms/kg; if necessary repeat injection every 1–2 minutes increasing

dose by 50–100 micrograms/kg until tachycardia terminated or max. single dose of 300 micrograms/kg given

Child 1 month–1 year 150 micrograms/kg; if necessary repeat injection every 1–2 minutes increasing the dose by 50–100 micrograms/kg until tachycardia terminated or max. single dose of 500 micrograms/kg given

Child 1–12 years 100 micrograms/kg; if necessary repeat injection every 1–2 minutes increasing dose by 50–100 micrograms/kg until tachycardia terminated or max. single dose of 500 micrograms/kg (max. 12 mg) given

Child 12–18 years initially 3 mg; if necessary followed by 6 mg after 1–2 minutes, and then by 12 mg after a further 1–2 minutes

Note In some children over 12 years 3-mg dose ineffective (e.g. if a small peripheral vein is used for administration) and higher initial dose sometimes used; however, those with *heart transplant* are **very sensitive** to the effects of adenosine, and should **not** receive higher initial doses. In children receiving dipyridamole reduce dose to a quarter of usual dose of adenosine

Administration by *rapid intravenous injection* over 2 seconds into central or large peripheral vein followed by rapid Sodium Chloride 0.9% flush; Injection solution may be diluted with Sodium Chloride 0.9% if required

Adenocor® (Sanofi-Aventis) ℗ℴ℧
Injection, adenosine 3 mg/mL in physiological saline, net price 2-mL vial = £4.45 (hosp. only)

Note Intravenous infusion of adenosine (*Adenoscan®*, Sanofi-Aventis) may be used in conjunction with radionuclide myocardial perfusion imaging in patients who cannot exercise adequately or for whom exercise is inappropriate—consult product literature

AMIODARONE HYDROCHLORIDE

Cautions liver-function and thyroid-function tests required before treatment and then every 6 months (see notes above for tests of thyroid function); hypokalaemia (measure serum-potassium concentration before treatment); pulmonary function tests and chest x-ray required before treatment; heart failure; severe bradycardia and conduction disturbances in excessive dosage; intravenous use may cause moderate and transient fall in blood pressure (circulatory collapse precipitated by rapid administration or overdosage) or severe hepato-cellular toxicity (monitor

transaminases closely); ECG monitoring and resuscitation facilities must be available during intravenous use; acute porphyria (section 9.8.2); avoid benzyl alcohol containing injections in neonates (see Excipients, p. 3); **interactions:** Appendix 1 (amiodarone)

Contra-indications *except in cardiac arrest:* sinus bradycardia, sino-atrial heart block; unless pacemaker fitted avoid in severe conduction disturbances or sinus node disease; thyroid dysfunction; iodine sensitivity; avoid *intravenous use* in severe respiratory failure, circulatory collapse, or

Cardiovascular system

2

▱ **AMIODARONE HYDROCHLORIDE** (*continued*)

severe arterial hypotension; avoid bolus injection in congestive heart failure or cardiomyopathy; avoid rapid loading after cardiac surgery

Pregnancy possible risk of neonatal goitre; use only if no alternative

Breast-feeding avoid; significant amount present in milk—risk of neonatal hypothyroidism from release of iodine

Side-effects nausea, vomiting, taste disturbances, raised serum transaminases (may require dose reduction or withdrawal if accompanied by acute liver disorders), jaundice; bradycardia (see Cautions); pulmonary toxicity (including pneumonitis and fibrosis); tremor, sleep disorders; hypothyroidism, hyperthyroidism; reversible corneal microdeposits (sometimes with night glare); phototoxicity, persistent slate-grey skin discoloration (see also notes above); *less commonly* onset or worsening of arrhythmia, conduction disturbances (see Cautions), peripheral neuropathy and myopathy (usually reversible on withdrawal); *very rarely* chronic liver disease including cirrhosis, sinus arrest, bronchospasm (in patients with severe respiratory failure), ataxia, benign intracranial hypertension, headache, vertigo, epididymo-orchitis, impotence, haemolytic or aplastic anaemia, thrombocytopenia, rash (including exfoliative dermatitis), hypersensitivity including vasculitis, alopecia, impaired vision due to optic neuritis or optic neuropathy (including blindness), anaphylaxis on rapid injection, also hypotension, respiratory distress syndrome, sweating, and hot flushes

Licensed use Not licensed for use in children under 3 years

Indication and dose

> Supraventricular and ventricular arrhythmias see notes above (initiated in hospital or under specialist supervision)
>
> • **By mouth**
>
> > **Neonate** initially 5–10 mg/kg twice daily for 7–10 days, then reduced to maintenance dose of 5–10 mg/kg once daily
> >
> > **Child 1 month–12 years** initially 5–10 mg/kg (max. 200 mg) twice daily for 7–10 days, then reduced to maintenance dose of 5–10 mg/kg once daily (max. 200 mg daily)
> >
> > **Child 12–18 years** 200 mg 3 times daily for 1 week then 200 mg twice daily for 1 week then usually 200 mg daily adjusted according to response
>
> • **By intravenous infusion**
>
> > **Neonate** initially 5 mg/kg over 30 minutes then 5 mg/kg over 30 minutes every 12–24 hours

> **Child 1 month–18 years** initially 5–10 mg/kg over 20 minutes–2 hours then *by continuous infusion* 300 micrograms/kg/hour, increased according to response to max. 1.5 mg/kg/hour; do not exceed 1.2 g in 24 hours

> Ventricular fibrillation or pulseless ventricular tachycardia refractory to defibrillation (see also section 2.3.1)
>
> • **By intravenous injection**
>
> > **Neonate** 5 mg/kg over at least 3 minutes
> >
> > **Child 1 month–18 years** 5 mg/kg (max. 300 mg) over at least 3 minutes

Administration intravenous administration via central venous catheter recommended if repeated or continuous infusion required, as infusion via peripheral veins may cause pain and inflammation.

For *intravenous infusion* dilute to a concentration of not less than 600 micrograms/mL with Glucose 5%; incompatible with Sodium Chloride infusion; avoid equipment containing the plasticizer di-2-ethylhexphthalate (DEHP).

For administration *by mouth*, tablets may be crushed and dispersed in water; injection solution should **not** be given orally (irritant)

Amiodarone (Non-proprietary) ℗ₒₘ

Tablets, amiodarone hydrochloride 100 mg, net price 28-tab pack = £1.38; 200 mg, 28-tab pack = £1.52. Label: 11

Injection, amiodarone hydrochloride 30 mg/mL, net price 10-mL prefilled syringe = £20.90
Excipients may include benzyl alcohol (avoid in neonates unless no safer alternative available, see Excipients, p. 3)

Sterile concentrate, amiodarone hydrochloride 50 mg/mL, net price 3-mL amp = £1.33, 6-mL amp = £2.86. For dilution and use as an infusion
Excipients may include benzyl alcohol (avoid in neonates unless no safer alternative available, see Excipients, p. 3)

◢ Extemporaneous formulations available see Extemporaneous Preparations, p. 8

Cordarone X® (Sanofi-Aventis) ℗ₒₘ

Tablets, scored, amiodarone hydrochloride 100 mg, net price 28-tab pack = £4.28; 200 mg, 28-tab pack = £6.99. Label: 11

Sterile concentrate, amiodarone hydrochloride 50 mg/mL, net price 3-mL amp = £1.33. For dilution and use as an infusion
Excipients include benzyl alcohol (avoid in neonates unless no safer alternative, see Excipients, p. 3)

◢ **FLECAINIDE ACETATE**

Cautions children with pacemakers (especially those who may be pacemaker dependent because stimulation threshold may rise appreciably); atrial fibrillation following heart surgery; monitor ECG and have resuscitation facilities available during

intravenous use; **interactions**: Appendix 1 (flecainide)

Contra-indications heart failure; abnormal left ventricular function; long-standing atrial fibrillation where conversion to sinus rhythm not attempted; haemodynamically significant valvu-

◁ **FLECAINIDE ACETATE** (*continued*)

lar heart disease; avoid in sinus node dysfunction, atrial conduction defects, second-degree or greater AV block, bundle branch block or distal block unless pacing rescue available

Hepatic impairment avoid or reduce dose in severe impairment; monitor plasma concentration (see pharmacokinetics below)

Renal impairment reduce dose by 25–50% if estimated glomerular filtration rate less than 35 mL/minute/1.73 m^2 and monitor plasma-flecainide concentration (see pharmacokinetics below)

Pregnancy used in pregnancy to treat maternal and fetal arrhythmias in specialist centres; toxicity reported in *animal* studies; infant hyperbilirubinaemia also reported

Breast-feeding significant amount present in milk but not known to be harmful

Side-effects oedema, pro-arrhythmic effects; dyspnoea; dizziness, asthenia, fatigue, fever; visual disturbances; *rarely* pneumonitis, hallucinations, depression, confusion, amnesia, dyskinesia, convulsions, peripheral neuropathy; *also reported* gastro-intestinal disturbances, anorexia, hepatic dysfunction, flushing, syncope, drowsiness, tremor, vertigo, headache, anxiety, insomnia, ataxia, paraesthesia, hypoaesthesia, anaemia, leucopenia, thrombocytopenia, corneal deposits, tinnitus, increased antinuclear antibodies, hypersensitivity reactions (including rash, urticaria, and photosensitivity), increased sweating

Pharmacokinetics plasma-flecainide concentration for optimal response 200–800 micrograms/litre; blood sample should be taken immediately before next dose

Licensed use Not licensed for use in children under 12 years

Indication and dose

> Resistant re-entry supraventricular tachycardia, ventricular ectopic beats or ventricular tachycardia, arrhythmias associated with accessory conduction pathways (e.g. Wolff-Parkinson-White syndrome), paroxysmal atrial fibrillation
> - By mouth
>> **Neonate** 2 mg/kg 2–3 times daily adjusted according to response and plasma-flecainide concentration
>>
>> **Child 1 month–12 years** 2 mg/kg 2–3 times daily adjusted according to response and plasma-flecainide concentration (max. 8 mg/kg/day or 300 mg daily)
>>
>> **Child 12–18 years** initially 50–100 mg twice daily; max. 300 mg daily (max. 400 mg daily for ventricular arrhythmias in heavily built children)

> - By slow intravenous injection or intravenous infusion
>> **Neonate** 1–2 mg/kg over 10–30 minutes; if necessary followed by continuous infusion at a rate of 100–250 micrograms/kg/hour until arrhythmia controlled; transfer to *oral* treatment as above
>>
>> **Child 1 month–12 years** 2 mg/kg over 10–30 minutes; if necessary followed by continuous infusion at a rate of 100–250 micrograms/kg/hour until arrhythmia controlled (max. cumulative dose 600 mg in 24 hours); transfer to *oral* treatment as above
>>
>> **Child 12–18 years** 2 mg/kg (max. 150 mg) over 10–30 minutes; if necessary followed by continuous infusion at a rate of 1.5 mg/kg/hour for 1 hour, then reduced to 100–250 micrograms/kg/hour until arrhythmia controlled (max. cumulative dose 600 mg in first 24 hours); transfer to *oral* treatment as above

Administration for administration *by mouth*, milk, infant formula, and dairy products may reduce absorption of flecainide—separate doses from feeds. Liquid has a local anaesthetic effect and should be given at least 30 minutes before or after food. Do not store liquid in refrigerator as precipitation occurs.

For *intravenous administration*, give initial dose over 30 minutes in children with sustained ventricular tachycardia or cardiac failure.

Dilute injection using Glucose 5%; concentrations of more than 300 micrograms/mL are unstable in chloride-containing solutions

Flecainide (Non-proprietary) ▣oM

Tablets, flecainide acetate 50 mg, net price 60-tab pack = £7.35; 100 mg, 60-tab pack = £11.38

Liquid, available from 'special-order' manufacturers or specialist importing companies, see p. 957

Tambocor® (3M) ▣oM

Tablets, flecainide acetate 50 mg, net price 60-tab pack = £13.25; 100 mg (scored), 60-tab pack = £19.00

Injection, flecainide acetate 10 mg/mL, net price 15-mL amp = £4.40

◀ **Modified release**

Tambocor® XL (Meda) ▣oM

Capsules, m/r, grey/pink, flecainide acetate 200 mg, net price 30-cap pack = £14.77. Label: 25

Dose

> Supraventricular arrhythmias
> - By mouth
>> **Child 12–18 years** 200 mg once daily
>> Note Not to be used to control arrhythmias in acute situations; children stabilised on 200 mg daily of immediate-release flecainide may be transferred to *Tambocor® XL*

▮ **LIDOCAINE HYDROCHLORIDE**

(Lignocaine hydrochloride)

Cautions lower doses in congestive heart failure and following cardiac surgery; monitor ECG; resuscitation facilities should be available; **interactions:** Appendix 1 (lidocaine)

Contra-indications sino-atrial disorders, all grades of atrioventricular block, severe myocardial depression; acute porphyria (section 9.8.2)

2

Cardiovascular system

◻ **LIDOCAINE HYDROCHLORIDE** (*continued*)

Hepatic impairment manufacturer advises caution—increased risk of side-effects

Renal impairment possible accumulation of lidocaine and active metabolite; manufacturers advise caution in severe impairment

Pregnancy crosses the placenta but not known to be harmful in *animal* studies—use if benefit outweighs risk

Breast-feeding present in milk but amount too small to be harmful

Side-effects dizziness, paraesthesia, or drowsiness (particularly if injection too rapid); other CNS effects include confusion, respiratory depression and convulsions; hypotension and bradycardia (may lead to cardiac arrest); *rarely* hypersensitivity reactions including anaphylaxis

Licensed use not licensed for use in children under 1 year

Indication and dose

Ventricular arrhythmias, pulseless ventricular tachycardia or ventricular fibrillation

• By intravenous or intraosseous injection, and intravenous infusion

Neonate 0.5–1 mg/kg by injection followed by infusion of 0.6–3 mg/kg/hour; if infusion not immediately available following initial injection, injection of 0.5–1 mg/kg may be repeated at intervals of not less than 5 minutes (to max. total dose 3 mg/kg)

Child 1 month–12 years 0.5–1 mg/kg by injection followed by infusion of 0.6–3 mg/kg/hour;

if infusion not immediately available following initial injection, injection of 0.5–1 mg/kg may be repeated at intervals of not less than 5 minutes (to max. total dose 3 mg/kg)

Child 12–18 years 50–100 mg by injection followed by infusion of 120 mg over 30 minutes *then* 240 mg over 2 hours *then* 60 mg/hour; reduce dose further if infusion continued beyond 24 hours; if infusion not immediately available following initial injection, injection of 50–100 mg may be repeated at intervals of not less than 5 minutes (to max. 300 mg in 1 hour)

Eye section 11.7

Local anaesthesia section 15.2

Administration for *intravenous infusion*, dilute with Glucose 5% or Sodium Chloride 0.9%

Lidocaine (Non-proprietary) ▣
Injection 2%, lidocaine hydrochloride 20 mg/mL, net price 2-mL amp = 27p; 5-mL amp = 27p; 10-mL amp = 60p; 20-mL amp = 61p

Infusion, lidocaine hydrochloride 0.1% (1 mg/mL) and 0.2% (2 mg/mL) in glucose intravenous infusion 5%. 500-mL containers

Minijet® Lignocaine (UCB Pharma) ▣
Injection, lidocaine hydrochloride 1% (10 mg/mL), net price 10-mL disposable syringe = £5.34; 2% (20 mg/mL), 5-mL disposable syringe = £5.20

2.4 Beta-adrenoceptor blocking drugs

Beta-adrenoceptor blocking drugs (beta-blockers) block the beta-adrenoceptors in the heart, peripheral vasculature, bronchi, pancreas, and liver.

Many beta-blockers are available but experience in children is limited to the use of only a few.

Differences between beta-blockers may affect choice. The water-soluble beta-blockers, atenolol and sotalol, are less likely to enter the brain and may therefore cause less sleep disturbance and nightmares. Water-soluble beta-blockers are excreted by the kidneys and dosage reduction is often necessary in renal impairment.

Some beta-blockers, such as atenolol, have an intrinsically longer duration of action and need to be given only once daily. Carvedilol and labetalol are beta-blockers which have, in addition, an arteriolar vasodilating action and thus lower peripheral resistance. Although carvedilol and labetalol possess both alpha- and beta-blocking properties, these drugs have no important advantages over other beta-blockers in the treatment of hypertension.

Beta-blockers slow the heart and can depress the myocardium; they are contraindicated in children with second- or third-degree heart block. Sotalol may prolong the QT interval, and it occasionally causes life-threatening ventricular arrhythmias (**important**: particular care is required to avoid hypokalaemia in children taking sotalol).

Beta-blockers can precipitate asthma and should usually be avoided in children with a history of asthma or bronchospasm. If there is no alternative, a child with well-controlled asthma can be treated for a co-existing condition (e.g. arrhythmia) with a cardioselective beta-blocker, which should be initiated with caution at a low dose by a specialist and the child monitored closely for adverse effects. Atenolol and metoprolol have less effect on the beta$_2$ (bronchial) receptors and are, therefore, relatively *cardioselective*, but they are not *cardiospecific*; they have a lesser effect on airways resistance but are not free of this side-effect.

Beta-blockers are also associated with fatigue, coldness of the extremities, and sleep disturbances with nightmares (may be less common with the water-soluble beta-blockers, see above).

Beta-blockers can affect carbohydrate metabolism causing hypoglycaemia or hyperglycaemia in children with or without diabetes; they can also interfere with metabolic and autonomic responses to hypoglycaemia thereby masking symptoms such as tachycardia. However, beta-blockers are not contra-indicated in diabetes, although the cardioselective beta-blockers (e.g. atenolol and metoprolol) may be preferred. Beta-blockers should be avoided altogether in those with frequent episodes of hypoglycaemia.

Pregnancy   Beta-blockers may cause intra-uterine growth restriction, neonatal hypoglycaemia, and bradycardia; the risk is greater in severe hypertension. The use of labetalol in maternal hypertension is not known to be harmful, except possibly in the first trimester. Information on the safety of carvedilol during pregnancy is lacking. If beta-blockers are used close to delivery, infants should be monitored for signs of beta-blockade (and alpha-blockade with labetalol or carvedilol). For the treatment of hypertension in pregnancy, see section 2.5.

Breast-feeding   Infants should be monitored as there is a risk of possible toxicity due to beta-blockade (and alpha-blockade with labetalol or carvedilol), but the amount of most beta-blockers present in milk is too small to affect infants. Atenolol and sotalol are present in milk in greater amounts than other beta-blockers. The manufacturer of esmolol advises avoidance if breast-feeding.

Hypertension   Beta-blockers are effective for reducing blood pressure (section 2.5), but their mode of action is not understood; they reduce cardiac output, alter baroceptor reflex sensitivity, and block peripheral adrenoceptors. Some beta-blockers depress plasma renin secretion. It is possible that a central effect may also partly explain their mode of action. Blood pressure can usually be controlled with relatively few side-effects. In general the dose of beta-blocker does not have to be high.

Labetalol may be given intravenously for *hypertensive emergencies* in children (section 2.5); however, care is needed to avoid dangerous hypotension or beta-blockade, particularly in neonates. **Esmolol** is also used intravenously for the treatment of hypertension particularly in the peri-operative period.

Beta-blockers can be used to control the pulse rate in children with *phaeochromocytoma* (section 2.5.4). However, they should never be used alone as beta-blockade without concurrent alpha-blockade may lead to a hypertensive crisis; phenoxybenzamine should always be used together with the beta-blocker.

Arrhythmias   In arrhythmias (section 2.3), beta-blockers act principally by attenuating the effects of the sympathetic system on automaticity and conductivity within the heart. They can be used alone or in conjunction with digoxin to control the ventricular rate in *atrial fibrillation*. Beta-blockers are also useful in the management of *supraventricular tachycardias* and *ventricular tachycardias* particularly to prevent recurrence of the tachycardia.

Esmolol is a relatively cardioselective beta-blocker with a very short duration of action, used intravenously for the short-term treatment of supraventricular arrhythmias and sinus tachycardia, particularly in the peri-operative period.

Sotalol is a non-cardioselective beta-blocker with additional class III anti-arrhythmic activity. Atenolol and sotalol suppress ventricular ectopic beats and non-sustained ventricular tachycardia (section 2.3.1). However, the pro-arrhythmic effects of sotalol, particularly in children with sick sinus syndrome, may prolong the QT interval and induce torsade de pointes.

Heart failure   Beta-blockers may produce benefit in heart failure by blocking sympathetic activity and the addition of a beta-blocker such as **carvedilol** to other treatment for heart failure may be beneficial. Treatment should be initiated by those experienced in the management of heart failure (see section 2.2 for details on heart failure).

2

Cardiovascular system

Cardiovascular system

2

Thyrotoxicosis Beta-blockers are used in the management of *thyrotoxicosis* including neonatal thyrotoxicosis; **propranolol** can reverse clinical symptoms within 4 days. Beta-blockers are also used for the pre-operative preparation for thyroidectomy; the thyroid gland is rendered less vascular, thus facilitating surgery (section 6.2.2).

Other uses In tetralogy of Fallot, esmolol or propranolol may be given intravenously in the initial management of *cyanotic spells*; propranolol is given by mouth for preventing cyanotic spells. If a severe cyanotic spell in a child with congenital heart disease persists despite optimal use of 100% oxygen, propranolol is given by intravenous infusion (for dose, see below). If cyanosis is still present after 10 minutes, sodium bicarbonate intravenous infusion is given in a dose of 1 mmol/kg to correct acidosis (or dose calculated according to arterial blood gas results); sodium bicarbonate 4.2% intravenous infusion is appropriate for a child under 1 year and sodium bicarbonate 8.4% intravenous infusion in children over 1 year. If blood-glucose concentration is less than 3 mmol/litre, glucose 10% intravenous infusion is given in a dose of 2 mL/kg (glucose 200 mg/kg) over 10 minutes, followed by morphine in a dose of 100 micrograms/kg by intravenous or intramuscular injection.

Beta-blockers are also used in the *prophylaxis of migraine* (section 4.7.4.2). Betaxolol, carteolol, levobunolol, and timolol are used topically in *glaucoma* (section 11.6).

� PROPRANOLOL HYDROCHLORIDE

Cautions see notes above; also avoid abrupt withdrawal; first-degree AV block; portal hypertension (risk of deterioration in liver function); diabetes (see also notes above); history of obstructive airways disease (introduce cautiously and monitor lung function—see also notes above); myasthenia gravis; symptoms of thyrotoxicosis may be masked (see also notes above); psoriasis; history of hypersensitivity—may increase sensitivity to allergens and result in more serious hypersensitivity response, also may reduce response to adrenaline (epinephrine); **interactions:** Appendix 1 (beta-blockers), **important:** verapamil interaction, see also p. 141

Contra-indications asthma (but see notes above), uncontrolled heart failure, marked bradycardia, hypotension, sick sinus syndrome, second- or third- degree AV block, cardiogenic shock, metabolic acidosis, severe peripheral arterial disease; phaeochromocytoma (apart from specific use with alpha-blockers, see also notes above)
Bronchospasm Beta-blockers, including those considered to be cardioselective, should usually be avoided in children with a history of asthma or bronchospasm. However, where there is no alternative a cardioselective beta-blocker can be given with caution under specialist supervision

Hepatic impairment reduce oral dose

Renal impairment manufacturer advises caution—dose reduction may be required

Pregnancy see notes above

Breast-feeding see notes above

Side-effects see notes above; also gastro-intestinal disturbances; bradycardia, heart failure, hypotension, conduction disorders, peripheral vasoconstriction (including exacerbation of intermittent claudication and Raynaud's phenomenon); bronchospasm (see above), dyspnoea; headache, fatigue, sleep disturbances, paraesthesia, dizziness, psychoses; sexual dysfunction; purpura, thrombocytopenia; visual disturbances; exacerbation of psoriasis, alopecia; *rarely* rashes and dry eyes (reversible on withdrawal); **over-**

dosage: see Emergency Treatment of Poisoning, p. 41

Licensed use not licensed for treatment of hypertension in children under 12 years

Indication and dose

Arrhythmias

• By mouth

> **Neonate** 250–500 micrograms/kg 3 times daily, adjusted according to response

> **Child 1 month–18 years** 250–500 micrograms/kg 3–4 times daily, adjusted according to response; max. 1 mg/kg 4 times daily, total daily dose not to exceed 160 mg daily

• By slow intravenous injection, with ECG monitoring

> **Neonate** 20–50 micrograms/kg repeated if necessary every 6–8 hours

> **Child 1 month–18 years** 25–50 micrograms/kg repeated every 6–8 hours if necessary

Hypertension

• By mouth

> **Neonate** initially, 250 micrograms/kg 3 times daily, increased if necessary to max. 2 mg/kg 3 times daily

> **Child 1 month–12 years** 0.25–1 mg/kg 3 times daily, increased at weekly intervals to max. 5 mg/kg daily

> **Child 12–18 years** initially 80 mg twice daily; increased at weekly intervals as required; maintenance 160–320 mg daily; slow-release preparations may be used for once daily administration

Tetralogy of Fallot

• By mouth

> **Neonate** 0.25–1 mg/kg 2–3 times daily, max. 2 mg/kg 3 times daily

⌐ PROPRANOLOL HYDROCHLORIDE (*continued*)

Child 1 month–12 years 0.25–1 mg/kg 3–4 times daily, max. 5 mg/kg daily

● **By slow intravenous injection with ECG monitoring**

Neonate initially 15–20 micrograms/kg (max. 100 micrograms/kg), repeated every 12 hours if necessary

Child 1 month–12 years initially 15–20 micrograms/kg (max. 100 micrograms/kg), repeated every 6–8 hours if necessary; higher doses rarely necessary

Migraine prophylaxis
● **By mouth**

Child 2–12 years 200–500 micrograms/kg 3 times daily; max. 4 mg/kg daily, usual dose 10–20 mg 2–3 times daily

Child 12–18 years 20–40 mg 2–3 times daily; maintenance 80–160 mg daily

Administration for *slow intravenous injection*, give over at least 3–5 minutes; rate of administration should not exceed 1 mg/minute. May be diluted with Sodium Chloride 0.9% or Glucose 5%. Incompatible with bicarbonate.

Note Excessive bradycardia can be countered with intravenous injection of atropine sulphate; for **overdosage** see Emergency Treatment of Poisoning, p. 41

Propranolol (Non-proprietary) ㏚
Tablets, propranolol hydrochloride 10 mg, net price 28 = 93p; 40 mg, 28 = 96p; 80 mg, 56 = £1.58; 160 mg, 56 = £3.13. Label: 8
Brands include *Angilol*®

Oral solution, propranolol hydrochloride 5 mg/5 mL, net price 150 mL = £12.50; 10 mg/5 mL, 150 mL = £16.45; 50 mg/5 mL, 150 mL = £19.98. Label: 8
Brands include *Syprol*®

Inderal® (AstraZeneca) ㏚
Injection, propranolol hydrochloride 1 mg/mL, net price 1-mL amp = 21p

◀Modified release
Note Modified-release preparations for once daily administration; use in older children only

Half-Inderal LA® (AstraZeneca) ㏚
Capsules, m/r, lavender/pink, propranolol hydrochloride 80 mg. Net price 28-cap pack = £5.40. Label: 8, 25
Note Modified-release capsules containing propranolol hydrochloride 80 mg also available; brands include *Bedranol SR*®, *Half Beta Prograne*®

Inderal-LA (AstraZeneca) ㏚
Capsules, m/r, lavender/pink, propranolol hydrochloride 160 mg. Net price 28-cap pack = £1.91. Label: 8, 25
Note Modified-release capsules containing propranolol hydrochloride 160 mg also available; brands include *Bedranol SR*®, *Beta-Prograne*®, *Slo-Pro*®

◢ ATENOLOL

Cautions see under Propranolol Hydrochloride
Contra-indications see under Propranolol Hydrochloride
Renal impairment initially use 50% of usual dose if estimated glomerular filtration rate 10–35 mL/minute/1.73 m^2; initially use 30–50% of usual dose if estimated glomerular filtration rate less than 10 mL/minute/1.73 m^2
Pregnancy see notes above
Breast-feeding see notes above
Side-effects see under Propranolol Hydrochloride
Licensed use not licensed for use in children under 12 years

Indication and dose
Hypertension
● **By mouth**

Neonate 0.5–2 mg/kg once daily; may be given in 2 divided doses

Child 1 month–12 years 0.5–2 mg/kg once daily (doses higher than 50 mg daily rarely necessary); may be given in 2 divided doses

Child 12–18 years 25–50 mg once daily (higher doses rarely necessary); may be given in 2 divided doses

Arrhythmias
● **By mouth**

Neonate 0.5–2 mg/kg once daily; may be given in 2 divided doses

Child 1 month–12 years 0.5–2 mg/kg once daily (max. 100 mg daily); may be given in 2 divided doses

Child 12–18 years 50–100 mg once daily; may be given in 2 divided doses

Atenolol (Non-proprietary) ㏚
Tablets, atenolol 25 mg, net price 28-tab pack = 89p; 50 mg, 28-tab pack = 91p; 100 mg, 28-tab pack = 92p. Label: 8
Brands include *Atenix*®

Tenormin® (AstraZeneca) ㏚
'25' tablets, f/c, atenolol 25 mg, net price 28-tab pack = £1.16. Label: 8
LS tablets, orange, f/c, scored, atenolol 50 mg, net price 28-tab pack = £2.04. Label: 8
Tablets, orange, f/c, scored, atenolol 100 mg, net price 28-tab pack = £3.46. Label: 8
Syrup, sugar-free, atenolol 25 mg/5 mL, net price 300 mL = £8.55. Label: 8

2

Cardiovascular system

CARVEDILOL

Cautions see under Propranolol Hydrochloride; monitor renal function during dose titration in children with heart failure who also have low blood pressure, renal impairment, ischaemic heart disease, or diffuse vascular disease

Contra-indications see under Propranolol Hydrochloride; acute or decompensated heart failure requiring intravenous inotropes

Hepatic impairment avoid

Pregnancy see notes above

Breast-feeding see notes above

Side-effects postural hypotension, dizziness, headache, fatigue, gastro-intestinal disturbances, bradycardia; occasionally diminished peripheral circulation, peripheral oedema and painful extremities, dry mouth, dry eyes, eye irritation or disturbed vision, impotence, disturbances of micturition, influenza-like symptoms; rarely angina, AV block, exacerbation of intermittent claudication or Raynaud's phenomenon; allergic skin reactions, exacerbation of psoriasis, nasal stuffiness, wheezing, depressed mood, sleep disturbances, paraesthesia, heart failure, changes in liver enzymes, thrombocytopenia, leucopenia also reported

Licensed use not licensed for use in children under 18 years

Indication and dose

Adjunct in heart failure (limited information available)

● By mouth

Child 2–18 years initially 50 micrograms/kg (max. 3.125 mg) twice daily, double dose at intervals of at least 2 weeks up to 350 micrograms/kg (max. 25 mg) twice daily

Carvedilol (Non-proprietary) [PoM]
Tablets, carvedilol 3.125 mg, net price 28-tab pack = £1.54; 6.25 mg, 28-tab pack = £1.98; 12.5 mg, 28-tab pack = £1.52; 25 mg, 28-tab pack = £1.99. Label: 8

Eucardic® (Roche) [PoM]
Tablets, scored, carvedilol 3.125 mg (pink), net price 28-tab pack = £7.27; 6.25 mg (yellow), 28-tab pack = £8.08; 12.5 mg (peach), 28-tab pack = £8.99; 25 mg, 28-tab pack = £11.22. Label: 8

ESMOLOL HYDROCHLORIDE

Cautions see under Propranolol Hydrochloride

Contra-indications see under Propranolol Hydrochloride

Renal impairment manufacturer advises caution

Pregnancy see notes above

Breast-feeding see notes above

Side-effects see under Propranolol Hydrochloride; infusion causes venous irritation and thrombophlebitis

Licensed use not licensed for use in children

Indication and dose

Arrhythmias, hypertensive emergencies (see also notes above and section 2.5)

● By intravenous administration

Child 1 month–18 years initially by *intravenous injection* over 1 minute 500 micrograms/kg then by *intravenous infusion* 50 micrograms/kg/minute for 4 minutes (rate reduced if low blood pressure or low heart rate); if inadequate response, repeat loading dose and increase

maintenance infusion by 50 micrograms/kg/minute increments; repeat until effective or max. infusion of 200 micrograms/kg/minute reached; doses over 300 micrograms/kg/minute not recommended

Tetralogy of Fallot

● By intravenous administration

Neonate initially by *intravenous injection* over 1–2 minutes 600 micrograms/kg then if necessary by *intravenous infusion* 300–900 micrograms/kg/minute

Administration dilute injection solution to a concentration of 10 mg/mL (20 mg/mL if fluid restricted) with Glucose 5% *or* Sodium Chloride 0.9% and give through central venous catheter; incompatible with bicarbonate

Brevibloc® (Baxter) [PoM]
Injection, esmolol hydrochloride 10 mg/mL, net price 10-mL vial = £7.79, 250-mL infusion bag = £89.69

LABETALOL HYDROCHLORIDE

Cautions see under Propranolol Hydrochloride; interferes with laboratory tests for catecholamines; liver damage (see below)

Liver damage Severe hepatocellular damage reported after both short-term and long-term treatment. Appropriate laboratory testing needed at first symptom of liver dysfunction and if laboratory evidence of damage (or if jaundice) labetalol should be stopped and not restarted

Contra-indications see under Propranolol Hydrochloride

Renal impairment dose reduction may be required

Pregnancy see notes above

Breast-feeding see notes above

Side-effects postural hypotension (avoid upright position during and for 3 hours after intravenous administration), tiredness, weakness, headache, rashes, scalp tingling, difficulty in micturition, epigastric pain, nausea, vomiting; liver damage (see above); rarely lichenoid rash

Licensed use not licensed for use in children

◁ **LABETALOL HYDROCHLORIDE** *(continued)*

Indication and dose

Hypertensive emergencies see also section 2.5
• **By intravenous infusion**

Neonate 500 micrograms/kg/hour adjusted at intervals of at least 15 minutes according to response; max. 4 mg/kg/hour

Child 1 month–12 years initially 0.5–1 mg/kg/hour adjusted at intervals of at least 15 minutes according to response; max. 3 mg/kg/hour

Child 12–18 years 30–120 mg/hour adjusted at intervals of at least 15 minutes according to response

Note Consult local guidelines. In hypertensive encephalopathy reduce blood pressure to normotensive level over 24–48 hours (more rapid reduction may lead to cerebral infarction, blindness, and death). If child fitting, reduce blood pressure rapidly, but not to normal levels

Hypertension
• **By mouth**

Child 1 month–12 years 1–2 mg/kg 3–4 times a day

Child 12–18 years initially 50–100 mg twice daily increased if required at intervals of 3–14 days to usual dose of 200–400 mg twice daily (3–4 divided doses if higher); max. 2.4 g daily

• **By intravenous injection**

Child 1 month–12 years 250–500 micrograms/kg as a single dose; max. 20 mg

Child 12–18 years 50 mg over at least 1 minute, repeated after 5 minutes if necessary; max. total dose 200 mg

Note Excessive bradycardia can be countered with intravenous injection of atropine sulphate; for **overdosage** see p. 41

Administration for *intravenous infusion*, dilute to a concentration of 1 mg/mL in Glucose 5% *or* Sodium Chloride and Glucose 5%; if fluid restricted may be given undiluted, preferably through a central venous catheter.

For administration *by mouth,* injection may be given orally with squash or juice

Labetalol Hydrochloride (Non-proprietary) PoM
Tablets, f/c, labetalol hydrochloride 100 mg, net price 56 = £9.74; 200 mg, 56 = £14.63; 400 mg, 56 = £19.02. Label: 8, 21

Trandate® (UCB Pharma) PoM
Tablets, all orange, f/c, labetalol hydrochloride 50 mg, net price 56-tab pack = £3.64; 100 mg, 56-tab pack = £4.01; 200 mg, 56-tab pack = £6.51; 400 mg, 56-tab pack = £9.05. Label: 8, 21

Injection, labetalol hydrochloride 5 mg/mL, net price 20-mL amp = £2.04

◢ Extemporaneous formulations available see Extemporaneous Preparations, p. 8

◢ **METOPROLOL TARTRATE**

Cautions see under Propranolol Hydrochloride
Contra-indications see under Propranolol Hydrochloride
Hepatic impairment reduce dose in severe impairment
Pregnancy see notes above
Breast-feeding see notes above
Side-effects see under Propranolol Hydrochloride
Licensed use not licensed for use in children
Indication and dose

Hypertension
• **By mouth**

Child 1 month–12 years initially 1 mg/kg twice daily, increased if necessary to max. 8 mg/kg (max. 400 mg) daily in 2–4 divided doses

Child 12–18 years initially 50–100 mg daily increased if necessary to 200 mg daily in 1–2 divided doses; max. 400 mg daily (but high doses rarely necessary)

Arrhythmias
• **By mouth**

Child 12–18 years usually 50 mg 2–3 times daily; up to 300 mg daily in divided doses if necessary

Metoprolol Tartrate (Non-proprietary) PoM
Tablets, metoprolol tartrate 50 mg, net price 28 = £1.33, 56 = £1.64; 100 mg, 28 = £1.70, 56 = £2.02. Label: 8

Lopresor® (Novartis) PoM
Tablets, f/c, scored, metoprolol tartrate 50 mg (pink), net price 56-tab pack = £2.57; 100 mg (blue), 56-tab pack = £6.68. Label: 8

◢ Extemporaneous formulations available see Extemporaneous Preparations, p. 8

◢ **SOTALOL HYDROCHLORIDE**

Cautions see under Propranolol Hydrochloride; correct hypokalaemia, hypomagnesaemia, or other electrolyte disturbances; severe or prolonged diarrhoea; reduce dose or discontinue if corrected QT interval exceeds 550 msec; **interactions:** Appendix 1 (beta-blockers), **important:** verapamil interaction see also p. 141

Contra-indications see under Propranolol Hydrochloride; congenital or acquired long QT syndrome; torsade de pointes

Renal impairment halve normal dose if estimated glomerular filtration rate 30–60 mL/minute/1.73 m^2; use one-quarter normal dose if estimated glomerular filtration rate 10–30 mL/minute/1.73 m^2; avoid if estimated glomerular filtration rate less than 10 mL/minute/1.73 m^2

2

Cardiovascular system

◻ **SOTALOL HYDROCHLORIDE** (*continued*)

Pregnancy see notes above

Breast-feeding see notes above

Side-effects see under Propranolol Hydrochloride; arrhythmogenic (pro-arrhythmic) effect (torsade de pointes—increased risk in females)

Licensed use not licensed for use in children under 12 years

Indication and dose

> Ventricular arrhythmias, life-threatening ventricular tachyarrhythmia and supraventricular arrhythmias initiated under specialist supervision and ECG monitoring and measurement of corrected QT interval
>
> • By mouth
>
>> Neonate initially 1 mg/kg twice daily, increased as necessary every 3–4 days to max. 4 mg/kg twice daily

> Atrial flutter, ventricular arrhythmias, life-threatening ventricular tachyarrhythmia and supraventricular arrhythmias initiated under specialist supervision and ECG monitoring and measurement of corrected QT interval
>
> • By mouth
>
>> Child 1 month–12 years initially 1 mg/kg twice daily, increased as necessary every 2–3 days to max. 4 mg/kg twice daily (max. 80 mg twice daily)

> Child 12–18 years initially 80 mg once daily *or* 40 mg twice daily, increased gradually at intervals of 2–3 days to usual dose 80–160 mg twice daily; higher doses of 480–640 mg daily for life-threatening ventricular arrhythmias under specialist supervision

Administration for administration *by mouth*, tablets may be crushed and dispersed in water

Note Excessive bradycardia can be countered with intravenous injection of atropine sulphate; for **overdosage** see Emergency Treatment of Poisoning, p. 41

Sotalol (Non-proprietary) PoM

Tablets, sotalol hydrochloride 40 mg, net price 56 = £1.29; 80 mg, 56-tab pack = £1.91; 160 mg, 28-tab pack = £2.08. Label: 8

Beta-Cardone® (UCB Pharma) PoM

Tablets, scored, sotalol hydrochloride 40 mg (green), net price 56-tab pack = £1.29; 80 mg (pink), 56-tab pack = £1.91; 200 mg, 28-tab pack = £2.40. Label: 8

Sotacor® (Bristol-Myers Squibb) PoM

Tablets, scored, sotalol hydrochloride 80 mg, net price 28-tab pack = £3.12. Label: 8

◢ Extemporaneous formulations available see Extemporaneous Preparations, p. 8

2.5 Hypertension

2.5.1 Vasodilator antihypertensive drugs and pulmonary hypertension

2.5.2 Centrally acting antihypertensive drugs

2.5.3 Adrenergic neurone blocking drugs

2.5.4 Alpha-adrenoceptor blocking drugs

2.5.5 Drugs affecting the renin-angiotensin system

Hypertension in children and adolescents can have a substantial effect on long-term health. Possible causes of hypertension (e.g. congenital heart disease, renal disease and endocrine disorders) and the presence of any complications (e.g. left ventricular hypertrophy) should be established. Treatment should take account of contributory factors and any factors that increase the risk of cardiovascular complications.

Serious hypertension is rare in *neonates* but it can present with signs of congestive heart failure; the cause is often renal and can follow embolic arterial damage.

Children (or their parents or carers) should be given advice on lifestyle changes to reduce blood pressure or cardiovascular risk; these include weight reduction (in obese children), reduction of dietary salt, reduction of total and saturated fat, increasing exercise, increasing fruit and vegetable intake, and not smoking.

Indications for antihypertensive therapy in children include symptomatic hypertension, secondary hypertension, hypertensive target-organ damage, diabetes mellitus, persistent hypertension despite lifestyle measures (see above), and pulmonary hypertension (section 2.5.1.2). The effect of antihypertensive treatment on growth and development is not known; treatment should be started only if benefits are clear.

Antihypertensive therapy should be initiated with a single drug at the lowest recommended dose; the dose can be increased until the target blood pressure is achieved. Once the highest recommended dose is reached, or sooner if the patient begins to experience side-effects, a second drug may be added if blood pressure is not controlled. If more than one drug is required, these should be given as separate products to allow dose adjustment of individual drugs, but fixed-dose combination products may be useful in adolescents if compliance is a problem.

Acceptable drug classes for use in children with hypertension include **ACE inhibitors** (section 2.5.5.1), **alpha-blockers** (section 2.5.4), **beta-blockers** (section 2.4), **calcium-channel blockers** (section 2.6.2), and **thiazide diuretics** (section 2.2.1). There is limited information on the use of **angiotensin-II receptor antagonists** (section 2.5.5.2) in children. Diuretics and beta-blockers have a long history of safety and efficacy in children. The newer classes of antihypertensive drugs, including ACE inhibitors and calcium-channel blockers have been shown to be safe and effective in short-term studies in children. Refractory hypertension may require additional treatment with agents such as **minoxidil** (section 2.5.1.1) or **clonidine** (section 2.5.2).

Other measures to reduce cardiovascular risk   **Aspirin** (section 2.9) may be used to reduce the risk of cardiovascular events; however, concerns about an increased risk of bleeding and Reye's syndrome need to be considered.

A **statin** can be of benefit in older children who have a high risk of cardiovascular disease and have hypercholesterolaemia (see section 2.12).

Hypertension in diabetes   Hypertension can occur in type 2 diabetes and treatment prevents both macrovascular and microvascular complications. ACE inhibitors (section 2.5.5.1) may be considered in children with diabetes and microalbuminaemia or proteinuric renal disease (see also section 6.1.5). Beta-blockers are best avoided in children with, or at a high risk of developing, diabetes, especially when combined with a thiazide diuretic.

Hypertension in renal disease   ACE inhibitors may be considered in children with micro-albuminuria or proteinuric renal disease (see also section 6.1.5). High doses of loop diuretics may be required. Specific cautions apply to the use of ACE inhibitors in renal impairment, see section 2.5.5.1, but ACE inhibitors may be effective. Dihydropyridine calcium-channel blockers may be added.

Hypertension in pregnancy   High blood pressure in pregnancy may usually be due to pre-existing essential hypertension or to pre-eclampsia. **Methyldopa** (BNF section 2.5.2) is safe in pregnancy. Beta-blockers are effective and safe in the third trimester. Modified-release preparations of **nifedipine** [unlicensed] are also used for hypertension in pregnancy. Intravenous administration of **labetalol** (section 2.4) can be used to control hypertensive crises; alternatively **hydralazine** (section 2.5.1.1) may be used by the intravenous route.

Hypertensive emergencies   Hypertensive emergencies in children may be accompanied by signs of hypertensive encephalopathy, including seizures. Controlled reduction in blood pressure over 72–96 hours is essential; rapid reduction can reduce perfusion leading to organ damage. Treatment should be initiated with intravenous drugs; once blood pressure is controlled, oral therapy can be started. It may be necessary to infuse fluids particularly during the first 12 hours to expand plasma volume should the blood pressure drop too rapidly.

Controlled reduction of blood pressure is achieved by intravenous administration of labetalol (section 2.4) or **sodium nitroprusside** (section 2.5.1.1). **Esmolol** (section 2.4) is useful for short-term use and has a short duration of action. **Nicardipine** (section 2.6.2) can be administered as a continuous intravenous infusion but it is not licensed for this use. In less severe cases, nifedipine capsules (section 2.6.2) can be used.

In resistant cases, **diazoxide** (section 2.5.1.1) is given intravenously, but it can cause sudden hypotension. Other antihypertensive drugs which can be given intravenously include hydralazine (section 2.5.1.1) and **clonidine** (section 2.5.2).

Hypertension in acute nephritis occurs as a result of sodium and water retention; it should be treated with sodium and fluid restriction, and with furosemide (section 2.2.2); antihypertensive drugs may be added if necessary.

For advice on short-term management of hypertensive episodes in phaeochromocytoma, see under Phaeochromocytoma, section 2.5.4.

2

Cardiovascular system

2.5.1 Vasodilator antihypertensive drugs and pulmonary hypertension

2.5.1.1 Vasodilator antihypertensives

Vasodilators have a potent hypotensive effect, especially when used in combination with a beta-blocker and a thiazide. **Important:** for a warning on the hazards of a very rapid fall in blood pressure, see Hypertensive Emergencies, p. 121.

Sodium nitroprusside is given by intravenous infusion to control severe hypertensive crisis when parenteral treatment is necessary. At low doses it reduces systemic vascular resistance and increases cardiac output; at high doses it can produce profound systemic hypotension—continuous blood pressure monitoring is therefore essential. Sodium nitroprusside may also be used to control paradoxical hypertension after surgery for coarctation of the aorta.

Diazoxide has also been used by intravenous injection in hypertensive emergencies; however it is not first-line therapy.

Hydralazine is given by mouth as an adjunct to other antihypertensives for the treatment of resistant hypertension but is rarely used; when used alone it causes tachycardia and fluid retention. The incidence of side-effects is lower if the dose is kept low, but systemic lupus erythematosus should be suspected if there is unexplained weight loss, arthritis, or any other unexplained ill health.

Minoxidil should be reserved for the treatment of severe hypertension resistant to other drugs. Vasodilatation is accompanied by increased cardiac output and tachycardia and children develop fluid retention. For this reason the addition of a beta-blocker and a diuretic (usually furosemide, in high dosage) are mandatory. Hypertrichosis is troublesome and renders this drug unsuitable for females.

Prazosin and **doxazosin** (section 2.5.4) have alpha-blocking and vasodilator properties.

DIAZOXIDE

Cautions during prolonged use monitor white cell and platelet count, and regularly assess growth, bone, and psychological development; **interactions:** Appendix 1 (diazoxide)

Renal impairment dose reduction may be required

Pregnancy prolonged use may produce alopecia, hypertrichosis, and impaired glucose tolerance in neonate; inhibits uterine activity during labour

Breast-feeding manufacturer advises avoid—no information available

Side-effects tachycardia, hypotension, hyperglycaemia, sodium and water retention; *rarely* cardiomegaly, hyperosmolar non-ketotic coma, leucopenia, thrombocytopenia, and hirsuitism

Licensed use intractable hypoglycaemia (section 6.1.4)

Indication and dose

> Hypertensive emergencies initiated on specialist advice
> • By intravenous injection
>> Child 1 month–18 years 1–3 mg/kg (max. 150 mg) as a single dose, repeat dose after 5–15 minutes until blood pressure controlled; max. 4 doses in 24 hours

> Resistant hypertension
> • By mouth
>> Neonate initially 1.7 mg/kg 3 times daily, adjusted according to response; usual max. 15 mg/kg daily
>> Child 1 month–18 years initially 1.7 mg/kg 3 times daily, adjusted according to response; usual max. 15 mg/kg daily

> Intractable hypoglycaemia section 6.1.4

Administration intravenous injection over 30 seconds. Do not dilute

Eudemine® (Goldshield) [PoM] ◢
Injection, diazoxide 15 mg/mL, net price 20-mL amp = £30.00

Tablets, section 6.1.4

◢ Extemporaneous formulations available see Extemporaneous Preparations, p. 8

HYDRALAZINE HYDROCHLORIDE

Cautions cerebrovascular disease; occasionally blood pressure reduction too rapid even with low parenteral doses; manufacturer advises test for antinuclear factor and for proteinuria every 6 months and check acetylator status before increasing dose, but evidence of clinical value unsatisfactory; **interactions:** Appendix 1 (hydralazine)

Contra-indications idiopathic systemic lupus erythematosus, severe tachycardia, high output heart failure, myocardial insufficiency due to mechanical obstruction, cor pulmonale; acute porphyria (section 9.8.2)

Hepatic impairment reduce dose

◁ **HYDRALAZINE HYDROCHLORIDE** (*continued*)

Renal impairment reduce dose if estimated glomerular filtration rate less than 30 mL/minute/1.73 m²

Pregnancy manufacturer advises avoid before third trimester; no reports of serious harm following use in third trimester

Breast-feeding present in milk but not known to be harmful; monitor infant

Side-effects tachycardia, palpitation, flushing, hypotension, fluid retention, gastro-intestinal disturbances; headache, dizziness; systemic lupus erythematosus-like syndrome after long-term therapy (especially in slow acetylator individuals); rarely rashes, fever, peripheral neuritis, polyneuritis, paraesthesia, arthralgia, myalgia, increased lacrimation, nasal congestion, dyspnoea, agitation, anxiety, anorexia; blood disorders (including leucopenia, thrombocytopenia, haemolytic anaemia), abnormal liver function, jaundice, raised plasma creatinine, proteinuria and haematuria reported

Licensed use not licensed for use in children

Indication and dose

> Hypertension
> • **By mouth**
>
> > **Neonate** 250–500 micrograms/kg every 8–12 hours increased as necessary to max. 2–3 mg/kg every 8 hours
> >
> > **Child 1 month–12 years** 250–500 micrograms/kg every 8–12 hours increased as necessary to max. 7.5 mg/kg daily (not exceeding 200 mg daily)
> >
> > **Child 12–18 years** 25 mg twice daily, increased to usual max. 50–100 mg twice daily
>
> • **By slow intravenous injection**
>
> > **Neonate** 100–500 micrograms/kg repeated every 4–6 hours as necessary; max. 3 mg/kg daily

> > **Child 1 month–12 years** 100–500 micrograms/kg repeated every 4–6 hours as necessary; max. 3 mg/kg daily (not exceeding 60 mg daily)
> >
> > **Child 12–18 years** 5–10 mg repeated every 4–6 hours as necessary
>
> • **By continuous intravenous infusion (preferred route in cardiac patients)**
>
> > **Neonate** 12.5–50 micrograms/kg/hour
> >
> > **Child 1 month–12 years** 12.5–50 micrograms/kg/hour; max. 3 mg/kg daily
> >
> > **Child 12–18 years** initially 3–9 mg/hour; max. 3 mg/kg daily

Administration for *intravenous injection*, initially reconstitute 20 mg with 1 mL Water for Injections, then dilute to a concentration of 0.5–1 mg/mL with Sodium Chloride 0.9% and administer over 5–20 minutes.

For *continuous intravenous infusion*, initially reconstitute 20 mg with 1 mL Water for Injections, then dilute with Sodium Chloride 0.9% *or* Ringer's solution. Incompatible with Glucose intravenous infusion.

For administration *by mouth*, diluted injection may be given orally

Hydralazine (Non-proprietary) ℙⓄⓂ
Tablets, hydralazine hydrochloride 25 mg, net price 56 = £11.96; 50 mg, 56 = £18.95

Apresoline® (Amdipharm) ℙⓄⓂ
Tablets, yellow, s/c, hydralazine hydrochloride 25 mg, net price 84-tab pack = £3.38
Excipients include gluten

Injection, powder for reconstitution, hydralazine hydrochloride, net price 20-mg amp = £2.19

◢ Extemporaneous formulations available see Extemporaneous Preparations, p. 8

◢ **MINOXIDIL**

Cautions see notes above; acute porphyria (section 9.8.2); **interactions**: Appendix 1 (vasodilator antihypertensives)

Contra-indications phaeochromocytoma

Renal impairment use with caution in significant impairment

Pregnancy neonatal hirsutism reported

Breast-feeding present in milk but not known to be harmful

Side-effects sodium and water retention; weight gain, peripheral oedema, tachycardia, hypertrichosis; reversible rise in creatinine and blood urea nitrogen; occasionally, gastro-intestinal disturbances, breast tenderness, rashes

Indication and dose

> Severe hypertension
> • **By mouth**
>
> > **Child 1 month–12 years** initially 200 micrograms/kg daily in 1–2 divided doses, increased in steps of 100–200 micrograms/kg daily at intervals of at least 3 days; max. 1 mg/kg daily
> >
> > **Child 12–18 years** initially 5 mg daily in 1–2 divided doses increased in steps of 5–10 mg at intervals of at least 3 days; max. 100 mg daily (seldom necessary to exceed 50 mg daily)

Loniten® (Pharmacia) ℙⓄⓂ
Tablets, scored, minoxidil 2.5 mg, net price 60-tab pack = £8.88; 5 mg, 60-tab pack = £15.83; 10 mg, 60-tab pack = £30.68

◢ Extemporaneous formulations available see Extemporaneous Preparations, p. 8

2

Cardiovascular system

◢ SODIUM NITROPRUSSIDE

Cautions hypothyroidism, hyponatraemia, impaired cerebral circulation, hypothermia; monitor blood pressure and blood-cyanide concentration, and if treatment exceeds 3 days also blood-thiocyanate concentration; avoid sudden withdrawal—terminate infusion over 15–30 minutes; **interactions:** Appendix 1 (nitroprusside)

Contra-indications severe vitamin B_{12} deficiency; Leber's optic atrophy; compensatory hypertension

Hepatic impairment use with caution; avoid in hepatic failure—cyanide or thiocyanate metabolites may accumulate

Renal impairment avoid prolonged use—cyanide or thiocyanate metabolites may accumulate

Pregnancy avoid prolonged use—potential for accumulation of cyanide in fetus

Breast-feeding no information available; caution advised due to thiocyanate metabolite

Side-effects associated with over rapid reduction in blood pressure (reduce infusion rate): headache, dizziness, nausea, retching, abdominal pain, perspiration, palpitation, anxiety, retrosternal discomfort; occasionally reduced platelet count, acute transient phlebitis
Cyanide Side-effects caused by excessive plasma concentration of the cyanide metabolite include tachycardia,

sweating, hyperventilation, arrhythmias, marked metabolic acidosis (discontinue and give antidote, see p. 44)

Licensed use not licensed for use in the UK

Indication and dose

Hypertensive emergencies
• By continuous infusion

> **Neonate** 500 nanograms/kg/minute then increased in steps of 200 nanograms/kg/minute as necessary to max. 8 micrograms/kg/minute (max. 4 micrograms/kg/minute if used for longer than 24 hours)

> **Child 1 month–18 years** 500 nanograms/kg/minute then increased in steps of 200 nanograms/kg/minute as necessary to max. 8 micrograms/kg/minute (max. 4 micrograms/kg/minute if used for longer than 24 hours)

Administration for *continuous intravenous infusion* in Glucose 5%, infuse *via* infusion device to allow precise control; protect infusion from light. For further details, consult product literature

Sodium Nitroprusside (Non-proprietary) PoM
Intravenous infusion, powder for reconstitution, sodium nitroprusside 10 mg/mL. For dilution and use as an infusion. Available from 'special-order' manufacturers or specialist importing companies, see p. 957

2.5.1.2 Pulmonary hypertension

Only pulmonary *arterial* hypertension is currently suitable for drug treatment. Pulmonary arterial hypertension includes persistent pulmonary hypertension of the newborn, idiopathic pulmonary arterial hypertension in children, and pulmonary hypertension related to congenital heart disease and cardiac surgery.

Some types of pulmonary hypertension are treated with vasodilator antihypertensive therapy and oxygen. Diuretics (section 2.2) may also have a role in children with right-sided heart failure.

Initial treatment of *persistent pulmonary hypertension of the newborn* involves the administration of **nitric oxide**; **epoprostenol** can be used until nitric oxide is available. Oral sildenafil may be helpful in less severe cases. Epoprostenol and sildenafil can cause profound systemic hypotension. In rare circumstances either **tolazoline** or **magnesium sulphate** can be given by intravenous infusion when nitric oxide and epoprostenol have failed.

Treatment of *idiopathic pulmonary arterial hypertension* is determined by acute vasodilator testing; drugs used for treatment include calcium-channel blockers (usually **nifedipine**, section 2.6.2), long-term intravenous **epoprostenol**, nebulised **iloprost**, **bosentan**, or **sildenafil**. Anticoagulation (usually with warfarin) may also be required to prevent secondary thrombosis.

Inhaled nitric oxide is a potent and selective pulmonary vasodilator. It acts on cyclic gaunosine monophosphate (cGMP) resulting in smooth muscle relaxation. Inhaled nitric oxide is used in the treatment of persistent pulmonary hypertension of the newborn, and may also be useful in other forms of arterial pulmonary hypertension. Dependency can occur with high doses and prolonged use; to avoid rebound pulmonary hypertension the drug should be withdrawn gradually, often with the aid of sildenafil.

Excess nitric oxide can cause methaemoglobinaemia; therefore, methaemoglobin concentration should be measured regularly, particularly in neonates.

Nitric oxide increases the risk of haemorrhage by inhibiting platelet aggregation, but it does not usually cause bleeding.

Epoprostenol (prostacyclin) is a prostaglandin and a potent vasodilator. It is used in the treatment of persistent pulmonary hypertension of the newborn, idiopathic pulmonary arterial hypertension, and in the acute phase following cardiac surgery. It is given by continuous 24-hour intravenous infusion.

Epoprostenol is a powerful inhibitor of platelet aggregation and there is a possible risk of haemorrhage. It is sometimes used as an antiplatelet in renal dialysis when heparins are unsuitable or contra-indicated. It can also cause serious systemic hypotension and, if withdrawn suddenly, can cause pulmonary hypertensive crisis.

Children on prolonged treatment can become tolerant to epoprostenol, and therefore require an increase in dose.

Iloprost is a synthetic analogue of epoprostenol and is efficacious when nebulised in adults with pulmonary arterial hypertension, but experience in children is limited. It is more stable than epoprostenol and has a longer half-life.

Bosentan is a dual endothelin receptor antagonist used orally in the treatment of idiopathic pulmonary arterial hypertension. The concentration of endothelin, a potent vasoconstrictor, is raised in sustained pulmonary hypertension.

Sildenafil, a vasodilator developed for the treatment of erectile dysfunction, is also used for pulmonary arterial hypertension. It is used either alone or as an adjunct to other drugs and has relatively few side-effects.

Sildenafil is a selective phosphodiesterase type-5 inhibitor. Inhibition of this enzyme in the lungs enhances the vasodilatory effects of nitric oxide and promotes relaxation of vascular smooth muscle.

Sildenafil has also been used in pulmonary hypertension for weaning children off inhaled nitric oxide following cardiac surgery, and less successfully in idiopathic pulmonary arterial hypertension.

Tolazoline is now rarely used to correct pulmonary artery vasospasm in pulmonary hypertension of the newborn as better alternatives are available (see above). Tolazoline is an alpha-blocker and produces both pulmonary and systemic vasodilation.

2

Cardiovascular system

BOSENTAN

Cautions not to be initiated if systemic systolic blood pressure is below 85 mmHg; monitor liver function before and at monthly intervals during treatment, and 2 weeks after dose increase (reduce dose or suspend treatment if liver enzymes raised significantly) — discontinue if symptoms of liver impairment (see Contra-indications below); monitor haemoglobin before and during treatment (monthly for first 4 months, then 3-monthly thereafter), withdraw treatment gradually; **interactions:** Appendix 1 (bosentan)

Contra-indications acute porphyria (section 9.8.2)

Hepatic impairment avoid in moderate and severe impairment

Pregnancy avoid (teratogenic in *animal* studies); effective contraception required during and for at least 3 months after administration (hormonal contraception not considered effective); monthly pregnancy tests advised

Breast-feeding manufacturer advises avoid—no information available

Side-effects gastro-intestinal disturbances, dry mouth, rectal haemorrhage, hepatic impairment (see Cautions, above); flushing, hypotension, palpitation, oedema, chest pain; dyspnoea; headache, dizziness, fatigue; back pain and pain in extremities; anaemia; hypersensitivity reactions (including rash, pruritus, and anaphylaxis)

Licensed use not licensed for use in children under 12 years

Indication and dose

Idiopathic pulmonary arterial hypertension
● By mouth

Child 3–18 years and body-weight 10–20 kg
initially 31.25 mg once daily increased after 4 weeks to 31.25 mg twice daily

Child 3–18 years and body-weight 20–40 kg
initially 31.25 mg twice daily increased after 4 weeks to 62.5 mg twice daily

Child 12–18 years and body-weight over 40 kg
initially 62.5 mg twice daily increased after 4 weeks to 125 mg twice daily; max. 250 mg twice daily

Administration Tablets may be cut, or suspended in water or non-acidic liquid. Suspension is stable at room-temperature (max. 25°C) for 24 hours

Tracleer® (Actelion) ▼ PoM
Tablets, f/c, orange, bosentan (as monohydrate) 62.5 mg, net price 56-tab pack = £1493.07; 125 mg, 56-tab pack = £1493.07

EPOPROSTENOL

Cautions anticoagulant monitoring required when given with anticoagulants; haemorrhagic diathesis; avoid abrupt withdrawal (see notes above); monitor blood pressure; concomitant use of drugs that increase risk of bleeding

◁ **EPOPROSTENOL** (continued)

Contra-indications severe left ventricular dysfunction; pulmonary veno-occlusive disease

Pregnancy manufacturer advises caution—no information available

Side-effects see notes above; gastro-intestinal disturbances, hypotension, bradycardia, tachycardia, pallor, flushing, sweating with higher doses; headache; lassitude, anxiety, agitation; dry mouth, jaw pain, chest pain; also reported, hyperglycaemia and injection-site reactions

Licensed use not licensed for use in children

Indication and dose

Persistent pulmonary hypertension of the newborn
• By continuous intravenous infusion

Neonate initially 2 nanograms/kg/minute adjusted according to response; usual max. 20 nanograms/kg/minute (rarely up to 40 nanograms/kg/minute)

Idiopathic pulmonary arterial hypertension
• By continuous intravenous infusion

Child 1 month–18 years initially 2 nanograms/kg/minute increased as necessary up to 40 nanograms/kg/minute

Administration reconstitute using the glycine buffer diluent provided to make a concentrate (pH 10.5); filter the concentrate using the filter pro-

vided. The concentrate can be administered via a central venous catheter, alternatively it may be diluted further either with the glycine buffer diluent or to a minimum concentration of 1.43 micrograms/mL with Sodium Chloride 0.9%. Solution stable for 12 hours at room temperature, although some units use for 24 hours and allow for loss of potency; solution stable for 24 hours if prepared in glycine buffer diluent only and administered via an ambulatory cold pouch system (to maintain solution at 2–8°C).
Neonatal intensive care, prepare a filtered concentrate of 10 micrograms/mL using the 500 microgram vial. *Neonate body-weight under 2 kg*, using the concentrate, dilute 150 micrograms/kg body-weight to a final volume of 50 mL with Sodium Chloride 0.9%; an intravenous infusion rate of 0.1 mL/hour provides a dose of 5 nanograms/kg/minute. *Neonate body-weight over 2 kg*, using the concentrate, dilute 60 micrograms/kg body-weight to a final volume of 50 mL with Sodium Chloride 0.9%; an intravenous infusion rate of 0.1 mL/hour provides a dose of 2 nanograms/kg/minute

Flolan® (GSK) (PoM)
Infusion, powder for reconstitution, epoprostenol (as sodium salt), net price 500-microgram vial (with diluent) = £62.05; 1.5-mg vial (▼) (with diluent) = £125.00

▌ **ILOPROST**

Cautions unstable pulmonary hypertension with advanced right heart failure; hypotension (do not initiate if systolic blood pressure below 85 mmHg); acute pulmonary infection; severe asthma; **interactions:** Appendix 1 (iloprost)

Contra-indications decompensated cardiac failure (unless under medical supervision); severe coronary heart disease; severe arrhythmias; congenital or acquired valvular defects of the myocardium; pulmonary veno-occlusive disease; conditions which increase risk of haemorrhage

Hepatic impairment dose may need to be halved in liver cirrhosis—initially 2.5 micrograms at intervals of at least 3 hours (max. 6 times daily), adjusted according to response

Pregnancy manufacturer advises avoid (toxicity in *animal* studies); effective contraception must be used during treatment

Breast-feeding manufacturer advises avoid—no information available

Side-effects vasodilatation, hypotension, syncope, cough, headache, throat or jaw pain; nausea, vomiting, diarrhoea, chest pain, dys-

pnoea, bronchospasm, and wheezing also reported

Licensed use not licensed for use in children under 18 years

Indication and dose

Idiopathic or familial pulmonary arterial hypertension
• By inhalation of nebulised solution

Child 8–18 years initial dose 2.5 micrograms increased to 5 micrograms for second dose, if tolerated maintain at 5 micrograms 6–9 times daily according to response; reduce to 2.5 micrograms 6–9 times daily if higher dose not tolerated

Raynaud's syndrome section 2.6.4.1

Ventavis® (Bayer Schering) (PoM)
Nebuliser solution, iloprost (as trometamol) 10 micrograms/mL, net price 30 × 1-mL (10 microgram) unit-dose vials = £407.94, 168 × 1-mL = £2284.49. For use with *Prodose®* (JHS) or *Venta-Neb®* (JHS) nebuliser

---

▌ **MAGNESIUM SULPHATE**

Cautions see section 9.5.1.3
Hepatic impairment see section 9.5.1.3
Renal impairment see section 9.5.1.3
Side-effects see section 9.5.1.3
Licensed use see section 9.5.1.3

Indication and dose

Persistent pulmonary hypertension of the newborn
• By intravenous infusion

Neonate initially 200 mg/kg over 20–30 minutes; if response occurs, then by continuous

◻ **MAGNESIUM SULPHATE (continued)**

intravenous infusion of 20–75 mg/kg/hour (to maintain plasma-magnesium concentration between 3.5–5.5 mmol/litre), given for up to 5 days

Severe acute asthma section 3.1

Torsade de pointes section 9.5.1.3

Neonatal hypocalcaemia section 9.5.1.3

Hypomagnesaemia section 9.5.1.3

Administration for *intravenous infusion*, dilute to a max. concentration of 100 mg/mL (200 mg/mL if fluid restricted) with Glucose 5% *or* Sodium Chloride 0.9%

Magnesium Sulphate (Non-proprietary) ᴾᵒᴹ
Injection, magnesium sulphate 50% (Mg²⁺ approx. 2 mmol/mL), net price 2-mL (1-g) amp= £2.80, 5-mL (2.5-g) amp = £3.00, 10-mL (5-g) amp = 96p; prefilled 10-mL (5-g) syringe = £4.95

◼ **SILDENAFIL**

Cautions hypotension (avoid if severe); intravascular volume depletion; left ventricular outflow obstruction; autonomic dysfunction; avoid abrupt withdrawal; other cardiovascular disease; pulmonary veno-occlusive disease; predisposition to priapism; anatomical deformation of the penis; bleeding disorders or active peptic ulceration; ocular disorders; initiate cautiously if child also on epoprostenol, iloprost, bosentan or nitric oxide; **interactions**: Appendix 1 (sildenafil)

Contra-indications recent history of stroke; history of non-arteritic anterior ischaemic optic neuropathy; hereditary degenerative retinal disorders; avoid concomitant use of nitrates

Hepatic impairment reduce dose if not tolerated in mild to moderate impairment; manufacturer advises avoid in severe impairment

Renal impairment reduce dose if not tolerated

Pregnancy manufacturer advises use only if potential benefit outweighs risk—no evidence of harm in *animal* studies

Breast-feeding manufacturer advises avoid—no information available

Side-effects gastro-intestinal disturbances, dry mouth; flushing, oedema; bronchitis, cough; headache, migraine, night sweats, paraesthesia, insomnia, anxiety, tremor, vertigo; fever, influenza-like symptoms; anaemia; back and limb pain, myalgia; visual disturbances, retinal haemorrhage, photophobia, painful red eyes; nasal congestion, epistaxis; cellulitis, alopecia; *less commonly* gynaecomastia, priapism; *also reported* rash, retinal vascular occlusion, non-arteritic anterior ischaemic optic neuropathy (discontinue if sudden visual impairment occurs), and sudden hearing loss (advise patient to seek medical help)

Licensed use not licensed for use in children under 18 years

Indication and dose

Pulmonary hypertension after cardiac surgery, weaning from nitric oxide, idiopathic pulmonary arterial hypertension, persistent pulmonary hypertension of the newborn
• By mouth

Neonate initially 250–500 micrograms/kg every 4–8 hours, adjusted according to response; max. 2 mg/kg every 6 hours; start with lower dose and frequency especially if used with other vasodilators (see Cautions above); withdraw gradually

Child 1 month– 18 years initially 250–500 micrograms/kg every 4–8 hours, adjusted according to response; max. 2 mg/kg every 6 hours; start with lower dose and frequency especially if used with other vasodilators (see Cautions above)

Administration tablet may be dissolved in water or blackcurrant drink and given by mouth or through a nasogastric tube

Viagra® (Pfizer) ᴾᵒᴹ ᴺᴴˢ
Tablets, all blue, f/c, sildenafil (as citrate), 25 mg, net price 4-tab pack = £16.59, 8-tab pack = £33.19; 50 mg, 4-tab pack = £19.34, 8-tab pack = £38.67; 100 mg, 4-tab pack = £23.50, 8-tab pack = £46.99

Revatio® (Pfizer) ▼ ᴾᵒᴹ
Tablets, f/c, sildenafil (as citrate), 20 mg, net price 90-tab pack = £373.50

◢ Extemporaneous formulations available see Extemporaneous Preparations, p. 8

◼ **TOLAZOLINE**

Cautions mitral stenosis; cardiotoxic accumulation may occur with continuous infusion, particularly in renal impairment—monitor blood pressure regularly for sustained systemic hypotension; **interactions**: Appendix 1 (alpha-blockers)

Contra-indications peptic ulcer disease

Renal impairment accumulates in renal impairment; risk of cardiotoxicity; lower doses may be necessary

Side-effects nausea, vomiting, diarrhoea, epigastric pain; flushing, tachycardia, cardiac arrhythmias; headache, shivering, sweating; oliguria, metabolic alkalosis, haematuria, blood dyscrasias (including thrombocytopenia); blotchy skin; at high doses severe hypotension, marked hypertension, renal failure, and haemorrhage reported

Licensed use not licensed for use in children

2

Cardiovascular system

⌐ **TOLAZOLINE** *(continued)*

Indication and dose

Correction of pulmonary vasospasm in neonates

• **By intravenous injection and continuous intravenous injection (maintenance)**

Neonate initially 1 mg/kg *by intravenous injection*
over 2–5 minutes, followed if necessary *by continuous intravenous infusion* of 200 micrograms/
kg/hour with careful blood pressure monitoring;
doses above 300 micrograms/kg/hour associated with cardiotoxicity and renal failure

• **By endotracheal administration**

Neonate 200 micrograms/kg

Administration for *continuous intravenous infusion*,
dilute with Glucose 5% *or* Sodium Chloride 0.9%.
Prepare a fresh solution every 24 hours.

For *endotracheal administration*, dilute with 0.5–
1 mL of Sodium Chloride 0.9%

Tolazoline (Non-proprietary)

Injection, tolazoline 25 mg/mL

Available from 'special-order' manufacturers or specialist
importing companies, see p. 957

2.5.2 **Centrally acting antihypertensive drugs**

Methyldopa, a centrally acting antihypertensive, is of little value in the management of refractory sustained hypertension in infants and children. On prolonged
use it is associated with fluid retention (which may be alleviated by concomitant
use of diuretics).

Methyldopa is effective for the management of hypertension in pregnancy (see
BNF section 2.5.2).

Clonidine is also a centrally acting antihypertensive but has the disadvantage that
sudden withdrawal may cause a hypertensive crisis. Clonidine is also used under
specialist supervision for pain management, sedation, and opioid withdrawal,
attention deficit hyperactivity disorder, and Tourette syndrome.

▌ **CLONIDINE HYDROCHLORIDE** ◢

Cautions must be withdrawn gradually to avoid
hypertensive crisis; Raynaud's syndrome or other
occlusive peripheral vascular disease; history of
depression; avoid in acute porphyria (section
9.8.2); **interactions:** Appendix 1 (clonidine)

Skilled tasks Drowsiness may affect performance of
skilled tasks (e.g. driving); effects of alcohol may be
enhanced

Pregnancy may lower fetal heart rate, but risk
should be balanced against risk of uncontrolled
maternal hypertension; avoid intravenous injection

Breast-feeding manufacturer advises avoid—
present in milk

Side-effects dry mouth, sedation, depression,
fluid retention, bradycardia, Raynaud's phenomenon, headache, dizziness, euphoria, nocturnal
unrest, rash, nausea, constipation, rarely impotence

Licensed use not licensed for use in children

Indication and dose

Severe hypertension
• **By mouth**

Child 2–18 years initially 0.5–1 microgram/kg 3
times daily, increased gradually if necessary;

max. 25 micrograms/kg daily in divided doses
(not exceeding 1.2 mg daily)

• **By slow intravenous injection**

Child 2–18 years 2–6 micrograms/kg (max.
300 micrograms) as a single dose

Administration for *intravenous injection*, give over
10–15 minutes; compatible with Sodium Chloride
0.9% *or* Glucose 5%.

For administration *by mouth*, tablets may be
crushed and dissolved in water

Catapres® (Boehringer Ingelheim) (PoM) ◢

Tablets, scored, clonidine hydrochloride 100 micrograms, net price 100-tab pack = £5.32; 300 micrograms, 100-tab pack = £12.39. Label: 3, 8

Injection, clonidine hydrochloride 150 micr-
ograms/mL, net price 1-mL amp = 28p

◢ Extemporaneous formulations available see
Extemporaneous Preparations, p. 8

2.5.3 **Adrenergic neurone blocking drugs**

Adrenergic neurone blocking drugs prevent the release of noradrenaline from
postganglionic adrenergic neurones. These drugs do not control supine blood
pressure and may cause postural hypotension. For this reason they have largely
fallen from use in adults and are rarely used in children.

2.5.4 Alpha-adrenoceptor blocking drugs

Doxazosin and **prazosin** have post-synaptic alpha-blocking and vasodilator properties and rarely cause tachycardia. They can, however, reduce blood pressure rapidly after the first dose and should be introduced with caution.

Alpha-blockers can be used with other antihypertensive drugs in the treatment of resistant hypertension.

DOXAZOSIN

Cautions care with initial dose (postural hypotension); pulmonary oedema due to aortic or mitral stenosis; cataract surgery (risk of intra-operative floppy iris syndrome); heart failure; **interactions:** Appendix 1 (alpha-blockers)

Driving May affect performance of skilled tasks e.g. driving

Contra-indications history of postural hypotension

Hepatic impairment use with caution; manufacturer advises avoid in severe impairment—no information available

Pregnancy no evidence of teratogenicity, manufacturers advise use only when potential benefit outweighs risk

Breast-feeding accumulates in milk in *animal* studies—manufacturer advises avoid

Side-effects gastro-intestinal disturbances; oedema, hypotension, postural hypotension, palpitation, tachycardia; dyspnoea, rhinitis, coughing; asthenia, fatigue, vertigo, dizziness, headache, paraesthesia, sleep disturbance, anxiety, depression; influenza-like symptoms; back pain, myalgia; *less commonly* weight changes; angina, myocardial infarction; hypoaesthesia, syncope, tremor, agitation, micturition disturbances, impotence, epistaxis, arthralgia, gout, tinnitus, hypersensitivity reactions (including pruritus, purpura, rash); *very rarely* cholestasis, hepatitis, jaundice, bradycardia, arrhythmias, bronchospasm, hot flushes, gynaecomastia, priapism, abnormal ejaculation, leucopenia, thrombocytopenia, blurred vision, and alopecia

Licensed use not licensed for use in children

Indication and dose

Hypertension (see notes above)

• By mouth

Child 6–12 years 500 micrograms once daily, increased at 1-week intervals to 2–4 mg daily

Child 12–18 years 1 mg daily, increased after 1–2 weeks to 2 mg once daily, and thereafter to 4 mg once daily if necessary; usual max. 4 mg daily (rarely up to 16 mg daily may be required)

Dysfunctional voiding section 7.4.1

Doxazosin (Non-proprietary) ▣ᴾᴼᴹ
Tablets, doxazosin (as mesilate) 1 mg, net price 28-tab pack = 99p; 2 mg, 28-tab pack = £1.05; 4 mg, 28-tab pack = £1.63. Counselling, initial dose, driving
Brands include *Doxadura*®

Cardura® (Pfizer) ▣ᴾᴼᴹ
Tablets, doxazosin (as mesilate) 1 mg, net price 28-tab pack = £10.56; 2 mg, 28-tab pack = £14.08. Counselling, initial dose, driving

◢ Extemporaneous formulations available see Extemporaneous Preparations, p. 8

◢ Modified-release
Note Children stabilised on immediate-release doxazosin can be transferred to the equivalent dose of modified-release doxazosin

Doxazosin (Non-proprietary) ▣ᴾᴼᴹ
Tablets, m/r, doxazosin (as mesilate) 4 mg, net price 28-tab pack = £6.33. Label: 25, counselling, initial dose, driving
Brands include *Doxadura*® XL, *Slocinx*® XL

Cardura® XL (Pfizer) ▣ᴾᴼᴹ
Tablets, m/r, doxazosin (as mesilate) 4 mg, net price 28-tab pack = £5.70; 8 mg, 28-tab pack = £9.98. Label: 25, counselling, initial dose, driving

PRAZOSIN

Cautions first dose may cause collapse due to hypotension (therefore should be taken on retiring to bed); cataract surgery (risk of intra-operative floppy iris syndrome); **interactions:** Appendix 1 (alpha-blockers)

Driving May affect performance of skilled tasks e.g. driving

Contra-indications not recommended for congestive heart failure due to mechanical obstruction (e.g. aortic stenosis)

Hepatic impairment start with low doses and adjust according to response

Renal impairment start with low doses in moderate to severe impairment; increase with caution

Pregnancy no evidence of teratogenicity; manufacturer advises use only when potential benefit outweighs risk

Breast-feeding present in milk; manufacturer advises use with caution

Side-effects gastro-intestinal disturbances; postural hypotension, oedema, palpitation; dyspnoea, nasal congestion; drowsiness, headache, depression, nervousness, vertigo; urinary frequency; weakness; blurred vision; *less commonly* tachycardia, insomnia, paraesthesia, sweating, impotence, arthralgia, eye disorders, tinnitus, epistaxis, allergic reactions including rash, pruritus, and urticaria; *rarely* pancreatitis, flushing,

◁ **PRAZOSIN** *(continued)*

vasculitis, bradycardia, hallucinations, worsening of narcolepsy, gynaecomastia, priapism, urinary incontinence, and alopecia

Licensed use not licensed for use in children under 12 years

Indication and dose

Hypertension (see notes above)
• By mouth

Child 1 month–12 years 10–15 micrograms/kg 2–4 times daily (initial dose at bedtime) increased gradually to max. 500 micrograms/kg daily in divided doses (not exceeding 20 mg daily)

Child 12–18 years 500 micrograms 2–3 times daily (initial dose at bedtime), increased after 3–7 days to 1 mg 2–3 times daily for a further 3–7 days; further increased gradually if necessary to max. 20 mg daily in divided doses

Congestive heart failure (but rarely used, see section 2.2)
• By mouth

Child 1 month–12 years 5 micrograms/kg twice daily (initial dose at bedtime), increased gradu-

ally to max. 100 micrograms/kg daily in divided doses

Child 12–18 years 500 micrograms 2–4 times daily (initial dose at bedtime), increasing to 4 mg daily in divided doses; maintenance 4–20 mg daily in divided doses

Administration for administration *by mouth*, tablets may be dispersed in water

Prazosin (Non-proprietary) [PoM]
Tablets, prazosin (as hydrochloride) 500 micrograms, net price 56-tab pack = £2.51; 1 mg, 56-tab pack = £3.23; 2 mg, 56-tab pack = £4.39; 5 mg, 56-tab pack = £8.75. Counselling, initial dose, driving

Hypovase® (Pfizer) [PoM]
Tablets, prazosin (as hydrochloride) 500 micrograms, net price 60-tab pack = £2.69; 1 mg, scored, 60-tab pack = £3.46. Counselling, initial dose, driving

---

Phaeochromocytoma

Long-term management of phaeochromocytoma involves surgery. However, surgery should not take place until there is adequate blockade of both alpha- and beta-adrenoceptors. Alpha-blockers are used in the short-term management of hypertensive episodes in phaeochromocytoma. Once alpha blockade is established, tachycardia can be controlled by the cautious addition of a beta-blocker (section 2.4); a cardioselective beta-blocker is preferred. There is no nationwide consensus on the optimal drug regimen or doses used for the management of phaeochromocytoma.

Phenoxybenzamine, a powerful alpha-blocker, is effective in the management of phaeochromocytoma but it has many side-effects. Phenoxybenzamine has also been used to lower severe systemic vascular resistance after cardiac surgery.

PHENOXYBENZAMINE HYDROCHLORIDE

Cautions congestive heart failure; severe ischaemic heart disease (see also Contra-indications); cerebrovascular disease (avoid if history of cerebrovascular accident); carcinogenic in *animals*; avoid in acute porphyria (section 9.8.2); avoid extravasation (irritant to tissues); avoid contact with skin (risk of contact sensitisation)

Contra-indications history of cerebrovascular accident; avoid infusion in hypovolaemia

Renal impairment use with caution

Pregnancy hypotension in newborn may occur

Breast-feeding may be present in milk

Side-effects postural hypotension with dizziness and marked compensatory tachycardia, lassitude, nasal congestion, miosis, inhibition of ejaculation; *rarely* gastro-intestinal disturbances; decreased sweating and dry mouth after intravenous infusion; idiosyncratic profound hypotension within few minutes of starting infusion; convulsions following rapid intravenous infusion also reported

Licensed use not licensed for use in children

Indication and dose

Hypertension in phaeochromocytoma
• By mouth

Child 1 month–18 years 0.5–1 mg/kg twice daily adjusted according to response

• By intravenous infusion

Child 1 month–18 years 0.5–1 mg/kg daily adjusted according to response; occasionally up to 2 mg/kg daily may be required; do not repeat dose within 24 hours

Severe vasoconstriction after cardiac surgery
• By intravenous infusion

Neonate initially 1 mg/kg then if necessary 500 micrograms/kg every 8–12 hours adjusted according to response

Child 1 month–18 years initially 1 mg/kg then if necessary 500 micrograms/kg every 8–12 hours adjusted according to response

◻ **PHENOXYBENZAMINE HYDROCHLORIDE (continued)**

Administration   for administration *by mouth*, capsules may be opened.

For *intravenous infusion*, dilute with Sodium Chloride 0.9% and give over at least 2 hours; max. 4 hours between dilution and completion of infusion

Phenoxybenzamine (Goldshield) [PoM]
Injection concentrate, phenoxybenzamine hydrochloride 50 mg/mL. To be diluted before use. Net price 2-mL amp = £57.14 (hosp. only)

Dibenyline® (Goldshield) [PoM]
Capsules, red/white, phenoxybenzamine hydrochloride 10 mg. Net price 30-cap pack = £10.84

2.5.5   Drugs affecting the renin-angiotensin system

2.5.5.1   Angiotensin-converting enzyme inhibitors
2.5.5.2   Angiotensin-II receptor antagonists

2.5.5.1   Angiotensin-converting enzyme inhibitors

Angiotensin-converting enzyme inhibitors (ACE inhibitors) inhibit the conversion of angiotensin I to angiotensin II. The main indications of ACE inhibitors in children are shown below. In infants and young children, captopril is often considered first.

Initiation under specialist supervision   Treatment with ACE inhibitors should be initiated under specialist supervision and with careful clinical monitoring in children.

Heart failure   ACE inhibitors have a valuable role in all grades of heart failure, usually combined with a loop diuretic (section 2.2). Potassium supplements and potassium-sparing diuretics should be discontinued before introducing an ACE inhibitor because of the risk of hyperkalaemia. In adults, a low dose of spironolactone may be beneficial in severe heart failure and can be used with an ACE inhibitor provided serum potassium is monitored carefully. Profound first-dose hypotension can occur when ACE inhibitors are introduced to children with heart failure who are already taking a high dose of a loop diuretic (see Cautions below). Temporary withdrawal of the loop diuretic reduces the risk, but can cause severe rebound pulmonary oedema.

Hypertension   ACE inhibitors may be considered for hypertension when thiazides and beta-blockers are contra-indicated, not tolerated, or fail to control blood pressure; they may be considered for hypertension in children with type 1 diabetes with nephropathy (see also section 6.1.5). ACE inhibitors can reduce blood pressure very rapidly in some patients particularly in those receiving diuretic therapy (see Cautions, below); the first dose should preferably be given at bedtime.

Diabetic nephropathy   For comment on the role of ACE inhibitors in the management of diabetic nephropathy, see section 6.1.5.

Renal effects   Renal function and electrolytes should be checked before starting ACE inhibitors (or increasing the dose) and monitored during treatment (more frequently if features mentioned below are present). Hyperkalaemia and other side-effects of ACE inhibitors are more common in children with impaired renal function and the dose may need to be reduced (see Renal Impairment, below).

Concomitant treatment with NSAIDs increases the risk of renal damage, and potassium-sparing diuretics (or potassium-containing salt substitutes) increase the risk of hyperkalaemia.

In children with severe bilateral renal artery stenosis (or severe stenosis of the artery supplying a single functioning kidney), ACE inhibitors reduce or abolish glomerular filtration and are likely to cause severe and progressive renal failure. They are therefore contra-indicated in children known to have these forms of critical renovascular disease.

ACE inhibitor treatment is unlikely to have an adverse effect on overall renal function in children with severe unilateral renal artery stenosis and a normal contralateral kidney, but glomerular filtration is likely to be reduced (or even abolished) in the affected kidney and the long-term consequences are unknown.

ACE inhibitors are therefore best avoided in those with known or suspected renovascular disease, unless the blood pressure cannot be controlled by other drugs. If they are used in these circumstances renal function needs to be monitored.

ACE inhibitors should also be used with particular caution in children who may have undiagnosed and clinically silent renovascular disease. ACE inhibitors are useful for the management of hypertension and proteinuria in children with nephritis. They are thought to have a beneficial effect by reducing intra-glomerular hypertension and protecting the glomerular capillaries and membrane.

Cautions ACE inhibitors need to be initiated with care in children receiving diuretics (**important:** see Concomitant Diuretics, below); first doses can cause hypotension especially in children taking high doses of diuretics, on a low-sodium diet, on dialysis, dehydrated, or with heart failure (see above). Discontinue if marked elevation of hepatic enzymes or jaundice (risk of hepatic necrosis). Renal function should be monitored before and during treatment. For use in pre-existing renovascular disease, see Renal Effects above. The risk of agranulocytosis is possibly increased in collagen vascular disease (blood counts recommended). ACE inhibitors should be used with care in children with severe or symptomatic aortic stenosis (risk of hypotension) and in hypertrophic cardiomyopathy. They should be used with care (or avoided) in those with a history of idiopathic or hereditary angioedema. Children with primary aldosteronism and Afro-Caribbean children may respond less well to ACE inhibitors. **Interactions:** Appendix 1 (ACE inhibitors).

Anaphylactoid reactions To prevent anaphylactoid reactions, ACE inhibitors should be avoided during dialysis with high-flux polyacrylonitrile membranes and during low-density lipoprotein apheresis with dextran sulphate; they should also be withheld before desensitisation with wasp or bee venom.

Concomitant diuretics ACE inhibitors can cause a very rapid fall in blood pressure in volume-depleted children; treatment should therefore be initiated with very low doses. In some children the diuretic dose may need to be reduced or the diuretic discontinued at least 24 hours beforehand (may not be possible in heart failure—risk of pulmonary oedema). If high-dose diuretic therapy cannot be stopped, close observation is recommended after administration of the first dose of ACE inhibitor, for at least 2 hours or until the blood pressure has stabilised.

Contra-indications ACE inhibitors are contra-indicated in children with hypersensitivity to ACE inhibitors (including angioedema) and in bilateral renovascular disease (see also above).

Renal impairment See Renal Effects above; start with low dose and adjust according to response.

Pregnancy ACE inhibitors should be avoided in pregnancy unless essential—they may adversely affect fetal and neonatal blood pressure control and renal function; skull defects and oligohydramnios have also been reported.

Side-effects ACE inhibitors can cause profound hypotension (see Cautions), renal impairment (see Renal Effects above), and a persistent dry cough. They can also cause angioedema (onset may be delayed; higher incidence reported in Afro-Caribbean patients), rash (which may be associated with pruritus and urticaria), pancreatitis, and upper respiratory-tract symptoms such as sinusitis, rhinitis, and sore throat. Gastro-intestinal effects reported with ACE inhibitors include nausea, vomiting, dyspepsia, diarrhoea, constipation, and abdominal pain. Altered liver function tests, cholestatic jaundice, hepatitis, fulminant hepatic necrosis, and hepatic failure have been reported—discontinue if marked elevation of hepatic enzymes or jaundice. Hyperkalaemia, hypoglycaemia and blood disorders including thrombocytopenia, leucopenia, neutropenia, and haemolytic anaemia have also been reported. Other reported side-effects include headache, dizziness, fatigue, malaise, taste disturbance, paraesthesia, bronchospasm, fever, serositis, vasculitis, myalgia, arthralgia, positive antinuclear antibody, raised erythrocyte sedimentation rate, eosinophilia, leucocytosis, and photosensitivity.

Neonates The neonatal response to treatment with ACE inhibitors is very variable, and some neonates develop profound hypotension with even small doses; a test-dose should be used initially and increased cautiously. Adverse effects such as apnoea, seizures, renal failure, and severe unpredictable hypotension are very common in the first month of life and it is therefore recommended that ACE inhibitors are avoided whenever possible, particularly in preterm neonates.

CAPTOPRIL

Cautions see notes above; acute porphyria (section 9.8.2)

Contra-indications see notes above

Renal impairment see notes above

Pregnancy see notes above

Breast-feeding avoid in first few weeks after delivery, particularly in preterm infants—risk of profound neonatal hypotension; can be used in older infant if essential but monitor infant's blood pressure

Side-effects see notes above; tachycardia, serum sickness, weight loss, stomatitis, maculopapular rash, photosensitivity, flushing and acidosis

Licensed use not licensed for use in children under 18 years

Indication and dose

Hypertension, heart failure, proteinuria in nephritis (under specialist supervision)
• By mouth

> **Neonate** (caution, see neonatal information above) test dose, 10–50 micrograms/kg (10 micrograms/kg in neonate less than 37 weeks post-menstrual age), monitor blood pressure carefully for 1–2 hours; if tolerated give 10–50 micrograms/kg 2–3 times daily increased as necessary to max. 2 mg/kg daily in divided doses (max. 300 micrograms/kg daily in divided doses in neonate less than 37 weeks post-menstrual age)

> **Child 1 month–12 years** test dose, 100 micrograms/kg (max. 6.25 mg), monitor blood pressure carefully for 1–2 hours; if tolerated give 100–300 micrograms/kg 2–3 times a day, increased as necessary to max. 6 mg/kg daily in divided doses (max. 4 mg/kg daily in divided doses for child 1 month–1 year)

> **Child 12–18 years** test dose, 100 micrograms/kg *or* 6.25 mg, monitor blood pressure carefully for 1–2 hours; if tolerated give 12.5–25 mg 2–3 times a day, increased as necessary to max. 150 mg daily in divided doses

Diabetic nephropathy (under specialist supervision)
• By mouth

> **Child 12–18 years** test dose, 100 micrograms/kg *or* 6.25 mg, monitor blood pressure carefully for 1–2 hours; if tolerated give 12.5–25 mg 2–3 times a day, increased as necessary to max. 150 mg daily in divided doses

Administration Administer under close supervision, see notes above. Give test dose whilst child supine. Tablets can be dispersed in water

Captopril (Non-proprietary) ⓅⓄⓂ
Tablets, captopril 12.5 mg, net price 56-tab pack = £1.44; 25 mg, 56-tab pack = £1.63; 50 mg, 56-tab pack = £2.17
Brands include *Ecopace®*, *Kaplon®*, *Tensopril®*

Liquid, various strengths available from 'special-order' manufacturers or specialist importing companies, see p. 957

Capoten® (Squibb) ⓅⓄⓂ
Tablets, captopril 25 mg, net price 28-tab pack = £5.37; 50 mg (scored), 56-tab pack = £18.33 (also available as *Acepril®*)

◢Extemporaneous formulations available see Extemporaneous Preparations, p. 8

ENALAPRIL MALEATE

Cautions see notes above

Contra-indications see notes above

Hepatic impairment monitor closely

Renal impairment see notes above

Pregnancy see notes above

Breast-feeding avoid in first few weeks after delivery, particularly in preterm infants—risk of profound neonatal hypotension; can be used in older infant if essential but monitor infant's blood pressure

Side-effects see notes above; also dyspnoea; depression, asthenia; blurred vision; *less commonly* dry mouth, peptic ulcer, anorexia, ileus; arrhythmias, palpitation, flushing; confusion, nervousness, drowsiness, insomnia, vertigo; impotence; muscle cramps; tinnitus; alopecia, sweating; hyponatraemia; *rarely* stomatitis, glossitis, Raynaud's syndrome, pulmonary infiltrates, allergic alveolitis, abnormal dreams, gynaecomastia, Stevens-Johnson syndrome, toxic epidermal necrolysis, exfoliative dermatitis, pemphigus; *very rarely* gastro-intestinal angioedema

Licensed use not licensed for use in children for congestive heart failure, proteinuria in nephritis or diabetic nephropathy; not licensed for use in children less than 20 kg for hypertension

Indication and dose

Hypertension, congestive heart failure, proteinuria in nephritis (under specialist supervision)
• By mouth

> **Neonate** (limited information) initially 10 micrograms/kg once daily, monitor blood pressure carefully for 1–2 hours, increased as necessary up to 500 micrograms/kg daily in 1–3 divided doses

> **Child 1 month–12 years** initially 100 micrograms/kg once daily, monitor blood pressure carefully for 1–2 hours, increased as necessary up to max. 1 mg/kg daily in 1–2 divided doses

> **Child 12–18 years** initially 2.5 mg once daily, monitor blood pressure carefully for 1–2 hours, usual maintenance dose 10–20 mg daily in 1–2 divided doses; max. 40 mg daily in 1–2 divided doses if body-weight over 50 kg

2

Cardiovascular system

◁ **ENALAPRIL MALEATE** (*continued*)

Diabetic nephropathy (under specialist supervision)
- **By mouth**

  Child 12–18 years initially 2.5 mg once daily, monitor blood pressure carefully for 1–2 hours, usual maintenance dose 10–20 mg daily in 1–2 divided doses; max. 40 mg daily in 1–2 divided doses if body-weight over 50 kg

Administration tablets may be crushed and suspended in water immediately before use

Enalapril Maleate (Non-proprietary) ℞
> Tablets, enalapril maleate 2.5 mg, net price 28-tab pack = £1.17; 5 mg, 28-tab pack = £1.04; 10 mg, 28-tab pack = £1.15; 20 mg, 28-tab pack = £1.27
> Brands include *Ednyt*®

> Liquid, various strengths available from 'special-order' manufacturers or specialist importing companies, see p. 957

Innovace® (MSD) ℞
> Tablets, enalapril maleate 2.5 mg, net price 28-tab pack = £5.35; 5 mg (scored), 28-tab pack = £7.51; 10 mg (red), 28-tab pack = £10.53; 20 mg (peach), 28-tab pack = £12.51

LISINOPRIL

Cautions see notes above
Contra-indications see notes above
Renal impairment see notes above
Pregnancy see notes above
Breast-feeding avoid—no information available
Side-effects see notes above; also *less commonly* tachycardia, palpitation, cerebrovascular accident, Raynaud's syndrome, confusion, mood changes, vertigo, sleep disturbances, asthenia, impotence; *rarely* dry mouth, gynaecomastia, alopecia, psoriasis; *very rarely* allergic alveolitis, pulmonary infiltrates, profuse sweating, pemphigus, Stevens-Johnson syndrome, and toxic epidermal necrolysis
Licensed use not licensed for use in children

Indication and dose

Hypertension, proteinuria in nephritis (under specialist supervision)
- **By mouth**

  Child 6–12 years initially 70 micrograms/kg (max. 5 mg) once daily, increased in intervals of 1–2 weeks to max. 600 micrograms/kg (*or* 40 mg) once daily

  Child 12–18 years initially 5 mg once daily; usual maintenance dose 10–20 mg once daily; max. 80 mg once daily

Diabetic nephropathy (under specialist supervision)
- **By mouth**

  Child 12–18 years initially 5 mg once daily; usual maintenance dose 10–20 mg once daily; max. 80 mg once daily

Heart failure (adjunct) (under specialist supervision)
- **By mouth**

  Child 12–18 years initially 2.5 mg once daily; increased in steps no greater than 10 mg at intervals of at least 2 weeks up to max. 35 mg once daily if tolerated

Lisinopril (Non-proprietary) ℞
> Tablets, lisinopril (as dihydrate) 2.5 mg, net price 28-tab pack = 92p; 5 mg, 28-tab pack = 97p; 10 mg, 28-tab pack = £1.05; 20 mg, 28-tab pack = £1.27

> Liquid, various strengths available from 'special-order' manufacturers or specialist importing companies, see p. 957

Zestril® (AstraZeneca) ℞
> Tablets, lisinopril (as dihydrate) 2.5 mg, net price 28-tab pack = £1.78; 5 mg (pink), 28-tab pack = £1.31; 10 mg (pink), 28-tab pack = £2.05; 20 mg (pink), 28-tab pack = £2.17

◢ Extemporaneous formulations available see Extemporaneous Preparations, p. 8

2.5.5.2 Angiotensin-II receptor antagonists

Losartan is a specific angiotensin-II receptor antagonist with many properties similar to those of the ACE inhibitors. However, unlike ACE inhibitors, losartan does not inhibit the breakdown of bradykinin and other kinins, and therefore does not appear to cause the persistent dry cough which commonly complicates ACE inhibitor therapy. It is therefore an alternative for children who have to discontinue an ACE inhibitor because of persistent cough.

Losartan can be used as an alternative to an ACE inhibitor in the management of hypertension; however, evidence for its use in children is very limited.

LOSARTAN POTASSIUM

Cautions renal artery stenosis (see also Renal Effects under ACE inhibitors, section 2.5.5.1); monitor plasma-potassium concentration (particularly in children with renal impairment); aortic or mitral valve stenosis; hypertrophic cardiomyopathy; severe heart failure; children with primary aldosteronism and Afro-Caribbean children, particularly those with left ventricular hypertrophy, may not benefit from losartan; **interactions**: Appendix 1 (angiotensin-II receptor antagonists)

▢ **LOSARTAN POTASSIUM** (*continued*)

Hepatic impairment manufacturer advises avoid—no information available

Renal impairment manufacturer advises avoid if estimated glomerular filtration rate less than 30 mL/minute/1.73m² —no information available

Pregnancy avoid unless essential—may adversely affect fetal and neonatal blood pressure control and renal function; skull defects and oligohydramnios reported

Breast-feeding avoid—no information available

Side-effects symptomatic hypotension including dizziness (particularly in children with intravascular volume depletion e.g. those taking high-dose diuretics); asthenia, fatigue, vertigo, hyperkalaemia; *less commonly* gastro-intestinal disturbances, angina, palpitation, oedema, dyspnoea, headache, sleep disorders, urticaria, pruritus, and rash; *rarely* hepatitis, atrial fibrillation, cerebrovascular accident, syncope, and paraesthesia; *also reported* pancreatitis, anaphylaxis, cough, depression, erectile dysfunction, anaemia, thrombocytopenia, hyponatraemia, arthralgia, myalgia, rhabdomyolysis, tinnitus, photosensitivity, and vasculitis (including Henoch-Schönlein purpura)

Indication and dose

Hypertension (under specialist supervision)

● **By mouth**

Child 6–18 years

Body-weight 20–50 kg initially 700 micrograms/kg (max. 25 mg) once daily (lower dose in intravascular volume depletion); adjusted according to response to max. 50 mg once daily

Body-weight 50 kg and over initially 50 mg once daily (initially 25 mg once daily in intravascular volume depletion); adjusted according to response to max. 1.4 mg/kg (max. 100 mg) once daily

Losartan Potassium (Non-proprietary)

Tablets, losartan potassium 12.5 mg, net price 28-tab pack = £7.28; 25 mg, 28-tab pack = £4.50; 50 mg, 28-tab pack = £3.50; 100 mg, 28-tab pack = £4.50

Cozaar® (MSD) ▼ [PoM]

Tablets, f/c, losartan potassium 12.5 mg (blue), net price 28-tab pack = £8.09; 25 mg (white), 28-tab pack = £16.18; 50 mg (white, scored), 28-tab pack = £12.80; 100 mg (white), 28-tab pack = £16.18

Oral suspension, losartan potassium 12.5 mg/5 mL when reconstituted with solvent provided, net price 200 mL (berry-citrus flavour) = £53.68

2.6 Nitrates, calcium-channel blockers, and other antianginal drugs

2.6.1 Nitrates
2.6.2 Calcium-channel blockers
2.6.3 Other antianginal drugs
2.6.4 Peripheral vasodilators and related drugs

Nitrates and calcium-channel blockers have a vasodilating and, consequently, blood-pressure lowering effect. Vasodilators can act in heart failure by arteriolar dilatation, which reduces both peripheral vascular resistance and left ventricular pressure during systole resulting in improved cardiac output. They can also cause venous dilatation, which results in dilatation of capacitance vessels, increase of venous pooling, and diminution of venous return to the heart (decreasing left ventricular end-diastolic pressure).

2.6.1 Nitrates

Nitrates are potent coronary vasodilators, but their principal benefit follows from a reduction in venous return which reduces left ventricular work. Unwanted effects such as flushing, headache, and postural hypotension may limit therapy, especially if the child is unusually sensitive to the effects of nitrates or is hypovolaemic.

For the use of glyceryl trinitrate in extravasation, see section 10.3.

Children receiving nitrates continuously throughout the day can develop tolerance (with reduced therapeutic effects). Reduction of blood-nitrate concentrations to low levels for 4 to 8 hours each day usually maintains effectiveness in such patients.

◢ **GLYCERYL TRINITRATE**

Cautions hypothyroidism; malnutrition; hypothermia; recent history of myocardial infarction; heart failure due to obstruction; hypoxaemia or other ventilation and perfusion abnormalities;

2 Cardiovascular system

◻ **GLYCERYL TRINITRATE** (*continued*)

susceptibility to angle-closure glaucoma; metal-containing transdermal systems should be removed before magnetic resonance imaging procedures, cardioversion, or diathermy; avoid abrupt withdrawal; monitor blood pressure and heart rate during infusion; tolerance (see notes above); **interactions:** Appendix 1 (nitrates)

Contra-indications hypersensitivity to nitrates; hypotensive conditions and hypovolaemia; hypertrophic cardiomyopathy; aortic stenosis; cardiac tamponade; constrictive pericarditis; mitral stenosis; toxic pulmonary oedema; head trauma; cerebral haemorrhage; cerebrovascular disease; marked anaemia

Hepatic impairment caution in severe impairment

Renal impairment manufacturers advise use with caution in severe impairment

Pregnancy not known to be harmful

Breast-feeding no information available—manufacturers advise use only if potential benefit outweighs risk

Side-effects postural hypotension, tachycardia (but paradoxical bradycardia also reported); throbbing headache, dizziness; *less commonly* nausea, vomiting, heartburn, flushing, syncope, temporary hypoxaemia, rash, application-site reactions with transdermal patches; *very rarely* angle-closure glaucoma

Injection Specific side-effects following injection (particularly if given too rapidly) include severe hypotension, diaphoresis, apprehension, restlessness, muscle twitching, retrosternal discomfort, palpitation, abdominal pain; prolonged administration has been associated with methaemoglobinaemia

Licensed use not licensed for use in children

Indication and dose

Hypertension during and after cardiac surgery, heart failure after cardiac surgery, coronary vasoconstriction in myocardial ischaemia, vasoconstriction in shock
• By continuous intravenous infusion

Neonate 0.2–0.5 micrograms/kg/minute, dose adjusted according to response; usual dose 1–3 micrograms/kg/minute; max. 10 micrograms/kg/minute

Child 1 month–18 years initially 0.2–0.5 micrograms/kg/minute, dose adjusted according to response, usual dose 1–3 micrograms/kg/minute; max. 10 micrograms/kg/minute (do not exceed 200 micrograms/minute)

Administration for *continuous intravenous infusion*, dilute to max. concentration of 400 micrograms/mL (but concentration of 1 mg/mL has been used via a central venous catheter) with Glucose 5% or Sodium Chloride 0.9%.

Glass or polyethylene apparatus is preferable; loss of potency will occur if PVC is used.

Neonatal intensive care, dilute 3 mg/kg body-weight to a final volume of 50 mL with infusion fluid; an intravenous infusion rate of 1 mL/hour provides a dose of 1 microgram/kg/minute

Glyceryl Trinitrate (Non-proprietary) ℗ₒₘ
Injection, glyceryl trinitrate 5 mg/mL. To be diluted before use. Net price 5-mL amp = £6.49; 10-mL amp = £12.98
Excipients may include ethanol, propylene glycol

Nitrocine® (UCB Pharma) ℗ₒₘ
Injection, glyceryl trinitrate 1 mg/mL. To be diluted before use or given undiluted with syringe pump. Net price 10-mL amp = £5.88; 50-mL bottle = £13.77
Excipients include propylene glycol

Nitronal® (Merck) ℗ₒₘ
Injection, glyceryl trinitrate 1 mg/mL. To be diluted before use or given undiluted with syringe pump. Net price 5-mL vial = £1.84; 50-mL vial = £15.06

2.6.2 Calcium-channel blockers

Calcium-channel blockers (less correctly called 'calcium-antagonists') interfere with the inward displacement of calcium ions through the slow channels of active cell membranes. They influence the myocardial cells, the cells within the specialised conducting system of the heart, and the cells of vascular smooth muscle. Thus, myocardial contractility may be reduced, the formation and propagation of electrical impulses within the heart may be depressed, and coronary or systemic vascular tone may be diminished.

Calcium-channel blockers differ in their predilection for the various possible sites of action and, therefore, their therapeutic effects are disparate, with much greater variation than those of beta-blockers. There are important differences between verapamil, diltiazem, and the dihydropyridine calcium-channel blockers (amlodipine, nicardipine, nifedipine, and nimodipine). Verapamil and diltiazem should usually be **avoided** in heart failure because they may further depress cardiac function and cause clinically significant deterioration.

Verapamil is used for the treatment of hypertension (section 2.5) and arrhythmias (section 2.3.2). However, it is no longer first-line treatment for arrhythmias in children because it has been associated with fatal collapse especially in infants under 1 year; adenosine is now recommended for first-line use.

Cardiovascular system (side label)

2 (side tab)

Verapamil is a highly negatively inotropic calcium channel-blocker and it reduces cardiac output, slows the heart rate, and may impair atrioventricular conduction. It may precipitate heart failure, exacerbate conduction disorders, and cause hypotension at high doses and should **not** be used with beta-blockers (see p. 141). Constipation is the most common side-effect.

Nifedipine relaxes vascular smooth muscle and dilates coronary and peripheral arteries. It has more influence on vessels and less on the myocardium than does verapamil, and unlike verapamil has no anti-arrhythmic activity. It rarely precipitates heart failure because any negative inotropic effect is offset by a reduction in left ventricular work. Short-acting formulations of nifedipine are not recommended for long-term management of hypertension; their use may be associated with large variations in blood pressure and reflex tachycardia. However, they may be used if a modified-release preparation delivering the appropriate dose is not available or if a child is unable to swallow (a liquid preparation may be prepared using capsules). Nifedipine may also be used for the management of angina due to coronary artery disease in Kawasaki disease or progeria and in the management of Raynaud's syndrome.

Nicardipine has similar effects to those of nifedipine and may produce less reduction of myocardial contractility; it is used to treat hypertensive crisis.

Amlodipine also resembles nifedipine and nicardipine in its effects and does not reduce myocardial contractility or produce clinical deterioration in heart failure. It has a longer duration of action and can be given once daily. Nifedipine and amlodipine are used for the treatment of hypertension. Side-effects associated with vasodilatation such as flushing and headache (which become less obtrusive after a few days), and ankle swelling (which may respond only partially to diuretics) are common.

Nimodipine is related to nifedipine but the smooth muscle relaxant effect preferentially acts on cerebral arteries. Its use is confined to prevention and treatment of vascular spasm following aneurysmal subarachnoid haemorrhage.

Diltiazem is a peripheral vasodilator and also has mild depressor effects on the myocardium. It is used in the treatment of Raynaud's syndrome.

Withdrawal   There is some evidence that sudden withdrawal of calcium-channel blockers may be associated with an exacerbation of myocardial ischaemia.

◢ AMLODIPINE

Cautions acute porphyria (but see section 9.8.2); **interactions:** Appendix 1 (calcium-channel blockers)

Contra-indications cardiogenic shock, significant aortic stenosis

Hepatic impairment may need dose reduction—half-life prolonged

Pregnancy no information available—manufacturer advises avoid, but risk to fetus should be balanced against risk of uncontrolled maternal hypertension

Breast-feeding manufacturer advises avoid—no information available

Side-effects abdominal pain, nausea; palpitation, flushing, oedema; headache, dizziness, sleep disturbances, fatigue; *less commonly* gastro-intestinal disturbances, dry mouth, taste disturbances, hypotension, syncope, chest pain, dyspnoea, rhinitis, mood changes, asthenia, tremor, paraesthesia, urinary disturbances, impotence, gynaecomastia, weight changes, myalgia, muscle cramps, back pain, arthralgia, visual disturbances, tinnitus, pruritus, rashes (including isolated reports of erythema multiforme), sweating, alopecia, purpura, and skin discolouration; *very rarely* gastritis, pancreatitis, hepatitis, jaundice, cholestasis, gingival hyperplasia, myocardial infarction, arrhythmias, tachycardia, vasculitis, coughing, peripheral neuropathy, hyperglycaemia, thrombocytopenia, angioedema, and urticaria

Licensed use not licensed for use in children under 6 years

Indication and dose

> Hypertension
> • By mouth
>
> **Child 1 month–12 years** initially 100–200 micrograms/kg once daily; if necessary increase at intervals of 1–2 weeks up to 400 micrograms/kg once daily; max. 10 mg once daily
>
> **Child 12–18 years** initially 5 mg once daily; if necessary increase at intervals of 1–2 weeks to max. 10 mg once daily

Administration tablets may be dispersed in water

Note Tablets from various suppliers may contain different salts (e.g. amlodipine besilate, amlodipine maleate, and amlodipine mesilate) but the strength is expressed in terms of amlodipine (base); tablets containing different salts are considered interchangeable

Amlodipine (Non-proprietary) (PoM)

Tablets, amlodipine (as maleate or as mesilate) 5 mg, net price 28-tab pack = £1.12; 10 mg, 28-tab pack = £1.26

Brands include Amlostin®

◻ **AMLODIPINE** *(continued)*

Istin® (Pfizer) [PoM]
Tablets, amlodipine (as besilate) 5 mg, net price 28-
tab pack = £11.08; 10 mg, 28-tab pack = £16.55

◢Extemporaneous formulations available see
Extemporaneous Preparations, p. 8

◢ DILTIAZEM HYDROCHLORIDE

Cautions heart failure or significantly impaired left
ventricular function, bradycardia (avoid if
severe); first degree AV block, or prolonged PR
interval; **interactions:** Appendix 1 (calcium-
channel blockers)

Contra-indications severe bradycardia, left
ventricular failure with pulmonary congestion,
second- or third-degree AV block (unless pacemaker fitted), sick sinus syndrome; acute porphyria (section 9.8.2)

Hepatic impairment reduce dose

Renal impairment start with smaller dose

Pregnancy avoid

Breast-feeding significant amount present in
milk—no evidence of harm but avoid unless no
safer alternative

Side-effects bradycardia, sino-atrial block, AV
block, palpitation, dizziness, hypotension,
malaise, asthenia, headache, hot flushes, gastro-
intestinal disturbances, oedema (notably of
ankles); rarely rashes (including erythema multiforme and exfoliative dermatitis), photosensitivity; hepatitis, gynaecomastia, gum hyperplasia,
extrapyramidal symptoms, depression reported

Licensed use not licensed for use in children

Indication and dose

> **Raynaud's syndrome**
> • **By mouth**
>> **Child 12–18 years** 30–60 mg 2–3 times daily

◢**Standard formulations**
Note These formulations are licensed as generics and there
is no requirement for brand name dispensing. Although their
means of formulation has called for the strict designation
'modified-release' their duration of action corresponds to
that of tablets requiring administration more frequently

Diltiazem (Non-proprietary) [PoM]
Tablets, m/r (but see note above), diltiazem
hydrochloride 60 mg, net price 84 = £2.81.
Label: 25
Brands include *Optil®*

Tildiem® (Sanofi-Aventis) [PoM]
Tablets, m/r (but see note above), off-white, diltiazem hydrochloride 60 mg, net price 90-tab pack =
£7.96. Label: 25

◢ NICARDIPINE HYDROCHLORIDE

Cautions congestive heart failure or significantly
impaired left ventricular function; avoid grapefruit juice (may affect metabolism); **interactions:**
Appendix 1 (calcium-channel blockers)

Contra-indications cardiogenic shock; advanced
aortic stenosis; acute porphyria (section 9.8.2)

Hepatic impairment half-life prolonged in severe
impairment—may need dose reduction

Renal impairment start with smaller dose

Pregnancy may inhibit labour; toxicity in *animal*
studies; manufacturer advises avoid, but risk to
fetus should be balanced against risk of uncontrolled maternal hypertension

Breast-feeding manufacturer advises avoid—no
information available

Side-effects dizziness, headache, peripheral
oedema, flushing, palpitation, nausea; also gastro-intestinal disturbances, drowsiness, insomnia,
tinnitus, hypotension, rashes, dyspnoea, paraesthesia, frequency of micturition; thrombocytopenia, depression and impotence reported

Licensed use not licensed for use in children

Indication and dose

> Hypertensive crisis
> • **By continuous intravenous infusion**
>> **Neonate** initially 500 nanograms/kg/minute,
>> adjusted according to response; usual mainte-
>> nance of 1–4 micrograms/kg/minute
>>
>> **Child 1 month–18 years** initially 500 nan-
>> ograms/kg/minute, adjusted according to
>> response; usual maintenance of 1–4 micr-
>> ograms/kg/minute (max. 250 micrograms/
>> minute)

Administration for *intravenous infusion*, dilute to a
concentration of 100 micrograms/mL with Glucose 5% *or* Sodium Chloride 0.9%; to minimise
peripheral venous irritation, change site of infusion every 12 hours

Cardene IV® [PoM]
Injection, nicardipine 2.5 mg/mL (10-mL ampoule)
Available from 'special-order' manufacturers or specialist
importing companies, see p. 957

◢ NIFEDIPINE

Cautions see notes above; also poor cardiac
reserve; heart failure or significantly impaired left
ventricular function (heart failure deterioration
observed); severe hypotension; diabetes mellitus;
avoid grapefruit juice (may affect metabolism);
acute porphyria (but see section 9.8.2); **interactions:** Appendix 1 (calcium-channel blockers)

Contra-indications cardiogenic shock; advanced
aortic stenosis

Hepatic impairment dose reduction may be
required in severe liver disease

Pregnancy may inhibit labour; manufacturer
advises avoid before week 20, but risk to fetus
should be balanced against risk of uncontrolled

◁ **NIFEDIPINE (continued)**

maternal hypertension; use only if other treatment options are not indicated or have failed

Breast-feeding amount too small to be harmful
but manufacturer advises avoid

Side-effects gastro-intestinal disturbance; hypotension, oedema, vasodilatation, palpitation;
headache, dizziness, lethargy, asthenia; *less commonly* tachycardia, hypotension, syncope, chills,
nasal congestion, dyspnoea, anxiety, sleep disturbance, vertigo, migraine, paraesthesia, tremor,
polyuria, dysuria, nocturia, erectile dysfunction,
epistaxis, myalgia, joint swelling, visual disturbance, sweating, and hypersensitivity reactions
(including angioedema, jaundice, pruritus, urticaria, and rash); *rarely* anorexia, gum hyperplasia,
mood disturbances, hyperglycaemia, male
infertility, purpura, and photosensitivity reactions; also reported dysphagia, intestinal
obstruction, intestinal ulcer, bezoar formation,
gynaecomastia, agranulocytosis, and anaphylaxis

Licensed use not licensed for use in children

Indication and dose

**Hypertensive crisis, acute angina in Kawasaki
disease or progeria**

• By mouth (see Administration, below)

Child 1 month–18 years 250–500 micrograms/
kg as a single dose

**Hypertension, angina in Kawasaki disease or
progeria**

• By mouth

Child 1 month–12 years 200–300 micrograms/
kg 3 times daily; max. 3 mg/kg daily *or* 90 mg
daily

Child 12–18 years 5–20 mg 3 times daily; max.
90 mg daily
Note Dose frequency depends on preparation used

Raynaud's syndrome

• By mouth

Child 2–18 years 2.5–10 mg 2–4 times daily;
start with low doses at night and increase gradually to avoid postural hypotension
Note Dose frequency depends on preparation used

Persistent hyperinsulinaemic hypoglycaemia
see also section 6.1.4

• By mouth

Neonates 100–200 micrograms/kg (max.
600 micrograms/kg) 4 times daily

Administration for rapid effect in *hypertensive crisis*
or *acute angina*, bite capsules and swallow liquid
or use liquid preparation if 5-mg or 10-mg dose
inappropriate; if liquid unavailable, extract contents of capsule via a syringe and use immediately—cover syringe with foil to protect contents
from light; capsule contents may be diluted with
water if necessary.

Modified-release tablets may be crushed—this
may alter the release profile; crushed tablets
should be administered within 30–60 seconds to
avoid significant loss of potency of drug

Nifedipine (Non-proprietary) [PoM]

Capsules, nifedipine 5 mg, net price 84-cap pack =
£4.20; 10 mg, 84-cap pack = £5.59
Dose

Give 3 times daily

Oral liquid, available from 'special-order' manufacturers or specialist importing companies, see
p. 957

Adalat® (Bayer Schering) [PoM]

Capsules, orange, nifedipine 5 mg, net price 90-cap
pack = £5.84; 10 mg, 90-cap pack = £7.44
Dose

Give 3 times daily

◢Modified release
Note Different versions of modified-release preparations
may not have the same clinical effect. To avoid confusion
between these different formulations of nifedipine, prescribers should specify the brand to be dispensed. Modified-
release formulations may not be suitable for dose titration in
hepatic disease

Adalat® LA (Bayer Schering) [PoM]

LA 20 tablets, m/r, f/c, pink, nifedipine 20 mg, net
price 28-tab pack = £5.06. Label: 25

LA 30 tablets, m/r, f/c, pink, nifedipine 30 mg, net
price 28-tab pack = £7.13. Label: 25

LA 60 tablets, m/r, f/c, pink, nifedipine 60 mg, net
price 28-tab pack = £9.31. Label: 25

Counselling Tablet membrane may pass through gastro-
intestinal tract unchanged, but being porous has no effect
on efficacy

Cautions dose form not appropriate for use in hepatic
impairment or where there is a history of oesophageal or
gastro-intestinal obstruction, decreased lumen diameter
of the gastro-intestinal tract, or inflammatory bowel disease (including Crohn's disease)

Dose

Give once daily

Adalat® Retard (Bayer Schering) [PoM]

Retard 10 tablets, m/r, f/c, grey-pink, nifedipine
10 mg, net price 56-tab pack = £7.48. Label: 25

Retard 20 tablets, m/r, f/c, grey-pink, nifedipine
20 mg, net price 56-tab pack = £8.98. Label: 25
Dose

Give twice daily

Adipine® MR (Chiesi) [PoM]

Tablets, m/r, nifedipine 10 mg (apricot), net price
56-tab pack = £5.73; 20 mg (pink), 56-tab pack =
£7.14. Label: 25
Dose

Give twice daily

Adipine® XL (Chiesi) [PoM]

Tablets, m/r, red, nifedipine 30 mg, net price 28-tab
pack = £5.66. Label: 25
Dose

Give once daily

Coracten SR® (UCB Pharma) [PoM]

Capsules, m/r, nifedipine 10 mg (grey/pink,
enclosing yellow pellets), net price 60-cap pack =

◻ **NIFEDIPINE** *(continued)*

£3.90; 20 mg (pink/brown, enclosing yellow pellets), 60-cap pack = £5.41. Label: 25

Dose
> Give twice daily

Coracten XL® (UCB Pharma) [PoM]
Capsules, m/r, nifedipine 30 mg (brown), net price 28-cap pack = £4.89; 60 mg (orange), 28-cap pack = £7.34. Label: 25

Dose
> Give once daily

Fortipine LA 40® (Goldshield) [PoM]
Tablets, m/r, red, nifedipine 40 mg, net price 30-tab pack = £9.60. Label: 21, 25

Dose
> Give 1–2 times daily

Hypolar® Retard 20 (Sandoz) [PoM]
Tablets, m/r, red, f/c, nifedipine 20 mg, net price 56-tab pack = £5.75. Label: 25

Dose
> Give twice daily

Nifedipress® MR (Dexcel) [PoM]
Tablets, m/r, pink, nifedipine 10 mg, net price 56-tab pack = £2.02; 20 mg, 56-tab pack = £2.02. Label: 25

Dose
> Give twice daily

Note Also available as *Calchan®* MR

Tensipine MR® (Genus) [PoM]
Tablets, m/r, pink-grey, nifedipine 10 mg, net price 56-tab pack = £4.30; 20 mg, 56-tab pack = £5.49. Label: 21, 25

Dose
> Give twice daily

Valni XL® (Winthrop) [PoM]
Tablets, m/r, red, nifedipine 30 mg, net price 28-tab pack = £7.29; 60 mg, 28-tab pack = £9.31. Label: 25

Cautions dose form not appropriate for use in hepatic impairment, or where there is a history of oesophageal or gastro-intestinal obstruction, decreased lumen diameter of the gastro-intestinal tract, inflammatory bowel disease, or ileostomy after proctocolectomy

Dose
> Give once daily

▰ NIMODIPINE

Cautions cerebral oedema or severely raised intracranial pressure; hypotension; avoid concomitant administration of nimodipine tablets and infusion, other calcium-channel blockers, or beta-blockers; concomitant nephrotoxic drugs; avoid grapefruit juice (may affect metabolism); **interactions**: Appendix 1 (calcium-channel blockers, alcohol (infusion only))

Contra-indications acute porphyria (section 9.8.2)

Hepatic impairment elimination reduced in cirrhosis—monitor blood pressure

Renal impairment manufacturer advises monitor renal function closely with intravenous administration

Pregnancy manufacturer advises use only if potential benefit outweighs risks

Breast-feeding manufacturer advises avoid—present in milk

Side-effects hypotension, variation in heart-rate, flushing, headache, gastro-intestinal disorders, nausea, sweating and feeling of warmth; thrombocytopenia and ileus reported

Licensed use not licensed for use in children

Indication and dose

> Treatment of vasospasm following subarachnoid haemorrhage under specialist advice only
> • By intravenous infusion
> **Child 1 month–12 years** initially 15 micrograms/kg/hour (max. 500 micrograms/hour) *or* initially 7.5 micrograms/kg/hour if blood pressure unstable; increase after 2 hours to 30 micrograms/kg/hour (max. 2 mg/hour) if no severe decrease in blood pressure; continue for at least 5 days (max. 14 days)

> **Child 12–18 years** initially 500 micrograms/hour (up to 1 mg/hour if body-weight over 70 kg and blood pressure stable), increase after 2 hours to 1–2 mg/hour if no severe fall in blood pressure; continue for at least 5 days (max. 14 days)

> Prevention of vasospasm following subarachnoid haemorrhage
> • By mouth
> **Child 1 month–18 years** 0.9–1.2 mg/kg (max. 60 mg) 6 times daily, starting within 4 days of haemorrhage and continued for 21 days

Administration for *continuous intravenous infusion*, administer undiluted *via* a Y-piece on a central venous catheter connected to a running infusion of Glucose 5%, Sodium Chloride 0.9%, *or* Compound Sodium Lactate; not to be added to an infusion container; incompatible with polyvinyl chloride giving sets or containers; protect infusion from light.

For administration *by mouth*, tablets may be crushed or halved but are light sensitive—administer immediately

Nimotop® (Bayer Schering) [PoM]
Tablets, yellow, f/c, nimodipine 30 mg, net price 100-tab pack = £37.33

Intravenous infusion, nimodipine 200 micrograms/mL; also contains ethanol 20% and macrogol '400' 17%. Net price 50-mL vial (with polyethylene infusion catheter) = £7.47

Note Polyethylene, polypropylene, or glass apparatus should be used; PVC should be avoided

▲ VERAPAMIL HYDROCHLORIDE

Cautions first-degree AV block; patients taking beta-blockers (**important:** see below); avoid grapefruit juice (may affect metabolism); **interactions:** Appendix 1 (calcium-channel blockers)

Verapamil and beta-blockers **Verapamil** injection should not be given to patients recently treated with beta-blockers because of the risk of hypotension and asystole. The suggestion that when verapamil injection has been given first, an interval of 30 minutes before giving a beta-blocker is sufficient has not been confirmed.

It may also be hazardous to give verapamil and a beta-blocker together by mouth (should only be contemplated if myocardial function well preserved).

Contra-indications hypotension, bradycardia, second- and third-degree AV block, sick sinus syndrome, cardiogenic shock, sino-atrial block; history of heart failure or significantly impaired left ventricular function, even if controlled by therapy; atrial flutter or fibrillation complicating syndromes associated with accessory conducting pathways (e.g. Wolff-Parkinson-White syndrome); acute porphyria (section 9.8.2)

Hepatic impairment oral dose may need to be reduced

Pregnancy may reduce uterine blood flow with fetal hypoxia; manufacturer advises avoid during first trimester unless absolutely necessary; may inhibit labour

Breast-feeding amount too small to be harmful

Side-effects constipation; *less commonly* nausea, vomiting, flushing, headache, dizziness, fatigue, ankle oedema; *rarely* allergic reactions (erythema, pruritus, urticaria, angioedema, Stevens-Johnson syndrome); myalgia, arthralgia, paraesthesia, erythromelalgia; increased prolactin concentration; gynaecomastia and gingival hyperplasia after long-term treatment; after intravenous administration or high doses, hypotension, heart failure, bradycardia, heart block, and asystole; hypersensitivity reactions involving reversibly raised liver function tests

Licensed use Modified release preparation not licensed for use in children

Indication and dose

Hypertension, prophylaxis of supraventricular arrhythmias under specialist advice only

• **By mouth**

   Child 1–2 years 20 mg 2–3 times daily

   Child 2–18 years 40–120 mg 2–3 times daily

Treatment of supraventricular arrhythmias

• **By intravenous injection over 2–3 minutes (with ECG and blood-pressure monitoring and under specialist advice)**

   Child 1–18 years 100–300 micrograms/kg (max. 5 mg) as a single dose, repeated after 30 minutes if necessary

Administration for *intravenous injection*, may be diluted with Glucose 5% *or* Sodium Chloride 0.9%; incompatible with solutions of pH greater than 6

Verapamil (Non-proprietary) ℗℗ℳ

Tablets, coated, verapamil hydrochloride 40 mg, net price 84-tab pack = £1.56; 80 mg, 84-tab pack = £1.83; 120 mg, 28-tab pack = £1.42; 160 mg, 56-tab pack = £28.20

Oral solution, verapamil hydrochloride 40 mg/ 5 mL, net price 150 mL = £36.90
Brands include *Zolvera*®

Cordilox® (Dexcel) ℗℗ℳ

Tablets, yellow, f/c, verapamil hydrochloride 40 mg, net price 84-tab pack = £1.50; 80 mg, 84-tab pack = £2.05; 120 mg, 28-tab pack = £1.15; 160 mg, 56-tab pack = £2.80

Injection, verapamil hydrochloride 2.5 mg/mL, net price 2-mL amp = £1.11

Securon® (Abbott) ℗℗ℳ

Injection, verapamil hydrochloride 2.5 mg/mL, net price 2-mL amp = £1.08

◀ Extemporaneous formulations available see Extemporaneous Preparations, p. 8

◀ Modified release

Half Securon SR® (Abbott) ℗℗ℳ

Tablets, m/r, f/c, verapamil hydrochloride 120 mg, net price 28-tab pack = £7.86. Label: 25

Dose

> Give once daily (doses above 240 mg daily, give 2–3 times daily)

Securon SR® (Abbott) ℗℗ℳ

Tablets, m/r, pale green, f/c, scored, verapamil hydrochloride 240 mg, net price 28-tab pack = £5.66. Label: 25

Dose

> Give once daily (doses above 240 mg daily, give 2–3 times daily)

Univer® (Cephalon) ℗℗ℳ

Capsules, m/r, verapamil hydrochloride 120 mg (yellow/dark blue), net price 28-cap pack = £4.96; 180 mg (yellow), 56-cap pack = £11.98; 240 mg (yellow/dark blue), 28-cap pack = £8.08. Label: 25

Dose

> Give once daily

Verapress MR® (Dexcel) ℗℗ℳ

Tablets, m/r, pale green, f/c, verapamil hydrochloride 240 mg, net price 28-tab pack = £6.04. Label: 25

Dose

> Give 1–2 times daily

Note Also available as *Cordilox*® MR

Vertab® SR 240 (Chiesi) ℗℗ℳ

Tablets, m/r, pale green, f/c, scored, verapamil hydrochloride 240 mg, net price 28-tab pack = £8.29. Label: 25

Dose

> Give 1–2 times daily

2

Cardiovascular system

Cardiovascular system (side)

2

2.6.3 Other antianginal drugs

Classification not used in *BNF for Children*.

2.6.4 Peripheral vasodilators and related drugs

Raynaud's syndrome consists of recurrent, long-lasting, and episodic vasospasm of the fingers and toes often associated with exposure to cold. Management includes avoidance of exposure to cold and stopping smoking (if appropriate). More severe symptoms may require vasodilator treatment, which is most often successful in primary Raynaud's syndrome. **Nifedipine** and **diltiazem** (section 2.6.2) are useful for reducing the frequency and severity of vasospastic attacks. In very severe cases, where digital infarction is likely, intravenous infusion of the prostacyclin analogue **iloprost** may be helpful.

Vasodilator therapy is not established as being effective for *chilblains* (section 13.13).

◢ ILOPROST

Cautions see section 2.5.1.2
Contra-indications see section 2.5.1.2
Side-effects see section 2.5.1.2
Licensed use not licensed for use in children

Indication and dose

Raynaud's syndrome see notes above
• By intravenous infusion
   Child 12–18 years initially 30 nanograms/kg/ hour, increased gradually to 60–120 nanograms/kg/hour given over 6 hours daily for 3–5 days

Pulmonary hypertension section 2.5.1.2

Administration for *intravenous infusion*, dilute to a concentration of 200 nanograms/mL with Glucose 5% or Sodium Chloride 0.9%; alternatively, may be diluted to a concentration of 2 micrograms/mL and given via syringe driver

Iloprost (Non-proprietary)
Concentrate for infusion, iloprost (as trometamol) 100 micrograms/mL
For dilution and use as an intravenous infusion
Note available on a named patient basis from Bayer Schering in 0.5 mL and 1 mL ampoules

2.7 Sympathomimetics

2.7.1 Inotropic sympathomimetics
2.7.2 Vasoconstrictor sympathomimetics
2.7.3 Cardiopulmonary resuscitation

The properties of sympathomimetics vary according to whether they act on alpha or on beta adrenergic receptors. Response to sympathomimetics can also vary considerably in children, particularly neonates. It is important to titrate the dose to the desired effect and to monitor the child closely.

2.7.1 Inotropic sympathomimetics

The cardiac stimulants **dobutamine** and **dopamine** act on beta$_1$ receptors in cardiac muscle and increase contractility with little effect on rate.

Dopamine has a variable, unpredictable, and dose dependent impact on vascular tone. Low dose infusion (2 micrograms/kg/minute) normally causes vasodilatation, but there is little evidence that this is clinically beneficial; moderate doses increase myocardial contractility and cardiac output in older children, but in neonates moderate doses may cause a reduction in cardiac output. High doses cause vasoconstriction and increase vascular resistance, and should therefore be used with caution following cardiac surgery, or where there is co-existing neonatal pulmonary hypertension.

In neonates the response to inotropic sympathomimetics varies considerably, particularly in those born prematurely; careful dose titration and monitoring are necessary.

Isoprenaline injection is available from 'special-order' manufacturers or specialist importing companies, see p. 957.

Shock   Shock is a medical emergency associated with a high mortality. The underlying causes of shock such as haemorrhage, sepsis or myocardial insufficiency should be corrected. Additional treatment is dependent on the type of shock.

Septic shock is associated with severe hypovolaemia (due to vasodilation and capillary leak) which should be corrected with crystalloids or colloids (section 9.2.2). If hypotension persists despite volume replacement, **dopamine** should be started. For shock refractory to treatment with dopamine, if cardiac output is high and peripheral vascular resistance is low (warm shock), **noradrenaline** (norepinephrine) (section 2.7.2) should be added *or* if cardiac output is low and peripheral vascular resistance is high (cold shock), **adrenaline** (epinephrine) (section 2.7.2) should be added. Additionally, in cold shock, a vasodilator such as **milrinone** (section 2.1.2), **glyceryl trinitrate** (section 2.6.1), or **sodium nitroprusside** (on specialist advice only) (section 2.5.1.1) can be used to reduce vascular resistance.

If the shock is resistant to volume expansion and catecholamines, and there is suspected or proven adrenal insufficiency, low dose **hydrocortisone** (section 6.3.2) can be used. ACTH-stimulated plasma-cortisol concentration should be measured; however, hydrocortisone can be started without such information.

Alternatively, if the child is resistant to catecholamines, and vascular resistance is low, **vasopressin** (section 6.5.2) can be added.

Neonatal septic shock can be complicated by the transition from fetal to neonatal circulation. Treatment to reverse right ventricular failure, by decreasing pulmonary artery pressures, is commonly needed in neonates with fluid-refractory shock and persistent pulmonary hypertension of the newborn (section 2.5.1.2). Rapid administration of fluid in neonates with patent ductus arteriosus may cause left-to-right shunting and congestive heart failure induced by ventricular overload.

In *cardiogenic shock*, the aim is to improve cardiac output and to reduce the afterload on the heart. If central venous pressure is low, cautious volume expansion with a colloid or crystalloid can be used. An inotrope such as **adrenaline** (epinephrine) (section 2.7.2) or **dopamine** should be given to increase cardiac output. **Dobutamine** is a peripheral vasodilator and is an alternative if hypotension is not significant.

Milrinone (section 2.1.2) has both inotropic and vasodilatory effects and can be used when vascular resistance is high. Alternatively, **glyceryl trinitrate** (2.6.1) or **sodium nitroprusside** (on specialist advice only) (section 2.5.1.1) can be used to reduce vasoconstriction.

Hypovolaemic shock should be treated with a crystalloid or colloid solution (or whole or reconstituted blood if source of hypovolaemia is haemorrhage) and further steps to improve cardiac output and decrease vascular resistance can be taken, as in cardiogenic shock.

The use of sympathomimetic inotropes and vasoconstrictors should preferably be confined to the intensive care setting and undertaken with invasive haemodynamic monitoring.

For advice on the management of anaphylactic shock, see section 3.4.3.

DOBUTAMINE

Cautions arrhythmias, acute myocardial infarction, acute heart failure, severe hypotension, marked obstruction of cardiac ejection (such as idiopathic hypertrophic subaortic stenosis); correct hypovolaemia before starting treatment; tolerance may develop with continuous infusions longer than 72 hours; hyperthyroidism; **interactions:** Appendix 1 (sympathomimetics)

Contra-indications phaeochromocytoma

Pregnancy no evidence of harm in *animal* studies—manufacturers advise use only if benefit outweighs risk

Breast-feeding manufacturers advise avoid—no information available

Side-effects nausea; hypotension, hypertension (marked increase in systolic blood pressure indicates overdose), arrhythmias, palpitation, chest pain; dyspnoea, bronchospasm; headache; fever; increased urinary urgency; eosinophilia; rash, phlebitis; *very rarely* myocardial infarction, hypokalaemia; *also reported* coronary artery spasm and thrombocytopenia

Licensed use strong sterile solution not licensed for use in children

Indication and dose

Inotropic support in low cardiac output states, after cardiac surgery, cardiomyopathies, shock
• By continuous intravenous infusion

Neonate initially 5 micrograms/kg/minute, adjusted according to response to 2–15 micrograms/kg/minute; max. 20 micrograms/kg/minute

2

Cardiovascular system

◁ **DOBUTAMINE** *(continued)*

Child 1 month–18 years initially 5 micrograms/kg/minute adjusted according to response to 2–20 micrograms/kg/minute

Administration for *continuous intravenous infusion*, using infusion pump, dilute to a concentration of 0.5–1 mg/mL (max. 5 mg/mL if fluid restricted) with Glucose 5% or Sodium Chloride 0.9%; infuse higher concentration solutions through central venous catheter only. Incompatible with bicarbonate and other strong alkaline solutions.
Neonatal intensive care, dilute 30 mg/kg body-weight to a final volume of 50 mL with infusion fluid; an intravenous infusion rate of 0.5 mL/hour provides a dose of 5 micrograms/kg/minute

Dobutamine (Non-proprietary) ℞
Injection, dobutamine (as hydrochloride) 5 mg/mL. To be diluted before use or given undiluted with syringe pump. Net price 50-mL vial = £7.50
Excipients may include sulphites

Strong sterile solution, dobutamine (as hydrochloride) 12.5 mg/mL. For dilution and use as an intravenous infusion. Net price 20-mL amp = £5.20
Excipients may include sulphites

DOPAMINE HYDROCHLORIDE

Cautions correct hypovolaemia; hyperthyroidism; **interactions**: Appendix 1 (sympathomimetics)

Contra-indications tachyarrhythmia, phaeochromocytoma

Pregnancy manufacturer advises use only if potential benefit outweighs risk

Side-effects nausea and vomiting, peripheral vasoconstriction, hypotension, hypertension, tachycardia

Licensed use not licensed for use in children under 12 years

Indication and dose

To correct the haemodynamic imbalance due to acute hypotension, shock, cardiac failure, adjunct following cardiac surgery
• By continuous intravenous infusion

Neonate initially 3 micrograms/kg/minute, adjusted according to response (max. 20 micrograms/kg/minute)

Child 1 month–18 years initially 5 micrograms/kg/minute adjusted according to response (max. 20 micrograms/kg/minute)

Administration for *continuous intravenous infusion*, dilute to a max. concentration of 3.2 mg/mL with Glucose 5% *or* Sodium Chloride 0.9%. Infuse higher concentrations through central venous catheter using a syringe pump to avoid extravasation and fluid overload. Incompatible with bicarbonate and other alkaline solutions.
Neonatal intensive care, dilute 30 mg/kg body-weight to a final volume of 50 mL with infusion fluid; an intravenous infusion rate of 0.3 mL/hour provides a dose of 3 micrograms/kg/minute

Dopamine (Non-proprietary) ℞
Sterile concentrate, dopamine hydrochloride 40 mg/mL, net price 5-mL amp = 90p; 160 mg/mL, net price 5-mL amp = £4.00. For dilution and use as an intravenous infusion

Intravenous infusion, dopamine hydrochloride 1.6 mg/mL in glucose 5% intravenous infusion, net price 250-mL container (400 mg) = £11.69. Available from 'special-order' manufacturers or specialist importing companies, p. 957

Select-A-Jet® Dopamine (UCB Pharma) ℞
Strong sterile solution, dopamine hydrochloride 40 mg/mL. For dilution and use as an intravenous infusion. Net price 5-mL vial = £5.51; 10-mL vial = £8.86

2.7.2 Vasoconstrictor sympathomimetics

Vasoconstrictor sympathomimetics raise blood pressure transiently by acting on alpha-adrenergic receptors to constrict peripheral vessels. They are sometimes used as an emergency method of elevating blood pressure where other measures have failed (see also section 2.7.1).

The danger of vasoconstrictors is that although they raise blood pressure they also reduce perfusion of vital organs such as the kidney.

Ephedrine is used to reverse hypotension caused by spinal and epidural anaesthesia.

Metaraminol is used as a vasopressor during cardiopulmonary bypass.

Phenylephrine causes peripheral vasoconstriction and increases arterial pressure.

Ephedrine, metaraminol and phenylephrine are rarely needed in children and should be used under specialist supervision.

Noradrenaline (norepinephrine) is reserved for children with low systemic vascular resistance that is unresponsive to fluid resuscitation following septic shock, spinal shock, and anaphylaxis.

Adrenaline (epinephrine) is mainly used for its inotropic action. Low doses (acting on beta receptors) cause systemic and pulmonary vasodilation, with some increase in heart rate and stroke volume and also an increase in contractility; high doses act predominantly on alpha receptors causing intense systemic vasoconstriction.

EPHEDRINE HYDROCHLORIDE

Cautions hyperthyroidism, diabetes mellitus, hypertension, susceptibility to angle-closure glaucoma, **interactions:** Appendix 1 (sympathomimetics)

Renal impairment use with caution

Pregnancy increased fetal heart rate reported with parenteral ephedrine

Breast-feeding irritability and disturbed sleep reported

Side-effects nausea, vomiting, anorexia; tachycardia (sometimes bradycardia), arrhythmias, anginal pain, vasoconstriction with hypertension, vasodilation with hypotension, dizziness and flushing; dyspnoea; headache, anxiety, restlessness, confusion, psychoses, insomnia, tremor; difficulty in micturition, urine retention; sweating, hypersalivation; changes in blood-glucose concentration; *very rarely* angle-closure glaucoma

Indication and dose

Reversal of hypotension from epidural and spinal anaesthesia
• By slow intravenous injection of a solution containing ephedrine hydrochloride 3 mg/mL

　Child 1–12 years 500–750 micrograms/kg *or* 17–25 mg/m^2 every 3–4 minutes according to response; max. 30 mg during episode

　Child 12–18 years 3–7.5 mg (max. 9 mg) repeated every 3–4 minutes according to response, max. 30 mg during episode

Nasal congestion section 12.2.2

Administration for *slow intravenous injection*, give via central venous catheter

Ephedrine Hydrochloride (Non-proprietary) ℗oM
Injection, ephedrine hydrochloride 3 mg/mL, net price 10-mL amp = £2.83; 30 mg/mL, net price 1-mL amp = 50p

METARAMINOL

Cautions see under Noradrenaline; longer duration of action than noradrenaline (norepinephrine), see below; cirrhosis; **interactions:** Appendix 1 (sympathomimetics)

Hypertensive response Metaraminol has a longer duration of action than noradrenaline, and an excessive vasopressor response may cause a prolonged rise in blood pressure

Contra-indications see under Noradrenaline

Pregnancy may reduce placental prefusion—manufacturer advises use only if potential benefit outweighs risk

Breast-feeding manufacturer advises caution—no information available

Side-effects see under Noradrenaline; tachycardia; fatal ventricular arrhythmia reported in Laennec's cirrhosis

Licensed use not licensed for use in children

Indication and dose

Acute hypotension
• By intravenous infusion
　Child 12–18 years 15–100 mg adjusted according to response

Emergency treatment of acute hypotension
• By intravenous administration
　Child 12–18 years initially by intravenous injection 0.5–5 mg, then by intravenous infusion 15–100 mg adjusted according to response

Administration for *intravenous infusion*, dilute to a concentration of 30–200 micrograms/mL with Glucose 5% *or* Sodium Chloride 0.9% and give through a central venous catheter

Metaraminol (Non-proprietary) ℗oM
Injection, metaraminol 10 mg (as tartrate)/mL. Available from 'special-order' manufacturers or specialist importing companies, see p. 957

NORADRENALINE/NOREPINEPHRINE

Cautions coronary, mesenteric, or peripheral vascular thrombosis; Prinzmetal's variant angina, hyperthyroidism, diabetes mellitus; hypoxia or hypercapnia; uncorrected hypovolaemia; extravasation at injection site may cause necrosis; **interactions:** Appendix 1 (sympathomimetics)

Contra-indications hypertension (monitor blood pressure and rate of flow frequently)

Pregnancy avoid—may reduce placental perfusion

Side-effects hypertension, headache, bradycardia, arrhythmias, peripheral ischaemia

Licensed use not licensed for use in children

Indication and dose

Acute hypotension (septic shock) or shock secondary to excessive vasodilation (as noradrenaline)
• By continuous intravenous infusion

　Neonate 20–100 nanograms (base)/kg/minute adjusted according to response; max. 1 microgram (base)/kg/minute

　Child 1 month–18 years 20–100 nanograms (base)/kg/minute adjusted according to response; max. 1 microgram (base)/kg/minute
　Note 1 mg of noradrenaline acid tartrate is equivalent to 500 micrograms of the base. Dose expressed as the base

2

Cardiovascular system

◯ **NORADRENALINE/NOREPINEPHRINE (continued)**

Administration for *continuous intravenous infusion*, dilute to a max. concentration of noradrenaline (base) 40 micrograms/mL (higher concentrations can be used if fluid-restricted) with Glucose 5% *or* Sodium Chloride and Glucose. Infuse through central venous catheter; discard if discoloured. Incompatible with bicarbonate or alkaline solutions.

Neonatal intensive care, dilute 600 micrograms (base)/kg body-weight to a final volume of 50 mL with infusion fluid; an intravenous infusion rate of 0.1 mL/hour provides a dose of 20 nanograms (base)/kg/minute

Noradrenaline/Norepinephrine (Non-proprietary)
PoM

Injection, noradrenaline acid tartrate 2 mg/mL (equivalent to noradrenaline base 1 mg/mL). For dilution before use. Net price 2-mL amp = £1.01, 4-mL amp = £1.50, 20-mL amp = £6.35
Excipients may include sodium metabisulphite

PHENYLEPHRINE HYDROCHLORIDE

Cautions see under Noradrenaline; longer duration of action than noradrenaline (norepinephrine), see below; coronary disease

Hypertensive response Phenylephrine has a longer duration of action than noradrenaline, and an excessive vasopressor response may cause a prolonged rise in blood pressure

Contra-indications see under Noradrenaline; severe hyperthyroidism

Pregnancy avoid if possible; malformations reported following use in first trimester; fetal hypoxia and bradycardia reported in late pregnancy and labour

Side-effects see under Noradrenaline; tachycardia or reflex bradycardia

Licensed use not licensed for use in children by intravenous infusion or injection

Indication and dose

Acute hypotension

- By subcutaneous or intramuscular injection (but intravenous injection preferred, see below)

  Child 1–12 years 100 micrograms/kg every 1–2 hours as needed (max. 5 mg)

  Child 12–18 years 2–5 mg, followed if necessary by further doses of 1–10 mg (max. initial dose 5 mg)

- By slow intravenous injection

  Child 1–12 years 5–20 micrograms/kg (max. 500 micrograms) repeated as necessary after at least 15 minutes

  Child 12–18 years 100–500 micrograms repeated as necessary after at least 15 minutes

- By intravenous infusion

  Child 1–16 years 100–500 nanograms/kg/minute, adjusted according to response

  Child 16–18 years initially up to 180 micrograms/minute reduced to 30–60 micrograms/minute according to response

Administration for *intravenous injection*, dilute to a concentration of 1 mg/mL with Water for Injections and administer slowly.

For *intravenous infusion*, dilute to a concentration of 20 micrograms/mL with Glucose 5% *or* Sodium Chloride 0.9% and administer as a continuous infusion via a central venous catheter using a controlled infusion device

Phenylephrine (Sovereign) PoM
Injection, phenylephrine hydrochloride 10 mg/mL (1%), net price 1-mL amp = £5.50

ADRENALINE/EPINEPHRINE

Cautions ischaemic heart disease, severe angina, obstructive cardiomyopathy, hypertension, arrhythmias, cerebrovascular disease; occlusive vascular disease, monitor blood pressure and ECG; cor pulmonale; organic brain damage, psychoneurosis; phaeochromocytoma; diabetes mellitus, hyperthyroidism; hypokalaemia, hypercalcaemia; susceptibility to angle-closure glaucoma; **interactions**: Appendix 1 (sympathomimetics)

Renal impairment manufacturers advise use with caution in severe impairment

Pregnancy may reduce placental perfusion and can delay second stage of labour; manufacturers advise use only if benefit outweighs risk

Breast-feeding present in milk but unlikely to be harmful as poor oral bioavailability

Side-effects nausea, vomiting, dry mouth, hypersalivation; arrhythmias, palpitation, syncope, angina, hypertension (risk of cerebral haemorrhage), cold extremities, pallor; dyspnoea, pulmonary oedema (on excessive dosage or extreme sensitivity); anxiety, tremor, restlessness, headache, weakness, dizziness, hallucinations; hyperglycaemia; difficulty in micturition, urinary retention; metabolic acidosis; hypokalaemia; mydriasis, angle-closure glaucoma; tissue necrosis at injection site and of extremities, liver and kidneys, sweating

Indication and dose

Acute hypotension

- By continuous intravenous infusion

  Neonate initially 100 nanograms/kg/minute adjusted according to response; higher doses up to 1.5 micrograms/kg/minute have been used in acute hypotension

  Child 1 month–18 years initially 100 nanograms/kg/minute adjusted according to response; higher doses up to 1.5 micrograms/kg/minute have been used in acute hypotension

Anaphylaxis section 3.4.3

◻ **ADRENALINE/EPINEPHRINE** (*continued*)

Administration for *continuous intravenous infusion*, dilute with Glucose 5% *or* Sodium Chloride 0.9% and give through a central venous catheter. Incompatible with bicarbonate and alkaline solutions.

Neonatal intensive care, dilute 3 mg/kg body-weight to a final volume of 50 mL with infusion fluid; an intravenous infusion rate of 0.1 mL/hour provides a dose of 100 nanograms/kg/minute

Note These infusions are usually made up with adrenaline 1 in 1000 (1 mg/mL) solution; this concentration of adrenaline is not licensed for intravenous administration

◢**Preparations**
Section 3.4.3

2.7.3 Cardiopulmonary resuscitation

The algorithms for cardiopulmonary resuscitation (see inside back cover) reflect the recommendations of the Resuscitation Council (UK); they cover paediatric basic life support, paediatric advanced life support, and newborn life support. The guidelines are available at www.resus.org.uk.

Paediatric advanced life support   Cardiopulmonary (cardiac) arrest in children is rare and frequently represents the terminal event of progressive shock or respiratory failure.

During cardiopulmonary arrest in children without intravenous access, the intraosseous route is chosen because it provides rapid and effective response; if circulatory access cannot be gained, the endotracheal tube can be used. When the endotracheal route is used ten times the intravenous dose should be used; the drug should be injected quickly down a narrow bore suction catheter beyond the tracheal end of the tube and then flushed in with 1 or 2 mL of sodium chloride 0.9%. The endotracheal route is useful for lipid-soluble drugs, including lidocaine, adrenaline, atropine, and naloxone. Drugs that are not lipid-soluble (e.g. sodium bicarbonate and calcium chloride) should **not** be administered by this route because they will injure the airways.

For the management of acute anaphylaxis see section 3.4.3.

2.8 Anticoagulants and protamine

2.8.1 Parenteral anticoagulants
2.8.2 Oral anticoagulants
2.8.3 Protamine sulphate

Although thrombotic episodes are uncommon in childhood, anticoagulants may be required in children with congenital heart disease; in children undergoing haemodialysis; for preventing thrombosis in children requiring chemotherapy and following surgery; and for systemic venous thromboembolism secondary to inherited thrombophilias, systemic lupus erythematosus, or indwelling central venous catheters.

2.8.1 Parenteral anticoagulants

Heparin

Heparin initiates anticoagulation rapidly but has a short duration of action. It is now often referred to as being **standard** or **unfractionated heparin** to distinguish it from the **low molecular weight heparins** (see p. 149), which have a longer duration of action. For children at high risk of bleeding, unfractionated heparin is more suitable than low molecular weight heparin because its effect can be terminated rapidly by stopping the infusion.

Heparins are used in both the treatment and prophylaxis of thromboembolic disease, mainly to prevent further clotting rather than to lyse existing clots—surgery or a thrombolytic drug may be necessary if a thrombus obstructs major vessels.

Treatment   For the initial treatment of thrombotic episodes unfractionated heparin is given as an intravenous loading dose, followed by continuous intravenous infusion (using an infusion pump) or by intermittent subcutaneous injection; the

2 Cardiovascular system

use of intermittent intravenous injection is no longer recommended. Alternatively, a low molecular weight heparin may be given for initial treatment. If an oral anticoagulant (usually warfarin, section 2.8.2) is also required, it may be started at the same time as the heparin (the heparin needs to be continued for at least 5 days and until the INR has been in the therapeutic range for 2 consecutive days). Laboratory monitoring of coagulation activity, preferably on a daily basis, involves determination of the activated partial thromboplastin time (APTT) (for unfractionated heparin only) or of the anti-Factor Xa concentration (for low molecular weight heparins). Local guidelines on recommended APTT for neonates and children should be followed.

Prophylaxis Low-dose unfractionated heparin by subcutaneous injection is used to prevent thrombotic episodes in 'high-risk' patients; laboratory monitoring of APTT or anti-Factor Xa concentration is also required in prophylactic regimens in children. Low molecular weight heparins, **aspirin** (section 2.9), and **warfarin** (section 2.8.2) can also be used for prophylaxis.

Pregnancy Heparins are used for the management of thromboembolic disease in pregnancy because they do not cross the placenta. Low molecular weight heparins are preferred because they have a lower risk of osteoporosis and of heparin-induced thrombocytopenia. Low molecular weight heparins are eliminated more rapidly in pregnancy, requiring alteration of the dosage regimen for drugs such as dalteparin, enoxaparin, and tinzaparin. Treatment should be stopped at the onset of labour and advice sought from a specialist on continuing therapy after birth.

Extracorporeal circuits Unfractionated heparin is also used in the maintenance of extracorporeal circuits in cardiopulmonary bypass and haemodialysis.

Haemorrhage If haemorrhage occurs it is usually sufficient to withdraw unfractionated or low molecular weight heparin, but if rapid reversal of the effects of the heparin is required, protamine sulphate (section 2.8.3) is a specific antidote (but only partially reverses the effects of low molecular weight heparins).

HEPARIN

Cautions see notes above; concomitant use of drugs that increase risk of bleeding; **interactions:** Appendix 1 (heparin)

Heparin-induced thrombocytopenia Clinically important heparin-induced thrombocytopenia is immune-mediated and does not usually develop until after 5–10 days; it can be complicated by thrombosis. Platelet counts should be measured just before treatment with unfractionated or low molecular weight heparin, and regular monitoring of platelet counts is recommended if given for longer than 4 days. Signs of heparin-induced thrombocytopenia include a 50% reduction of platelet count, thrombosis, or skin allergy. If heparin-induced thrombocytopenia is strongly suspected or confirmed, the heparin should be **stopped** and an alternative anticoagulant, such as danaparoid, should be given. Ensure platelet counts return to normal range in those who require warfarin

Hyperkalaemia Inhibition of aldosterone secretion by unfractionated or low molecular weight heparin can result in hyperkalaemia; patients with diabetes mellitus, chronic renal failure, acidosis, raised plasma-potassium concentration, or those taking potassium-sparing drugs seem to be more susceptible. The risk appears to increase with duration of therapy and plasma-potassium concentration should be measured in children at risk of hyperkalaemia before starting the heparin and monitored regularly thereafter, particularly if treatment is to be continued for longer than 7 days

Contra-indications haemophilia and other haemorrhagic disorders, thrombocytopenia (including history of heparin-induced thrombocytopenia), recent cerebral haemorrhage, severe hypertension; peptic ulcer; after major trauma or recent surgery to eye or nervous system; acute bacterial endocarditis; spinal or epidural anaesthesia with treatment doses of unfractionated or low molecular weight heparin; hypersensitivity to unfractionated or low molecular weight heparin

Hepatic impairment risk of bleeding increased—reduce dose or avoid in severe impairment (including oesophageal varices)

Renal impairment risk of bleeding increased in severe impairment—dose may need to be reduced

Pregnancy does not cross the placenta; maternal osteoporosis reported after prolonged use; multidose vials may contain benzyl alcohol—some manufacturers advise avoid; see also notes above

Breast-feeding not excreted in milk due to high molecular weight

Side-effects haemorrhage (see notes above), thrombocytopenia (see Cautions), rarely rebound hyperlipidaemia following unfractionated heparin withdrawal, priapism, hyperkalaemia (see Cautions), osteoporosis (risk lower with low molecular weight heparins), alopecia on prolonged use, injection-site reactions, skin necrosis, and hypersensitivity reactions (including urticaria, angioedema, and anaphylaxis)

Licensed use Some preparations licensed for use in children

Indication and dose

Maintenance of neonatal umbilical arterial catheter
• By intravenous infusion

Neonate 0.5 units/hour

◻ **HEPARIN** *(continued)*

Treatment of thrombotic episodes
- **By intravenous administration**

  Neonate initially 75 units/kg (50 units/kg if under 35 weeks post-menstrual age) *by intravenous injection*, then *by continuous intravenous infusion* 25 units/kg/hour, adjusted according to APTT

  Child 1 month–1 year initially 75 units/kg *by intravenous injection*, then *by continuous intravenous infusion* 25 units/kg/hour, adjusted according to APTT

  Child 1–18 years initially 75 units/kg *by intravenous injection*, then *by continuous intravenous infusion* 20 units/kg/hour, adjusted according to APTT

- **By subcutaneous injection**

  Child 1 month–18 years 250 units/kg twice daily, adjusted according to APTT

Prophylaxis of thrombotic episodes
- **By subcutaneous injection**

  Child 1 month–18 years 100 units/kg (max. 5000 units) twice daily, adjusted according to APTT

Prevention of clotting in extracorporeal circuits consult product literature

Administration for *continuous intravenous infusion*, dilute with Glucose 5% *or* Sodium Chloride 0.9%. *Maintenance of neonatal umbilical arterial catheter*, dilute 50 units to a final volume of 50 mL with Sodium Chloride 0.45% *or* use ready-made bag containing 500 units in 500 mL Sodium Chloride 0.9%; infuse at 0.5 mL/hour.
Neonatal intensive care (treatment of thrombosis), dilute 1250 units/kg body-weight to a final volume of 50 mL with infusion fluid; an intravenous infusion rate of 1 mL/hour provides a dose of 25 units/kg/hour

Heparin Sodium (Non-proprietary) ℗ₒ𝔐
Injection, heparin sodium 1000 units/mL, net price 1-mL amp = 50p, 5-mL amp = £1.25, 5-mL vial = £1.25, 10-mL amp = £2.15, 20-mL amp = £3.54; 5000 units/mL, 1-mL amp = 97p, 5-mL amp = £2.53, 5-mL vial = £2.82; 25 000 units/mL, 0.2-mL amp = £1.25, 1-mL amp = £2.57, 5-mL vial = £3.68
Excipients may include benzyl alcohol (avoid in neonates, see Excipients, p. 3)

Heparin Calcium (Non-proprietary) ℗ₒ𝔐
Injection, heparin calcium 25 000 units/mL, net price 0.2-mL amp = £1.30

2

Cardiovascular system

Low molecular weight heparins

Dalteparin, **enoxaparin**, and **tinzaparin** are low molecular weight heparins used for treatment and prophylaxis of thrombotic episodes in children (see also Heparin, p. 147). Their duration of action is longer than that of unfractionated heparin and in adults and older children *once-daily subcutaneous* dosage is sometimes possible; however, younger children require relatively higher doses (possibly due to larger volume of distribution, altered heparin pharmacokinetics, or lower plasma concentrations of antithrombin) and twice daily dosage is sometimes necessary. Low molecular weight heparins are convenient to use, especially in children with poor venous access. Routine monitoring of anti-Factor Xa activity is not usually required except in neonates; monitoring may also be necessary in severely ill children and those with renal or hepatic impairment.

Haemorrhage   See under Heparin.

Hepatic impairment   Reduce dose in severe impairment—risk of bleeding may be increased.

Pregnancy   Not known to be harmful, low molecular weight heparins do not cross the placenta; see also Heparin, p. 148.

Breast-feeding   Due to the relatively high molecular weight of these drugs and inactivation in the gastro-intestinal tract, passage into breast-milk and absorption by the nursing infant are likely to be negligible; however manufacturers advise avoid.

◼ **DALTEPARIN SODIUM**

Cautions see under Heparin and notes above
Contra-indications see under Heparin
Hepatic impairment see notes above
Renal impairment risk of bleeding may be increased—dose reduction and monitoring of anti-Factor Xa may be required; use of unfractionated heparin may be preferable
Pregnancy see notes above; also multidose vial contains benzyl alcohol—manufacturer advises avoid

Breast-feeding see notes above
Side-effects see under Heparin
Licensed use not licensed for use in children

Indication and dose

  Treatment of thrombotic episodes
  - **By subcutaneous injection**

    Neonate 100 units/kg twice daily

◻ DALTEPARIN SODIUM (continued)

Child 1 month–12 years 100 units/kg twice daily

Child 12–18 years 200 units/kg (max. 18 000 units) once daily, if increased risk of bleeding reduced to 100 units/kg twice daily

Treatment of venous thromboembolism in pregnancy
• By subcutaneous injection

Child 12–18 years early pregnancy body-weight under 50 kg, 5000 units twice daily; body-weight 50–70 kg, 6000 units twice daily; body-weight 70–90 kg, 8000 units twice daily; body-weight over 90 kg, 10 000 units twice daily

Prophylaxis of thrombotic episodes
• By subcutaneous injection

Neonate 100 units/kg once daily

Child 1 month–12 years 100 units/kg once daily

Child 12–18 years 2500–5000 units once daily

Fragmin® (Pharmacia) [PoM]
Injection (single-dose syringe), dalteparin sodium 12 500 units/mL, net price 2500-unit (0.2-mL) syringe = £1.86; 25 000 units/mL, 5000-unit (0.2-mL) syringe = £2.82, 7500-unit (0.3-mL) syringe = £4.23, 10 000-unit (0.4-mL) syringe = £5.65, 12 500-unit (0.5-mL) syringe = £7.06, 15 000-unit (0.6-mL) syringe = £8.47, 18 000-unit (0.72-mL) syringe = £10.16

Injection, dalteparin sodium 2500 units/mL (for subcutaneous or intravenous use), net price 4-mL (10 000-unit) amp = £5.12; 10 000-units/mL (for subcutaneous or intravenous use), 1-mL (10 000-unit) amp = £5.12; 25 000 units/mL (for subcutaneous use only), 4-mL (100 000-unit) vial = £48.66
Excipients include benzyl alcohol (in 100 000-unit/4 mL multidose vial) (avoid in neonates, see, p. 3)

Injection (graduated syringe), dalteparin sodium 10 000 units/mL, net price 1-mL (10 000-unit) syringe = £5.65

◼ ENOXAPARIN SODIUM

Cautions see under Heparin and notes above
Contra-indications see under Heparin
Hepatic impairment see notes above
Renal impairment risk of bleeding may be increased; reduce dose if estimated glomerular filtration rate less than 30 mL/minute/1.73 m²; monitoring of anti-Factor Xa may be required; use of unfractionated heparin may be preferable
Pregnancy see notes above
Breast-feeding see notes above
Side-effects see under Heparin
Licensed use not licensed for use in children

Indication and dose

Treatment of thrombotic episodes
• By subcutaneous injection

Neonate 1.5–2 mg/kg twice daily

Child 1–2 months 1.5 mg/kg twice daily

Child 2 months–18 years 1 mg/kg twice daily

Treatment of venous thromboembolism in pregnancy
• By subcutaneous injection

Child 12–18 years early pregnancy body-weight under 50 kg, 40 mg (4000 units) twice daily; body-weight 50–70 kg, 60 mg (6000 units) twice daily; body-weight 70–90 kg, 80 mg (8000 units) twice daily; body-weight over 90 kg, 100 mg (10 000 units) twice daily

Prophylaxis of thrombotic episodes
• By subcutaneous injection

Neonate 750 micrograms/kg twice daily

Child 1–2 months 750 micrograms/kg twice daily

Child 2 months–18 years 500 micrograms/kg twice daily; max. 40 mg daily

Clexane® (Sanofi-Aventis) [PoM]
Injection, enoxaparin sodium 100 mg/mL, net price 20-mg (0.2-mL, 2000-units) syringe = £3.03, 40-mg (0.4-mL, 4000-units) syringe = £4.04, 60-mg (0.6-mL, 6000-units) syringe = £4.57, 80-mg (0.8-mL, 8000-units) syringe = £5.19, 100-mg (1-mL, 10 000-units) syringe = £6.43, 300-mg (3-mL, 30 000-units) vial (Clexane® Multi-Dose) = £21.33; 150 mg/mL (Clexane® Forte), 120-mg (0.8-mL, 12 000-units) syringe = £9.77, 150-mg (1-mL, 15 000-units) syringe = £11.10
Excipients include benzyl alcohol (in 300 mg multidose vials) (avoid in neonates, see, p. 3)

◼ TINZAPARIN SODIUM

Cautions see under Heparin and notes above
Contra-indications see under Heparin
Hepatic impairment see notes above
Renal impairment risk of bleeding may be increased—dose reduction and monitoring of anti-Factor Xa may be required; unfractionated heparin may be preferable
Pregnancy see notes above; also vials contain benzyl alcohol—manufacturer advises avoid
Breast-feeding see notes above

Side-effects see under Heparin
Licensed use not licensed for use in children

Indication and dose

Treatment of thrombotic episodes
• By subcutaneous injection

Child 1–2 months 275 units/kg once daily

Child 2 months–1 year 250 units/kg once daily

Child 1–5 years 240 units/kg once daily

◻ **TINZAPARIN SODIUM** (*continued*)

Child 5–10 years 200 units/kg once daily

Child 10–18 years 175 units/kg once daily

Treatment of venous thromboembolism in pregnancy
• By subcutaneous injection

Child 12–18 years 175 units/kg once daily (based on early pregnancy body-weight)

Prophylaxis of thrombotic episodes
• By subcutaneous injection

Child 1 month–18 years 50 units/kg once daily

Innohep® (LEO) [PoM]

Injection, tinzaparin sodium 10 000 units/mL, net price 2500-unit (0.25-mL) syringe = £1.98, 3500-unit (0.35-mL) syringe = £2.77, 4500-unit (0.45-mL) syringe = £3.56, 20 000-unit (2-mL) vial = £10.56

Injection, tinzaparin sodium 20 000 units/mL, net price 0.5-mL (10 000-unit) syringe = £8.63, 0.7-mL (14 000-unit) syringe = £12.08, 0.9-mL (18 000-unit) syringe = £15.53, 2-mL (40 000-unit) vial = £34.20
Excipients include benzyl alcohol (in vials) (avoid in neonates, see Excipients, p. 3), sulphites (in 20 000 units/mL vial and syringe)

Heparinoids

Danaparoid is a heparinoid that has a role in children who develop heparin-induced thrombocytopenia, providing they have no evidence of cross-reactivity.

▌ DANAPAROID SODIUM

Cautions recent bleeding or risk of bleeding; concomitant use of drugs that increase risk of bleeding; antibodies to heparins (risk of antibody-induced thrombocytopenia)

Contra-indications haemophilia and other haemorrhagic disorders, thrombocytopenia (unless patient has heparin-induced thrombocytopenia), recent cerebral haemorrhage, severe hypertension, active peptic ulcer (unless this is the reason for operation), diabetic retinopathy, acute bacterial endocarditis, spinal or epidural anaesthesia with treatment doses of danaparoid

Hepatic impairment caution in moderate impairment (increased risk of bleeding); avoid in severe impairment unless the child has heparin-induced thrombocytopenia and no alternative available

Renal impairment use with caution in moderate impairment; increased risk of bleeding (monitor anti-Factor Xa activity); avoid in severe impairment unless child has heparin-induced thrombocytopenia and no alternative available

Pregnancy manufacturer advises avoid—limited information available but not known to be harmful

Breast-feeding amount probably too small to be harmful but manufacturer advises avoid

Side-effects haemorrhage; hypersensitivity reactions (including rash)

Licensed use not licensed for use in children

Indication and dose

Thromboembolic disease in children with history of heparin-induced thrombocytopenia
• By intravenous administration

Neonate initially 30 units/kg *by intravenous injection* then *by continuous intravenous infusion* 1.2–2 units/kg/hour adjusted according to coagulation activity

Child 1 month–16 years initially 30 units/kg (max. 1250 units if body-weight under 55 kg, 2500 units if over 55 kg) *by intravenous injection* then *by continuous intravenous infusion* 1.2–2 units/kg/hour adjusted according to coagulation activity

Child 16–18 years initially 2500 units (1250 units if body-weight under 55 kg, 3750 units if over 90 kg) *by intravenous injection* then *by continuous intravenous infusion* 400 units/hour for 2 hours, *then* 300 units/hour for 2 hours, *then* 200 units/hour for 5 days adjusted according to coagulation activity

Administration for *intravenous infusion*, dilute with Glucose 5% *or* Sodium Chloride 0.9%

Orgaran® (Organon) [PoM]
Injection, danaparoid sodium 1250 units/mL, net price 0.6-mL amp (750 units) = £27.19

▌ Heparin flushes

The use of heparin flushes should be kept to a minimum. For maintaining patency of peripheral venous catheters, sodium chloride 0.9% injection is as effective as heparin flushes. The role of heparin flushes in maintaining patency of arterial and central venous catheters is unclear.

Heparin Sodium (Non-proprietary) [PoM]
Solution, heparin sodium 10 units/mL, net price 5-mL amp = 91p; 100 units/mL, 2-mL amp = 83p
Excipients may include benzyl alcohol (avoid in neonates, see Excipients, p. 3)

2

Cardiovascular system

Epoprostenol

Epoprostenol (prostacyclin) can be given to inhibit platelet aggregation during renal dialysis when heparins are unsuitable or contra-indicated. For its use in pulmonary hypertension, see section 2.5.1.2. It is a potent vasodilator and therefore its side-effects include flushing, headache, and hypotension.

2.8.2 Oral anticoagulants

Oral anticoagulants antagonise the effects of vitamin K and take at least 48 to 72 hours for the anticoagulant effect to develop fully; if an immediate effect is required, unfractionated or low molecular weight heparin must be given concomitantly.

Uses Warfarin is the drug of choice for the treatment of systemic thromboembolism in children (not neonates) after initial heparinisation. It may also be used occasionally for the treatment of intravascular or intracardiac thrombi. Warfarin is used prophylactically in those with chronic atrial fibrillation, dilated cardiomyopathy, certain forms of reconstructive heart surgery, mechanical prosthetic heart valves, and some forms of hereditary thrombophilia (e.g. homozygous protein C deficiency).

Unfractionated or a low molecular weight heparin (section 2.8.1) is usually preferred for the prophylaxis of venous thromboembolism in children undergoing surgery; alternatively warfarin can be continued in selected children currently taking warfarin and who are at a high risk of thromboembolism (seek expert advice).

Dose The base-line prothrombin time should be determined but the initial dose should not be delayed whilst awaiting the result.

An induction dose is usually given over 4 days (see under Warfarin Sodium below). The subsequent maintenance dose depends on the prothrombin time, reported as INR (international normalised ratio) and should be taken at the same time each day. The following indications and target INRs[1] for **adults** take into account recommendations of the British Society for Haematology[2];

- INR 2.5 for treatment of deep-vein thrombosis and pulmonary embolism (including those associated with antiphospholipid syndrome or for recurrence in patients no longer receiving warfarin), for atrial fibrillation, cardioversion (higher target values, such as an INR of 3, can be used for up to 4 weeks before the procedure to avoid cancellations due to low INR; anticoagulation should continue for at least 4 weeks following the procedure), dilated cardiomyopathy, mural thrombus, symptomatic inherited thrombophilia, coronary artery thrombosis (if anticoagulated), and paroxysmal nocturnal haemoglobinuria;

- INR 3.5 for recurrent deep-vein thrombosis and pulmonary embolism (in patients currently receiving warfarin with INR above 2);

- For mechanical prosthetic heart valves, the recommended target INR depends on the type and location of the valve. Generally, a target INR of 3 is recommended for mechanical aortic valves, and 3.5 for mechanical mitral valves.

Monitoring It is essential that the INR be determined daily or on alternate days in early days of treatment, *then* at longer intervals (depending on response[3]) *then* up to every 12 weeks.

Haemorrhage The main adverse effect of all oral anticoagulants is haemorrhage. Checking the INR and omitting doses when appropriate is essential; if the anticoagulant is stopped but not reversed, the INR should be measured 2–3 days later to ensure that it is falling. The following recommendations are based on the result of the INR and whether there is major or minor bleeding; the recommendations apply to **adults** taking warfarin:

- Major bleeding—stop warfarin; give phytomenadione (vitamin K₁) 5–10 mg by slow intravenous injection; give dried prothrombin complex (factors II, VII, IX,

1. An INR which is within 0.5 units of the target value is generally satisfactory; larger deviations require dosage adjustment. Target values (rather than ranges) are now recommended.
2. Guidelines on Oral Anticoagulation (warfarin): third edition—2005 update. Br J Haematol 2005; **132**: 277–285.
3. Change in child's clinical condition, particularly associated with liver disease, intercurrent illness, or drug administration, necessitates more frequent testing. See also **interactions**, Appendix 1 (warfarin). Major changes in diet (especially involving salads and vegetables) and in alcohol consumption may also affect warfarin control.

and X—section 2.11) 30–50 units/kg (if dried prothrombin complex unavailable, fresh frozen plasma 15 mL/kg can be given but is less effective)

- INR > 8.0, no bleeding or minor bleeding—stop warfarin and give phytomenadione (vitamin K_1) 2.5–5 mg by mouth using the intravenous preparation orally [unlicensed use], or 0.5–1 mg by slow intravenous injection (if complete reversal required 5–10 mg by slow intravenous injection); repeat dose of phytomenadione if INR still too high after 24 hours; restart warfarin when INR < 5.0

- INR 5.0–8.0, no bleeding—stop warfarin; minor bleeding—stop warfarin and give phytomenadione (vitamin K_1) 1–2.5 mg by mouth using the intravenous preparation orally [unlicensed use]; restart warfarin when INR < 5.0

- Unexpected bleeding at therapeutic levels—always investigate possibility of underlying cause e.g. unsuspected renal or gastro-intestinal tract pathology

Pregnancy   Oral anticoagulants are teratogenic and should not be given in the first trimester of pregnancy. Adolescents at risk of pregnancy should be warned of this danger since stopping warfarin before the sixth week of gestation may largely avoid the risk of fetal abnormality. Oral anticoagulants cross the placenta with risk of congenital malformations, and placental, fetal, or neonatal haemorrhage, especially during the last few weeks of pregnancy and at delivery. Therefore, if at all possible, oral anticoagulants should be avoided in pregnancy, especially in the first and third trimesters. Difficult decisions may have to be made, particularly in those with prosthetic heart valves or with a history of recurrent venous thrombosis, pulmonary embolism, or atrial fibrillation.

Babies of mothers taking warfarin at the time of delivery need to be offered immediate prophylaxis with at least 100 micrograms/kg of intramuscular phytomenadione (vitamin K_1), see section 9.6.6.

Dietary differences   Infant formula is supplemented with vitamin K, which makes formula-fed infants resistant to warfarin; they may therefore need higher doses. In contrast breast milk contains low concentrations of vitamin K making breast-fed infants more sensitive to warfarin.

Treatment booklets   Anticoagulant treatment booklets should be issued to children or their carers, and are available for distribution to local healthcare professionals from Health Authorities and from:
3M Security Printing and Systems Limited
Gorse Street
Chadderton
Oldham, OL9 9QH.
Tel: 0845 610 1112
nhsforms@spsl.uk.com

These booklets include advice for children or their carers on anticoagulant treatment, an alert card to be carried by the patient at all times, and a section for recording of INR results and dosage information. Electronic copies are also available at www.npsa.nhs.uk/nrls/alerts-and-directives/alerts/anticoagulant.

WARFARIN SODIUM

Cautions   see notes above; also recent surgery; concomitant use of drugs that increase risk of bleeding; bacterial endocarditis (increased risk of bleeding; use only if warfarin otherwise indicated); **interactions:** Appendix 1 (warfarin)

Contra-indications   peptic ulcer, severe hypertension

Hepatic impairment   avoid in severe impairment, especially if prothrombin time already prolonged

Renal impairment   use with caution (avoid in severe impairment)

Pregnancy   see notes above

Breast-feeding   not present in milk in significant amounts; no evidence of harm; see also notes above

Side-effects   haemorrhage—see notes above; other side-effects reported include hypersensitivity, rash, alopecia, diarrhoea, unexplained drop in haematocrit, 'purple toes', skin necrosis, jaundice, hepatic dysfunction; also nausea, vomiting, and pancreatitis

Licensed use   not licensed for use in children

Indication and dose

Treatment and prophylaxis of thrombotic episodes
- By mouth

Neonate (under specialist advice) 200 micrograms/kg as a single dose on first day, reduced to 100 micrograms/kg once daily for following 3

◻ **WARFARIN SODIUM** (*continued*)

days (but if INR still below 1.4 use 200 micrograms/kg once daily, or if INR above 3 use 50 micrograms/kg once daily, if INR above 3.5 omit dose); then adjusted according to INR, usual maintenance 100–300 micrograms/kg once daily (may need up to 400 micrograms/kg once daily especially if bottle fed—see notes above)

Child 1 month–18 years 200 micrograms/kg (max. 10 mg) as a single dose on first day, reduced to 100 micrograms/kg (max. 5 mg) once daily for following 3 days (but if INR still below 1.4 use 200 micrograms/kg (max. 10 mg) once daily, or if INR above 3 use 50 micrograms/kg (max. 2.5 mg) once daily, or if INR above 3.5 omit dose); then adjusted according to

INR, usual maintenance 100–300 micrograms/kg once daily (may need up to 400 micrograms/kg once daily especially if bottle fed—see notes above)

Note Induction dose may need to be altered according to condition (e.g. abnormal liver function tests, cardiac failure), concomitant interacting drugs, and if baseline INR above 1.3

Warfarin (Non-proprietary) PoM
Tablets, warfarin sodium 500 micrograms (white), net price 28-tab pack = £1.60; 1 mg (brown), 28-tab pack = £1.06; 3 mg (blue), 28-tab pack = £1.10; 5 mg (pink), 28-tab pack = £1.21. Label: 10, anticoagulant card
Brands include *Marevan*®

◢Extemporaneous formulations available see Extemporaneous Preparations, p. 8

2.8.3 Protamine sulphate

Protamine sulphate is used to treat overdosage of unfractionated or low molecular weight heparin. The long half-life of low molecular weight heparins should be taken into consideration when determining the dose of protamine sulphate; the effects of low molecular weight heparins can persist for up to 24 hours after administration. Excessive doses of protamine sulphate can have an anticoagulant effect.

PROTAMINE SULPHATE
(Protamine Sulfate)

Cautions see above; also monitor activated partial thromboplastin time or other appropriate blood clotting parameters; if increased risk of allergic reaction to protamine (includes previous treatment with protamine or protamine insulin, allergy to fish, and adolescent males who are infertile)

Side-effects nausea, vomiting, lassitude, flushing, hypotension, hypertension, bradycardia, dyspnoea, rebound bleeding, back pain; hypersensitivity reactions (including angioedema, anaphylaxis) and pulmonary oedema reported

Indication and dose

Overdosage with intravenous injection or intravenous infusion of unfractionated heparin
• **By intravenous injection** (rate not exceeding 5 mg/minute)
    Child 1 month–18 years *to neutralise each 100 units of unfractionated heparin*, 1 mg if less than 30 minutes lapsed since overdose, 500–750 micrograms if 30–60 minutes lapsed, 375–500 micrograms if 60–120 minutes lapsed, 250–375 micrograms if over 120 minutes lapsed; max. 50 mg

Overdosage with subcutaneous injection of unfractionated heparin
• **By intravenous injection and intravenous infusion**
    Child 1 month–18 years 1 mg neutralises approx. 100 units of unfractionated heparin; give 50–100% of the total dose by *intravenous injection* (rate not exceeding 5 mg/minute), then give any remainder of dose by *intravenous infusion* over 8–16 hours; max. total dose 50 mg

Overdosage with subcutaneous injection of low molecular weight heparin
• **By intermittent intravenous injection** (rate not exceeding 5 mg/minute) **or by continuous intravenous infusion**
    Child 1 month–18 years 1 mg neutralises approx. 100 units low molecular weight heparin (consult product literature of low molecular weight heparin for details); max. 50 mg

Administration may be diluted if necessary with Sodium Chloride 0.9%

Protamine Sulphate (Non-proprietary) PoM
Injection, protamine sulphate 10 mg/mL, net price 5-mL amp = £1.43, 10-mL amp = £4.15

2.9 Antiplatelet drugs

Antiplatelet drugs decrease platelet aggregation and inhibit thrombus formation in the arterial circulation, because in faster-flowing vessels, thrombi are composed mainly of platelets with little fibrin.

Aspirin has limited use in children because it has been associated with Reye's syndrome. Aspirin-containing preparations should not be given to children and adolescents under 16 years, unless specifically indicated, such as for Kawasaki syndrome (see below), for prophylaxis of clot formation after cardiac surgery, or for prophylaxis of stroke in children at high risk.

If aspirin causes dyspepsia, or if the child is at a high risk of gastro-intestinal bleeding, a proton pump inhibitor (section 1.3.5) or a H$_2$-receptor antagonist (section 1.3.1) can be added.

Dipyridamole is also used as an antiplatelet drug to prevent clot formation after cardiac surgery and may be used with specialist advice for treatment of persistent coronary artery aneurysms in Kawasaki syndrome.

Kawasaki syndrome   Initial treatment is with high-dose aspirin and a single dose of intravenous normal immunoglobulin (p. 763); this combination has an additive anti-inflammatory effect resulting in faster resolution of fever and a decreased incidence of coronary artery complications. After the acute phase, when the patient is afebrile, aspirin is continued at a lower dose to prevent coronary artery abnormalities.

ASPIRIN (antiplatelet)
(Acetylsalicylic Acid)

Cautions   asthma; uncontrolled hypertension; previous peptic ulceration (but manufacturers may advise avoidance of low-dose aspirin in history of peptic ulceration); concomitant use of drugs that increase risk of bleeding; G6PD deficiency (section 9.1.5); **interactions:** Appendix 1 (aspirin)

Contra-indications   children under 16 years (risk of Reye's syndrome) unless for indications below; active peptic ulceration; haemophilia and other bleeding disorders

Hypersensitivity Aspirin and other NSAIDs are **contra-indicated** in history of hypersensitivity to aspirin or any other NSAID—which includes those in whom attacks of asthma, angioedema, urticaria, or rhinitis have been precipitated by aspirin or any other NSAID

Hepatic impairment   avoid in severe impairment—increased risk of gastro-intestinal bleeding

Renal impairment   use with caution (avoid in severe impairment); sodium and water retention; deterioration in renal function; increased risk of gastro-intestinal bleeding

Pregnancy   use with caution during third trimester; impaired platelet function and risk of haemorrhage; delayed onset and increased duration of labour with increased blood loss; avoid analgesic doses if possible in last few weeks (low doses probably not harmful); with high doses, closure of fetal ductus arteriosus *in utero* and possibly persistent pulmonary hypertension of newborn; kernicterus in jaundiced neonates

Breast-feeding   avoid—possible risk of Reye's syndrome; regular use of high doses could impair platelet function and produce hypoprothrombinaemia in infant if neonatal vitamin K stores low

Side-effects   bronchospasm; gastro-intestinal haemorrhage (occasionally major), also other haemorrhage (e.g. subconjunctival)

Licensed use   Not licensed for use in children under 16 years

Indication and dose

Kawasaki syndrome
- By mouth

Neonate initially 8 mg/kg 4 times daily for 2 weeks *or* until afebrile, followed by 5 mg/kg once daily for 6–8 weeks; if no evidence of coronary lesions after 8 weeks, discontinue treatment or seek expert advice

Child 1 month–12 years initially 7.5–12.5 mg/kg 4 times daily for 2 weeks or until afebrile, then 2–5 mg/kg once daily for 6–8 weeks; if no evidence of coronary lesions after 8 weeks, discontinue treatment or seek expert advice

Antiplatelet, prevention of thrombus formation after cardiac surgery
- By mouth

Neonate 1–5 mg/kg once daily

Child 1 month–12 years 1–5 mg/kg (usual max. 75 mg) once daily

Child 12–18 years 75 mg once daily

Aspirin (Non-proprietary) [PoM]
Dispersible tablets, aspirin 75 mg, net price 28 = 86p; 300 mg, 100-tab pack = £6.13 Label: 13, 21, 32

Tablets, e/c, aspirin 75 mg, net price 28-tab pack = 98p; 56-tab pack = £1.11; 300 mg, 100-tab pack = £4.72. Label: 5, 25, 32
Brands include *Micropirin®*

Suppositories, available from 'special-order' manufacturers or specialist importing companies, see p. 957

Caprin® (Pinewood) [PoM]
Tablets, e/c, pink, aspirin 75 mg, net price 28-tab pack = £1.55, 56-tab pack = £3.08, 100-tab pack = £5.24; 300 mg, 100-tab pack = £4.89. Label: 5, 25, 32

Nu-Seals® Aspirin (Alliance) [PoM]
Tablets, e/c, aspirin 75 mg, net price 56-tab pack = £3.12; 300 mg, 100-tab pack = £4.15. Label: 5, 25, 32

2

Cardiovascular system

DIPYRIDAMOLE

Cautions aortic stenosis, left ventricular outflow obstruction, heart failure; may exacerbate migraine; hypotension; myasthenia gravis (risk of exacerbation); concomitant use of drugs that increase risk of bleeding; coagulation disorders; **interactions:** Appendix 1 (dipyridamole)

Pregnancy not known to be harmful

Breast-feeding manufacturers advise use only if essential—small amount present in milk

Side-effects gastro-intestinal effects, dizziness, myalgia, throbbing headache, hypotension, hot flushes and tachycardia; hypersensitivity reactions such as rash, urticaria, severe bronchospasm and angioedema; increased bleeding during or after surgery; thrombocytopenia reported

Licensed use not licensed for use in children

Indication and dose

Kawasaki syndrome
 • By mouth
   Child 1 month–12 years 1 mg/kg 3 times daily

Prevention of thrombus formation after cardiac surgery
 • By mouth
   Child 1 month–12 years 2.5 mg/kg twice daily
   Child 12–18 years 100–200 mg 3 times daily

Administration injection solution can be given orally

Dipyridamole (Non-proprietary) [PoM]
Tablets, coated, dipyridamole 25 mg, net price 84 = £2.86; 100 mg, 84 = £3.09. Label: 22

Oral suspension, dipyridamole 50 mg/5 ml, net price 150 mL = £37.47

Persantin® (Boehringer Ingelheim) [PoM]
Tablets, both s/c, dipyridamole 25 mg (orange), net price 84-tab pack = £1.49; 100 mg, 84-tab pack = £4.16. Label: 22

Injection, dipyridamole 5 mg/mL, net price 2-mL amp = 12p

2.10 Myocardial infarction and fibrinolysis

2.10.1 Management of myocardial infarction
2.10.2 Fibrinolytic drugs

2.10.1 Management of myocardial infarction

This section is not included in *BNF for Children*.

2.10.2 Fibrinolytic drugs

Fibrinolytic drugs act as thrombolytics by activating plasminogen to form plasmin, which degrades fibrin and so breaks up thrombi.

Alteplase, streptokinase, and urokinase are used in children to dissolve intravascular thrombi and unblock occluded arteriovenous shunts, catheters, and indwelling central lines blocked with fibrin clots. Treatment should be started as soon as possible after a clot has formed and discontinued once a pulse in the affected limb is detected, or the shunt or catheter unblocked.

The safety and efficacy of treatment remains uncertain, especially in neonates. A fibrinolytic drug is probably only appropriate where arterial occlusion threatens ischaemic damage; an anticoagulant may stop the clot getting bigger. Alteplase is the preferred fibrinolytic in children and neonates; there is less risk of adverse effects including allergic reactions.

Cautions Thrombolytic drugs should be used with caution if there is a risk of bleeding including that from venepuncture or invasive procedures. They should also be used with caution in external chest compression, pregnancy (see individual drugs), hypertension, other conditions in which thrombolysis might give rise to embolic complications such as enlarged left atrium with atrial fibrillation (risk of dissolution of clot and subsequent embolisation), and recent or concurrent use of drugs that increase the risk of bleeding.

Contra-indications Thrombolytic drugs are contra-indicated in recent haemorrhage, trauma, or surgery (including dental extraction), coagulation defects, bleeding diatheses, aortic dissection, aneurysm, coma, history of cerebrovascular disease especially recent events or with any residual disability, recent symptoms of possible peptic ulceration, heavy vaginal bleeding, severe hypertension, active pulmonary disease with cavitation, acute pancreatitis, pericarditis, bacterial endocarditis, severe liver disease, and oesophageal varices; also in the case of streptokinase, previous allergic reactions to streptokinase.

Prolonged persistence of antibodies to streptokinase can reduce the effectiveness of subsequent treatment; therefore, streptokinase should not be used again beyond 4 days of first administration. Streptokinase should also be avoided in children who have had streptococcal infection in the last 12 months.

Hepatic impairment Thrombolytic drugs should be avoided in severe hepatic impairment as there is an increased risk of bleeding.

Pregnancy Thrombolytic drugs can possibly lead to premature separation of the placenta in the first 18 weeks of pregnancy. There is also a risk of maternal haemorrhage throughout pregnancy and post-partum, and also a theoretical risk of fetal haemorrhage throughout pregnancy.

Side-effects Side-effects of thrombolytics are mainly bleeding, nausea, and vomiting. Reperfusion can cause cerebral and pulmonary oedema. Hypotension can also occur and can usually be controlled by elevating the patient's legs, or by reducing the rate of infusion or stopping it temporarily. Back pain, fever, and convulsions have been reported. Bleeding is usually limited to the site of injection, but intracerebral haemorrhage or bleeding from other sites can occur. Serious bleeding calls for discontinuation of the thrombolytic and may require administration of coagulation factors and antifibrinolytic drugs (e.g. tranexamic acid). Thrombolytics can cause allergic reactions (including rash, flushing and uveitis) and anaphylaxis has been reported (for details of management see Allergic Emergencies, section 3.4.3). Guillain-Barré syndrome has been reported rarely after streptokinase treatment.

ALTEPLASE

(rt-PA, tissue-type plasminogen activator)

Cautions see notes above; in children who have had an *acute stroke*, monitor for intracranial haemorrhage and monitor blood pressure

Contra-indications see notes above; in children who have had an *acute stroke*, convulsion accompanying stroke, severe stroke, history of stroke in children with diabetes, stroke in last 3 months, hypoglycaemia, hyperglycaemia

Hepatic impairment see notes above

Pregnancy see notes above

Side-effects see notes above; also risk of cerebral bleeding increased in acute stroke

Licensed use not licensed for use in children

Indication and dose

Intravascular thrombosis doses may vary—consult local guidelines

• **By intravenous infusion**

Neonate 100–500 micrograms/kg/hour for 3–6 hours; use ultrasound assessment to monitor effect before considering a second course of treatment

Child 1 month–18 years 100–500 micrograms/kg/hour for 3–6 hours; max. 100 mg total daily

dose; use ultrasound assessment to monitor effect before considering a second course of treatment

Occluded arteriovenous shunts, catheters, and indwelling central lines

• **By injection direct into catheter or central line**

Child 1 month–18 years using 1 mg/mL solution, instill up to 2 mL according to dead-space of catheter or central line; aspirate lysate after 4 hours; flush with Sodium Chloride 0.9%

Administration for *intravenous infusion*, dissolve in Water for Injections to a concentration of 1 mg/mL or 2 mg/mL and infuse intravenously; alternatively dilute further in Sodium Chloride 0.9% to a concentration of not less than 200 micrograms/mL; not to be diluted in Glucose

Actilyse® (Boehringer Ingelheim) [PoM]
Injection, powder for reconstitution, alteplase 10 mg (5.8 million units)/vial, net price per vial (with diluent) = £120.00; 20 mg (11.6 million units)/vial (with diluent and transfer device) = £180.00; 50 mg (29 million units)/vial (with diluent, transfer device, and infusion bag) = £300.00

STREPTOKINASE

Cautions see notes above

Contra-indications see notes above

Hepatic impairment see notes above

Pregnancy see notes above

Side-effects see notes above

Licensed use not licensed for use in children under 18 years

Indication and dose

Intravascular thrombosis

• **By intravenous infusion**

Child 1 month–12 years initially 2500–4000 units/kg over 30 minutes, followed by

continuous intravenous infusion of 500–1000 units/kg/hour for up to 3 days until reperfusion occurs

Child 12–18 years initially 250 000 units over 30 minutes, followed by *continuous intravenous infusion* of 100 000 units/hour for up to 3 days until reperfusion occurs

Administration reconstitute with Sodium Chloride 0.9%, then dilute further with Glucose 5% or Sodium Chloride 0.9% after reconstitution. Monitor fibrinogen concentration closely; if fibrinogen concentration less than 1 g/litre, stop streptokinase infusion and start unfractionated

◁ **STREPTOKINASE (continued)**

heparin; restart streptokinase once fibrinogen concentration reaches 1 g/litre

Streptase® (CSL Behring) [PoM]
Injection, powder for reconstitution, streptokinase, net price 250 000-unit vial = £15.91; 750 000-unit vial = £41.72; 1.5 million-unit vial = £83.44 (hosp. only)

▌UROKINASE

Cautions see notes above
Contra-indications see notes above
Hepatic impairment see notes above
Pregnancy see notes above
Side-effects see notes above
Licensed use not licensed for use in children

Indication and dose

Intravascular thrombosis
• **By intravenous injection and infusion**

Neonate 4400 units/kg as a single dose *by intravenous injection* in 15 mL diluent, followed by 4400 units/kg/hour *by intravenous infusion* for 6–12 hours, adjusted according to response

Child 1 month–18 years 4400 units/kg as a single dose *by intravenous injection* in 15 mL diluent, followed by 4400 units/kg/hour *by intravenous infusion* for 6–12 hours, adjusted according to response

Occluded arteriovenous shunts, catheters, and indwelling central lines
• **By injection directly into catheter or central line**

Neonate 5000–10 000 units in sodium chloride 0.9% to fill catheter dead-space **only**; leave for 2–4 hours then aspirate the lysate; flush with sodium chloride 0.9%

Child 1 month–18 years 5000–10 000 units in sodium chloride 0.9% to fill catheter dead-space **only**; leave for 2–4 hours then aspirate the lysate; flush with sodium chloride 0.9%

Administration may be diluted, after reconstitution, with Sodium Chloride 0.9%

Syner-KINASE® (Syner-Med) [PoM]
Injection, powder for reconstitution, urokinase, net price 10 000-unit vial = £35.95; 25 000-unit vial = £45.95; 100 000-unit vial = £112.95
Note 50 000-unit vial and 250 000-unit vial also available from 'special-order' manufacturers or specialist importing companies, see p. 957

▌2.11 Antifibrinolytic drugs and haemostatics

Fibrin dissolution can be impaired by the administration of **tranexamic acid**, which inhibits fibrinolysis. It can be used to prevent bleeding or treat bleeding associated with excessive fibrinolysis (e.g. in prostatectomy, bladder surgery, in dental extraction in children with haemophilia, and in traumatic hyphaema) and in the management of menorrhagia. Tranexamic acid may also be used in hereditary angioedema (section 3.4.3), epistaxis, and thrombolytic overdose.

Desmopressin (section 6.5.2) is used in the management of mild to moderate haemophilia and von Willebrands' disease. It is also used for testing fibrinolytic response.

▌TRANEXAMIC ACID

Cautions massive haematuria (avoid if risk of ureteric obstruction); not for use in disseminated intravascular coagulation; irregular menstrual bleeding (establish cause before initiating therapy); regular liver function tests in long-term treatment of hereditary angioedema
Contra-indications thromboembolic disease
Renal impairment reduce dose in mild to moderate impairment; avoid in severe impairment
Pregnancy no evidence of teratogenicity in *animal* studies; manufacturer advises use only if potential benefit outweighs risk—crosses the placenta
Breast-feeding small amount present in milk—antifibrinolytic effect in infant unlikely
Side-effects nausea, vomiting, diarrhoea (reduce dose); *rarely* disturbances in colour vision (discontinue), thromboembolic events, allergic skin reactions; giddiness and hypotension on *rapid intravenous injection*
Licensed use Licensed for inhibition of fibrinolysis

Indication and dose

Inhibition of fibrinolysis, hereditary angioedema
• **By mouth**

Child 1 month–18 years 15–25 mg/kg (max. 1.5 g) 2–3 times daily

• **By intravenous injection over at least 10 minutes**

Child 1 month–18 years 10 mg/kg (max. 1 g) 2–3 times daily

• **By continuous intravenous infusion**

Child 1 month–18 years 45 mg/kg over 24 hours

2 Cardiovascular system

◻ **TRANEXAMIC ACID** (*continued*)

Prevention of excessive bleeding after dental procedures (e.g. in haemophilia)

• **By intravenous injection (pre-operatively) and by mouth (post-operatively)**

Child 6–18 years 10 mg/kg (max. 1.5 g) *by intravenous injection* pre-operatively, followed by 15–25 mg/kg (max. 1.5 g) 2–3 times daily *by mouth* for up to 8 days

• **Mouthwash 5% solution (specialist use only)**

Child 6–18 years rinse mouth with 5–10 mL 4 times daily for 2 days; not to be swallowed
Note Mouthwash available only as extemporaneously prepared preparation, see Extemporaneous Preparations, p. 8

Menorrhagia

• **By mouth**

Child 12–18 years 1 g 3–4 times daily for up to 4 days; max. 4 g daily (initiate when menstruation has started)

Administration for *intravenous administration*, dilute with Glucose 5% *or* Sodium Chloride 0.9%

Tranexamic acid (Non-proprietary) PoM
Tablets, tranexamic acid 500 mg, net price 60-tab pack = £7.26

Cyklokapron® (Meda) PoM
Tablets, f/c, scored, tranexamic acid 500 mg, net price 60-tab pack = £14.30

Cyklokapron® (Pfizer) PoM
Injection, tranexamic acid 100 mg/mL, net price 5-mL amp = £1.55

Blood products

These products should be used on the advice of a haematologist.

▍ DRIED PROTHROMBIN COMPLEX

(Human Prothrombin Complex)

Dried prothrombin complex is prepared from human plasma by a suitable fractionation technique, and contains factor IX, together with variable amounts of factors II, VII, and X

Cautions risk of thrombosis; disseminated intravascular coagulation; history of myocardial infarction or coronary heart disease; postoperative use; vaccination against hepatitis A (p. 743) and hepatitis B (p. 745) may be required

Contra-indications angina; recent myocardial infarction (except in life-threatening haemorrhage following overdosage of oral anticoagulants, and before induction of fibrinolytic therapy); history of heparin-induced thrombocytopenia

Hepatic impairment monitor closely (risk of thromboembolic complications)

Side-effects thrombotic events (including disseminated intravascular coagulation); *rarely* headache; *very rarely* pyrexia, antibody formation, hypersensitivity reactions (including anaphylaxis); nephrotic syndrome also reported

Indication and dose

Treatment and peri-operative prophylaxis of haemorrhage in congenital deficiency of factors II, VII, IX, or X if purified specific coagulation factors not available; treatment and peri-operative prophylaxis of haemorrhage in acquired deficiency of factors II, VII, IX, or X (e.g. during warfarin treatment—see section 2.8.2)

Consult haematologist

Available from CSL Behring (*Beriplex® P/N*), Octapharma (*Octaplex®*)

▍ FACTOR VIIa (RECOMBINANT)

Eptacog alfa (activated)

Cautions risk of thrombosis or disseminated intravascular coagulation

Side-effects *very rarely* nausea, thrombotic events (including myocardial infarction and cerebrovascular accident), coagulation disorders, fever, pain, and allergic reactions including rash

Indication and dose

Treatment and prophylaxis of haemorrhage in haemophilia A or B with inhibitors to factors VIII or IX, acquired haemophilia, factor VII deficiency, or Glanzmann's thrombasthenia

Consult haematologist

Available from Novo Nordisk (*NovoSeven®* ▼)

▍ FACTOR VIII FRACTION, DRIED

(Human Antihaemophilic Fraction, Dried)

Dried factor VIII fraction is prepared from human plasma by a suitable fractionation technique; it may also contain varying amounts of von Willebrand factor

Cautions monitor for development of factor VIII inhibitors; intravascular haemolysis after large or frequently repeated doses in patients with blood groups A, B, or AB—less likely with high potency concentrates; vaccination against hepatitis A (p. 743) and hepatitis B (p. 745) may be required (not necessary with recombinant preparation)

Side-effects gastro-intestinal disturbances, taste disturbances; flushing, palpitation; dyspnoea, coughing; headache, dizziness, paraesthesia, drowsiness; blurred vision; antibody formation; hypersensitivity reactions including hypotension, angioedema, chills, fever, urticaria, and anaphylaxis

2

Cardiovascular system

◻ **FACTOR VIII FRACTION, DRIED** (*continued*)

Indication and dose

Treatment and prophylaxis of haemorrhage in congenital factor VIII deficiency (haemophilia A), acquired factor VIII deficiency, or von Willebrand's disease

Consult haematologist

Available from Biotest UK (*Haemoctin*® ▼), CSL Behring (*Haemate*® *P*), BPL (*Optivate*®; *8Y*®), Grifols (*Alphanate*®;

Fanhdi®), Octapharma (*Octanate*®; *Wilate*® ▼); *Haemoctin*®, *Optivate*®, *Fanhdi*®, and *Octanate*® are not indicated for use in von Willebrand's disease

Note Preparation of recombinant human antihaemophilic factor VIII (octocog alfa) available from CSL Behring (*Helixate*® *NexGen*), Baxter (*Advate*®), Bayer (*Kogenate*® *Bayer*); preparation of recombinant human antihaemophilic factor VIII (moroctocog alfa) available from Wyeth (*ReFacto AF*® ▼); octocog alfa and moroctocog alfa are not indicated for use in von Willebrand's disease

---

◼ FACTOR VIII INHIBITOR BYPASSING FRACTION

Preparations with factor VIII inhibitor bypassing activity are prepared from human plasma

Cautions vaccination against hepatitis A (p. 743) and hepatitis B (p. 745) may be required

Contra-indications disseminated intravascular coagulation

Side-effects thrombosis, disseminated intravascular coagulation, myocardial infarction; paraesthesia; pyrexia; hypersensitivity reactions including hypotension, flushing, urticaria, rash, and anaphylaxis

Indication and dose

Treatment and prophylaxis of haemorrhage in congenital factor VIII deficiency (haemophilia A) and factor VIII inhibitors; treatment of haemorrhage in non-haemophiliac children with acquired factor VIII inhibitors

Consult haematologist

Available from Baxter (*FEIBA*®)

◼ FACTOR IX FRACTION, DRIED

Dried factor IX fraction is prepared from human plasma by a suitable fractionation technique; it may also contain clotting factors II, VII, and X

Cautions risk of thrombosis—principally with former low purity products; vaccination against hepatitis A (p. 743) and hepatitis B (p. 745) may be required (not necessary with recombinant preparation)

Contra-indications disseminated intravascular coagulation

Side-effects gastro-intestinal disturbances; headache, dizziness; allergic reactions including chills, fever

Indication and dose

Treatment and prophylaxis of haemorrhage in congenital factor IX deficiency (haemophilia B)

Consult haematologist

Available from CSL Behring (*Mononine*®), BPL (*Replenine*®-*VF*, Dried Factor IX Fraction), Grifols (*AlphaNine*®)

Note Preparation of recombinant coagulation factor IX (nonacog alfa) available from Wyeth (*BeneFIX*®)

◼ FACTOR XIII FRACTION, DRIED
(Human Fibrin-stabilising Factor, Dried)

Cautions vaccination against hepatitis A (p. 743) and hepatitis B (p. 745) may be required

Side-effects *rarely* allergic reactions and fever

Indication and dose

Congenital factor XIII deficiency

Consult haematologist

Available from CSL Behring (*Fibrogammin*® *P*)

◼ FRESH FROZEN PLASMA

Fresh frozen plasma is prepared from the supernatant liquid obtained by centrifugation of one donation of whole blood

Cautions need for compatibility; vaccination against hepatitis A (p. 743) and hepatitis B (p. 745) may be required

Contra-indications circulatory overload; avoid use as a volume expander

Side-effects allergic reactions including chills, fever, bronchospasm; acute respiratory distress syndrome

Indication and dose

Replacement of coagulation factors or other plasma proteins where their concentration or functional activity is critically reduced

Consult haematologist

Available from Regional Blood Transfusion Services and BPL

Note Children under 16 years should only receive methylthioninium chloride (methylene blue) treated preparations to minimise the risk of vCJD transmission

Note A preparation of solvent/detergent treated human plasma (frozen) from pooled donors is available from Octapharma (*Octaplas*®) but must not be used in children under 16 years

PROTEIN C CONCENTRATE

Protein C is prepared from human plasma

Cautions hypersensitivity to heparins; vaccination against hepatitis A (p. 743) and hepatitis B (p. 745) may be required

Side-effects *very rarely* fever, bleeding, dizziness, and hypersensitivity reactions

Indication and dose

Congenital protein C deficiency
   Consult haematologist

Available from Baxter (*Ceprotin*®)

2.12 Lipid-regulating drugs

Atherosclerosis begins in childhood and raised serum-cholesterol in children is associated with cardiovascular disease in adulthood. Lowering the cholesterol, without hindering growth and development in children and adolescents, should reduce the risk of cardiovascular disease in later life.

The risk factors for developing cardiovascular disease include raised serum cholesterol concentration, smoking, hypertension, impaired glucose tolerance, male sex, ethnicity, obesity, triglyceride concentration, chronic kidney disease, and a family history of cardiovascular disease. Heterozygous familial hypercholesterolaemia is the most common cause of raised serum cholesterol in children; homozygous familial hypercholesterolaemia is very rare and its specialised management is not covered in *BNF for Children*. Familial hypercholesterolaemia can lead to a greater risk of early coronary heart disease and should be managed by a specialist.

Secondary causes of hypercholesterolaemia should be addressed, these include obesity, diet, diabetes mellitus, hypothyroidism (see below), nephrotic syndrome, obstructive biliary disease, glycogen storage disease, and drugs such as corticosteroids.

Management   The aim of management of hypercholesterolaemia is to reduce the risk of atherosclerosis while ensuring adequate growth and development. Children with hypercholesterolaemia (or their carers) should receive advice on appropriate lifestyle changes such as improved diet, increased exercise, weight reduction, and not smoking; hypertension should also be managed appropriately (section 2.5). Drug therapy may also be necessary and is discussed below.

Hypothyroidism Children with hypothyroidism should receive adequate thyroid replacement therapy before their requirement for lipid-regulating treatment is assessed because correction of hypothyroidism itself may resolve the lipid abnormality. Untreated hypothyroidism increases the risk of myositis with lipid-regulating drugs.

Drug treatment in heterozygous familial hypercholesterolaemia Lifestyle modifications alone are unlikely to lower cholesterol concentration adequately in heterozygous familial hypercholesterolaemia and drug treatment is often required. Lipid-regulating drugs should be considered by the age of 10 years. The decision to initiate drug treatment will depend on the child's age, the age of onset of coronary heart disease within the family, and the presence of other cardiovascular risk factors. In children with a family history of coronary heart disease in early adulthood, drug treatment before the age of 10 years, and a combination of lipid-regulating drugs may be necessary.

Drug treatment in secondary hypercholesterolaemia If 6–12 months of dietary and other lifestyle interventions has failed to lower cholesterol concentration adequately, drug treatment may be indicated in children 10 years and older (rarely necessary in younger children) who are at a high risk of developing cardiovascular disease.

Choice of drugs   Experience in the use of lipid-regulating drugs in children is limited and they should be initiated on specialist advice.

Statins are the drugs of first choice in children and are generally well tolerated; atorvastatin and simvastatin are the preferred statins. Other lipid-regulating drugs can be used if statins are ineffective or are not tolerated.

2

Cardiovascular system

Ezetimibe can be used alone when statins are not tolerated, or in combination with a statin when a high-dose statin fails to control cholesterol concentration adequately.

Bile acid sequestrants are also available but tolerability of and compliance with these drugs is poor, and their use is declining.

Evidence for the use of a **fibrate** (**bezafibrate** or **fenofibrate**) in children is limited; fibrates should be considered only if dietary intervention and treatment with a statin and a bile acid sequestrant is unsuccessful or contra-indicated.

In hypertriglyceridaemia which cannot be controlled by very strict diet, omega-3 fatty acid compounds can be considered.

Statins

The statins (**atorvastatin**, **fluvastatin**, **pravastatin**, and **simvastatin**) competitively inhibit 3-hydroxy-3-methylglutaryl coenzyme A (HMG CoA) reductase, an enzyme involved in cholesterol synthesis, especially in the liver. They are more effective than other classes of drugs in lowering LDL-cholesterol but less effective than the fibrates in reducing triglycerides. Statins also increase concentrations of HDL-cholesterol.

Statins reduce cardiovascular disease events and total mortality in adults, irrespective of the initial cholesterol concentration.

Cautions Hypothyroidism should be managed adequately before starting treatment with a statin (see Hypothyroidism, p. 161). Statins should be used with caution in those with a history of liver disease or with a high alcohol intake—see also Hepatic Impairment, below. There is little information available on a rational approach to liver-function monitoring; however, a NICE guideline[1] suggests that liver enzymes should be measured before treatment, and repeated within 3 months and at 12 months of starting treatment, unless indicated at other times by signs or symptoms suggestive of hepatotoxicity. Those with serum transaminases that are raised, but less than 3 times the upper limit of the reference range, should **not** be routinely excluded from statin therapy. Those with serum transaminases of more than 3 times the upper limit of the reference range should discontinue statin therapy. Statins should be used with caution in those with risk factors for myopathy or rhabdomyolysis; children or their carers should be advised to report unexplained muscle pain (see Muscle Effects below). Creatine kinase concentration should be measured in children before treatment and if unexplained muscle pain occurs. Statins should be avoided in acute porphyria (section 9.8.2). **Interactions**: Appendix 1 (statins).

Hepatic impairment Statins should be used with caution in those with a history of liver disease and avoided in active liver disease or when there are unexplained persistent elevations in serum transaminases.

Pregnancy Statins should be avoided in pregnancy as congenital anomalies have been reported and the decreased synthesis of cholesterol possibly affects fetal development. Adequate contraception is required during treatment and for 1 month afterwards.

Breast-feeding The manufacturers of atorvastatin, fluvastatin, and simvastatin advise avoiding use in mothers who are breast-feeding as there is no information available. The manufacturers of pravastatin advise against use in breast-feeding mothers as a small amount of drug is present in breast milk.

Side-effects Statins can cause various muscular side-effects, including myopathy, myositis, and rhabdomyolysis. Muscular effects are rare but often significant (see Muscle Effects below). Statins can cause gastro-intestinal disturbances, and very rarely pancreatitis. They can also cause altered liver function tests, and rarely hepatitis and jaundice; hepatic failure has been reported very rarely. Other side-effects include sleep disturbance, headache, dizziness, depression, paraesthesia, hypoaesthesia, asthenia, peripheral neuropathy, amnesia, fatigue, sexual dysfunction, thrombocytopenia, arthralgia, visual disturbance, alopecia, and hypersensitivity reactions (including rash, pruritus, urticaria, and very rarely lupus erythematosus-like reactions). In very rare cases statins can cause inter-

1. NICE clinical guideline 67 (May 2008). Lipid Modification—Cardiovascular risk assessment and the modification of blood lipids for the primary and secondary prevention of cardiovascular disease

stitial lung disease; if children develop symptoms such as dyspnoea, cough, and weight loss, they should seek medical attention.

Muscle effects Myalgia, myositis, myopathy, and rarely rhabdomyolysis have been reported with the statins; if myopathy is suspected and creatine kinase is markedly elevated (more than 5 times upper limit of reference range), treatment should be discontinued; in children at high risk of muscle effects, a statin should not be started if creatine kinase is elevated. Children at high risk of myopathy include those with a personal or family history of muscular disorders, previous history of muscular toxicity or liver disease; the risk may be increased in those with renal impairment and possibly in those with hypothyroidism (see Hypothyroidism, p. 161). There is also an increased incidence of myopathy if the statins are given at a high dose or with a fibrate, with lipid-lowering doses of nicotinic acid or with drugs that increase the plasma-statin concentration, such as ciclosporin; close monitoring of liver function and, if symptomatic, of creatine kinase is required in patients receiving these drugs. Rhabdomyolysis with acute renal impairment secondary to myoglobinuria has also been reported.

Counselling　Advise children or their carers to report promptly unexplained muscle pain, tenderness, or weakness.

ATORVASTATIN

Cautions　see notes above; also haemorrhagic stroke

Hepatic impairment　see notes above

Pregnancy　see notes above

Breast-feeding　see notes above

Side-effects　see notes above; also chest pain; back pain; pruritus; *less commonly* anorexia, malaise, weight gain, hypoglycaemia, hyperglycaemia, and tinnitus; *rarely* cholestatic jaundice and peripheral oedema; *very rarely* taste disturbances, gynaecomastia, hearing loss, Stevens-Johnson syndrome, and toxic epidermal necrolysis

Indication and dose

Hyperlipidaemia including familial hypercholesterolaemia

• By mouth

Child 10–17 years initially 10 mg once daily, increased if necessary, at intervals of at least 4 weeks to usual max. 20 mg once daily (max. 80 mg once daily in homozygous familial hypercholesterolaemia)

Child 17–18 years initially 10 mg once daily, increased if necessary, at intervals of at least 4 weeks to max. 80 mg once daily

Note Reduced dose required with concomitant ciclosporin, clarithromycin, or itraconazole—seek specialist advice

Lipitor® (Pfizer) PoM
Tablets, all f/c, atorvastatin (as calcium trihydrate) 10 mg, net price 28-tab pack = £13.00; 20 mg, 28-tab pack = £24.64; 40 mg, 28-tab pack = £24.64; 80 mg, 28-tab pack = £28.21. Counselling, muscle effects, see notes above

FLUVASTATIN

Cautions　see notes above

Hepatic impairment　see notes above

Pregnancy　see notes above

Breast-feeding　see notes above

Side-effects　see notes above; also *very rarely* vasculitis

Indication and dose

Heterozygous familial hypercholesterolaemia

• By mouth

Child 9–18 years initially 20 mg daily in the evening, adjusted in steps of 20 mg daily at intervals of at least 6 weeks; max. 80 mg daily (40 mg twice daily)

Fluvastatin (Non-proprietary) PoM
Capsules, fluvastatin (as sodium salt) 20 mg, net price 28-cap pack = £8.41; 40 mg, 28-cap pack = £9.97. Counselling, muscle effects, see notes above

Lescol® (Novartis) PoM
Capsules, fluvastatin (as sodium salt) 20 mg (brown/yellow), net price 28-cap pack = £15.26; 40 mg (brown/orange), 28-cap pack = £15.26, 56-cap pack = £30.53. Counselling, muscle effects, see notes above

PRAVASTATIN SODIUM

Cautions　see notes above

Hepatic impairment　see notes above

Renal impairment　start with lower doses in moderate to severe impairment

Pregnancy　see notes above

Breast-feeding　see notes above

Side-effects　see notes above; *less commonly* abnormal urination (including dysuria, nocturia, and frequency); *very rarely* fulminant hepatic necrosis

Licensed use　licensed in children over 8 years for familial hypercholesterolaemia

Indication and dose

Hyperlipidaemia including familial hypercholesterolaemia

• By mouth

Child 8–14 years 10 mg once daily at night, adjusted at intervals of at least 4 weeks to max. 20 mg once daily at night

2

Cardiovascular system

◁ **PRAVASTATIN SODIUM** (*continued*)

Child 14–18 years 10 mg once daily at night, adjusted at intervals of at least 4 weeks to max. 40 mg once daily at night

Pravastatin (Non-proprietary) PoM

Tablets, pravastatin sodium 10 mg, net price 28-tab pack = £1.83; 20 mg, 28-tab pack = £2.22; 40 mg, 28-tab pack = £3.02.

Counselling muscle effects, see notes above

Lipostat® (Squibb) PoM

Tablets, all yellow, pravastatin sodium 10 mg, net price 28-tab pack = £14.46; 20 mg, 28-tab pack = £26.53; 40 mg, 28-tab pack = £26.53. Counselling, muscle effects, see notes above

SIMVASTATIN

Cautions see notes above

Hepatic impairment see notes above

Renal impairment doses above 10 mg daily should be used with caution if estimated glomerular filtration rate less than 30 mL/minute/1.73 m²

Pregnancy see notes above

Breast-feeding see notes above

Side-effects see notes above; also *rarely* anaemia

Licensed use not licensed for use in children

Indication and dose

Hyperlipidaemia including familial hypercholesterolaemia

• By mouth

Child 5–10 years initially 10 mg at night increased, if necessary, at intervals of at least 4 weeks to max. 20 mg at night

Child 10–18 years initially 10 mg at night increased, if necessary, at intervals of at least 4 weeks to max. 40 mg at night

Note Reduced dose required with concomitant ciclosporin, danazol, fibrates (except fenofibrate), amiodarone, diltiazem, or verapamil—seek specialist advice

Simvastatin (Non-proprietary) PoM

Tablets, simvastatin 10 mg, net price 28-tab pack = 95p; 20 mg, 28-tab pack = £1.02; 40 mg, 28-tab pack = £1.40; 80 mg, 28-tab pack = £3.27. Counselling, muscle effects, see notes above
Brands include *Simvador®*

Zocor® (MSD) PoM

Tablets, all f/c, simvastatin 10 mg (peach), net price 28-tab pack = £18.03; 20 mg (tan), 28-tab pack = £29.69; 40 mg (red), 28-tab pack = £29.69; 80 mg (red), 28-tab pack = £29.69. Counselling, muscle effects, see notes above

Bile acid sequestrants

Colestyramine (cholestyramine) and **colestipol** are bile acid sequestrants used in the management of hypercholesterolaemia. They act by binding bile acids, preventing their reabsorption; this promotes hepatic conversion of cholesterol into bile acids; the resultant increased LDL-receptor activity of liver cells increases the clearance of LDL-cholesterol from the plasma. Thus both compounds effectively reduce LDL-cholesterol but can aggravate hypertriglyceridaemia. Bile acid sequestrants are not well tolerated and compliance with treatment is poor, therefore they are rarely used in children.

Cautions Bile acid sequestrants interfere with the absorption of fat-soluble vitamins; supplements of vitamins A, D, K, and folic acid may be required when treatment is prolonged and the child's growth and development should be monitored. **Interactions:** Appendix 1 (bile acid sequestrants).

Pregnancy and breast-feeding Bile acid sequestrants should be used with caution as although the drugs are not absorbed, they may cause fat-soluble vitamin deficiency on prolonged use.

Side-effects As bile acid sequestrants are not absorbed, gastro-intestinal side-effects predominate. Constipation is common, but diarrhoea has occurred, as have nausea, vomiting, and gastro-intestinal discomfort. Hypertriglyceridaemia may be aggravated. An increased bleeding tendency has been reported due to hypoprothrombinaemia associated with vitamin K deficiency.

Counselling Other drugs should be taken at least 1 hour before or 4–6 hours after bile acid sequestrants to reduce possible interference with absorption.

COLESTYRAMINE

(Cholestyramine)

Cautions see notes above

Contra-indications complete biliary obstruction (not likely to be effective)

Pregnancy see notes above

Breast-feeding see notes above

◻ **COLESTYRAMINE** (*continued*)

Side-effects see notes above; intestinal obstruction reported rarely and hyperchloraemic acidosis reported on prolonged use

Licensed use licensed in children over 6 years to reduce cholesterol; see also section 1.9.2

Indication and dose

> Familial hypercholesterolaemia
>
> • By mouth
>
>> **Child 6–12 years** initially 4 g once daily increased to 4 g up to 3 times daily according to response
>>
>> **Child 12–18 years** initially 4 g once daily increased by 4 g at weekly intervals to 12–24 g daily in 1–4 divided doses, then adjusted according to response; max. 36 g daily

> Cholestatic pruritus section 1.9.2

> Diarrhoea section 1.9.2

Administration The contents of each sachet should be mixed with at least 150 mL of water or other suitable liquid such as fruit juice, skimmed milk, thin soups, and pulpy fruits with a high moisture content; total daily dose may be given as a single dose if tolerated

Colestyramine (Non-proprietary) ⟨PoM⟩
Powder, sugar-free, colestyramine (anhydrous) 4 g/sachet, net price 50-sachet pack = £16.40.
Label: 13, counselling, avoid other drugs at same time (see notes above)
Excipients may include aspartame (section 9.4.1)

Questran® (Bristol-Myers Squibb) ⟨PoM⟩
Powder, colestyramine (anhydrous) 4 g/sachet, net price 50-sachet pack = £10.97. Label: 13, counselling, avoid other drugs at same time (see notes above)
Excipients include sucrose 3.79 g/sachet

Questran Light® (Bristol-Myers Squibb) ⟨PoM⟩
Powder, sugar-free, colestyramine (anhydrous) 4 g/sachet, net price 50-sachet pack = £16.47.
Label: 13, counselling, avoid other drugs at same time (see notes above)
Excipients include aspartame (section 9.4.1)

COLESTIPOL HYDROCHLORIDE

Cautions see notes above

Pregnancy see notes above

Breast-feeding see notes above

Side-effects see notes above

Licensed use not licensed for use in children

Indication and dose

> Familial hypercholesterolaemia
>
> • By mouth
>
>> **Child 12–18 years** initially 5 g 1–2 times daily increased if necessary in 5-g increments at intervals of 1 month to max. of 30 g daily in 1–2 divided doses

Administration the contents of each sachet should be mixed with at least 100 mL of water or other suitable liquid such as fruit juice, skimmed milk, thin soups, cereals, yoghurt, and pulpy fruits with a high moisture content; total daily dose may be given as a single dose if tolerated

Colestid® (Pharmacia) ⟨PoM⟩
Granules, yellow, colestipol hydrochloride 5 g/sachet, net price 30 sachets = £15.05. Label: 13, counselling, avoid other drugs at same time (see notes above)

Colestid Orange, granules, yellow/orange, colestipol hydrochloride 5 g/sachet, with aspartame, net price 30 sachets = £15.05. Label: 13, counselling, avoid other drugs at same time (see notes above)

Ezetimibe

Ezetimibe inhibits the intestinal absorption of cholesterol. It is given in combination with a statin or alone if a statin is inappropriate. If ezetimibe is used in combination with a statin, there is an increased risk of rhabdomyolysis (see also Muscle Effects, p. 163)

EZETIMIBE

Cautions interactions: Appendix 1 (ezetimibe)

Hepatic impairment avoid in moderate and severe impairment—may accumulate

Pregnancy manufacturer advises use only if potential benefit outweighs risk—no information available

Breast-feeding manufacturer advises avoid—present in milk in *animal* studies

Side-effects gastro-intestinal disturbances; headache, fatigue; myalgia; *rarely* arthralgia, hypersensitivity reactions (including rash, angioedema, and anaphylaxis), hepatitis; *very rarely* pancreatitis, cholelithiasis, cholecystitis, thrombocytopenia, raised creatine kinase, myopathy, and rhabdomyolysis

Indication and dose

> Adjunct to dietary measures and statin treatment in primary hypercholesterolaemia and homozygous familial hypercholesterolaemia (ezetimibe alone in primary hypercholesterolaemia if statin inappropriate or not tolerated); adjunct to dietary measures in homozygous sitosterolaemia
>
> • By mouth
>
>> **Child 10–18 years** 10 mg once daily

◁ **EZETIMIBE (continued)**

Ezetrol® (MSD, Schering-Plough) ⓅⓄⓂ
Tablets, ezetimibe 10 mg, net price 28-tab pack =
£26.31

Fibrates

Bezafibrate and **fenofibrate** act mainly by decreasing serum triglycerides; they have variable effects on LDL-cholesterol. Fibrates may reduce the risk of coronary heart disease in those with low HDL-cholesterol or with raised triglycerides.

Fibrates can cause a myositis-like syndrome, especially in children with impaired renal function. Also, combination of a fibrate with a statin increases the risk of muscle effects (especially rhabdomyolysis) and should be used with caution (see Muscle Effects, p. 163).

There is limited evidence to support their use in children and they should only be considered if treatment with a statin and a bile acid sequestrant is unsuccessful or contra-indicated.

BEZAFIBRATE

Cautions correct hypothyroidism before initiating treatment (see Lipid-regulating Drugs, p. 161); see under Myotoxicity below; **interactions:** Appendix 1 (fibrates)

Contra-indications hypoalbuminaemia, primary biliary cirrhosis, gall bladder disease, nephrotic syndrome

Hepatic impairment avoid in severe liver disease

Renal impairment reduce dose if estimated glomerular filtration rate 15–60 mL/minute/ 1.73 m²; avoid if estimated glomerular filtration rate less than 15 mL/minute/1.73 m²

Myotoxicity Special care needed in patients with renal disease, as progressive increases in serum-creatinine concentration or failure to follow dosage guidelines may result in myotoxicity (rhabdomyolysis); discontinue if myotoxicity suspected or creatine kinase concentration increases significantly

Pregnancy manufacturers advise avoid—embryotoxicity in *animal* studies

Breast-feeding manufacturer advises avoid—no information available

Side-effects gastro-intestinal disturbances, anorexia; *less commonly* cholestasis, weight gain, dizziness, headache, fatigue, drowsiness, renal impairment, raised serum creatinine (unrelated to renal impairment), erectile dysfunction, myotoxicity (with myasthenia or myalgia)—particular risk in renal impairment (see Cautions), urticaria, pruritus, photosensitivity reactions; *very rarely* gallstones, hypoglycaemia, anaemia, leucopenia, thrombocytopenia, increased platelet count, alopecia, Stevens-Johnson syndrome, and toxic epidermal necrolysis

Licensed use not licensed for use in children

Indication and dose

> **Hyperlipidaemia including familial hyper-cholesterolaemia** (on specialist advice only)
> • By mouth
> **Child 10–18 years** 200 mg once daily adjusted according to response to max. 200 mg 3 times daily

Bezafibrate (Non-proprietary) ⓅⓄⓂ
Tablets, bezafibrate 200 mg, net price 100-tab pack = £8.82. Label: 21

Bezalip® (Actavis) ⓅⓄⓂ
Tablets, f/c, bezafibrate 200 mg, net price 100-tab pack = £8.79. Label: 21

FENOFIBRATE

Cautions see under Bezafibrate; liver function tests recommended every 3 months for first year (discontinue treatment if significantly raised)

Contra-indications gall bladder disease; photosensitivity to ketoprofen

Hepatic impairment avoid in severe impairment

Renal impairment reduce dose if estimated glomerular filtration rate less than 60 mL/minute/1.73 m²; avoid if estimated glomerular filtration rate less than 15 mL/minute/1.73 m²

Myotoxicity Special care needed in patients with renal disease, as progressive increases in serum-creatinine concentration or failure to follow dosage guidelines may result in myotoxicity (rhabdomyolysis); discontinue if myotoxicity suspected or creatine kinase concentration increases significantly

Pregnancy manufacturer advises avoid—embryotoxicity in animal studies

Breast-feeding manufacturer advises avoid—no information available

Side-effects see under Bezafibrate; also *very rarely* hepatitis, pancreatitis, and interstitial pneumopathies

Licensed use *Lipantil® Micro 67* is licensed for use in children with hypercholesterolaemia

Indication and dose

> **Hyperlipidaemias including familial hyper-cholesterolaemia** (on specialist advice only)
> • By mouth
> **Child 4–15 years** 1 capsule/20 kg body-weight daily
>
> **Child 15–18 years** initially 3 capsules daily in divided doses; usual range 2–4 capsules daily

◁ **FENOFIBRATE** (*continued*)

Lipantil® (Solvay) PoM
  Lipantil® Micro 67 capsules, yellow, fenofibrate
  (micronised) 67 mg, net price 90-cap pack = £23.30.
  Label: 21

2.13 Local sclerosants

Classification not used in *BNF for Children*.

2.14 Drugs affecting the ductus arteriosus

Closure of the ductus arteriosus

Patent ductus arteriosus is a frequent problem in premature neonates with respiratory distress syndrome. Substantial left-to-right shunting through the ductus arteriosus may increase the risk of intraventricular haemorrhage, necrotising enterocolitis, bronchopulmonary dysplasia, and possibly death.

Indometacin or ibuprofen can be used to close the ductus arteriosus. **Indometacin** has been used for many years and is effective but it reduces cerebral blood flow, and causes a transient fall in renal and gastro-intestinal blood flow. **Ibuprofen** may also be used; it has little effect on renal function (there may be a small reduction in sodium excretion) when used in doses for closure of the ductus arteriosus; gastro-intestinal problems are uncommon.

If drug treatment fails to close the ductus arteriosus, surgery may be indicated.

IBUPROFEN

Cautions may mask symptoms of infection; monitor for bleeding; monitor gastro-intestinal function; allergic disorders; **interactions:** Appendix 1 (NSAIDs)

Contra-indications life-threatening infection; active bleeding especially intracranial or gastro-intestinal; thrombocytopenia or coagulation defects; marked unconjugated hyperbilirubinaemia; known or suspected necrotising enterocolitis; pulmonary hypertension

Hepatic impairment increased risk of gastro-intestinal bleeding and fluid retention; avoid in severe liver disease

Renal impairment use lowest effective dose and monitor renal function; sodium and water retention; deterioration in renal function possibly leading to renal failure; avoid if possible in severe impairment

Side-effects intestinal perforation; intraventricular haemorrhage; ischaemic brain injury; bronchopulmonary dysplasia, pulmonary haemorrhage; thrombocytopenia, neutropenia, oliguria, haematuria, fluid retention, hyponatr-

aemia; *less commonly* gastro-intestinal haemorrhage; hypoxaemia

Licensed use Orphan licence for the injection for closure of ductus arteriosus in premature neonates less than 34 weeks gestational age

Indication and dose

Closure of ductus arteriosus
• By slow intravenous injection

  Neonate initially 10 mg/kg as a single dose followed at 24-hour intervals by 2 doses of 5 mg/kg; course may be repeated after 48 hours if necessary

Mild to moderate pain, pain and inflammation of soft tissue injuries and rheumatic disease, pyrexia section 10.1.1

Administration for *slow intravenous injection*, give over 15 minutes, preferably undiluted. May be diluted with Glucose 5% or Sodium Chloride 0.9%

Pedea® (Orphan Europe) PoM
  Intravenous solution, ibuprofen 5 mg/mL, net price 4 × 2-mL vials = £263.00

INDOMETACIN

Cautions see notes above; also may mask symptoms of infection; may reduce urine output by 50% or more (monitor carefully—see also under Anuria or Oliguria, below) and precipitate renal impairment especially if extracellular volume

depleted, heart failure, sepsis, or concomitant use of nephrotoxic drugs; may induce hyponatraemia; inhibition of platelet aggregation (monitor for bleeding); **interactions:** Appendix 1 (NSAIDs)

2 Cardiovascular system

◻ **INDOMETACIN (continued)**

Contra-indications untreated infection, bleeding (especially with active intracranial haemorrhage or gastro-intestinal bleeding); thrombocytopenia, coagulation defects, necrotising enterocolitis

Hepatic impairment increased risk of gastro-intestinal bleeding and fluid retention; avoid in severe impairment

Renal impairment use lowest effective dose and monitor renal function; sodium and water retention; deterioration in renal function possibly leading to renal failure; avoid if possible in severe impairment

Anuria or oliguria If anuria or marked oliguria (urinary output less than 0.6 mL/kg/hour), delay further doses until renal function returns to normal

Side-effects haemorrhagic, renal, gastro-intestinal, metabolic, and coagulation disorders; pulmonary hypertension, intracranial bleeding, fluid retention, and exacerbation of infection

Indication and dose

Closure of ductus arteriosus
• By intravenous infusion over 20–30 minutes

> Neonate under 48 hours initially 200 micrograms/kg as a single dose followed by (if urine output adequate) 2 doses of 100 micrograms/kg

at intervals of 12–24 hours; course may be repeated after 48 hours if necessary

> Neonate 2–7 days initially 200 micrograms/kg as a single dose followed by (if urine output adequate) 2 doses of 200 micrograms/kg at intervals of 12–24 hours; course may be repeated after 48 hours if necessary

> Neonate over 7 days initially 200 micrograms/kg as a single dose followed by (if urine output adequate) 2 doses of 250 micrograms/kg at intervals of 12–24 hours; course may be repeated after 48 hours if necessary
> Note In some units by intravenous infusion initially 100 micrograms/kg (200 micrograms/kg if symptomatic) then 100 micrograms/kg every 24 hours for 5 further doses

Pain and inflammation in rheumatic disease
section 10.1.1

Administration for intravenous infusion dilute each vial with 1–2 mL Sodium Chloride 0.9% or Water for Injections

Indocid PDA® (IDIS) [PoM]
Injection, powder for reconstitution, indometacin (as sodium trihydrate), net price 3 × 1-mg vials = £43.50 (hosp. only)

Maintenance of patency

In the newborn with duct-dependent congenital heart disease it is often necessary to maintain the patency of the ductus arteriosus whilst awaiting surgery.

Alprostadil (prostaglandin E1) and **dinoprostone** (prostaglandin E2) are potent vasodilators that are effective for maintaining the patency of the ductus arteriosus. They are usually given by continuous intravenous infusion, but oral dosing of dinoprostone is still used in some centres.

During the infusion of a prostaglandin, the newborn requires careful monitoring of heart rate, blood pressure, respiratory rate, and core body temperature. In the event of complications such as apnoea, profound bradycardia, or severe hypotension, the infusion should be temporarily stopped and the complication dealt with; the infusion should be restarted at a lower dose. Recurrent or prolonged apnoea may require ventilatory support in order for the prostaglandin infusion to continue.

ALPROSTADIL

Cautions see notes above; also history of haemorrhage; avoid in hyaline membrane disease; monitor arterial pressure, respiratory rate, heart rate, temperature, and venous blood pressure in arm and leg; facilities for intubation and ventilation must be immediately available; **interactions:** Appendix 1 (alprostadil)

Side-effects apnoea (particularly in neonates under 2 kg), flushing, bradycardia, hypotension, tachycardia, cardiac arrest, oedema, diarrhoea, fever, convulsions, disseminated intravascular coagulation, hypokalaemia; cortical proliferation of long bones; weakening of the wall of the ductus arteriosus and pulmonary artery may follow prolonged use; gastric-outlet obstruction reported

Indication and dose

Maintaining patency of the ductus arteriosus
• By continuous intravenous infusion

> Neonate initially 5 nanograms/kg/minute, adjusted according to response in steps of 5 nanograms/kg/minute; max. 100 nanograms/kg/minute (but associated with increased side-effects)

Note Alprostadil doses in BNFC may differ from those in product literature

Administration dilute 150 micrograms/kg body-weight to a final volume of 50 mL with Glucose 5% or Sodium Chloride 0.9%; an intravenous infusion rate of 0.1 mL/hour provides a dose of 5 nanograms/kg/minute. Undiluted solution must not come into contact with the barrel of the plastic syringe; add the required volume of alprostadil to a volume of infusion fluid in the syringe and then make up to final volume

◯ **ALPROSTADIL (continued)**

Prostin VR® (Pharmacia) PoM
Intravenous solution, alprostadil 500 micrograms/
mL in alcohol. For dilution and use as an infusion.
Net price 1–mL amp = £75.19 (hosp.only)

▌ DINOPROSTONE

Cautions see notes above; also history of
haemorrhage; avoid in hyaline membrane disease; monitor arterial oxygenation, heart rate,
temperature, and blood pressure in arm and leg;
facilities for intubation and ventilation must be
immediately available; **interactions**: Appendix 1
(prostaglandins)

Hepatic impairment manufacturer advises avoid

Renal impairment manufacturer advises avoid

Side-effects nausea, vomiting, diarrhoea; flushing, bradycardia, hypotension, cardiac arrest;
respiratory depression and apnoea, particularly
with high doses and in low birth-weight neonates,
bronchospasm; pyrexia and raised white blood
cell count, shivering; local reactions, erythema; if
used for longer than 5 days, gastric outlet
obstruction; cortical hyperostosis (prolonged use)

Licensed use not licensed for use in children

Indication and dose

> Maintaining patency of the ductus arteriosus
> • By continuous intravenous infusion
>
> > **Neonate** initially 5 nanograms/kg/minute,
> > increased as necessary in 5 nanogram/kg/min-
> > ute increments to 20 nanograms/kg/minute
> > Note Doses up to 100 nanograms/kg/minute have
> > been used but are associated with increased side-
> > effects

> • By mouth
>
> > **Neonate** 20–25 micrograms/kg every 1–2 hours
> > doubled if necessary; if treatment continues for
> > more than 1 week gradually reduce the dose

Administration for *continuous intravenous infusion*,
dilute to a concentration of 1 microgram/mL with
Glucose 5% *or* Sodium Chloride 0.9%.

For administration *by mouth*, injection solution
can be given orally; dilute with water

Prostin® E2 (Pharmacia) PoM
Intravenous solution, for dilution and use as an
infusion, dinoprostone 1 mg/mL, net price 0.75-mL
amp = £8.52; 10 mg/mL, 0.5-mL amp = £18.40
(both hosp. only)

◀ Extemporaneous formulations available see
Extemporaneous Preparations, p. 8

2

Cardiovascular system

3 Respiratory system

This chapter includes advice on the drug management of the following:

    acute asthma, p. 171

    anaphylaxis, p. 202

    angioedema, p. 205

    chronic asthma, p. 173

    croup, p. 175

3.1 Bronchodilators

Asthma

Drugs used in the management of asthma include beta$_2$ agonists (section 3.1.1), antimuscarinic bronchodilators (section 3.1.2), theophylline (section 3.1.3), corticosteroids (section 3.2), cromoglicate and nedocromil (section 3.3.1), leukotriene receptor antagonists (section 3.3.2), and in specialist centres, omalizumab (section 3.4.2).

For tables outlining the management of chronic asthma and management of acute asthma, see p. 173 and p. 174.

Administration of drugs for asthma

Inhalation   This route delivers the drug directly to the airways; the dose required is smaller than when given by mouth and side-effects are reduced. See Inhaler devices, section 3.1.5.

Solutions for nebulisation for use in acute severe asthma are administered over 5–10 minutes from a nebuliser, usually driven by oxygen in hospital. See Nebulisers, section 3.1.5.

Oral   Systemic side-effects occur more frequently when a drug is given orally rather than by inhalation. Oral corticosteroids, theophylline, and leukotriene receptor antagonists are sometimes required for the management of asthma. Oral administration of a beta$_2$ agonist is generally not recommended for children, but may be necessary in infants and young children unable to use an inhaler device.

Parenteral   Drugs such as beta$_2$ agonists, corticosteroids, and aminophylline can be given by injection in acute severe asthma when drug administration by nebulisation is inadequate or inappropriate; in these circumstances the child should generally be treated in a high-dependency or intensive care unit.

Pregnancy and breast-feeding

Women with asthma should be closely monitored during pregnancy. Well-controlled asthma has no important effects on pregnancy, labour, or the fetus. Drugs for asthma should preferably be administered by inhalation to minimise fetal drug exposure. Inhaled drugs, theophylline, and prednisolone can be taken as normal during pregnancy and breast-feeding. Women planning to become pregnant should be counselled about the importance of taking their asthma medication regularly to maintain good control.

Severe acute exacerbations of asthma can have an adverse effect on pregnancy and should be treated promptly in hospital with conventional therapy, including nebulisation of a beta$_2$ agonist, and oral or parenteral administration of a corticosteroid; prednisolone is the preferred corticosteroid for oral administration since very little of the drug reaches the fetus. Oxygen should be given immediately to maintain an arterial oxygen saturation of 94–98% and prevent maternal and fetal hypoxia. An intravenous beta$_2$ agonist, aminophylline, or magnesium sulphate can be used during pregnancy if necessary; parenteral beta$_2$ agonists can affect the myometrium, see BNF section 7.1.3.

Management of acute asthma[1]

> **Important**
> Regard each emergency consultation as being for **severe acute asthma** until shown otherwise.
>
> Failure to respond adequately **at any time** requires immediate transfer to hospital.

---

1. Advice on the management of acute asthma is based on the recommendations of the British Thoracic Society and Scottish Intercollegiate Guidelines Network (updated June 2009); updates available at www.brit-thoracic.org.uk

3 Respiratory system

Severe acute asthma can be fatal and must be treated promptly and energetically. Treatment of severe acute asthma is safer in hospital where resuscitation facilities are immediately available. Treatment should **never** be delayed for investigations, children should **never** be sedated, and the possibility of a pneumothorax should be considered. If the child's condition deteriorates despite pharmacological treatment, urgent transfer to a paediatric intensive care unit should be arranged. For a table outlining the management of severe acute asthma, see Management of acute asthma p. 174.

Mild to moderate acute asthma Administer a **short-acting beta$_2$ agonist** using a pressurised metered-dose inhaler with a spacer device; for a child under 3 years use a close-fitting facemask. Give 1 puff every 15–30 seconds up to a maximum of 10 puffs; repeat dose after 10–20 minutes if necessary.

Give **prednisolone** by mouth, child under 12 years 1–2 mg/kg (max. 40 mg) once daily for up to 3 days, or longer if necessary; if the child has been taking an oral corticosteroid for more than a few days, give prednisolone 2 mg/kg (max. 60 mg) once daily. For children 12–18 years, give prednisolone 40–50 mg daily for at least 5 days.

If response is poor or if a relapse occurs within 3–4 hours, transfer child **immediately** to hospital for assessment and further treatment.

Children under 18 months often respond poorly to bronchodilators; nebulised beta$_2$ agonists have been associated with mild (but occasionally severe) paradoxical bronchospasm and transient worsening of oxygen saturation; response to prednisolone may also be poor in this age group.

Severe or life-threatening acute asthma Start treatment below and transfer **immediately** to hospital. Administer high-flow **oxygen** (section 3.6) using a close-fitting face mask or nasal prongs.

Treat severe or life-threatening acute exacerbations of asthma with an inhaled **short-acting beta$_2$ agonist** (as above). Treatment of life-threatening asthma should be initiated with nebulised salbutamol 2.5 mg or terbutaline 5 mg (via an oxygen-driven nebuliser if available); nebulised doses may be doubled for children over 5 years. Repeat the dose every 20–30 minutes or as necessary, then reduce the frequency on improvement.

Give **prednisolone** by mouth, child under 12 years 1–2 mg/kg (max. 40 mg) once daily for up to 3 days, or longer if necessary; if the child has been taking an oral corticosteroid for more than a few days, give prednisolone 2 mg/kg (max. 60 mg) once daily. For children 12–18 years, give prednisolone 40–50 mg daily for at least 5 days. If oral administration is not possible, use intravenous **hydrocortisone** (preferably as sodium succinate) 4 mg/kg (child under 2 years max. 25 mg, 2–5 years 50 mg, 5–18 years 100 mg) every 6 hours.

If response is poor, add nebulised **ipratropium bromide** (child under 12 years 250 micrograms, 12–18 years 500 micrograms) every 20–30 minutes for the first 2 hours, then every 4–6 hours as necessary.

If the condition does not respond or is life-threatening, transfer the child to an intensive care unit and treat with a parenteral **short-acting beta$_2$ agonist** (e.g. salbutamol, section 3.1.1.1) or parenteral **aminophylline** (section 3.1.3). Children over 2 years with severe acute asthma may be helped by intravenous infusion of **magnesium sulphate** 40 mg/kg (max. 2 g) over 20 minutes (section 9.5.1.3), but evidence of benefit is limited.

Follow-up in all cases Episodes of acute asthma should be regarded as a failure of preventive therapy. A careful history should be taken to establish the reason for the exacerbation. Inhaler technique should be checked and regular treatment should be reviewed in accordance with the Management of Chronic Asthma table, p. 173. Children or their carers should be given an asthma action plan aimed at preventing relapse, optimising treatment, and preventing delay in seeking assistance in future exacerbations. If possible, follow-up within 48 hours should be arranged with the general practitioner or appropriate primary care health professional. Children should also be reviewed in a paediatric asthma clinic within one month of the exacerbation.

Management of chronic asthma

Important   Start at **step most appropriate** to initial severity; before initiating a new drug consider whether diagnosis is correct, check compliance and inhaler technique, and eliminate trigger factors for acute exacerbations

Child 5–18 years

Step 1: occasional relief bronchodilator
Inhaled short-acting beta$_2$ agonist as required (up to once daily)
Note Move to step 2 if needed more than twice a week, or if night-time symptoms more than once a week, or if exacerbation in the last 2 years

Step 2: regular inhaled preventer therapy
Inhaled short-acting beta$_2$ agonist as required
plus
Regular standard-dose[1] inhaled corticosteroid (alternatives[2] are considerably less effective)

Step 3: inhaled corticosteroid + inhaled long-acting beta$_2$ agonist
Inhaled short-acting beta$_2$ agonist as required
plus
Regular standard-dose[1] inhaled corticosteroid
plus
Regular inhaled long-acting beta$_2$ agonist (salmeterol *or* formoterol)
If asthma not controlled
Increase dose of inhaled corticosteroid to upper end of standard dose range[1]
and
Either stop long-acting beta$_2$ agonist if of no benefit
Or continue long-acting beta$_2$ agonist if of some benefit
If asthma still not controlled and long-acting beta$_2$ agonist stopped, add one of

  Leukotriene receptor antagonist
  Modified-release oral theophylline
  Modified-release oral beta$_2$ agonist

Step 4: high-dose inhaled corticosteroid + regular bronchodilators
Inhaled short-acting beta$_2$ agonist as required
with
Regular high-dose[3] inhaled corticosteroid
plus
Inhaled long-acting beta$_2$ agonist (if of benefit)
plus
A 6-week sequential therapeutic trial of one or more of

  Leukotriene receptor antagonist
  Modified-release oral theophylline
  Modified-release oral beta$_2$ agonist

Step 5: regular corticosteroid tablets
Refer to respiratory paediatrician
Inhaled short-acting beta$_2$ agonist as required
with
Regular high-dose[3] inhaled corticosteroid
and
One or more long-acting bronchodilators (see step 4)
plus
Regular prednisolone tablets (as single daily dose)
Note In addition to regular prednisolone, continue high-dose inhaled corticosteroid (in exceptional cases may exceed licensed doses)

Stepping down
Review treatment every 3 months; if control achieved stepwise reduction may be possible; reduce dose of *inhaled* corticosteroid slowly (consider reduction every 3 months, decreasing dose by up to 50% each time) to the lowest dose which controls asthma

Child under 5 years[4]

Step 1: occasional relief bronchodilator
Short-acting beta$_2$ agonist as required (not more than once daily)
Note Preferably by inhalation (less effective and more side-effects when given as tablets or syrup)
Move to step 2 if needed more than twice a week, or if night-time symptoms more than once a week, or if exacerbation in the last 2 years

Step 2: regular preventer therapy
Inhaled short-acting beta$_2$ agonist as required
plus
Regular standard-dose[1] inhaled corticosteroid
Or leukotriene receptor antagonist if inhaled corticosteroid cannot be used

Step 3: add-on therapy
Child under 2 years:
Refer to respiratory paediatrician
Child 2–5 years:
Inhaled short-acting beta$_2$ agonist as required
plus
Regular standard-dose[1] inhaled corticosteroid
plus
Leukotriene receptor antagonist

Step 4: persistent poor control
Refer to respiratory paediatrician

Stepping down
Regularly review need for treatment

1. **Standard doses** of inhaled corticosteroids
   Beclometasone dipropionate or **budesonide**:
   Child under 12 years 100–200 micrograms twice daily;
   Child 12–18 years 100–400 micrograms twice daily.
   Fluticasone propionate:
   Child 4–12 years 50–100 micrograms twice daily;
   Child 12–18 years 50–200 micrograms twice daily.
   Mometasone furoate (given through a dry powder inhaler):
   Child 12–18 years 200 micrograms twice daily
   Note Doses of inhaled corticosteroids here are for CFC-free metered-dose inhalers given through a large-volume spacer; dose adjustments may be required for some inhaler devices, see under individual preparations section 3.2.

2. Alternatives to inhaled corticosteroid are leukotriene receptor antagonists, theophylline, inhaled nedocromil, or inhaled cromoglicate

3. **High doses** of inhaled corticosteroids
   Beclometasone dipropionate or **budesonide**:
   Child 5–12 years 200–400 micrograms twice daily;
   Child 12–18 years 0.4–1 mg twice daily.
   Fluticasone propionate:
   Child 5–12 years 100–200 micrograms twice daily;
   Child 12–18 years 200–500 micrograms twice daily.
   Mometasone furoate (given through a dry powder inhaler):
   Child 12–18 years up to 400 micrograms twice daily.
   Note Doses of inhaled corticosteroids here are for CFC-free metered-dose inhalers given through a large-volume spacer; dose adjustments may be required for some inhaler devices, see under individual preparations section 3.2.
   Failure to achieve control with these doses is unusual, see also Side-effects of Inhaled Corticosteroids, section 3.2

4. Lung-function measurements cannot be used to guide management in those under 5 years

Advice on the management of chronic asthma is based on the recommendations of the British Thoracic Society and Scottish Intercollegiate Guidelines Network (updated June 2009); updates available at www.brit-thoracic.org.uk

3

Respiratory system

Management of acute asthma

Respiratory system

3

> **Important**   The assessment of acute asthma in early childhood can be difficult. Children with severe or life-threatening acute asthma may not be distressed and may not have all of these abnormalities; the presence of any should alert the doctor. Regard each emergency consultation as being for **severe acute asthma** until shown otherwise

Moderate acute asthma	Severe acute asthma	Life-threatening acute asthma
• Able to talk • Respiration (breaths/minute) Child 2–5 years ≤ 40, 5–12 years ≤ 30, 12–18 years < 25 • Pulse (beats/minute) Child 2–5 years ≤ 140, 5–12 years ≤ 125, 12–18 years < 110 • Arterial oxygen saturation ≥ 92% • Peak flow Child 5–12 years ≥ 50% of predicted or best, 12–18 years > 50% *Treat at home or in surgery and assess response to treatment*	• Child under 12 years too breathless to talk or feed, 12–18 years cannot complete sentences in one breath • Use of accessory breathing muscles • Respiration (breaths/minute) Child 2–5 years > 40, 5–12 years > 30, 12–18 years ≥ 25 • Pulse (beats/minute) Child 2–5 years > 140, 5–12 years >125, 12–18 years ≥ 110 • Arterial oxygen saturation Child under 12 years < 92%, 12–18 years ≥ 92% • Peak flow Child 5–12 years < 50% of predicted or best, 12–18 years 33–50% *Start treatment below and send immediately to hospital*	• Silent chest, cyanosis, poor respiratory effort • Arrhythmia, hypotension • Exhaustion, altered consciousness, agitation, confusion • Arterial oxygen saturation <92% • Peak flow < 33% of predicted or best *Start treatment below and send immediately to hospital; consult with senior medical staff and refer to paediatric intensive care*
Treatment • Inhaled **short-acting beta₂ agonist** via a large-volume spacer (and a close-fitting face mask if child under 3 years) or oxygen-driven nebuliser (if available); give 2–10 puffs of **salbutamol** 100 micrograms/metered inhalation each inhaled separately, and repeat at 10–20 minute intervals if necessary *or* give nebulised **salbutamol**, Child under 5 years 2.5 mg, 5–12 years 2.5–5 mg, 12–18 years 5 mg *or* **terbutaline** Child under 5 years 5 mg, 5–12 years 5–10 mg, 12–18 years 10 mg, and repeat at 20–30 minute intervals if necessary • **Prednisolone** by mouth Child under 12 years 1–2 mg/kg (max. 40 mg) daily for up to 3 days or longer if necessary; if the child has been taking an oral corticosteroid for more than a few days, give prednisolone 2 mg/kg (max. 60 mg); Child 12–18 years 40–50 mg daily for at least 5 days *Monitor response for 15–30 minutes* *If response is poor or a relapse occurs in 3–4 hours, send immediately to hospital for assessment and further treatment*	**Treatment** • High-flow **oxygen** (if available) • Inhaled **short-acting beta₂ agonist** via a large-volume spacer (and a close-fitting face mask if child under 3 years) or oxygen-driven nebuliser (if available); give 2–10 puffs of **salbutamol** 100 micrograms/metered inhalation each inhaled separately, and repeat at 10–20 minute intervals or as necessary *or* give nebulised **salbutamol**, Child under 5 years 2.5 mg, 5–12 years 2.5–5 mg, 12–18 years 5 mg *or* **terbutaline** Child under 5 years 5 mg, 5–12 years 5–10 mg, 12–18 years 10 mg, and repeat at 20–30 minute intervals as necessary • **Prednisolone** by mouth as for moderate acute asthma *or* intravenous **hydrocortisone** (preferably as sodium succinate) 4 mg/kg (Child under 2 years max. 25 mg, 2–5 years 50 mg, 5–18 years 100 mg) until conversion to oral prednisolone is possible *Monitor response for 15–30 minutes* *If response is poor:* • Inhaled **ipratropium bromide** via oxygen-driven nebuliser (if available), Child under 12 years, 250 micrograms, 12–18 years, 500 micrograms repeated every 20–30 minutes for the first 2 hours, then every 4–6 hours as necessary *Refer those who fail to respond and require ventilatory support to a paediatric intensive care or high-dependency unit* • Consider intravenous **beta₂ agonists**, **aminophylline**, or **magnesium sulphate** [unlicensed indication] only after consultation with senior medical staff	**Treatment** • High-flow **oxygen** (if available) • Inhaled **short-acting beta₂ agonist** via oxygen-driven nebuliser (if available); give **salbutamol**, Child under 5 years 2.5 mg, 5–12 years 2.5–5 mg, 12–18 years 5 mg, *or* **terbutaline**, Child under 5 years 5 mg, 5–12 years 5–10 mg, 12–18 years 10 mg, and repeat as necessary; reserve **intravenous beta₂ agonists** for those in whom inhaled therapy cannot be used reliably or there is no current effect • **Prednisolone** by mouth as for moderate acute asthma *or* intravenous **hydrocortisone** (preferably as sodium succinate) 4 mg/kg (Child under 2 years, max. 25 mg, 2–5 years 50 mg, 5–18 years 100 mg) every 6 hours until conversion to oral prednisolone is possible • Inhaled **ipratropium bromide** via oxygen-driven nebuliser (if available), Child under 12 years 250 micrograms, 12–18 years 500 micrograms repeated every 20–30 minutes for the first 2 hours, then every 4–6 hours as necessary *Monitor response for 15–30 minutes* *If response is poor:* • Consider intravenous **beta₂ agonists**, **aminophylline**, or **magnesium sulphate** [unlicensed indication] only after consultation with senior medical staff

---

Follow up in all cases

Monitor symptoms and peak flow. Set up asthma action plan and check inhaler technique with child and carer
Review by general practitioner or appropriate primary care health professional within 48 hours; see also, p. 172

Advice on the management of acute asthma is based on the recommendations of the British Thoracic Society and Scottish Intercollegiate Guidelines Network (updated June 2009); updates available at www.brit-thoracic.org.uk

Croup

Mild croup is largely self-limiting, but treatment with a single dose of a corticosteroid (e.g. **dexamethasone** 150 micrograms/kg) by mouth is of benefit.

Severe croup (or mild croup that might cause complications) calls for hospital admission—a single dose of either dexamethasone 150 micrograms/kg or prednisolone 1–2 mg/kg, can be administered by mouth before transfer to hospital. In hospital, dexamethasone 150 micrograms/kg (by mouth or by injection) or budesonide 2 mg by nebulisation (section 3.2) will often reduce symptoms; the dose may be repeated after 12 hours if necessary.

For severe croup not effectively controlled with corticosteroid treatment, nebulised **adrenaline** (section 3.4.3) solution 1 in 1000 (1 mg/mL) can be given with close clinical monitoring in a dose of 400 micrograms/kg (max. 5 mg) repeated after 30 minutes if necessary (the dose may be diluted with sterile sodium chloride 0.9% solution). The effects of nebulised adrenaline last 2–3 hours; the child needs to be carefully monitored for recurrence of the obstruction.

3.1.1 Adrenoceptor agonists
(Sympathomimetics)

3.1.1.1 Selective beta$_2$ agonists

3.1.1.2 Other adrenoceptor agonists

The selective beta$_2$ agonists (selective beta$_2$-adrenoceptor agonists, selective beta$_2$ stimulants) such as salbutamol or terbutaline are the safest and most effective short-acting beta$_2$ agonists for the treatment of asthma.

Adrenaline (epinephrine), which has both alpha- and beta-adrenoceptor agonist properties, is used in the emergency management of acute allergic and anaphylactic reactions (section 3.4.3); it is also used as a nebuliser solution to treat severe croup.

3.1.1.1 Selective beta$_2$ agonists

Selective beta$_2$ agonists produce bronchodilation. A short-acting beta$_2$ agonist is used for immediate relief of asthma symptoms while a long-acting beta$_2$ agonist is used in addition to an inhaled corticosteroid in children requiring prophylactic treatment.

Short-acting beta$_2$ agonists   Mild to moderate symptoms of asthma respond rapidly to the inhalation of a selective short-acting beta$_2$ agonist such as **salbutamol** or **terbutaline**. If beta$_2$ agonist inhalation is needed more often than once daily, prophylactic treatment should be considered, using a stepped approach as outlined in the Management of Chronic Asthma, p. 173. Regular treatment with an inhaled short-acting beta$_2$ agonist is less effective than 'as required' inhalation and is not appropriate prophylactic treatment.

A short-acting beta$_2$ agonist inhaled immediately before exertion reduces *exercise-induced asthma*; however, frequent exercise-induced asthma probably reflects poor overall control and calls for reassessment of asthma treatment.

Long-acting beta$_2$ agonists   **Formoterol** (eformoterol) and **salmeterol** are longer-acting beta$_2$ agonists which are administered by inhalation. Added to regular inhaled corticosteroid treatment, they have a role in the long-term control of chronic asthma (see Management of Chronic Asthma, p. 173) and they can be useful in nocturnal asthma. Salmeterol should not be used for the relief of an asthma attack; it has a slower onset of action than salbutamol or terbutaline. Formoterol is licensed for short-term symptom relief and for the prevention of exercise-induced bronchospasm; its speed of onset of action is similar to that of salbutamol.

Combination inhalers that contain a long-acting beta$_2$ agonist and a corticosteroid (section 3.2) ensure that long-acting beta$_2$ agonists are not used alone, but reduce the flexibility to adjust the dose of each component.

3 Respiratory system

CHM advice
To ensure safe use, the CHM has advised that for the management of chronic asthma, long-acting beta$_2$ agonists (formoterol and salmeterol) should:

- be added only if regular use of standard-dose inhaled corticosteroids has failed to control asthma adequately;
- not be initiated in patients with rapidly deteriorating asthma;
- be introduced at a low dose and the effect monitored before considering dose increase;
- be discontinued in the absence of benefit;
- be reviewed as clinically appropriate: stepping down therapy should be considered when good long-term asthma control has been achieved.

Children and their carers should be advised to report any deterioration in symptoms following initiation of treatment with a long-acting beta$_2$ agonist, see Management of Chronic Asthma, p. 173.

Management of Chronic Asthma, see p. 173
Management of Acute Asthma, see p. 171
For guidance on the use of inhalers and spacer devices, see section 3.1.5

Inhalation A *pressurised metered-dose inhaler* is an effective method of drug administration in mild to moderate chronic asthma; to deliver the drug effectively particularly in children under 12 years, a spacer device should be used (see also NICE guidance, section 3.1.5). When a pressurised metered-dose inhaler with a spacer is unsuitable or inconvenient, a *dry-powder inhaler* or *breath-actuated inhaler* may be used instead if the child is able to use the device effectively. At recommended inhaled doses the duration of action of salbutamol and terbutaline is about 3 to 5 hours and for salmeterol and formoterol is about 12 hours. The **dose**, the frequency, and the maximum number of inhalations in 24 hours of the beta$_2$ agonist should be **stated explicitly** to the child and the child's carer. High doses of beta$_2$ agonists can be dangerous in some children (see Cautions, below). Excessive use is usually an indication of **inadequately controlled** asthma and should be managed with a prophylactic drug such as an inhaled corticosteroid. The child and the child's carer should be advised to seek medical advice when the prescribed dose of beta$_2$ agonist fails to provide the usual degree of symptomatic relief because this usually indicates a worsening of the asthma and the child may require alternative medication (see Management of Chronic Asthma, p. 173).

Children and their carers should be advised to follow manufacturers' instructions on the care and cleansing of inhaler devices.

Nebuliser (or respirator) solutions of salbutamol and terbutaline are used for the treatment of severe acute asthma both in hospital and in general practice. Children with a severe attack of asthma should have oxygen if possible during nebulisation since beta$_2$ agonists can increase arterial hypoxaemia, see also section 3.1.5.

Oral Oral preparations of beta$_2$ agonists may be used for children if an inhaler device cannot be used but inhaled beta$_2$ agonists are more effective and have fewer side-effects. A modified-release formulation of salbutamol may be of value in nocturnal asthma as an alternative to modified-release theophylline preparations (section 3.1.3), but an inhaled long-acting beta$_2$ agonist is preferable.

Parenteral Beta$_2$ agonists can be given intravenously in children with severe or life-threatening acute asthma. Chronic asthma unresponsive to stepwise treatment (see Management of Chronic Asthma, p. 173) may benefit from continuous subcutaneous infusion of a beta$_2$ agonist, but this should be used only under the supervision of a respiratory specialist; the evidence of benefit is uncertain and it may be difficult to withdraw such treatment once started.

Cautions Beta$_2$ agonists should be used with caution in diabetes—monitor blood glucose (risk of ketoacidosis, especially when a beta$_2$ agonist is given intravenously). Beta$_2$ agonists should be used with caution in hyperthyroidism, cardiovascular disease, arrhythmias, susceptibility to QT-interval prolongation, and hypertension. **Interactions:** Appendix 1 (sympathomimetics, beta$_2$).

Hypokalaemia Potentially serious hypokalaemia may result from beta$_2$ agonist therapy. Particular caution is required in severe asthma, because this effect may be potentiated by concomitant treatment with theophylline and its derivatives, corticosteroids, and diuretics, and by hypoxia. Plasma-potassium concentration should therefore be monitored in severe asthma.

Side-effects Side-effects of the beta$_2$ agonists include fine tremor (particularly in the hands), nervous tension, headache, peripheral dilatation and palpitation. Other side-effects include tachycardia, arrhythmias, peripheral vasodilation, myocardial ischaemia, and disturbances of sleep and behaviour. Muscle cramps and hypersensitivity reactions including paradoxical bronchospasm (occasionally severe), urticaria, angioedema, hypotension, and collapse have also been reported. High doses of beta$_2$ agonists are associated with hypokalaemia (see Hypokalaemia, above).

FORMOTEROL FUMARATE

(Eformoterol fumarate)

Cautions see notes above

Pregnancy see p. 171

Breast-feeding see p. 171

Side-effects see notes above; nausea, dizziness, rash, taste disturbances, and pruritus also reported

Indication and dose

Reversible airways obstruction (including nocturnal asthma and prevention of exercise-induced bronchospasm) in patients requiring long-term regular bronchodilator therapy see also Management of Chronic Asthma, p. 173; for dose see preparations below

Counselling Advise children and carers not to exceed prescribed dose, and to follow manufacturer's directions; if a previously effective dose of inhaled formoterol fails to provide adequate relief, a doctor's advice should be obtained as soon as possible

Formoterol (Non-proprietary) PoM

Dry powder for inhalation, formoterol fumarate 12 micrograms/metered inhalation, net price 120-dose unit = £24.11. Counselling, dose

Brands include *Easyhaler® Formoterol*

Dose

Chronic asthma

- By inhalation of powder

Child 6–18 years 12 micrograms twice daily, increased to 24 micrograms twice daily in more severe airways obstruction

Atimos Modulite® (Chiesi) ▼ PoM

Aerosol inhalation, formoterol fumarate 12 micrograms/metered inhalation, net price 100-dose unit = £30.06. Counselling, dose

Excipients include HFA-134a (a non-CFC propellant)

Dose

Chronic Asthma

- By aerosol inhalation

Child 12–18 years 12 micrograms twice daily, increased to max. 24 micrograms twice daily in more severe airways obstruction

Foradil® (Novartis) PoM

Dry powder for inhalation, formoterol fumarate 12 micrograms/capsule, net price 60-cap pack (with inhaler device) = £30.06. Counselling, dose

Dose

Chronic asthma

- By inhalation of powder

Child 5–18 years 12 micrograms twice daily, increased to 24 micrograms twice daily in more severe airways obstruction

Oxis® (AstraZeneca) PoM

Turbohaler®(= dry powder inhaler), formoterol fumarate 6 micrograms/inhalation, net price 60-dose unit = £24.80; 12 micrograms/inhalation, 60-dose unit = £24.80. Counselling, dose

Dose

Chronic asthma

- By inhalation of powder

Child 6–18 years 6–12 micrograms 1–2 times daily; occasionally up to 48 micrograms daily may be needed (max. single dose 12 micrograms); reassess treatment if additional doses required on more than 2 days a week

Relief of bronchospasm

- By inhalation of powder

Child 6–18 years 6–12 micrograms

Prevention of exercise-induced bronchospasm

- By inhalation of powder

Child 6–18 years 6–12 micrograms before exercise

◢Compound preparations

For **compound preparations** containing formoterol, see section 3.2

SALBUTAMOL

(Albuterol)

Cautions see notes above

Pregnancy see p. 171

Breast-feeding see p. 171

Side-effects see notes above

Licensed use not licensed for use in hyperkalaemia; syrup not licensed for use in children under 2 years; modified-release tablets not licensed for use in children under 3 years; injection not licensed for use in children; *Pulvinal®*

◻ **SALBUTAMOL** *(continued)*

Salbutamol not licensed for use in children under 6 years

Indication and dose

Acute asthma

• **By aerosol or nebulised solution inhalation**
See Management of Acute Asthma, p. 171

• **By intravenous injection over 5 minutes (see also Management of Acute Asthma, p. 171)**
Child 1 month–2 years 5 micrograms/kg as a single dose

Child 2–18 years 15 micrograms/kg (max. 250 micrograms) as a single dose

• **By continuous intravenous infusion**
Child 1 month–18 years 1–2 micrograms/kg/minute, adjusted according to response and heart rate up to 5 micrograms/kg/minute; doses above 2 micrograms/kg/minute should be given in an intensive care setting

Exacerbations of reversible airways obstruction (including nocturnal asthma) and prevention of allergen- or exercise-induced bronchospasm, see also Management of Chronic Asthma, p. 173

• **By aerosol inhalation**
Child 1 month–18 years 100–200 micrograms (1–2 puffs); for persistent symptoms up to 4 times daily

• **By inhalation of powder**
(for *Asmasal Clickhaler®*, *Salbulin Novolizer®*, and *Ventolin Accuhaler®* doses, see under preparations)
Child 5–12 years 200 micrograms; for persistent symptoms up to 4 times daily

Child 12–18 years 200–400 micrograms; for persistent symptoms up to 4 times daily

• **By mouth (but use by inhalation preferred)**
Child 1 month–2 years 100 micrograms/kg (max. 2 mg) 3–4 times daily

Child 2–6 years 1–2 mg 3–4 times daily

Child 6–12 years 2 mg 3–4 times daily

Child 12–18 years 4 mg (sensitive patients initially 2 mg) 3–4 times daily; max. single dose 8 mg (but unlikely to provide extra benefit or to be tolerated)

Severe hyperkalaemia (section 9.2.1.1)
• **By intravenous injection over 5 minutes**
Neonate 4 micrograms/kg as a single dose; repeat if necessary

Child 1 month–18 years 4 micrograms/kg as a single dose; repeat if necessary

• **By inhalation of nebulised solution (but intravenous injection preferred)**
Neonate 2.5–5 mg as a single dose; repeat if necessary

Child 1 month–18 years 2.5–5 mg as a single dose; repeat if necessary

Administration for *continuous intravenous infusion*, dilute to a concentration of 200 micrograms/mL

with Glucose 5% *or* Sodium Chloride 0.9%; if fluid-restricted, can be given undiluted through central venous catheter

For *intravenous injection*, dilute to a concentration of 50 micrograms/mL with Glucose 5%, Sodium Chloride 0.9%, *or* Water for injections

For *nebulisation*, dilute nebuliser solution with a suitable volume of sterile Sodium Chloride 0.9% solution according to nebuliser type and duration of administration; salbutamol and ipratropium bromide solutions are compatible and can be mixed for nebulisation

◢Oral

Salbutamol (Non-proprietary) ▣ᴘᴏᴹ
Tablets, salbutamol (as sulphate) 2 mg, net price 28-tab pack = £13.33; 4 mg, 28-tab pack = £12.32

Oral solution, salbutamol (as sulphate) 2 mg/5 mL, net price 150 mL = £1.60
Brands include *Salapin®* (sugar-free)

Ventmax® SR (Chiesi) ▣ᴘᴏᴹ
Capsules, m/r, salbutamol (as sulphate) 4 mg (green/grey), net price 56-cap pack = £8.24; 8 mg (white), 56-cap pack = £9.88. Label: 25

Dose
Chronic asthma (but see notes above)
• **By mouth**
Child 3–12 years 4 mg twice daily
Child 12–18 years 8 mg twice daily

Ventolin® (A&H) ▣ᴘᴏᴹ
Syrup, sugar-free, salbutamol (as sulphate) 2 mg/5 mL, net price 150 mL = 60p

◢Parenteral

Ventolin® (A&H) ▣ᴘᴏᴹ
Injection, salbutamol (as sulphate) 500 micrograms/mL, net price 1-mL amp = 38p

Solution for intravenous infusion, salbutamol (as sulphate) 1 mg/mL. Dilute before use. Net price 5-mL amp = £2.48

◢Inhalation

Counselling Advise children and carers not to exceed prescribed dose and to follow manufacturer's directions; if a previously effective dose of inhaled salbutamol fails to provide at least 3 hours relief, a doctor's advice should be obtained as soon as possible.

Salbutamol (Non-proprietary) ▣ᴘᴏᴹ
Aerosol inhalation, salbutamol (as sulphate) 100 micrograms/metered inhalation, net price 200-dose unit = £2.99. Counselling, dose
Excipients include HFA-134a (a non-CFC propellant)
Brands include *Salamol®*

Dry powder for inhalation, salbutamol 100 micrograms/metered inhalation, net price 200-dose unit = £3.46; 200 micrograms/metered inhalation, 100-dose unit = £4.85, 200-dose unit = £6.92. Counselling, dose
Brands include *Easyhaler® Salbutamol*, *Pulvinal® Salbutamol*

Inhalation powder, *hard capsule* (for use with *Cyclohaler®* device), salbutamol 200 micrograms, net price 120-cap pack = £8.99; 400 micrograms, 120-cap pack = £12.99. Counselling, dose
Brands include *Salbutamol Cyclocaps®*

⊿ SALBUTAMOL (continued)

Nebuliser solution, salbutamol (as sulphate) 1 mg/
mL, net price 20 × 2.5 mL (2.5 mg) = £1.91; 2 mg/
mL, 20 × 2.5 mL (5 mg) = £3.82. May be diluted
with sterile sodium chloride 0.9%
Brands include *Salamol Steri-Neb®*

Airomir® (IVAX) [PoM]

Aerosol inhalation, salbutamol (as sulphate)
100 micrograms/metered inhalation, net price 200-
dose unit = £1.97. Counselling, dose
Excipients include HFA-134a (a non-CFC propellant)

Autohaler (breath-actuated aerosol inhalation),
salbutamol (as sulphate) 100 micrograms/metered
inhalation, net price 200-dose unit = £6.02. Counselling, dose
Excipients include HFA-134a (a non-CFC propellant),

Asmasal Clickhaler® (UCB Pharma) [PoM]

Dry powder for inhalation, salbutamol (as sulphate)
95 micrograms/metered inhalation, net price 200-
dose unit = £5.65. Counselling, dose

Dose

Acute bronchospasm
- By inhalation of powder
  Child 5–18 years 1–2 puffs; for persistent symptoms
  up to 4 times daily (but see also Management of
  Chronic Asthma, p. 173)

Prophylaxis of allergen- or exercise-induced bron-
chospasm
- By inhalation of powder
  Child 5–18 years 1–2 puffs

Salamol Easi-Breathe® (IVAX) [PoM]

Aerosol inhalation , salbutamol 100 micrograms/
metered inhalation, net price 200-dose breath-
actuated unit = £6.30. Counselling, dose
Excipients include HFA-134a (a non-CFC propellant)

Salbulin Novolizer® (Meda) [PoM]

Dry powder for inhalation, salbutamol (as sulphate)
100 micrograms/metered inhalation, net price

refillable 200-dose unit = £4.95; 200-dose refill =
£2.75. Counselling, dose

Dose

Acute bronchospasm
- By inhalation of powder
  Child 6–12 years 100–200 micrograms; for persistent
  symptoms up to 400 micrograms daily (but see also
  Management of Chronic Asthma, p. 173)

  Child 12–18 years 100–200 micrograms; for persistent symptoms up to 800 micrograms daily (but see
  also Management of Chronic Asthma, p. 173)

Prophylaxis of allergen- or exercise-induced bron-
chospasm
- By inhalation of powder
  Child 6–12 years 100–200 micrograms
  Child 12–18 years 200 micrograms

Ventolin® (A&H) [PoM]

Accuhaler® (dry powder for inhalation), disk containing 60 blisters of salbutamol (as sulphate)
200 micrograms/blister with *Accuhaler®* device, net
price = £4.92. Counselling, dose

Dose

Acute bronchospasm
- By inhalation of powder
  Child 5–18 years 200 micrograms; for persistent
  symptoms up to 4 times daily but see also Management of Chronic Asthma, p. 173

Prophylaxis of allergen- or exercise-induced bron-
chospasm
- By inhalation of powder
  Child 5–18 years 200 micrograms

Evohaler® *aerosol inhalation*, salbutamol (as sulphate) 100 micrograms/metered inhalation, net
price 200-dose unit = £1.50. Counselling, dose
Excipients include HFA-134a (a non-CFC propellant)

Nebules® (for use with nebuliser), salbutamol (as
sulphate) 1 mg/mL, net price 20 × 2.5 mL (2.5 mg)
= £1.68; 2 mg/mL, 20 × 2.5 mL (5 mg) = £2.83. May
be diluted with sterile sodium chloride 0.9%

Respirator solution (for use with a nebuliser or
ventilator), salbutamol (as sulphate) 5 mg/mL. Net
price 20 mL = £2.18 (hosp. only). May be diluted
with sterile sodium chloride 0.9%

SALMETEROL

Note Not for immediate relief of acute attacks; existing
corticosteroid therapy should not be reduced or withdrawn

Cautions see notes above

Pregnancy see p. 171

Breast-feeding see p. 171

Side-effects see notes above; nausea, dizziness,
arthralgia, and rash also reported

Indication and dose

Reversible airways obstruction (including
nocturnal asthma and prevention of exercise-
induced bronchospasm) in patients requiring
long-term regular bronchodilator therapy see
also Management of Chronic Asthma, p. 173

- By inhalation
  Child 5–12 years 50 micrograms (2 puffs or 1
  blister) twice daily

Child 12–18 years 50 micrograms (2 puffs or 1
blister) twice daily; up to 100 micrograms (4
puffs or 2 blisters) twice daily in more severe
airways obstruction
Counselling Advise children and carers that salmeterol should **not** be used for relief of acute attacks,
not to exceed prescribed dose, and to follow manufacturer's directions; if a previously effective dose of
inhaled salmeterol fails to provide adequate relief, a
doctor's advice should be obtained as soon as possible

Serevent® (A&H) [PoM]

Accuhaler® (dry powder for inhalation), disk containing 60 blisters of salmeterol (as xinafoate)
50 micrograms/blister with *Accuhaler®* device, net
price = £29.26. Counselling, dose

3

Respiratory system

◻ **SALMETEROL (continued)**

Evohaler® aerosol inhalation▼, salmeterol (as xinafoate) 25 micrograms/metered inhalation, net price 120-dose unit = £29.26. Counselling, dose
Excipients include HFA-134a (a non-CFC propellant)

Diskhaler® (dry powder for inhalation), disks containing 4 blisters of salmeterol (as xinafoate) 50 micrograms/blister, net price 15 disks with *Dis-khaler*® device = £35.79, 15-disk refill = £35.15. Counselling, dose

◢**Compound preparations**
For **compound preparations** containing salmeterol, see section 3.2

TERBUTALINE SULPHATE

Cautions see notes above
Pregnancy see p. 171
Breast-feeding see p. 171
Side-effects see notes above
Licensed use tablets not licensed for use in children under 7 years; injection not licensed for use in children under 2 years

Indication and dose

Acute asthma
- **By inhalation of nebulised solution**
  see Management of Acute Asthma, p. 171

- **By subcutaneous or slow intravenous injection**
  Child 2–15 years 10 micrograms/kg (max. 300 micrograms) up to 4 times daily
  Child 15–18 years 250–500 micrograms up to 4 times daily

- **By continuous intravenous infusion**
  Child 1 month–18 years initially 2–4 micrograms/kg as a loading dose, then 1–10 micrograms/kg/hour according to response and heart rate (doses above 10 micrograms/kg/hour with close monitoring)

Exacerbations of reversible airways obstruction (including nocturnal asthma) and prevention of exercise-induced bronchospasm see Management of Chronic Asthma, p. 173
- **By inhalation of powder**
  Child 5–18 years 500 micrograms (1 inhalation) up to 4 times daily (for occasional use only)

- **By mouth (but not recommended)**
  Child 1 month–7 years 75 micrograms/kg (max. 2.5 mg) 3 times daily
  Child 7–15 years 2.5 mg 2–3 times daily

Child 15–18 years initially 2.5 mg 3 times daily, increased if necessary to 5 mg 3 times daily

Administration For *continuous intravenous infusion*, dilute to a concentration of 5 micrograms/mL with Glucose 5% or Sodium Chloride 0.9%; if fluid-restricted, dilute to a concentration of 100 micrograms/mL
For *nebulisation*, dilute nebuliser solution with sterile Sodium Chloride 0.9% solution according to nebuliser type and duration of administration; terbutaline and ipratropium bromide solutions are compatible and may be mixed for nebulisation.

◢**Oral and parenteral**
Bricanyl® (AstraZeneca) ⒫ⓄⓂ
Tablets, scored, terbutaline sulphate 5 mg, net price 100-tab pack = £4.09

Syrup, sugar-free, terbutaline sulphate 1.5 mg/5 mL, net price 100 mL = £2.00

Injection, terbutaline sulphate 500 micrograms/mL, net price 1-mL amp = 30p; 5-mL amp = £1.40

◢**Inhalation**
Counselling Advise children and carers not to exceed prescribed dose and to follow manufacturer's directions; if a previously effective dose of inhaled terbutaline fails to provide at least 3 hours relief, a doctor's advice should be obtained as soon as possible

Bricanyl® (AstraZeneca) ⒫ⓄⓂ
Turbohaler® (= dry powder inhaler), terbutaline sulphate 500 micrograms/metered inhalation, net price 100-dose unit = £6.92. Counselling, dose

Respules® (= single-dose units for nebulisation), terbutaline sulphate 2.5 mg/mL, net price 20 × 2-mL units (5-mg) = £4.04

3.1.1.2 **Other adrenoceptor agonists**

Adrenaline (epinephrine) injection (1 in 1000) is used in the emergency treatment of acute allergic and anaphylactic reactions (section 3.4.3), in angioedema (section 3.4.3), and in cardiopulmonary resuscitation (section 2.7.3). Adrenaline solution (1 in 1000) is used by nebulisation in the management of severe croup (section 3.1).

3.1.2 **Antimuscarinic bronchodilators**

Ipratropium by nebulisation can be added to other standard treatment in life-threatening acute asthma or if acute asthma fails to improve with standard therapy (see Management of Acute Asthma, p. 171). Ipratropium can be used to provide short-term relief in chronic asthma, but short-acting beta₂ agonists act more quickly and are preferred.

The aerosol inhalation of ipratropium has a maximum effect 30–60 minutes after use; its duration of action is 3 to 6 hours.

IPRATROPIUM BROMIDE

Cautions risk of glaucoma (see below), bladder outflow obstruction; **interactions:** Appendix 1 (antimuscarinics)

Glaucoma *Acute angle-closure glaucoma* reported with nebulised ipratropium, particularly when given with nebulised salbutamol (and possibly other beta₂ agonists); care needed to protect the child's eyes from nebulised drug or from drug powder

Pregnancy see p. 171

Breast-feeding see p. 171

Side-effects dry mouth; *less commonly* nausea and headache; *rarely* constipation, tachycardia, palpitation, paradoxical bronchospasm, urinary retention, blurred vision, angle-closure glaucoma, and hypersensitivity reactions including rash, urticaria, and angioedema

Indication and dose

Acute asthma
- **By inhalation of nebulised solution**
  See Management of Acute Asthma, section 3.1

Reversible airways obstruction see notes above
- **By aerosol inhalation**
  Child 1 month–6 years 20 micrograms 3 times daily

  Child 6–12 years 20–40 micrograms 3 times daily

  Child 12–18 years 20–40 micrograms 3–4 times daily

- **By inhalation of powder**
  Child 12–18 years 40 micrograms 3–4 times daily (dose may be doubled in less responsive condition)

Counselling Advise child and carer not to exceed prescribed dose and to follow manufacturer's directions

Rhinitis section 12.2.2

Ipratropium Bromide (Non-proprietary) [PoM]
Nebuliser solution, ipratropium bromide 250 micrograms/mL, net price 20 × 1-mL (250-microgram) unit-dose vials = £6.75, 60 × 1-mL = £21.78; 20 × 2-mL (500-microgram) = £7.43, 60 × 2-mL = £26.97

Atrovent® (Boehringer Ingelheim) [PoM]
Aerocaps® (dry powder for inhalation; for use with *Atrovent Aerohaler®*), green, ipratropium bromide 40 micrograms, net price pack of 100 caps with *Aerohaler®* = £14.53; 100 caps = £10.53. Counselling, dose
Note One *Atrovent Aerocap®* is equivalent to 2 puffs of *Atrovent®* metered aerosol inhalation

Aerosol inhalation ▼, ipratropium bromide 20 micrograms/metered inhalation, net price 200-dose unit = £5.05. Counselling, dose
Excipients include HFA-134a (a non-CFC propellant)

Nebuliser solution, isotonic, ipratropium bromide 250 micrograms/mL, net price 20 × 1-mL unit-dose vials = £4.14, 60 × 1-mL vials = £12.44; 20 × 2-mL vials = £4.87, 60 × 2-mL vials = £14.59

Ipratropium Steri-Neb® (IVAX) [PoM]
Nebuliser solution, isotonic, ipratropium bromide 250 micrograms/mL, net price 20 × 1-mL (250-microgram) unit-dose vials = £8.72; 20 × 2-mL (500-microgram) = £9.94

Respontin® (A&H) [PoM]
Nebuliser solution, isotonic, ipratropium bromide 250 micrograms/mL, net price 20 × 1-mL (250-microgram) unit-dose vials = £4.87; 20 × 2-mL (500-microgram) = £5.72

3.1.3 Theophylline

Theophylline is a xanthine used as a bronchodilator in asthma, see Management of Chronic Asthma p. 173. It may have an additive effect when used in conjunction with small doses of beta₂ agonists; the combination may increase the risk of side-effects, including hypokalaemia (see p. 177).

Theophylline is given by injection as **aminophylline**, a mixture of theophylline with ethylenediamine, which is 20 times more soluble than theophylline alone. Aminophylline injection is needed rarely for severe acute asthma (see Management of Acute Asthma p. 174). It must be given by **very slow** intravenous injection (over at least 20 minutes) or by intravenous infusion; it is too irritant for intramuscular use. Intravenous aminophylline may be used as a respiratory stimulant in neonates with apnoea, but **caffeine**, a xanthine derivative, (section 3.5.1) is usually preferred. Measurement of plasma-theophylline concentration may be helpful and is **essential** if a loading dose of aminophylline is to be given to children who are already taking theophylline, because serious side-effects such as convulsions and arrhythmias can occasionally precede other symptoms of toxicity.

Theophylline is metabolised in the liver. The plasma-theophylline concentration is *increased* in heart failure, cirrhosis, viral infections, and by drugs that inhibit its metabolism. The plasma-theophylline concentration is *decreased* in smokers and by drugs that induce its metabolism. For interactions of theophylline, see Appendix 1.

Plasma-theophylline concentration   In most individuals a plasma-theophylline concentration of 10–20 mg/litre (55–110 micromol/litre) is required for satisfactory bronchodilation, but a lower concentration of 5–15 mg/litre may be effective. Adverse effects can occur within the range 10–20 mg/litre and both the frequency and severity increase if the concentration exceeds 20 mg/litre. In neonates, toxic symptoms sometimes occur when the plasma-theophylline concentration exceeds 14 mg/litre (78 micromol/litre). If theophylline is used in the treatment of *neonatal apnoea*, the usual target range is 8–12 mg/litre (44–66 micromol/litre).

Plasma-theophylline concentration is measured 5 days after starting oral treatment and at least 3 days after any dose adjustment. A blood sample should be taken 1–2 hours after an oral dose (after 4–6 hours in the case of a modified-release preparation). If aminophylline is given intravenously, a blood sample should be taken 4–6 hours after starting treatment.

◢ THEOPHYLLINE

Cautions   see notes above; also cardiac disease, hypertension, hyperthyroidism; peptic ulcer; epilepsy; fever; hypokalaemia risk, p. 177; avoid in acute porphyria (section 9.8.2); monitor plasma-theophylline concentration (see notes above); **interactions**: Appendix 1 (theophylline) and notes above

Hepatic impairment   reduce dose

Pregnancy   neonatal irritability and apnoea reported; see also, p. 171

Breast-feeding   present in milk—irritability in infant reported; modified-release preparations preferable; see also, p. 171

Side-effects   tachycardia, palpitation, nausea and other gastro-intestinal disturbances, headache, CNS stimulation, insomnia, arrhythmias, and convulsions especially if given rapidly by intravenous injection; **overdosage**: see Emergency Treatment of Poisoning, p. 43

Licensed use   *Slo-Phyllin*® capsules not licensed for use in children under 2 years

Indication and dose

Chronic asthma
see under preparations below and Management of Chronic Asthma p. 173
Note Plasma-theophylline concentration for optimum response 10–20 mg/litre (55–110 micromol/litre); narrow margin between therapeutic and toxic dose, see also notes above

◢ Modified release

Note The rate of absorption from modified-release preparations can vary between different brands. The Council of the Royal Pharmaceutical Society of Great Britain advises pharmacists that if a general practitioner prescribes a modified-release oral theophylline preparation without specifying an brand name, the pharmacist should contact the prescriber and agree the brand to be dispensed. Additionally, it is essential that a child discharged from hospital should be maintained on the brand on which that child was stabilised as an in-patient.

Nuelin SA® (3M)
SA tablets, m/r, theophylline 175 mg. Net price 60-tab pack = £3.19. Label: 21, 25
Dose
Chronic asthma
• By mouth
Child 6–12 years 175 mg every 12 hours
Child 12–18 years 175–350 mg every 12 hours

SA 250 tablets, m/r, scored, theophylline 250 mg. Net price 60-tab pack = £4.46. Label: 21, 25
Dose
Chronic asthma
• By mouth
Child 6–12 years 125–250 mg every 12 hours
Child 12–18 years 250–500 mg every 12 hours

Slo-Phyllin® (Merck Serono)
Capsules, m/r, theophylline 60 mg (white/clear, enclosing white pellets), net price 56-cap pack = £2.76; 125 mg (brown/clear, enclosing white pellets), 56-cap pack = £3.48; 250 mg (blue/clear, enclosing white pellets), 56-cap pack = £4.34. Label: 25, or counselling, see below
Dose
Chronic asthma
• By mouth
Child 6 months–2 years (body-weight under 10 kg) 12 mg/kg every 12 hours
Child 2–6 years (body-weight over 10 kg) 60–120 mg every 12 hours
Child 6–12 years 125–250 mg every 12 hours
Child 12–18 years 250–500 mg every 12 hours
Administration Contents of the capsule (enteric-coated granules) may be sprinkled on to a spoonful of soft food (e.g. yoghurt) and swallowed without chewing

Uniphyllin Continus® (Napp)
Tablets, m/r, scored, theophylline 200 mg, net price 56-tab pack = £3.00; 300 mg, 56-tab pack = £4.77; 400 mg, 56-tab pack = £5.42. Label: 25
Dose
Chronic asthma
• By mouth
Child 2–12 years 9 mg/kg (up to 200 mg) every 12 hours; some children with chronic asthma may require 10–16 mg/kg (max. 400 mg) every 12 hours
Child 12–18 years 200 mg every 12 hours, increased according to response to 400 mg every 12 hours
Note May be appropriate to give larger evening or morning dose to achieve optimum therapeutic effect when symptoms most severe; in children whose night or daytime symptoms persist despite other therapy, who are not currently receiving theophylline, total daily requirement may be added as a single evening or morning dose

Respiratory system

3

■ AMINOPHYLLINE

Note Aminophylline is a stable mixture or combination of theophylline and ethylenediamine; the ethylenediamine confers greater solubility in water

Cautions see under Theophylline; also rapid intravenous injection can cause arrhythmias

Hepatic impairment see under Theophylline

Pregnancy see under Theophylline

Breast-feeding see under Theophylline

Side-effects see under Theophylline; also allergy to ethylenediamine can cause urticaria, erythema, and exfoliative dermatitis

Licensed use *Minijet® Aminophylline* not licensed for use in children under 6 months

Indication and dose

To avoid excessive dosage in obese children, dose should be calculated on the basis of ideal weight for height

Chronic asthma (see also Management of Chronic Asthma, p. 173)
● **By mouth**
See under preparations below

Severe acute asthma not previously treated with theophylline (with close monitoring; see also Management of Acute Asthma, section 3.1)
● **By intravenous injection over at least 20 minutes**
Child 1 month–18 years 5 mg/kg (max. 500 mg) then by intravenous infusion

Severe acute asthma (with close monitoring; see also Management of Acute Asthma, section 3.1)
● **By intravenous infusion**
Child 1 month–12 years 1 mg/kg/hour adjusted according to plasma-theophylline concentration
Child 12–18 years 500–700 micrograms/kg/hour adjusted according to plasma-theophylline concentration

Note Plasma-theophylline concentration for optimum response in asthma 10–20 mg/litre (55–110 micromol/litre); narrow margin between therapeutic and toxic dose,

see also notes above on plasma-theophylline concentration; children taking oral theophylline or *aminophylline* should not normally receive intravenous aminophylline unless plasma-theophylline concentration is available to guide dosage; loading dose adjusted on the basis that each 600 micrograms/kg *aminophylline* will increase plasma-theophylline concentration by 1 mg/litre

Neonatal apnoea (but see notes above)
● **By intravenous injection over 20 minutes**
Neonate initially 6 mg/kg, then 2.5 mg/kg every 12 hours (increased if necessary to 3.5 mg/kg every 12 hours)

Note Plasma-theophylline concentration for optimum response in neonatal apnoea 8–12 mg/litre (44–66 micromol/litre), see also notes above

Administration For *intravenous infusion*, dilute to a concentration of 1 mg/mL with Glucose 5% *or* Sodium Chloride 0.9%

Aminophylline (Non-proprietary) PoM
Injection, aminophylline 25 mg/mL, net price 10-mL amp = 90p
Brands include *Minijet® Aminophylline*

Injection, aminophylline 2 mg/mL, 20-mL amp; 5 mg/mL, 20-mL amp
Available from 'special-order' manufacturers or specialist importing companies, see p. 957

◢ Modified release

Note Advice about modified-release theophylline preparations on p. 182 also applies to modified-release aminophylline preparations

Phyllocontin Continus® (Napp)
Tablets, m/r, yellow, f/c, aminophylline hydrate 225 mg, net price 56-tab pack = £2.44. Label: 25
Dose
Chronic asthma (see also Management of Chronic Asthma, p. 173)
● **By mouth**
Child body-weight over 40 kg initially 1 tablet twice daily, increased after 1 week to 2 tablets twice daily according to plasma-theophylline concentration

Note Brands of modified-release tablets containing aminophylline 225 mg include *Norphyllin® SR*

3.1.4 Compound bronchodilator preparations

In general, children are best treated with single-ingredient preparations, such as a selective beta₂ agonist (section 3.1.1.1) or ipratropium bromide (section 3.1.2), so that the dose of each drug can be adjusted. This flexibility is lost with compound bronchodilator preparations.

3.1.5 Peak flow meters, inhaler devices, and nebulisers

Peak flow meters

Peak flow meters may be used to assess lung function in children over 5 years with asthma, but symptom monitoring is the most reliable assessment of asthma control. They are best used for short periods to assess the severity of asthma and to monitor response to treatment; continuous use of peak flow meters may detract from compliance with inhalers.

Standard Range Peak Flow Meter

Conforms to standard EN 13826

AirZone®, range 60–720 litres/minute, net price = £4.50, replacement mouthpiece = 38p (Clement Clarke)

MicroPeak®, range 60–800 litres/minute, net price = £6.50, replacement mouthpiece = 38p (Micro Medical)

Mini-Wright®, range 60–800 litres/minute, net price = £6.86, replacement mouthpiece = 38p (Clement Clarke)

Personal Best®, range 60–800 litres/minute, net price = £6.86, replacement mouthpiece = 25p (Respironics)

Piko-1®, range 15–999 litres/minute, net price = £9.50, replacement mouthpiece = 38p (nSPIRE Health)

Pinnacle®, range 60–900 litres/minute, net price = £6.50 (Fyne Dynamics)

Pocketpeak®, range 60–800 litres/minute, net price = £6.53, replacement mouthpiece = 38p (nSPIRE Health)

Vitalograph®, range 50–800 litres/minute, net price = £4.50 (a child's peak flow meter is also available), replacement mouthpiece = 40p (Vitalograph)

Vitalograph asma-1®, range 0–999 litres/minute, net price = £9.50, replacement mouthpiece = 40p (Vitalograph)

Note Readings from new peak flow meters are often lower than those obtained from old Wright-scale peak flow meters and the correct recording chart should be used

Low Range Peak Flow Meter

Compliant to standard EN 13826 except for scale range

Mini-Wright®, range 30–400 litres/minute, net price = £6.90, replacement mouthpiece = 38p (Clement Clarke)

Pocketpeak®, range 50–400 litres/minute, net price = £6.53, replacement mouthpiece = 38p (nSPIRE Health)

Note Readings from new peak flow meters are often lower than those obtained from old Wright-scale peak flow meters and the correct recording chart should be used

Drug delivery devices

Inhaler devices   A *pressurised metered-dose inhaler* is an effective method of drug administration in mild to moderate chronic asthma; to deliver the drug effectively, a spacer device should also be used (see also NICE guidance, below). By the age of 3 years, a child can usually be taught to use a spacer device without a mask. As soon as a child is able to use the mouthpiece, then this is the preferred delivery system.

Dry powder inhalers may be useful in children over 5 years, who are unwilling or unable to use a pressurised metered-dose inhaler with a spacer device; *breath-actuated inhalers* may be useful in older children if they are able to use the device effectively. The child or child's carer should be instructed carefully on the use of the inhaler. It is important to check that the inhaler is being used correctly; poor inhalation technique may be mistaken for a lack of response to the drug.

On changing from a pressurised metered-dose inhaler to a dry powder inhaler, the child may notice a lack of sensation in the mouth and throat previously associated with each actuation; coughing may occur more frequently following use of a dry-powder inhaler.

CFC-free metered-dose inhalers should be cleaned **weekly** according to the manufacturer's instructions.

> NICE guidance
>
> Inhaler devices for children with chronic asthma (children under 5 years, August 2000; children 5–15 years, March 2002)
>
> A child's needs, ability to develop and maintain effective technique, and likelihood of good compliance should govern the choice of inhaler and spacer device; only then should cost be considered.
>
> For children aged under 5 years:
>
> - corticosteroid and bronchodilator therapy should be delivered by pressurised metered-dose inhaler **and** spacer device, with a facemask if necessary;
>
> - if this is not effective, and depending on the child's condition, nebulised therapy may be considered and, in children over 3 years, a dry powder inhaler may also be considered [but see notes above].
>
> For children aged 5–15 years:
>
> - corticosteroid therapy should be routinely delivered by a pressurised metered-dose inhaler **and** spacer device;
>
> - children and their carers should be trained in the use of the chosen device; suitability of the device should be reviewed at least annually. Inhaler technique and compliance should be monitored.

Spacer devices   Spacer devices are particularly useful for infants, for children with poor inhalation technique, or for nocturnal asthma, because the device reduces the need for coordination between actuation of a pressurised metered-dose inhaler and inhalation. The spacer device reduces the velocity of the aerosol

3 Respiratory system

and subsequent impaction on the oropharynx and allows more time for evaporation of the propellant so that a larger proportion of the particles can be inhaled and deposited in the lungs. Smaller-volume spacers may be more manageable for pre-school children and infants. The spacer device used must be compatible with the prescribed metered-dose inhaler.

Use and care of spacer devices   The suitability of the spacer device should be carefully assessed; opening the one-way valve is dependent on the child's inspiratory flow. Some devices can be tipped to 45° to open the valve during inhaler actuation and inspiration to assist the child.

Inhalation from the spacer device should follow the actuation as soon as possible because the drug aerosol is very short-lived. The total dose (which may be more than a single puff) should be administered as single actuations (with tidal breathing for 10–20 seconds or 5–6 breaths for each actuation) for children with good inspiratory flow. Larger doses may be necessary for a child with acute bronchospasm; for guidance on the Management of Acute Asthma, see section 3.1.

The device should be cleansed once a month by washing in mild detergent and then allowed to dry in air without rinsing; the mouthpiece should be wiped clean of detergent before use. Some manufacturers recommend more frequent cleaning, but this should be avoided since any electrostatic charge may affect drug delivery. Spacer devices should be replaced every 6–12 months.

Able Spacer® (Clement Clarke)
Spacer device, small-volume device. For use with all pressurised (aerosol) inhalers, net price standard device = £4.20; with infant, child or adult mask = £6.86

AeroChamber® Plus (GSK)
Spacer device, medium-volume device. For use with all pressurised (aerosol) inhalers, net price standard device (blue) = £4.47, with mask (blue) = £7.45; infant device (orange) with mask = £7.45; child device (yellow) with mask = £7.45

Babyhaler® (A&H) NHS
Spacer device, paediatric use with *Flixotide®*, *Seretide®*, *Serevent®*, and *Ventolin®* inhalers, net price = £11.34

Haleraid® (A&H)
Inhalation aid, device to place over pressurised (aerosol) inhalers to allow strength in hands is impaired (e.g. arthritis). For use with *Flixotide®*, *Seretide®*, *Serevent®*, and *Ventolin®* inhalers. Available as *Haleraid®-120* for 120-dose inhalers and *Haleraid®-200* for 200-dose inhalers, net price = 80p

NebuChamber® (AstraZeneca)
Spacer device, for use with *Pulmicort®* aerosol inhalers, net price = £8.56.

Optichamber® (Respironics)
Spacer device, for use with all pressurised (aerosol) inhalers, net price = £4.28; with small, medium or large mask = £7.00

PARI Vortex Spacer® (Pari) NHS
Spacer device, medium-volume device. For use with all pressurised (aerosol) inhalers, net price with mouthpiece = £6.07 NHS; with mask for infant or child = £7.91; adult mask = £9.97 NHS

Pocket Chamber® (nSPIRE Health)
Spacer device, small-volume device. For use with all pressurised (aerosol) inhalers, net price = £4.18; with infant, small, medium, or large mask = £9.75

Volumatic® (A&H)
Spacer inhaler, large-volume device. For use with *Clenil Modulite®*, *Flixotide®*, *Seretide®*, *Serevent®*, and *Ventolin®* inhalers, net price = £2.77; with paediatric mask = £2.77

Nebulisers

> In England and Wales nebulisers and compressors are not available on the NHS (but they are free of VAT); some nebulisers (but not compressors) are available on form GP10A in Scotland (for details consult Scottish Drug Tariff).
>
> For details of jet nebulisers, home compressors with nebulisers, and compressors, see current BNF.

A nebuliser converts a solution of a drug into an aerosol for inhalation. It is used to deliver higher doses of drug to the airways than is usual with standard inhalers. The main indications for use of a nebuliser are:

- to deliver a beta₂ agonist or ipratropium to a child with an *acute exacerbation* of asthma or of airways obstruction;

- to deliver *prophylactic medication* to a child unable to use other conventional devices;

- to deliver an antibacterial (such as colistin or tobramycin) to a child with chronic purulent infection (as in cystic fibrosis or bronchiectasis);

- to deliver budesonide to a child with severe croup;

- to deliver pentamidine for the prophylaxis and treatment of pneumocystis pneumonia to a child with AIDS.

The proportion of a nebuliser solution that reaches the lungs depends on the type of nebuliser and although it can be as high as 30% it is more frequently close to

10% and sometimes below 10%. The remaining solution is left in the nebuliser as residual volume or it is deposited in the mouthpiece and tubing. The extent to which the nebulised solution is deposited in the airways or alveoli depends on particle size. Particles with a median diameter of 1–5 microns are deposited in the airways and are therefore appropriate for asthma whereas a particle size of 1–2 microns is needed for alveolar deposition of pentamidine to combat pneumocystis infection. The type of nebuliser is therefore chosen according to the deposition required and according to the viscosity of the solution (antibacterial solutions usually being more viscous).

Some jet nebulisers are able to increase drug output during inspiration and hence increase efficiency.

Nebulised bronchodilators are appropriate for children with chronic persistent asthma or those with severe acute asthma. In chronic asthma, nebulised bronchodilators should only be used to relieve persistent daily wheeze (see Management of Chronic Asthma table, p. 173). The use of nebulisers in chronic persistent asthma should be considered only:

- after a review of the diagnosis and use of current inhaler devices;
- if the airflow obstruction is significantly reversible by bronchodilators without unacceptable side-effects;
- if the child does not benefit from use of conventional inhaler device, such as pressurised metered-dose inhaler plus spacer;
- if the child is complying with the prescribed dose and frequency of anti-inflammatory treatment including regular use of high-dose inhaled corticosteroid.

When a nebuliser is prescribed, the child or child's carer must:

- have clear instructions from doctor, specialist nurse or pharmacist on the use of the nebuliser (and on peak-flow monitoring—see notes above);
- be instructed not to treat acute attacks without also seeking medical help;
- have regular follow up with doctor or specialist nurse.

Jet nebulisers are more widely used than ultrasonic nebulisers. Most jet nebulisers require an optimum flow rate of 6–8 litres/minute and in hospital can be driven by piped air or oxygen; in acute asthma the nebuliser should always be driven by oxygen. Domiciliary oxygen cylinders do not provide an adequate flow rate therefore an electrical compressor is required for domiciliary use.

> Safe practice
> The Department of Health has reminded users of the need to use the correct grade of tubing when connecting a nebuliser to a medical gas supply or compressor.

For a list of available devices see BNF (section 3.1.5).

Nebuliser diluent

Nebulisation may be carried out using an undiluted nebuliser solution or it may require dilution beforehand. The usual diluent is sterile sodium chloride 0.9% (physiological saline).

Sodium Chloride (Non-proprietary) ⓟⓞⓜ
Nebuliser solution, sodium chloride 0.9%, net price
20×2.5 mL = £11.50
Brands include *Saline Steripoule®*, *Saline Steri-Neb®*

3.2 Corticosteroids

Corticosteroids are effective in the management of *asthma*; they reduce airway inflammation.

An inhaled corticosteroid is used regularly for prophylaxis of asthma when a child requires a beta₂ agonist more than twice a week, or if symptoms disturb sleep more than once a week, or if the child has suffered exacerbations in the last 2 years requiring a systemic corticosteroid or a nebulised bronchodilator (see Management of Chronic Asthma, p. 173).

In adults, current or previous smoking reduces the effectiveness of inhaled corticosteroids and higher doses may be necessary.

Corticosteroid inhalers must be used regularly for maximum benefit; alleviation of symptoms usually occurs 3 to 7 days after initiation but may take longer. **Beclometasone dipropionate** (beclomethasone dipropionate), **budesonide, fluticasone propionate,** and **mometasone furoate** appear to be equally effective. A spacer device should be used for administering inhaled corticosteroids in children under 15 years (see NICE guidance, section 3.1.5); a spacer device is also useful in children over 15 years, particularly if high doses are required.

In children 12–18 years using an inhaled corticosteroid and a long-acting beta$_2$ agonist for the prophylaxis of asthma, but who are poorly controlled, (see step 3 of the Management of Chronic Asthma table, p. 173) *Symbicort*® (budesonide with formoterol) may be used as a reliever (instead of a short-acting beta$_2$ agonist), in addition to its regular use for the prophylaxis of asthma [unlicensed]. *Symbicort*® can also be used in this way in children 12–18 years using an inhaled corticosteroid with a dose greater than 400 micrograms beclometasone dipropionate daily[1], but who are poorly controlled [unlicensed] (see step 2 of the Management of Chronic Asthma table, p. 173). When starting this treatment, the total regular dose of inhaled corticosteroid should not be reduced. Children and their carers must be carefully instructed on the appropriate dose and management of exacerbations before initiating this treatment, preferably by a respiratory specialist. Children using budesonide with formoterol as a reliever once a day or more should have their treatment reviewed regularly; see also Side-effects below. This management approach has not been investigated with combination inhalers containing other corticosteroids and long-acting beta$_2$ agonists.

High doses of inhaled corticosteroids can be prescribed for children who respond only partially to standard doses of an inhaled corticosteroid and a long-acting beta$_2$ agonist or to other long-acting bronchodilators (see Management of Chronic Asthma, p. 173). High doses should be continued only if there is clear benefit over the lower dose. The recommended maximum dose of an inhaled corticosteroid should not generally be exceeded; however, if a higher dose is required it should be initiated and supervised by a respiratory paediatrician. The use of high doses of an inhaled corticosteroid can minimise the requirement for an oral corticosteroid.

Cautions of inhaled corticosteroids   Systemic therapy may be required during periods of stress, such as during severe infections, or when airways obstruction or mucus prevent drug access to smaller airways; **interactions**: Appendix 1 (corticosteroids).

Paradoxical bronchospasm   The potential for paradoxical bronchospasm (calling for discontinuation and alternative therapy) should be borne in mind—mild bronchospasm may be prevented by inhalation of a short-acting beta$_2$ agonist beforehand (or by transfer from an aerosol inhalation to a dry powder inhalation if suitable).

CFC-free inhalers   Chlorofluorocarbon (CFC) propellants in pressurised aerosol inhalers are being replaced by hydrofluoroalkane (HFA) propellants. Carers of children and children receiving CFC-free pressurised metered-dose inhalers should be reassured about the efficacy of the new inhalers and counselled that the aerosol may feel and taste different; any difficulty with the new inhaler should be discussed with the doctor, asthma nurse specialist, or pharmacist.

Doses for corticosteroid CFC-free inhalers may be different from those that contain CFCs, see also MHRA/CHM advice below.

> **MHRA/CHM advice (July 2008)**
> Beclometasone dipropionate CFC-free pressurised metered-dose inhalers (*Qvar*® and *Clenil Modulite*®) are **not** interchangeable and should be prescribed by brand name; *Qvar*® has extra-fine particles, is more potent than traditional beclometasone dipropionate CFC-containing inhalers, and is approximately twice as potent as *Clenil Modulite*®.

1. For standard doses of other inhaled corticosteroids, see Management of Chronic Asthma table, p. 173

Respiratory system

Side-effects of inhaled corticosteroids Inhaled corticosteroids have considerably fewer systemic effects than oral corticosteroids, but adverse effects have been reported.

High doses of inhaled corticosteroids (see Management of Chronic Asthma, p. 173) used for prolonged periods can induce adrenal suppression. Inhaled corticosteroids have occasionally been associated with adrenal crisis and coma in children; excessive doses should be **avoided**. Children using high doses of inhaled corticosteroids should be under the supervision of a paediatrician for the duration of the treatment; they should be given a 'steroid card' (section 6.3.2) and specific written advice to consider corticosteroid replacement during an episode of stress, such as a severe intercurrent illness or an operation.

In adults, bone mineral density is sometimes reduced following long-term inhalation of higher doses of corticosteroids, predisposing patients to osteoporosis (section 6.6). It is, therefore, sensible to ensure that the dose of an inhaled corticosteroid is no higher than necessary to keep a child's asthma under good control.

Growth restriction associated with systemic corticosteroid therapy does not seem to occur with recommended doses of inhaled corticosteroids; although initial growth velocity may be reduced, there appears to be no effect on achieving normal adult height. However, the height of children receiving prolonged treatment with inhaled corticosteroid should be monitored; if growth is slowed, referral to a paediatrician should be considered.

Hoarseness and candidiasis of the mouth or throat have been reported, usually only with high doses (see also below). Hypersensitivity reactions (including rash and angioedema) have been reported rarely. Other side-effects that have very rarely been reported include paradoxical bronchospasm, anxiety, depression, sleep disturbances, and behavioural changes including hyperactivity and irritability.

Candidiasis The risk of oral candidiasis can be reduced by using a spacer device with the corticosteroid inhaler; rinsing the mouth with water (or cleaning the child's teeth) after inhalation of a dose may also be helpful. Antifungal oral suspension or lozenges (section 12.3.2) can be used to treat oral candidiasis while continuing corticosteroid therapy.

Oral An acute attack of asthma should be treated with a short course (3–5 days) of oral corticosteroid, see Management of Acute Asthma, p. 171. The dose can usually be stopped abruptly in a mild exacerbation of asthma (see also Withdrawal of Corticosteroids, section 6.3.2) but it should be reduced gradually in children with poorer asthma control, to reduce the possibility of serious relapse.

In chronic continuing asthma, when the response to other drugs has been inadequate, longer term administration of an oral corticosteroid may be necessary; in such cases high doses of an inhaled corticosteroid should be continued to minimise oral corticosteroid requirements.

An oral corticosteroid should normally be taken as a single dose in the morning to reduce the disturbance to circadian cortisol secretion. Dosage should always be titrated to the lowest dose that controls symptoms. Some clinicians use alternate-day dosing of an oral corticosteroid.

Parenteral For the use of hydrocortisone injection in the emergency treatment of acute severe asthma, see Management of Acute Asthma, p. 171.

BECLOMETASONE DIPROPIONATE
(Beclomethasone Dipropionate)

Cautions see notes above

Pregnancy see p. 171

Breast-feeding see p. 171

Side-effects see notes above

Licensed use *Becodisk*-400, *Clenil Modulite*-200 and -250, and *Qvar* are not licensed for use in children under 12 years

Indication and dose

> Prophylaxis of asthma
>
> see Management of Chronic Asthma, p. 173
> Important for *Asmabec Clickhaler*, *Becodisks*, and *Qvar* doses, see under preparations below

Beclometasone (Non-proprietary) ℗oM

Aerosol inhalation, beclometasone dipropionate 50 micrograms/metered inhalation, net price 200-dose unit = £3.05; 100 micrograms/metered inhalation, 200-dose unit = £5.42; 200 micrograms/metered inhalation, 200-dose unit = £16.58;

◁ **BECLOMETASONE DIPROPIONATE** (*continued*)

250 micrograms/metered inhalation, 200-dose unit = £12.41. Label: 8, counselling, dose; also 10 and steroid card with high doses
Excipients include CFC propellants

Dry powder for inhalation, beclometasone dipropionate 100 micrograms/metered inhalation, net price 100-dose unit = £5.36; 200 micrograms/metered inhalation, 200-dose unit = £9.89, 200-dose unit = £15.60; 400 micrograms/metered inhalation, 100-dose unit = £19.61. Label: 8, counselling, dose; also 10 and steroid card with high doses
Brands include *Pulvinal® Beclometasone Dripropionate, Easyhaler® Beclometasone Dipropionate*

Inhalation powder, hard capsule (for use with *Cyclohaler®* device), beclometasone dipropionate 100 micrograms, net price 120-cap pack = £15.99; 200 micrograms, 120-cap pack = £25.00; 400 micrograms, 120-cap pack = £32.25. Label: 8, counselling, dose; also 10 and steroid card with high doses
Brands include *Beclometasone Cyclocaps®*

Asmabec Clickhaler® (UCB Pharma) [PoM]
Dry powder for inhalation, beclometasone dipropionate 50 micrograms/metered inhalation, net price 200-dose unit = £6.42; 100 micrograms/metered inhalation, 200-dose unit = £9.43; 250 micrograms/metered inhalation, 100-dose unit = £11.83. Label: 8, counselling, dose; also 10 and steroid card with high doses

Dose
Prophylaxis of asthma
• **By inhalation of powder**
    Child 6–12 years 50–200 micrograms twice daily, adjusted as necessary
    Child 12–18 years 100–400 micrograms twice daily, adjusted as necessary; max. 1 mg twice daily

Becodisks® (A&H) [PoM]
Dry powder for inhalation, disks containing 8 blisters of beclometasone dipropionate 100 micrograms/blister, net price 15 disks with *Diskhaler®* device = £11.53, 15-disk refill = £10.97; 200 micrograms/blister, 15 disks with *Diskhaler®* device = £21.98, 15-disk refill = £21.41; 400 micrograms/blister, 15 disks with *Diskhaler®* device = £43.38, 15-disk refill = £42.83. Label: 8, counselling, dose; also 10 and steroid card with high doses

Dose
Prophylaxis of asthma
• **By inhalation of powder**
    Child 5–12 years 100–200 micrograms twice daily, adjusted as necessary
    Child 12–18 years 400–800 micrograms twice daily, adjusted as necessary

Clenil Modulite® (Chiesi) [PoM]
Aerosol inhalation, beclometasone dipropionate 50 micrograms/metered inhalation, net price 200-dose unit = £3.70; 100 micrograms/metered inhalation = £7.42; 200 micrograms/metered inhalation

= £16.17; 250 micrograms/metered inhalation = £16.29. Label: 8, counselling, dose; also 10 and steroid card with high doses
Excipients include HFA-134a (a non-CFC propellant)

Dose
Prophylaxis of asthma
• **By aerosol inhalation**
    Child 2–12 years 100–200 micrograms twice daily
    Child 12–18 years 200–400 micrograms twice daily adjusted as necessary up to 1 mg twice daily

Note *Clenil Modulite®* is not interchangeable with other CFC-free beclometasone dipropionate inhalers; the MHRA has advised (July 2008) that CFC-free beclometasone dipropionate inhalers should be prescribed by brand name, see p. 187
Dental prescribing on NHS *Clenil Modulite®* 50 micrograms/metered inhalation may be prescribed

Qvar® (IVAX) [PoM]
Aerosol inhalation, beclometasone dipropionate 50 micrograms/metered inhalation, net price 200-dose unit = £7.87; 100 micrograms/metered inhalation, 200-dose unit = £17.21. Label: 8, counselling, dose; also 10 and steroid card with high doses
Excipients include HFA-134a (a non-CFC propellant)

Autohaler® (breath-actuated aerosol inhalation), beclometasone dipropionate 50 micrograms/metered inhalation, net price 200-dose unit = £7.87; 100 micrograms/metered inhalation, 200-dose unit = £17.21. Label: 8, counselling, dose; also 10 and steroid card with high doses
Excipients include HFA-134a (a non-CFC propellant)

Easi-Breathe® (breath-actuated aerosol inhalation), beclometasone dipropionate 50 micrograms/metered inhalation, net price 200-dose = £7.74; 100 micrograms/metered inhalation, 200-dose = £16.95. Label: 8, counselling, dose; also 10 and steroid card with high doses
Excipients include HFA-134a (a non-CFC propellant)

Dose
Prophylaxis of asthma
• **By aerosol inhalation**
    Child 12–18 years 50–200 micrograms twice daily, increased if necessary to max. 400 micrograms twice daily

Important When switching a child with well-controlled asthma from another corticosteroid inhaler, initially a 100-microgram metered dose of *Qvar®* should be prescribed for:
•   200–250 micrograms of beclometasone dipropionate or budesonide
•   100 micrograms of fluticasone propionate
When switching a child with poorly controlled asthma from another corticosteroid inhaler, initially a 100-microgram metered dose of *Qvar®* should be prescribed for 100 micrograms of beclometasone dipropionate, budesonide, or fluticasone propionate; the dose of *Qvar®* should be adjusted according to response

Note *Qvar®* is not interchangeable with other CFC-free beclometasone dipropionate inhalers; the MHRA has advised (July 2008) that beclometasone dipropionate CFC-free inhalers should be prescribed by brand name, see p. 187

◼ **BUDESONIDE**

Cautions see notes above
Pregnancy see p. 171
Breast-feeding see p. 171
Side-effects see notes above

Licensed use *Pulmicort®* nebuliser solution not licensed for use in children under 3 months; not licensed for use in bronchopulmonary dysplasia;

3
Respiratory system

◻ **BUDESONIDE (continued)**

Symbicort® not licensed for use in children for asthma maintenance and reliever therapy

Indication and dose

> **Prophylaxis of asthma** see Management of Chronic Asthma, p. 173, and preparations below

> **Croup**
> • **By inhalation of nebuliser suspension**
> **Child over 1 month** 2 mg as single dose or in 2 divided doses separated by 30 minutes; dose may be repeated after 12 hours if necessary

> **Bronchopulmonary dysplasia with assisted ventilation**
> • **By aerosol inhalation**
> **Neonate** 400 micrograms twice daily
>
> **Child 1–4 months** 400 micrograms twice daily

> **Bronchopulmonary dysplasia with sponta-neous respiration**
> • **By inhalation of nebuliser suspension**
> **Neonate** 500 micrograms twice daily
>
> **Child 1–4 months** 500 micrograms twice daily; for severe symptoms in child body-weight 2.5 kg or over, 1 mg twice daily

Administration For *aerosol inhalation* in ventilated babies with bronchopulmonary dysplasia, use medium-volume spacer (section 3.1.5) attached directly to endotracheal tube; hand-ventilate through spacer, using a bag system; inflate chest 10 times between activations of inhaler

Budesonide (Non-proprietary) PoM
Dry powder for inhalation, budesonide 100 micr-ograms/metered inhalation, net price 200-dose unit = £9.25; 200 micrograms/metered inhalation 200-dose unit = £18.50; 400 micrograms/metered inhalation 100-dose unit = £18.50. Label: 8, coun-selling, dose; also 10 and steroid card with high doses
Brands include *Easyhaler® Budesonide*

Inhalation powder, hard capsule (for use with *Cyclohaler®* device), budesonide 200 micrograms, net price 100-cap pack = £15.48; 400 micrograms, 50-cap pack = £15.48. Label: 8, counselling, dose; also 10 and steroid card with high doses
Brands include *Budesonide Cyclocaps®*

Dose
> **Prophylaxis of asthma**
> • **By inhalation of powder**
> **Child 6–12 years** 100–400 micrograms twice daily, adjusted as necessary; alternatively, in mild to mod-erate asthma, 200–400 micrograms as a single dose each evening if stabilised on daily dose given in 2 divided doses
>
> **Child 12–18 years** 100–800 micrograms twice daily, adjusted as necessary; alternatively, in mild to mod-erate asthma, 200–400 micrograms as a single dose each evening if stabilised on daily dose given in 2 divided doses (max. 800 micrograms)

Budelin Novolizer® (Meda) PoM
Dry powder for inhalation, budesonide 200 micr-ograms, net price refillable inhaler device and 100-dose cartridge = £14.86; 100-dose refill cartridge =

£9.59. Label: 8, counselling, dose; also 10 and steroid card with high doses

Dose
> **Prophylaxis of asthma**
> • **By inhalation of powder**
> **Child 6–12 years** 200–400 micrograms twice daily, adjusted as necessary; alternatively, in mild to mod-erate asthma, 200–400 micrograms as a single dose each evening if stabilised on daily dose given in 2 divided doses
>
> **Child 12–18 years** 200–800 micrograms twice daily, adjusted as necessary; alternatively, in mild to mod-erate asthma, 200–400 micrograms as a single dose each evening if stabilised on daily dose given in 2 divided doses (max. 800 micrograms)

Pulmicort® (AstraZeneca) PoM
Aerosol inhalation ▼, budesonide 100 micrograms/ metered inhalation, net price 120-dose unit = £9.60; 200 micrograms/metered inhalation, net price 120-dose unit = £13.20. Label: 8, counselling, dose, change to CFC-free inhaler; also 10 and steroid card with high doses
Excipients include HFA–134a (a non-CFC propellant)

Dose
> **Prophylaxis of asthma**
> • **By aerosol inhalation**
> **Child 2–12 years** 100–400 micrograms twice daily, adjusted as necessary
>
> **Child 12–18 years** 100–400 micrograms twice daily, adjusted as necessary; max. 800 micrograms twice daily

Turbohaler® (= dry powder inhaler), budesonide 100 micrograms/metered inhalation, net price 200-dose unit = £18.50; 200 micrograms/metered inhalation, 100-dose unit = £18.50; 400 micr-ograms/metered inhalation, 50-dose unit = £18.50. Label: 8, counselling, dose; also 10 and steroid card with high doses

Dose
> **Prophylaxis of asthma**
> • **By inhalation of powder**
> **Child 6–12 years** 100–400 micrograms twice daily, adjusted as necessary; alternatively, in mild to mod-erate asthma, 200–400 micrograms as a single dose each evening if stabilised on daily dose given in 2 divided doses
>
> **Child 12–18 years** 100–800 micrograms twice daily, adjusted as necessary; alternatively, in mild to mod-erate asthma, 200–400 micrograms as a single dose each evening if stabilised on daily dose given in 2 divided doses (max. 800 micrograms)

Respules® (= single-dose units for nebulisation), budesonide 250 micrograms/mL, net price 20 × 2-mL (500-microgram) unit = £32.00; 500 micr-ograms/mL, 20 × 2-mL (1-mg) unit = £44.64. May be diluted with sterile sodium chloride 0.9%. Label: 8, counselling, dose, 10, steroid card

Dose
> **Prophylaxis of asthma**
> • **By inhalation of nebuliser suspension**
> **Child 3 months–12 years** initially 0.5–1 mg twice daily, reduced to 250–500 micrograms twice daily
>
> **Child 12–18 years** initially 1–2 mg twice daily, reduced to 0.5–1 mg twice daily

Respiratory system

3

◌ **BUDESONIDE (***continued***)**

◢ Compound preparations

For prescribing information on formoterol fumarate, see section 3.1.1.1

Symbicort® (AstraZeneca) [PoM]

Symbicort 100/6 Turbohaler® (= dry powder inhaler), budesonide 100 micrograms, formoterol fumarate 6 micrograms/metered inhalation, net price 120-dose unit = £33.00. Label: 8, counselling, dose

Dose

Asthma, maintenance therapy
● By inhalation of powder
  Child 6–12 years 2 puffs twice daily reduced to 1 puff once daily if control maintained
  Child 12–18 years 1–2 puffs twice daily reduced to 1 puff once daily if control maintained

Asthma, maintenance and reliever therapy (but see notes above, p. 186)
● By inhalation of powder
  Child 12–18 years 2 puffs daily in 1–2 divided doses; for relief of symptoms, 1 puff as needed up to max. 6 puffs at a time; max. 8 puffs daily

Symbicort 200/6 Turbohaler® (= dry powder inhaler), budesonide 200 micrograms, formoterol fumarate 6 micrograms/metered inhalation, net price 120-dose unit = £38.00. Label: 8, counselling, dose; also 10 and steroid card with high doses

Dose

Asthma, maintenance therapy
● By inhalation of powder
  Child 12–18 years 1–2 puffs twice daily reduced in well-controlled asthma to 1 puff once daily

Asthma, maintenance and reliever therapy (but see notes above, p. 186)
● By inhalation of powder
  Child 12–18 years 2 puffs daily in 1–2 divided doses, increased if necessary to 2 puffs twice daily; for relief of symptoms, 1 puff as needed up to max. 6 puffs at a time; max. 8 puffs daily

Symbicort 400/12 Turbohaler® (= dry powder inhaler), budesonide 400 micrograms, formoterol fumarate 12 micrograms/metered inhalation, net price 60-dose unit = £38.00. Label: 8, counselling, dose; also 10 and steroid card with high doses

Dose

Asthma, maintenance therapy
● By inhalation of powder
  Child 12–18 years 1 puff twice daily; may be reduced in well-controlled asthma to 1 puff once daily

▊ CICLESONIDE

Cautions see notes above
Pregnancy see p. 171
Breast-feeding see p. 171
Side-effects see notes above

Indication and dose

Prophylaxis of asthma
● By aerosol inhalation
  Child 12–18 years 160 micrograms daily as a single dose reduced to 80 micrograms daily if control maintained

Alvesco® (Nycomed) [PoM]

Aerosol inhalation, ciclesonide 80 micrograms/metered inhalation, net price 120-dose unit = £28.56; 160 micrograms/metered inhalation, 60-dose unit = £16.80, 120-dose unit = £33.60. Label: 8, counselling, dose
Excipients include HFA-134a (a non-CFC propellant)

▊ FLUTICASONE PROPIONATE

Cautions see notes above
Pregnancy see p. 171
Breast-feeding see p. 171
Side-effects see notes above; also *very rarely* dyspepsia, hyperglycaemia, and arthralgia

Indication and dose

Prophylaxis of asthma see Management of Chronic Asthma, p. 173, and preparations below

Flixotide® (A&H) [PoM]

Accuhaler® (dry powder for inhalation), disk containing 60 blisters of *fluticasone propionate* 50 micrograms/blister with *Accuhaler®* device, net price = £6.38; 100 micrograms/blister with *Accuhaler®* device = £8.93; 250 micrograms/blister with *Accuhaler®* device = £21.26; 500 micrograms/blister with *Accuhaler®* device = £36.14. Label: 8, counselling, dose; also 10 and steroid card with high doses

Dose

Prophylaxis of asthma
● By inhalation of powder
  Child 5–16 years 50–100 micrograms twice daily adjusted as necessary; max. 200 micrograms twice daily

  Child 16–18 years 100–500 micrograms twice daily, adjusted as necessary; max. 1 mg twice daily (doses above 500 micrograms twice daily initiated by a specialist)

Diskhaler® (dry powder for inhalation), fluticasone propionate 100 micrograms/blister, net price 15 disks of 4 blisters with *Diskhaler®* device = £12.71, 15-disk refill = £12.18; 250 micrograms/blister, 15 disks of 4 blisters with *Diskhaler®* device = £24.11, 15-disk refill = £23.58; 500 micrograms/blister, 15 disks of 4 blisters with *Diskhaler®* device = £40.05, 15-disk refill = £39.52. Label: 8, counselling, dose; also 10 and steroid card with high doses

Dose

Prophylaxis of asthma
● By inhalation of powder
  Child 5–16 years 100–200 micrograms twice daily

  Child 16–18 years 100–500 micrograms twice daily adjusted as necessary; max. 1 mg twice daily (doses above 500 micrograms twice daily initiated by a specialist)

Evohaler® *aerosol inhalation*, fluticasone propionate 50 micrograms/metered inhalation, net price 120-dose unit = £5.44; 125 micrograms/metered inhalation, 120-dose unit = £21.26; 250 micrograms/

3

Respiratory system

◻ **FLUTICASONE PROPIONATE** (*continued*)

metered inhalation, 120-dose unit = £36.14.
Label: 8, counselling, dose, change to CFC-free
inhaler; also 10 and steroid card with high doses
Excipients include HFA-134a (a non-CFC propellant)

Dose

Prophylaxis of asthma
• **By aerosol inhalation**
  Child 4–16 years 50–100 micrograms twice daily
  adjusted as necessary; max. 200 micrograms twice
  daily

  Child 16–18 years 100–500 micrograms twice daily
  adjusted as necessary; max. 1 mg twice daily (doses
  above 500 micrograms twice daily initiated by a specialist)

Nebules® (= single-dose units for nebulisation)
fluticasone propionate 250 micrograms/mL, net
price 10 × 2-mL (500-microgram) unit = £9.34;
1 mg/mL, 10 × 2-mL (2-mg) unit = £37.35. May be
diluted with sterile sodium chloride 0.9%. Label: 8,
counselling, dose, 10, steroid card

Dose

Prophylaxis of asthma
• **By inhalation of nebuliser suspension**
  Child 4–16 years 1 mg twice daily

  Child 16–18 years 0.5–2 mg twice daily

◢ Compound preparations
For prescribing information on salmeterol, see
section 3.1.1.1

Seretide® (A&H) [PoM]
Seretide 100 Accuhaler® (dry powder for inhalation), disk containing 60 blisters of fluticasone
propionate 100 micrograms, salmeterol (as xinafoate) 50 micrograms/blister with *Accuhaler®* device,
net price = £31.19. Label: 8, counselling, dose

Dose

Prophylaxis of asthma
• **By inhalation of powder**
  Child 5–18 years 1 blister twice daily, reduced to 1
  blister once daily if control maintained

Seretide 250 Accuhaler® (dry powder for inhalation), disk containing 60 blisters of fluticasone
propionate 250 micrograms, salmeterol (as xinafoate) 50 micrograms/blister with *Accuhaler®* device,
net price = £35.00. Label: 8, counselling, dose, 10,
steroid card

Dose

Prophylaxis of asthma
• **By inhalation of powder**
  Child 12–18 years 1 blister twice daily

Seretide 500 Accuhaler® (dry powder for inhalation), disk containing 60 blisters of fluticasone
propionate 500 micrograms, salmeterol (as xinafoate) 50 micrograms/blister with *Accuhaler®* device,
net price = £40.92. Label: 8, counselling, dose, 10,
steroid card

Dose

Prophylaxis of asthma
• **By inhalation of powder**
  Child 12–18 years 1 blister twice daily

Seretide 50 Evohaler® (aerosol inhalation), fluticasone propionate 50 micrograms, salmeterol (as
xinafoate) 25 micrograms/metered inhalation, net
price 120-dose unit = £18.00. Label: 8, counselling,
dose, change to CFC-free inhaler
Excipients include HFA-134a (a non-CFC propellant)

Dose

Prophylaxis of asthma
• **By aerosol inhalation**
  Child 5–18 years 2 puffs twice daily, reduced to 2 puffs
  once daily if control maintained

Seretide 125 Evohaler® (aerosol inhalation), fluticasone propionate 125 micrograms, salmeterol
(as xinafoate) 25 micrograms/metered inhalation,
net price 120-dose unit = £35.00. Label: 8, counselling, dose, change to CFC-free inhaler, 10,
steroid card
Excipients include HFA-134a (a non-CFC propellant)

Dose

Prophylaxis of asthma
• **By aerosol inhalation**
  Child 12–18 years 2 puffs twice daily

Seretide 250 Evohaler® (aerosol inhalation), fluticasone propionate 250 micrograms, salmeterol
(as xinafoate) 25 micrograms/metered inhalation,
net price 120-dose unit = £59.48. Label: 8, counselling, dose, change to CFC-free inhaler, 10,
steroid card
Excipients include HFA-134a (a non-CFC propellant)

Dose

Prophylaxis of asthma
• **By aerosol inhalation**
  Child 12–18 years 2 puffs twice daily

▮ **MOMETASONE FUROATE**

Cautions see notes above

Pregnancy see p. 171

Breast-feeding see p. 171

Side-effects see notes above; also pharyngitis,
headache; *less commonly* palpitation

Indication and dose

Prophylaxis of asthma see also Management of
Chronic Asthma, p. 173
• **By inhalation of powder**
  Child 12–18 years 200–400 micrograms as a
  single dose in the evening or in 2 divided doses;
  dose increased to 400 micrograms twice daily if
  necessary

Asmanex® (Schering-Plough) ▼ [PoM]
Twisthaler (= dry powder inhaler), mometasone
furoate 200 micrograms/metered inhalation, net
price 30-dose unit = £15.70, 60-dose unit = £23.54;
400 micrograms/metered inhalation, 30-dose unit
= £21.78, 60-dose unit = £36.05. Label: 8, counselling, dose, 10, steroid card

Note The *Scottish Medicines Consortium* has advised
(November 2003) that *Asmanex®* is restricted for use
following failure of first-line inhaled corticosteroids

3.3 Cromoglicate and related therapy and leukotriene receptor antagonists

3.3.1 Cromoglicate and related therapy

3.3.2 Leukotriene receptor antagonists

3.3.1 Cromoglicate and related therapy

The mode of action of **sodium cromoglicate** and **nedocromil** is not completely understood; they may be of value as *prophylaxis* in asthma with an allergic basis, but the evidence for benefit of sodium cromoglicate in children is contentious. Prophylaxis with cromoglicate or nedocromil is less effective than with inhaled corticosteroids (see Management of Chronic Asthma, p. 173).

Nedocromil may be of some benefit in the prophylaxis of exercise-induced asthma.

For the use of sodium cromoglicate and nedocromil in allergic conjunctivitis see section 11.4.2; sodium cromoglicate is used also in allergic rhinitis (section 12.2.1) and allergy-related diarrhoea (section 1.5.4).

SODIUM CROMOGLICATE

(Sodium Cromoglycate)

Cautions discontinue if eosinophilic pneumonia occurs

Pregnancy see p. 171

Breast-feeding see p. 171

Side-effects coughing, transient bronchospasm, and throat irritation; *very rarely* hypersensitivity reactions (including angioedema); rhinitis and headache also reported

Indication and dose

Prophylaxis of asthma (see also Management of Chronic Asthma, p. 173)

• By aerosol inhalation

Child 5–18 years 10 mg (2 puffs) 4 times daily, increased if necessary to 6–8 times daily; an additional dose may also be taken before exercise; maintenance, 5 mg (1 puff) 4 times daily

Food allergy section 1.5.4

Allergic conjunctivitis section 11.4.2

Allergic rhinitis section 12.2.1

Intal® CFC-free inhaler (Sanofi-Aventis) (PoM)
Aerosol inhalation, sodium cromoglicate 5 mg/metered inhalation, net price 112-dose unit = £14.84. Label: 8
Excipients include HFA-227 (a non-CFC propellant)

NEDOCROMIL SODIUM

Pregnancy see p. 171

Breast-feeding see p. 171

Side-effects see under Sodium Cromoglicate; also headache, nausea, vomiting, dyspepsia and abdominal pain; bitter taste (masked by mint flavour)

Licensed use not licensed for use in children under 6 years

Indication and dose

Prophylaxis of asthma (but see notes above)

Counselling Regular use is necessary

• By aerosol inhalation

Child 5–18 years 4 mg (2 puffs) 4 times daily, when control achieved may be possible to reduce to twice daily

Allergic conjunctivitis section 11.4.2

Tilade CFC-free inhaler® (Sanofi-Aventis) ▼ (PoM)
Aerosol inhalation, mint-flavoured, nedocromil sodium 2 mg/metered inhalation. Net price 112-dose unit = £39.94. Label: 8
Excipients include HFA-227 (a non-CFC propellant)

3.3.2 Leukotriene receptor antagonists

The leukotriene receptor antagonists, **montelukast** and **zafirlukast**, block the effects of cysteinyl leukotrienes in the airways; they can be used in children for the management of chronic asthma with an inhaled corticosteroid or as an alternative if an inhaled corticosteroid cannot be used (see Management of Chronic Asthma, p. 173). Montelukast has not been shown to be more effective than a standard dose of inhaled corticosteroid, but the two drugs appear to have an additive effect.

3

Respiratory system

The leukotriene receptor antagonists may be of benefit in exercise-induced asthma and in those with concomitant rhinitis, but they are less effective in children with severe asthma who are also receiving high doses of other drugs.

Churg-Strauss syndrome   Churg-Strauss syndrome has occurred very rarely in association with the use of leukotriene receptor antagonists; in many of the reported cases the reaction followed the reduction or withdrawal of oral cortico-steroid therapy. Prescribers should be alert to the development of eosinophilia, vasculitic rash, worsening pulmonary symptoms, cardiac complications, or peripheral neuropathy.

Pregnancy   There is limited evidence for the safe use of leukotriene receptor antagonists during pregnancy; however, they can be taken as normal in women who have shown a significant improvement in asthma not achievable with other drugs before becoming pregnant, see also p. 171.

MONTELUKAST

Cautions interactions: Appendix 1 (leukotriene receptor antagonists)

Pregnancy manufacturer advises avoid unless essential; see also notes above

Breast-feeding manufacturer advises avoid unless essential

Side-effects abdominal pain, thirst; hyperkinesia (in young children), headache; *very rarely* Churg-Strauss syndrome (see notes above); dry mouth, diarrhoea, dyspepsia, nausea, vomiting, hepatic disorders, palpitation, oedema, increased bleeding, epistaxis, hypersensitivity reactions (including anaphylaxis, angioedema, and skin reactions), depression, tremor, asthenia, dizziness, hallucinations, suicidal thoughts and behaviour, paraesthesia, hypoaesthesia, sleep disturbances, abnormal dreams, agitation, aggression, seizures, pyrexia, arthralgia, and myalgia also reported

Indication and dose

Prophylaxis of asthma see notes above and Management of Chronic Asthma, p. 173
• By mouth
    Child 6 months–6 years 4 mg once daily in the evening
    Child 6–15 years 5 mg once daily in the evening
    Child 15–18 years 10 mg once daily in the evening

Symptomatic relief of seasonal allergic rhinitis in children with asthma
• By mouth
    Child 15–18 years 10 mg once daily in the evening

Singulair® (MSD) PoM
Chewable tablets, pink, cherry-flavoured, montelukast (as sodium salt) 4 mg, net price 28-tab pack = £25.69; 5 mg, 28-tab pack = £25.69. Label: 23, 24
Excipients include aspartame equivalent to phenylalanine 674 micrograms/4-mg tablet and 842 micrograms/5-mg tablet (section 9.4.1)

Granules, montelukast (as sodium salt) 4 mg, net price 28-sachet pack = £25.69. Counselling, administration
Counselling Granules may be swallowed whole or mixed with cold food (but not fluid) and taken immediately

Tablets, beige, f/c, montelukast (as sodium salt) 10 mg, net price 28-tab pack = £26.97
Note The *Scottish Medicines Consortium* has advised (June 2007) that *Singulair®* chewable tablets and granules are restricted for use as an alternative to low-dose inhaled corticosteroids for children 2–14 years with mild persistent asthma who have not recently had serious asthma attacks that required oral corticosteroid use, and who are not capable of using inhaled corticosteroids; *Singulair®* chewable tablets and granules should be initiated by a specialist in paediatric asthma

ZAFIRLUKAST

Cautions interactions: Appendix 1 (leukotriene receptor antagonists)
Hepatic disorders Children or their carers should be told how to recognise development of liver disorder and advised to seek medical attention if symptoms or signs such as persistent nausea, vomiting, malaise or jaundice develop

Hepatic impairment manufacturer advises avoid

Renal impairment manufacturer advises caution in moderate to severe impairment

Pregnancy manufacturer advises use only if potential benefit outweighs risk; see also notes above

Breast-feeding present in milk—manufacturer advises avoid

Side-effects gastro-intestinal disturbances; headache; *rarely* bleeding disorders, hypersensitivity reactions including angioedema and skin reactions, arthralgia, myalgia, hepatitis, hyperbilirubinaemia, thrombocytopenia; *very rarely* Churg-Strauss syndrome (see notes above), agranulocytosis

Indication and dose

Prophylaxis of asthma see notes above and Management of Chronic Asthma, p. 173
• By mouth
    Child 12–18 years 20 mg twice daily

Accolate® (AstraZeneca) PoM
Tablets, f/c, zafirlukast 20 mg, net price 56-tab pack = £17.75. Label: 23

3.4 Antihistamines, immunotherapy, and allergic emergencies

3.4.1 Antihistamines
3.4.2 Allergen immunotherapy
3.4.3 Allergic emergencies

3.4.1 Antihistamines

Antihistamines (histamine H_1-receptor antagonists) are classified as *sedating* or *non-sedating*, according to their relative potential for CNS depression. Antihistamines differ in their duration of action, incidence of drowsiness, and antimuscarinic effects; the response to an antihistamine may vary from child to child (see Side-effects, p. 196). Either a sedating or a non-sedating antihistamine may be used to treat an acute allergic reaction; for conditions with more persistent symptoms, a non-sedating antihistamine should be used regularly.

Oral antihistamines are used in the treatment of nasal allergies, particularly seasonal allergic rhinitis (hay fever), and may be of some value in vasomotor rhinitis; rhinorrhoea and sneezing is reduced, but antihistamines are usually less effective for nasal congestion. Antihistamines are used topically to treat allergic reactions in the eye (section 11.4.2) and in the nose (section 12.2.1). Topical application of antihistamines to the skin is not recommended (section 13.3).

An oral antihistamine may be used to prevent urticaria, and for the treatment of acute urticarial rashes, pruritus, insect bites, and stings. Antihistamines are also used in the management of nausea and vomiting (section 4.6), of migraine (section 4.7.4.1), and the adjunctive management of anaphylaxis and angioedema (section 3.4.3).

Sedating antihistamines are occasionally useful when insomnia is associated with urticaria and pruritus (section 4.1.1). Most of the sedating antihistamines are relatively short acting, but promethazine may be effective for up to 12 hours. **Alimemazine** (trimeprazine) and **promethazine** have a more sedative effect than **chlorphenamine** (chlorpheniramine) and **cyclizine** (section 4.6). Chlorphenamine is used as an adjunct to adrenaline (epinephrine) in the emergency treatment of anaphylaxis and angioedema (section 3.4.3).

The *non-sedating* antihistamine **cetirizine** is safe and effective in children; it causes less sedation and psychomotor impairment than the sedating antihistamines. Other non-sedating antihistamines that are used in children include **desloratadine** (an active metabolite of loratadine), **fexofenadine** (an active metabolite of terfenadine), **levocetirizine** (an isomer of cetirizine), **loratadine**, and **mizolastine**. Most non-sedating antihistamines are long-acting (usually 12–24 hours). There is little evidence that desloratadine or levocetirizine confer any additional benefit—they should be reserved for children who cannot tolerate other therapies.

Cautions and contra-indications   Antihistamines should be used with caution in children with epilepsy. Most antihistamines should be avoided in acute porphyria, but some are thought to be safe (see section 9.8.2). Sedating antihistamines should not be given to children under 2 years, except on specialist advice, because the safety of such use has not been established. Sedating antihistamines have significant antimuscarinic activity—they should **not** be used in neonates and should be used with caution in children with urinary retention, glaucoma, or pyloroduodenal obstruction. **Interactions:** see Appendix 1 (antihistamines).

Hepatic impairment   Sedating antihistamines should be avoided in children with severe liver disease—increased risk of coma.

Pregnancy   Most manufacturers of antihistamines advise avoiding their use during pregnancy; however there is no evidence of teratogenicity, except for hydroxyzine and loratadine where toxicity has been reported with high doses in *animal* studies. The use of sedating antihistamines in the latter part of the third trimester may cause adverse effects in neonates such as irritability, paradoxical excitability, and tremor.

Breast-feeding   Most antihistamines are present in breast milk in varying amounts; although not known to be harmful, most manufacturers advise avoiding their use in mothers who are breast-feeding.

3

Respiratory system

Side-effects Drowsiness is a significant side-effect with most of the older antihistamines although paradoxical stimulation may occur rarely in children, especially with high doses. Drowsiness may diminish after a few days of treatment and is considerably less of a problem with the newer antihistamines (see also notes above). Side-effects that are more common with the older antihistamines include headache, psychomotor impairment, and antimuscarinic effects such as urinary retention, dry mouth, blurred vision, and gastro-intestinal disturbances. Other rare side-effects of antihistamines include hypotension, palpitation, arrhythmias, extrapyramidal effects, dizziness, confusion, depression, sleep disturbances, tremor, convulsions, hypersensitivity reactions (including bronchospasm, angioedema, anaphylaxis, rashes, and photosensitivity reactions), blood disorders, and liver dysfunction.

Non-sedating antihistamines

Skilled tasks Although drowsiness is rare, children and their carers should be advised that it can occur and may affect performance of skilled tasks (e.g. cycling or driving); alcohol should be avoided.

ACRIVASTINE

Cautions see notes above

Contra-indications see notes above; also hypersensitivity to triprolidine

Renal impairment avoid in severe impairment

Pregnancy see notes above

Breast-feeding see notes above

Side-effects see notes above

Indication and dose

Symptomatic relief of allergy such as hay fever, chronic idiopathic urticaria
- By mouth
  Child 12–18 years 8 mg 3 times daily

Acrivastine (Non-proprietary)
Capsules, acrivastine 8 mg, net price 12-cap pack = £2.59, 24-cap pack = £4.49. Counselling, skilled tasks
Brands include *Benadryl® Allergy Relief*

CETIRIZINE HYDROCHLORIDE

Cautions see notes above

Contra-indications see notes above

Renal impairment use half normal dose if estimated glomerular filtration rate less than 30 mL/minute/1.73 m²

Pregnancy see notes above

Breast-feeding see notes above

Side-effects see notes above

Licensed use not licensed for use in children under 6 years except for use in children 2–6 years for treatment of seasonal allergic rhinitis

Indication and dose

Symptomatic relief of allergy such as hay fever, chronic idiopathic urticaria, atopic dermatitis
- By mouth
  Child 1–2 years 250 micrograms/kg twice daily

Child 2–6 years 5 mg once daily *or* 2.5 mg twice daily

Child 6–18 years 10 mg once daily *or* 5 mg twice daily

Cetirizine (Non-proprietary)
Tablets, cetirizine hydrochloride 10 mg, net price 30-tab pack = £1.01. Counselling, skilled tasks

Dental prescribing on NHS Cetirizine 10 mg tablets may be prescribed

Oral solution, cetirizine hydrochloride 5 mg/5 mL, net price 200 mL = £2.42. Counselling, skilled tasks

DESLORATADINE

Note Desloratadine is a metabolite of loratadine

Cautions see notes above

Contra-indications see notes above; also hypersensitivity to loratadine

Renal impairment use with caution in severe impairment

Pregnancy see notes above

Breast-feeding see notes above

Side-effects see notes above; *rarely* myalgia; *very rarely* hallucinations

Indication and dose

Symptomatic relief of allergy such as hay fever, chronic idiopathic urticaria
- By mouth
  Child 1–6 years 1.25 mg once daily
  Child 6–12 years 2.5 mg once daily
  Child 12–18 years 5 mg once daily

◻ **DESLORATADINE** (*continued*)

Neoclarityn® (Schering-Plough) [PoM]
Tablets, blue, f/c, desloratadine 5 mg, net price 30-tab pack = £6.90. Counselling, skilled tasks

Oral solution, desloratadine 2.5 mg/5 mL, net price 100 mL (bubblegum-flavour) = £6.90, 150 mL = £10.35. Counselling, skilled tasks
Excipients include propylene glycol (see Excipients p. 3)

FEXOFENADINE HYDROCHLORIDE

Note Fexofenadine is a metabolite of terfenadine
Cautions see notes above
Contra-indications see notes above
Pregnancy see notes above
Breast-feeding see notes above
Side-effects see notes above

Indication and dose

> Symptomatic relief of seasonal allergic rhinitis
> * **By mouth**
>
>   Child 6–12 years 30 mg twice daily
>
>   Child 12–18 years 120 mg once daily

> Symptomatic relief of chronic idiopathic urticaria
> * **By mouth**
>
>   Child 12–18 years 180 mg once daily

Fexofenadine (Non-proprietary) [PoM]
Tablets, f/c, fexofenadine hydrochloride 120 mg, net price 30-tab pack = £4.30; 180 mg, 30-tab pack = £5.18. Label: 5, counselling, skilled tasks

Telfast® (Sanofi-Aventis) [PoM]
Tablets, f/c, peach, fexofenadine hydrochloride 30 mg, net price 60-tab pack = £5.46; 120 mg, 30-tab pack = £5.99; 180 mg, 30-tab pack = £7.58. Label: 5, counselling, skilled tasks

LEVOCETIRIZINE HYDROCHLORIDE

Note Levocetirizine is an isomer of cetirizine
Cautions see notes above
Contra-indications see notes above
Renal impairment estimated glomerular filtration rate 30–50 mL/minute/1.73 m², reduce dose frequency to alternate days; estimated glomerular filtration rate 10–30 mL/minute/1.73 m², reduce dose frequency to every 3 days; estimated glomerular filtration rate less than 10 mL/minute/1.73 m², avoid
Pregnancy see notes above
Breast-feeding see notes above
Side-effects see notes above; *very rarely* weight gain
Licensed use tablets not licensed for use in children under 6 years

Indication and dose

> Symptomatic relief of allergy such as hay fever, urticaria
> * **By mouth**
>
>   Child 2–6 years 1.25 mg twice daily
>
>   Child 6–18 years 5 mg once daily

Xyzal® (UCB Pharma) [PoM]
Tablets, f/c, levocetirizine hydrochloride 5 mg, net price 30-tab pack = £4.39. Counselling, skilled tasks

Oral solution, levocetirizine hydrochloride 2.5 mg/5 mL, net price 200 mL = £6.00. Counselling, skilled tasks

LORATADINE

Cautions see notes above
Contra-indications see notes above
Hepatic impairment reduce dose frequency to alternate days in severe impairment
Pregnancy manufacturer advises avoid—toxicity in *animal* studies with high doses; see notes above
Breast-feeding see notes above
Side-effects see notes above

Indication and dose

> Symptomatic relief of allergy such as hay fever, chronic idiopathic urticaria
> * **By mouth**
>
>   Child 2–12 years
>
>   Body-weight under 30 kg 5 mg once daily
>
>   Body-weight over 30 kg 10 mg once daily
>
>   Child 12–18 years 10 mg once daily

Loratadine (Non-proprietary)
Tablets, loratadine 10 mg, net price 30-tab pack = £1.29. Counselling, skilled tasks

Dental prescribing on NHS Loratadine 10 mg tablets may be prescribed

Syrup, loratadine 5 mg/5 mL, net price 100 mL = £2.84. Counselling, skilled tasks

MIZOLASTINE

Cautions see notes above
Contra-indications see notes above; also susceptibility to QT-interval prolongation (including cardiac disease and hypokalaemia)

Hepatic impairment manufacturer recommends avoid in significant hepatic impairment
Pregnancy see notes above
Breast-feeding see notes above

3

Respiratory system

◁ **MIZOLASTINE** (*continued*)

Side-effects see notes above; weight gain; anxiety, asthenia; *less commonly* arthralgia and myalgia

Indication and dose

Symptomatic relief of allergy such as hay fever, urticaria
- By mouth

  Child 12–18 years 10 mg once daily

Mizollen® (Sanofi-Aventis) [PoM]

Tablets, m/r, f/c, scored, mizolastine 10 mg, net price 30-tab pack = £5.77. Label: 25, counselling, skilled tasks

---

RUPATADINE

Cautions see notes above; also susceptibility to QT-interval prolongation (including cardiac disease and hypokalaemia)

Hepatic impairment manufacturer advises avoid—no information available

Renal impairment manufacturer advises avoid—no information available

Pregnancy manufacturer advises caution—limited information available; see also notes above

Breast-feeding manufacturer advises caution; see also notes above

Side-effects see notes above; also asthenia; *less commonly* pyrexia, irritability, increased appetite, arthralgia, and myalgia

Indication and dose

Symptomatic relief of allergic rhinitis and chronic idiopathic urticaria
- By mouth

  Child 12–18 years 10 mg once daily

Rupafin® (GSK) ▼ [PoM]

Tablets, salmon, rupatadine (as fumarate) 10 mg, net price 30-tab pack = £5.00. Counselling, skilled tasks

---

Sedating antihistamines

Skilled tasks Drowsiness may affect performance of skilled tasks (e.g. cycling or driving); sedating effects enhanced by alcohol.

ALIMEMAZINE TARTRATE
(Trimeprazine tartrate)

Cautions see notes above

Contra-indications see notes above

Hepatic impairment see notes above

Renal impairment avoid

Pregnancy see notes above

Breast-feeding see notes above

Side-effects see notes above

Licensed use not licensed for use in children under 2 years

Indication and dose

Urticaria, pruritus
- By mouth

  Child 6 months–2 years 250 micrograms/kg (max. 2.5 mg) 3–4 times daily—specialist use only

  Child 2–5 years 2.5 mg 3–4 times daily

  Child 5–12 years 5 mg 3–4 times daily

  Child 12–18 years 10 mg 2–3 times daily, in severe cases up to max. 100 mg daily

Premedication section 15.1.4
- By mouth

  Child 2–7 years up to max. 2 mg/kg 1–2 hours before operation

Alimemazine (Non-proprietary) [PoM]

Tablets, blue, f/c, alimemazine tartrate 10 mg, net price 28-tab pack = £4.28. Label: 2

Syrup, alimemazine tartrate 7.5 mg /5 mL, net price 100 mL = £4.88; 30 mg/5 mL, 100-mL = £6.86. Label: 2

CHLORPHENAMINE MALEATE
(Chlorpheniramine maleate)

Cautions see notes above

Contra-indications see notes above

Hepatic impairment see notes above

Pregnancy see notes above

Breast-feeding see notes above

Side-effects see notes above; also exfoliative dermatitis and tinnitus reported; injections may cause transient hypotension or CNS stimulation and may be irritant

Licensed use *syrup* not licensed for use in children under 1 year; *tablets* not licensed for use in children under 6 years; *injection* not licensed for use in neonates

Indication and dose

Symptomatic relief of allergy such as hay fever, urticaria
- By mouth

  Child 1 month–2 years 1 mg twice daily

⌂ **CHLORPHENAMINE MALEATE (continued)**

Child 2–6 years 1 mg every 4–6 hours, max. 6 mg daily

Child 6–12 years 2 mg every 4–6 hours, max. 12 mg daily

Child 12–18 years 4 mg every 4–6 hours, max. 24 mg daily

Emergency treatment of anaphylactic reactions, symptomatic relief of allergy
• By intramuscular or intravenous injection

Child under 6 months 250 micrograms/kg (max. 2.5 mg), repeated if required up to 4 times in 24 hours

Child 6 months–6 years 2.5 mg, repeated if required up to 4 times in 24 hours

Child 6–12 years 5 mg, repeated if required up to 4 times in 24 hours

Child 12–18 years 10 mg, repeated if required up to 4 times in 24 hours

Administration for *intravenous injection*, give over 1 minute; if small dose required, dilute with Sodium Chloride 0.9%

Chlorphenamine (Non-proprietary)
Tablets, chlorphenamine maleate 4 mg, net price 28 = £1.09. Label: 2

Dental prescribing on NHS Chlorphenamine tablets may be prescribed

Oral solution, chlorphenamine maleate 2 mg/5 mL, net price 150 mL = £2.34. Label: 2

Dental prescribing on NHS Chlorphenamine oral solution may be prescribed

Injection ⟨PoM⟩¹, chlorphenamine maleate 10 mg/mL, net price 1-mL amp = £1.62
1. ⟨PoM⟩ restriction does not apply where administration is for saving life in emergency

Piriton® (GSK Consumer Healthcare)
Tablets, yellow, scored, chlorphenamine maleate 4 mg, net price 28 = £1.62. Label: 2

Syrup, chlorphenamine maleate 2 mg/5 mL, net price 150 mL = £2.39. Label: 2

HYDROXYZINE HYDROCHLORIDE

Cautions see notes above
Contra-indications see notes above
Hepatic impairment reduce daily dose by one-third; see also notes above
Renal impairment reduce daily dose by half
Pregnancy toxicity in *animal* studies with high doses; see also notes above
Breast-feeding see notes above
Side-effects see notes above
Licensed use *Ucerax®* syrup not licensed for use in children under 1 year

Indication and dose
Pruritus
• By mouth
Child 6 months–6 years initially 5–15 mg at night, increased if necessary to 50 mg daily in 3–4 divided doses

Child 6–12 years initially 15–25 mg at night, increased if necessary to 50–100 mg daily in 3–4 divided doses

Child 12–18 years initially 25 mg at night, increased if necessary to 100 mg in 3–4 divided doses

Atarax® (Alliance) ⟨PoM⟩
Tablets, both f/c, hydroxyzine hydrochloride 10 mg (orange), net price 84-tab pack = £2.18; 25 mg (green), 28-tab pack = £1.17. Label: 2

Ucerax® (UCB Pharma) ⟨PoM⟩
Tablets ⟨JHS⟩, f/c, scored, hydroxyzine hydrochloride 25 mg, net price 25-tab pack = £1.22. Label: 2
Syrup, hydroxyzine hydrochloride 10 mg/5 mL. Net price 200-mL pack = £1.78. Label: 2

KETOTIFEN

Cautions see notes above
Contra-indications see notes above
Hepatic impairment see notes above
Pregnancy see notes above
Breast-feeding see notes above
Side-effects see notes above; also irritability, nervousness; *less commonly* cystitis; *rarely* weight gain; *very rarely* Stevens-Johnson syndrome

Indication and dose
Symptomatic relief of allergy such as allergic rhinitis
• By mouth
Child 3–18 years 1 mg twice daily

Zaditen® (Novartis) ⟨PoM⟩
Tablets, scored, ketotifen (as hydrogen fumarate) 1 mg, net price 60-tab pack = £10.75. Label: 2, 21
Elixir, ketotifen (as hydrogen fumarate), 1 mg/5 mL, net price 300 mL (strawberry-flavoured) = £12.73. Label: 2, 21

PROMETHAZINE HYDROCHLORIDE

Cautions see notes above
Contra-indications see notes above; severe coronary artery disease

Hepatic impairment see notes above
Renal impairment use with caution
Pregnancy see notes above

◁ **PROMETHAZINE HYDROCHLORIDE** (*continued*)

Breast-feeding   see notes above
Side-effects   see notes above; also restlessness

Indication and dose

Symptomatic relief of allergy such as hay fever, insomnia associated with urticaria and pruritus
• **By mouth**
   Child 2–5 years 5 mg twice daily *or* 5–15 mg at night
   Child 5–10 years 5–10 mg twice daily *or* 10–25 mg at night
   Child 10–18 years 10–20 mg 2–3 times daily *or* 25 mg at night increased to 25 mg twice daily if necessary

Sedation section 4.1.1

Nausea and vomiting section 4.6

Phenergan® (Sanofi-Aventis)
   Tablets, both blue, f/c, promethazine hydrochloride 10 mg, net price 56-tab pack = £2.85; 25 mg, 56-tab pack = £4.34. Label: 2

Dental prescribing on NHS May be prescribed as Promethazine Hydrochloride Tablets 10 mg or 25 mg

   Elixir, golden, promethazine hydrochloride 5 mg/5 mL. Net price 100 mL = £2.67. Label: 2

Dental prescribing on NHS May be prescribed as Promethazine Hydrochloride Oral Solution 5 mg/5 mL

3.4.2 Allergen immunotherapy

Immunotherapy using allergen vaccines containing house dust mite, animal dander (cat or dog), or extracts of grass and tree pollen can improve symptoms of asthma and allergic rhino-conjunctivitis in children. A vaccine containing extracts of wasp and bee venom is used to reduce the risk of severe anaphylaxis and systemic reactions in children with hypersensitivity to wasp and bee stings. An oral preparation of grass pollen extract (*Grazax®*) is also licensed for grass pollen induced rhinitis and conjunctivitis. Children requiring immunotherapy must be referred to a hospital specialist for accurate allergy diagnosis, assessment, and treatment.

> In view of concerns about the safety of desensitising vaccines, it is recommended that they are used by specialists and only for the following indications:
> • seasonal allergic hay fever (caused by pollen) that has not responded to anti-allergic drugs;
> • hypersensitivity to wasp and bee venoms.
> Desensitising vaccines should generally be avoided or used with particular care in children with asthma.

Desensitising vaccines should be avoided in pregnant women, in children under 5 years, and in those taking beta-blockers (adrenaline will be ineffective if a hypersensitivity reaction occurs), or ACE inhibitors (risk of severe anaphylactoid reactions).

Hypersensitivity reactions to immunotherapy (especially to wasp and bee venom extracts) can be life-threatening; bronchospasm usually develops within 1 hour and anaphylaxis within 30 minutes of injection. Therefore, facilities for cardio-pulmonary resuscitation must be immediately available and the child needs to be monitored for at least 1 hour after injection. If symptoms or signs of hypersensitivity develop (e.g. rash, urticaria, bronchospasm, faintness), **even when mild**, the child should be observed until these have **resolved completely**. The first dose of oral grass pollen extract (*Grazax®*) should be taken under medical supervision and the child should be monitored for 20–30 minutes.

For details of the management of anaphylactic shock, see section 3.4.3.

Each set of allergen extracts usually contains vials for the administration of graded amounts of allergen. Maintenance sets containing vials at the highest strength are also available. Product literature must be consulted for details of allergens, vial strengths, and administration.

BEE AND WASP ALLERGEN EXTRACTS

Cautions   see notes above and consult product literature
Contra-indications   see notes above and consult product literature

Pregnancy   avoid
Side-effects   consult product literature

◻ BEE AND WASP ALLERGEN EXTRACTS (*continued*)

Indication and dose

Hypersensitivity to wasp or bee venom (see notes above)

• By subcutaneous injection
  Consult product literature

Pharmalgen® (ALK-Abelló) [PoM]

Bee venom extract (*Apis mellifera*) or wasp venom extract (*Vespula* spp.). Net price initial treatment set = £59.77 (bee), £73.28 (wasp); maintenance treatment set = £69.54 (bee), £89.45 (wasp)

◼ GRASS AND TREE POLLEN EXTRACTS

Cautions see notes above and consult product literature

Contra-indications see notes above and consult product literature

Pregnancy avoid

Side-effects consult product literature

Indication and dose

Treatment of seasonal allergic hay fever due to grass or tree pollen (see notes above)

  See under preparations, below

Pollinex® (Allergy) [PoM]

Grasses and rye or tree pollen extract, net price initial treatment set (3 vials) and extension course treatment (1 vial) = £450.00

Dose

• By subcutaneous injection
  Consult product literature

◀Grass pollen extract

Grazax® (ALK-Abelló) ▼ [PoM]

Oral lyophilisates (= freeze-dried tablets), grass pollen extract 75 000 units, net price 30-tab pack = £67.50. Counselling, administration

Dose

• By mouth
  Child 5–18 years 1 tablet daily; start treatment at least 4 months before start of pollen season and continue for up to 3 years

  Counselling Tablets should be placed under the tongue and allowed to disperse. Advise not to eat or drink for 5 minutes after taking the tablet

Omalizumab

Omalizumab is a monoclonal antibody that binds to immunoglobulin E (IgE). It is licensed for use as additional therapy in children over 6 years with proven IgE-mediated sensitivity to inhaled allergens, whose severe persistent allergic asthma cannot be controlled adequately with high-dose inhaled corticosteroid together with a long-acting beta$_2$ agonist. Omalizumab should be initiated by physicians experienced in the treatment of severe persistent asthma.

Churg-Strauss syndrome has occurred rarely in patients given omalizumab; the reaction is usually associated with the reduction or withdrawal of oral corticosteroid therapy. Churg-Strauss syndrome can present as eosinophilia, vasculitic rash, cardiac complications, worsening pulmonary symptoms, or peripheral neuropathy. Hypersensitivity reactions can also occur immediately following treatment with omalizumab or sometimes more than 24 hours after the first injection.

For details on the management of anaphylactic shock, see section 3.4.3.

> **NICE guidance**
>
> Omalizumab for severe persistent allergic asthma (November 2007)
> Omalizumab is recommended as additional therapy for the prophylaxis of severe persistent allergic asthma in children over 12 years, who cannot be controlled adequately with high-dose inhaled corticosteroids and long-acting beta$_2$ agonists in addition to leukotriene receptor antagonists, theophylline, oral corticosteroids, oral beta$_2$ agonists, and smoking cessation where clinically appropriate. The following conditions apply:
>
> • confirmation of IgE-mediated allergy to a perennial allergen by clinical history and allergy skin testing;
>
> • either 2 or more severe exacerbations of asthma requiring hospital admission within the previous year, or 3 or more severe exacerbations of asthma within the previous year, at least one of which required hospital admission, and a further 2 which required treatment or monitoring in excess of the patient's usual regimen, in an accident and emergency unit.
>
> Omalizumab should be initiated and monitored by a physician experienced in both allergy and respiratory medicine in a specialist centre, and discontinued at 16 weeks in patients who have not shown an adequate response to therapy.

3

Respiratory system

▌ **OMALIZUMAB**

Cautions autoimmune disease; susceptibility to helminth infections—discontinue if infection does not respond to anthelmintic

Hepatic impairment manufacturer advises caution—no information available

Renal impairment manufacturer advises caution—no information available

Pregnancy manufacturer advises avoid unless essential; no evidence of teratogenicity in *animal* studies

Breast-feeding manufacturer advises avoid—present in milk in *animal* studies

Side-effects headache; injection-site reactions; *less commonly* nausea, diarrhoea, dyspepsia, flushing, fatigue, dizziness, drowsiness, paraesthesia, influenza-like symptoms, photosensitivity, hypersensitivity reactions (including hypotension, bronchospasm, laryngoedema, rash, pruritus, serum sickness, and anaphylaxis); Churg-Strauss syndrome (see notes above), thrombocytopenia, arthralgia, myalgia, and alopecia also reported

Indication and dose

Prophylaxis of severe persistent allergic asthma (see notes above)

● By subcutaneous injection

Child 6–18 years according to immunoglobulin E concentration and body-weight, consult product literature

Xolair® (Novartis) ▼ PoM

Injection, powder for reconstitution, omalizumab, net price 150-mg vial = £256.15 (with solvent)
Excipients include sucrose 108 mg/vial

3.4.3 Allergic emergencies

Adrenaline (epinephrine) provides physiological reversal of the immediate symptoms (such as laryngeal oedema, bronchospasm, and hypotension) associated with hypersensitivity reactions such as *anaphylaxis* and *angioedema*.

Anaphylaxis

Anaphylactic shock requires prompt treatment of *laryngeal oedema, bronchospasm, and hypotension*. Atopic individuals are particularly susceptible. Insect stings are a recognised risk (in particular wasp and bee stings). Latex and certain foods, including eggs, fish, cows' milk protein, peanuts, sesame, shellfish, soy, and tree nuts may also precipitate anaphylaxis. Medicinal products particularly associated with anaphylaxis include blood products, vaccines, allergen immunotherapy preparations, antibacterials, aspirin and other NSAIDs, and neuromuscular blocking drugs. In the case of drugs, anaphylaxis is more likely after parenteral administration; resuscitation facilities must always be available when giving injections associated with special risk. Refined arachis (peanut) oil, which may be present in some medicinal products, is unlikely to cause an allergic reaction—nevertheless it is wise to check the full formula of preparations which may contain allergenic fats or oils.

Treatment of anaphylaxis

First-line treatment includes:

● securing the airway, restoration of blood pressure (laying the child flat and raising the legs, or in the recovery position if unconscious or nauseous and at risk of vomiting);

● administering **adrenaline** (epinephrine) by **intramuscular** injection (for doses see Intramuscular Adrenaline, p. 203); the dose should be repeated if necessary at 5-minute intervals according to blood pressure, pulse, and respiratory function [**important**: possible need for *intravenous route using dilute solution* (Adrenaline 1 in 10 000), see Intravenous Adrenaline p. 203];

● administering high-flow **oxygen** (section 3.6) and **intravenous fluids** (section 9.2.2);

● administering an antihistamine, such as **chlorphenamine** (chlorpheniramine), by slow intravenous injection or intramuscular injection (section 3.4.1) as adjunctive treatment given after adrenaline injection and the antihistamine continued orally for 24 to 48 hours according to clinical response to prevent relapse.

Continuing respiratory deterioration requires further treatment with **bronchodilators** including inhaled or intravenous salbutamol (see p. 177), inhaled ipratropium (see p. 181), intravenous aminophylline (see p. 183), or intravenous magnesium sulphate [unlicensed indication] (see Management of Acute Asthma, p. 171). In addition to oxygen, assisted respiration and possibly emergency tracheotomy may be necessary.

Respiratory system

3

An intravenous corticosteroid (section 6.3.2) such as **hydrocortisone** (as sodium succinate) is of secondary value in the initial management of anaphylactic shock because the onset of action is delayed for several hours, but should be given to prevent further deterioration in severely affected children and continued for 24–48 hours according to clinical response.

When a child is so ill that there is doubt as to the adequacy of the circulation, the initial injection of adrenaline may need to be given as a *dilute solution by the intravenous route*, or by the intraosseous route if venous access is difficult—for details of cautions, dose and strength, see under Intravenous Adrenaline (Epinephrine), below.

Some children with severe allergy to insect stings or foods are encouraged to carry prefilled adrenaline syringes for *self-administration* during periods of risk.

Children who are suspected of having had an anaphylactic reaction should be referred to a specialist for specific allergy diagnosis; avoidance of the allergen is the principal treatment.

Intramuscular adrenaline (epinephrine)

The *intramuscular route* is the *first choice route* for the administration of adrenaline in the management of anaphylactic shock. Adrenaline has a rapid onset of action after intramuscular administration and in the shocked patient its absorption from the intramuscular site is faster and more reliable than from the subcutaneous site. The intravenous route should be reserved for extreme emergency when there is doubt about the adequacy of the circulation; for details of cautions, dose and strength see Intravenous Adrenaline (Epinephrine), below.

Children with severe allergy, or their carers, should ideally be instructed in the self-administration of adrenaline by intramuscular injection (for details see Self-administration of Adrenaline (Epinephrine), p. 204).

Prompt injection of adrenaline is of paramount importance. The following adrenaline doses are based on the revised recommendations of the Working Group of the Resuscitation Council (UK).

Dose of *intramuscular* injection of adrenaline (epinephrine) for anaphylactic shock		
Age range	Dose	Volume of adrenaline **1 in 1000** (1 mg/mL)
Under 6 years	150 micrograms	0.15 mL[1]
6–12 years	300 micrograms	0.3 mL
12–18 years	500 micrograms	0.5 mL[2]
These doses may be repeated several times if necessary at 5-minute intervals according to blood pressure, pulse and respiratory function.		

1. Use suitable syringe for measuring small volume
2. 300 micrograms (0.3 mL) if child is small or prepubertal

Intravenous adrenaline (epinephrine)

Intravenous adrenaline should be given only by those experienced in its use, in a setting where patients can be carefully monitored; it should be given to children only when intravenous access is already available.

Where the child is severely ill and there is real doubt about adequacy of the circulation and absorption from the intramuscular injection site, adrenaline may be given by **slow** *intravenous injection*. Children may respond to as little as 1 microgram/kg (0.01 mL/kg) of the dilute 1 in 10 000 adrenaline injection by **slow** *intravenous injection* over several minutes, repeated according to response. A single dose of adrenaline by intravenous injection should not exceed 50 micrograms; if multiple doses are required consider giving adrenaline by slow intravenous *infusion*. Great vigilance is needed to ensure that the *correct strength* of adrenaline injection is used; anaphylactic shock kits need to make a *very clear distinction* between the 1 in 10 000 strength and the 1 in 1000 strength. It is also important that, where intramuscular injection might still succeed, time should not be wasted seeking intravenous access.

For reference to the use of the intravenous route for *acute hypotension*, see section 2.7.2.

3 Respiratory system

Respiratory system

3

Self-administration of adrenaline (epinephrine)

Children at considerable risk of anaphylaxis need to carry (or have available) adrenaline at all times and the child, or child's carers, need to be *instructed in advance* how to inject it. Packs for self-administration need to be **clearly labelled with instructions** on how to administer adrenaline (intramuscularly, preferably at the midpoint of the outer thigh, through light clothing if necessary). It is important to ensure that an adequate supply is provided to treat symptoms until medical assistance is available.

Adrenaline for administration by intramuscular injection is available in 'auto-injectors' (e.g. *Anapen®* or *EpiPen®*), pre-assembled syringes fitted with a needle suitable for very rapid administration (if necessary by a bystander or a healthcare provider if it is the only preparation available). A syringe delivering 300 micrograms of adrenaline is recommended for a child over 30 kg. A syringe delivering 150 micrograms of adrenaline is recommended for a child 15–30 kg, but on the basis of a dose of 10 micrograms/kg, 300 micrograms may be more appropriate for some children.

ADRENALINE/EPINEPHRINE

Cautions for cautions in non-life-threatening situations, see section 2.7.2

Interactions Severe anaphylaxis in children on non-cardioselective beta-blockers may not respond to adrenaline injection calling for intravenous injection of salbutamol (see section 3.1.1.1); furthermore, adrenaline may cause severe hypertension and bradycardia in those receiving non-cardioselective beta-blockers. Other **interactions**, see Appendix 1 (sympathomimetics).

Renal impairment section 2.7.2

Pregnancy section 2.7.2

Breast-feeding section 2.7.2

Side-effects section 2.7.2

Licensed use auto-injector delivering 150-microgram dose of adrenaline not licensed for use in children body-weight under 15 kg

Indication and dose

Emergency treatment of acute anaphylaxis, angioedema
- By intramuscular injection (preferably midpoint in anterolateral thigh) of 1 in 1000 (1 mg/mL) solution
  See notes and table above

Acute anaphylaxis when there is doubt as to the adequacy of the circulation
- By slow intravenous injection of 1 in 10 000 (100 micrograms/mL) solution (extreme caution—specialist use only)
  See notes above

Safe Practice Intravenous route should be used with **extreme care** by specialists only, see notes above

Croup (section 3.1)
- By inhalation of nebulised solution of adrenaline 1 in 1000 (1 mg/mL)

  Child 1 month–12 years 400 micrograms/kg (max. 5 mg), repeated after 30 minutes if necessary

  Administration For nebulisation, dilute adrenaline 1 in 1000 solution with sterile sodium chloride 0.9% solution

Acute hypotension, low cardiac output section 2.7.2

Cardiopulmonary resuscitation section 2.7.3

◢ Intramuscular or subcutaneous
¹**Adrenaline/Epinephrine 1 in 1000** (Non-proprietary) PoM

　Injection, adrenaline (as acid tartrate) 1 mg/mL, net price 0.5-mL amp = 49p; 1-mL amp = 51p
Excipients include sulphites

¹**Minijet® Adrenaline 1 in 1000** (UCB Pharma) PoM
　Injection, adrenaline (as hydrochloride) 1 in 1000 (1 mg/mL). Net price 1 mL (with 25 gauge × 0.25 inch needle for subcutaneous injection) = £10.79, 1 mL (with 21 gauge × 1.5 inch needle for intramuscular injection) = £6.36 (both disposable syringes)
Excipients include sulphites

◢ Intravenous
Extreme caution, see notes above

Adrenaline/Epinephrine 1 in 10 000, Dilute (Non-proprietary) PoM
　Injection, adrenaline (as acid tartrate) 100 micrograms/mL, 10-mL amp, 1-mL and 10-mL prefilled syringe
Excipients include sulphites

Minijet® Adrenaline 1 in 10 000 (UCB Pharma) PoM
　Injection, adrenaline (as hydrochloride) 1 in 10 000 (100 micrograms/mL), net price 3-mL prefilled syringe = £6.27; 10-mL prefilled syringe = £6.15
Excipients include sulphites

◢ Intramuscular injection for self-administration
Anapen® (Lincoln Medical) PoM
　Anapen® 500 (delivering a single dose of adrenaline 500 micrograms), adrenaline 1.7 mg/mL, net price 1.05-mL auto-injector device = £30.67
Excipients include sulphites
Note 0.75 mL of the solution remains in the auto-injector device after use
Dose
　Acute anaphylaxis
　- By intramuscular injection
　　Child 12–18 years body-weight over 60 kg 500 micrograms repeated after 10–15 minutes if necessary

1. PoM restriction does not apply to adrenaline injection 1 mg/mL where administration is for saving life in emergency

◁ **ADRENALINE/EPINEPHRINE (continued)**

[1]Anapen® 300 (delivering a single dose of adrenaline 300 micrograms), adrenaline 1 mg/mL (1 in 1000), net price 1.05-mL auto-injector device = £30.67
Excipients include sulphites
Note 0.75 mL of the solution remains in the auto-injector device after use

Dose

Acute anaphylaxis
• **By intramuscular injection**
  Child body-weight over 30 kg 300 micrograms repeated after 10–15 minutes as necessary

Anapen® 150 (delivering a single dose of adrenaline 150 micrograms), adrenaline 500 micrograms/mL (1 in 2000), net price 1.05-mL auto-injector device = £30.67
Excipients include sulphites
Note 0.75 mL of the solution remains in the auto-injector device after use

Dose

Acute anaphylaxis
• **By intramuscular injection**
  Child body-weight under 15 kg 150 micrograms repeated after 10–15 minutes as necessary
  Child body–weight 15–30 kg 150 micrograms (but on the basis of a dose of 10 micrograms/kg, 300 micrograms may be more appropriate for some children) repeated after 10–15 minutes as necessary

EpiPen® (ALK-Abelló) [PoM]
[1]EpiPen® Auto-injector 0.3 mg (delivering a single dose of adrenaline 300 micrograms), adrenaline 1 mg/mL (1 in 1000), net price 2-mL auto-injector device = £29.15
Excipients include sulphites
Note 1.7 mL of the solution remains in the auto-injector device after use

Dose

Acute anaphylaxis
• **By intramuscular injection**
  Child body-weight over 30 kg 300 micrograms repeated after 5–15 minutes as necessary

Epipen® Jr Auto-injector 0.15 mg (delivering a single dose of adrenaline 150 micrograms), adrenaline 500 micrograms/mL (1 in 2000), net price 2-mL auto-injector device = £29.18
Excipients include sulphites
Note 1.7 mL of the solution remains in the auto-injector device after use

Dose

Acute anaphylaxis
• **By intramuscular injection**
  Child body-weight under 15 kg 150 micrograms repeated after 5–15 minutes as necessary
  Child body-weight 15–30 kg 150 micrograms (but on the basis of a dose of 10 micrograms/kg, 300 micrograms may be more appropriate for some children) repeated after 5–15 minutes as necessary

3 Respiratory system

Angioedema

Angioedema is dangerous if *laryngeal oedema* is present. In this circumstance adrenaline (epinephrine) injection and oxygen should be given as described under Anaphylaxis (see above); antihistamines and corticosteroids should also be given (see again above). Tracheal intubation may be necessary. In some children with laryngeal oedema, adrenaline 1 in 1000 (1 mg/mL) solution may be given by nebuliser. However, nebulised adrenaline cannot be relied upon for a systemic effect—intramuscular adrenaline should be used.

Hereditary angioedema   The administration of C1-esterase inhibitor (in fresh frozen plasma or in partially purified form) may terminate acute attacks of *hereditary angioedema*, but is not practical for long-term prophylaxis; it can also be used for short-term prophylaxis before surgery or dental procedures [unlicensed indication]. **Tranexamic acid** (section 2.11) is used for short-term or long-term prophylaxis of hereditary angioedema; short-term prophylaxis is started several days before planned procedures which may trigger an acute attack of hereditary angioedema (e.g. dental work) and continued for 2–5 days afterwards. **Danazol** [unlicensed indication, see BNF section 6.7.2] is best avoided in children because of its androgenic effects but it can be used for short-term prophylaxis of hereditary angioedema.

▌ C1-ESTERASE INHIBITOR

Cautions vaccination against hepatitis A (p. 743) and hepatitis B (p. 745) may be required

Pregnancy manufacturer advises avoid unless essential

Breast-feeding manufacturer advises use only if potential benefit outweighs risk—no information available

Side-effects *rarely* injection-site reactions, hypersensitivity reactions (including anaphylaxis)

Licensed use not licensed for short-term prophylaxis of hereditary angioedema

Indication and dose

Acute attacks of hereditary angioedema, short-term prophylaxis of hereditary angioedema before surgery or dental procedures
• **By slow intravenous injection or intravenous infusion (specialist use only)**
  Neonate 20 units/kg
  Child 1 month–18 years 20 units/kg

---

1. [PoM] restriction does not apply to adrenaline injection 1 mg/mL where administration is for saving life in emergency

◁ **C1-ESTERASE INHIBITOR** (*continued*)

Berinert® (CSL Behring) ▼ [PoM]
Injection, powder for reconstitution C1-esterase
inhibitor, net price 500-unit vial = £550.00
Electrolytes Na⁺ 2.1 mmol/10 mL-vial

3.5 Respiratory stimulants and pulmonary surfactants

3.5.1 Respiratory stimulants
3.5.2 Pulmonary surfactants

3.5.1 Respiratory stimulants

Respiratory stimulants (analeptic drugs), such as caffeine and doxapram, should
only be given under **expert supervision** in hospital; it is important to rule out any
underlying disorder, such as seizures, hypoglycaemia, or infection, causing respiratory exhaustion before starting treatment with a respiratory stimulant.

Caffeine (as caffeine base) is licensed for the treatment of apnoea in preterm
neonates; it is used in preference to theophylline (section 3.1.3). Caffeine can also
be used to stimulate ventilation, or assist extubation in ventilated infants. Caffeine
has fewer adverse effects and a longer half-life than theophylline in neonates. It is
well absorbed when given orally; intravenous treatment is rarely necessary.
Plasma-caffeine concentration should be measured if the child has previously
been treated with theophylline. The therapeutic range for plasma-caffeine concentration is usually 10–20 mg/litre (50–100 micromol/litre), but a concentration
of 25–35 mg/litre (130–180 micromol/litre) may be required (section 3.1.3).

Doxapram may be given by continuous intravenous infusion or by mouth for
preterm neonates and infants who continue to have troublesome apnoea despite
treatment with caffeine. When given by continuous intravenous infusion, blood
pressure monitoring and frequent measurement of arterial blood gas and pH are
necessary to ensure correct dosage.

CAFFEINE

Cautions gastro-oesophageal reflux; cardiovascular disease; monitor plasma-caffeine concentration (see notes above); monitor closely for 1 week
after stopping treatment

Side-effects hypertension, tachycardia; irritability, restlessness; hypoglycaemia, hyperglycaemia;
fluid and electrolyte imbalance

Licensed use not licensed for use as an adjunct to
extubation in pre-term neonates

Indication and dose

> Note Dose expressed as caffeine base

> **Neonatal apnoea, adjunct to extubation in pre-
> term neonates**
> • **By mouth, expressed as caffeine base**
>
> **Neonate** initially 10 mg/kg, then 2.5–5 mg/kg
> once daily starting 24 hours after initial dose
> (some neonates may require 10 mg/kg/day)

> • **By intravenous infusion, expressed as caffeine
> base**
>
> **Neonate** initially 10 mg/kg over 30 minutes,
> then 2.5–5 mg/kg over 10 minutes once daily
> starting 24 hours after initial dose (some neo-
> nates may require 10 mg/kg/day)

> Safe practice When prescribing, always state dose in
> terms of caffeine base
> Caffeine base 1 mg = caffeine *citrate* 2 mg

Administration caffeine injection may be administered *by mouth* or *by intravenous infusion*

Caffeine (Non-proprietary) [PoM]
Injection, caffeine 5 mg/mL, net price 1-mL amp =
£4.44
Electrolytes Na⁺ < 0.5 mmol/amp

◢ **Caffeine citrate preparations**
Caffeine citrate oral liquid available from 'special-
order' manufacturers or specialist importing companies, see p. 957

DOXAPRAM HYDROCHLORIDE

Cautions impaired cardiac reserve; risk of QT
interval prolongation; **interactions**: Appendix 1
(doxapram)

Contra-indications severe hypertension, thyrotoxicosis, epilepsy, physical obstruction of respiratory tract

Hepatic impairment use with caution

Pregnancy no evidence of harm, but manufacturer advises avoid unless benefit outweighs risk

Side-effects perineal warmth, dizziness, sweating, moderate increase in blood pressure and
heart rate; hyperexcitability; high doses may
cause convulsions; oral dose may cause slowed
gastric emptying

◁ **DOXAPRAM HYDROCHLORIDE** (*continued*)

Licensed use not licensed for use in children

Indication and dose

Neonatal apnoea (see notes above)

• **By intravenous infusion**

Neonate initially 2.5 mg/kg over 5–10 minutes, then by *continuous intravenous infusion* 300 microgram/kg/hour adjusted according to response, up to max. 1.5 mg/kg/hour

• **By mouth** (after initial intravenous dose)

Neonate 6 mg/kg 4 times daily

Administration for *intravenous infusion*, dilute injection solution (20 mg/mL) to a concentration of 1 mg/mL with Glucose 5% *or* Sodium Chloride 0.9%

For administration *by mouth*, dilute doxapram injection solution with Glucose 5% if necessary

Dopram® (Chiesi) (PoM)
Injection, doxapram hydrochloride 20 mg/mL. Net price 5-mL amp = £3.00

Intravenous infusion, doxapram hydrochloride 2 mg/mL in glucose 5%. Net price 500-mL bottle = £21.33

3.5.2 Pulmonary surfactants

Pulmonary surfactants derived from animal lungs, **beractant** and **poractant alfa** are used to prevent and treat respiratory distress syndrome (hyaline membrane disease) in preterm neonates. Prophylactic use of a pulmonary surfactant may reduce the need for mechanical ventilation and is more effective than 'rescue treatment' in preterm neonates of 29 weeks or less post-menstrual age.

Pulmonary surfactants may also be of benefit in neonates with meconium aspiration syndrome or intrapartum streptococcal infection.

Pulmonary immaturity with surfactant deficit is the commonest reason for respiratory failure in the neonate, especially in those of less than 30 weeks postmenstrual age. Betamethasone (section 6.3.2) given to the mother (at least 12 hours but preferably 48 hours) before delivery substantially enhances pulmonary maturity in the neonate.

Cautions Continuous monitoring is required to avoid hyperoxaemia caused by rapid improvement in arterial oxygen concentration.

Side-effects Pulmonary haemorrhage has been rarely associated with pulmonary surfactants, especially in more preterm neonates. Obstruction of the endotracheal tube by mucous secretions has also been reported.

BERACTANT

Cautions see notes above

Side-effects see notes above

Licensed use licensed for use in respiratory distress syndrome in newborn premature infants, birth-weight over 700 g, and as prophylaxis in neonates less than 32 weeks post-menstrual age

Indication and dose

Treatment of respiratory distress syndrome in preterm neonate; prophylaxis of respiratory distress syndrome in preterm neonate

• **By endotracheal tube**

Neonate phospholipid 100 mg/kg equivalent to a volume of 4 mL/kg, preferably within 8 hours of birth; may be repeated within 48 hours at intervals of at least 6 hours for up to 4 doses

Survanta® (Abbott) (PoM)
Suspension, beractant (bovine lung extract) providing phospholipid 25 mg/mL, with lipids and proteins, net price 8-mL vial = £306.43

PORACTANT ALFA

Cautions see notes above

Side-effects see notes above

Licensed use licensed for use in respiratory distress syndrome in newborn premature infants, birth-weight over 700 g, and as prophylaxis in neonates 24–32 weeks post-menstrual age

Indication and dose

Treatment of respiratory distress syndrome or hyaline membrane disease in preterm neonate; prophylaxis of respiratory distress syndrome in preterm neonate

• **By endotracheal tube**

Neonate *treatment*, 100–200 mg/kg; further doses of 100 mg/kg may be repeated 12 hours later and after further 12 hours if still intubated; max. total dose 300–400 mg/kg; *prophylaxis,*

3

Respiratory system

◁ **PORACTANT ALFA** (*continued*)

100–200 mg/kg soon after birth (preferably within 15 minutes); further doses of 100 mg/kg may be repeated 6–12 hours later and after further 12 hours if still intubated; max. total dose 300–400 mg/kg

Curosurf® (Chiesi) [PoM]
Suspension, poractant alfa (porcine lung phospholipid fraction) 80 mg/mL, net price 1.5-mL vial = £298.74; 3-mL vial = £580.64

3.6 Oxygen

Oxygen should be regarded as a drug. It is prescribed for hypoxaemic patients to increase alveolar oxygen tension and decrease the work of breathing. The concentration of oxygen required depends on the condition being treated; administration of an inappropriate concentration of oxygen may have serious or even fatal consequences. High concentrations of oxygen can cause pulmonary epithelial damage (bronchopulmonary dysplasia), convulsions, and retinal damage, especially in preterm neonates.

Oxygen is probably the most common drug used in medical emergencies. It should be prescribed initially to achieve a normal or near-normal oxygen saturation. In most acutely ill children with an expected or known normal or low arterial carbon dioxide (P_aCO_2), oxygen saturation should be maintained above 92%; some clinicians may aim for a target of 94–98%. In some clinical situations, such as carbon monoxide poisoning, (see also Emergency Treatment of Poisoning, p. 45), it is more appropriate to aim for the highest possible oxygen saturation until the child is stable. Hypercapnic respiratory failure is rare in children; in those children at risk, a lower oxygen saturation target of 88–92% is indicated, see below.

High concentration oxygen therapy is safe in uncomplicated cases of conditions such as pneumonia, pulmonary embolism, pulmonary fibrosis, shock, severe trauma, sepsis, or anaphylaxis. In such conditions, low arterial oxygen (P_aO_2) is usually associated with low or normal arterial carbon dioxide (P_aCO_2) and there is little risk of hypoventilation and carbon dioxide retention.

In severe acute asthma, the arterial carbon dioxide (P_aCO_2) is usually subnormal, but as asthma deteriorates it may rise steeply. These patients usually require a high concentration of oxygen and if the arterial carbon dioxide (P_aCO_2) remains high despite treatment, intermittent positive pressure ventilation needs to be considered urgently.

Oxygen should not be given to neonates except under expert supervision. Particular care is required in preterm neonates because of the risk of hyperoxia (see above).

Low concentration oxygen therapy (controlled oxygen therapy) is reserved for children at risk of hypercapnic respiratory failure, which is more likely in children with:

- advanced cystic fibrosis;
- advanced non-cystic fibrosis bronchiectasis;
- severe kyphoscoliosis or severe ankylosing spondylitis;
- severe lung scarring caused by tuberculosis;
- neuromuscular disorders with respiratory weakness, especially if on home ventilation;
- an overdose of opioids, benzodiazepines, or other drugs causing respiratory depression.

Until blood gases can be measured, initial oxygen should be given using a controlled concentration of 28% or less, titrated towards a target concentration of 88–92%. The aim is to provide the child with enough oxygen to achieve an acceptable arterial oxygen tension without worsening carbon dioxide retention and respiratory acidosis.

Domiciliary oxygen   Oxygen should only be prescribed for use in the home after careful evaluation in hospital by a respiratory care specialist. Children and their carers should be advised of the risks of continuing to smoke when receiving oxygen, including the risk of fire. Smoking cessation therapy (section 4.10) should be tried before home oxygen prescription.

Long-term oxygen therapy

The aim of long-term oxygen therapy is to maintain oxygen saturation of at least 92%. Children (especially those with chronic neonatal lung disease) often require supplemental oxygen, either for 24-hours a day or during periods of sleep; many children are eventually weaned off long-term oxygen therapy as their condition improves.

Long-term oxygen therapy should be considered for children with conditions such as:

- bronchopulmonary dysplasia (chronic neonatal lung disease);
- congenital heart disease with pulmonary hypertension;
- pulmonary hypertension secondary to pulmonary disease;
- idiopathic pulmonary hypertension;
- sickle-cell disease with persistent nocturnal hypoxia;
- interstitial lung disease and obliterative bronchiolitis;
- cystic fibrosis;
- obstructive sleep apnoea syndrome;
- neuromuscular or skeletal disease requiring non-invasive ventilation;
- pulmonary malignancy or other terminal disease with disabling dyspnoea.

Increased respiratory depression is seldom a problem in children with stable respiratory failure treated with low concentrations of oxygen although it may occur during exacerbations; children and their carers should be warned to call for medical help if drowsiness or confusion occurs.

Short-burst oxygen therapy

Oxygen is occasionally prescribed for short-burst (intermittent) use for episodes of breathlessness.

Ambulatory oxygen therapy

Ambulatory oxygen is prescribed for children on long-term oxygen therapy who need to be away from home on a regular basis.

Oxygen therapy equipment

Under the NHS oxygen may be supplied as **oxygen cylinders**. Oxygen flow can be adjusted by means of an oxygen flow meter. Oxygen delivered from a cylinder should be passed through a humidifier if used for long periods.

Oxygen concentrators are more economical for children who require oxygen for long periods, and in England and Wales can be ordered on the NHS on a regional tendering basis (see below). A concentrator is recommended for a child who requires oxygen for more than 8 hours a day (or 21 cylinders per month). Exceptionally, if a higher concentration of oxygen is required the output of 2 oxygen concentrators can be combined using a 'Y' connection.

A nasal cannula is usually preferred to a face mask for long-term oxygen therapy from an oxygen concentrator. Nasal cannulas can, however, cause dermatitis and mucosal drying in sensitive individuals.

Giving oxygen by nasal cannula allows the child to talk, eat, and drink, but the concentration is not controlled and the method may not be appropriate for acute respiratory failure. When oxygen is given through a nasal cannula at a rate of 1–2 litres/minute the inspiratory oxygen concentration is usually low, but it varies with ventilation and can be high if the child is underventilating.

Arrangements for supplying oxygen

The following services may be ordered in England and Wales:

- emergency oxygen;
- short-burst (intermittent) oxygen therapy;
- long-term oxygen therapy;
- ambulatory oxygen.

The type of oxygen service (or combination of services) should be ordered on a Home Oxygen Order Form (HOOF); the amount of oxygen required (hours per day) and flow rate should be specified. The supplier will determine the appro-

3

Respiratory system

priate equipment to be provided. Special needs or preferences should be specified on the HOOF.

The clinician should obtain the patient's consent to pass on the patient's details to the supplier and the fire brigade. The supplier will contact the patient to make arrangements for delivery, installation, and maintenance of the equipment. The supplier will also train the patient to use the equipment.

The clinician should send order forms to the supplier by facsimile (see below); a copy of the HOOF should be sent to the Primary Care Trust or Local Health Board. The supplier will continue to provide the service until a revised order is received, or until notified that the patient no longer requires the home oxygen service.

HOOF and further instructions are available at www.bprs.co.uk/oxygen.html.

Eastern England	BOC Medical *to order:* Tel: 0800 136 603 Fax: 0800 169 9989
North East South West	Air Liquide *to order:* Tel: 0808 202 2229 Fax: 0191 497 4340
South London South East Coast South Central	Air Liquide *to order:* Tel: 0500 823 773 Fax: 0800 781 4610
North West Yorkshire and Humberside East Midlands West Midlands North London Wales	Air Products *to order:* Tel: 0800 373 580 Fax: 0800 214 709

In **Scotland**, refer the child for assessment by a paediatric respiratory consultant. If the need for a concentrator is confirmed the consultant will arrange for the provision of a concentrator through the Common Services Agency. In **Northern Ireland** oxygen concentrators and cylinders should be prescribed on form HS21; oxygen concentrators are supplied by a local contractor. In **Scotland** and **Northern Ireland**, prescriptions for oxygen cylinders and accessories can be dispensed by pharmacies contracted to provide domiciliary oxygen services.

3.7 Mucolytics

Mucolytics, such as **carbocisteine** and **mecysteine**, are used to facilitate mucociliary clearance and expectoration by reducing sputum viscosity but evidence of efficacy is limited.

Dornase alfa is a genetically engineered version of a naturally occurring human enzyme which cleaves extracellular deoxyribonucleic acid (DNA); it is used to reduce sputum viscosity in children with cystic fibrosis. Dornase alfa is administered by inhalation using a jet nebuliser (section 3.1.5), usually once daily at least 1 hour before physiotherapy; however, alternate-day therapy may be as effective as daily treatment. Not all children benefit from treatment with dornase alfa; improvement occurs within 2 weeks, but in more severely affected children a trial of 6–12 weeks may be required.

Nebulised **hypertonic sodium chloride** solution may improve mucociliary clearance in children with cystic fibrosis.

Mesna (*Mistabron®*, available from 'special-order' manufacturers or specialist importing companies, see p. 957) is used in some children with cystic fibrosis when other mucolytics have failed to reduce sputum viscosity; 3–6 mL of a 20% solution is nebulised twice daily.

Acetylcysteine has been used to treat meconium ileus in neonates and distal intestinal obstruction syndrome in children with cystic fibrosis, but evidence of efficacy is lacking. *Gastrografin®* (section 1.6.5), or a bowel cleansing preparation containing macrogols (section 1.6.5), is usually more effective. Acetylcysteine may be used as a mucolytic to prevent further obstruction.

ACETYLCYSTEINE

Cautions history of peptic ulceration; asthma

Side-effects hypersensitivity-like reactions including rashes and anaphylaxis

Licensed use not licensed for use in meconium ileus or for distal intestinal obstructive syndrome in children with cystic fibrosis

Indication and dose

Meconium ileus (but see notes above)
* By mouth

NEONATE 200–400 mg up to 3 times daily if necessary

Treatment of distal intestinal obstructive syndrome (but see notes above)
* By mouth

Child 1 month–2 years 0.4–3 g as a single dose

Child 2–7 years 2–3 g as a single dose

Child 7–18 years 4–6 g as a single dose

Prevention of distal intestinal obstruction syndrome
* By mouth

Child 1 month–2 years 100–200 mg 3 times daily

Child 2–12 years 200 mg 3 times daily

Child 12–18 years 200–400 mg 3 times daily

Administration For *oral* administration, use oral granules, *or* dilute injection solution (200 mg/mL) to a concentration of 50 mg/mL; orange or blackcurrant juice or cola drink may be used as a diluent to mask the bitter taste

Acetylcysteine (Non-proprietary) PoM
Oral granules, acetylcysteine 100 mg/sachet; 200 mg/sachet. Label: 13
Available from 'special-order' manufacturers or specialist importing companies, see p. 957

◢Injection
See Emergency treatment of poisoning, p. 37

CARBOCISTEINE

Cautions history of peptic ulceration

Contra-indications active peptic ulceration

Pregnancy manufacturer advises avoid in first trimester

Breast-feeding no information available

Side-effects *rarely* gastro-intestinal bleeding; hypersensitivity reactions (including rash and anaphylaxis) also reported

Indication and dose

Reduction of sputum viscosity
* By mouth

Child 2–5 years 62.5–125 mg 4 times daily

Child 5–12 years 250 mg 3 times daily

Child 12–18 years initially 2.25 g daily in divided doses, then 1.5 g daily in divided doses as condition improves

Carbocisteine (Sanofi-Aventis) PoM
Capsules, carbocisteine 375 mg, net price 120-cap pack = £16.03
Brands include *Mucodyne®*

Oral liquid, carbocisteine 125 mg/5 mL, net price 300 mL = £4.39; 250 mg/5 mL, 300 mL = £5.61
Brands include *Mucodyne® Paediatric* 125 mg/5 mL (cherry- and raspberry-flavoured) and *Mucodyne®* 250 mg/5 mL (cinnamon- and rum-flavoured)

DORNASE ALFA

Phosphorylated glycosylated recombinant human deoxyribonuclease 1 (rhDNase)

Pregnancy no evidence of teratogenicity; manufacturer advises use only if potential benefit outweighs risk

Breast-feeding amount probably too small to be harmful—manufacturer advises caution

Side-effects pharyngitis, voice changes, chest pain; occasionally laryngitis, rashes, urticaria, conjunctivitis

Indication and dose

Management of cystic fibrosis patients with a forced vital capacity (FVC) of greater than 40% of predicted to improve pulmonary function
* By inhalation of nebulised solution (by jet nebuliser)

Child 5–18 years 2500 units (2.5 mg) once daily

Pulmozyme® (Roche) PoM
Nebuliser solution, dornase alfa 1000 units (1 mg)/mL. Net price 2.5-mL (2500 units) vial = £16.88

Note For use undiluted with jet nebulisers only; ultrasonic nebulisers are unsuitable

MECYSTEINE HYDROCHLORIDE

(Methyl Cysteine Hydrochloride)

Cautions history of peptic ulceration

Pregnancy manufacturer advises avoid

Breast-feeding manufacturer advises avoid

Indication and dose

Reduction of sputum viscosity
* By mouth

Child 5–12 years 100 mg 3 times daily

Child 12–18 years 200 mg 4 times daily for 2 days, then 200 mg 3 times daily for 6 weeks, then 200 mg twice daily

Visclair® (Ranbaxy)
Tablets, yellow, s/c, e/c, mecysteine hydrochloride 100 mg, net price 100= £15.44. Label: 5, 22, 25

3 Respiratory system

Hypertonic sodium chloride

Nebulised hypertonic sodium chloride solution (3–7 %) is used to mobilise lower respiratory tract secretions in mucous consolidation (e.g. cystic fibrosis).

MucoClear® 6% (Pari)
Nebuliser solution, sodium chloride 6%, net price 20 × 4 ml = £12.98; 60 × 4 ml = £29.98

Dose
• By inhalation of nebulised solution
  Child 4 mL twice daily

3.8 Aromatic inhalations

Inhalations containing volatile substances such as eucalyptus oil are traditionally used to relieve congestion and ease breathing. Although the vapour may contain little of the additive, it encourages deliberate inspiration of warm moist air which is often comforting. Boiling water should not be used for inhalations owing to the risk of scalding.

Strong aromatic decongestants (applied as rubs or to pillows) are not recommended for infants under the age of 3 months. **Sodium chloride 0.9%** solution given as nasal drops can be used to liquefy mucous secretions and relieve nasal congestion in infants and young children.

Benzoin Tincture, Compound, BP
(Friars' Balsam)
Tincture, balsamic acids approx. 4.5%. Label: 15

Dose
Nasal congestion
• By inhalation
  Add one teaspoonful to a pint of hot, **not** boiling, water and inhale the vapour

Menthol and Eucalyptus Inhalation, BP 1980
Inhalation, racementhol or levomenthol 2 g, eucalyptus oil 10 mL, light magnesium carbonate 7 g, water to 100 mL

Dose
Nasal congestion
• By inhalation
  Add one teaspoonful to a pint of hot, **not** boiling, water and inhale the vapour

Dental prescribing on the NHS May be prescribed as Menthol and Eucalyptus Inhalation BP, 1980

3.9 Cough preparations

3.9.1 Cough suppressants
3.9.2 Expectorant and demulcent cough preparations

3.9.1 Cough suppressants

Cough may be a symptom of an underlying disorder such as asthma (section 3.1), gastro-oesophageal reflux disease (section 1.1), or rhinitis (section 12.2.1), which should be addressed before prescribing cough suppressants. Cough may be associated with smoking or environmental pollutants. Cough can also result from bronchiectasis including that associated with cystic fibrosis; cough can also have a significant habit component. There is little evidence of any significant benefit from the use of cough suppressants in children with acute cough in ambulatory settings. Cough suppressants may cause sputum retention and this can be harmful in children with bronchiectasis.

The use of cough suppressants containing **pholcodine** or similar opioid analgesics is not generally recommended in children and should be avoided in children under 6 years, see MHRA/CHM advice below.

Sedating antihistamines (section 3.4.1) are used as the cough suppressant component of many compound cough preparations on sale to the public; all tend to cause drowsiness which may reflect their main mode of action.

> **MHRA/CHM advice (March 2008 and February 2009)**
> Children under 6 years should not be given over-the-counter cough and cold medicines containing the following ingredients:
> - brompheniramine, chlorphenamine, diphenhydramine, doxylamine, promethazine, or triprolidine (antihistamines);
> - dextromethorphan or pholcodine (cough suppressants);
> - guaifenesin or ipecacuanha (expectorants);
> - phenylephrine, pseudoephedrine, ephedrine, oxymetazoline, or xylometazoline (decongestants).
>
> Over-the-counter cough and cold medicines can be considered for children aged 6–12 years after basic principles of best care have been tried, but treatment should be restricted to five days or less. Children should not be given more than 1 cough or cold preparation at a time because different brands may contain the same active ingredient; care should be taken to give the correct dose.

PHOLCODINE

Cautions may cause sputum retention

Hepatic impairment see Codeine Phosphate, section 4.7.2

Renal impairment see Codeine Phosphate, section 4.7.2

Pregnancy see Codeine Phosphate, section 4.7.2

Breast-feeding see Codeine Phosphate, section 4.7.2

Side-effects nausea, sputum retention, constipation

Indication and dose

Dry or painful cough (but not generally recommended for children, see notes above)
- By mouth
  Child 6–12 years 2–5 mg 3–4 times daily
  Child 12–18 years 5–10 mg 3–4 times daily

Pholcodine Linctus, BP
Linctus (= oral solution), pholcodine 5 mg/5 mL in a suitable flavoured vehicle, containing citric acid monohydrate 1%. Net price 100 mL = 44p
Brands include *Pavacol-D*® (sugar-free), *Galenphol*® (sugar-free)

Pholcodine Linctus, Strong, BP
Linctus (= oral solution), pholcodine 10 mg/5 mL in a suitable flavoured vehicle, containing citric acid monohydrate 2%. Net price 100 mL = 38p
Brands include *Galenphol*®

Galenphol® (Thornton & Ross)
Paediatric linctus (= oral solution), orange, sugar-free, pholcodine 2 mg/5 mL. Net price 90-mL pack = £1.11

3.9.2 Expectorant and demulcent cough preparations

Simple linctus and other demulcent cough preparations containing soothing substances, such as syrup or glycerol, may temporarily relieve a dry irritating cough. These preparations have the advantage of being harmless and inexpensive and sugar-free versions are available.

Expectorants are claimed to promote expulsion of bronchial secretions but there is no evidence that any drug can specifically facilitate expectoration.

Compound cough preparations for children are on sale to the public but should not be used in children under 6 years; the rationale for some is dubious. Care should be taken to give the correct dose and to not use more than one preparation at a time, see MHRA/CHM advice above.

Simple Linctus, Paediatric, BP
Linctus (= oral solution), citric acid monohydrate 0.625% in a suitable vehicle with an anise flavour. Net price 100 mL = 72p
A sugar-free version is also available

Dose
Cough
- By mouth
  Child 1 month–12 years 5–10 mL 3–4 times daily

Simple Linctus, BP
Linctus (= oral solution), citric acid monohydrate 2.5% in a suitable vehicle with an anise flavour. Net price 100 mL = 42p
A sugar-free version is also available

Dose
Cough
- By mouth
  Child 12–18 years 5 mL 3–4 times daily

3.10 Systemic nasal decongestants

Nasal congestion in children due to allergic or vasomotor rhinitis should be treated with oral antihistamines (section 3.4.1), topical nasal preparations containing corticosteroids (section 12.2.1), or topical decongestants (section 12.2.2).

There is little evidence to support the use of systemic decongestants in children.

Pseudoephedrine has few sympathomimetic effects, and is commonly combined with other ingredients (including antihistamines) in preparations intended for the relief of cough and cold symptoms but it should not be used in children under 6 years, see MHRA/CHM advice, p. 213.

PSEUDOEPHEDRINE HYDROCHLORIDE

Cautions hypertension, heart disease, diabetes, hyperthyroidism, raised intra-ocular pressure; **interactions:** Appendix 1 (sympathomimetics)

Contra-indications treatment with MAOI within previous 2 weeks

Hepatic impairment manufacturer advises caution in severe impairment

Renal impairment manufacturer advises caution in moderate to severe impairment

Pregnancy defective closure of the abdominal wall (gastrochisis) reported very rarely in newborns after first trimester exposure

Breast-feeding amount too small to be harmful

Side-effects tachycardia, anxiety, restlessness, insomnia; *rarely* hallucinations, rash; urinary retention also reported

Indication and dose

Congestion of mucous membranes of upper respiratory tract
- By mouth
  Child 6–12 years 30 mg 3–4 times daily
  Child 12–18 years 60 mg 3–4 times daily

¹**Galpseud®** (Thornton & Ross) ◢
Tablets, pseudoephedrine hydrochloride 60 mg, net price 20 = £1.06

Linctus, orange, sugar-free, pseudoephedrine hydrochloride 30 mg/5 mL, net price 100 mL = 69p

¹**Sudafed®** (McNeil) ◢
Tablets, red, f/c, pseudoephedrine hydrochloride 60 mg, net price 24 = £2.12

Elixir, red, pseudoephedrine hydrochloride 30 mg/5 mL, net price 100 mL = £1.55

---

1. Can be sold to the public provided no more than 720 mg of pseudoephedrine salts are supplied, and ephedrine base (or salts) are not supplied at the same time; for details see *Medicines, Ethics and Practice*, No. 33, London, Pharmaceutical Press, 2009 (and subsequent editions as available)

4 Central nervous system

4 Central nervous system

4.1 Hypnotics and anxiolytics

4.1.1 Hypnotics
4.1.2 Anxiolytics
4.1.3 Barbiturates

Most anxiolytics ('sedatives') will induce sleep when given at night and most hypnotics will sedate when given during the day. Hypnotics and anxiolytics should be reserved for short courses to alleviate acute conditions after causal factors have been established.

The role of drug therapy in the management of anxiety disorders in children and adolescents is uncertain; drug therapy should be initiated only by specialists after psychosocial interventions have failed. Benzodiazepines and tricyclic antidepressants have been used but adverse effects may be problematic.

Skilled tasks Hypnotics and anxiolytics may impair judgement and increase reaction time, and so affect ability to drive or perform skilled tasks; they increase the effects of alcohol. Moreover the hangover effects of a night dose may impair performance on the following day.

> **Important**
> 1. Benzodiazepines are indicated for the short-term relief (two to four weeks only) of anxiety that is severe, disabling or causing the child unacceptable distress, occurring alone or in association with insomnia or short-term psychosomatic, organic, or psychotic illness.
> 2. The use of benzodiazepines to treat short-term 'mild' anxiety is inappropriate.
> 3. Benzodiazepines should be used to treat insomnia only when it is severe, disabling, or causing the child extreme distress.

4.1.1 Hypnotics

The prescribing of hypnotics to children, except for occasional use such as for sedation for procedures (section 15.1.4), is not justified. There is a risk of habituation with prolonged use. Problems settling children at night should be managed with behavioural therapy.

Dental procedures Some anxious children may benefit from the use of a hypnotic the night before the dental appointment. Hypnotics do not relieve pain, and if pain interferes with sleep an appropriate analgesic should be given.

Chloral and derivatives

Chloral hydrate and derivatives were formerly popular hypnotics for children. **Triclofos** causes fewer gastro-intestinal disturbances than chloral hydrate.

Chloral hydrate and triclofos are now mainly used for sedation during diagnostic procedures (section 15.1.4) and in intensive care units. These drugs accumulate on prolonged use.

CHLORAL HYDRATE

Cautions reduce dose in debilitated; avoid prolonged use (and abrupt withdrawal thereafter); avoid contact with skin and mucous membranes; **interactions**: Appendix 1 (anxiolytics and hypnotics)

Skilled tasks Drowsiness may persist the next day and affect performance of skilled tasks (e.g. driving); effects of alcohol enhanced

Contra-indications severe cardiac disease; gastritis; acute porphyria (section 9.8.2)

Hepatic impairment can precipitate coma; reduce dose in mild to moderate hepatic impairment; avoid in severe impairment

Renal impairment avoid in severe impairment

Pregnancy avoid

Breast-feeding sedation in infant—avoid

Side-effects gastric irritation (nausea and vomiting reported), abdominal distention, flatulence, headache, tolerance, dependence, excitement, delirium (especially on abrupt withdrawal), ketonuria, and rash

Licensed use not licensed for sedation for painless procedures

Indication and dose

Insomnia (but not recommended)
- By mouth or by rectum (if oral route not available)

   Child 1 month–12 years 30–50 mg/kg (max. 1 g) at night

   Child 12–18 years 0.5–1 g (max. 2 g) at night

Sedation for painless procedures
- By mouth or by rectum (if oral route not available)

   Neonate 30–50 mg/kg 45–60 minutes before procedure; doses up to 100 mg/kg may be used with respiratory monitoring

   Child 1 month–12 years 30–50 mg/kg (max. 1 g) 45–60 minutes before procedure; higher doses up to 100 mg/kg (max. 2 g) may be used

   Child 12–18 years 1–2 g 45–60 minutes before procedure

Administration for administration *by mouth* dilute liquid with plenty of water or juice to mask unpleasant taste.

Chloral Mixture, BP 2000 PoM
(Chloral Oral Solution)
Mixture, chloral hydrate 500 mg/5 mL in a suitable vehicle. Available from 'special-order' manufacturers or specialist importing companies, see p. 957

◻ **CHLORAL HYDRATE** (*continued*)

Chloral Elixir, Paediatric, BP 2000 PoM
(Chloral Oral Solution, Paediatric)
Elixir, chloral hydrate 200 mg/5 mL (4%) in a suitable vehicle with a black currant flavour. Available from 'special-order' manufacturers or specialist importing companies, see p. 957

Chloral Hydrate (Non-proprietary) PoM
Suppositories, chloral hydrate 25 mg, 50 mg, 60 mg, 100 mg, 200 mg, 500 mg. Available from 'special-order' manufacturers or specialist importing companies, see p. 957

◢ Cloral betaine

Welldorm® (Alphashow) PoM
Tablets, blue-purple, f/c, cloral betaine 707 mg (≡ chloral hydrate 414 mg), net price 30-tab pack = £12.10. Label: 19, 27

Dose

> Short-term treatment of insomnia
> • By mouth
> **Child 12–18 years** 1–2 tablets with water or milk at bedtime, max. 5 tablets (chloral hydrate 2 g) daily

Elixir, red, chloral hydrate 143.3 mg/5 mL, net price 150-mL pack = £8.70. Label: 19, 27

Dose

> Short-term treatment of insomnia
> • By mouth
> **Child 2–12 years** 1–1.75 mL/kg (chloral hydrate 30–50 mg/kg) with water or milk at bedtime; max. 35 mL (chloral hydrate 1 g) daily
> **Child 12–18 years** 15–45 mL (chloral hydrate 0.4–1.3 g) with water or milk at bedtime; max. 70 mL (chloral hydrate 2 g) daily

---

◢ **TRICLOFOS SODIUM**

Cautions avoid prolonged use (and abrupt withdrawal thereafter); **interactions**: Appendix 1 (anxiolytics and hypnotics)

Skilled tasks Drowsiness may persist the next day and affect performance of skilled tasks (e.g. driving); effects of alcohol enhanced

Contra-indications cardiac disease; gastritis; acute porphyria (section 9.8.2)

Hepatic impairment can precipitate coma

Renal impairment start with small doses in severe impairment, increased cerebral sensitivity

Pregnancy avoid

Breast-feeding avoid

Side-effects abdominal distension, flatulence, gastric irritation including nausea and vomiting, dependence, malaise, ataxia, drowsiness, headache, lightheadedness, vertigo, confusion, paranoia, excitement, nightmares, delirium (especially on abrupt withdrawal), ketonuria, blood disorders, skin reactions, and urticaria

Licensed use not licensed for sedation for painless procedures

Indication and dose

> Insomnia (but not recommended)
> • By mouth
> **Child 1 month–1 year** 25–30 mg/kg at night
> **Child 1–5 years** 250–500 mg at night
> **Child 6–12 years** 0.5–1 g at night
> **Child 12–18 years** 1–2 g at night

> Sedation for painless procedures
> • By mouth
> **Neonate** 25–30 mg/kg 45–60 minutes before procedure
> **Child 1 month–18 years** 30–50 mg/kg (max. 2 g) 45–60 minutes before procedure; higher doses up to 100 mg/kg (max. 2 g) may be used but respiratory monitoring is required

Triclofos Oral Solution, BP PoM
(Triclofos Elixir)
Oral solution, triclofos sodium 500 mg/5 mL, net price 300 mL = £28.23. Label: 19

Antihistamines

Some **antihistamines** (section 3.4.1) such as promethazine are used for occasional insomnia in adults; their prolonged duration of action can often cause drowsiness the following day. The sedative effect of antihistamines may diminish after a few days of continued treatment; antihistamines are associated with headache, psychomotor impairment and antimuscarinic effects.

The use of antihistamines as hypnotics in children is not usually justified.

◢ **PROMETHAZINE HYDROCHLORIDE** ◿

Cautions see notes in section 3.4.1

Contra-indications see Promethazine Hydrochloride, section 3.4.1

Hepatic impairment see notes in section 3.4.1

Renal impairment use with caution

Pregnancy see notes in section 3.4.1

Breast-feeding see notes in section 3.4.1

Side-effects see Promethazine Hydrochloride, section 3.4.1

4
Central nervous system

□ **PROMETHAZINE HYDROCHLORIDE (continued)**

Licensed use not licensed for use in children under 2 years

Indication and dose

Sedation (short-term use)
- By mouth
  Child 2–5 years 15–20 mg
  Child 5–10 years 20–25 mg
  Child 10–18 years 25–50 mg

Sedation in intensive care
- By mouth or by slow intravenous injection or by deep intramuscular injection
  Child 1 month–12 years 0.5–1 mg/kg (max. 25 mg) 4 times daily, adjusted according to response
  Child 12–18 years 25–50 mg 4 times daily, adjusted according to response

Allergy and urticaria section 3.4.1

Nausea and vomiting section 4.6

[1]**Promethazine** (Non-proprietary) PoM
Injection, promethazine hydrochloride 25 mg/mL, net price 1-mL amp = 68p, 2-mL amp = £1.20
1. PoM restriction does not apply where administration is for saving life in emergency

[1]**Phenergan®** (Sanofi-Aventis) PoM
Injection, promethazine hydrochloride 25 mg/mL, net price 1-mL amp = 67p
1. PoM restriction does not apply where administration is for saving life in emergency

◢**Oral preparations**
Section 3.4.1

Melatonin

Melatonin is a pineal hormone which may affect sleep pattern. Clinical experience suggests that when appropriate behavioural sleep interventions fail, melatonin may be of value for treating sleep onset insomnia and delayed sleep phase syndrome in children with conditions such as visual impairment, cerebral palsy, attention deficit hyperactivity disorder, autism, and learning difficulties. It is also sometimes used before magnetic resonance imaging (MRI), computed tomography (CT), or EEG investigations. Little is known about its long-term effects in children, and there is uncertainty as to the effect on other circadian rhythms including endocrine or reproductive hormone secretion. Treatment with melatonin should be initiated and supervised by a specialist, but may be continued by general practitioners under a shared-care arrangement. The need for continuing melatonin therapy should be reviewed every 6 months.

Melatonin is available as a modified-release tablet (*Circadin®*) and also as unlicensed formulations. *Circadin®* is licensed for the short-term treatment of primary insomnia in adults over 55 years. Unlicensed immediate-release preparations may be more suitable for children; the manufacturer should be specified in the shared-care guideline because of variability in clinical effect of unlicensed formulations.

MELATONIN

Cautions autoimmune disease (manufacturer advises avoid—no information available); **interactions**: Appendix 1 (melatonin)

Hepatic impairment clearance of melatonin reduced—manufacturer advises avoid

Renal impairment no information available—caution

Pregnancy no information available—avoid

Breast-feeding present in milk—avoid

Side-effects abdominal pain, constipation, dry mouth, weight gain, drowsiness, dizziness, migraine, asthenia, sleep disorders, restlessness, nervousness, irritability, and sweating; *rarely* flatulence, halitosis, hypersalivation, vomiting, hypertriglyceridaemia, aggression, agitation, fatigue, impaired memory, mood changes, hot flushes, priapism, increased libido, leucopenia, thrombocytopenia, muscle cramp, lacrimation, visual disturbances, and skin reactions

Licensed use not licensed for use in children

Indication and dose

Sleep onset insomnia and delayed sleep phase syndrome (see notes above)
- By mouth
  Child 1 month–18 years initially 2–3 mg increased if necessary after 1–2 weeks to 4–6 mg; max. 10 mg daily

Circadin® (Lundbeck) ▼ PoM
Tablets, m/r, melatonin 2 mg, net price 21-tab pack = £10.77. Label: 2, 21, 25
Note Other formulations of melatonin are available from 'special-order' manufacturers or specialist importing companies, see p. 957

4.1.2 Anxiolytics

Anxiolytic treatment should be used in children only to relieve acute anxiety (and related insomnia) caused by fear (e.g. before surgery, section 15.1.4.1).

Anxiolytic treatment should be limited to the lowest possible dose for the shortest possible time (see p. 215).

Buspirone

Buspirone is thought to act at specific serotonin ($5HT_{1A}$) receptors; safety and efficacy in children have yet to be determined.

4.1.3 Barbiturates

Classification not used in *BNF for Children*.

4.2 Drugs used in psychoses and related disorders

4.2.1 Antipsychotic drugs
4.2.2 Antipsychotic depot injections
4.2.3 Antimanic drugs

Advice on doses of antipsychotic drugs above *BNF for Children* upper limit

1. Consider alternative approaches including adjuvant therapy.
2. Bear in mind risk factors, including obesity.
3. Consider potential for drug interactions—see **interactions**: Appendix 1 (antipsychotics).
4. Carry out ECG to exclude untoward abnormalities such as prolonged QT interval; repeat ECG periodically and reduce dose if prolonged QT interval or other adverse abnormality develops.
5. Increase dose slowly and not more often than once weekly.
6. Carry out regular pulse, blood pressure, and temperature checks; ensure that patient maintains adequate fluid intake.
7. Consider high-dose therapy to be for limited period and review regularly; abandon if no improvement after 3 months (return to standard dosage).

Important When prescribing an antipsychotic for administration on an emergency basis, the intramuscular dose should be **lower** than the corresponding oral dose (owing to absence of first-pass effect), particularly if the child is very active (increased blood flow to muscle considerably increases the rate of absorption). The prescription should specify the dose for **each route** and should **not** imply that the same dose can be given by mouth or by intramuscular injection. The dose of antipsychotic for emergency use should be reviewed at least **daily**.

4.2.1 Antipsychotic drugs

There is little information on the efficacy and safety of antipsychotic drugs in children and adolescents and much of the information available has been extrapolated from adult data; in particular, little is known about the long-term effects of antipsychotic drugs on the developing nervous system. Antipsychotic drugs should be initiated and managed under the close supervision of an appropriate specialist.

Antipsychotic drugs are also known as 'neuroleptics' and (misleadingly) as 'major tranquillisers'. Antipsychotic drugs generally tranquillise without impairing consciousness and without causing paradoxical excitement but they should not be regarded merely as tranquillisers. For conditions such as schizophrenia the tranquillising effect is of secondary importance.

In the short term they are used to calm disturbed children whatever the underlying psychopathology, which may be schizophrenia, brain damage, mania, toxic delirium, or agitated depression. Antipsychotic drugs are used to alleviate severe anxiety but this too should be a short-term measure.

Schizophrenia   Antipsychotic drugs relieve psychotic symptoms such as thought disorder, hallucinations, and delusions, and prevent relapse. Although they are usually less effective in apathetic withdrawn children, they sometimes appear to have an activating influence. Children with acute schizophrenia generally respond better than those with chronic symptoms. Children should receive antipsychotic drugs for 4–6 weeks before the drug is deemed ineffective.

Long-term treatment of a child with a definite diagnosis of schizophrenia may be necessary even after the first episode of illness in order to prevent the manifest illness from becoming chronic. Withdrawal of drug treatment requires careful surveillance because children who appear well on medication may suffer a disastrous relapse if treatment is withdrawn inappropriately. In addition the need for continuation of treatment may not become immediately evident because relapse is often delayed for several weeks after cessation of treatment.

Antipsychotic drugs are considered to act by interfering with dopaminergic transmission in the brain by blocking dopamine D_2 receptors, which may give rise to the extrapyramidal effects described below, and also to hyperprolactinaemia. Antipsychotic drugs may also affect cholinergic, alpha-adrenergic, histaminergic, and serotonergic receptors.

Choice of drug is influenced by the potential for side-effects and is often guided by individual circumstances e.g. the psychological effects of potential weight gain. The drugs most commonly used in children are haloperidol, risperidone, and olanzapine.

Cautions Assess child for movement disorders before starting treatment. Monitor neurological parameters, bowel habit, pulse, and blood pressure. Regular clinical monitoring of endocrine function should be considered when children are taking an antipsychotic known to increase prolactin levels; this includes measuring weight and height, assessing sexual maturation, and monitoring menstrual function. Children with schizophrenia should have physical health monitoring (including cardiovascular disease risk assessment) at least once per year.

Antipsychotic drugs should be used with **caution** in children with cardiovascular disease; an ECG may be required (see individual drug monographs), particularly if physical examination identifies cardiovascular risk factors, if there is a personal history of cardiovascular disease, or if the child is being admitted as an inpatient. Antipsychotic drugs should also be used with caution in children with epilepsy (and conditions predisposing to epilepsy), depression, myasthenia gravis (avoid chlorpromazine, pericyazine and prochlorperazine in these conditions) or a susceptibility to angle-closure glaucoma. Caution is also required in severe respiratory disease and in children with a history of jaundice or who have blood dyscrasias (perform blood counts if unexplained infection or fever develops). As photosensitisation may occur with higher dosages, children should avoid direct sunlight. **Interactions:** Appendix 1 (antipsychotics).

Contra-indications Antipsychotic drugs may be **contra-indicated** in comatose states, CNS depression, and phaeochromocytoma.

Skilled tasks Drowsiness may affect performance of skilled tasks (e.g. driving or operating machinery), especially at start of treatment; effects of alcohol are enhanced.

Withdrawal There is a high risk of relapse if medication is stopped after 1–2 years. Withdrawal of antipsychotic drugs after long-term therapy should always be gradual and closely monitored to avoid the risk of acute withdrawal syndromes or rapid relapse. Children should be monitored regularly for signs and symptoms of relapse for 2 years after withdrawal of antipsychotic medication.

Hepatic impairment All antipsychotics can precipitate coma if used in hepatic impairment; phenothiazines are hepatotoxic.

Renal impairment Start with small doses of antipsychotic drugs in severe renal impairment because of increased cerebral sensitivity. Pericyazine should be avoided in renal impairment.

Pregnancy Extrapyramidal effects have been reported occasionally in the neonate when antipsychotic drugs are taken during the third trimester of pregnancy.

Breast-feeding Although the amount present in milk is probably too small to be harmful, *animal* studies indicate possible adverse effects of antipsychotic medicines on the developing nervous system. Treatment with antipsychotics whilst breast-feeding should be avoided unless absolutely necessary.

Side-effects   Extrapyramidal symptoms are the most troublesome. They occur most frequently with the piperazine phenothiazines (such as perphenazine, prochlorperazine, and trifluoperazine), the butyrophenones (such as haloperidol), and the depot preparations. They are easy to recognise but cannot be predicted accurately because they depend on the dose, the type of drug, and on individual susceptibility.

Extrapyramidal symptoms consist of:

- *parkinsonian symptoms* (including tremor), which may appear gradually (but less commonly than in adults);

- *dystonia* (abnormal face and body movements) and *dyskinesia*, which appear after only a few doses;

- *akathisia* (restlessness), which characteristically occurs after large initial doses and may resemble an exacerbation of the condition being treated; and

- *tardive dyskinesia* (rhythmic, involuntary movements of tongue, face, and jaw), which usually develops on long-term therapy or with high dosage, but it may develop on short-term treatment with low doses—short-lived tardive dyskinesia may occur after withdrawal of the drug.

Parkinsonian symptoms remit if the drug is withdrawn and may be suppressed by the administration of **antimuscarinic** drugs (section 4.9.2). However, routine administration of such drugs is not justified because not all children are affected and because they may unmask or worsen tardive dyskinesia.

Tardive dyskinesia is of particular concern because it may be irreversible on withdrawing therapy and treatment is usually ineffective. However, some manufacturers suggest that drug withdrawal at the earliest signs of tardive dyskinesia (fine vermicular movements of the tongue) may halt its full development. Tardive dyskinesia may occur and treatment must be carefully and regularly reviewed.

Hypotension and interference with temperature regulation are dose-related side-effects.

Neuroleptic malignant syndrome (hyperthermia, fluctuating level of consciousness, muscle rigidity, and autonomic dysfunction with pallor, tachycardia, labile blood pressure, sweating, and urinary incontinence) is a rare but potentially fatal side-effect of some antipsychotic drugs. Discontinuation of the antipsychotic is essential because there is no proven effective treatment, but cooling, bromocriptine, and dantrolene have been used. The syndrome, which usually lasts for 5–7 days after drug discontinuation, may be unduly prolonged if depot preparations have been used.

Other side-effects include: drowsiness; apathy; agitation, excitement and insomnia; convulsions; dizziness; headache; confusion; gastro-intestinal disturbances; nasal congestion; antimuscarinic symptoms (such as dry mouth, constipation, difficulty with micturition, and blurred vision; *very rarely* angle-closure glaucoma); cardiovascular symptoms (such as hypotension, tachycardia, and arrhythmias); ECG changes (cases of sudden death have occurred); endocrine effects such as menstrual disturbances, galactorrhoea, gynaecomastia, impotence, and weight gain; blood dyscrasias (such as agranulocytosis and leucopenia), photosensitisation, contact sensitisation and rashes, and jaundice (including cholestatic); corneal and lens opacities, and purplish pigmentation of the skin, cornea, conjunctiva, and retina.

Overdosage: for poisoning with phenothiazines and related compounds, see Emergency Treatment of Poisoning, p. 42.

Classification of antipsychotics   The **phenothiazine** derivatives can be divided into 3 main groups.

Group 1: chlorpromazine, levomepromazine (methotrimeprazine), and promazine, generally characterised by pronounced sedative effects and moderate antimuscarinic and extrapyramidal side-effects.

Group 2: pericyazine and pipotiazine, generally characterised by moderate sedative effects, marked antimuscarinic effects, but fewer extrapyramidal side-effects than groups 1 or 3.

Group 3: perphenazine, prochlorperazine, and trifluoperazine, generally characterised by fewer sedative effects, fewer antimuscarinic effects, but more pronounced extrapyramidal side-effects than groups 1 and 2.

Drugs of other chemical groups resemble the phenothiazines of *group 3* in their clinical properties. They include the **butyrophenones** (e.g. haloperidol); **diphenylbutylpiperidines** (e.g. pimozide); **thioxanthenes** (flupentixol and zuclopenthixol); and the **substituted benzamides** (e.g. sulpiride).

For details of the newer antipsychotic drugs amisulpride, aripiprazole, clozapine, olanzapine, quetiapine, and risperidone, see under Atypical Antipsychotic Drugs, p. 226.

Choice   As indicated above, the various drugs differ somewhat in predominant actions and side-effects. Selection is influenced by the degree of sedation required and the child's susceptibility to extrapyramidal side-effects. However, the differences between antipsychotic drugs are less important than the great variability in response; moreover, tolerance to secondary effects such as sedation usually develops. The atypical antipsychotic drugs may be appropriate if extrapyramidal side-effects are a particular concern (see under Atypical Antipsychotic Drugs, p. 226). **Clozapine** is used for schizrenia when other antipsychotic drugs are ineffective or not tolerated.

Prescribing of more than one antipsychotic drug at the same time is **not** recommended; it may constitute a hazard and there is no significant evidence that side-effects are minimised.

Chlorpromazine is associated with a wide range of adverse effects, including marked sedation.

Pimozide is less sedating than chlorpromazine. Although pimozide is licensed for use in children, it is not used because of the risk of serious cardiac side-effects (see ECG Monitoring, p. 225).

Sulpiride in high doses controls florid positive symptoms, but in lower doses it has an alerting effect on patients with apathetic withdrawn schizophrenia.

Haloperidol and **trifluoperazine** are also licensed for use in children but their use is limited by the high incidence of extrapyramidal symptoms. Haloperidol may be preferred for the rapid control of hyperactive psychotic states; it causes less hypotension than chlorpromazine.

Other uses   Nausea and vomiting (section 4.6), choreas, motor tics, and intractable hiccup.

Equivalent doses of oral antipsychotic drugs	
These equivalences are intended **only** as an approximate guide; individual dosage instructions should **also** be checked; children should be carefully monitored after **any** change in medication	
Antipsychotic drug	Daily dose
Chlorpromazine	100 mg
Clozapine	50 mg
Haloperidol	2–3 mg
Pimozide	2 mg
Risperidone	0.5–1 mg
Sulpiride	200 mg
Trifluoperazine	5 mg
Important These equivalences must **not** be extrapolated beyond the max. dose for the drug. Higher doses require careful titration in specialist units and the equivalences shown here may not be appropriate	

Dosage
After an initial period of stabilisation, the total daily oral dose of antipsychotic drugs can be given as a single dose in most children. For advice on doses above the *BNF for Children* upper limit, see p. 219.

CHLORPROMAZINE HYDROCHLORIDE

Warning Owing to the risk of contact sensitisation, pharmacists, nurses, and other health workers should avoid direct contact with chlorpromazine; tablets should not be crushed and solutions should be handled with care

Cautions   see notes above; also children should remain supine, with blood pressure monitoring

for 30 minutes after intramuscular injection; dose adjustment may be necessary if smoking started or stopped during treatment

Contra-indications   see notes above; hypothyroidism

◻ **CHLORPROMAZINE HYDROCHLORIDE** (*continued*)

Hepatic impairment see notes above
Renal impairment see notes above
Pregnancy see notes above
Breast-feeding see notes above
Side-effects see notes above; also hyperglycaemia; intramuscular injection may cause hypotension and tachycardia

Indication and dose

> **Childhood schizophrenia and other psychoses** (under specialist supervision)
> • **By mouth**
>> **Child 1–6 years** 500 micrograms/kg every 4–6 hours adjusted according to response (max. 40 mg daily)
>> **Child 6–12 years** 10 mg 3 times daily, adjusted according to response (max. 75 mg daily)
>> **Child 12–18 years** 25 mg 3 times daily (*or* 75 mg at night), adjusted according to response, to usual maintenance dose of 75–300 mg daily (but up to 1 g daily may be required)

> **Relief of acute symptoms of psychoses** (under specialist supervision) but see also Cautions and Side-effects
> • **By deep intramuscular injection**
>> **Child 1–6 years** 500 micrograms/kg every 6–8 hours (max. 40 mg daily)
>> **Child 6–12 years** 500 micrograms/kg every 6–8 hours (max. 75 mg daily)
>> **Child 12–18 years** 25–50 mg every 6–8 hours

> **Induction of hypothermia (to prevent shivering)** (under specialist supervision)
> • **By deep intramuscular injection**
>> **Child 1–12 years** initially 0.5–1 mg/kg, followed by maintenance 500 micrograms/kg every 4–6 hours
>> **Child 12–18 years** 25–50 mg every 6–8 hours

Chlorpromazine (Non-proprietary) ℗ₒₘ
Tablets, coated, chlorpromazine hydrochloride 25 mg, 28-tab pack = £2.74; 50 mg, 28-tab pack = £3.26; 100 mg, 28-tab pack = £3.41. Label: 2, 11
Brands include *Chloractil*®

Oral solution, chlorpromazine hydrochloride 25 mg/5 mL, net price 150 mL = £1.50, 100 mg/5 mL, 150 mL = £3.76. Label: 2, 11

Injection, chlorpromazine hydrochloride 25 mg/mL, net price 1-mL amp = 60p; 2-mL amp = 63p

Largactil® (Sanofi-Aventis) ℗ₒₘ
Injection, chlorpromazine hydrochloride 25 mg/mL. Net price 2-mL amp = 60p

▲ **HALOPERIDOL**

Cautions see notes above; also subarachnoid haemorrhage and metabolic disturbances such as hypokalaemia, hypocalcaemia, or hypomagnesaemia; dose adjustment may be necessary if smoking started or stopped during treatment
Contra-indications see notes above; QT-interval prolongation (avoid concomitant administration of drugs that prolong QT interval); bradycardia
Hepatic impairment see notes above
Renal impairment see notes above
Pregnancy see notes above
Breast-feeding see notes above
Side-effects see notes above, but less sedating and fewer antimuscarinic or hypotensive symptoms; pigmentation and photosensitivity reactions rare; extrapyramidal symptoms, particularly dystonic reactions and akathisia especially in thyrotoxic patients; weight loss; *less commonly* dyspnoea; oedema; *rarely* bronchospasm; hypoglycaemia; inappropriate antidiuretic hormone secretion; venous thromboembolism, Stevens-Johnson syndrome, toxic epidermal necrolysis, and hypothermia also reported
Licensed use not licensed for use in children for nausea and vomiting in palliative care

Indication and dose

> **Schizophrenia and other psychoses, mania, short-term adjunctive management of psychomotor agitation, excitement and violent or dangerously impulsive behaviour** (under specialist supervision)
> • **By mouth**
>> **Child 12–18 years** initially 0.5–3 mg 2–3 times daily *or* 3–5 mg 2–3 times daily in severely affected or resistant disease; in resistant schizophrenia up to 30 mg daily may be needed; adjusted according to response to lowest effective maintenance dose (as low as 5–10 mg daily)

> **Motor tics (including Tourette syndrome)** (under specialist supervision)
> • **By mouth**
>> **Child 5–12 years** 12.5–25 micrograms/kg twice daily, adjusted according to response up to 10 mg daily
>> **Child 12–18 years** 1.5 mg 3 times daily, adjusted according to response up to 10 mg daily

> **Nausea and vomiting in palliative care**
> • **By mouth**
>> **Child 12–18 years** 1.5 mg once daily at night, increased to 1.5 mg twice daily if necessary; max. 5 mg twice daily
> • **By continuous intravenous or subcutaneous infusion**
>> **Child 1 month–12 years** 25–85 micrograms/kg over 24 hours
>> **Child 12–18 years** 1.5–5 mg over 24 hours

Haloperidol (Non-proprietary) ℗ₒₘ
Tablets, haloperidol 500 micrograms, net price 28-tab pack = 91p; 1.5 mg, 28-tab pack = £1.49; 5 mg, 28-tab pack = £2.52; 10 mg, 28-tab pack = £4.70; 20 mg, 28-tab pack = £11.95. Label: 2

Dozic® (Rosemont) ℗ₒₘ
Oral liquid, sugar-free, haloperidol 1 mg/mL, net price 100-mL pack = £6.86. Label: 2

4
Central nervous system

◻ **HALOPERIDOL (continued)**

Haldol® (Janssen-Cilag) PoM
Tablets, both scored, haloperidol 5 mg (blue), net price 100-tab pack = £7.35; 10 mg (yellow), 100-tab pack = £14.37. Label: 2

Oral liquid, sugar-free, haloperidol 2 mg/mL, net price 100-mL pack (with pipette) = £4.54. Label: 2

Injection, haloperidol 5 mg/mL, net price 1-mL amp = 29p

Serenace® (IVAX) PoM
Capsules, green, haloperidol 500 micrograms, net price 30-cap pack = 98p. Label: 2

Tablets, haloperidol 1.5 mg, net price 30-tab pack = £1.37; 5 mg (pink), 30-tab pack = £3.95; 10 mg (pale pink), 30-tab pack = £6.76. Label: 2

Oral liquid, sugar-free, haloperidol 2 mg/mL, net price 500-mL pack = £34.48. Label: 2

LEVOMEPROMAZINE
(Methotrimeprazine)

Cautions see notes above; children receiving large initial doses should remain supine

Contra-indications see notes above

Hepatic impairment see notes above

Renal impairment see notes above

Pregnancy see notes above

Breast-feeding see notes above

Side-effects see notes above; occasionally raised erythrocyte sedimentation rate occurs

Indication and dose

> Restlessness and confusion in palliative care
> * By continuous subcutaneous infusion
>   **Child 1–12 years** 0.35–3 mg/kg over 24 hours
>   **Child 12–18 years** 12.5–200 mg over 24 hours

> Nausea and vomiting in palliative care
> * By continuous intravenous or subcutaneous infusion
>   **Child 1 month–12 years** 100–400 micrograms/kg over 24 hours
>   **Child 12–18 years** 5–25 mg over 24 hours

Administration for administration by *subcutaneous infusion* dilute with a suitable volume of Sodium Chloride 0.9%

Nozinan® (Archimedes) PoM
Tablets, scored, levomepromazine maleate 25 mg, net price 84-tab pack = £20.26. Label: 2

Injection, levomepromazine hydrochloride 25 mg/mL, net price 1-mL amp = £2.01

PERICYAZINE
(Periciazine)

Cautions see notes above

Contra-indications see notes above

Hepatic impairment see notes above

Renal impairment see notes above

Pregnancy see notes above

Breast-feeding see notes above

Side-effects see notes above; more sedating; hypotension common when treatment initiated; respiratory depression

Licensed use tablets not licensed for use in children

Indication and dose

> Schizophrenia, psychoses (severe mental or behavioural disorders only) (under specialist supervision)
> * By mouth
>   **Child 1–12 years** initially 500 micrograms daily for 10-kg child, increased by 1 mg for each additional 5 kg to max. total daily dose of 10 mg; dose may be gradually increased according to response but maintenance should not exceed twice initial dose
>   **Child 12–18 years** initially 25 mg 3 times daily increased at weekly intervals by steps of 25 mg according to response; usual max. 100 mg 3 times daily; total daily dose may alternatively be given in 2 divided doses

Pericyazine (Non-proprietary) PoM
Tablets, yellow, scored, pericyazine 2.5 mg, net price 84-tab pack = £9.23; 10 mg, 84-tab pack = £24.95. Label: 2

Syrup forte, brown, pericyazine 10 mg/5 mL, net price 100-mL pack = £12.08. Label: 2

PERPHENAZINE

Cautions see notes above; hypothyroidism

Contra-indications see notes above

Hepatic impairment see notes above

Renal impairment see notes above

Pregnancy see notes above

Breast-feeding see notes above

Side-effects see notes above; less sedating; extrapyramidal symptoms, especially dystonia, more frequent, particularly at high dosage; *rarely* systemic lupus erythematosus

Indication and dose

> Schizophrenia and other psychoses, mania, short-term adjunctive management of anxiety, severe psychomotor agitation, excitement, violent or dangerously impulsive behaviour (under specialist supervision)
> * By mouth
>   **Child 14–18 years** initially 4 mg 3 times daily adjusted according to the response; max. 24 mg daily

4 Central nervous system

◁ **PERPHENAZINE (continued)**

Fentazin® (Goldshield) PoM
Tablets, both s/c, perphenazine 2 mg, net price
100-tab pack = £22.38; 4 mg, 100-tab pack =
£26.34. Label: 2

PIMOZIDE

Cautions see notes above
ECG monitoring Following reports of sudden unexplained
death, an ECG is recommended before treatment. It is
also recommended that patients taking pimozide should
have an annual ECG (if the QT interval is prolonged,
treatment should be reviewed and either withdrawn or
dose reduced under close supervision) and that pimozide
should **not** be given with other antipsychotic drugs
(including depot preparations), tricyclic antidepressants
or other drugs which prolong the QT interval, such as
certain antimalarials, anti-arrhythmic drugs and certain
antihistamines and should **not** be given with drugs which
cause electrolyte disturbances (especially diuretics)

Contra-indications see notes above; history of
arrhythmias or congenital QT prolongation

Hepatic impairment see notes above

Renal impairment see notes above

Pregnancy see notes above

Breast-feeding see notes above

Side-effects see notes above; less sedating; serious arrhythmias, venous thromboembolism,
glycosuria, and *rarely*, hyponatraemia reported

Licensed use not licensed for use in Tourette
syndrome

Indication and dose

Schizophrenia (under specialist supervision)
● By mouth
Child 12–18 years initially 1 mg daily, increased
according to response in steps of 2–4 mg at
intervals of not less than 1 week; usual dose
range 2–20 mg daily

Tourette syndrome (under specialist supervision)
● By mouth
Child 2–12 years 1–4 mg daily
Child 12–18 years 2–10 mg daily

Orap® (Janssen-Cilag) PoM
Tablets, scored, green, pimozide 4 mg, net price
100-tab pack = £27.41. Label: 2

SULPIRIDE

Cautions see notes above; also excited, agitated,
or aggressive children (even low doses may
aggravate symptoms)

Contra-indications see notes above; also acute
porphyria (section 9.8.2)

Hepatic impairment see notes above

Renal impairment see notes above

Pregnancy see notes above

Breast-feeding see notes above

Side-effects see notes above; also hepatitis and
venous thromboembolism

Licensed use not licensed for use in Tourette
syndrome

Indication and dose

Schizophrenia (under specialist supervision)
● By mouth
Child 14–18 years 200–400 mg twice daily;
max. 800 mg daily in predominantly negative
symptoms, dose increased to max. 2.4 g daily in
mainly positive symptoms

Tourette syndrome (under specialist supervision)
● By mouth
Child 2–12 years 50–400 mg twice daily
Child 12–18 years 100–400 mg twice daily

Sulpiride (Non-proprietary) PoM
Tablets, sulpiride 200 mg, net price 30-tab pack =
£8.51; 56-tab pack = £6.46; 400 mg, 30-tab pack =
£12.42. Label: 2

Dolmatil® (Sanofi-Aventis) PoM
Tablets, both scored, sulpiride 200 mg, net price
100-tab pack = £13.31; 400 mg (f/c), 100-tab pack
= £34.87. Label: 2

Sulpor® (Rosemont) PoM
Oral solution, sugar-free, lemon- and aniseed-fla-
voured, sulpiride 200 mg/5 mL, net price 150 mL =
£25.38. Label: 2

TRIFLUOPERAZINE

Cautions see notes above

Contra-indications see notes above

Hepatic impairment see notes above

Renal impairment see notes above

Pregnancy see notes above

Breast-feeding see notes above

Side-effects see notes above; extrapyramidal
symptoms more frequent, especially at doses
exceeding 6 mg daily; pancytopenia; thrombocytopenia; hyperthermia; anorexia; muscle weakness

Indication and dose

Schizophrenia and other psychoses, short-term
adjunctive management of psychomotor agitation, excitement and violent or dangerously
impulsive behaviour (under specialist supervision)
● By mouth
Child 12–18 years initially 5 mg twice daily,
increased by 5 mg daily after 1 week, then at
intervals of 3 days, according to response

4

Central nervous system

◻ **TRIFLUOPERAZINE** (*continued*)

Short-term adjunctive management of severe anxiety (under specialist supervision)
• By mouth

Child 3–6 years up to 500 micrograms twice daily

Child 6–12 years up to 2 mg twice daily

Child 12–18 years 1–2 mg twice daily, increased if necessary to 3 mg twice daily

Antiemetic section 4.6

Trifluoperazine (Non-proprietary) ℗ₒₘ
Tablets, coated, trifluoperazine (as hydrochloride) 1 mg, net price 100-tab pack = £6.10; 5 mg, 100-tab pack = £5.32. Label: 2

Oral solution, trifluoperazine (as hydrochloride) 5 mg/5 mL, net price 150-mL pack = £9.49. Label: 2

Stelazine® (Goldshield) ℗ₒₘ
Tablets, blue, f/c, trifluoperazine (as hydrochloride) 1 mg, net price 112-tab pack = £3.43; 5 mg, 112-tab pack = £4.89. Label: 2

Syrup, sugar-free, yellow, trifluoperazine (as hydrochloride) 1 mg/5 mL, net price 200-mL pack = £2.95. Label: 2

Atypical antipsychotic drugs

The 'atypical antipsychotic' drugs **amisulpride, aripiprazole, clozapine, olanzapine, quetiapine,** and **risperidone** may be better tolerated than other antipsychotic drugs; extrapyramidal symptoms may be less frequent than with older antipsychotic drugs.

Clozapine, olanzapine, and quetiapine cause little or no elevation of prolactin concentration; when changing from other antipsychotic drugs, a reduction in prolactin may increase fertility.

Clozapine is used for the treatment of schizophrenia only in children unresponsive to, or intolerant of, conventional antipsychotic drugs. It can cause agranulocytosis and its use is restricted to patients registered with a clozapine Patient Monitoring Service (see under Clozapine).

Cautions and contra-indications While atypical antipsychotic drugs have not generally been associated with clinically significant prolongation of the QT interval, they should be used with care if prescribed with other drugs that increase the QT interval. Atypical antipsychotic drugs should be used with caution in children with cardiovascular disease, or a history of epilepsy; **interactions:** Appendix 1 (antipsychotics).

Skilled tasks Atypical antipsychotic drugs may affect performance of skilled tasks (e.g. driving); effects of alcohol are enhanced.

Withdrawal Withdrawal of antipsychotic drugs after long-term therapy should always be gradual and closely monitored to avoid the risk of acute withdrawal syndromes or rapid relapse.

Side-effects Side-effects of the atypical antipsychotic drugs include weight gain, dizziness, postural hypotension (especially during initial dose titration) which may be associated with syncope or reflex tachycardia in some children, extrapyramidal symptoms (usually mild and transient and which respond to dose reduction or to an antimuscarinic drug), and occasionally tardive dyskinesia on long-term administration (discontinue drug on appearance of early signs). Hyperglycaemia and sometimes diabetes can occur, particularly with clozapine, olanzapine and risperidone; monitoring weight and plasma-glucose concentration may identify the development of hyperglycaemia. Neuroleptic malignant syndrome has been reported rarely. Hypersalivation associated with clozapine therapy can be treated with hyoscine hydrobromide (p. 252), provided that the patient is not at particular risk from the additive antimuscarinic side-effects of hyoscine and clozapine.

AMISULPRIDE

Cautions see notes above
Contra-indications see notes above; phaeochromocytoma, prolactin-dependent tumours
Renal impairment halve dose if estimated glomerular filtration rate 30–60 mL/minute/1.73 m²; use one-third dose if estimated glomerular filtra-

tion rate 10–30 mL/minute/1.73 m²; no information available if estimated glomerular filtration rate less than 10 mL/minute/1.73 m²
Pregnancy avoid
Breast-feeding avoid—no information available

⌂ **AMISULPRIDE (continued)**

Side-effects see notes above; also insomnia, anxiety, agitation, drowsiness, gastro-intestinal disorders such as constipation, nausea, vomiting, and dry mouth; hyperprolactinaemia; *occasionally* bradycardia; *rarely* seizures

Indication and dose

> **Acute psychotic episode** (under specialist supervision)
> • By mouth
> **Child 15–18 years** 200–400 mg twice daily adjusted according to response; max. 1.2 g daily

> **Predominantly negative symptoms** (under specialist supervision)
> • By mouth
> **Child 15–18 years** 50–300 mg daily

Amisulpride (Non-proprietary) ℗ₒₘ
Tablets, amisulpride 50 mg, net price 60-tab pack = £12.04; 100 mg, 60-tab pack = £32.39; 200 mg, 60-tab pack = £25.48; 400 mg, 60-tab pack = £111.29. Label: 2

Solian® (Sanofi-Aventis) ℗ₒₘ
Tablets, scored, amisulpride 50 mg, net price 60-tab pack = £22.76; 100 mg, 60-tab pack = £35.29; 200 mg, 60-tab pack = £58.99, 400 mg, 60-tab pack = £117.97. Label: 2

Solution, 100 mg/mL, net price 60 mL (caramel flavour) = £33.76. Label: 2

ARIPIPRAZOLE

Cautions see notes above; cerebrovascular disease

Contra-indications see notes above

Hepatic impairment use with caution in severe impairment

Pregnancy use only if potential benefit outweighs risk—no information available

Breast-feeding avoid—present in milk in *animal* studies

Side-effects see notes above; gastro-intestinal disturbances; tachycardia; fatigue, insomnia, agitation, akathesia, drowsiness, restlessness, tremor, headache, asthenia; blurred vision; *less commonly* depression; *very rarely* anorexia, dysphagia, oropharangeal spasm, laryngospasm, hepatitis, jaundice, hypersalivation, pancreatitis, oedema, thromboembolism, arrhythmias, bradycardia, hypertension, chest pain, anxiety, speech disorder, suicidal ideation, seizures, hyponatraemia, stiffness, myalgia, rhabdomyolysis, priapism, urinary retention and incontinence, blood disorders, sweating, alopecia, photosensitivity reactions, rash, and impaired temperature regulation

Licensed use not licensed for use in children under 15 years; not licensed for treating mania in children

Indication and dose

> **Schizophrenia and mania** (under specialist supervision)
> • By mouth
> **Child 13–18 years** 2 mg once daily, increased to 5 mg once daily after 2 days, then further increased to 10 mg once daily after a further 2 days; further increased if necessary in steps of 5 mg to max. 30 mg daily

Abilify® (Bristol-Myers Squibb) ℗ₒₘ
Tablets, aripiprazole 5 mg (blue), net price 28-tab pack = £97.67; 10 mg (pink), 28-tab pack = £97.67; 15 mg (yellow), 28-tab pack = £97.67; 30 mg (pink), 28-tab pack = £195.33. Label: 2

Orodispersible tablets, aripiprazole 10 mg (pink), net price 28-tab pack = £97.67; 15 mg (yellow), 28-tab pack = £97.67. Label: 2, counselling, administration
Excipients include aspartame (section 9.4.1)
Counselling Tablets should be placed on the tongue and allowed to dissolve, or be dispersed in water and swallowed

Oral solution, aripiprazole 1 mg/mL, net price 150 mL with measuring cup = £104.64. Label: 2

CLOZAPINE

Cautions see notes above; monitor leucocyte and differential blood counts (see Agranulocytosis, below); susceptibility to angle-closure glaucoma; taper off other antipsychotics before starting; close medical supervision during initiation (risk of collapse because of hypotension); dose adjustment may be necessary if smoking started or stopped during treatment
Withdrawal On planned withdrawal reduce dose over 1–2 weeks to avoid risk of rebound psychosis. If abrupt withdrawal necessary observe child carefully

Agranulocytosis Neutropenia and potentially fatal agranulocytosis reported. Leucocyte and differential blood counts must be normal before starting; monitor counts every week for 18 weeks then at least every 2 weeks and if clozapine continued and blood count stable after 1 year at least every 4 weeks (and 4 weeks after

discontinuation); if leucocyte count below 3000/mm³ or if absolute neutrophil count below 1500/mm³ discontinue permanently and refer to haematologist. Patients who have a low white blood cell count because of benign ethnic neutropenia may be started on clozapine with the agreement of a haematologist. Avoid drugs which depress leucopoiesis; children (or carers) should report immediately symptoms of infection, especially influenza-like illness
Myocarditis and cardiomyopathy Fatal myocarditis (most commonly in first 2 months) and cardiomyopathy reported.

• Perform physical examination and take full medical history before starting;

• Specialist examination required if cardiac abnormalities or history of heart disease found—clozapine initiated only in absence of severe heart disease and if benefit outweighs risk;

4 Central nervous system

◻ **CLOZAPINE** (*continued*)

- Persistent tachycardia especially in first 2 months should prompt observation for other indicators for myocarditis or cardiomyopathy;
- If myocarditis or cardiomyopathy suspected clozapine should be stopped and child evaluated urgently by cardiologist;
- Discontinue permanently in clozapine-induced myocarditis or cardiomyopathy

Gastro-intestinal obstruction Reactions resembling gastro-intestinal obstruction reported. Clozapine should be used cautiously with drugs which cause constipation (e.g. antimuscarinic drugs) or in children with history of colonic disease or bowel surgery. Monitor for constipation and prescribe laxative if required

Contra-indications severe cardiac disorders (e.g. myocarditis; see Cautions); history of neutropenia or agranulocytosis (see Cautions); bone-marrow disorders; paralytic ileus (see Cautions); alcoholic and toxic psychoses; history of circulatory collapse; drug intoxication; coma or severe CNS depression; uncontrolled epilepsy

Hepatic impairment monitor hepatic function regularly; avoid in symptomatic or progressive liver disease or hepatic failure

Renal impairment avoid in severe impairment

Pregnancy use with caution

Breast-feeding avoid

Side-effects see notes above; also constipation (see Cautions), hypersalivation, dry mouth, nausea, vomiting, anorexia; tachycardia, ECG changes, hypertension; drowsiness, dizziness, headache, tremor, seizures, fatigue, impaired temperature regulation; urinary incontinence and retention; leucopenia, eosinophilia, leucocytosis; blurred vision; sweating; *less commonly* agranulocytosis (**important**: see Cautions); *rarely* dysphagia, hepatitis, cholestatic jaundice, pancreatitis, circulatory collapse, arrhythmia, myocarditis (**important**: see Cautions), pericarditis, thromboembolism, agitation, confusion, delirium, anaemia; *very rarely* parotid gland enlargement, intestinal obstruction (see Cautions), cardiomyopathy, myocardial infarction, respiratory depression, priapism, interstitial nephritis, thrombocytopenia, thrombocythaemia, hypertriglyceridaemia, hypercholesterolaemia, hyperlipidaemia, fulminant hepatic necrosis, angle-closure glaucoma, and skin reactions

Licensed use not licensed for use in children under 16 years

Indication and dose

Schizophrenia in children unresponsive to, or intolerant of, conventional antipsychotic drugs (under specialist supervision)

- **By mouth**

  Child 12–18 years 12.5 mg once or twice on first day then 25–50 mg on second day then increased gradually (if well tolerated) in steps of 25–50 mg daily over 14–21 days up to 300 mg daily in divided doses (larger dose at night, up to 200 mg daily may be taken as a single dose at bedtime); if necessary may be further increased in steps of 50–100 mg once (preferably) or twice weekly; usual dose 200–450 mg daily (max. 900 mg daily)

  Note *Restarting* after *interval of more than 2 days*, 12.5 mg once or twice on first day (but may be feasible to increase more quickly than on initiation)—extreme caution if previous respiratory or cardiac arrest with initial dosing

Clozaril® (Novartis) ▣ᴾᴼᴹ
Tablets, yellow, clozapine 25 mg (scored), net price 28-tab pack = £6.17, 84-tab pack (hosp. only) = £18.49; 100 mg, 28-tab pack = £24.64, 84-tab pack (hosp. only) = £73.92. Label: 2, 10, patient information leaflet

Note Child, prescriber, and supplying pharmacist must be registered with the Clozaril Patient Monitoring Service—takes several days to do this

Denzapine® (Merz) ▣ᴾᴼᴹ
Tablets, yellow, scored, clozapine 25 mg, net price 28-tab pack = £6.17, 84-tab pack = £18.49; 50 mg, 50-tab pack = £22.00; 100 mg, 28-tab pack = £24.64, 84-tab pack = £73.92; 200 mg, 50-tab pack = £88.00. Label: 2, 10, patient information leaflet

Suspension, clozapine 50 mg/mL, net price 100 mL = £44.00. Label: 2, 10, patient information leaflet, counselling, administration

Counselling Shake well for 90 seconds when dispensing or if visibly settled; otherwise shake well for 10 seconds before use

Note May be diluted in water

Note Child, prescriber, and supplying pharmacist must be registered with the Denzapine Patient Monitoring Service—takes several days to do this

Zaponex® (TEVA UK) ▣ᴾᴼᴹ
Tablets, yellow, scored, clozapine 25 mg, net price 84-tab pack = £8.28; 100 mg, 84-tab pack = £33.88. Label: 2, 10, patient information leaflet

Note Child, prescriber, and supplying pharmacist must be registered with the Zaponex Treatment Access System—takes several days to do this

▰ OLANZAPINE

Cautions see notes above; also susceptibility to angle-closure glaucoma, paralytic ileus, diabetes mellitus (risk of exacerbation or ketoacidosis), low leucocyte or neutrophil count, bone-marrow depression, hyper-eosinophilic disorders, myeloproliferative disease; dose adjustment may be necessary if smoking started or stopped during treatment

Hepatic impairment initial dose 5 mg daily, increased slowly

Renal impairment initial dose 5 mg daily, increased slowly

Pregnancy use only if potential benefit outweighs risk; neonatal lethargy, tremor and hypertonia reported when used in third trimester

Breast-feeding avoid—present in milk

Side-effects see notes above; also mild, transient antimuscarinic effects; drowsiness, speech difficulty, abnormal gait, hallucinations, akathisia, asthenia, increased appetite, increased body temperature, raised triglyceride concentration,

◻ **OLANZAPINE** (*continued*)

oedema, hyperprolactinaemia (but clinical manifestations rare); urinary incontinence; eosinophilia; *less commonly* hypotension, bradycardia,
QT interval prolongation, and photosensitivity;
rarely seizures, leucopenia, and rash; *very rarely*
hepatitis, pancreatitis, thromboembolism, hypercholesterolaemia, hypothermia, urinary retention, priapism, thrombocytopenia, neutropenia,
rhabdomyolysis, and angle-closure glaucoma;
with injection, injection-site reactions, sinus pause,
hypoventilation

Licensed use not licensed for use in children

Indication and dose

> Schizophrenia, combination therapy for mania
> (under specialist supervision)
> • By mouth
>> **Child 12–18 years** initially 5–10 mg daily
>> adjusted to usual range of 5–20 mg daily; doses
>> greater than 10 mg daily only after reassess-
>> ment; max. 20 mg daily

> **Monotherapy for mania** (under specialist super-
> vision)
> • By mouth
>> **Child 12–18 years** 15 mg daily adjusted to usual
>> range of 5–20 mg daily; doses greater than
>> 15 mg only after reassessment; max. 20 mg daily

Note When one or more factors present that might result
in slower metabolism (e.g. female gender, non-smoker)
consider lower initial dose and more gradual dose
increase

Zyprexa® (Lilly) PoM
Tablets, f/c, olanzapine 2.5 mg, net price 28-tab
pack = £21.85; 5 mg, 28-tab pack = £43.70; 7.5 mg,
56-tab pack = £131.10; 10 mg, 28-tab pack =
£79.45, 15 mg (blue), 28-tab pack = £119.18; 20 mg
(pink), 28-tab pack = £158.90. Label: 2

Orodispersible tablet (*Velotab®*), yellow, olanzapine 5 mg, net price 28-tab pack = £48.07; 10 mg,
28-tab pack = £87.40; 15 mg, 28-tab pack =
£131.10; 20 mg, 28-tab pack = £174.79. Label: 2,
counselling, administration
Excipients include aspartame (section 9.4.1)

Counselling *Velotab®* may be placed on the tongue and
allowed to dissolve or dispersed in water, orange juice,
apple juice, milk, or coffee

◼ **QUETIAPINE**

Cautions see notes above; cerebrovascular disease

Hepatic impairment for *immediate-release tablets*,
initially 25 mg daily, increased daily in steps of
25–50 mg

Pregnancy use only if potential benefit outweighs
risk

Breast-feeding avoid—no information available

Side-effects see notes above; also drowsiness,
dyspepsia, constipation, dry mouth, hypertension, mild asthenia, rhinitis, tachycardia, irritability; leucopenia, neutropenia and occasionally
eosinophilia reported; elevated plasma-triglycer-
ide and cholesterol concentrations, hypothyroidism; possible QT interval prolongation; restless
legs syndrome; *rarely* oedema; *very rarely* priapism

Licensed use not licensed for use in children

Indication and dose

> Schizophrenia (under specialist supervision)
> • By mouth
>> **Child 12–18 years** initially 25 mg twice daily
>> adjusted in steps of 25–50 mg according to
>> response; max. 750 mg daily

Seroquel® (AstraZeneca) PoM
Tablets, f/c, quetiapine (as fumarate) 25 mg
(peach), net price 60-tab pack = £33.83; 100 mg
(yellow), 60-tab pack = £113.10; 150 mg (pale yellow), 60-tab pack = £113.10; 200 mg (white), 60-tab
pack = £113.10; 300 mg (white), 60-tab pack =
£170.00. Label: 2

◀ **Modified release**
Seroquel® XL (AstraZeneca) PoM
Tablets, m/r, quetiapine (as fumarate) 50 mg
(peach), net price 60-tab pack = £67.66; 200 mg
(yellow), 60-tab pack = £113.10; 300 mg (pale yellow), 60-tab pack = £170.00; 400 mg (white), 60-tab
pack = £226.20. Label: 2, 23, 25
Dose
> Schizophrenia (under specialist supervision)
> • By mouth
>> **Child 12–18 years** initially 50 mg once daily adjusted
>> in steps of 50 mg daily according to response, usual
>> dose 400–800 mg once daily; max. 800 mg once daily
>> **Note** Patients can be switched from immediate-release
>> to modified-release tablets at the equivalent daily
>> dose; to maintain clinical response, dose titration may
>> be required

◼ **RISPERIDONE**

Cautions see notes above; hyperprolactinaemia,
prolactin-dependent tumours; dehydration;
family history of sudden cardiac death (perform
ECG); avoid in acute porphyria (section 9.8.2)

Hepatic impairment initial and subsequent oral
doses should be halved

Renal impairment initial and subsequent oral
doses should be halved

Pregnancy use only if potential benefit outweighs
risk; extrapyramidal effects reported in neonate
when taken in third trimester

Breast-feeding use only if potential benefit outweighs risk—small amount present in milk

Side-effects see notes above; also gastro-intestinal disturbances (including diarrhoea, constipation, nausea and vomiting, dyspepsia, abdominal pain), dry mouth; dyspnoea; drowsiness,
asthenia, tremor, sleep disturbances, agitation,

◻ **RISPERIDONE** (*continued*)

anxiety, headache; urinary incontinence; hyper-prolactinaemia (*less commonly* galactorrhoea, menstrual disturbances, gynaecomastia); arthralgia, myalgia; abnormal vision; epistaxis; rash; *less commonly* anorexia, ECG changes, hypoaesthesia, impaired concentration, sexual dysfunction, blood disorders, tinnitus, angio-edema; *rarely* intestinal obstruction, pancreatitis, jaundice, seizures, hyponatraemia, abnormal temperature regulation; oedema and priapism also reported

Licensed use not licensed for use in children under 15 years for psychoses; not licensed for use in autism

Indication and dose

Acute and chronic psychoses (under specialist supervision)
● By mouth
   Child 12–18 years 2 mg in 1–2 divided doses on first day *then* 4 mg in 1–2 divided doses on second day (slower titration appropriate in some children); usual dose range 4–6 mg daily; doses above 10 mg daily only if benefit considered to outweigh risk (max. 16 mg daily)

Short-term treatment (up to 6 weeks) of persistent aggression in conduct disorder (under specialist supervision)
● By mouth
   Child 5–18 years and body-weight under 50 kg initially 250 micrograms once daily increased according to response in steps of 250 micrograms on alternate days; usual dose 500 micrograms daily (up to 750 micrograms once daily has been required)
   Child 5–18 years and body-weight over 50 kg initially 500 micrograms once daily increased according to response in steps of 500 micrograms on alternate days; usual dose 1 mg daily (up to 1.5 mg once daily has been required)

Short-term treatment of severe aggression in autism (under specialist supervision)
● By mouth
   Child over 5 years and 15–20 kg 250 micrograms daily increased if necessary after at least 4 days to 500 micrograms daily; thereafter

increased by 250 micrograms daily at 2-week intervals to max. 1 mg daily

   Child over 20 kg 500 micrograms daily increased if necessary after at least 4 days to 1 mg daily; thereafter increased by 500 micrograms daily at 2-week intervals; max. daily dose 2.5 mg if under 45 kg; max. daily dose 3 mg if over 45 kg

Risperidone (Non-proprietary) ▼ PoM
Tablets, risperidone 500 micrograms, net price 20-tab pack = £1.06; 1 mg, 20-tab pack = £1.36, 60-tab pack = £2.13; 2 mg, 60-tab pack = £3.03; 3 mg, 60-tab pack = £3.40; 4 mg, 60-tab pack = £43.50; 6 mg, 28-tab pack = £32.10. Label: 2

Orodispersible tablets, risperidone 0.5 mg, net price 28-tab pack = £8.37; 1 mg, 28-tab pack = £18.39; 2 mg, 28-tab pack = £33.30. Label: 2, counselling, administration
Counselling Tablets should be placed on the tongue, allowed to dissolve and swallowed

Liquid, risperidone 1 mg/mL, net price 100-mL pack = £53.90. Label: 2, counselling, use of dose syringe
Note Liquid may be diluted with any non-alcoholic drink, except tea

Risperdal® (Janssen-Cilag) ▼ PoM
Tablets, f/c, scored, risperidone 500 micrograms (brown-red), net price 20-tab pack = £6.78; 1 mg (white), 20-tab pack = £11.16, 60-tab pack = £33.48; 2 mg (orange), 60-tab pack = £66.01; 3 mg (yellow), 60-tab pack = £97.07; 4 mg (green), 60-tab pack = £128.14; 6 mg (yellow), 28-tab pack = £90.60. Label: 2

Orodispersible tablets (*Quicklet®*), pink, risperidone 500 micrograms, net price 28-tab pack = £10.98; 1 mg, 28-tab pack = £17.67; 2 mg, 28-tab pack = £33.31; 3 mg, 28-tab pack = £48.38; 4 mg, 28-tab pack = £62.31. Label: 2, counselling, administration
Excipients include aspartame (section 9.4.1)

Counselling Tablets should be placed on the tongue, allowed to dissolve and swallowed

Liquid, risperidone 1 mg/mL, net price 100-mL pack = £53.93. Label: 2, counselling, use of dose syringe
Note Liquid may be diluted with any non-alcoholic drink, except tea

4.2.2 Antipsychotic depot injections

There is limited information on the use of antipsychotic depot injections in children and use should be restricted to specialist centres.

4.2.3 Antimanic drugs

Antimanic drugs are used in mania to control acute attacks and to prevent recurrence of episodes of mania or hypomania. Long-term treatment of bipolar disorder should continue for at least two years from the last manic episode and up to five years if the patient has risk factors for relapse.

An antidepressant drug (section 4.3) may also be required for the treatment of co-existing depression, but should be avoided in patients with rapid-cycling bipolar disorder, recent history of hypomania, or rapid mood fluctuations.

Benzodiazepines

Use of benzodiazepines (section 4.1) may be helpful in the initial stages of treatment for behavioural disturbance or agitation; they should not be used for long periods because of the risk of dependence.

Antipsychotic drugs

Atypical antipsychotic drugs (normally **olanzapine**, **quetiapine**, or **risperidone**) (section 4.2.1) are useful in acute episodes of mania and hypomania; if the response to antipsychotic drugs is inadequate, lithium or valproate may be added. An antipsychotic drug may be used concomitantly with lithium or valproate in the initial treatment of severe acute mania.

Atypical antipsychotics are the treatment of choice for the long-term management of bipolar disorder in children and adolescents; if the patient has frequent relapses or continuing functional impairment, consider concomitant therapy with lithium or valproate. An atypical antipsychotic which causes less weight gain and does not increase prolactin levels is preferred.

When discontinuing antipsychotics, the dose should be reduced gradually over at least 4 weeks if the child is continuing on other antimanic drugs; if the child is not continuing on other antimanic drugs, or has a history of manic relapse, a withdrawal period of up to 3 months is required.

High doses of haloperidol may be hazardous when used with lithium; irreversible toxic encephalopathy has been reported.

Carbamazepine

Carbamazepine (section 4.8.1) may be used under specialist supervision for the prophylaxis of bipolar disorder (manic-depressive disorder) in children unresponsive to a combination of other prophylactic drugs; it seems to be particularly effective in those with rapid-cycling manic-depressive illness (4 or more affective episodes per year). The dose of carbamazepine should not normally be increased if an acute episode of mania occurs. When stopping treatment with carbamazepine, reduce the dose gradually over a period of at least 4 weeks.

Valproate

Valproic acid (as the semisodium salt) is licensed in adults for the treatment of manic episodes associated with bipolar disorder. Sodium valproate (section 4.8.1) is unlicensed for the treatment of bipolar disorder.

Valproate can be used for the prophylaxis of bipolar disorder [unlicensed use]; however, it should not normally be prescribed for women of child-bearing potential. In patients with frequent relapse or continuing functional impairment, consider switching therapy to lithium or an atypical antipsychotic, or adding lithium or an atypical antipsychotic to valproate. If a patient taking valproate experiences an acute episode of mania that is not ameliorated by increasing the valproate dose, consider concomitant therapy with olanzapine, quetiapine, or risperidone. When stopping valproate reduce the dose gradually over at least 4 weeks.

Lithium

Lithium salts are used in the prophylaxis and treatment of mania, in the prophylaxis of bipolar disorder (manic-depressive disorder), as concomitant therapy with antidepressant medication in children who have had an incomplete response to treatment for acute depression in bipolar disorder, and in the prophylaxis of recurrent depression (unipolar illness or unipolar depression).

Lithium is used to treat acute episodes of mania in children who have responded to lithium before and whose symptoms are not severe.

The decision to give prophylactic lithium usually requires specialist advice, and must be based on careful consideration of the likelihood of recurrence in the individual child, and the benefit of treatment weighed against the risks. The full prophylactic effect of lithium may not occur for six to twelve months after the initiation of therapy. An atypical antipsychotic or valproate (given alone or as adjunctive therapy with lithium) are alternative prophylactic treatments in patients who experience frequent relapses or continuing functional impairment. Long-term use of lithium has been associated with thyroid disorders and mild cognitive and memory impairment. Long-term treatment should therefore be undertaken only with careful assessment of risk and benefit, and with monitoring of thyroid function at baseline and every 6 months (more often if there is evidence of deterioration). Renal function should be monitored at baseline and every 6 months thereafter (more often if there is evidence of deterioration or the patient has other risk factors, such as starting ACE inhibitors, NSAIDs, or diuretics). The need for continued therapy should be assessed regularly and children should be maintained on lithium after 3–5 years only if benefit persists.

Serum concentrations Lithium salts have a narrow therapeutic/toxic ratio and should not be prescribed unless facilities for monitoring serum-lithium concentrations are available. There seem few if any reasons for preferring one or other of the salts of lithium available. Doses are adjusted to achieve a serum-lithium concentration of 0.6–1 mmol/litre on samples taken 12 hours after the preceding dose. A target serum-lithium concentration of 0.8–1 mmol/litre is recommended for acute episodes of mania, and for patients who have previously relapsed or have sub-syndromal symptoms. It is important to determine the optimum range for each individual child. Serum-lithium monitoring should be performed weekly after initiation and after each dose change until levels are stable, then every 3 months thereafter.

Overdosage, usually with serum-lithium concentration of over 1.5 mmol/litre, may be fatal and toxic effects include tremor, ataxia, dysarthria, nystagmus, renal impairment, and convulsions. If these potentially hazardous signs occur, treatment should be stopped, serum-lithium concentrations redetermined, and steps taken to reverse lithium toxicity. In mild cases withdrawal of lithium and administration of sodium and fluid will reverse the toxicity. A serum-lithium concentration in excess of 2 mmol/litre requires urgent treatment as described under Emergency Treatment of Poisoning, p. 42.

Interactions Lithium toxicity is made worse by sodium depletion, therefore concurrent use of diuretics (particularly thiazides) is hazardous and should be avoided. For other **interactions** with lithium, see Appendix 1 (lithium).

Withdrawal While there is no clear evidence of withdrawal or rebound psychosis, abrupt discontinuation of lithium increases the risk of relapse. If lithium is to be discontinued, the dose should be reduced gradually over a period of at least 4 weeks (preferably over a period of up to 3 months). Children and carers should be warned of the risk of relapse if lithium is discontinued abruptly. If lithium is stopped or has to be discontinued abruptly, consider changing therapy to an atypical antipsychotic or valproate.

Lithium treatment packs
A lithium treatment pack should be given to all patients on initiation of treatment with lithium. The pack consists of a patient information booklet, lithium alert card, and a record book for tracking serum-lithium concentration. Prescribers and pharmacists should check that blood tests are being monitored regularly and that it is safe to issue a repeat prescription or dispense the prescribed lithium.

Packs may be purchased from 3M

Tel: 0845 610 1112
nhsforms@spsl.uk.com

LITHIUM CARBONATE

Cautions measure serum-lithium concentration regularly (every 3 months on stabilised regimens), measure renal function and thyroid function every 6 months on stabilised regimens and advise children and carers to seek attention if symptoms of hypothyroidism develop (females are at greater risk) e.g. lethargy, feeling cold; maintain adequate sodium and fluid intake; test renal function before initiating and if evidence of toxicity, avoid in cardiac disease, and conditions with sodium imbalance such as Addison's disease; reduce dose or discontinue in diarrhoea,

vomiting, and intercurrent infection (especially if sweating profusely); psoriasis (risk of exacerbation); diuretic treatment, myasthenia gravis; surgery (section 15.1); if possible avoid abrupt withdrawal (see notes above); **interactions:** Appendix 1 (lithium)

Counselling Children should maintain adequate fluid intake and avoid dietary changes which reduce or increase sodium intake; lithium treatment packs are available (see above)

□ **LITHIUM CARBONATE** (*continued*)

Renal impairment avoid if possible or reduce dose and closely monitor serum-lithium concentration

Pregnancy avoid if possible in first trimester (risk of teratogenicity, including cardiac abnormalities); dose requirements increased in second and third trimesters (but on delivery, return abruptly to normal); close monitoring of serum-lithium concentration advised (risk of toxicity in neonate)

Breast-feeding present in milk and risk of toxicity in infant—avoid

Side-effects gastro-intestinal disturbances, fine tremor, renal impairment (particularly impaired urinary concentration and polyuria), polydipsia, leucocytosis; also weight gain and oedema (may respond to dose reduction); hyperparathyroidism and hypercalcaemia reported; signs of intoxication are blurred vision, increasing gastro-intestinal disturbances (anorexia, vomiting, diarrhoea), muscle weakness, increased CNS disturbances (mild drowsiness and sluggishness increasing to giddiness with ataxia, coarse tremor, lack of co-ordination, dysarthria), and require withdrawal of treatment; with severe **overdosage** (serum-lithium concentration above 2 mmol/litre) hyperreflexia and hyperextension of limbs, convulsions, toxic psychoses, syncope, renal failure, circulatory failure, coma, and occasionally, death; goitre, raised antidiuretic hormone concentration, hypothyroidism, hypokalaemia, ECG changes, and kidney changes may also occur; see also Emergency Treatment of Poisoning, p. 42

Indication and dose

Treatment and prophylaxis of mania, bipolar disorder, recurrent depression (see also notes above), aggressive or self-mutilating behaviour
• **By mouth**
See under preparations below, adjusted to achieve a serum-lithium concentration of 0.6–1 mmol/litre 12 hours after a dose on days 4–7 of treatment, then every week until dosage has remained constant for 4 weeks and every 3 months thereafter; doses are initially divided throughout the day, but once daily administra-

tion is preferred when serum-lithium concentration stabilised
Note Preparations vary widely in bioavailability; changing the preparation requires the same precautions as initiation of treatment

Camcolit® (Norgine) [PoM]
Camcolit 250® tablets, f/c, scored, lithium carbonate 250 mg (Li+ 6.8 mmol), net price 100-tab pack = £3.09 Label: 10, lithium card, counselling, see above

Camcolit 400® tablets, m/r, f/c, scored, lithium carbonate 400 mg (Li+ 10.8 mmol), net price 100-tab pack = £4.13. Label: 10, lithium card, 25, counselling, see above
Dose
Treatment
• By mouth
(See above for advice on bioavailability and serum-lithium monitoring)
Child 12–18 years initially 1–1.5 g daily

Prophylaxis
• By mouth
(See above for advice on bioavailability and serum-lithium monitoring)
Child 12–18 years initially 300–400 mg daily

Liskonum® (GSK) [PoM]
Tablets, m/r, f/c, scored, lithium carbonate 450 mg (Li+ 12.2 mmol), net price 60-tab pack = £2.88. Label: 10, lithium card, 25, counselling, see above
Dose
Treatment
• By mouth
(See above for advice on bioavailability and serum-lithium monitoring)
Child 12–18 years initially 225–675 mg twice daily

Prophylaxis
• By mouth
(See above for advice on bioavailability and serum-lithium monitoring)
Child 12–18 years initially 225–450 mg twice daily

4 Central nervous system

■ **LITHIUM CITRATE**

Cautions see under Lithium Carbonate and notes above
Counselling Patients should maintain an adequate fluid intake and should avoid dietary changes which might reduce or increase sodium intake; lithium treatment cards are available from pharmacies (see above)

Side-effects see under Lithium Carbonate and notes above

Licensed use not licensed for use in children

Indication and dose
See under Lithium Carbonate and notes above
• **By mouth**
Adjust to achieve serum-lithium concentration of 0.6–1 mmol/litre as described under Lithium Carbonate above
Note Preparations vary widely in bioavailability; changing the preparation requires the same precautions as initiation of treatment

Li-Liquid® (Rosemont) [PoM]
Oral solution, lithium citrate 509 mg/5 mL (Li+ 5.4 mmol/5 mL), yellow, net price 150-mL pack = £5.79; 1.018 g/5 mL (Li+ 10.8 mmol/5 mL), orange, 150-mL pack = £11.58. Label: 10, lithium card, counselling, see above
Note 5-mL dose of 509 mg/5 mL oral solution is equivalent to 200 mg lithium carbonate

Priadel® (Sanofi-Aventis) [PoM]
Liquid, sugar-free, lithium citrate 520 mg/5 mL (approx. Li+ 5.4 mmol/5 mL), net price 150-mL pack = £5.61. Label: 10, lithium card, counselling, see above
Note 5-mL dose is equivalent to 200 mg lithium carbonate

4.3 Antidepressant drugs

4.3.1 Tricyclic antidepressant drugs
4.3.2 Monoamine-oxidase inhibitors
4.3.3 Selective serotonin re-uptake inhibitors
4.3.4 Other antidepressant drugs

Depression in children should be managed by an appropriate specialist and treatment should involve psychological therapy.

The major classes of antidepressant drugs include the tricyclics and related antidepressant drugs (section 4.3.1), the selective serotonin re-uptake inhibitors (SSRIs) (section 4.3.3), and the monoamine oxidase inhibitors (MAOIs).

Antidepressant drugs should not be used routinely in mild depression, and psychological therapy should be considered initially; however, a trial of antidepressant therapy may be considered in cases refractory to psychological treatments or those associated with psychosocial or medical problems. Drug treatment of mild depression may also be considered in children with a history of moderate or severe depression.

Choice of antidepressant drug should be based on the individual child's requirements, including the presence of concomitant disease, existing therapy, suicide risk, and previous response to antidepressant therapy.

When drug treatment of depression is considered necessary in children, the SSRIs should be considered first-line treatment; following a safety and efficacy review, **fluoxetine** is licensed to treat depression in children.

Tricyclic antidepressant drugs should be avoided for the treatment of depression in children.

St John's wort (*Hypericum perforatum*) is a popular herbal remedy on sale to the public for treating mild depression in adults. It should not be used for the treatment of depression in children because St John's wort can induce drug metabolising enzymes and a number of important interactions with conventional drugs have been identified, see Appendix 1 (St John's wort). Furthermore, the amount of active ingredient varies between different preparations of St John's wort and switching from one to another can change the degree of enzyme induction. If a child stops taking St John's wort, concentrations of interacting drugs may increase, leading to toxicity. Other antidepressant drugs should not be used with St John's wort because of the potential for interaction.

Hyponatraemia and antidepressant therapy
Hyponatraemia (possibly due to inappropriate secretion of antidiuretic hormone) has been associated with all types of antidepressants; however, it has been reported more frequently with SSRIs than with other antidepressant drugs. Hyponatraemia should be considered in all children who develop drowsiness, confusion, or convulsions while taking an antidepressant drug.

Suicidal behaviour and antidepressant therapy
The use of antidepressant drugs has been linked with suicidal thoughts and behaviour. Where necessary, children should be monitored for suicidal behaviour, self-harm, and hostility, particularly at the beginning of treatment or if the dose is changed.

Withdrawal Withdrawal effects on stopping treatment with antidepressant drugs are usually mild and self-limiting, but in some cases may be severe. Gastro-intestinal symptoms of nausea, vomiting, and anorexia, accompanied by headache, giddiness, 'chills', and insomnia, and sometimes by hypomania, panic-anxiety, and extreme motor restlessness may occur if an antidepressant is stopped suddenly after regular administration for 8 weeks or more. The dose should preferably be reduced gradually over about 4 weeks, or longer if withdrawal symptoms emerge (6 months in children who have been on long-term maintenance treatment). SSRIs have been associated with a specific withdrawal syndrome (section 4.3.3).

Anxiety   Management of *acute anxiety* in children with drug treatment is contentious (section 4.1.2). For *chronic anxiety* (of longer than 4 weeks' duration), it may be appropriate to use an antidepressant drug before a benzodiazepine.

4.3.1   Tricyclic antidepressant drugs

> Studies have shown that tricyclic antidepressants are not effective for treating depression in children.

For reference to the role of some tricyclic antidepressant drugs in some forms of *neuralgia*, see section 4.7.3, and in *nocturnal enuresis* in children, see section 7.4.2.

Dosage   It is important to use doses that are sufficiently high for effective treatment but not so high as to cause toxic effects. Low doses should be used for initial treatment.

In most children the long half-life of tricyclic antidepressant drugs allows **once-daily** administration, usually at night; the use of modified-release preparations is therefore unnecessary.

Cautions   Tricyclic antidepressant drugs should be used with caution in children with cardiovascular disease (see also Contra-indications, below); because of the risk of arrhythmias, children with concomitant conditions such as hyperthyroidism and phaeochromocytoma should be treated with care. Care is also needed in children with epilepsy and diabetes.

Tricyclic antidepressant drugs have antimuscarinic activity, and therefore caution is needed in children with chronic constipation, urinary retention, or those with a susceptibility to angle-closure glaucoma. Tricyclic antidepressant drugs should be used with caution in children with a significant risk of suicide, or a history of psychosis or bipolar disorder, because antidepressant therapy may aggravate these conditions; treatment should be stopped if the child enters a manic phase.

Skilled tasks   Drowsiness may affect the performance of skilled tasks (e.g. driving); effects of alcohol enhanced.

Contra-indications   Tricyclic antidepressants are contra-indicated in arrhythmias (particularly heart block), and in the manic phase of bipolar disorder. Avoid treatment with tricyclic antidepressant drugs in acute porphyria (section 9.8.2).

Hepatic impairment   The sedative effects of tricyclic antidepressant drugs are increased in children with hepatic impairment. They should be avoided in severe liver disease.

Breast-feeding   The amount of tricyclic antidepressants secreted into breast milk is too small to be harmful. However, most manufacturers advise that tricyclic antidepressants should be avoided during breast-feeding.

Side-effects   Arrhythmias and heart block occasionally follow the use of tricyclic antidepressants, particularly amitriptyline, and may be a factor in the sudden death of children with cardiac disease; other cardiovascular side-effects include postural hypotension, tachycardia, and ECG changes.

Central nervous system side-effects are common, and include anxiety, dizziness, agitation, confusion, sleep disturbances, irritability, and paraesthesia; drowsiness is associated with some of the tricyclic antidepressants. Convulsions, hallucinations, delusions, mania, and hypomania may occur (see also under Cautions, above), and, *rarely*, extrapyramidal symptoms including tremor and dysarthria.

Antimuscarinic side-effects include dry mouth, blurred vision (*very rarely* precipitation of angle-closure glaucoma), constipation (*rarely* leading to paralytic ileus), and urinary retention.

Endocrine effects include breast enlargement, galactorrhoea, and gynaecomastia. Sexual dysfunction may occur. Changes in blood sugar, increased appetite, and weight gain can accompany treatment with tricyclic antidepressant drugs, but anorexia and weight loss are also seen. Hepatic and haematological reactions may occur. Hyponatraemia has been associated with antidepressant treatment

4

Central nervous system

(see Hyponatraemia and Antidepressant Therapy, p. 234). Other class side-effects include nausea, vomiting, taste disturbance, tinnitus, rash, urticaria, pruritus, photosensitivity, alopecia, and sweating.

Neuroleptic malignant syndrome (section 4.2.1) may, *very rarely*, occur in the course of antidepressant drug treatment.

Suicidal behaviour has been linked with antidepressant drugs (see p. 234).

Overdosage Limited quantities of tricyclic antidepressant drugs should be prescribed at any one time because their cardiovascular and epileptogenic effects are dangerous in overdosage. In particular, overdosage with **amitriptyline** is associated with a relatively high rate of fatality. For advice on overdosage see Emergency Treatment of Poisoning, p. 40.

Withdrawal If possible tricyclic antidepressant drugs should be withdrawn slowly (see also section 4.3).

AMITRIPTYLINE HYDROCHLORIDE

Cautions see notes above; see section 7.4.2 for additional nocturnal enuresis warnings; **interactions**: Appendix 1 (antidepressants, tricyclic)

Contra-indications see notes above

Hepatic impairment see notes above

Pregnancy use only if potential benefit outweighs risk

Breast-feeding see notes above

Side-effects see notes above; also abdominal pain, stomatitis, palpitation, oedema, hypertension, restlessness, fatigue, mydriasis, and increased intra-ocular pressure; **overdosage**: see Emergency Treatment of Poisoning, p. 40 (high rate of fatality—see Overdosage, above)

Licensed use not licensed for use in neuropathic pain

Indication and dose

Depression (but see notes above)
- By mouth

   Child 16–18 years 10–25 mg 3 times daily (total daily dose may alternatively be given as a single dose at bedtime) increased gradually as necessary to 150–200 mg daily

Nocturnal enuresis
- By mouth

   Child 6–11 years 10–20 mg at night

   Child 11–16 years 25–50 mg at night

   Note Max. period of treatment (including gradual withdrawal) 3 months—full physical examination before further course, see also section 7.4.2

Neuropathic pain in palliative care
- By mouth

   Child 2–12 years initially 200–500 micrograms/kg (max. 25 mg) once daily at night, increased if necessary; max. 1 mg/kg twice daily on specialist advice

   Child 12–18 years initially 10–25 mg once daily at night, increased gradually if necessary to usual dose 75 mg at night; higher doses on specialist advice

Amitriptyline (Non-proprietary) PoM

Tablets, coated, amitriptyline hydrochloride 10 mg, net price 28 = £1.03; 25 mg, 28 = £1.04; 50 mg, 28 = £1.18. Label: 2

Oral solution, amitriptyline hydrochloride 25 mg/5 mL, net price 150 mL = £13.95; 50 mg/5 mL, 150 mL = £14.79. Label: 2

DOXEPIN

Cautions see notes above

Contra-indications see notes above

Hepatic impairment see notes above

Renal impairment use with caution

Pregnancy caution—limited information available

Breast-feeding see notes above; accumulation of doxepin metabolite may cause sedation and respiratory depression

Side-effects see notes above; also abdominal pain, stomatitis, diarrhoea, flushing, and oedema

Indication and dose

Depressive illness, particularly where sedation is required (but see notes above)
- By mouth

   Child 12–18 years initially 75 mg daily in divided doses *or* as a single dose at bedtime, adjusted according to response; usual maintenance 30–300 mg daily (doses above 100 mg given in 3 divided doses)

Sinepin® (Marlborough) PoM

Capsules, doxepin (as hydrochloride) 25 mg, net price 28-cap pack = £3.77; 50 mg, 28-cap pack = £5.71. Label: 2

IMIPRAMINE HYDROCHLORIDE

Cautions see notes above

Contra-indications see notes above

Hepatic impairment see notes above

Renal impairment use with caution in severe impairment

Pregnancy tachycardia, irritability, and muscle spasms reported in neonates when used in third trimester

Breast-feeding see notes above

Side-effects see notes above; also palpitation, flushing, restlessness, headache, fatigue; *very rarely* abdominal pain, stomatitis, diarrhoea, hypertension, oedema, cardiac decompensation, allergic alveolitis, aggression, myoclonus, peripheral vasospasm, and mydriasis

Licensed use not licensed for use for attention deficit hyperactivity disorder

Indication and dose

Nocturnal enuresis
- **By mouth**

  Child 6–8 years 25 mg at bedtime

  Child 8–11 years 25–50 mg at bedtime

  Child 11–18 years 50–75 mg at bedtime
  Note Max. period of treatment (including gradual withdrawal) 3 months—full physical examination before further course, see also section 7.4.2

Attention deficit hyperactivity disorder (under specialist supervision)
- **By mouth**

  Child 6–18 years 10–30 mg twice daily

Imipramine (Non-proprietary) PoM
Tablets, coated, imipramine hydrochloride 10 mg, net price 28-tab pack = £1.66; 25 mg, 28-tab pack = £1.71. Label: 2

NORTRIPTYLINE

Cautions see notes above; manufacturer advises plasma-nortriptyline concentration monitoring if dose above 100 mg daily, but evidence of practical value uncertain

Contra-indications see notes above

Hepatic impairment see notes above

Pregnancy use only if potential benefit outweighs risk

Breast-feeding see notes above

Side-effects see notes above; also abdominal pain, stomatitis, diarrhoea, hypertension, oedema, flushing, restlessness, fatigue, and mydriasis

Indication and dose

Depression (but see notes above)
- **By mouth**

  Child 12–18 years low dose initially increased as necessary to 30–50 mg daily in divided doses *or* as a single dose (max. 150 mg daily)

Nocturnal enuresis
- **By mouth**

  Child 6–8 years 10 mg at night

  Child 8–11 years 10–20 mg at night

  Child 11–18 years 25–35 mg at night
  Note Max. period of treatment (including gradual withdrawal) 3 months—full physical examination and ECG before further course, see also section 7.4.2

Allegron® (King) PoM
Tablets, nortriptyline (as hydrochloride) 10 mg, net price 100-tab pack = £12.06; 25 mg (orange, scored), 100-tab pack = £24.02. Label: 2

4

Central nervous system

4.3.2 Monoamine-oxidase inhibitors (MAOIs)

Classification not used in *BNF for Children*.

4.3.3 Selective serotonin re-uptake inhibitors

Citalopram, escitalopram, fluoxetine, fluvoxamine, paroxetine, and **sertraline** selectively inhibit the re-uptake of serotonin (5-hydroxytryptamine, 5-HT); they are termed selective serotonin re-uptake inhibitors (SSRIs).

> **Depressive illness in children and adolescents**
> The balance of risks and benefits for the treatment of depressive illness in individuals under 18 years is considered unfavourable for the SSRIs **citalopram, escitalopram, paroxetine**, and **sertraline**, and for **mirtazapine** and **venlafaxine**. Clinical trials have failed to show efficacy and have shown an increase in harmful outcomes. However, it is recognised that specialists may sometimes decide to use these drugs in response to individual clinical need; children and adolescents should be monitored carefully for suicidal behaviour, self-harm or hostility, particularly at the beginning of treatment. Only **fluoxetine** has been shown in clinical trials to be effective for treating depressive illness in children and adolescents. However, it is possible that, in common with the other SSRIs, it is associated with a small risk of self-harm and suicidal thoughts. Overall, the balance of risks and benefits for fluoxetine in the treatment of depressive illness in individuals under 18 years is considered favourable, but children and adolescents must be carefully monitored as above.

Cautions   SSRIs should be used with caution in children with epilepsy (avoid if poorly controlled, discontinue if convulsions develop), cardiac disease, diabetes mellitus, susceptibility to angle-closure glaucoma, a history of mania or bleeding disorders (especially gastro-intestinal bleeding), and if used together with other drugs that increase the risk of bleeding. They should also be used with caution in those receiving concurrent electroconvulsive therapy (prolonged seizures reported with fluoxetine). SSRIs may also impair performance of skilled tasks (e.g. driving). **Interactions:** Appendix 1 (antidepressants, SSRI).

Withdrawal   Gastro-intestinal disturbances, headache, anxiety, dizziness, paraesthesia, electric shock sensation in the head, tinnitus, sleep disturbances, fatigue, influenza-like symptoms, and sweating are the most common features of abrupt withdrawal of an SSRI or marked reduction of the dose; palpitation and visual disturbances can occur less commonly. The dose should be tapered over a few weeks to avoid these effects. It may be necessary to withdraw treatment over a longer period; consider obtaining specialist advice if symptoms persist.

Contra-indications   SSRIs should not be used if the child enters a manic phase.

Pregnancy   Manufacturers advise that SSRIs should not be used during pregnancy unless the potential benefit outweighs the risk. If SSRIs are used during the third trimester there is a risk of neonatal withdrawal symptoms, particularly with fluoxetine.

Side-effects   SSRIs are less sedating and have fewer antimuscarinic and cardiotoxic effects than tricyclic antidepressant drugs (section 4.3.1). Side-effects of the SSRIs include gastro-intestinal effects (dose-related and fairly common—include nausea, vomiting, dyspepsia, abdominal pain, diarrhoea, constipation), anorexia with weight loss (increased appetite and weight gain also reported) and hypersensitivity reactions including rash (consider discontinuation—may be sign of impending serious systemic reaction, possibly associated with vasculitis), urticaria, angioedema, anaphylaxis, arthralgia, myalgia and photosensitivity; other side-effects include dry mouth, nervousness, anxiety, headache, insomnia, tremor, dizziness, asthenia, hallucinations, drowsiness, convulsions (see Cautions above), galactorrhoea, sexual dysfunction, urinary retention, sweating, hypomania or mania (see Cautions above), movement disorders and dyskinesias, visual disturbances, hyponatraemia (see Hyponatraemia and Antidepressant Therapy, p. 234), and bleeding disorders including ecchymoses and purpura. Suicidal behaviour has been linked with antidepressants, see p. 234. Angle-closure glaucoma may very rarely be precipitated by treatment with SSRIs.

◢ CITALOPRAM

Cautions   see notes above

Contra-indications   see notes above

Hepatic impairment   use doses at lower end of range

Renal impairment   no information available for estimated glomerular filtration rate less than 20 mL/minute/1.73 m^2

Pregnancy   see notes above

Breast-feeding   present in milk—avoid

Side-effects   see notes above; also palpitation, tachycardia, postural hypotension, coughing, yawning, confusion, impaired concentration, malaise, amnesia, migraine, paraesthesia, abnormal dreams, taste disturbance, increased saliva-

◁ CITALOPRAM (*continued*)

tion, rhinitis, tinnitus, polyuria, micturition disorders, euphoria

Licensed use not licensed for use in children

Indication and dose

> Major depression (but see Depressive Illness in Children and Adolescents, above)
> • **By mouth as tablets**
> **Child 12–18 years** initially 10 mg once daily, increased if necessary to 20 mg once daily over 2–4 weeks; max. 60 mg once daily
> • **By mouth as oral drops**
> **Child 12–18 years** initially 8 mg once daily increased if necessary to 16 mg once daily over 2–4 weeks; max. 48 mg once daily

Citalopram (Non-proprietary) PoM

Tablets, citalopram (as hydrobromide) 10 mg, net price 28-tab pack = £1.15; 20 mg, 28-tab pack =

£1.32; 40 mg, 28-tab pack = £1.54. Counselling, driving

Oral drops, citalopram (as hydrochloride) 40 mg/mL, net price 15-mL pack = £19.66. Counselling, driving, administration

Note 4 drops (8 mg) can be considered equivalent in therapeutic effect to 10-mg tablet
Mix with water, orange juice, or apple juice before taking

Cipramil® (Lundbeck) PoM

Tablets, f/c, citalopram (as hydrobromide) 10 mg, net price 28-tab pack = £8.97; 20 mg (scored), 28-tab pack = £14.91; 40 mg, 28-tab pack = £25.20. Counselling, driving

Oral drops, sugar-free, citalopram (as hydrochloride) 40 mg/mL, net price 15-mL pack = £20.16. Counselling, driving, administration

Note 4 drops (8 mg) can be considered equivalent in therapeutic effect to 10-mg tablet
Mix with water, orange juice, or apple juice before taking

▮ FLUOXETINE

Cautions see notes above

Contra-indications see notes above

Hepatic impairment reduce dose or increase dose interval

Pregnancy see notes above

Breast-feeding present in breast milk, avoid

Side-effects see notes above; also vasodilatation, postural hypotension, pharyngitis, dyspnoea, chills, taste disturbances, sleep disturbances, euphoria, confusion, yawning, impaired concentration, changes in blood sugar, alopecia, urinary frequency; *rarely* pulmonary inflammation and fibrosis; *very rarely* hepatitis, toxic epidermal necrolysis, and neuroleptic malignant syndrome-like event

Indication and dose

> Major depression
> • **By mouth**
> **Child 8–18 years** 10 mg once daily increased after 1–2 weeks if necessary, max. 20 mg once daily
> **Long duration of action** Consider the long half-life of fluoxetine when adjusting dosage (or in overdosage)

Fluoxetine (Non-proprietary) PoM

Capsules, fluoxetine (as hydrochloride) 20 mg, net price 30-cap pack = £1.15; 60 mg, 30-cap pack = £60.35. Counselling, driving
Brands include *Oxactin*®

Liquid, fluoxetine (as hydrochloride) 20 mg/5 mL, net price 70 mL = £6.22. Counselling, driving
Brands include *Prozep*®

Prozac® (Lilly) PoM

Capsules, fluoxetine (as hydrochloride) 20 mg (green/yellow), net price 30-cap pack = £5.00. Counselling, driving

Liquid, fluoxetine (as hydrochloride) 20 mg/5 mL, net price 70 mL = £11.12. Counselling, driving

▮ FLUVOXAMINE MALEATE

Cautions see notes above

Contra-indications see notes above

Hepatic impairment start with low dose

Renal impairment start with low dose

Pregnancy see notes above

Breast-feeding present in milk—avoid

Side-effects see notes above; palpitation, tachycardia (may also cause bradycardia); *rarely* postural hypotension, confusion, ataxia, paraesthesia, malaise, taste disturbance, neuroleptic malignant syndrome-like event, abnormal liver function tests, usually symptomatic (discontinue treatment)

Indication and dose

> Obsessive-compulsive disorder
> • **By mouth**
> **Child 8–18 years** initially 25 mg daily increased if necessary in steps of 25 mg every 4–7 days according to response (total daily doses above 50 mg in 2 divided doses); max. 100 mg twice daily
> **Note** If no improvement in obsessive-compulsive disorder within 10 weeks, treatment should be reconsidered

Fluvoxamine (Non-proprietary) PoM

Tablets, fluvoxamine maleate 50 mg, net price 60-tab pack = £7.31; 100 mg, 30-tab pack = £8.63. Counselling, driving

◁ **FLUVOXAMINE MALEATE** (*continued*)

Faverin® (Solvay) PoM
Tablets, f/c, scored, fluvoxamine maleate 50 mg, net price 60-tab pack = £17.10; 100 mg, 30-tab pack = £17.10. Counselling, driving

SERTRALINE

Cautions see notes above

Contra-indications see notes above

Hepatic impairment reduce dose or increase dose interval in mild or moderate impairment; avoid in severe impairment

Renal impairment use with caution

Pregnancy see notes above

Breast-feeding not known to be harmful but consider discontinuing breast-feeding

Side-effects see notes above; pancreatitis, hepatitis, jaundice, liver failure, stomatitis, palpitation, hypertension, hypercholesterolaemia, tachycardia, postural hypotension, bronchospasm, amnesia, paraesthesia, aggression, hypoglycaemia, hypothyroidism, hyperprolactinaemia, urinary incontinence, menstrual irregularities, leucopenia, and tinnitus also reported

Licensed use not licensed for use in children for depression

Indication and dose

Obsessive-compulsive disorder
● By mouth
Child 6–12 years initially 25 mg daily increased to 50 mg daily after 1 week, further increased if necessary in steps of 50 mg at intervals of at least 1 week; max. 200 mg daily

Child 12–18 years initially 50 mg daily increased if necessary in steps of 50 mg over several weeks; usual range 50–200 mg daily

Major depression (but see Depressive Illness in Children and Adolescents, above)
● By mouth
Child 12–18 years initially 50 mg once daily increased if necessary in steps of 50 mg daily at intervals of at least a week; max. 200 mg once daily

Sertraline (Non-proprietary) PoM
Tablets, sertraline (as hydrochloride) 50 mg, net price 28-tab pack = £1.34; 100 mg, 28-tab pack = £1.59. Counselling, driving

Lustral® (Pfizer) PoM
Tablets, both f/c, sertraline (as hydrochloride) 50 mg (scored), net price 28-tab pack = £17.82; 100 mg, 28-tab pack = £29.16. Counselling, driving

4.3.4 Other antidepressant drugs

Classification not used in *BNF for Children*.

4.4 CNS stimulants and other drugs for attention deficit hyperactivity disorder

CNS stimulants should be prescribed for children with severe and persistent symptoms of *attention deficit hyperactivity disorder* (ADHD), when the diagnosis has been confirmed by a specialist; children with moderate symptoms of ADHD can be treated with CNS stimulants when psychological interventions have been unsuccessful or are unavailable. Prescribing of CNS stimulants may be continued by general practitioners under a shared-care arrangement. Treatment of ADHD often needs to be continued into adolescence, and may need to be continued into adulthood.

Drug treatment of ADHD should be part of a comprehensive treatment programme. The choice of medication should take into consideration co-morbid conditions (such as tic disorders, Tourette syndrome, and epilepsy), the adverse effect profile, potential for drug misuse, and preferences of the child and carers. **Methylphenidate** and **atomoxetine** are used for the management of ADHD; **dexamfetamine** (dexamphetamine) is an alternative in children who do not respond to these drugs.

The need to continue drug treatment for ADHD should be reviewed at least annually. This may involve suspending treatment.

A tricyclic antidepressant such as **imipramine** (section 4.3.1) is sometimes used in the treatment of ADHD; it should not be prescribed concomitantly with a CNS stimulant.

Modafinil is used for the treatment of daytime sleepiness associated with narcolepsy; dependence with long-term use cannot be excluded and it should therefore be used with caution.

Dexamfetamine and methylphenidate [both unlicensed] are also used to treat narcolepsy.

ATOMOXETINE

Cautions cardiovascular disease including hypertension and tachycardia; structural cardiac abnormalities; monitor growth; QT-interval prolongation (avoid concomitant administration of drugs that prolong QT-interval); psychosis or mania; history of seizures; aggressive behaviour, hostility, or emotional lability; susceptibility to angle-closure glaucoma; **interactions:** Appendix 1 (atomoxetine)

Hepatic disorders Following rare reports of hepatic disorders, children and carers should be advised of the risk and be told how to recognise symptoms; prompt medical attention should be sought in case of abdominal pain, unexplained nausea, malaise, darkening of the urine or jaundice

Suicidal ideation Following reports of suicidal thoughts and behaviour, children and carers should be informed about the risk and told to report clinical worsening, suicidal thoughts or behaviour, irritability, agitation, or depression

Hepatic impairment halve dose in moderate impairment; quarter dose in severe impairment; see also Hepatic Disorders above

Pregnancy no information available; avoid unless potential benefit outweighs risk

Breast-feeding avoid—present in milk in *animal* studies

Side-effects anorexia, dry mouth, nausea, vomiting, abdominal pain, constipation, dyspepsia, flatulence; palpitation, tachycardia, increased blood pressure, postural hypotension, hot flushes; sleep disturbance, dizziness, headache, fatigue, lethargy, depression, psychotic or manic symptoms, aggression, hostility, emotional lability, drowsiness, anxiety, irritability, tremor, rigors; urinary retention, prostatitis, sexual dysfunction, menstrual disturbances; mydriasis, conjunctivitis; dermatitis, pruritus, rash, sweating; *less commonly* suicidal ideation (see Suicidal Ideation, above), cold extremities; *very rarely* hepatic disorders (see Hepatic Disorders, above), seizures, Raynaud's phenomenon, and angle-closure glaucoma

Licensed use doses above 100 mg daily not licensed

Indication and dose

Attention deficit hyperactivity disorder initiated by specialist

• By mouth

Child over 6 years (body-weight under 70 kg) initially 500 micrograms/kg daily for 7 days, increased according to response; usual maintenance dose 1.2 mg/kg daily, but may be increased to 1.8 mg/kg daily (max. 120 mg daily) under the direction of a specialist

Child over 6 years (body-weight over 70 kg) initially 40 mg daily for 7 days, increased according to response; usual maintenance dose 80 mg daily, but may be increased to max. 120 mg daily under the direction of a specialist

Note Total daily dose may be given *either* as a single dose in the morning *or* in 2 divided doses with last dose no later than early evening

Strattera® (Lilly) ▼ PoM
Capsules, atomoxetine (as hydrochloride) 10 mg (white), net price 7-cap pack = £15.62, 28-cap pack = £62.46; 18 mg (gold/white), 7-cap pack = £15.62, 28-cap pack = £62.46; 25 mg (blue/white), 7-cap pack = £15.62, 28-cap pack = £62.46; 40 mg (blue), 7-cap pack = £15.62, 28-cap pack = £62.46; 60 mg (blue/gold), 28-cap pack = £62.46; 80 mg (brown/white), 28-cap pack = £83.28. Label: 3

DEXAMFETAMINE SULPHATE

(Dexamphetamine sulphate)

Cautions anorexia; mild hypertension (contra-indicated if moderate or severe)—monitor blood pressure; psychosis or bipolar disorder; monitor for aggressive behaviour or hostility during initial treatment; history of epilepsy (discontinue if convulsions occur); tics and Tourette syndrome (use with caution)—discontinue if tics occur; monitor growth (see also below); susceptibility to angle-closure glaucoma; avoid abrupt withdrawal; data on safety and efficacy of long-term use not complete; acute porphyria (see section 9.8.2); **interactions:** Appendix 1 (sympathomimetics)

Growth restriction Monitor height and weight as growth restriction may occur during prolonged therapy (drug-free periods may allow catch-up in growth but withdraw slowly to avoid inducing depression or renewed hyperactivity).

Contra-indications cardiovascular disease including moderate to severe hypertension, structural cardiac abnormalities, hyperexcitability or agitated states, hyperthyroidism, history of drug or alcohol abuse

Skilled tasks May affect performance of skilled tasks (e.g. driving); effects of alcohol unpredictable

Renal impairment use with caution

Pregnancy avoid (retrospective evidence of uncertain significance suggesting possible embryotoxicity)

Breast-feeding significant amount in milk—avoid

Side-effects insomnia, restlessness, irritability and excitability, night terrors, euphoria, tremor, dizziness, aggression, paranoia, anxiety, depression, confusion, fatigue, headache; seizures (see also Cautions); dependence and tolerance, psychosis; anorexia, gastro-intestinal symptoms, growth restriction (see also Cautions); dry mouth, sweating, tachycardia (and anginal pain), palpitation, myocardial infarction, hypotension, hypertension; impotence; visual disturbances; alopecia, rash; cardiomyopathy reported with chronic use; cardiovascular collapse; cerebral

◁ **DEXAMFETAMINE SULPHATE** (*continued*)

vasculitis; central stimulants have provoked choreoathetoid movements and dyskinesia, tics and Tourette syndrome in predisposed individuals (see also Cautions); *very rarely* angle-closure glaucoma; **overdosage:** see Emergency Treatment of Poisoning, p. 43

Indication and dose

> Refractory attention deficit hyperactivity disorder initiated by specialist
> - By mouth
>   **Child 6–18 years** initially 5–10 mg once daily, increased if necessary at weekly intervals by

5 mg; usual max. 1 mg/kg daily, up to 20 mg (40 mg daily has been required in some children); maintenance dose given in 2–4 divided doses

Administration tablets can be halved

Dexedrine® (UCB Pharma) ⒸⒹ
Tablets, scored, dexamfetamine sulphate 5 mg. Net price 28-tab pack = £3.00. Counselling, driving

METHYLPHENIDATE HYDROCHLORIDE

Cautions monitor for psychiatric disorders and monitor growth every 6 months; measure blood pressure and heart rate at baseline and then every 6 months; anxiety or agitation; tics or a family history of Tourette syndrome; epilepsy (discontinue if increased seizure frequency); avoid abrupt withdrawal; **interactions:** Appendix 1 (sympathomimetics)

Contra-indications severe depression, suicidal ideation; anorexia nervosa; drug or alcohol dependence; psychosis; uncontrolled bipolar disorder; hyperthyroidism; cardiovascular disease (including heart failure, cardiomyopathy, severe hypertension, and arrhythmias), structural cardiac abnormalities; phaeochromocytoma

Pregnancy limited experience—avoid unless potential benefit outweighs risk

Breast-feeding limited information available—avoid

Side-effects abdominal pain, nausea, vomiting, diarrhoea, dyspepsia, dry mouth, anorexia, reduced weight gain; tachycardia, palpitation, arrhythmias, changes in blood pressure; tics (*very rarely* Tourette syndrome), insomnia, nervousness, asthenia, depression, irritability, aggression, headache, drowsiness, dizziness, movement disorders; fever, arthralgia; rash, pruritus, alopecia; growth restriction; *less commonly* constipation, abnormal dreams, confusion, suicidal ideation, urinary frequency, haematuria, muscle cramps, epistaxis; *rarely* sweating and visual disturbances; *very rarely* hepatic dysfunction, cerebral arteritis, psychosis, seizures, neuroleptic malignant syndrome, tolerance and dependence, blood disorders including leucopenia and thrombocytopenia, exfoliative dermatitis, and erythema multiforme

Licensed use not licensed for use in children under 6 years; doses over 60 mg daily not licensed; doses of *Concerta®* XL over 54 mg daily not licensed

Indication and dose

> Attention deficit hyperactivity disorder initiated by specialist
> - By mouth
>   **Child 4–6 years** 2.5 mg twice daily increased if necessary at weekly intervals by 2.5 mg daily to max. 1.4 mg/kg daily in 2–3 divided doses; discontinue if no response after 1 month

> **Child 6–18 years** initially 5 mg 1–2 times daily, increased if necessary at weekly intervals by 5–10 mg daily; licensed max. 60 mg daily in 2–3 divided doses but may be increased to 2.1 mg/kg daily in 2–3 divided doses (max. 90 mg daily) under the direction of a specialist; discontinue if no response after 1 month
> **Evening dose** If effect wears off in evening (with rebound hyperactivity) a dose at bedtime may be appropriate (establish need with trial bedtime dose)
> **Note** Treatment may be started using a modified-release preparation

Administration *Equasym®* and *Ritalin®* tablets may be halved; contents of *Equasym XL®* capsules can be sprinkled on a tablespoon of apple sauce, then swallowed immediately without chewing

Methylphenidate Hydrochloride (Non-proprietary) ⒸⒹ
Tablets, methylphenidate hydrochloride 5 mg, net price 30-tab pack = £2.67; 10 mg, 30-tab pack = £5.80; 20 mg, 30-tab pack = £9.59
Brands include *Equasym®*, *Medikinet®*

Ritalin® (Novartis) ⒸⒹ
Tablets, scored, methylphenidate hydrochloride 10 mg, net price 30-tab pack = £5.57

◢**Modified release**

Concerta® XL (Janssen-Cilag) ⒸⒹ
Tablets, m/r, methylphenidate hydrochloride 18 mg (yellow), net price 30-tab pack = £31.19; 27 mg (grey), 30-tab pack = £36.81; 36 mg (white), 30-tab pack = £42.45. Label: 25

Counselling Tablet membrane may pass through gastro-intestinal tract unchanged
Cautions dose form not appropriate for use in dysphagia or if gastro-intestinal lumen restricted

Dose
> - By mouth
>   **Child 6–18 years** initially 18 mg once daily (in the morning), increased if necessary at weekly intervals by 18 mg according to response; licensed max. 54 mg once daily, but may be increased to 2.1 mg/kg daily (max. 108 mg daily) under the direction of a specialist; discontinue if no response after 1 month
>   **Note** Total daily dose of 15 mg of standard-release formulation is considered equivalent to *Concerta®* XL 18 mg once daily

Equasym XL® (Shire) ⒸⒹ
Capsules, m/r, methylphenidate hydrochloride 10 mg (white/green), net price 30-cap pack = £25.00; 20 mg (white/blue), 30-cap pack = £30.00;

◻ **METHYLPHENIDATE HYDROCHLORIDE (continued)**

30 mg (white/brown), 30-cap pack = £35.00.
Label: 25

Dose

• **By mouth**

Child 6–18 years initially 10 mg once daily in the morning before breakfast, increased gradually at weekly intervals if necessary; licensed max. 60 mg daily, but may be increased to 2.1 mg/kg daily (max. 90 mg daily) under the direction of a specialist; discontinue if no response after 1 month

Medikinet XL® (Flynn) CD

Capsules, m/r, methylphenidate hydrochloride 10 mg (lilac/white), net price 28-cap pack = £20.18;

20 mg (lilac), 28-cap pack = £26.91; 30 mg (purple/light grey), 28-cap pack = £31.39; 40 mg (purple/grey), 28-cap pack = £43.20. Label: 25

Dose

• **By mouth**

Child 6–18 years 10 mg once daily in the morning with breakfast, adjusted at weekly intervals according to response; licensed max. 60 mg daily, but may be increased to 2.1 mg/kg daily (max. 90 mg daily) under the direction of a specialist; discontinue if no response after 1 month

Note Contents of capsule can be sprinkled on a tablespoon of apple sauce (then swallowed immediately without chewing)

▌ **MODAFINIL**

Cautions monitor blood pressure and heart rate in hypertension (see Contra-indications); possibility of dependence; **interactions**: Appendix 1 (modafinil)

Contra-indications moderate to severe uncontrolled hypertension, arrhythmia; history of left ventricular hypertrophy, of cor pulmonale, or of clinically significant stimulant-induced mitral-valve prolapse (including ischaemic ECG changes, chest pain and arrhythmias)

Hepatic impairment halve dose in severe impairment

Renal impairment halve dose in severe impairment

Pregnancy avoid

Breast-feeding avoid—present in milk in *animal* studies

Side-effects dry mouth, appetite changes, gastro-intestinal disturbances (including nausea, diarrhoea, constipation, and dyspepsia), abdominal pain; tachycardia, vasodilation, chest pain, palpitation; headache (uncommonly migraine), anxiety, sleep disturbances, dizziness, depression, confusion, paraesthesia, asthenia; visual disturbances; *less commonly* mouth ulcers, glossitis, pharyngitis, dysphagia, taste disturbance, increased thirst, hypertension, hypotension, bradycardia, arrhythmia, peripheral oedema, hypercholesterolaemia, rhinitis, dyspnoea, agita-

tion, dyskinesia, amnesia, emotional lability, abnormal dreams, tremor, decreased libido, weight changes, hyperglycaemia, urinary frequency, menstrual disturbances, eosinophilia, leucopenia, myasthenia, muscle cramps, dry eye, sinusitis, epistaxis, myalgia, arthralgia, acne, sweating, rash, and pruritus; *very rarely* psychosis, mania, Stevens-Johnson syndrome, and toxic epidermal necrolysis

Licensed use not licensed for use in children under 12 years

Indication and dose

Narcolepsy

• **By mouth**

Child 5–12 years initially 100 mg daily in the morning, dose adjusted according to response to 100–400 mg daily *either* in 2 divided doses morning and at noon *or* as a single dose in the morning

Child 12–18 years 200 mg daily, *either* in 2 divided doses morning and at noon *or* as a single dose in the morning, dose adjusted according to response to 200–400 mg daily in 2 divided doses *or* as a single dose

Provigil® (Cephalon) ▼ PoM

Tablets, modafinil 100 mg, net price 30-tab pack = £53.62; 200 mg, 30-tab pack = £107.25

---

4 Central nervous system

4.5 **Drugs used in the treatment of obesity**

Obesity is associated with many health problems including cardiovascular disease, diabetes mellitus, gallstones, and osteoarthritis. Factors that aggravate obesity may include depression, other psychosocial problems, and some drugs.

The main treatment of the obese individual is a suitable diet, carefully explained to the individual or carer, with appropriate support and encouragement; increased physical activity should also be encouraged. If appropriate, smoking cessation (while maintaining body weight) may be worthwhile before attempting supervised weight loss, since cigarette smoking may be more harmful than obesity.

Obesity should be managed in an appropriate setting by staff who have been trained in the management of obesity in children; the individual or carer should receive advice on diet and lifestyle modification and should be monitored for changes in weight as well as in blood pressure, blood lipids, and other associated conditions.

NICE has recommended (December 2006) that drug treatment should only be considered for obese children after dietary, exercise, and behavioural approaches have been started, and who have associated conditions such as orthopaedic problems or sleep apnoea; treatment is intended both to facilitate weight loss and to maintain reduced weight. Initial treatment should involve a 6–12 month trial of orlistat, with regular reviews of effectiveness, tolerance, and adherence.

Choice **Orlistat**, a lipase inhibitor, reduces the absorption of dietary fat. Some weight loss in those taking orlistat probably results from a reduction in fat intake to avoid severe gastro-intestinal effects including steatorrhoea. Vitamin supplementation (especially of vitamin D) may be considered if there is concern about deficiency of fat-soluble vitamins.

Thyroid hormones have no place in the treatment of obesity except in biochemically proven hypothyroid children. The use of diuretics, chorionic gonadotrophin, or amphetamines is not appropriate for weight reduction.

4.6 Drugs used in nausea and vertigo

Antiemetics should be prescribed only when the cause of vomiting is known because otherwise they may delay diagnosis. Antiemetics are unnecessary and sometimes harmful when the cause can be treated, such as in diabetic ketoacidosis, or in digoxin or antiepileptic overdose.

If antiemetic drug treatment is indicated, the drug is chosen according to the aetiology of vomiting.

Antihistamines are effective against nausea and vomiting resulting from many underlying conditions. There is no evidence that any one antihistamine is superior to another but their duration of action and incidence of adverse effects (drowsiness and antimuscarinic effects) differ.

The **phenothiazines** are dopamine antagonists and act centrally by blocking the chemoreceptor trigger zone. They may be considered for the prophylaxis and treatment of nausea and vomiting associated with diffuse neoplastic disease, radiation sickness, and the emesis caused by drugs such as opioids, general anaesthetics, and cytotoxics. **Prochlorperazine**, **perphenazine**, and **trifluoperazine** are less sedating than **chlorpromazine**; severe dystonic reactions sometimes occur with phenothiazines (see below). Some phenothiazines are available as rectal suppositories, which can be useful in children with persistent vomiting or with severe nausea; for children over 12 years prochlorperazine can also be administered as a buccal tablet which is placed between the upper lip and the gum.

Droperidol is a butyrophenone, structurally related to haloperidol, which blocks dopamine receptors in the chemoreceptor trigger zone.

Other antipsychotic drugs including **haloperidol** and **levomepromazine** (methotrimeprazine) (section 4.2.1) are also used for the relief of nausea in palliative care (see p. 27 and p. 28).

Metoclopramide is an effective antiemetic and its activity closely resembles that of the phenothiazines. Metoclopramide also acts directly on the gastro-intestinal tract and it may be superior to the phenothiazines for emesis associated with gastroduodenal, hepatic, and biliary disease. In postoperative nausea and vomiting, metoclopramide has limited efficacy. For the role of metoclopramide in cytotoxic-induced nausea and vomiting see section 8.1.

> **Acute dystonic reactions**
> Phenothiazines and metoclopramide can all induce acute dystonic reactions such as facial and skeletal muscle spasms and oculogyric crises; children (especially girls, young women, and those under 10 kg) are particularly susceptible. With metoclopramide, dystonic effects usually occur shortly after starting treatment and subside within 24 hours of stopping it. An antimuscarinic drug such as procyclidine (section 4.9.2) is used to abort dystonic attacks.

Domperidone acts at the chemoreceptor trigger zone; it has the advantage over metoclopramide and the phenothiazines of being less likely to cause central effects such as sedation and dystonic reactions because it does not readily cross the blood-brain barrier. For the role of domperidone in cytotoxic-induced nausea and vomiting see section 8.1. Domperidone is also used to treat vomiting due to emergency hormonal contraception (section 7.3.5).

Granisetron and **ondansetron** are specific $5HT_3$ antagonists which block $5HT_3$ receptors in the gastro-intestinal tract and in the CNS. They are of value in the management of nausea and vomiting in children receiving cytotoxics and in postoperative nausea and vomiting.

Nabilone is a synthetic cannabinoid with antiemetic properties. It may be used for nausea and vomiting caused by cytotoxic chemotherapy that is unresponsive to conventional antiemetics. Side-effects such as drowsiness and dizziness occur frequently with standard doses.

Dexamethasone (section 6.3.2) has antiemetic effects. For the role of dexa-methasone in cytotoxic-induced nausea and vomiting see section 8.1.

Vomiting during pregnancy

Nausea in the first trimester of pregnancy is generally mild and does not require drug therapy. On rare occasions if vomiting is severe, short-term treatment with an antihistamine, such as **promethazine**, may be required. **Prochlorperazine** or **metoclopramide** may be considered as second-line treatments. If symptoms do not settle in 24 to 48 hours then specialist opinion should be sought. Hyperemesis gravidarum is a more serious condition, which requires intravenous fluid and electrolyte replacement and sometimes nutritional support. Supplementation with thiamine must be considered in order to reduce the risk of Wernicke's encephalopathy.

Postoperative nausea and vomiting

The incidence of postoperative nausea and vomiting depends on many factors including the anaesthetic used, and the type and duration of surgery. The aim is to prevent postoperative nausea and vomiting from occurring. Drugs used include some **phenothiazines** (e.g. prochlorperazine), **droperidol**, **metoclopramide**, **$5HT_3$ antagonists**, **antihistamines** (such as cyclizine), and **dexamethasone**. A combination of two antiemetic drugs acting at different sites may be needed in resistant postoperative nausea and vomiting.

Opioid-induced nausea and vomiting

Cyclizine, ondansetron, and prochlorperazine are used to relieve opioid-induced nausea and vomiting; ondansetron has the advantage of not producing sedation.

Motion sickness

Antiemetics should be given to prevent motion sickness rather than after nausea or vomiting develop. The most effective drug for the prevention of motion sickness is **hyoscine hydrobromide**. For children over 10 years old, a transder-mal hyoscine patch provides prolonged activity but it needs to be applied several hours before travelling. The sedating antihistamines are slightly less effective against motion sickness, but are generally better tolerated than hyoscine. If a sedative effect is desired **promethazine** is useful, but generally a slightly less sedating antihistamine such as **cyclizine** or **cinnarizine** is preferred. The $5HT_3$ antagonists, domperidone, metoclopramide, and the phenothiazines (except the antihistamine phenothiazine promethazine) are **ineffective** in motion sickness.

Other vestibular disorders

Management of vestibular diseases is aimed at treating the underlying cause as well as treating symptoms of the balance disturbance and associated nausea and vomiting.

Antihistamines (such as cinnarizine), and **phenothiazines** (such as prochlorper-azine) are effective for prophylaxis and treatment of nausea and vertigo resulting from vestibular disorders; however, when nausea and vertigo are associated with middle ear surgery, treatment can be difficult.

Cytotoxic chemotherapy

For the management of nausea and vomiting induced by cytotoxic chemotherapy, see section 8.1.

4 Central nervous system

Central nervous system

4

Palliative care

For the management of nausea and vomiting in palliative care, see p. 27 and p. 28.

Migraine

For the management of nausea and vomiting associated with migraine, see p. 270.

Antihistamines

CINNARIZINE

Cautions section 3.4.1

Contra-indications section 3.4.1

Hepatic impairment section 3.4.1

Renal impairment use with caution—no information available

Pregnancy section 3.4.1

Breast-feeding section 3.4.1

Side-effects section 3.4.1; also *rarely* weight gain, sweating, lichen planus, and lupus-like skin reactions

Indication and dose

Relief of symptoms of vestibular disorders
• By mouth
Child 5–12 years 15 mg 3 times daily
Child 12–18 years 30 mg 3 times daily

Motion sickness
• By mouth
Child 5–12 years 15 mg 2 hours before travel then 7.5 mg every 8 hours during journey if necessary
Child 12–18 years 30 mg 2 hours before travel then 15 mg every 8 hours during journey if necessary

Cinnarizine (Non-proprietary)
Tablets, cinnarizine 15 mg, net price 84-tab pack = £17.67. Label: 2

Stugeron® (Janssen-Cilag)
Tablets, scored, cinnarizine 15 mg, net price 15-tab pack = £1.55, 100-tab pack = £3.35. Label: 2

CYCLIZINE

Cautions section 3.4.1; severe heart failure; may counteract haemodynamic benefits of opioids; **interactions:** Appendix 1 (antihistamines)
Skilled tasks Drowsiness may affect performance of skilled tasks (e.g. driving); effects of alcohol enhanced

Contra-indications section 3.4.1

Hepatic impairment section 3.4.1

Pregnancy section 3.4.1

Breast-feeding use with caution—no information available

Side-effects section 3.4.1

Licensed use tablets not licensed for use in children under 6 years; injection not licensed for use in children

Indication and dose

Nausea and vomiting of known cause; nausea and vomiting associated with vestibular disorders and palliative care
• By mouth or by intravenous injection over 3–5 minutes
Child 1 month–6 years 0.5–1 mg/kg up to 3 times daily; max. single dose 25 mg
Child 6–12 years 25 mg up to 3 times daily
Child 12–18 years 50 mg up to 3 times daily

• By rectum
Child 2–6 years 12.5 mg up to 3 times daily
Child 6–12 years 25 mg up to 3 times daily
Child 12–18 years 50 mg up to 3 times daily

• By continuous intravenous or subcutaneous infusion
Child 1 month–2 years 3 mg/kg over 24 hours
Child 2–5 years 50 mg over 24 hours
Child 6–12 years 75 mg over 24 hours
Child 12–18 years 150 mg over 24 hours

Administration for administration *by mouth*, tablets may be crushed

Valoid® (Amdipharm)
Tablets, scored, cyclizine hydrochloride 50 mg, net price 100-tab pack = £7.41. Label: 2

Injection PoM, cyclizine lactate 50 mg/mL, net price 1-mL amp = 52p

Cyclizine (Non-proprietary)
Suppositories, 12.5 mg, 25 mg, 50 mg, 100 mg. Available from 'special-order' manufacturers or specialist importing companies, see p. 957

PROMETHAZINE HYDROCHLORIDE

Cautions see notes in section 3.4.1

Contra-indications see Promethazine Hydrochloride, section 3.4.1

Hepatic impairment see notes in section 3.4.1

Renal impairment use with caution

Pregnancy see notes in section 3.4.1

Breast-feeding see notes in section 3.4.1

Side-effects see Promethazine Hydrochloride, section 3.4.1 but more sedating

Indication and dose

Nausea and vomiting
• By mouth
Child 2–5 years 5 mg at bedtime on night before travel, repeat following morning if necessary

▱ **PROMETHAZINE HYDROCHLORIDE** (*continued*)

Child 5–10 years 10 mg at bedtime on night before travel, repeat following morning if necessary

Child 10–18 years 20–25 mg at bedtime on night before travel, repeat following morning if necessary

Allergy and urticaria section 3.4.1

Sedation section 4.1.1

◀**Preparations**
Section 3.4.1

◢ **PROMETHAZINE TEOCLATE**

Cautions section 3.4.1
Contra-indications section 3.4.1
Hepatic impairment section 3.4.1
Renal impairment use with caution
Pregnancy section 3.4.1
Breast-feeding section 3.4.1
Side-effects section 3.4.1
Licensed use not licensed to treat vomiting of pregnancy

Indication and dose

Nausea, vomiting, labyrinthine disorders
• By mouth
Child 5–10 years 12.5–37.5 mg daily
Child 10–18 years 25–75 mg daily (max. 100 mg)

Motion sickness prevention
• By mouth
Child 5–10 years 12.5 mg at bedtime on night before travel *or* 12.5 mg 1–2 hours before travel
Child 10–18 years 25 mg at bedtime on night before travel *or* 25 mg 1–2 hours before travel

Severe vomiting during pregnancy
• By mouth
25 mg at bedtime increased if necessary to max. 100 mg daily (but see also Vomiting During Pregnancy, p. 245)

Avomine® (Manx)
Tablets, scored, promethazine teoclate 25 mg, net price 10-tab pack = £1.13; 28-tab pack = £3.13. Label: 2

Phenothiazines and related drugs

◢ **CHLORPROMAZINE HYDROCHLORIDE**

Cautions see Chlorpromazine Hydrochloride, section 4.2.1
Contra-indications see notes in section 4.2.1
Hepatic impairment see notes in section 4.2.1
Renal impairment see notes in section 4.2.1
Pregnancy see notes in section 4.2.1
Breast-feeding see notes in section 4.2.1
Side-effects see Chlorpromazine Hydrochloride, section 4.2.1

Indication and dose

Nausea and vomiting of terminal illness (where other drugs are unsuitable)
• By mouth
Child 1–6 years 500 micrograms/kg every 4–6 hours; max. 40 mg daily

Child 6–12 years 500 micrograms/kg every 4–6 hours; max. 75 mg daily
Child 12–18 years 10–25 mg every 4–6 hours
• By deep intramuscular injection
Child 1–6 years 500 micrograms/kg every 6–8 hours; max. 40 mg daily
Child 6–12 years 500 micrograms/kg every 6–8 hours; max. 75 mg daily
Child 12–18 years initially 25 mg then 25–50 mg every 3–4 hours until vomiting stops

◀**Preparations**
Section 4.2.1

◢ **DROPERIDOL**

Cautions section 4.2.1; also chronic obstructive pulmonary disease or respiratory failure; electrolyte disturbances; history of alcohol abuse; continuous pulse oximetry required if risk of ventricular arrhythmia—continue for 30 minutes following administration; **interactions**: Appendix 1 (droperidol)

Contra-indications section 4.2.1; QT-interval prolongation (avoid concomitant administration of drugs that prolong QT interval); hypokalaemia; hypomagnesaemia; bradycardia

Hepatic impairment max. 625 micrograms repeated every 6 hours as required
Renal impairment max. 625 micrograms repeated every 6 hours as required
Pregnancy section 4.2.1
Breast-feeding limited information available—avoid repeated administration
Side-effects section 4.2.1; also anxiety, cardiac arrest, hallucinations, and inappropriate secretion of antidiuretic hormone

4

Central nervous system

◻ DROPERIDOL (*continued*)

Indication and dose

Prevention and treatment of postoperative nausea and vomiting
- By intravenous injection

  Child 2–18 years 20–50 micrograms/kg (max. 1.25 mg) 30 minutes before the end of surgery, repeated every 6 hours as necessary

Xomolix® (ProStrakan) ▼ PoM
Injection, droperidol 2.5 mg/mL, net price 1-mL amp = £3.94

PERPHENAZINE

Cautions see notes in section 4.2.1
Contra-indications see notes in section 4.2.1
Hepatic impairment see notes in section 4.2.1
Renal impairment see notes in section 4.2.1
Pregnancy see notes in section 4.2.1
Breast-feeding see notes in section 4.2.1
Side-effects see Perphenazine, section 4.2.1; extrapyramidal symptoms

Indication and dose

Severe nausea and vomiting unresponsive to other antiemetics
- By mouth

  Child 14–18 years 4 mg 3 times daily, adjusted according to response, max. 24 mg daily

◢ Preparations
Section 4.2.1

PROCHLORPERAZINE

Cautions section 4.2.1; hypotension more likely after intramuscular injection
Contra-indications section 4.2.1
Hepatic impairment section 4.2.1
Renal impairment section 4.2.1
Pregnancy section 4.2.1
Breast-feeding section 4.2.1
Side-effects section 4.2.1; extrapyramidal symptoms, particularly dystonias, more frequent; respiratory depression may occur in susceptible children
Licensed use injection not licensed for use in children

Indication and dose

Prevention and treatment of nausea and vomiting
- By mouth

  Child 1–12 years and over 10 kg 250 micrograms/kg 2–3 times daily

  Child 12–18 years 5–10 mg, repeated if necessary up to 3 times daily

- By intramuscular injection

  Child 2–5 years, 1.25–2.5 mg, repeated if necessary up to 3 times daily

  Child 5–12 years 5–6.25 mg, repeated if necessary up to 3 times daily

  Child 12–18 years 12.5 mg, repeated if necessary up to 3 times daily

Note Doses are expressed as prochlorperazine maleate or mesilate; 1 mg prochlorperazine maleate ≡ 1 mg prochlorperazine mesilate

Prochlorperazine (Non-proprietary) PoM
Tablets, prochlorperazine maleate 5 mg, net price 28 = £1.45, 84 = £3.81. Label: 2

Injection, prochlorperazine mesilate 12.5 mg/mL, net price 1-mL amp = 52p

Stemetil® (Sanofi-Aventis) PoM
Tablets, prochlorperazine maleate 5 mg (off-white), net price 84-tab pack = £5.94. Label: 2

Syrup, straw-coloured, prochlorperazine mesilate 5 mg/5 mL, net price 100-mL pack = £3.34. Label: 2

Injection, prochlorperazine mesilate 12.5 mg/mL, net price 1-mL amp = 52p

◢ Buccal preparation
Buccastem® (Alliance) PoM
Tablets (buccal), pale yellow, prochlorperazine maleate 3 mg, net price 5 × 10-tab pack = £4.91. Label: 2, counselling, administration, see under Dose below

Dose
- By mouth
  Child 12–18 years 1–2 tablets twice daily; tablets are placed high between upper lip and gum and left to dissolve

TRIFLUOPERAZINE

Cautions see notes in section 4.2.1
Contra-indications see notes in section 4.2.1
Hepatic impairment see notes in section 4.2.1
Renal impairment see notes in section 4.2.1
Pregnancy see notes in section 4.2.1
Breast-feeding see notes in section 4.2.1
Side-effects see Trifluoperazine section 4.2.1

Indication and dose

Severe nausea and vomiting unresponsive to other antiemetics
- By mouth

  Child 3–5 years up to 500 micrograms twice daily

  Child 6–12 years up to 2 mg twice daily

◻ **TRIFLUOPERAZINE** (*continued*)

Child 12–18 years 1–2 mg twice daily; max. 3 mg twice daily

◀**Preparations**
Section 4.2.1

▰▰▰ **Domperidone and metoclopramide**

◢ **DOMPERIDONE**

Cautions children; **interactions**: Appendix 1 (domperidone)

Contra-indications prolactinaemia; if increased gastro-intestinal motility harmful

Hepatic impairment avoid

Renal impairment reduce dose in renal impairment

Pregnancy use only if potential benefit outweighs risk

Breast-feeding amount too small to be harmful

Side-effects *rarely* gastro-intestinal disturbances (including cramps), and hyperprolactinaemia; *very rarely* ventricular arrhythmias, agitation, seizures, extrapyramidal effects, headache, and rashes; also reported QT-interval prolongation

Indication and dose

Nausea and vomiting
• By mouth

Child over 1 month and body-weight up to 35 kg 250–500 micrograms/kg 3–4 times daily; max. 2.4 mg/kg in 24 hours

Body-weight 35 kg and over 10–20 mg 3–4 times daily, max. 80 mg daily

• By rectum

Body-weight 15–35 kg 30 mg twice daily

Body-weight over 35 kg 60 mg twice daily

Gastro-intestinal stasis section 1.2

¹**Domperidone** (Non-proprietary) ℞
Tablets, 10 mg (as maleate), net price 30-tab pack = £1.30; 100-tab pack = £2.39

Suspension, domperidone 5 mg/5 mL, net price 200-mL pack = £7.22

1. Domperidone can be sold to the public for children over 16 years (provided packs do not contain more than 200 mg) for the relief of postprandial symptoms of excessive fullness, nausea, epigastric bloating and belching occasionally accompanied by epigastric discomfort and heartburn, and for the relief of nausea and vomiting of less than 48 hours duration (max. single dose 10 mg, max. daily dose 40 mg)

Motilium® (Sanofi-Aventis) ℞
Tablets, f/c, domperidone 10 mg (as maleate), net price 30-tab pack = £2.71; 100-tab pack = £9.04

Suppositories, domperidone 30 mg, net price 10 = £3.06

◢ **METOCLOPRAMIDE HYDROCHLORIDE**

Cautions atopic allergy (including asthma); may mask underlying disorders such as cerebral irritation; epilepsy; acute porphyria (section 9.8.2); **interactions**: Appendix 1 (metoclopramide)

Contra-indications gastro-intestinal obstruction, perforation or haemorrhage; 3–4 days after gastro-intestinal surgery; phaeochromocytoma

Hepatic impairment reduce dose

Renal impairment avoid or use small dose in severe impairment; increased risk of extrapyramidal reactions

Pregnancy not known to be harmful but manufacturer advises use only when compelling reasons

Breast-feeding small amount present in milk; avoid

Side-effects extrapyramidal effects (see p. 244), hyperprolactinaemia, occasionally tardive dyskinesia on prolonged administration; also reported anxiety, confusion, drowsiness, restlessness, diarrhoea, depression, neuroleptic malignant syndrome, rashes, pruritus, oedema; cardiac conduction abnormalities reported following intravenous administration; *rarely* methaemoglobinaemia (more severe in G6PD deficiency)

Licensed use not licensed for use in neonates as a prokinetic

Indication and dose

Severe intractable vomiting of known cause, vomiting associated with radiotherapy and cytotoxics, aid to gastro-intestinal intubation, as a prokinetic in neonates
• By mouth, or by intramuscular injection or by intravenous injection over 1–2 minutes

Neonate 100 micrograms/kg every 6–8 hours (by mouth or by intravenous injection only)

Child 1 month–1 year and body-weight up to 10 kg 100 micrograms/kg (max. 1 mg) twice daily

Child 1–3 years and body-weight 10–14 kg 1 mg 2–3 times daily

Child 3–5 years and body-weight 15–19 kg 2 mg 2–3 times daily

Child 5–9 years and body-weight 20–29 kg 2.5 mg 3 times daily

Child 9–18 years and body-weight 30–60 kg 5 mg 3 times daily

Child 15–18 years and body-weight over 60 kg 10 mg 3 times daily

Note Daily dose of metoclopramide should not normally exceed 500 micrograms/kg

4

Central nervous system

△ **METOCLOPRAMIDE HYDROCHLORIDE (continued)**

Premedication in diagnostic procedures
- **By mouth as a single dose 5–10 minutes before examination**

  Child 1 month–3 years and body-weight up to 14 kg 100 micrograms/kg, max. 1 mg

  Child 3–5 years and body-weight 15–19 kg 2 mg

  Child 5–9 years and body-weight 20–29 kg 2.5 mg

  Child 9–15 years and body-weight 30–60 kg 5 mg

  Child 15–18 years and body-weight over 60 kg 10 mg

Metoclopramide (Non-proprietary) PoM
  Tablets, metoclopramide hydrochloride 10 mg, net price 28-tab pack = £1.00

Oral solution, metoclopramide hydrochloride 5 mg/5 mL, net price 150-mL pack = £3.63. Counselling, use of pipette

Note Sugar-free versions are available and can be ordered by specifying 'sugar-free' on the prescription

Injection, metoclopramide hydrochloride 5 mg/mL, net price 2-mL amp = 26p

Maxolon® (Amdipharm) PoM
  Tablets, scored, metoclopramide hydrochloride 10 mg, net price 84-tab pack = £5.24

  Injection, metoclopramide hydrochloride 5 mg/mL, net price 2-mL amp = 27p

◢Compound preparations (for migraine)
  Section 4.7.4.1

5HT₃ antagonists

GRANISETRON

Cautions QT-interval prolongation (avoid concomitant administration of drugs that prolong QT interval)

Pregnancy use only when compelling reasons—no information available

Breast-feeding avoid—no information available

Side-effects constipation, nausea, diarrhoea, vomiting, abdominal pain; headache, drowsiness, asthenia; fever; *rarely* hepatic dysfunction, chest pain, arrhythmia; *very rarely* anorexia, dizziness, insomnia, agitation, movement disorders, rash

Licensed use sterile solution not licensed for use in children under 2 years

Indication and dose

Treatment and prevention of nausea and vomiting induced by cytotoxic chemotherapy or radiotherapy
- **By mouth**

  Child 12–18 years 1–2 mg within 1 hour before start of treatment, then 1 mg twice daily during treatment (total daily dose may alternatively be given as a single dose); when intravenous infusion also used, max. combined total 9 mg in 24 hours

- **By intravenous infusion**

  Child 1 month–12 years prevention, 40 micrograms/kg (max. 3 mg) before start of cytotoxic therapy; treatment, 40 micrograms/kg (max.

3 mg) repeated within 24 hours if necessary (not less than 10 minutes after initial dose)

- **By intravenous injection or by intravenous infusion**

  Child 12–18 years prevention, 3 mg before start of cytotoxic therapy (up to 2 additional 3-mg doses may be given within 24 hours); treatment, 3 mg repeated if necessary (doses must not be given less than 10 minutes apart). max. 9 mg in 24 hours

Administration for *intravenous infusion*, dilute 3 mL in 10–30 mL Glucose 5% *or* Sodium Chloride 0.9%, *or* Compound Sodium Lactate; give over 5 minutes

Granisetron (Non-proprietary) PoM
  Tablets, granisetron (as hydrochloride) 1 mg, net price 10-tab pack = £65.49

  Injection, granisetron (as hydrochloride) 1 mg/mL, for dilution before use, net price 1-mL amp = £1.60, 3-mL amp = £4.80

Kytril® (Roche) PoM
  Tablets, f/c, granisetron (as hydrochloride) 1 mg, net price 10-tab pack = £62.94; 2 mg, 5-tab pack = £62.94

  Injection, granisetron (as hydrochloride) 1 mg/mL, for dilution before use, net price 1-mL amp = £8.26, 3-mL amp = £24.78

ONDANSETRON

Cautions QT-interval prolongation (avoid concomitant administration of drugs that prolong QT interval); subacute intestinal obstruction; adenotonsillar surgery

Hepatic impairment reduce dose in moderate or severe impairment

Pregnancy no information available; avoid unless potential benefit outweighs risk

Breast-feeding present in milk in *animal* studies—avoid

Side-effects constipation; headache; flushing; injection-site reactions; *less commonly* hiccups, hypotension, bradycardia, chest pain, arrhythmias, movement disorders, seizures; *on intravenous administration*, *rarely* dizziness, transient visual disturbances (*very rarely* transient blindness)

◁ ONDANSETRON *(continued)*

Licensed use oral and parenteral preparations not licensed for use in children under 6 months for the treatment of chemotherapy-induced nausea and vomiting or children under 1 month for the prevention and treatment of post-operative nausea and vomiting; not licensed for radiotherapy-induced nausea and vomiting in children

Indication and dose

Prevention and treatment of chemotherapy- and radiotherapy-induced nausea and vomiting
• **By intravenous infusion over 15 minutes**
Child 6 months–18 years *either* 5 mg/m^2 immediately before chemotherapy (max. single dose 8 mg), then give by mouth, *or* 150 micrograms/kg immediately before chemotherapy (max. single dose 8 mg) repeated every 4 hours for 2 further doses, then give by mouth; max. total daily dose 32 mg

• **By mouth following intravenous administration**
Child 6 months–18 years

Body surface area less than 0.6 m^2 *or* body-weight 10 kg or less 2 mg every 12 hours for up to 5 days (max. total daily dose 32 mg)

Body surface area 0.6 m^2 or greater *or* body-weight over 10 kg 4 mg every 12 hours for up to 5 days (max. total daily dose 32 mg)

Treatment and prevention of postoperative nausea and vomiting
• **By slow intravenous injection over at least 30 seconds**
Child 1 month–18 years 100 micrograms/kg (max. 4 mg), as a single dose before, during, or after induction of anaesthesia

Administration for *intravenous infusion*, dilute to a concentration of 320–640 micrograms/mL with Glucose 5% *or* Sodium Chloride 0.9% *or* Ringer's Solution; give over at least 15 minutes

Ondansetron (Non-proprietary) ℞
Tablets, ondansetron (as hydrochloride) 4 mg, net price 30-tab pack = £87.81; 8 mg, 10-tab pack = £58.52
Brands include *Ondemet*®

Injection, ondansetron (as hydrochloride) 2 mg/mL, net price 2-mL amp = £5.39, 4-mL amp = £10.79
Brands include *Ondemet*®

Zofran® (GSK) ℞
Tablets, yellow, f/c, ondansetron (as hydrochloride) 4 mg, net price 30-tab pack = £107.91; 8 mg, 10-tab pack = £71.94

Oral lyophilisates (*Zofran Melt*®), ondansetron 4 mg, net price 10-tab pack = £35.97; 8 mg, 10-tab pack = £71.94. Counselling, administration
Excipients include aspartame (section 9.4.1)

Counselling Tablets should be placed on the tongue, allowed to disperse and swallowed

Syrup, sugar-free, strawberry-flavoured, ondansetron (as hydrochloride) 4 mg/5 mL, net price 50-mL pack = £35.97

Injection, ondansetron (as hydrochloride) 2 mg/mL, net price 2-mL amp = £5.99; 4-mL amp = £11.99

Cannabinoid

NABILONE

Cautions history of psychiatric disorder; hypertension; heart disease; adverse effects on mental state can persist for 48–72 hours after stopping; **interactions**: Appendix 1 (nabilone)
Skilled tasks Drowsiness may affect performance of skilled tasks (e.g. driving); effects of alcohol enhanced

Hepatic impairment avoid in severe impairment

Pregnancy avoid unless essential

Breast-feeding avoid—no information available

Side-effects drowsiness, vertigo, euphoria, dry mouth, ataxia, visual disturbance, concentration difficulties, sleep disturbance, dysphoria, hypotension, headache and nausea; also confusion, disorientation, hallucinations, psychosis, depression, decreased coordination, tremors, tachycardia, decreased appetite, and abdominal pain
Behavioural effects Children and carers should be made aware of possible changes of mood and other adverse behavioural effects

Licensed use not licensed for use in children

Indication and dose

Nausea and vomiting caused by cytotoxic chemotherapy, unresponsive to conventional antiemetics (under close observation, preferably in hospital setting)
• **By mouth**
Consult local treatment protocol for details

Nabilone (Valeant) ℅
Capsules, blue/white, nabilone 1 mg, net price 20-cap pack = £125.84. Label: 2, counselling, behavioural effects

4

Central nervous system

Hyoscine

HYOSCINE HYDROBROMIDE

(Scopolamine Hydrobromide)

Cautions section 1.2; also epilepsy

Skilled tasks Drowsiness may affect performance of skilled tasks (e.g. driving) and may persist for up to 24 hours or longer after removal of patch; effects of alcohol enhanced

Contra-indications section 1.2

Hepatic impairment use with caution

Renal impairment use with caution

Pregnancy use only if potential benefit outweighs risk; injection may depress neonatal respiration

Breast-feeding amount too small to be harmful

Side-effects section 1.2

Licensed use not licensed for use in excessive respiratory secretions or hypersalivation associated with clozapine therapy

Indication and dose

Motion sickness

* By mouth

  Child 4–10 years 75–150 micrograms 30 minutes before start of journey, repeated every 6 hours if required; max. 3 doses in 24 hours

  Child 10–18 years 150–300 micrograms 30 minutes before start of journey, repeated every 6 hours if required; max. 3 doses in 24 hours

* By topical application

  Child 10–18 years apply 1 patch (1 mg) to hairless area of skin behind ear 5–6 hours before journey; replace if necessary after 72 hours, siting replacement patch behind the other ear

Excessive respiratory secretions

* By mouth or by sublingual administration

  Child 2–12 years 10 micrograms/kg, max. 300 micrograms 4 times daily

  Child 12–18 years 300 micrograms 4 times daily

* By transdermal route

  Child 1 month–3 years 250 micrograms every 72 hours (quarter of a patch)

  Child 3–10 years 500 micrograms every 72 hours (half a patch)

  Child 10–18 years 1 mg every 72 hours (one patch)

* By subcutaneous injection, intravenous injection, intravenous infusion, or subcutaneous infusion

  See Prescribing in Palliative Care, p. 27 and p. 28

Hypersalivation associated with clozapine therapy

* By mouth

  Child 12–18 years 300 micrograms up to 3 times daily; max. 900 micrograms daily

Premedication section 15.1.3

Administration *patch* applied to hairless area of skin behind ear; if less than whole patch required **either** cut with scissors along full thickness ensuring membrane is not peeled away **or** cover portion to prevent contact with skin
For administration *by mouth*, injection solution may be given orally

Joy-Rides® (GSK Consumer Healthcare)
Tablets, chewable, hyoscine hydrobromide 150 micrograms, net price 12-tab pack = £1.49. Label: 2, 24

Kwells® (Bayer Consumer Care)
Tablets, chewable, hyoscine hydrobromide 150 micrograms (*Kwells® Kids*), net price 12-tab pack = £1.67; 300 micrograms, 12-tab pack = £1.67. Label: 2

Scopoderm TTS® (Novartis Consumer Health) PoM
Patch, self-adhesive, pink, releasing hyoscine approx. 1 mg/72 hours when in contact with skin. Net price 2 = £4.30. Label: 19, counselling, see below

Counselling Explain accompanying instructions to child and carer, in particular emphasise advice to wash hands after handling and to wash application site after removing, and to use one patch at a time

4.7 Analgesics

4.7.1	Non-opioid analgesics
4.7.2	Opioid analgesics
4.7.3	Neuropathic pain
4.7.4	Antimigraine drugs

The non-opioid drugs (section 4.7.1), paracetamol and ibuprofen (and other NSAIDs), are particularly suitable for pain in musculoskeletal conditions, whereas the opioid analgesics (section 4.7.2) are more suitable for moderate to severe pain, particularly of visceral origin.

Pain in palliative care   For advice on pain relief in palliative care, see p. 24.

Pain in sickle-cell disease   The pain of mild sickle-cell crises is managed with paracetamol, an NSAID (section 10.1.1), codeine, or dihydrocodeine. Severe crises may require the use of morphine or diamorphine; concomitant use of an

(side margin) 4 Central nervous system

NSAID may potentiate analgesia and allow lower doses of the opioid to be used. A mixture of nitrous oxide and oxygen (*Entonox*®, *Equanox*®) may also be used.

Dental and orofacial pain   Analgesics should be used judiciously in dental care as a **temporary** measure until the cause of the pain has been dealt with.

Dental pain of inflammatory origin, such as that associated with pulpitis, apical infection, localised osteitis (dry socket) or pericoronitis is usually best managed by treating the infection, providing drainage, restorative procedures, and other local measures. Analgesics provide temporary relief of pain (usually for about 1 to 7 days) until the causative factors have been brought under control. In the case of pulpitis, intra-osseous infection or abscess, reliance on analgesics alone is usually inappropriate.

Similarly the pain and discomfort associated with acute problems of the oral mucosa (e.g. acute herpetic gingivostomatitis, erythema multiforme) may be relieved by **benzydamine** (p. 663) or topical anaesthetics until the cause of the mucosal disorder has been dealt with. However, where a child is febrile, the antipyretic action of **paracetamol** (p. 254) or **ibuprofen** (p. 613) is often helpful.

The *choice* of an analgesic for dental purposes should be based on its suitability for the child. Most dental pain is relieved effectively by non-steroidal anti-inflammatory drugs (NSAIDs) e.g. ibuprofen (section 10.1.1). **Paracetamol** has analgesic and antipyretic effects but no anti-inflammatory effect.

Opioid analgesics (section 4.7.2) such as **dihydrocodeine** act on the central nervous system and are traditionally used for *moderate to severe pain*. However, opioid analgesics are relatively ineffective in dental pain and their side-effects can be unpleasant.

Combining a non-opioid with an opioid analgesic can provide greater relief of pain than either analgesic given alone. However, this applies only when an adequate dose of each analgesic is used. Most combination analgesic preparations have not been shown to provide greater relief of pain than an adequate dose of the non-opioid component given alone. Moreover, combination preparations have the disadvantage of an increased number of side-effects.

Any analgesic given before a dental procedure should have a low risk of increasing postoperative bleeding. In the case of pain after the dental procedure, taking an analgesic before the effect of the local anaesthetic has worn off can improve control. Postoperative analgesia with ibuprofen is usually continued for about 24 to 72 hours.

Dysmenorrhoea   Paracetamol or a NSAID (section 10.1.1) will generally provide adequate relief of pain from dysmenorrhoea. Alternatively use of a combined hormonal contraceptive in adolescent girls may prevent the pain.

4.7.1 Non-opioid analgesics

Paracetamol has analgesic and antipyretic properties but no demonstrable anti-inflammatory activity; unlike opioid analgesics, it does not cause respiratory depression and is less irritant to the stomach than the NSAIDs. **Overdosage** with paracetamol is particularly dangerous as it may cause hepatic damage which is sometimes not apparent for 4 to 6 days (see Emergency Treatment of Poisoning, p. 36).

Non-steroidal anti-inflammatory analgesics (NSAIDs, section 10.1.1) are particularly useful for the treatment of children with chronic disease accompanied by pain and inflammation. Some of them are also used in the short-term treatment of mild to moderate pain including transient musculoskeletal pain but paracetamol is now often preferred. They are also suitable for the relief of pain in *dysmenorrhoea* and to treat pain caused by *secondary bone tumours*, many of which produce lysis of bone and release prostaglandins (see Prescribing in Palliative Care, p. 24). Due to an association with Reye's syndrome (section 2.9), **aspirin** should be avoided in children under 16 years except in Kawasaki syndrome or for its antiplatelet action (section 2.9). NSAIDs are also used for peri-operative analgesia (section 15.1.4.2).

Dental and orofacial pain   Most dental pain is relieved effectively by NSAIDs (section 10.1.1).

Paracetamol is less irritant to the stomach than NSAIDs. Paracetamol is a suitable analgesic for children; sugar-free versions can be requested by specifying 'sugar-free' on the prescription.

For further information on the management of dental and orofacial pain, see notes above, p. 253.

Compound analgesic preparations

Compound analgesic preparations that contain a simple analgesic (such as aspirin or paracetamol) with an opioid component reduce the scope for effective titration of the individual components in the management of pain of varying intensity.

Compound analgesic preparations containing paracetamol or aspirin with a *low dose* of an opioid analgesic (e.g. 8 mg of codeine phosphate per compound tablet) may be used in older children but the advantages have not been substantiated. The low dose of the opioid may be enough to cause opioid side-effects (in particular, constipation) and can complicate the treatment of **overdosage** (see p. 39) yet may not provide significant additional relief of pain.

A *full dose* of the opioid component (e.g. 60 mg codeine phosphate) in compound analgesic preparations effectively augments the analgesic activity but is associated with the full range of opioid side-effects (including nausea, vomiting, severe constipation, drowsiness, respiratory depression, and risk of dependence on long-term administration). For details of the **side-effects** of opioid analgesics, see p. 256.

PARACETAMOL
(Acetaminophen)

Cautions alcohol dependence; high risk of liver toxicity with high doses; **interactions:** Appendix 1 (paracetamol)

Hepatic impairment dose-related toxicity—avoid large doses; reduce *infusion* dose in hepatic impairment to max. 3 g daily

Renal impairment increase *infusion* dose interval to every 6 hours if estimated glomerular filtration rate less than 30 mL/minute/1.73m^2

Pregnancy not known to be harmful

Breast-feeding amount too small to be harmful

Side-effects side-effects rare, but rashes, blood disorders (including thrombocytopenia, leucopenia, neutropenia) reported; hypotension, flushing, and tachycardia also reported on infusion; **important:** liver damage (and less frequently renal damage) following **overdosage**, see Emergency Treatment of Poisoning, p. 36

Licensed use not licensed for use in children under 2 months by mouth; doses for severe symptoms not licensed; co-codamol 8/500 tablets not licensed for use in children under 12 years

Indication and dose

Pain; pyrexia with discomfort
• By mouth

Neonate 28–32 weeks postmenstrual age 20 mg/kg as a single dose then 10–15 mg/kg every 8–12 hours as necessary; max. 30 mg/kg daily in divided doses

Neonate over 32 weeks postmenstrual age 20 mg/kg as a single dose then 10–15 mg/kg every 6–8 hours as necessary; max. 60 mg/kg daily in divided doses

Child 1–3 months 30–60 mg every 8 hours as necessary

Child 3–12 months 60–120 mg every 4–6 hours (max. 4 doses in 24 hours)

Child 1–6 years 120–250 mg every 4–6 hours (max. 4 doses in 24 hours)

Child 6–12 years 250–500 mg every 4–6 hours (max. 4 doses in 24 hours)

Child 12–18 years 500 mg every 4–6 hours

• By rectum

Neonate 28–32 weeks postmenstrual age 20 mg/kg as a single dose then 15 mg/kg every 12 hours as necessary; max. 30 mg/kg daily in divided doses

Neonate over 32 weeks postmenstrual age 30 mg/kg as a single dose then 20 mg/kg every 8 hours as necessary; max. 60 mg/kg daily in divided doses

Child 1–3 months 30–60 mg every 8 hours as necessary

Child 3–12 months 60–125 mg every 4–6 hours as necessary (max. 4 doses in 24 hours)

Child 1–5 years 125–250 mg every 4–6 hours as necessary (max. 4 doses in 24 hours)

Child 5–12 years 250–500 mg every 4–6 hours as necessary (max. 4 doses in 24 hours)

Child 12–18 years 500 mg every 4–6 hours

• By intravenous infusion over 15 minutes

Neonate 7.5 mg/kg every 4–6 hours; max. 30 mg/kg daily

Child body-weight under 10 kg 7.5 mg/kg every 4–6 hours; max. 30 mg/kg daily

Child body-weight 10–50 kg 15 mg/kg every 4–6 hours; max. 60 mg/kg daily

Child body-weight over 50 kg 1 g every 4–6 hours; max. 4 g daily

◁ **PARACETAMOL** *(continued)*

Severe pain; severe pyrexia (but see Cautions)

● **By mouth**

Child 1–3 months 20–30 mg/kg as a single dose then 15–20 mg/kg every 6–8 hours; max. 60 mg/kg daily in divided doses

Child 3–12 months 20–30 mg/kg as a single dose then 15–20 mg/kg every 6–8 hours; max. 90 mg/kg daily in divided doses

Child 1–6 years 20–30 mg/kg as a single dose then 15–20 mg/kg every 6–8 hours; max. 90 mg/kg daily in divided doses

Child 6–12 years 20–30 mg/kg (max. 1 g) as a single dose then 15–20 mg/kg every 6–8 hours; max. 90 mg/kg (max. 4 g) daily in divided doses

Child 12–18 years 1 g every 4–6 hours (max. 4 doses in 24 hours)

● **By rectum**

Child 1–3 months 30 mg/kg as a single dose then 15–20 mg/kg every 6–8 hours; max. 60 mg/kg daily in divided doses

Child 3–12 months 30–40 mg/kg as a single dose then 15–20 mg/kg every 6–8 hours; max. 90 mg/kg daily in divided doses

Child 1–6 years 30–40 mg/kg as a single dose then 15–20 mg/kg every 6–8 hours; max. 90 mg/kg daily in divided doses

Child 6–12 years 30–40 mg/kg (max. 1 g) as a single dose then 15–20 mg/kg every 6–8 hours; max. 90 mg/kg (max. 4 g) daily in divided doses

Child 12–18 years 1 g every 4–6 hours (max. 4 doses in 24 hours)

Post-immunisation pyrexia in infants (see also p. 734)

● **By mouth**

Child 2–3 months 60 mg as a single dose repeated once after 6 hours if necessary

Paracetamol (Non-proprietary)

Tablets and caplets [PoM]¹, paracetamol 500 mg, net price 16-tab pack = 17p, 32-tab pack = £1.02, 100-tab pack = £1.72. Label: 29, 30
Brands include *Panadol*® [JHS]

Dental prescribing on NHS Paracetamol Tablets may be prescribed

Capsules [PoM]¹, paracetamol 500 mg, net price 32-cap pack = £1.07. Label: 29, 30
Brands include *Panadol Capsules*® [JHS]

Soluble tablets (= Dispersible tablets) [PoM]², paracetamol 500 mg, net price 60-tab pack = £4.02. Label: 13, 29, 30
Brands include *Panadol Soluble*® [JHS] (contains Na⁺ 18.6 mmol/tablet), *Paracetamol Seltzer*® (contains Na⁺ 16.9 mmol/tablet)

Dental prescribing on NHS Paracetamol Soluble Tablets 500 mg may be prescribed

Paediatric soluble tablets (= Paediatric dispersible tablets), paracetamol 120 mg, net price 16-tab pack = 89p. Label: 13, 30
Brands include *Disprol*® Soluble Paracetamol [JHS]

Oral suspension 120 mg/5 mL (= Paediatric Mixture), paracetamol 120 mg/5 mL, net price 100 mL = 42p. Label: 30

Note BP directs that when Paediatric Paracetamol Oral Suspension or Paediatric Paracetamol Mixture is prescribed Paracetamol Oral Suspension 120 mg/5 mL should be dispensed; sugar-free versions can be ordered by specifying 'sugar-free'on the prescription
Brands include *Calpol*® Paediatric, *Calpol*® Paediatric sugar-free, *Disprol*® Paediatric, *Medinol*® Paediatric sugar-free, *Panadol*® sugar-free

Oral suspension 250 mg/5 mL (= Mixture), paracetamol 250 mg/5 mL, net price 100 mL = 66p. Label: 30
Brands include *Calpol*® 6 Plus [JHS], *Medinol*® Over 6 [JHS]

Dental prescribing on NHS Paracetamol Oral Suspension may be prescribed

Suppositories, paracetamol 60 mg, net price 10 = £9.96; 125 mg, 10 = £11.50; 250 mg, 10 = £23.00; 500 mg, 10 = £35.79. Label: 30
Brands include *Alvedon*®

Note Other strengths available from 'special-order' manufacturers or specialist importing companies, see p. 957

Panadol OA® (GSK) [PoM]

Tablets, f/c, paracetamol 1000 mg, net price 100-tab pack = £3.30. Label: 30

Dose

Pain, pyrexia

● **By mouth**

Child 12–18 years 1 tablet up to 4 times daily, not more often than every 4 hours

Perfalgan® (Bristol-Myers Squibb) ▼ [PoM]

Intravenous infusion, paracetamol 10 mg/mL, net price 50-mL vial = £1.44, 100-mL vial = £1.59

Administration give undiluted or dilute to a concentration of 1 mg/mL in Glucose 5% *or* Sodium Chloride 0.9%; use within 1 hour of dilution

◁ **Co-codamol 8/500**

When co-codamol tablets, dispersible (or effervescent) tablets, or capsules are prescribed and **no strength is stated**, tablets, dispersible (or effervescent) tablets, or capsules, respectively, containing codeine phosphate **8 mg** and paracetamol **500 mg** should be dispensed.

²**Co-codamol 8/500** (Non-proprietary) [PoM] ◁

Tablets, co-codamol 8/500 (codeine phosphate 8 mg, paracetamol 500 mg), net price 30-tab pack = £1.05. Label: 29, 30
Brands include *Panadeine*® [JHS]

Dose

Pain, pyrexia

● **By mouth**

Child 6–12 years ½–1 tablet every 4–6 hours; max. 4 tablets daily

Child 12–18 years 1–2 tablets every 4–6 hours; max. 8 tablets daily

1. Can be sold to the public provided packs contain no more than 32 capsules or tablets; pharmacists can sell multiple packs up to a total quantity of 100 capsules or tablets in justifiable circumstances; for details see *Medicines, Ethics and Practice*, No. 33, London, Pharmaceutical Press, 2009 (and subsequent editions as available)
2. Can be sold to the public under certain circumstances; for exemptions see *Medicines, Ethics and Practice*, No. 33, London, Pharmaceutical Press, 2009 (and subsequent editions as available)

◁ **PARACETAMOL** (*continued*)

Effervescent *or* dispersible tablets, co-codamol 8/500 (codeine phosphate 8 mg, paracetamol 500 mg), net price 100-tab pack = £4.62. Label: 13, 29, 30

Brands include *Paracodol®* ⟨NHS⟩

Note The Drug Tariff allows tablets of co-codamol labelled 'dispersible' to be dispensed against an order for 'effervescent' and *vice versa*

Dose

Pain, pyrexia
• **By mouth**
  Child 6–12 years ½–1 tablet in water every 4–6 hours; max. 4 tablets daily

Child 12–18 years 1–2 tablets in water every 4–6 hours; max. 8 tablets daily

Capsules, co-codamol 8/500 (codeine phosphate 8 mg, paracetamol 500 mg), net price 10-cap pack = £1.10, 20-cap pack = £1.66. Label: 29, 30

Brands include *Paracodol®* ⟨NHS⟩

Dose

Pain, pyrexia
• **By mouth**
  Child 12–18 years 1–2 capsules every 4 hours; max. 8 capsules daily

4.7.2 Opioid analgesics

Opioid analgesics are usually used to relieve moderate to severe pain particularly of visceral origin. Repeated administration may cause tolerance, but this is no deterrent in the control of pain in terminal illness, for guidelines see Prescribing in Palliative Care, p. 24. Regular use of a potent opioid may be appropriate for certain cases of chronic non-malignant pain; treatment should be supervised by a specialist and the child should be assessed at regular intervals.

Cautions Opioids should be used with caution in children with impaired respiratory function and asthma (avoid during an acute attack), hypotension, shock, obstructive or inflammatory bowel disorders, diseases of the biliary tract, and convulsive disorders. A reduced dose is recommended in hypothyroidism or adrenocortical insufficiency. Repeated use of opioid analgesics is associated with the development of psychological and physical dependence; although this is rarely a problem with therapeutic use, caution is advised if prescribing for patients with a history of drug dependence. Avoid abrupt withdrawal after long-term treatment. Transdermal preparations (fentanyl or buprenorphine patches) are not suitable for acute pain or in those children whose analgesic requirements are changing rapidly, because the long time to steady state prevents rapid titration of the dose.

Palliative care In the control of pain in terminal illness, the cautions listed above should not necessarily be a deterrent to the use of opioid analgesics.

Contra-indications Opioid analgesics should be avoided in children with acute respiratory depression, and when there is a risk of paralytic ileus. They are also contra-indicated in conditions associated with raised intracranial pressure, and in head injury (opioid analgesics interfere with pupillary responses vital for neurological assessment). Comatose children should not be treated with opioid analgesics.

Hepatic impairment Opioid analgesics may precipitate coma in children with hepatic impairment; avoid use or reduce dose.

Renal impairment The effects of opioid analgesia are increased and prolonged and there is increased cerebral sensitivity when children with renal impairment are treated with opioid analgesics; avoid use or reduce dose.

Pregnancy Respiratory depression and withdrawal symptoms can occur in the neonate if opioid analgesics are used during delivery; also gastric stasis and inhalation pneumonia has been reported in the mother if opioid analgesics are used during labour.

Side-effects Opioid analgesics share many side-effects, although qualitative and quantitative differences exist. The most common side-effects include nausea and vomiting (particularly in initial stages), constipation, dry mouth and biliary spasm; larger doses produce muscle rigidity, hypotension and respiratory depression (for reversal of opioid-induced respiratory depression, see section 15.1.7); neonates, particularly if preterm, may be more susceptible. Other common side-effects of opioid analgesics include bradycardia, tachycardia, palpitation, oedema, postural hypotension, hallucinations, vertigo, euphoria, dysphoria, mood changes, dependence, dizziness, confusion, drowsiness, sleep disturbances, headache, sexual dysfunction, difficulty with micturition, urinary retention, ureteric spasm, miosis, visual disturbances, sweating, flushing, rash, urticaria, and pruritus. **Overdosage:** see Emergency Treatment of Poisoning, p. 39.

Interactions See Appendix 1 (opioid analgesics) (**important:** special hazard with *pethidine and possibly other opioids* and MAOIs).

Skilled tasks Drowsiness may affect performance of skilled tasks (e.g. driving); effects of alcohol enhanced.

Strong opioids **Morphine** remains the most valuable opioid analgesic for severe pain although it frequently causes nausea and vomiting. It is the standard against which other opioid analgesics are compared. In addition to relief of pain, morphine also confers a state of euphoria and mental detachment.

Morphine is the opioid of choice for the oral treatment of *severe pain in palliative care.* It is given regularly every 4 hours (or every 12 or 24 hours as modified-release preparations). For guidelines on dosage adjustment in palliative care, see p. 24.

Buprenorphine has both opioid agonist and antagonist properties and may precipitate withdrawal symptoms, including pain, in children dependent on other opioids. It has abuse potential and may itself cause dependence. It has a much longer duration of action than morphine and sublingually is an effective analgesic for 6 to 8 hours. Unlike most opioid analgesics, the effects of buprenorphine are only partially reversed by naloxone. It is used rarely in children.

Diamorphine (heroin) is a powerful opioid analgesic. It may cause less nausea and hypotension than morphine. In *palliative care* the greater solubility of diamorphine allows effective doses to be injected in smaller volumes and this is important in the emaciated child.

Diamorphine is sometimes given by the intranasal route to treat acute pain in children, for example, in accident and emergency units; however, as yet, there is limited safety and efficacy data to support this practice.

Alfentanil, fentanyl and **remifentanil** are used by injection for intra-operative analgesia (section 15.1.4.3). Fentanyl is available in a transdermal drug delivery system as a self-adhesive patch which is changed every 72 hours.

Methadone is less sedating than morphine and acts for longer periods. In prolonged use, methadone should not be administered more often than twice daily to avoid the risk of accumulation and opioid overdosage. Methadone may be used instead of morphine when excitation (or exacerbation of pain) occurs with morphine. Methadone may also be used to treat children with neonatal abstinence syndrome (section 4.10).

Papaveretum should not be used in children; morphine is easier to prescribe and less prone to error with regard to the strength and dose.

Pethidine produces prompt but short-lasting analgesia; it is less constipating than morphine, but even in high doses is a less potent analgesic. Its use in children is not recommended. Pethidine is used for analgesia in labour; however, other opioids, such as morphine or diamorphine, are often preferred for obstetric pain.

Tramadol is used in older children and produces analgesia by two mechanisms: an opioid effect and an enhancement of serotonergic and adrenergic pathways. It has fewer of the typical opioid side-effects (notably, less respiratory depression, less constipation and less addiction potential); psychiatric reactions have been reported.

Weak opioids **Codeine** is used for the relief of mild to moderate pain but is too constipating for long-term use.

Dihydrocodeine has an analgesic efficacy similar to that of codeine; doses may be given every 4 hours.

Dose Doses of opioids may need to be **adjusted individually** according to the degree of analgesia and side-effects; response to opioids varies widely, particularly in the neonatal period. Opioid overdosage can have serious consequences and the dose should be calculated and **checked with care.**

Postoperative analgesia A combination of opioid and non-opioid analgesics is used to treat postoperative pain (section 15.1.4.2). The use of intra-operative opioids affects the prescribing of postoperative analgesics. A postoperative opioid analgesic should be given with care since it may potentiate any residual respir-

4

Central nervous system

atory depression (for the treatment of opioid-induced respiratory depression, see section 15.1.7).

Morphine is used most widely. **Tramadol** is not as effective in severe pain as other opioid analgesics. **Buprenorphine** may antagonise the analgesic effect of previously administered opioids and is generally not recommended. **Pethidine** is unsuitable for post-operative pain because it is metabolised to norpethidine which may accumulate, particularly in neonates and in renal impairment; norpethidine stimulates the central nervous system and may cause convulsions.

Opioids are also given epidurally [unlicensed route] in the postoperative period but are associated with side-effects such as pruritus, urinary retention, nausea and vomiting; respiratory depression can be delayed, particularly with morphine.

For details of patient-controlled analgesia (PCA) and nurse-controlled analgesia (NCA) to relieve postoperative pain, consult hospital protocols. Formulations specifically designed for PCA are available (*Pharma-Ject® Morphine Sulphate*).

Dental and orofacial pain   Opioid analgesics are **relatively ineffective** in dental pain. Like other opioids, **dihydrocodeine** often causes nausea and vomiting which limits its value in dental pain; if taken for more than a few doses it is also liable to cause constipation. Dihydrocodeine is not very effective in post-operative dental pain.

For the management of dental and orofacial pain, see p. 253.

Addicts   Although caution is necessary, addicts (and ex-addicts) may be treated with analgesics in the same way as other people when there is a real clinical need. Doctors do not require a special licence to prescribe opioid analgesics for addicts for relief of pain due to organic disease or injury.

Dependence and withdrawal   Psychological dependence rarely occurs when opioids are used for pain relief but tolerance can develop during long-term treatment; they should be withdrawn gradually to avoid abstinence symptoms. For information on the treatment of neonatal abstinence syndrome, see section 4.10.

BUPRENORPHINE

Cautions   see notes above; also impaired consciousness; effects only partially reversed by naloxone

Contra-indications   see notes above; also myasthenia gravis

Hepatic impairment   see notes above

Renal impairment   see notes above

Pregnancy   see notes above

Breast-feeding   avoid unless essential—may inhibit lactation; contra-indicated in the treatment of opioid dependence

Side-effects   see notes above; can induce mild withdrawal symptoms in children dependent on opioids; also diarrhoea, abdominal pain, anorexia, dyspepsia; vasodilatation; dyspnoea; paraesthesia, asthenia, fatigue, agitation, anxiety; *less commonly* flatulence, taste disturbance, hypertension, syncope, hypoxia, wheezing, cough, restlessness, depersonalisation, dysarthria, impaired memory, hypoaesthesia, tremor, influenza-like symptoms, pyrexia, rhinitis, rigors, muscle cramp, myalgia, tinnitus, dry eye, and dry skin; *rarely* paralytic ileus, dysphagia, diverticulitis, impaired concentration, and psychosis; *very rarely* retching, hyperventilation, hiccups, and muscle fasciculation

Licensed use   sublingual tablets not licensed for use in children under 6 years; injection not licensed for use in children under 6 months

Indication and dose

Moderate to severe pain

• By sublingual administration

    Child body-weight 16–25 kg 100 micrograms every 6–8 hours

    Child body-weight 25–37.5 kg 100–200 micrograms every 6–8 hours

    Child body-weight 37.5–50 kg 200–300 micrograms every 6–8 hours

    Child body-weight over 50 kg 200–400 micrograms every 6–8 hours

• By intramuscular or by slow intravenous injection

    Child 6 months–12 years 3–6 micrograms/kg every 6–8 hours, max. 9 micrograms/kg

    Child 12–18 years 300–600 micrograms every 6–8 hours

Administration   for administration *by mouth*, tablets may be halved

Temgesic® (Schering-Plough) ⒸⒹ
Tablets (sublingual), buprenorphine (as hydrochloride), 200 micrograms, net price 50-tab pack = £5.23; 400 micrograms, 50-tab pack = £10.46. Label: 2, 26

Injection, buprenorphine (as hydrochloride) 300 micrograms/mL, net price 1-mL amp = 48p

CODEINE PHOSPHATE

Cautions see notes above; also cardiac arrhythmias; myasthenia gravis; acute abdomen; gallstones

Variation in metabolism The capacity to metabolise codeine can vary considerably between individuals and lead to either reduced therapeutic effect or marked increase in side-effects

Contra-indications see notes above

Hepatic impairment see notes above

Renal impairment see notes above

Pregnancy see notes above

Breast-feeding amount usually too small to be harmful; however, mothers vary considerably in their capacity to metabolise codeine—risk of morphine overdose in infant

Side-effects see notes above; also abdominal pain, anorexia, seizures, malaise, hypothermia, and muscle fasciculation; pancreatitis also reported

Licensed use tablets not licensed for use in children; injection not licensed for use in children under 1 year

Indication and dose

Mild to moderate pain

- **By mouth or by rectum or by subcutaneous injection or by intramuscular injection**

  Neonate 0.5–1 mg/kg every 4–6 hours

  Child 1 month–12 years 0.5–1 mg/kg every 4–6 hours, max. 240 mg daily

  Child 12–18 years 30–60 mg every 4–6 hours, max. 240 mg daily

Codeine Phosphate (Non-proprietary)

Tablets [PoM], codeine phosphate 15 mg, net price 28 = £1.19; 30 mg, 28 = £1.51; 60 mg, 28 = £1.98. Label: 2

Syrup [PoM], codeine phosphate 25 mg/5 mL. Net price 100 mL = 90p. Label: 2

Injection [CD], codeine phosphate 60 mg/mL. Net price 1-mL amp = £2.44

DIAMORPHINE HYDROCHLORIDE

(Heroin Hydrochloride)

Cautions see notes above; also severe diarrhoea; toxic psychosis, CNS depression; severe cor pulmonale

Contra-indications see notes above; also delayed gastric emptying; phaeochromocytoma

Hepatic impairment see notes above

Renal impairment see notes above

Pregnancy see notes above

Breast-feeding therapeutic doses unlikely to affect infant; withdrawal symptoms in infants of dependent mothers; breast-feeding not best method of treating dependence in offspring

Side-effects see notes above; also anorexia, taste disturbance; syncope; asthenia, raised intracranial pressure; myocardial infarction also reported

Licensed use intranasal route not licensed

Indication and dose

Acute or chronic pain

- **By mouth**

  Child 1 month–12 years 100–200 micrograms/kg (max. 10 mg) every 4 hours as necessary

  Child 12–18 years 5–10 mg every 4 hours as necessary

- **By intravenous administration**

  Neonate (ventilated) initially *by intravenous injection* over 30 minutes, 50 micrograms/kg then *by continuous intravenous infusion*, 15 micrograms/kg/hour

  Neonate (non-ventilated) *by continuous intravenous infusion* 2.5–7 micrograms/kg/hour

  Child 1 month–12 years *by continuous intravenous infusion* 12.5–25 micrograms/kg/hour

- **By intravenous injection**

  Child 1–3 months 20 micrograms/kg every 6 hours as necessary

  Child 3–6 months 25–50 micrograms/kg every 6 hours as necessary

  Child 6–12 months 75 micrograms/kg every 4 hours as necessary

  Child 1–12 years 75–100 micrograms/kg every 4 hours as necessary

  Child 12–18 years 2.5–5 mg every 4 hours as necessary

- **By continuous subcutaneous infusion**
  See Prescribing in Palliative Care, p. 24

- **By subcutaneous or by intramuscular injection**

  Child 12–18 years 5 mg every 4 hours as necessary

Acute pain in an emergency setting; short painful procedures

- **Intranasally (but see p. 257)**

  Child over 10 kg 100 micrograms/kg, max. 10 mg

Administration for *intravenous infusion*, dilute in Glucose 5% *or* Sodium Chloride 0.9%; Glucose 5% is preferable

For *intranasal* administration, diamorphine powder should be dissolved in sufficient volume of Water for Injections to provide the requisite dose in 0.2 mL of solution; use solution immediately after preparation

Diamorphine (Non-proprietary) [CD]

Tablets, diamorphine hydrochloride 10 mg. Net price 100-tab pack = £14.76. Label: 2

Injection, powder for reconstitution, diamorphine hydrochloride. Net price 5-mg amp = £2.76, 10-mg amp = £3.43, 30-mg amp = £3.65, 100-mg amp = £10.16, 500-mg amp = £44.52

◀ Extemporaneous formulations available see Extemporaneous Preparations, p. 8

4

Central nervous system

▐ DIHYDROCODEINE TARTRATE

Cautions see notes above; also pancreatitis; severe cor pulmonale

Contra-indications see notes above

Hepatic impairment see notes above

Renal impairment see notes above

Pregnancy see notes above

Breast-feeding use only if potential benefit outweighs risk

Side-effects see notes above; also paralytic ileus, abdominal pain, and paraesthesia

Licensed use most preparations not licensed for use in children under 4 years

Indication and dose

> Moderate to severe pain
> • By mouth or by intramuscular injection or by subcutaneous injection
>> **Child 1–4 years** 500 micrograms/kg every 4–6 hours
>>
>> **Child 4–12 years** 0.5–1 mg/kg (max. 30 mg) every 4–6 hours
>>
>> **Child 12–18 years** 30 mg (max. 50 mg by intramuscular or deep subcutaneous injection) every 4–6 hours

Dihydrocodeine (Non-proprietary)

Tablets [PoM], dihydrocodeine tartrate 30 mg, net price 28-tab pack = £1.59. Label: 2

Dental prescribing on NHS Dihydrocodeine Tablets 30 mg may be prescribed

Oral solution [PoM], dihydrocodeine tartrate 10 mg/5 mL, net price 150 mL = £3.08. Label: 2

Injection [CD], dihydrocodeine tartrate 50 mg/mL, net price 1-mL amp = £2.64

DF 118 Forte® (Martindale) [PoM]

Tablets, dihydrocodeine tartrate 40 mg, net price 100-tab pack = £11.51. Label: 2

Dose

> Severe pain
> • By mouth
>> **Child 12–18 years** 40–80 mg 3 times daily; max. 240 mg daily

▲Modified release

DHC Continus® (Napp) [PoM]

Tablets, m/r, dihydrocodeine tartrate 60 mg, net price 56-tab pack = £5.28; 90 mg, 56-tab pack = £8.66; 120 mg, 56-tab pack = £11.11. Label: 2, 25

Dose

> Chronic severe pain
> • By mouth
>> **Child 12–18 years** 60–120 mg every 12 hours

▐ FENTANYL

Cautions see notes above; also diabetes mellitus, impaired consciousness, cerebral tumour, myasthenia gravis

> Transdermal fentanyl
> **Fever or external heat** Monitor patients using patches for increased side-effects if fever present (increased absorption possible); avoid exposing application site to external heat (may also increase absorption)
> **Respiratory depression** Risk of fatal respiratory depression, particularly in patients not previously treated with a strong opioid analgesic; manufacturer recommends use only in opioid tolerant patients

Contra-indications see notes above

Hepatic impairment see notes above

Renal impairment see notes above

Pregnancy see notes above

Breast-feeding monitor infant for opioid-induced side-effects; manufacturer advises avoid

Side-effects see notes above; also abdominal pain, anorexia, dyspepsia, mouth ulcer, taste disturbance, dry mouth; vasodilatation; apnoea; anxiety; myoclonus; *less commonly* flatulence, diarrhoea, laryngospasm, dyspnoea, hypoventilation, depersonalisation, dysarthria, amnesia, incoordination, paraesthesia, malaise, agitation, tremor, and muscle weakness; *rarely* hiccups and arrhythmia; *very rarely* paralytic ileus, haemoptysis, psychosis, and seizures; shock, asystole, pyrexia, ataxia, and muscle fasciculation also reported; *with patches*, local reactions such as rash, erythema, and itching reported

Licensed use lozenges not licensed for use in children

Indication and dose

> Severe chronic pain
> • By transdermal route
>> **Child 2–16 years currently treated** with strong opioid analgesic, initial dose based on previous 24-hour opioid requirement (consult product literature)
>>
>> **Child 16–18 years** child **not currently treated** with strong opioid analgesic (but see Cautions, p. 256), one '12' or '25 micrograms/hour' patch replaced after 72 hours; child **currently treated** with strong opioid analgesic, initial dose based on previous 24-hour opioid requirement (consult product literature)
>>
>> **Dose adjustment** When starting, evaluation of the analgesic effect should **not** be made before the system has been worn for 24 hours (to allow for the gradual increase in plasma-fentanyl concentration)—previous analgesic therapy should be phased out gradually from time of first patch application; if necessary dose should be adjusted at 72-hour intervals in steps of 12–25 micrograms/hour. More than one patch may be used at a time for doses greater than 100 micrograms/hour (but applied at *same time* to avoid confusion)—consider additional or alternative analgesic therapy if dose required exceeds 300 micrograms/hour (**important**: it may take up to 25 hours for the plasma-fentanyl concentration to decrease by 50%—replacement opioid therapy should be initiated at a low dose and increased gradually).
>>
>> **Long duration of action** In view of the long duration of action, children who have had severe side-effects should be monitored for up to 24 hours after patch removal

> Breakthrough pain and premedication analgesia, see under preparation below

◁ **FENTANYL** (*continued*)

Peri-operative analgesia section 15.1.4.3

Conversion (from oral morphine to transdermal fentanyl), see Prescribing in Palliative Care, p. 25

Administration For *patches*, apply to dry, non-irritated, non-irradiated, non-hairy skin on torso or upper arm, removing after 72 hours and siting replacement patch on a different area (avoid using the same area for several days).

◢**Lozenges**

Actiq® (Flynn) CD

Lozenge, (with oromucosal applicator), fentanyl (as citrate) 200 micrograms, net price 3 = £17.86, 30 = £178.55; 400 micrograms, 3 = £17.86, 30 = £178.55; 600 micrograms, 3 = £17.86, 30 = £178.55; 800 micrograms, 3 = £17.86, 30 = £178.55; 1.2 mg, 3 = £17.86, 30 = £178.55; 1.6 mg, 3 = £17.86, 30 = £178.55. Label: 2

Dose

> Breakthrough pain
> * **By transmucosal application** (lozenge with oromucosal applicator)
>   **Child 2–18 years** (over 10 kg body-weight) 15–20 micrograms/kg as a single dose; max. dose 400 micrograms
>   **Note** If more than 4 episodes of breakthrough pain each day, adjust dose of background analgesic

> Premedication analgesia
> * **By transmucosal application** (lozenge with oromucosal applicator)
>   **Child 2–18 years** (over 10 kg body-weight) 15–20 micrograms/kg as a single dose; max. 400 micrograms

◢**Patches**

Prescriptions Prescriptions for fentanyl patches can be written to show the strength in terms of the release rate and it is acceptable to write '*Fentanyl 25 patches*' to prescribe patches that release fentanyl 25 micrograms per hour. The dosage should be expressed in terms of the interval between applying a patch and replacing it with a new one, e.g. '*one patch to be applied every 72 hours*'. The total quantity of patches should be written in words and figures.

Fentanyl (Non-proprietary) CD

Patches, self-adhesive, fentanyl, '12' patch (releasing approx. 12 micrograms/hour for 72 hours), net price 5 = £18.11; '25' patch (releasing approx. 25 micrograms/hour for 72 hours), 5 = £25.89; '50' patch (releasing approx. 50 micrograms/hour for 72 hours), 5 = £48.36; '75' patch (releasing approx. 75 micrograms/hour for 72 hours), 5 = £67.41; '100' patch (releasing approx. 100 micrograms/hour for 72 hours), 5 = £83.09. Label: 2, counselling, administration

Brands include *Fentalis®* , *Matrifen®*, *Mezolar®*, *Osmanil®*, *Tilofyl®*, *Victanyl®*

Durogesic DTrans® (Janssen-Cilag) CD

Patches, self-adhesive, transparent, fentanyl, '12' patch (releasing approx. 12 micrograms/hour for 72 hours), net price 5 = £18.11; '25' patch (releasing approx. 25 micrograms/hour for 72 hours), 5 = £25.89; '50' patch (releasing approx. 50 micrograms/hour for 72 hours), 5 = £48.36; '75' patch (releasing approx. 75 micrograms/hour for 72 hours), 5 = £67.41; '100' patch (releasing approx. 100 micrograms/hour for 72 hours), 5 = £83.09. Label: 2, counselling, administration

▰ HYDROMORPHONE HYDROCHLORIDE

Cautions see notes above; also pancreatitis; toxic psychosis

Contra-indications see notes above; also acute abdomen

Hepatic impairment see notes above

Renal impairment see notes above

Pregnancy see notes above

Breast-feeding avoid—no information available

Side-effects see notes above; also paralytic ileus, peripheral oedema, seizures, asthenia, dyskinesia, agitation, and tremor

Indication and dose

> Severe pain in cancer
> * **By mouth**
>   **Child 12–18 years** 1.3 mg every 4 hours, increased if necessary according to severity of pain

Administration Swallow whole capsule or sprinkle contents on soft food

Palladone® (Napp) CD

Capsules, hydromorphone hydrochloride 1.3 mg (orange/clear), net price 56-cap pack = £8.82; 2.6 mg (red/clear), 56-cap pack = £17.64. Label: 2, counselling, see below

◢**Modified release**

Palladone® SR (Napp) CD

Capsules, m/r, hydromorphone hydrochloride 2 mg (yellow/clear), net price 56-cap pack = £20.98; 4 mg (pale blue/clear), 56-cap pack = £28.75; 8 mg (pink/clear), 56-cap pack = £56.08; 16 mg (brown/clear), 56-cap pack = £106.53; 24 mg (dark blue/clear), 56-cap pack = £159.82. Label: 2, counselling, see below

Dose

> Severe pain in cancer
> * **By mouth**
>   **Child 12–18 years** 4 mg every 12 hours, increased if necessary according to severity of pain

Counselling Swallow whole or open capsule and sprinkle contents on soft food

▰ METHADONE HYDROCHLORIDE

Cautions see notes above; also myasthenia gravis; history of cardiac conduction abnormalities, family history of sudden death (ECG monitoring recommended; see also QT Interval Prolongation, below)

QT interval prolongation Children with the following risk factors for QT interval prolongation should be carefully

monitored while taking methadone: heart or liver disease, electrolyte abnormalities, or concomitant treatment with drugs that can prolong QT interval; children requiring more than 100 mg daily should also be monitored

Contra-indications see notes above; also phaeochromocytoma

Hepatic impairment see notes above

262 4.7.2 Opioid analgesics

BNFC 2010–2011

◻ **METHADONE HYDROCHLORIDE (continued)**

Renal impairment see notes above

Pregnancy see notes above

Breast-feeding withdrawal symptoms in infant; breast-feeding permissible during maintenance but dose should be as low as possible and infant monitored to avoid sedation

Side-effects see notes above; also QT interval prolongation; torsade de pointes, hypothermia, restlessness, raised intracranial pressure, dysmenorrhoea, dry eyes, and hyperprolactinaemia

Licensed use not licensed for use in children

Indication and dose

> Neonatal opioid withdrawal dose may vary, consult local guidelines
>
> • By mouth
>
>> **Neonate** initially 100 micrograms/kg increased by 50 micrograms/kg every 6 hours until symptoms are controlled; for maintenance, total daily dose that controls symptoms given in 2 divided doses; to withdraw, reduce dose over 7–10 days

Methadone (Non-proprietary) ㏅
Oral solution 1 mg/mL, methadone hydrochloride 1 mg/mL, net price 30 mL = 62p, 50 mL = £1.04, 100 mL = £1.31, 500 mL = £9.28. Label: 2
Brands include *Eptadone®*, *Metharose®* (sugar-free), *Physeptone* (also as sugar-free)

> **Safe Practice** This preparation is 2½ times the strength of Methadone Linctus; many preparations of this strength are licensed for opioid dependence only but some are also licensed for analgesia in severe pain

MORPHINE SALTS

Cautions see notes above; also pancreatitis, myasthenia gravis, cardiac arrhythmias, severe cor pulmonale

Contra-indications see notes above; also delayed gastric emptying, acute abdomen; heart failure secondary to chronic lung disease; phaeochromocytoma

Hepatic impairment see notes above

Renal impairment see notes above

Pregnancy see notes above

Breast-feeding therapeutic doses unlikely to affect infant; withdrawal symptoms in infants of dependent mothers; breast-feeding not best method of treating dependence in offspring

Side-effects see notes above; also paralytic ileus, abdominal pain, anorexia, dyspepsia, exacerbation of pancreatitis, taste disturbance; hypertension, hypothermia, syncope, bronchospasm, inhibition of cough reflex; restlessness, seizures, paraesthesia, asthenia, malaise, disorientation, excitation, agitation, delirium, raised intracranial pressure; amenorrhoea, myoclonus, muscle fasciculation, and rhabdomyolysis

Licensed use *Oramorph®* solution not licensed for use in children under 1 year; *Oramorph®* unit dose vials not licensed for use in children under 6 years; *Sevredol®* tablets not licensed for use in children under 3 years; *MST Continus®* preparations licensed to treat children with cancer pain (age-range not specified by manufacturer); *MXL®* capsules not licensed for use in children under 1 year

Indication and dose

> Pain
>
> • By subcutaneous injection
>
>> **Neonate** initially 100 micrograms/kg every 6 hours, adjusted according to response
>>
>> **Child 1–6 months** initially 100–200 micrograms/kg every 6 hours, adjusted according to response
>>
>> **Child 6 months–2 years** initially 100–200 micrograms/kg every 4 hours, adjusted according to response
>>
>> **Child 2–12 years** initially 200 micrograms/kg every 4 hours, adjusted according to response
>>
>> **Child 12–18 years** initially 2.5–10 mg every 4 hours, adjusted according to response
>
> • By intravenous injection over at least 5 minutes
>
>> **Neonate** initially 50 micrograms/kg every 6 hours, adjusted according to response
>>
>> **Child 1–6 months** initially 100 micrograms/kg every 6 hours, adjusted according to response
>>
>> **Child 6 months–12 years** initially 100 micrograms/kg every 4 hours, adjusted according to response
>>
>> **Child 12–18 years** initially 2.5 mg every 4 hours, adjusted according to response
>
> • By intravenous administration
>
>> **Neonate** initially *by intravenous injection* (over at least 5 minutes) 50 micrograms/kg then *by continuous intravenous infusion* 5–20 micrograms/kg/hour adjusted according to response
>>
>> **Child 1–6 months** initially *by intravenous injection* (over at least 5 minutes) 100 micrograms/kg then *by continuous intravenous infusion* 10–30 micrograms/kg/hour adjusted according to response
>>
>> **Child 6 months–12 years** initially *by intravenous injection* (over at least 5 minutes) 100 micrograms/kg then *by continuous intravenous infusion* 20–30 micrograms/kg/hour adjusted according to response
>>
>> **Child 12–18 years** initially *by intravenous injection* (over at least 5 minutes) 2.5–10 mg then *by continuous intravenous infusion* 20–30 micrograms/kg/hour adjusted according to response

Central nervous system **4**

◻ **MORPHINE SALTS (continued)**

* By mouth or by rectum

Child 1–3 months initially 50–100 micrograms/kg every 4 hours, adjusted according to response

Child 3–6 months 100–150 micrograms/kg every 4 hours, adjusted according to response

Child 6–12 months 200 micrograms/kg every 4 hours, adjusted according to response

Child 1–2 years initially 200–300 micrograms/kg every 4 hours, adjusted according to response

Child 2–12 years initially 200–300 micrograms/kg every 4 hours, adjusted according to response

Child 12–18 years initially 5–20 mg every 4 hours, adjusted according to response

* By continuous subcutaneous infusion

Child 1–3 months 10 micrograms/kg/hour, adjusted according to response

Child 3 months–18 years 20 micrograms/kg/hour, adjusted according to response

---

Neonatal opioid withdrawal under specialist supervision

* By mouth

Neonate initially 40 micrograms/kg every 4 hours until symptoms controlled; increase dose if necessary; reduce frequency gradually over 6–10 days, and stop when 40 micrograms/kg once daily achieved; dose may vary, consult local guidelines

---

Administration for *continuous intravenous infusion*, dilute with Glucose 5% or 10% *or* Sodium Chloride 0.9%

Neonatal intensive care, dilute 2.5 mg/kg body-weight to a final volume of 50 mL with infusion fluid; an intravenous infusion rate of 0.1 mL/hour provides a dose of 5 micrograms/kg/hour

◢ **Oral solutions**

Note For advice on transfer from oral solutions of morphine to modified-release preparations of morphine, see Prescribing in Palliative Care, p. 24

Morphine Oral Solutions

PoM or CD

Oral solutions of morphine can be prescribed by writing the formula:
Morphine hydrochloride 5 mg
Chloroform water to 5 mL

Note The proportion of morphine hydrochloride may be altered when specified by the prescriber; if above 13 mg per 5 mL the solution becomes CD. For sample prescription see Controlled Drugs and Drug Dependence, p. 11. It is usual to adjust the strength so that the dose volume is 5 or 10 mL.

Oramorph® (Boehringer Ingelheim)

Oramorph® oral solution PoM, morphine sulphate 10 mg/5 mL, net price 100-mL pack = £1.78; 300-mL pack = £4.95; 500-mL pack = £7.47. Label: 2

Oramorph® concentrated oral solution CD, sugar-free, morphine sulphate 100 mg/5 mL, net price 30-mL pack = £4.98; 120-mL pack = £18.59 (both with calibrated dropper). Label: 2

◢ **Tablets**

Sevredol® (Napp) CD

Tablets, f/c, scored, morphine sulphate 10 mg (blue), net price 56-tab pack = £5.61; 20 mg (pink), 56-tab pack = £11.21; 50 mg (pale green), 56-tab pack = £28.02. Label: 2

◢ **Modified-release 12-hourly oral preparations**

MST Continus® (Napp) CD

Tablets, m/r, f/c, morphine sulphate 5 mg (white), net price 60-tab pack = £3.29; 10 mg (brown), 60-tab pack = £5.26; 15 mg (green), 60-tab pack = £9.61; 30 mg (purple), 60-tab pack = £12.65; 60 mg (orange), 60-tab pack = £24.68; 100 mg (grey), 60-tab pack = £39.07; 200 mg (green), 60-tab pack = £78.16. Label: 2, 25

Suspension (= sachet of granules to mix with water), m/r, pink, morphine sulphate 20 mg/sachet, net price 30-sachet pack = £24.58; 30 mg/sachet, 30-sachet pack = £25.54; 60 mg/sachet, 30-sachet pack = £51.09; 100 mg/sachet, 30-sachet pack = £85.15; 200 mg/sachet pack, 30-sachet pack = £170.30. Label: 2, 13

Dose
* By mouth

Every 12 hours, dose adjusted according to daily morphine requirements; for further advice on determining dose, see Prescribing in Palliative Care, p. 24; dosage requirements should be reviewed if the brand is altered

Note Prescriptions must also specify 'tablets' or 'suspension' (i.e. 'MST Continus tablets' or 'MST Continus suspension')

◢ **Modified-release 24-hourly oral preparations**

MXL® (Napp) CD

Capsules, m/r, morphine sulphate 30 mg (light blue), net price 28-cap pack = £10.91; 60 mg (brown), 28-cap pack = £14.95; 90 mg (pink), 28-cap pack = £22.04; 120 mg (green), 28-cap pack = £29.15; 150 mg (blue), 28-cap pack = £36.43; 200 mg (red-brown), 28-cap pack = £46.15. Label: 2, counselling, see below

Dose
* By mouth

Every 24 hours, dose adjusted according to daily morphine requirements; for further advice on determining dose, see Prescribing in Palliative Care, p. 24; dosage requirements should be reviewed if the brand is altered

Counselling Swallow whole or open capsule and sprinkle contents on soft food

Note Prescriptions must also specify 'capsules' (i.e. 'MXL capsules')

◢ **Suppositories**

Morphine (Non-proprietary) CD

Suppositories, morphine hydrochloride or sulphate 10 mg, net price 12 = £10.68; 15 mg, 12 = £8.58; 20 mg, 12 = £33.22; 30 mg, 12 = £12.45. Label: 2

Note Both the strength of the suppositories and the morphine salt contained in them must be specified by the prescriber

Morphine sulphate 5 mg suppositories available from 'special-order' manufacturers or specialist importing companies, see p. 957

4

Central nervous system

◻ **MORPHINE SALTS** (*continued*)

◢**Injections**

Morphine Sulphate (Non-proprietary) CD

Injection, morphine sulphate 10, 15, 20, and 30 mg/mL, net price 1- and 2-mL amp (all) = 72p–£1.40

Intravenous infusion, morphine sulphate 1 mg/mL, net price 50-mL vial = £5.00; 2 mg/mL, 50-mL vial = £5.89

Minijet® Morphine Sulphate (UCB Pharma) CD

Injection, morphine sulphate 1 mg/mL, net price 10-mL disposable syringe = £8.34

◢**Injection with antiemetic**

Caution Not recommended in palliative care, see Nausea and Vomiting, p. 27

Cyclimorph® (Amdipharm) CD

Cyclimorph-10® Injection, morphine tartrate 10 mg, cyclizine tartrate 50 mg/mL. Net price 1-mL amp = £1.75

Dose

Moderate to severe pain (short-term use only)
● **By subcutaneous, intramuscular, or intravenous injection**

Child 12–18 years 1 mL, repeated not more often than every 4 hours, max. 3 doses in any 24-hour period

Cyclimorph-15® Injection, morphine tartrate 15 mg, cyclizine tartrate 50 mg/mL. Net price 1-mL amp = £1.82

Dose

Moderate to severe pain (short-term use only)
● **By subcutaneous, intramuscular, or intravenous injection**

Child 12–18 years 1 mL, repeated not more often than every 4 hours, max. 3 doses in any 24-hour period

---

◢ OXYCODONE HYDROCHLORIDE

Cautions see notes above; also toxic psychosis; pancreatitis

Contra-indications see notes above; also acute abdomen; delayed gastric emptying; chronic constipation; cor pulmonale; acute porphyria (section 9.8.2)

Hepatic impairment avoid in moderate or severe impairment; see also notes above

Renal impairment avoid if estimated glomerular filtration rate less than 10 mL/minute/1.73m²; see also notes above

Pregnancy see notes above

Breast-feeding present in milk—avoid

Side-effects see notes above; also diarrhoea, abdominal pain, anorexia, dyspepsia; bronchospasm, dyspnoea, impaired cough reflex; asthenia, anxiety; chills; muscle fasciculation; *less commonly* paralytic ileus, gastritis, flatulence, dysphagia, taste disturbance, belching, hiccups, vasodilatation, supraventricular tachycardia, syncope, amnesia, hypoaesthesia, restlessness, seizures, pyrexia, amenorrhoea, hypotonia, paraesthesia, disorientation, malaise, agitation, speech disorder, tremor, and dry skin

Licensed use not licensed for use in children

Indication and dose

Moderate to severe pain in palliative care (see also Prescribing in Palliative Care, p. 25)
● **By mouth**

Child 1 month–12 years initially 200 micrograms/kg (up to 5 mg) every 4–6 hours, dose increased if necessary according to severity of pain

Child 12–18 years initially 5 mg every 4–6 hours, dose increased if necessary according to severity of pain

Oxynorm® (Napp) CD

Capsules, oxycodone hydrochloride 5 mg (orange/beige), net price 56-cap pack = £11.59; 10 mg (white/beige), 56-cap pack = £23.19; 20 mg (pink/beige), 56-cap pack = £46.38. Label: 2

Liquid (= oral solution), sugar-free, oxycodone hydrochloride 5 mg/5 mL, net price 250 mL = £9.85. Label: 2

Concentrate (= concentrated oral solution), sugar-free, oxycodone hydrochloride 10 mg/mL, net price 120 mL = £47.32. Label: 2

◢**Modified release**

OxyContin® (Napp) CD

Tablets, f/c, m/r, oxycodone hydrochloride 5 mg (blue), net price 28-tab pack = £12.71; 10 mg (white), 56-tab pack = £25.41; 20 mg (pink), 56-tab pack = £50.82; 40 mg (yellow), 56-tab pack = £101.67; 80 mg (green), 56-tab pack = £203.35. Label: 2, 25

Dose

Moderate to severe pain in palliative care
● **By mouth**

Child 8–12 years initially, 5 mg every 12 hours, increased if necessary according to severity of pain

Child 12–18 years initially, 10 mg every 12 hours, increased if necessary according to severity of pain

---

◢ PAPAVERETUM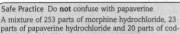

Safe Practice Do **not** confuse with papaverine

A mixture of 253 parts of morphine hydrochloride, 23 parts of papaverine hydrochloride and 20 parts of codeine hydrochloride

To avoid confusion, the figures of 7.7 mg/mL or 15.4 mg/mL should be used for prescribing purposes

Cautions see notes above; supraventricular tachycardia

Contra-indications see notes above; heart failure secondary to chronic lung disease; phaeochromocytoma

Hepatic impairment see notes above

Renal impairment see notes above

◁ **PAPAVERETUM** (*continued*)

Pregnancy see notes above

Breast-feeding see Morphine

Side-effects see notes above; also hypothermia

Indication and dose

> Premedication, postoperative analgesia, severe chronic pain
> • **By subcutaneous or intramuscular injection**
>
> > **Neonate** 115 micrograms/kg repeated every 4 hours if necessary
> >
> > **Child 1–12 months** 154 micrograms/kg repeated every 4 hours if necessary
> >
> > **Child 1–6 years** 1.93–3.85 mg repeated every 4 hours if necessary

> > **Child 6–12 years** 3.85–7.7 mg repeated every 4 hours if necessary
> >
> > **Child 12–18 years** 7.7–15.4 mg repeated every 4 hours if necessary
>
> • **By intravenous injection**
>
> > Generally 25–50% of the corresponding subcutaneous or intramuscular dose

Papaveretum (Non-proprietary) ⒸⒹ ◢
Injection, papaveretum 15.4 mg/mL (providing the equivalent of 10 mg of anhydrous morphine/mL), net price 1-mL amp = £1.64

▀ **PETHIDINE HYDROCHLORIDE**

Cautions see notes above; not suitable for severe continuing pain; accumulation of metabolites may result in neurotoxicity; myasthenia gravis; cardiac arrhythmias, severe cor pulmonale

Contra-indications see notes above; phaeochromocytoma

Hepatic impairment see notes above

Renal impairment see notes above

Pregnancy see notes above

Breast-feeding present in milk but not known to be harmful

Side-effects see notes above; also restlessness, tremor, and hypothermia; convulsions reported in **overdosage**

Indication and dose

> Obstetric analgesia
> • **By subcutaneous or by intramuscular injection**
>
> > **Child 12–18 years** 1 mg/kg (max.100 mg), repeated 1–3 hours later if necessary; max. 400 mg in 24 hours

Pethidine (Non-proprietary) ⒸⒹ
Injection, pethidine hydrochloride 50 mg/mL, net price 1-mL amp = 53p, 2-mL amp = 56p; 10 mg/mL, 5-mL amp = £3.17, 10-mL amp = £2.18

▀ **TRAMADOL HYDROCHLORIDE**

Cautions see notes above; impaired consciousness; excessive bronchial secretions; not suitable as substitute in opioid-dependent patients
  General anaesthesia Not recommended for analgesia during potentially light planes of general anaesthesia (possibly increased intra-operative recall reported)

Contra-indications see notes above; uncontrolled epilepsy

Hepatic impairment see notes above

Renal impairment see notes above

Pregnancy embryotoxic in *animal* studies—manufacturer advises avoid; see also notes above

Breast-feeding amount probably too small to be harmful, but manufacturer advises avoid

Side-effects see notes above; also diarrhoea; fatigue; *less commonly* retching, gastritis, and flatulence; *rarely* anorexia, syncope, hypertension, bronchospasm, dyspnoea, wheezing, seizures, paraesthesia, and muscle weakness; blood disorders also reported

Licensed use not licensed for use in children under 12 years

Indication and dose

> Moderate to severe pain
> • **By mouth**
>
> > **Child 12–18 years** 50–100 mg not more often than every 4 hours; total of more than 400 mg daily not usually required

> • **By intravenous injection (over 2–3 minutes) or by intravenous infusion or by intramuscular injection**
>
> > **Child 12–18 years** 50–100 mg every 4–6 hours

> Postoperative pain
> • **By intravenous injection (over 2–3 minutes)**
>
> > **Child 12–18 years** 100 mg initially then 50 mg every 10–20 minutes if necessary up to total max. 250 mg (including initial dose) in first hour, *then* 50–100 mg every 4–6 hours; max. 600 mg daily

Administration for *intravenous infusion*, dilute with Glucose 5% *or* Sodium Chloride 0.9% *or* Compound Sodium Lactate *or* Ringer's Solution

Tramadol Hydrochloride (Non-proprietary) ⒫ⓞⓜ
Capsules, tramadol hydrochloride 50 mg, net price 30-cap pack = £1.54, 100-cap pack = £2.66. Label: 2
Brands include *Tramake®*

Injection, tramadol hydrochloride 50 mg/mL, net price 2-mL amp = 98p

Zamadol® (Meda) ⒫ⓞⓜ
Capsules, tramadol hydrochloride 50 mg, net price 100-cap pack = £8.00. Label: 2

4

Central nervous system

◁ **TRAMADOL HYDROCHLORIDE** (*continued*)

Orodispersible tablets (*Zamadol Melt*®), tramadol hydrochloride 50 mg, net price 60-tab pack = £7.12. Label: 2, counselling, administration
Excipients include aspartame (section 9.4.1)

Counselling *Zamadol Melt*® should be sucked and then swallowed. May also be dispersed in water

Injection, tramadol hydrochloride 50 mg/mL, net price 2-mL amp = £1.10

Zydol® (Grünenthal) [PoM]
Capsules, green/yellow, tramadol hydrochloride 50 mg, net price 30-cap pack = £3.22, 100-cap pack = £10.71. Label: 2

Soluble tablets, tramadol hydrochloride 50 mg, net price 20-tab pack = £2.95, 100-tab pack = £13.95. Label: 2, 13

Injection, tramadol hydrochloride 50 mg/mL, net price 2-mL amp = 90p

◢**Modified-release 12-hourly preparations**
Larapam® **SR** (Sandoz) [PoM]
Tablets, m/r, tramadol hydrochloride 100 mg, net price 60-tab pack = £17.55; 150 mg, 60-tab pack = £27.35; 200 mg, 60-tab pack = £36.50. Label: 2, 25

Dose

> Moderate to severe pain
> • By mouth
>> **Child 12–18 years** initially 100 mg twice daily increased if necessary; usual max. 200 mg twice daily

Mabron® (Morningside) [PoM]
Tablets, m/r, tramadol hydrochloride 100 mg, net price 60-tab pack = £18.26; 150 mg, 60-tab pack = £27.39; 200 mg, 60-tab pack = £36.52. Label: 2, 25

Dose

> Moderate to severe pain
> • By mouth
>> **Child 12–18 years** 100 mg twice daily increased if necessary; usual max. 200 mg twice daily

Maxitram SR® (Chiesi) [PoM]
Capsules, m/r, tramadol hydrochloride 50 mg (white), net price 60-cap pack = £4.55; 100 mg (yellow), 60-cap pack = £12.14; 150 mg (yellow), 60-cap pack = £18.21; 200 mg (yellow), 60-cap pack = £24.28. Label: 2, 25

Dose

> Moderate to severe pain
> • By mouth
>> **Child 12–18 years** initially 100 mg twice daily increased if necessary; usual max. 200 mg twice daily

Tramquel SR® (Meda) [PoM]
Capsules, m/r, tramadol hydrochloride 50 mg (dark green), net price 60-cap pack = £7.64; 100 mg (white), 60-cap pack = £15.28; 150 mg (dark green), 60-cap pack = £22.92; 200 mg (yellow), 60-cap pack = £30.55. Label: 2, counselling, administration

Dose

> Moderate to severe pain
> • By mouth
>> **Child 12–18 years** 50–100 mg twice daily increased if necessary; usual max. 200 mg twice daily

Administration Swallow whole or open capsule and swallow contents immediately without chewing

Zamadol® **SR** (Meda) [PoM]
Capsules, m/r, tramadol hydrochloride 50 mg (green), net price 60-cap pack = £7.64; 100 mg, 60-cap pack = £15.28; 150 mg (dark green), 60-cap pack = £22.92; 200 mg (yellow), 60-cap pack = £30.55. Label: 2, counselling, administration

Dose

> Moderate to severe pain
> • By mouth
>> **Child 12–18 years** 50–100 mg twice daily increased if necessary to 150–200 mg twice daily; total of more than 400 mg daily not usually required

Administration Swallow whole or open capsule and swallow contents immediately without chewing

Zeridame® **SR** (Actavis) [PoM]
Tablets, m/r, tramadol hydrochloride 100 mg, net price 60-tab pack = £18.26; 150 mg, 60-tab pack = £27.39; 200 mg, 60-tab pack = £36.52. Label: 2, 25

Dose

> Moderate to severe pain
> • By mouth
>> **Child 12–18 years** 100 mg twice daily, increased if necessary; usual max. 200 mg twice daily

Zydol SR® (Grünenthal) [PoM]
Tablets, m/r, f/c, tramadol hydrochloride 100 mg, net price 60-tab pack = £18.26; 150 mg (beige), 60-tab pack = £27.39; 200 mg (orange), 60-tab pack = £36.52. Label: 2, 25

Dose

> Moderate to severe pain
> • By mouth
>> **Child 12–18 years** 100 mg twice daily increased if necessary to 150–200 mg twice daily; total of more than 400 mg daily not usually required

◢**Modified-release 24-hourly preparations**
Tradorec XL® (MSD) [PoM]
Tablets, m/r, tramadol hydrochloride 100 mg, net price 30-tab pack = £14.10; 200 mg, 30-tab pack = £14.98; 300 mg, 30-tab pack = £22.47. Label: 2, 25

Dose

> Moderate to severe pain
> • By mouth
>> **Child 12–18 years** initially 100 mg once daily, increased if necessary to max. 400 mg once daily

Zamadol® **24hr** (Meda) [PoM]
Tablets, f/c, m/r, tramadol hydrochloride 150 mg, net price 28-tab pack = £10.70; 200 mg, 28-tab pack = £14.26; 300 mg, 28-tab pack = £21.39; 400 mg, 28-tab pack = £28.51. Label: 2, 25

Dose

> Moderate to severe pain
> • By mouth
>> **Child 12–18 years** initially 150 mg once daily increased if necessary; max. 400 mg once daily

Zydol XL® (Grünenthal) [PoM]
Tablets, m/r, f/c, tramadol hydrochloride 150 mg, net price 30-tab pack = £12.18; 200 mg, 30-tab pack

◻ **TRAMADOL HYDROCHLORIDE** (*continued*)

= £17.98; 300 mg, 30-tab pack = £24.94; 400 mg, 30-tab pack = £32.47. Label: 2, 25

Dose

Moderate to severe pain
• By mouth
  Child 12–18 years 150 mg once daily increased if necessary; more than 400 mg once daily not usually required

◀**With paracetamol**

Tramacet (Grünenthal) PoM
Tablets, f/c, yellow, tramadol hydrochloride 37.5 mg, paracetamol 325 mg, net price 60-tab pack = £9.68. Label: 2, 25, 29, 30

Effervescent tablets, pink, tramadol hydrochloride 37.5 mg, paracetamol 325 mg, net price 60-tab pack = £9.68. Label: 2, 13, 29, 30 (contains Na$^+$ 7.8 mmol/tablet)

Dose

Moderate to severe pain
• By mouth
  Child 12–18 years 2 tablets not more than every 6 hours; max. 8 tablets daily

4.7.3 Neuropathic pain

Neuropathic pain, which occurs as a result of damage to neural tissue, includes *postherpetic neuralgia, phantom limb pain, complex regional pain syndrome* (reflex sympathetic dystrophy, causalgia) *compression neuropathies, peripheral neuropathies* (e.g. due to diabetes, haematological malignancies, rheumatoid arthritis, alcoholism, drug misuse), *trauma, central pain* (e.g. pain following stroke, spinal cord injury and syringomyelia) and *idiopathic neuropathy.* The pain occurs in an area of sensory deficit and may be described as burning, shooting or scalding and is often accompanied by pain that is evoked by a non-noxious stimulus (allodynia).

Neuropathic pain is generally managed with a tricyclic antidepressant such as amitriptyline (p. 236) or antiepileptic drugs such as carbamazepine (p. 274). Neuropathic pain may respond only partially to opioid analgesics. Nerve blocks, transcutaneous electrical nerve stimulation (TENS) and, in selected cases, central electrical stimulation may help. Many children with chronic neuropathic pain require multidisciplinary management, including physiotherapy and psychological support. A corticosteroid may help to relieve pressure in compression neuropathy and thereby reduce pain.

For the management of neuropathic pain in *palliative care*, see p. 25.

Chronic facial pain   Chronic oral and facial pain including persistent idiopathic facial pain (also termed 'atypical facial pain') and temporomandibular dysfunction (previously termed temporomandibular joint pain dysfunction syndrome) may call for prolonged use of analgesics or for other drugs. Tricyclic antidepressants (section 4.3.1) may be useful for facial pain [unlicensed indication], but are not on the Dental Practitioners' List. Disorders of this type require specialist referral and psychological support to accompany drug treatment. Children on long-term therapy need to be monitored both for progress and for side-effects.

4.7.4 Antimigraine drugs

4.7.4.1 Treatment of acute migraine
4.7.4.2 Prophylaxis of migraine
4.7.4.3 Cluster headache and the trigeminal autonomic cephalalgias

4.7.4.1 Treatment of acute migraine

Treatment of a migraine attack should be guided by response to previous treatment and the severity of the attacks. A **simple analgesic** such as paracetamol (preferably in a soluble or dispersible form) or an NSAID, usually ibuprofen, is often effective; concomitant **antiemetic** treatment may be required. If treatment with an analgesic is inadequate, an attack may be treated with a specific antimigraine compound such as the 5HT$_1$ agonist **sumatriptan**. **Ergot alkaloids** are associated with many side-effects and should be avoided.

Excessive use of acute treatments for migraine (opioid and non-opioid analgesics, 5HT$_1$ agonists, and ergotamine) is associated with medication-overuse headache (analgesic-induced headache); therefore, increasing consumption of these medicines needs careful management.

4 Central nervous system

| Analgesics |

ANALGESICS

◢Paracetamol
Section 4.7.1

◢Non-steroidal anti-inflammatory drugs (NSAIDs)
Section 10.1.1

◢With antiemetics

Migraleve® (McNeil) ◢

Tablets, all f/c, *pink tablets*, buclizine hydrochloride 6.25 mg, paracetamol 500 mg, codeine phosphate 8 mg; *yellow tablets*, paracetamol 500 mg, codeine phosphate 8 mg, net price 48-tab *Migraleve* [PoM] (32 pink + 16 yellow) = £5.10; 48 pink (*Migraleve Pink*) = £5.56. Label: 2, (*Migraleve Pink*), 17, 30

Dose

> Treatment of acute migraine
> • By mouth
> > **Child under 10 years** only under close medical supervision
> >
> > **Child 10–14 years** 1 pink tablet at onset of attack, or if it is imminent then 1 yellow tablet every 4 hours if necessary; max. 1 pink and 3 yellow tablets in 24 hours

> **Child 14–18 years** 2 pink tablets at onset of attack, or if it is imminent, then 2 yellow tablets every 4 hours if necessary; max. in 24 hours 2 pink and 6 yellow

Paramax® (Sanofi-Aventis) [PoM]

Tablets, scored, paracetamol 500 mg, metoclopramide hydrochloride 5 mg, net price 42-tab pack = £9.64. Label: 17, 30

Sachets, effervescent powder, sugar-free, the contents of 1 sachet = 1 tablet; to be dissolved in ¼ tumblerful of liquid before administration, net price 42-sachet pack = £12.52. Label: 13, 17, 30

Dose

> Treatment of acute migraine
> • By mouth
> > **Child 12–18 years** 1 at onset of attack then 1 every 4 hours when necessary to max. of 3 in 24 hours (max. dose of metoclopramide 500 micrograms/kg daily)
> >
> > **Important** Metoclopramide can cause **severe extrapyramidal effects** (for further details, see p. 244 and p. 249)

| 5HT$_1$ agonists |

5HT$_1$ agonists are used in the treatment of acute migraine attacks; treatment of children should be initiated by a specialist. The 5HT$_1$ agonists ('triptans') act on the 5HT (serotonin) 1B/1D receptors and they are therefore sometimes referred to as 5HT$_{1B/1D}$-receptor agonists. A 5HT$_1$ agonist may be used during the established headache phase of an attack and is the preferred treatment in those who fail to respond to conventional analgesics.

Sumatriptan and **zolmitriptan** are used for migraine in children. They may also be of value in cluster headache (see also section 4.7.4.3).

Cautions 5HT$_1$ agonists are recommended as monotherapy and should not be taken concurrently with other therapies for acute migraine; see also **interactions**: Appendix 1 (5HT$_1$ agonists).

SUMATRIPTAN

Cautions see under 5HT$_1$ agonists above; pre-existing cardiac disease; history of seizures; sensitivity to sulphonamides; **interactions**: Appendix 1 (5HT$_1$ agonists)
> Skilled tasks Drowsiness may affect performance of skilled tasks (e.g. driving)

Contra-indications vasospasm; previous cerebrovascular accident or transient ischaemic attack; peripheral vascular disease; moderate and severe hypertension

Hepatic impairment reduce dose of oral therapy; avoid in severe impairment

Renal impairment caution

Pregnancy limited experience—avoid unless potential benefit outweighs risk

Breast-feeding present in milk but amount probably too small to be harmful; withhold breast-feeding for 12 hours

Side-effects nausea, vomiting; sensations of tingling, heat, heaviness, pressure, or tightness of any part of the body (including throat and chest—discontinue if intense, may be due to coronary

vasoconstriction or to anaphylaxis), transient increase in blood pressure, flushing, drowsiness, dizziness, weakness; *very rarely* ischaemic colitis, hypotension, bradycardia or tachycardia, palpitation, arrhythmias, myocardial infarction, Raynaud's syndrome, seizures, tremor, dystonia, nystagmus, and visual disturbances; nasal irritation and epistaxis with nasal spray

Licensed use tablets and injection not licensed for use in children; not licensed for treating cluster headache in children

Indication and dose

> Treatment of acute migraine
> • By mouth
> > **Child 6–10 years** 25 mg as a single dose, repeated once after at least 2 hours if migraine recurs
> >
> > **Child 10–12 years** 50 mg as a single dose, repeated once after at least 2 hours if migraine recurs

◁ **SUMATRIPTAN (continued)**

Child 12–18 years 50–100 mg as a single dose, repeated once after at least 2 hours if migraine recurs

• **By subcutaneous injection (using auto-injector)**

Child 10–18 years 6 mg as a single dose, repeated once after at least 1 hour if migraine recurs; max. 12 mg in 24 hours

• **Intranasally**

Child 12–18 years 10–20 mg as a single dose, repeated once after at least 2 hours if migraine recurs; max. 40 mg in 24 hours

Treatment of acute cluster headache
• **By subcutaneous injection (using auto-injector)**

Child 10–18 years 6 mg as a single dose, repeated once after at least 1 hour if headache recurs; max. 12 mg in 24 hours

• **Intranasally**

Child 12–18 years 10 mg as a single dose, repeated once after at least 2 hours if headache recurs; max. 20 mg in 24 hours

Note Child not responding to initial dose should not take second dose for same attack

¹**Sumatriptan** (Non-proprietary) PoM
Tablets, sumatriptan (as succinate) 50 mg, net price 6-tab pack = £1.94; 100 mg, 6-tab pack = £2.69. Label: 3, 10, patient information leaflet
1. Sumatriptan 50 mg tablets can be sold to the public to treat previously diagnosed migraine; max. daily dose 100 mg

Imigran® (GSK) PoM
Tablets, sumatriptan (as succinate) 50 mg, net price 6-tab pack = £26.54; 100 mg, 6-tab pack = £42.90. Label: 3, 10, patient information leaflet

Injection, sumatriptan (as succinate) 12 mg/mL (= 6 mg/0.5-mL syringe), net price, treatment pack (2 × 0.5-mL prefilled syringes and auto-injector) = £42.47; refill pack 2 × 0.5-mL prefilled cartridges = £40.41. Label: 3, 10, patient information leaflet

Nasal spray, sumatriptan 10 mg/0.1-mL actuation, net price 2 unit-dose spray device = £11.80; 20 mg/ 0.1-mL actuation, 2 unit-dose spray device = £11.80, 6 unit-dose spray device = £35.39. Label: 3, 10, patient information leaflet

Imigran Radis® (GSK) PoM
Tablets, f/c, sumatriptan (as succinate) 50 mg (pink), net price 6-tab pack = £23.90; 100 mg (white), 6-tab pack = £42.90. Label: 3, 10, patient information leaflet

---

■ **ZOLMITRIPTAN**

Cautions see under 5HT₁ agonists above; should not be taken within 12 hours of any other 5HT₁ agonist; **interactions**: Appendix 1 (5HT₁ agonists)

Contra-indications vasospasm; Wolff-Parkinson-White syndrome or arrhythmias associated with accessory cardiac conduction pathways; previous cerebrovascular accident or transient ischaemic attack; ischaemic heart disease; uncontrolled hypertension

Hepatic impairment max. 5 mg in 24 hours in moderate or severe impairment

Pregnancy limited experience—avoid unless potential benefit outweighs risk

Breast-feeding use with caution—present in milk in *animal* studies

Side-effects abdominal pain, dry mouth, nausea, vomiting; palpitations, sensations of tingling, heat, heaviness, pressure, or tightness of any part of the body (including throat and chest—discontinue if intense, may be due to coronary vasoconstriction or to anaphylaxis); dizziness, headache, paraesthesia, asthenia; muscle weakness; *less commonly* tachycardia, transient increases in blood pressure, polyuria; *rarely* angioedema, urticaria; *very rarely* gastro-intestinal and splenic infarction, ischaemic colitis, angina pectoris, myocardial infarction; *with nasal spray*, taste disturbance, epistaxis, and nasal irritation

Licensed use not licensed for use in children

Indication and dose
Treatment of acute migraine
• **By mouth**

Child 12–18 years 2.5 mg, repeated after not less than 2 hours if migraine recurs (if response unsatisfactory after 3 attacks consider increasing dose to 5 mg or switching to alternative treatment); max. 10 mg in 24 hours

• **Intranasally**

Child 12–18 years 5 mg (1 spray) into 1 nostril, repeated after not less than 2 hours if migraine recurs; max. 10 mg in 24 hours

Treatment of acute cluster headache
• **Intranasally**

Child 12–18 years 5 mg (1 spray) into 1 nostril, repeated after not less than 2 hours if headache recurs; max. 10 mg in 24 hours

Zomig® (AstraZeneca) PoM
Tablets, f/c, yellow, zolmitriptan 2.5 mg, net price 6-tab pack = £18.00, 12-tab pack = £36.00

Orodispersible tablets (*Zomig Rapimelt®*), zolmitriptan 2.5 mg, net price 6-tab pack = £17.90; 5 mg, 6-tab pack = £22.80. Counselling, administration

Counselling *Zomig Rapimelt®* should be placed on the tongue, allowed to disperse and swallowed
Excipients include aspartame equivalent to phenylalanine 2.81 mg/tablet (section 9.4.1)

Nasal spray, zolmitriptan 5 mg/0.1-mL unit-dose spray device, net price 6 unit-dose sprays = £36.50

Central nervous system

4

Antiemetics

Antiemetics (section 4.6), including **metoclopramide**, **domperidone**, phenothiazines, and antihistamines, relieve the nausea associated with migraine attacks. Antiemetics may be given by intramuscular injection or rectally if vomiting is a problem. Metoclopramide and domperidone have the added advantage of promoting gastric emptying and normal peristalsis; a single dose should be given at the onset of symptoms (**important:** for warnings relating to extrapyramidal effects of metoclopramide see p. 244 and p. 249).

4.7.4.2 Prophylaxis of migraine

Where migraine attacks are frequent, possible provoking factors such as stress should be sought; combined oral contraceptives may also provoke migraine. Preventive treatment should be considered if migraine attacks interfere with school and social life, particularly for children who:

- suffer at least two attacks a month;
- suffer an increasing frequency of headaches;
- suffer significant disability despite suitable treatment for migraine attacks;
- cannot take suitable treatment for migraine attacks.

In children it is often possible to stop prophylaxis after a period of treatment.

Propranolol (section 2.4) may be effective in preventing migraine in children but it is contra-indicated in those with asthma. Side-effects such as depression and postural hypotension can further limit its use.

Pizotifen, an antihistamine and serotonin antagonist, taken at night or twice daily, may also be used but its efficacy in children has not been clearly established. Common side-effects include drowsiness and weight gain.

Topiramate (section 4.8.1) is licensed for migraine prophylaxis. Treatment should be supervised by a specialist.

PIZOTIFEN

Cautions urinary retention; susceptibility to angle-closure glaucoma; history of epilepsy; **interactions:** Appendix 1 (pizotifen)

Skilled tasks Drowsiness may affect performance of skilled tasks (e.g. driving); effects of alcohol enhanced

Renal impairment use with caution

Pregnancy avoid unless potential benefit outweighs risk

Breast-feeding amount probably too small to be harmful but manufacturer advises avoid

Side-effects antimuscarinic effects, nausea, dizziness, drowsiness, increased appetite and weight gain; *less commonly* constipation; *rarely* anxiety, aggression, paraesthesia, hallucination, depression, arthralgia, myalgia; *very rarely* seizures, angle-closure glaucoma; CNS stimulation may occur

Licensed use *Sanomigran®* elixir and 500-microgram tablets not licensed for use in children under 2 years; 1.5-mg tablets not licensed for use in children

Indication and dose

Prophylaxis of migraine

- By mouth

Child 5–10 years initially 500 micrograms at night increased according to response up to 500 micrograms 3 times daily; max. single dose at night 1 mg; max. 1.5 mg in 24 hours

Child 10–12 years initially 1 mg at night increased according to response up to 500 micrograms 3 times daily; max. single dose at night 1 mg; max. 1.5 mg in 24 hours

Child 12–18 years initially 1.5 mg at night increased according to response to 1.5 mg 3 times daily; max. single dose 3 mg; max. 4.5 mg in 24 hours

Pizotifen (Non-proprietary) [PoM]
Tablets, pizotifen (as hydrogen malate), 500 micrograms, net price 28-tab pack = £1.36; 1.5 mg, 28-tab pack = £2.16. Label: 2

Sanomigran® (Novartis) [PoM]
Tablets, both ivory-yellow, s/c, pizotifen (as hydrogen malate), 500 micrograms, net price 60-tab pack = £2.57; 1.5 mg, 28-tab pack = £4.28. Label: 2

Elixir, pizotifen (as hydrogen malate) 250 micrograms/5 mL, net price 300 mL = £4.51. Label: 2

Cluster headache rarely responds to standard analgesics. **Sumatriptan** given by subcutaneous injection is the drug of choice for the *treatment* of cluster headache. If an injection is unsuitable, sumatriptan nasal spray or **zolmitriptan** nasal spray may be used. Treatment should be initiated by a specialist. Alternatively, 100% **oxygen** at a rate of 10–15 litres/minute for 10–20 minutes is useful in aborting an attack.

The other trigeminal autonomic cephalalgias, paroxysmal hemicrania (sensitive to indometacin), and short-lasting unilateral neuralgiform headache attacks with conjunctival injection and tearing, are seen rarely and are best managed by a specialist.

4.8 Antiepileptics

4.8.1 Control of epilepsy

The decision about when to start treatment with an antiepileptic drug and the choice of medication depend on frequency of seizures, neurological findings, the identification of an epilepsy syndrome, and the wishes of the child and carers. For the majority of children, epilepsy is controlled with a single antiepileptic drug.

The object of treatment is to prevent the occurrence of seizures by maintaining an effective dose of one or more antiepileptic drugs. Careful adjustment of doses is necessary, starting with low doses and increasing gradually until seizures are controlled or there are significant adverse effects.

When choosing an antiepileptic drug to use, the seizure type, concomitant medication, co-morbidity, age, and sex should be taken into account. For women of child-bearing age, see Pregnancy and Breast-feeding, p. 273.

The frequency of administration is often determined by the plasma half-life, and should be kept as low as possible to encourage better adherence. Most antiepileptics, when used in usual dosage, may be given twice daily. Lamotrigine, phenobarbital and phenytoin, which have long half-lives, can be given as a daily dose at bedtime. However, with large doses, some antiepileptics may need to be given 3 times daily to avoid adverse effects associated with high peak plasma-drug concentrations. Young children metabolise antiepileptics more rapidly than adults and therefore require more frequent doses and a higher amount per kilogram body-weight.

Management   When monotherapy with a first-line antiepileptic drug has failed, monotherapy with a second drug should be tried; the diagnosis should be checked before starting an alternative drug if the first drug showed lack of efficacy. The change from one antiepileptic drug to another should be cautious, slowly withdrawing the first drug only when the new regimen has been established. Combination therapy with 2 or more antiepileptic drugs may be necessary, but the concurrent use of antiepileptic drugs increases the risk of adverse effects and drug interactions (see below). If combination therapy does not bring about worthwhile benefits, revert to the regimen (monotherapy or combination therapy) that provided the best balance between tolerability and efficacy.

Interactions   Interactions between antiepileptics are complex and may increase toxicity without a corresponding increase in antiepileptic effect. Interactions are usually caused by *hepatic enzyme induction* or *hepatic enzyme inhibition*; *displacement from protein binding sites* is not usually a problem. These interactions are highly variable and unpredictable.

For interactions of antiepileptic drugs, see Appendix 1; for advice on hormonal contraception and enzyme-inducing drugs, see section 7.3.1 and section 7.3.2.

Significant interactions that occur **between antiepileptics** that may affect dosing requirements are as follows:

> **Note** Check each drug for possible interactions when two or more antiepileptic drugs are used

Carbamazepine
often lowers plasma concentration of clobazam, clonazepam, lamotrigine, an active metabolite of oxcarbazepine, and of phenytoin (but may also raise phenytoin concentration), tiagabine, topiramate, and valproate

sometimes lowers plasma concentration of ethosuximide, and primidone (but tendency for corresponding increase in plasma-phenobarbital concentration)

Ethosuximide
sometimes raises plasma concentration of phenytoin

Lamotrigine
sometimes raises plasma concentration of an active metabolite of carbamazepine (but evidence is conflicting)

Oxcarbazepine
sometimes lowers plasma concentration of carbamazepine (but may raise concentration of an active metabolite of carbamazepine)

sometimes raises plasma concentration of phenytoin

often raises plasma concentration of phenobarbital

Phenobarbital *or* Primidone
often lowers plasma concentration of carbamazepine, clonazepam, lamotrigine, an active metabolite of oxcarbazepine and of phenytoin (but may also raise phenytoin concentration), tiagabine, and valproate

sometimes lowers plasma concentration of ethosuximide

Phenytoin
often lowers plasma concentration of clonazepam, carbamazepine, lamotrigine, an active metabolite of oxcarbazepine, and of tiagabine, topiramate, and valproate

often raises plasma concentration of phenobarbital

sometimes lowers plasma concentration of ethosuximide, and primidone (by increasing conversion to phenobarbital)

Rufinamide
sometimes raises plasma concentration of phenytoin

Stiripentol
often raises plasma concentration of carbamazepine, clobazam, phenobarbital, and phenytoin

Topiramate
sometimes raises plasma concentration of phenytoin

Valproate
sometimes lowers plasma concentration of an active metabolite of oxcarbazepine

often raises plasma concentration of an active metabolite of carbamazepine, and of lamotrigine, primidone, phenobarbital, and phenytoin (but may also lower)

sometimes raises plasma concentration of ethosuximide, and primidone (and tendency for significant increase in plasma-phenobarbital concentration)

Vigabatrin
often lowers plasma concentration of phenytoin

sometimes lowers plasma concentration of phenobarbital and primidone

Withdrawal Antiepileptics should be withdrawn under specialist supervision. Abrupt withdrawal, particularly of the barbiturates and benzodiazepines, should be avoided because this may precipitate severe rebound seizures. Reduction in dosage should be gradual and, in the case of barbiturates, the withdrawal process may take months.

The decision to withdraw antiepileptics from a seizure-free child, and its timing, depends on individual circumstances such as the type of epilepsy and its cause. Even in children who have been seizure-free for several years, there is a significant risk of seizure recurrence on drug withdrawal.

Drugs should be gradually withdrawn over at least 2–3 months by reducing the daily dose by 10–25% at intervals of 1–2 weeks. Benzodiazepines may need to be withdrawn over 6 months or longer.

In children receiving several antiepileptic drugs, only one drug should be withdrawn at a time.

Monitoring Routine measurement of plasma concentrations of antiepileptic drugs is not usually justified, because the target concentration ranges are arbitrary and often vary between individuals. However, plasma-drug concentrations may be measured in children with worsening seizures, status epilepticus, suspected non-compliance, or suspected toxicity. Similarly, haematological and biochemical monitoring should only be undertaken if clinically indicated.

Driving Older children with epilepsy may drive a motor vehicle (but not a large goods or passenger carrying vehicle) provided that they have been seizure-free for one year or, if subject to attacks only while asleep, have established a 3-year period of asleep attacks without awake attacks. Those affected by drowsiness should not drive or operate machinery.

Guidance issued by the Drivers Medical Unit of the Driver and Vehicle Licensing Agency (DVLA) recommends that patients should be advised not to drive during medication changes or withdrawal of antiepileptic drugs, and for 6 months afterwards.

Patients who have had a first or single epileptic seizure must not drive for 6 months (5 years in the case of large goods or passenger carrying vehicles) after the event; driving may then be resumed, provided the patient has been assessed by a specialist as fit to drive because no abnormality was detected on investigation.

Pregnancy and breast-feeding There is an increased risk of teratogenicity associated with the use of antiepileptic drugs (especially if the young woman takes two or more antiepileptic drugs). However, the benefit of antiepileptic treatment usually outweighs the potential teratogenic risk, and treatment should not be stopped during pregnancy without discussing with a specialist (see also under individual drugs). In view of the increased risk of neural tube and other defects associated, in particular, with **carbamazepine, lamotrigine, oxcarbazepine, phenytoin**, and **valproate**, women taking antiepileptic drugs who *may become pregnant* should be **informed of the possible consequences**. Those who *wish to become pregnant* should be referred to an appropriate specialist for advice. Young women who become pregnant should be **counselled** and offered **antenatal screening** (including alpha-fetoprotein measurement and a second trimester ultrasound scan).

To counteract the risk of neural tube defects adequate folate supplements are advised for women before and during pregnancy; to prevent recurrence of neural tube defects, women should receive folic acid 5 mg daily (section 9.1.2)—this dose may also be appropriate for women receiving antiepileptic drugs.

The concentration of antiepileptic drugs in the blood can change during pregnancy, particularly in the later stages. The dose of antiepileptic drugs should be monitored carefully during pregnancy and after birth, and adjustments made on a clinical basis.

Routine injection of vitamin K (section 9.6.6) at birth effectively counteracts any antiepileptic-associated risk of neonatal haemorrhage.

Breast-feeding is acceptable with all antiepileptic drugs taken in normal doses, with the possible exception of the barbiturates and some of the more recently introduced antiepileptics (see under individual drugs).

Partial seizures with or without secondary generalisation

Carbamazepine, lamotrigine, oxcarbazepine, and **sodium valproate** are the drugs of choice for partial (focal) seizures; second-line drugs include clobazam, gabapentin, levetiracetam, tiagabine, and topiramate.

Generalised seizures

Tonic-clonic seizures The drugs of choice for tonic-clonic seizures are **carbamazepine, lamotrigine, levetiracetam**, and **sodium valproate**. For children who have tonic-clonic seizures as part of the syndrome of primary generalised epilepsy, **sodium valproate** is the drug of choice. Second-line drugs include clobazam, oxcarbazepine, and topiramate.

4

Central nervous system

Absence seizures Ethosuximide and **sodium valproate** are the drugs of choice in typical absence seizures; **lamotrigine** can be used if these are unsuitable. Sodium valproate is also highly effective in treating the generalised tonic-clonic seizures which may co-exist with absence seizures in idiopathic primary generalised epilepsy.

Myoclonic seizures Myoclonic seizures (myoclonic jerks) occur in a variety of syndromes, and response to treatment varies considerably. **Sodium valproate** is the drug of choice and clobazam, clonazepam, ethosuximide, lamotrigine, levetiracetam, or topiramate are second-line drugs for treating myoclonic seizures.

Atypical absence, atonic, and tonic seizures *Atypical absence* and *atonic seizures* may be managed with **sodium valproate**, **lamotrigine**, or **ethosuximide**. *Tonic seizures* may be treated with **sodium valproate**. Second-line drugs for atypical absence, atonic, and tonic seizures include clobazam, clonazepam, levetiracetam, and topiramate; tonic seizures may rarely be aggravated by benzodiazepines.

Epilepsy syndromes

Infantile spasms Vigabatrin is the drug of choice for infantile spasms associated with tuberous sclerosis. In spasms of other causes, high doses of corticosteroids such as **prednisolone** (section 6.3.2) or **tetracosactide** (section 6.5.1) may be more effective. Second-line alternatives include clobazam, clonazepam, sodium valproate, and topiramate; nitrazepam is used but it is sedating.

Lennox-Gastaut syndrome Lamotrigine, **sodium valproate**, and **topiramate** are first-line drugs for treating Lennox-Gastaut syndrome. Clobazam, clonazepam, ethosuximide, levetiracetam, and rufinamide are also used.

Landau-Kleffner syndrome Prednisolone, **lamotrigine**, and **sodium valproate** are commonly used to treat Landau-Kleffner syndrome. Alternatives include clobazam, levetiracetam and topiramate.

Neonatal seizures Seizures can occur before delivery, but they are most common up to 24 hours after birth. Seizures in neonates occur as a result of biochemical disturbances, inborn errors of metabolism, hypoxic ischaemic encephalopathy, drug withdrawal, severe jaundice (kernicterus), meningitis, stroke, or cerebral haemorrhage or malformation.

Seizures caused by biochemical imbalance and those in neonates with inherited abnormal pyridoxine or biotin metabolism should be corrected by treating the underlying cause (section 9.6.2). Seizures caused by drug withdrawal following intra-uterine exposure are treated with a drug withdrawal regimen.

Phenobarbital may be preferred when there is a risk of seizure recurrence in neonates; phenytoin is an alternative. The benzodiazepines (clonazepam, diazepam, lorazepam, and midazolam) and rectal paraldehyde may be useful in the management of seizures which are likely to be brief with little risk of recurrence.

Severe myoclonic epilepsy of infancy Stiripentol is licensed to treat severe myoclonic epilepsy of infancy (Dravet Syndrome).

Carbamazepine and oxcarbazepine

Carbamazepine is a drug of choice for simple and complex partial seizures and for tonic-clonic seizures secondary to a focal discharge. It can exacerbate myoclonic and absence seizures. It is essential to initiate carbamazepine therapy at a low dose and build this up slowly in small increments every 3–7 days. Reversible blurring of vision, dizziness, and unsteadiness are dose-related, and may be dose-limiting. These side-effects may be reduced by altering the timing of medication; use of modified-release tablets also significantly lessens the incidence of dose-related side-effects.

Oxcarbazepine may be used for the treatment of partial seizures with or without secondary generalised tonic-clonic seizures. Oxcarbazepine induces hepatic enzymes to a lesser extent than carbamazepine.

CARBAMAZEPINE

Cautions cardiac disease (see also Contra-indications); skin reactions (see also Blood, Hepatic, or Skin disorders, below and under Side-effects); test for HLA-B*1502 allele in individuals of Han Chinese or Thai origin (avoid unless no alternative—risk of Stevens-Johnson syndrome in the pre-

◻ **CARBAMAZEPINE** (*continued*)

sence of HLA-B*1502 allele); history of haematological reactions to other drugs; manufacturer recommends blood counts and hepatic and renal function tests (but evidence of practical value unsatisfactory); may exacerbate absence and myoclonic seizures; consider vitamin D supplementation in patients that are immobilised for long periods or who have inadequate sun exposure or dietary intake of calcium; susceptibility to angle-closure glaucoma; cross-sensitivity reported with oxcarbazepine, and with phenytoin; avoid abrupt withdrawal; **interactions:** see p. 271 and Appendix 1 (carbamazepine)

Blood, hepatic, or skin disorders Children or their carers should be told how to recognise signs of blood, liver, or skin disorders, and advised to seek immediate medical attention if symptoms such as fever, sore throat, rash, mouth ulcers, bruising, or bleeding develop. Carbamazepine should be withdrawn immediately in cases of aggravated liver dysfunction or acute liver disease. Leucopenia which is severe, progressive, or associated with clinical symptoms requires withdrawal (if necessary under cover of suitable alternative).

Contra-indications AV conduction abnormalities (unless paced); history of bone marrow depression, acute porphyria (section 9.8.2)

Hepatic impairment metabolism impaired in advanced liver disease; see also Blood, Hepatic, or Skin Disorders, above

Renal impairment use with caution

Pregnancy see Pregnancy and Breast-feeding, p. 273

Breast-feeding amount probably too small to be harmful but monitor infant for possible adverse reactions; see also Pregnancy and Breast-feeding, p. 273

Side-effects nausea and vomiting, dizziness, drowsiness, headache, ataxia, confusion and agitation, visual disturbances (especially diplopia and often associated with peak plasma concentrations); constipation or diarrhoea, anorexia; mild transient generalised erythematous rash may occur in a large number of children (withdraw if worsens or is accompanied by other symptoms); leucopenia and other blood disorders (including thrombocytopenia, agranulocytosis and aplastic anaemia); other side-effects include cholestatic jaundice, vanishing bile duct syndrome, hepatitis and acute renal failure, Stevens-Johnson syndrome, toxic epidermal necrolysis, alopecia, thromboembolism, arthralgia, fever, proteinuria, lymph node enlargement, cardiac conduction disturbances (sometimes arrhythmias), dyskinesias, paraesthesia, depression, impotence (and impaired male fertility), gynaecomastia, galactorrhoea, aggression, activation of psychosis; *very rarely* angle-closure glaucoma; photosensitivity, pulmonary hypersensitivity (with dyspnoea and pneumonitis), hyponatraemia, oedema, and disturbances of bone metabolism (with osteomalacia) also reported (see Cautions); suicidal ideation; suppositories may cause occasional rectal irritation

Pharmacokinetics plasma concentration for optimum response 4–12 mg/litre (20–50 micromol/litre) measured after 1–2 weeks

Licensed use *suppositories* not licensed for use in trigeminal neuralgia or prophylaxis of bipolar disorder

Indication and dose

Partial and generalised tonic-clonic seizures, trigeminal neuralgia, prophylaxis of bipolar disorder

• **By mouth**

Child 1 month–12 years initially 5 mg/kg at night or 2.5 mg/kg twice daily, increased as necessary by 2.5–5 mg/kg every 3–7 days; usual maintenance dose 5 mg/kg 2–3 times daily; doses up to 20 mg/kg daily have been used

Child 12–18 years initially 100–200 mg 1–2 times daily, increased slowly to usual maintenance dose 200–400 mg 2–3 times daily; in some cases doses up to 1.8 g daily may be needed

• **By rectum**

Child 1 month–18 years use approx. 25% more than the oral dose (max. 250 mg) up to 4 times daily

Note Different preparations may vary in bioavailability; to avoid reduced effect or excessive side-effects, it may be prudent to avoid changing the formulation (see also notes above on how side-effects may be reduced)

Administration Oral liquid has been used rectally—should be retained for at least 2 hours (but may have laxative effect)

Carbamazepine (Non-proprietary) [PoM]
Tablets, carbamazepine 100 mg, net price 28 = £6.02; 200 mg, 28 = £5.53; 400 mg, 28 = £6.59. Label: 3, 8, counselling, blood, hepatic or skin disorder symptoms (see above), driving (see notes above)
Brands include *Epimaz*®
Dental prescribing on NHS Carbamazepine Tablets may be prescribed

Tegretol® (Novartis) [PoM]
Tablets, scored, carbamazepine 100 mg, net price 84-tab pack = £2.43; 200 mg, 84-tab pack = £4.50; 400 mg, 56-tab pack = £5.90. Label: 3, 8, counselling, blood, hepatic or skin disorder symptoms (see above), driving (see notes above)

Chewtabs, orange, carbamazepine 100 mg, net price 56-tab pack = £3.72; 200 mg, 56-tab pack = £6.92. Label: 3, 8, 21, 24, counselling, blood, hepatic or skin disorder symptoms (see above), driving (see notes above)

Liquid, sugar-free, carbamazepine 100 mg/5 mL. Net price 300-mL pack = £7.20. Label: 3, 8, counselling, blood, hepatic or skin disorder symptoms (see above), driving (see notes above)

Suppositories, carbamazepine 125 mg, net price 5 = £9.45; 250 mg, 5 = £12.60. Label: 3, 8, counselling, blood, hepatic or skin disorder symptoms (see above), driving (see notes above)

Dose

Epilepsy for short-term use (max. 7 days) when oral therapy temporarily not possible

Note Suppositories of 125 mg may be considered to be approximately equivalent in therapeutic effect to tablets of 100 mg but final adjustment should always depend on clinical response (plasma concentration monitoring recommended); max. dose *by rectum* 250 mg 4 times daily

Central nervous system

4

◁ **CARBAMAZEPINE** (*continued*)

◢**Modified release**

Carbagen® SR (Generics) ℞

Tablets, m/r, f/c, scored, carbamazepine 200 mg, net price 56-tab pack = £4.88; 400 mg, 56-tab pack = £9.63. Label: 3, 8, 25, counselling, blood, hepatic or skin disorder symptoms (see above), driving (see notes above)

Dose

> **Child 5–18 years** as above; total daily dose given in 1–2 divided doses

Tegretol® Retard (Novartis) ℞

Tablets, m/r, scored, carbamazepine 200 mg (beige-orange), net price 56-tab pack = £5.30; 400 mg (brown-orange), 56-tab pack = £10.44. Label: 3, 8, 25, counselling, blood, hepatic or skin disorder symptoms (see above), driving (see notes above)

Dose

> **Child 5–18 years** as above; total daily dose given in 2 divided doses

> **Administration** *Tegretol® Retard* tablets can be halved but should not be chewed

OXCARBAZEPINE

Cautions hypersensitivity to carbamazepine; avoid abrupt withdrawal; hyponatraemia (monitor plasma-sodium concentration in patients at risk), heart failure (monitor body-weight), cardiac conduction disorders; avoid in acute porphyria (section 9.8.2); **interactions**: see p. 271 and Appendix 1 (oxcarbazepine)

Blood, hepatic, or skin disorders Children or their carers should be told how to recognise signs of blood, liver, or skin disorders, and advised to seek immediate medical attention if symptoms such as lethargy, confusion, muscular twitching, fever, sore throat, rash, blistering, mouth ulcers, bruising, or bleeding develop

Hepatic impairment caution in severe impairment—no information available

Renal impairment halve initial dose if estimated glomerular filtration rate less than 30 mL/minute/1.73 m², increase according to response at intervals of at least 1 week

Pregnancy risk of teratogenesis including increased risk of neural tube defects; see also Pregnancy and Breast-feeding, p. 273

Breast-feeding amount probably too small to be harmful but manufacturer advises avoid; see also Pregnancy and Breast-feeding, p. 273

Side-effects nausea, vomiting, constipation, diarrhoea, abdominal pain, dizziness, headache, drowsiness, agitation, amnesia, asthenia, ataxia, confusion, impaired concentration, depression, tremor, hyponatraemia, acne, alopecia, rash, nystagmus, visual disorders including diplopia; *less commonly* urticaria, leucopenia; *very rarely* hepatitis, pancreatitis, arrhythmias, blood disorders, systemic lupus erythematosus, Stevens-Johnson syndrome, and toxic epidermal necrolysis; hypertension and hypothyroidism also reported; suicidal ideation

Indication and dose

> Monotherapy and adjunctive therapy of partial seizures with or without secondary generalised tonic-clonic seizures
>
> • By mouth
>
> > **Child 6–18 years** initially 4–5 mg/kg (max. 300 mg) twice daily, increased according to response in steps of up to 5 mg/kg twice daily at weekly intervals (usual maintenance dose for adjunctive therapy 15 mg/kg twice daily); max. 23 mg/kg twice daily

> **Note** In adjunctive therapy the dose of concomitant antiepileptics may need to be reduced when using high doses of oxcarbazepine

Oxcarbazepine (Non-proprietary) ℞

Tablets, oxcarbazepine 150 mg, net price 50-tab pack = £9.91; 300 mg, 50-tab pack = £20.14; 600 mg, 50-tab pack = £40.18. Label: 3, 8, counselling, blood, hepatic or skin disorders (see above), driving (see notes above)

Trileptal® (Novartis) ℞

Tablets, f/c, scored, oxcarbazepine 150 mg (green), net price 50-tab pack = £10.00; 300 mg (yellow), 50-tab pack = £20.00; 600 mg (pink), 50-tab pack = £40.00. Label: 3, 8, counselling, blood, hepatic or skin disorders (see above), driving (see notes above)

Oral suspension, sugar-free, oxcarbazepine 300 mg/5 mL, net price 250 mL (with oral syringe) = £40.00. Label: 3, 8, counselling, blood, hepatic or skin disorders (see above), driving (see notes above)

Excipients include propylene glycol (see Excipients, p. 3)

Ethosuximide

Ethosuximide is used in typical absence seizures; it may also be used in myoclonic seizures and in atypical absence, atonic, and tonic seizures.

ETHOSUXIMIDE

Cautions avoid abrupt withdrawal; avoid in acute porphyria (section 9.8.2); **interactions**: see p. 271 and Appendix 1 (ethosuximide)

Blood disorders Children or their carers should be told how to recognise signs of blood disorders, and advised to seek immediate medical attention if symptoms such as fever, sore throat, mouth ulcers, bruising, or bleeding develop

Hepatic impairment use with caution

Renal impairment use with caution

Pregnancy low teratogenic risk; see also Pregnancy and Breast-feeding, p. 273

Breast-feeding present in milk but not known to be harmful; see also Pregnancy and Breast-feeding, p. 273

◁ **ETHOSUXIMIDE** (*continued*)

Side-effects gastro-intestinal disturbances (including nausea, vomiting, diarrhoea, abdominal pain, and anorexia), weight loss; *less frequently* headache, fatigue, drowsiness, dizziness, hiccup, ataxia, mild euphoria, irritability, aggression, and impaired concentration; *rarely* tongue swelling, sleep disturbances, night terrors, depression, psychosis, photophobia, dyskinesia, increased libido, vaginal bleeding, myopia, gingival hypertrophy, and rash; also reported, hyperactivity, increase in seizure frequency, blood disorders such as leucopenia, agranulocytosis, pancytopenia, and aplastic anaemia (blood counts required if features of infection), systemic lupus erythematosus, and Stevens-Johnson syndrome; suicidal ideation

Indication and dose

Absence seizures, atypical absence, myoclonic seizures

• By mouth

Child 1 month–6 years initially 5 mg/kg (max. 125 mg) twice daily, increased gradually over 2– 3 weeks up to maintenance dose of 10–20 mg/ kg (max. 500 mg) twice daily; total daily dose may rarely be given in 3 divided doses

Child 6–18 years initially 250 mg twice daily, increased by 250 mg at intervals of 4–7 days to usual dose of 500–750 mg twice daily; occasionally up to 1 g twice daily may be needed

Ethosuximide (Non-proprietary) [PoM]
Capsules, ethosuximide 250 mg, net price 56-cap pack = £38.23. Label: 8, counselling, blood disorders (see above), driving (see notes above)

Emeside® (Chemidex) [PoM]
Syrup, black currant, ethosuximide 250 mg/5 mL, net price 200-mL pack = £6.60. Label: 8, counselling, blood disorders (see above), driving (see notes above)

Zarontin® (Pfizer) [PoM]
Syrup, yellow, ethosuximide 250 mg/5 mL, net price 200-mL pack = £4.31. Label: 8, counselling, blood disorders (see above), driving (see notes above)

Gabapentin

Gabapentin is used as adjunctive therapy for the treatment of partial seizures with or without secondary generalisation; it can be used as monotherapy in children over 12 years.

GABAPENTIN

Cautions avoid abrupt withdrawal (may cause anxiety, insomnia, nausea, pain, and sweating— taper off over at least 1 week); diabetes mellitus, false positive readings with some urinary protein tests; **interactions**: Appendix 1 (gabapentin)

Renal impairment reduce dose if estimated glomerular filtration rate less than 80 mL/minute/1.73 m²; consult product literature

Pregnancy toxicity in *animal* studies; see also Pregnancy and Breast-feeding, p. 273

Breast-feeding present in milk—manufacturer advises use only if potential benefit outweighs risk; see also Pregnancy and Breast-feeding, p. 273

Side-effects diarrhoea, dry mouth, dyspepsia, nausea, vomiting, constipation, abdominal pain, flatulence, appetite changes, gingivitis, weight gain; hypertension, vasodilation, oedema; dyspnoea, cough, rhinitis; confusion, depression, hostility, sleep disturbances, headache; dizziness, anxiety, amnesia, ataxia, dysarthria, nystagmus, tremor, asthenia, paraesthesia, hyperkinesia; influenza-like symptoms; impotence, urinary incontinence; leucopenia; myalgia, arthralgia; diplopia, amblyopia; rash, purpura, pruritus, acne; *rarely* pancreatitis, hepatitis, jaundice, palpitation, hallucinations, movement disorders, thrombocytopenia, blood-glucose fluctuations in patients with diabetes, tinnitus, acute renal failure, Stevens-Johnson syndrome, and alopecia; suicidal ideation

Licensed use not licensed for use in children under 6 years; not licensed at doses over 50 mg/ kg daily in children under 12 years

Indication and dose

Adjunctive treatment of partial seizures with or without secondary generalisation

• By mouth

Child 2–6 years 10 mg/kg once daily on day 1, then 10 mg/kg twice daily on day 2, then 10 mg/kg 3 times daily on day 3, increased according to response to usual dose of 30– 70 mg/kg daily in 3 divided doses

Child 6–12 years 10 mg/kg once daily (max. 300 mg) on day 1, then 10 mg/kg (max. 300 mg) twice daily on day 2, then 10 mg/kg (max. 300 mg) 3 times daily on day 3; usual dose 25– 35 mg/kg daily in 3 divided doses; max. 70 mg/ kg daily in 3 divided doses

Child 12–18 years 300 mg once daily on day 1, then 300 mg twice daily on day 2, then 300 mg 3 times daily on day 3 *or* initially 300 mg 3 times daily on day 1; then increased according to response in steps of 300 mg daily (in 3 divided doses) every 2–3 days; usual dose 0.9–3.6 g daily in 3 divided doses

Monotherapy for partial seizures with or without secondary generalisation

• By mouth

Child 12–18 years 300 mg once daily on day 1, then 300 mg twice daily on day 2, then 300 mg 3 times daily on day 3 *or* initially 300 mg 3 times

△ **GABAPENTIN (continued)**

daily on day 1; then increased according to
response in steps of 300 mg daily (in 3 divided
doses) every 2–3 days; usual dose 0.9–3.6 g
daily in 3 divided doses

Note Some children may not tolerate daily increments;
longer intervals (up to weekly) may be more appropriate

Administration capsules can be opened but the
bitter taste is difficult to mask

Gabapentin (Non-proprietary) [PoM]
Capsules, gabapentin 100 mg, net price 100-cap
pack = £3.94; 300 mg, 100-cap pack = £5.52;
400 mg, 100-cap pack = £5.91. Label: 3, 5, 8,
counselling, driving (see notes above)

Tablets, gabapentin 600 mg, net price 100-tab pack
= £41.06; 800 mg, 100-tab pack= £54.19. Label: 3,
5, 8, counselling, driving (see notes above)

Neurontin® (Pfizer) [PoM]
Capsules, gabapentin 100 mg (white), net price
100-cap pack = £18.29; 300 mg (yellow), 100-cap
pack = £42.40; 400 mg (orange), 100-cap pack =
£49.06. Label: 3, 5, 8, counselling, driving (see notes
above)

Tablets, f/c, gabapentin 600 mg, net price 100-tab
pack = £84.80; 800 mg, 100-tab pack = £98.13.
Label: 3, 5, 8, counselling, driving (see notes above)

Lacosamide

Lacosamide is licensed for adjunctive treatment of partial seizures with or
without secondary generalisation.

The *Scottish Medicines Consortium* (p. 4) has advised (January 2009) that lacosamide (*Vimpat®*) is accepted for restricted use within NHS Scotland as adjunctive
treatment for partial seizures with or without secondary generalisation in patients
from 16 years. It is restricted for specialist use in refractory epilepsy.

LACOSAMIDE

Cautions conduction problems or severe cardiac
disease (increased risk of PR-interval prolongation); **interactions:** Appendix 1 (lacosamide)

Contra-indications second- or third-degree AV
block

Hepatic impairment caution in severe impairment—no information available

Renal impairment caution; max. 250 mg daily if
estimated glomerular filtration rate is less than
30 mL/minute/1.73 m²

Pregnancy manufacturer advises avoid unless
potential benefit outweighs risk; see also
Pregnancy and Breast-feeding, p. 273

Breast-feeding manufacturer advises avoid—
present in milk in *animal* studies; see also
Pregnancy and Breast-feeding, p. 273

Side-effects nausea, vomiting, flatulence, constipation; dizziness, headache, depression, diplopia,
nystagmus, impaired coordination, impaired
memory, cognitive disorder, drowsiness, tremor,
asthenia, fatigue; pruritus; *less commonly* PR-
interval prolongation; suicidal ideation

Indication and dose

**Adjunctive treatment of partial seizures with or
without secondary generalisation**
- By intravenous infusion over 15–60 minutes
  (for up to 5 days) or by mouth

  Child 16–18 years initially 50 mg twice daily,
  increased in steps of 50 mg twice daily every
  week to max. 200 mg twice daily

Administration for *intravenous infusion*, give undiluted or dilute with Glucose 5% *or* Sodium
Chloride 0.9%

Vimpat® (UCB Pharma) ▼ [PoM]
Tablets, f/c, lacosamide 50 mg (pink), net price 14-
tab pack = £9.01; 100 mg (yellow), 14-tab pack =
£18.02, 56-tab pack = £72.08; 150 mg (salmon), 14-
tab pack = £27.03, 56-tab pack £108.12; 200 mg
(blue), 56-tab pack = £144.16. Label: 8, counselling,
driving (see notes above)

Syrup, lacosamide 15 mg/mL, net price 200 mL =
£38.61. Label: 8, counselling, driving (see notes
above)
Excipients include aspartame (section 9.4.1)

Intravenous infusion, lacosamide 10 mg/mL net
price 200-mg vial = £29.70
Electrolytes Na⁺ 2.6 mmol/200-mg vial

Lamotrigine

Lamotrigine is an antiepileptic for partial seizures, primary and secondary
generalised tonic-clonic seizures, and for typical absence seizures; however,
efficacy may not be maintained in all children treated for typical absence seizures.
It may be tried for atypical absence, atonic, and tonic seizures. Lamotrigine may
cause serious skin rash; dose recommendations should be adhered to closely.

Lamotrigine is used either as sole treatment or as an adjunct to treatment with
other antiepileptic drugs. Valproate increases plasma-lamotrigine concentration
whereas the enzyme inducing antiepileptics reduce it; care is therefore required in
choosing the appropriate initial dose and subsequent titration. Where the poten-

tial for interaction is not known, treatment should be initiated with lower doses such as those used with valproate.

◣ LAMOTRIGINE

Cautions closely monitor and consider withdrawal if rash, fever, or signs of hypersensitivity syndrome develop; avoid abrupt withdrawal (taper off over 2 weeks or longer) unless serious skin reaction occurs; myoclonic seizures (may be exacerbated); **interactions:** see p. 271 and Appendix 1 (lamotrigine)

Blood disorders The CSM has advised prescribers to be alert for symptoms and signs suggestive of bone-marrow failure such as anaemia, bruising, or infection. Aplastic anaemia, bone-marrow depression, and pancytopenia have occurred rarely

Hepatic impairment halve dose in moderate impairment; quarter dose in severe impairment

Renal impairment caution in renal failure; metabolite may accumulate; consider reducing maintenance dose in significant impairment

Pregnancy risk of teratogenesis; see also Pregnancy and Breast-feeding, p. 273

Breast-feeding present in milk, but limited data suggest no harmful effect on infant; see also Pregnancy and Breast-feeding, p. 273

Side-effects rash (see Skin Reactions, below); hypersensitivity syndrome (possibly including rash, fever, facial oedema, lymphadenopathy, hepatic dysfunction, blood disorders, disseminated intravascular coagulation, and multi-organ dysfunction); nausea, vomiting, diarrhoea, hepatic dysfunction; headache, fatigue, dizziness, sleep disturbances, tremor, movement disorders, agitation, confusion, hallucinations, occasional increase in seizure frequency; blood disorders (including leucopenia, thrombocytopenia, pancytopenia—see Blood Disorders, above); arthralgia; lupus erythematosus-like effect; photosensitivity; nystagmus, diplopia, blurred vision, conjunctivitis; suicidal ideation

Skin reactions Serious skin reactions including Stevens-Johnson syndrome and toxic epidermal necrolysis (rarely with fatalities) have developed especially in children; most rashes occur in the first 8 weeks. Rash is sometimes associated with hypersensitivity syndrome (see Side-effects, above) and is more common in patients with history of allergy or rash from other antiepileptic drugs. Consider withdrawal if rash or signs of hypersensitivity syndrome develop. Factors associated with increased risk of serious skin reactions include concomitant use of valproate, initial lamotrigine dosing higher than recommended, and more rapid dose escalation than recommended.

Counselling Warn children and their carers to see their doctor immediately if rash or signs or symptoms of hypersensitivity syndrome develop

Indication and dose

Monotherapy and adjunctive treatment of partial seizures and primary and secondary generalised tonic-clonic seizures; seizures associated with Lennox-Gastaut syndrome

• By mouth

Adjunctive therapy of seizures *with valproate*

Child 2–12 years initially 150 micrograms/kg once daily for 14 days (those weighing under 13 kg may receive 2 mg on alternate days for first 14 days) then 300 micrograms/kg once daily for further 14 days, thereafter increased by max. of 300 micrograms/kg daily every 7–14 days; usual maintenance 1–5 mg/kg daily in 1–2 divided doses (max. single dose 100 mg)

Child 12–18 years initially 25 mg on alternate days for 14 days then 25 mg daily for further 14 days, thereafter increased by max. 25–50 mg daily every 7–14 days; usual maintenance 100–200 mg daily in 1–2 divided doses

Adjunctive therapy of seizures (with enzyme inducing drugs) *without valproate*

Child 2–12 years initially 300 micrograms/kg twice daily for 14 days then 600 micrograms/kg twice daily for further 14 days, thereafter increased by max. 1.2 mg/kg daily every 7–14 days; usual maintenance 2.5–7.5 mg/kg (max. single dose 200 mg) twice daily

Child 12–18 years initially 50 mg daily for 14 days then 50 mg twice daily for further 14 days, thereafter increased by max. 100 mg daily every 7–14 days; usual maintenance 100–200 mg twice daily (up to 700 mg daily has been required)

Adjunctive therapy of seizures (without enzyme inducing drugs) *without valproate*

Child 2–12 years initially 300 micrograms/kg daily in 1–2 divided doses for 14 days then 600 micrograms/kg daily in 1–2 divided doses for further 14 days, thereafter increased by max. 600 micrograms/kg daily every 7–14 days; usual maintenance 1–10 mg/kg daily in 1–2 divided doses; max. 200 mg daily

Child 12–18 years initially 25 mg daily for 14 days, increased to 50 mg daily for further 14 days, then increased by max. 50–100 mg daily every 7–14 days; usual maintenance 100–200 mg daily in 1–2 divided doses

Monotherapy of seizures

Child 12–18 years initially 25 mg daily for 14 days, increased to 50 mg daily for further 14 days, then increased by max. 50–100 mg daily every 7–14 days; usual maintenance as monotherapy, 100–200 mg daily in 1–2 divided doses (up to 500 mg daily has been required)

Monotherapy of typical absence seizures

• By mouth

Child 2–12 years initially 300 micrograms/kg daily in 1–2 divided doses for 14 days, then 600 micrograms/kg daily in 1–2 divided doses for further 14 days, thereafter increased by max. 600 micrograms/kg daily every 7–14 days; usual maintenance 1–10 mg/kg daily in 1–2 divided doses; (up to 15 mg/kg daily has been required)

Note Dose titration should be repeated if restarting after interval of more than 5 days

Safe Practice Do not confuse the different combinations; see also notes above

4

Central nervous system

◁ **LAMOTRIGINE** *(continued)*

Lamotrigine (Non-proprietary) PoM
Tablets, lamotrigine 25 mg, net price 56-tab pack = £2.77; 50 mg, 56-tab pack = £3.73; 100 mg, 56-tab pack = £5.39; 200 mg, 30-tab pack = £27.53, 56-tab pack = £9.63. Label: 8, counselling, driving (see notes above), skin reactions (see above)

Dispersible tablets, lamotrigine 5 mg, net price 28-tab pack = £2.67; 25 mg, 56-tab pack = £3.41; 100 mg, 56-tab pack = £6.50. Label: 8, 13, counselling, driving (see notes above), skin reactions (see above)

Lamictal® (GSK) PoM
Tablets, yellow, lamotrigine 25 mg, net price 21-tab pack ('*Valproate Add-on therapy' Starter Pack*) = £7.35, 42-tab pack ('*Monotherapy' Starter Pack*) = £14.70, 56-tab pack = £19.61; 50 mg, 42-tab pack ('*Non-valproate Add-on therapy' Starter Pack*) = £25.01, 56-tab pack = £33.35; 100 mg, 56-tab pack = £57.53; 200 mg, 56-tab pack = £97.79. Label: 8, counselling, driving (see notes above), skin reactions (see above)

Dispersible tablets, chewable, lamotrigine 2 mg, net price 30-tab pack = £10.45; 5 mg, 28-tab pack = £7.82; 25 mg, 56-tab pack = £19.61; 100 mg, 56-tab pack = £57.53. Label: 8, 13, counselling, driving (see notes above), skin reactions (see above)

Levetiracetam

Levetiracetam is used for monotherapy and adjunctive treatment of partial seizures with or without secondary generalisation, and for adjunctive treatment of myoclonic seizures and generalised tonic-clonic seizures.

LEVETIRACETAM

Cautions avoid abrupt withdrawal; **interactions:** Appendix 1 (levetiracetam)

Hepatic impairment halve dose in severe hepatic impairment if estimated glomerular filtration rate less than 60 mL/minute/1.73 m^2

Renal impairment reduce dose if estimated glomerular filtration rate less than 80 mL/minute/1.73 m^2 (consult product literature)

Pregnancy toxicity in *animal* studies—manufacturer advises use only if potential benefit outweighs risk; see also Pregnancy and Breast-feeding, p. 273

Breast-feeding present in milk—manufacturer advises avoid; see also Pregnancy and Breast-feeding, p. 273

Side-effects nausea, vomiting, dyspepsia, diarrhoea, abdominal pain, anorexia, weight changes; cough; drowsiness, asthenia, amnesia, ataxia, seizures, dizziness, headache, tremor, hyperkinesia, depression, emotional lability, insomnia, anxiety, impaired balance and attention, aggression, irritability; thrombocytopenia; myalgia; visual disturbances; pruritus, rash; *also reported* pancreatitis, hepatic dysfunction, confusion, psychosis, hallucinations, suicidal ideation, paraesthesia, leucopenia, pancytopenia, and alopecia

Indication and dose

Monotherapy of partial seizures with or without secondary generalisation
- By mouth or by intravenous infusion

Child 16–18 years initially 250 mg once daily increased after 1 week to 250 mg twice daily; thereafter, increased according to response in steps of 250 mg twice daily every 2 weeks; max. 1.5 g twice daily

Adjunctive therapy of partial seizures with or without secondary generalisation
- By mouth

Child 1–6 months initially 7 mg/kg once daily, increased gradually by max. 7 mg/kg twice daily every 2 weeks; max. 21 mg/kg twice daily

Child 6 months–18 years, body-weight under 50 kg initially 10 mg/kg once daily, increased gradually by max. 10 mg/kg twice daily every 2 weeks; max. 30 mg/kg twice daily

Child 12–18 years, body-weight over 50 kg initially 250 mg twice daily, increased gradually by 500 mg twice daily every 2 weeks; max. 1.5 g twice daily

- By intravenous infusion

Child 4–18 years, body-weight under 50 kg initially 10 mg/kg once daily, increased gradually by max. 10 mg/kg twice daily every 2 weeks; max. 30 mg/kg twice daily

Child 12–18 years, body-weight over 50 kg initially 250 mg twice daily, increased gradually by 500 mg twice daily every 2 weeks; max. 1.5 g twice daily

Adjunctive therapy of myoclonic seizures and tonic-clonic seizures
- By mouth or by intravenous infusion

Child 12–18 years, body-weight under 50 kg initially 10 mg/kg once daily, increased gradually by max. 10 mg/kg twice daily every 2 weeks; max. 30 mg/kg twice daily

Child 12–18 years, body-weight over 50 kg initially 250 mg twice daily, increased gradually by 500 mg twice daily every 2 weeks; max. 1.5 g twice daily

Administration for *intravenous infusion*, dilute requisite dose with at least 100 mL Glucose 5% *or* Sodium Chloride 0.9%; give over 15 minutes
For administration of *oral solution*, requisite dose may be diluted in a glass of water

Keppra® (UCB Pharma) PoM
Tablets, f/c, levetiracetam 250 mg (blue), net price 60-tab pack = £29.70; 500 mg (yellow), 60-tab pack = £52.30; 750 mg (orange), 60-tab pack = £89.10; 1 g (white), 60-tab pack = £101.10. Label: 8

Oral solution, sugar-free, levetiracetam 100 mg/mL, net price 300 mL = £71.00. Label: 8

◁ **LEVETIRACETAM** (*continued*)

Concentrate for intravenous infusion, levetiracetam 100 mg/mL. For dilution before use. Net price
5-mL vial = £13.50
Electrolytes Na⁺ <0.5 mmol/vial

Phenobarbital and other barbiturates

Phenobarbital (phenobarbitone) is effective for tonic-clonic, partial seizures and
neonatal seizures but may cause behavioural disturbances and hyperkinesia. It
may be tried for atypical absence, atonic, and tonic seizures. Rebound seizures
may be a problem on withdrawal. Monitoring plasma concentrations is less useful
than with other drugs because tolerance occurs.

Primidone is largely converted to phenobarbital and this is probably responsible
for its antiepileptic action. It is used rarely in children.

PHENOBARBITAL
(Phenobarbitone)

Cautions see also notes above; debilitated; respiratory depression (avoid if severe); avoid abrupt
withdrawal (dependence with prolonged use);
history of drug and alcohol abuse; consider vitamin D supplementation in patients that are
immobilised for long periods or who have
inadequate sun exposure or dietary intake of
calcium; avoid in acute porphyria (see section
9.8.2); **interactions:** see p. 271 and Appendix 1
(barbiturates)

Hepatic impairment may precipitate coma; avoid
in severe impairment

Renal impairment use with caution

Pregnancy congenital malformation; see also
Pregnancy and Breast-feeding, p. 273

Breast-feeding avoid if possible; drowsiness may
occur; see also Pregnancy and Breast-feeding,
p. 273

Side-effects hepatitis, cholestasis; hypotension;
respiratory depression; drowsiness, lethargy,
depression, ataxia, behavioural disturbances,
nystagmus, irritability, hallucinations, impaired
memory and cognition, hyperactivity; osteomalacia (see Cautions); megaloblastic anaemia (may
be treated with folic acid), agranulocytosis,
thrombocytopenia; allergic skin reactions; *very
rarely* Stevens-Johnson syndrome and toxic epidermal necrolysis; suicidal ideation; **overdosage:**
see Emergency Treatment of Poisoning, p. 35

Pharmacokinetics trough plasma concentration
for optimum response 15–40 mg/litre (60–
180 micromol/litre)

Indication and dose

All forms of epilepsy except absence seizures

• **By mouth or by intravenous injection**

> **Neonate** initially 20 mg/kg *by slow intravenous
> injection* then 2.5–5 mg/kg once daily either *by*

slow intravenous injection or *by mouth*; dose and
frequency adjusted according to response

• **By mouth**

> **Child 1 month–12 years** initially 1–1.5 mg/kg
> twice daily, increased by 2 mg/kg daily as
> required; usual maintenance dose 2.5–4 mg/kg
> once or twice daily

> **Child 12–18 years** 60–180 mg once daily

Status epilepticus section 4.8.2

Note For therapeutic purposes phenobarbital and phenobarbital sodium may be considered equivalent in effect

Administration for administration *by mouth*,
tablets may be crushed

For *intravenous injection*, dilute to a concentration
of 20 mg/mL with Water for Injections; give over
20 minutes (no faster than 1 mg/kg/minute)

Phenobarbital (Non-proprietary) Ⓒ🄳
Tablets, phenobarbital 15 mg, net price 28-tab pack
= 85p; 30 mg, 28-tab pack = £1.06; 60 mg, 28-tab
pack = 66p. Label: 2, 8, counselling, driving (see
notes above)

Elixir, phenobarbital 15 mg/5 mL in a suitable flavoured vehicle, containing alcohol 38%, net price
100 mL = 77p. Label: 2, 8, counselling, driving (see
notes above)

Note Some hospitals supply **alcohol-free** formulations of
varying phenobarbital strengths

Injection, phenobarbital sodium 200 mg/mL in
propylene glycol 90% and water for injections 10%,
net price 1-mL amp = £2.00

Note Must be diluted before intravenous administration
(see Administration)

PRIMIDONE

Cautions see Phenobarbital; **interactions:** see
p. 271 and Appendix 1 (primidone)

Hepatic impairment reduce dose, may precipitate
coma

Renal impairment see Phenobarbital

Pregnancy see Phenobarbital

Breast-feeding see Phenobarbital

Side-effects see Phenobarbital; also nausea and
visual disturbances; *less commonly* vomiting,
headache, and dizziness; *rarely* arthralgia

Pharmacokinetics monitor plasma concentrations of derived phenobarbital. Optimum range as
for phenobarbital

4

Central nervous system

Central nervous system 4

△ **PRIMIDONE** (*continued*)

Indication and dose

All forms of epilepsy except absence seizures
(but see notes above)
• By mouth

Child under 2 years initially 125 mg daily at
bedtime, increased by 125 mg every 3 days
according to response; usual maintenance, 125–
250 mg twice daily

Child 2–5 years initially 125 mg daily at bedtime, increased by 125 mg every 3 days
according to response; usual maintenance, 250–
375 mg twice daily

Child 5–9 years initially 125 mg daily at bedtime, increased by 125 mg every 3 days
according to response; usual maintenance, 375–
500 mg twice a day

Child 9–18 years initially 125 mg daily at bedtime, increased by 125 mg every 3 days to
250 mg twice daily, then increased according to
response by 250 mg every 3 days to max.
750 mg twice daily

Mysoline® (Acorus) PoM
Tablets, scored, primidone 250 mg, net price 100-
tab pack = £12.60. Label: 2, 8, counselling, driving
(see notes above)

Phenytoin

Phenytoin is effective for tonic-clonic, partial, and neonatal seizures but it may
worsen myoclonus. It has a narrow therapeutic index and the relationship
between dose and plasma concentration is non-linear; small dosage increases
in some children may produce large rises in plasma concentrations with acute
toxic side-effects. Monitoring of plasma concentration can assist dosage adjustment. A few missed doses or a small change in drug absorption may result in a
marked change in plasma concentration.

Phenytoin may cause coarse facies, acne, hirsutism, and gingival hyperplasia and
so may be particularly undesirable in adolescent patients.

When only parenteral administration is possible, **fosphenytoin** (section 4.8.2), a
pro-drug of phenytoin, may be convenient to give. Whereas phenytoin can be
given intravenously only, fosphenytoin may also be given by intramuscular
injection.

PHENYTOIN

Cautions see notes above; avoid abrupt withdrawal; manufacturer recommends blood counts
(but evidence of practical value unsatisfactory);
consider vitamin D supplementation in patients
that are immobilised for long periods or who have
inadequate sun exposure or dietary intake of
calcium; avoid in acute porphyria (section 9.8.2);
interactions: see p. 271 and Appendix 1 (phenytoin)

Blood or skin disorders Children and their carers should
be told how to recognise signs of blood or skin disorders,
and advised to seek immediate medical attention if
symptoms such as fever, sore throat, rash, mouth ulcers,
bruising, or bleeding develop. Leucopenia which is severe,
progressive, or associated with clinical symptoms
requires withdrawal (if necessary under cover of suitable
alternative)

Hepatic impairment reduce dose

Pregnancy congenital malformations; changes in
plasma-protein binding make interpretation of
plasma-phenytoin concentrations difficult—
monitor unbound fraction; see also Pregnancy
and Breast-feeding, p. 273

Breast-feeding small amounts present in milk,
but not known to be harmful; see also Pregnancy
and Breast-feeding, p. 273

Side-effects nausea, vomiting, constipation;
insomnia, transient nervousness, tremor, paraesthesia, dizziness, headache, anorexia; gingival
hypertrophy and tenderness (maintain good oral
hygiene); rash (discontinue; if mild reintroduce
cautiously but discontinue immediately if recurrence), acne, hirsutism, coarse facies; *rarely*

hepatoxicity, peripheral neuropathy, dyskinesia,
lymphadenopathy, osteomalacia (see Cautions),
blood disorders (including megaloblastic anaemia (may be treated with folic acid), leucopenia,
thrombocytopenia, and aplastic anaemia), polyarteritis nodosa, lupus erythematosus, Stevens-
Johnson syndrome, and toxic epidermal necrolysis; also reported pneumonitis and interstitial
nephritis; suicidal ideation; *with excessive dosage*
nystagmus, diplopia, slurred speech, ataxia, confusion, and hyperglycaemia

Pharmacokinetics therapeutic plasma-phenytoin
concentrations reduced in first 3 months of life
because of reduced protein binding

Trough plasma concentration for optimum
response:

Neonate–3 months, 6–15 mg/litre (25–60 micr-
omol/litre)

Child 3 months–18 years, 10–20 mg/litre (40–
80 micromol/litre)

Licensed use licensed for use in children (age
range not specified by manufacturer)

Indication and dose

All forms of epilepsy except absence seizures
• By intravenous injection (over 20–30 minutes)
and by mouth

Neonate initial loading dose *by slow intravenous
injection* (section 4.8.2) 18 mg/kg then *by mouth*
2.5–5 mg/kg twice daily adjusted according to
response and plasma-phenytoin concentration
(usual max. 7.5 mg/kg twice daily)

◁ **PHENYTOIN** (*continued*)

• **By mouth**

Child 1 month–12 years initially 1.5–2.5 mg/kg
twice daily, then adjusted according to response
and plasma-phenytoin concentration to 2.5–
5 mg/kg twice daily (usual max. 7.5 mg/kg
twice daily *or* 300 mg daily)

Child 12–18 years initially 75–150 mg twice
daily then adjusted according to response and
plasma-phenytoin concentration to 150–200 mg
twice daily (usual max. 300 mg twice daily)

**Status epilepticus, acute symptomatic seizures
associated with head trauma or neurosurgery**
section 4.8.2

Administration for administration *by mouth*, interrupt enteral feeds for at least 1–2 hours before
and after giving phenytoin; give with water to
enhance absorption

For administration by *intravenous injection* and
intravenous infusion, see p. 294

Phenytoin (Non-proprietary) PoM
Tablets , coated, phenytoin sodium 100 mg, net
price 28-tab pack = £30.00. Label: 8, counselling,
administration, blood or skin disorder symptoms
(see above), driving (see notes above)

Note On the basis of single dose tests there are no
clinically relevant differences in bioavailability between
available phenytoin sodium tablets and capsules but there

may be a pharmacokinetic basis for maintaining the same
brand of phenytoin in some patients

Epanutin® (Pfizer) PoM
Capsules , phenytoin sodium 25 mg (white/purple),
net price 28-cap pack = 66p; 50 mg (white/pink),
28-cap pack = 67p; 100 mg (white/orange), 84-cap
pack = £2.83; 300 mg (white/green), 28-cap pack =
£2.83. Label: 8, counselling, administration, blood
or skin disorder symptoms (see above), driving (see
notes above)

Infatabs® (= chewable tablets), yellow, scored,
phenytoin 50 mg, net price 112 = £7.38. Label: 8,
24, counselling, blood or skin disorder symptoms
(see above), driving (see notes above)

Note Contain phenytoin 50 mg (as against phenytoin
sodium) therefore care is needed on changing to capsules
or tablets containing phenytoin sodium

Suspension , red, phenytoin 30 mg/5 mL, net price
500 mL = £4.27. Label: 8, counselling, administration, blood or skin disorder symptoms (see above),
driving (see notes above)

Note Suspension of phenytoin 90 mg in 15 mL may be
considered to be approximately equivalent in therapeutic
effect to capsules or tablets containing phenytoin sodium
100 mg, but nevertheless care is needed in making
changes

◢**Parenteral preparations**
Section 4.8.2

Rufinamide

Rufinamide is licensed for the adjunctive treatment of seizures in Lennox-Gastaut
syndrome.

The *Scottish Medicines Consortium* (p. 4) has advised (October 2008) that rufinamide (*Inovelon®*) is accepted for restricted use within NHS Scotland as adjunctive
therapy in the treatment of seizures associated with Lennox-Gastaut syndrome in
patients 4 years and above. It is restricted for use when alternative traditional
antiepileptic drugs are unsatisfactory.

RUFINAMIDE

Cautions closely monitor and consider withdrawal if rash, fever, or other signs of hypersensitivity syndrome (see Side-effects) develop;
avoid abrupt withdrawal; **interactions:** see p. 271
and Appendix 1 (rufinamide)

Hepatic impairment caution and careful dose
titration in mild to moderate impairment; avoid in
severe impairment

Pregnancy manufacturer advises avoid unless
potential benefit outweighs risk—toxicity in *animal* studies; effective contraception must be used
during treatment; see also Pregnancy and Breast-
feeding, p. 273

Breast-feeding manufacturer advises avoid—no
information available; see also Pregnancy and
Breast-feeding, p. 273

Side-effects nausea, vomiting, constipation,
diarrhoea, dyspepsia, abdominal pain; rhinitis,
epistaxis; weight loss, anorexia, dizziness, headache, drowsiness, insomnia, anxiety, fatigue,
increase in seizure frequency, impaired coordination, hyperactivity, tremor, gait disturbances;
influenza-like symptoms; oligomenorrhoea; back

pain; nystagmus, diplopia, blurred vision; rash,
and acne; hypersensitivity syndrome (possibly
including rash, fever, lymphadenopathy, hepatic
dysfunction, haematuria, and multi-organ dysfunction) also reported

Hypersensitivity syndrome Serious hypersensitivity
syndrome (see above) has developed especially in children and upon initiation of therapy; consider withdrawal if
rash or signs or symptoms of hypersensitivity syndrome
develop

Counselling Warn children and their carers to seek
immediate medical attention if signs or symptoms of
hypersensitivity syndrome develop

Indication and dose

**Adjunctive treatment of seizures in Lennox-
Gastaut syndrome**
• **By mouth**

Child 4–18 years body-weight less than 30 kg,
initially 100 mg twice daily increased according
to response in steps of 100 mg twice daily up to
every 2 days; max. 500 mg twice daily (max.
300 mg twice daily if adjunctive therapy *with
valproate*)

◁ **RUFINAMIDE** *(continued)*

Child 4–18 years body-weight over 30 kg, initially 200 mg twice daily increased according to response in steps of 200 mg twice daily up to every 2 days; body-weight 30–50 kg max. 900 mg twice daily; body-weight 50–70 kg max. 1.2 g twice daily; body-weight over 70 kg max. 1.6 g twice daily

Administration Tablets may be crushed and given in half a glass of water

Inovelon® (Eisai) ▼ PoM
Tablets, pink, f/c, scored, rufinamide 100 mg, net price 10-tab pack = £8.58; 200 mg, 60-tab pack = £51.48; 400 mg, 60-tab pack = £85.80. Label: 21, counselling, driving (see notes above), hypersensitivity syndrome (see above)

Stiripentol

Stiripentol is licensed for use in combination with clobazam and valproate as adjunctive therapy of refractory generalised tonic-clonic seizures in children with severe myoclonic epilepsy in infancy (Dravet Syndrome). It should be used under specialist supervision.

STIRIPENTOL

Cautions perform full blood count and liver function tests prior to initiating treatment and every 6 months thereafter; monitor growth; **interactions:** Appendix 1 (stiripentol)

Contra-indications history of psychosis

Hepatic impairment avoid—no information available

Renal impairment avoid—no information available

Pregnancy manufacturer advises use only if potential benefit outweighs risk; see also Pregnancy and Breast-feeding, p. 273

Breast-feeding present in milk in *animal* studies; see also Pregnancy and Breast-feeding, p. 273

Side-effects nausea, vomiting; aggression, anorexia, ataxia, drowsiness, dystonia, hyperexcitability, hyperkinesia, hypotonia, irritability, sleep disorders, weight loss; neutropenia; *less commonly* fatigue, photosensitivity, rash, and urticaria

Indication and dose

Severe myoclonic epilepsy in infancy
● By mouth

Child 3–18 years initially 10 mg/kg in 2–3 divided doses; titrate dose over minimum of 3 days to max. 50 mg/kg/day in 2–3 divided doses

Diacomit® (Alan Pharmaceuticals) PoM
Capsules, stiripentol 250 mg (pink), net price 60-cap pack = £284.00; 500 mg (white), 60-cap pack = £493.00. Label: 1, 8, 21, counselling, administration

Powder, stiripentol 250 mg, net price 60-sachet pack = £284.00; 500 mg, 60-sachet pack = £493.00. Label: 1, 8, 13, 21, counselling, administration
Excipients include aspartame (section 9.4.1)

Counselling Do not take with milk, diary products, carbonated drinks, fruit juice, or with food or drink that contains caffeine

---

Tiagabine

Tiagabine is used as adjunctive treatment for partial seizures, with or without secondary generalisation.

TIAGABINE

Cautions avoid in acute porphyria (section 9.8.2); avoid abrupt withdrawal; **interactions:** Appendix 1 (tiagabine)
Driving May impair performance of skilled tasks (e.g. driving)

Hepatic impairment initial maintenance dose 5–10 mg 1–2 times daily in mild to moderate impairment; avoid in severe impairment

Pregnancy no evidence of teratogenicity in *animal* studies, but manufacturer advises use only if potential benefit outweighs risk; see also Pregnancy and Breast-feeding, p. 273

Breast-feeding manufacturer advises use only if potential benefit outweighs risk; see also Pregnancy and Breast-feeding, p. 273

Side-effects diarrhoea; dizziness, tiredness, nervousness, tremor, impaired concentration, emotional lability, speech impairment; *rarely* confusion, depression, drowsiness, psychosis, nonconvulsive status epilepticus, bruising, and visual disturbances; suicidal ideation; leucopenia also reported

Indication and dose

Adjunctive treatment *with enzyme-inducing drugs* for partial seizures with or without secondary generalisation not satisfactorily controlled by other antiepileptics
● By mouth

Child 12–18 years initially 5 mg twice daily for 1 week then increased at weekly intervals in steps of 5–10 mg daily; usual maintenance dose 30–45 mg daily in 2–3 divided doses (doses above 30 mg daily given in 3 divided doses)

◁ **TIAGABINE** (*continued*)

Adjunctive treatment *with non-enzyme-inducing drugs* for partial seizures with or without secondary generalisation not satisfactorily controlled by other antiepileptics

• By mouth

Child 12–18 years initially 5 mg twice daily for 1 week then increased at weekly intervals in steps of 5–10 mg daily; initial maintenance dose 15–

30 mg daily in 2–3 divided doses (doses above 30 mg daily given in 3 divided doses)

Gabitril® (Cephalon) PoM
Tablets, f/c, tiagabine (as hydrochloride) 5 mg, net price 100-tab pack = £41.68; 10 mg, 100-tab pack = £83.36; 15 mg, 100-tab pack = £125.04. Label: 21

Topiramate

Topiramate can be given alone or as adjunctive treatment in generalised tonic-clonic seizures or partial seizures with or without secondary generalisation. It can also be used as adjunctive treatment for seizures associated with Lennox-Gastaut syndrome. Topiramate is also licensed for prophylaxis of migraine (section 4.7.4.2).

TOPIRAMATE

Cautions avoid abrupt withdrawal; ensure adequate hydration (especially if predisposition to nephrolithiasis or in strenuous activity or warm environment); avoid in acute porphyria (section 9.8.2); **interactions:** see p. 271 and Appendix 1 (topiramate)

Important Topiramate has been associated with acute myopia with secondary angle-closure glaucoma, typically occurring within 1 month of starting treatment. Choroidal effusions resulting in anterior displacement of the lens and iris have also been reported. If raised intra-ocular pressure occurs:

• seek specialist ophthalmological advice;

• use appropriate measures to reduce intra-ocular pressure;

• stop topiramate as rapidly as feasible

Hepatic impairment use with caution—clearance may be reduced

Renal impairment longer time to steady-state plasma concentration

Pregnancy manufacturer advises avoid unless potential benefit outweighs risk—toxicity in *animal* studies; see also Pregnancy and Breast-feeding, p. 273

Breast-feeding manufacturer advises avoid—present in milk; see also Pregnancy and Breast-feeding, p. 273

Side-effects nausea, abdominal pain, dyspepsia, diarrhoea, dry mouth, taste disturbances, weight loss, anorexia; paraesthesia, hypoaesthesia, headache, fatigue, dizziness, speech disorder, drowsiness, insomnia, impaired memory and concentration, anxiety, depression; visual disturbances; *less commonly* suicidal ideation; *rarely* reduced sweating, metabolic acidosis, and alopecia; *very rarely* leucopenia, thrombocytopenia, and serious skin reactions

Indication and dose

Monotherapy of generalised tonic-clonic seizures or partial seizures with or without secondary generalisation

• By mouth

Child 6–16 years initially 0.5–1 mg/kg at night for 1 week then increased in steps of 250–500 micrograms/kg twice daily at intervals of 1–

2 weeks; usual dose 1.5–3 mg/kg twice daily; max. 7.5 mg/kg twice daily

Child 16–18 years initially 25 mg at night for 1 week then increased in steps of 12.5–25 mg twice daily at intervals of 1–2 weeks; usual dose 50 mg twice daily; max. 200 mg twice daily

Adjunctive treatment of generalised tonic-clonic seizures or partial seizures with or without secondary generalisation, adjunctive treatment of seizures in Lennox-Gastaut syndrome

• By mouth

Child 2–16 years initially 25 mg at night for 1 week then increased in steps of 0.5–1.5 mg/kg twice daily at intervals of 1–2 weeks; usual dose 2.5–4.5 mg/kg twice daily; max. 7.5 mg/kg twice daily

Child 16–18 years initially 25 mg at night for 1 week then increased in steps of 12.5–25 mg twice daily at intervals of 1–2 weeks; usual dose 100–200 mg twice daily; max. 400 mg twice daily

Migraine prophylaxis

• By mouth

Child 16–18 years initially 25 mg daily at night for 1 week then increased in steps of 25 mg daily at intervals of 1 week; usual dose 50–100 mg daily in 2 divided doses

Note If child cannot tolerate titration regimens recommended above then smaller steps or longer interval between steps may be used

Topamax® (Janssen-Cilag) ▼ PoM
Tablets, f/c, topiramate 25 mg, net price 60-tab pack = £19.68; 50 mg (light yellow), 60-tab pack = £32.33; 100 mg (yellow), 60-tab pack = £57.91; 200 mg (salmon), 60-tab pack = £112.46. Label: 3, 8, counselling, driving (see notes above)

Sprinkle capsules, topiramate 15 mg, net price 60-cap pack = £15.09; 25 mg, 60-cap pack = £22.63; 50 mg, 60-cap pack = £37.18. Label: 3, 8, counselling, administration, driving (see notes above)

Counselling Swallow whole or open capsule and sprinkle contents on soft food

4

Central nervous system

Central nervous system

4

Valproate

Valproate (as either sodium valproate or valproic acid) is effective in controlling tonic-clonic seizures, particularly in primary generalised epilepsy. It is a drug of choice in primary generalised epilepsy, generalised absences and myoclonic seizures, and can be tried in atypical absence, atonic, and tonic seizures. Valproate should generally be avoided in children under 2 years especially if they are on other antiepileptics, but may be required in infants with continuing epileptic tendency. Sodium valproate has widespread metabolic effects, and may have dose-related side-effects.

Valproic acid (as semisodium valproate) is licensed in adults for acute mania associated with bipolar disorder.

SODIUM VALPROATE

Cautions see notes above; monitor liver function before therapy and during first 6 months especially in children most at risk (see also below); measure full blood count and ensure no undue potential for bleeding before starting and before surgery; systemic lupus erythematosus; false-positive urine tests for ketones; avoid sudden withdrawal; consider vitamin D supplementation in patients that are immobilised for long periods or who have inadequate sun exposure or dietary intake of calcium; **interactions:** see p. 271 and Appendix 1 (valproate)

Liver toxicity Liver dysfunction (including fatal hepatic failure) has occurred in association with valproate (especially in children under 3 years and in those with metabolic or degenerative disorders, organic brain disease or severe seizure disorders associated with mental retardation) usually in first 6 months and usually involving multiple antiepileptic therapy. Raised liver enzymes during valproate treatment are usually transient but children should be reassessed clinically and liver function (including prothrombin time) monitored until return to normal—discontinue if abnormally prolonged prothrombin time (particularly in association with other relevant abnormalities)

Blood or hepatic disorders Children and their carers should be told how to recognise signs of blood or liver disorders and advised to seek immediate medical attention if symptoms develop

Pancreatitis Children and their carers should be told how to recognise signs and symptoms of pancreatitis and advised to seek immediate medical attention if symptoms such as abdominal pain, nausea, or vomiting develop; discontinue if pancreatitis is diagnosed

Contra-indications family history of severe hepatic dysfunction; acute porphyria (section 9.8.2)

Hepatic impairment avoid if possible—hepatotoxicity and hepatic failure may occasionally occur (usually in first 6 months); avoid in active liver disease; see also under Cautions

Renal impairment reduce dose; adjust dosage according to free serum valproic acid concentration

Pregnancy increased risk of congenital malformations and developmental delay (counselling and screening advised—**important**: see also Pregnancy and Breast-feeding, p. 273); neonatal bleeding (related to hypofibrinaemia) and neonatal hepatotoxicity also reported

Breast-feeding amount too small to be harmful; see also Pregnancy and Breast-feeding, p. 273

Side-effects nausea, gastric irritation, diarrhoea; weight gain; hyperammonaemia, thrombocytopenia; transient hair loss (regrowth may be curly); *less frequently* increased alertness, aggression, hyperactivity, behavioural disturbances, ataxia, tremor, and vasculitis; *rarely* hepatic dysfunction (see under Cautions; withdraw treatment immediately if persistent vomiting and abdominal pain, anorexia, jaundice, oedema, malaise, drowsiness, or loss of seizure control), lethargy, drowsiness, confusion, stupor, hallucinations, menstrual disturbances, anaemia, leucopenia, pancytopenia, hearing loss, and rash; *very rarely* pancreatitis (see under Cautions), peripheral oedema, increase in bleeding time, extrapyramidal symptoms, encephalopathy, coma, gynaecomastia, Fanconi's syndrome, hirsutism, enuresis, hyponatraemia, acne, toxic epidermal necrolysis, and Stevens-Johnson syndrome; suicidal ideation; reduced bone mineral density (see Cautions)

Indication and dose

All forms of epilepsy

• By mouth or by rectum

Neonate initially 20 mg/kg once daily; usual maintenance dose 10 mg/kg twice daily

Child 1 month–12 years initially 5–7.5 mg/kg twice daily; usual maintenance dose 12.5–15 mg/kg twice daily (up to 30 mg/kg twice daily in infantile spasms; monitor clinical chemistry and haematological parameters if dose exceeds 20 mg/kg twice daily)

Child 12–18 years initially 300 mg twice daily increased in steps of 200 mg daily at 3-day intervals; usual maintenance dose 0.5–1 g twice daily; max. 1.25 g twice daily

• By intravenous injection over 3–5 minutes

Neonate 10 mg/kg twice daily

Child 1 month–18 years 10 mg/kg twice daily **Note** If switching from oral therapy to intravenous therapy, the intravenous dose should be the same as the established oral dose

• By continuous intravenous infusion

Child 1 month–12 years initially 10 mg/kg *by intravenous injection* then *by continuous intravenous infusion* 20–40 mg/kg daily

Child 12–18 years initially 10 mg/kg *by intravenous injection* then up to max. 2.5 g daily *by continuous intravenous infusion* **Note** If switching from oral therapy to intravenous therapy, the intravenous dose should be the same as the established oral dose

Administration for *rectal administration*, sodium valproate oral solution may be given rectally and

◁ **SODIUM VALPROATE** (*continued*)

retained for 15 minutes (may require dilution with water to prevent rapid expulsion).

For *intravenous injection*, may be diluted in Glucose 5% *or* Sodium Chloride 0.9%.

For *continuous intravenous infusion*, dilute injection solution with Glucose 5% *or* Sodium Chloride 0.9%

◢**Oral**

Sodium Valproate (Non-proprietary) ᴾᵒᴹ

Tablets (crushable), scored, sodium valproate 100 mg, net price 100 = £5.60. Label: 8, counselling, pancreatitis, blood or hepatic disorder symptoms (see above), driving (see notes above)

Tablets, e/c, sodium valproate 200 mg, net price 100-tab pack = £5.35; 500 mg, 100-tab pack = £11.31. Label: 5, 8, 25, counselling, pancreatitis, blood, or hepatic disorder symptoms (see above), driving (see notes above)
Brands include *Orlept*®

Oral solution, sodium valproate 200 mg/5 mL, net price 300 mL = £6.13. Label: 8, counselling, pancreatitis, blood, or hepatic disorder symptoms (see above), driving (see notes above)
Brands include *Orlept*® (sugar-free)

Epilim® (Sanofi-Aventis) ᴾᵒᴹ

Tablets (crushable), scored, sodium valproate 100 mg, net price 100 = £5.60. Label: 8, counselling, pancreatitis, blood or hepatic disorder symptoms (see above), driving (see notes above)

Tablets, both e/c, lilac, sodium valproate 200 mg, net price 100 = £7.70; 500 mg, 100 = £19.25. Label: 5, 8, 25, counselling, pancreatitis, blood or hepatic disorder symptoms (see above), driving (see notes above)

Liquid, red, sugar-free, sodium valproate 200 mg/5 mL, net price 300-mL pack = £9.33. Label: 8, counselling, pancreatitis, blood or hepatic disorder symptoms (see above), driving (see notes above)

Syrup, red, sodium valproate 200 mg/5 mL, net price 300-mL pack = £7.78. Label: 8, counselling, pancreatitis, blood or hepatic disorder symptoms (see above), driving (see notes above)

◢**Modified release**

Epilim Chrono® (Sanofi-Aventis) ᴾᵒᴹ

Tablets, m/r, lilac, sodium valproate 200 mg (as sodium valproate and valproic acid), net price 100-tab pack = £11.65; 300 mg, 100-tab pack = £17.47; 500 mg, 100-tab pack = £29.10. Label: 8, 25, counselling, pancreatitis, blood or hepatic disorder symptoms (see above), driving (see notes above)

Dose

> **Child body-weight over 20 kg** as above, total daily dose given in 1–2 divided doses

Epilim Chronosphere® (Sanofi-Aventis) ᴾᵒᴹ

Granules, m/r, sodium valproate 50 mg (as sodium valproate and valproic acid), net price 30-sachet

pack = £30.00; 100 mg, 30-sachet pack = £30.00; 250 mg, 30-sachet pack = £30.00; 500 mg, 30-sachet pack = £30.00; 750 mg, 30-sachet pack = £30.00; 1000 mg, 30-sachet pack = £30.00. Label: 8, 25, counselling, administration, pancreatitis, blood or hepatic disorder symptoms (see above), driving (see notes above)

Dose

> **Child** as above, total daily dose given in 1–2 divided doses

Counselling Granules may be mixed with cold food or drink and swallowed immediately without chewing

Episenta® (Beacon) ᴾᵒᴹ

Capsules, enclosing m/r granules, sodium valproate 150 mg, net price 100-cap pack = £5.70; 300 mg, 100-cap pack = £10.90. Label: 8, 25, counselling, administration, pancreatitis, blood or hepatic disorder symptoms (see above), driving (see notes above)

Dose

> **Child** as above, total daily dose given in 1–2 divided doses

Counselling Contents of capsule may be mixed with cold food or drink and swallowed immediately without chewing

Granules, m/r, sodium valproate 500 mg, net price 100-sachet pack = £18.00; 1 g, 100-sachet pack = £35.50. Label: 8, 25, counselling, administration, pancreatitis, blood or hepatic disorder symptoms (see above), driving (see notes above)

Dose

> **Child** as above, total daily dose given in 1–2 divided doses

Counselling Granules may be mixed with cold food or drink and swallowed immediately without chewing

◢**Parenteral**

Epilim® **Intravenous** (Sanofi-Aventis) ᴾᵒᴹ

Injection, powder for reconstitution, sodium valproate, net price 400-mg vial (with 4-mL amp water for injections) = £11.58

Episenta® (Beacon) ᴾᵒᴹ

Injection, sodium valproate 100 mg/mL, net price 3-mL amp = £7.00, 10-mL amp = £23.33

◢**Valproic acid**

Convulex® (Pharmacia) ᴾᵒᴹ

Capsules, e/c, valproic acid 150 mg, net price 100-cap pack = £3.68; 300 mg, 100-cap pack = £7.35; 500 mg, 100-cap pack = £12.25. Label: 8, 25, counselling, pancreatitis, blood or hepatic disorder symptoms (see above), driving (see notes above)

Dose

> **Child** as for sodium valproate, total daily dose given in 2–4 divided doses

Equivalence to sodium valproate Manufacturer advises that *Convulex*® has a 1:1 dose relationship with products containing sodium valproate, but nevertheless care is needed in making changes

4
Central nervous system

Vigabatrin

For partial epilepsy with or without secondary generalisation, **vigabatrin** is given in combination with other antiepileptic treatment; its use is restricted to children in whom all other combinations are inadequate or are not tolerated. It can be used as sole therapy in the management of infantile spasms.

About one-third of those treated with vigabatrin have suffered visual field defects; counselling and **careful monitoring** for this side-effect are required (see also Visual Field Defects under Cautions below). Vigabatrin has prominent behavioural side-effects in some children.

VIGABATRIN

Cautions closely monitor neurological function; avoid sudden withdrawal (taper off over 2–4 weeks); history of psychosis, depression or behavioural problems; absence seizures (may be exacerbated); **interactions:** see p. 271 and Appendix 1 (vigabatrin)

Visual field defects Vigabatrin is associated with visual field defects. The CSM has advised that onset of symptoms varies from 1 month to several years after starting. In most cases, visual field defects have persisted despite discontinuation, and further deterioration after discontinuation cannot be excluded. Product literature advises visual field testing before treatment and at 6-month intervals. Children and their carers should be warned to report any new visual symptoms that develop and those with symptoms should be referred for an urgent ophthalmological opinion. Gradual withdrawal of vigabatrin should be considered.

Contra-indications visual field defects

Renal impairment consider reduced dose or increased dose interval if estimated glomerular filtration rate less than 60 mL/minute/1.73 m²

Pregnancy congenital anomalies reported—manufacturer advises avoid unless potential benefit outweighs risk; see also Pregnancy and Breast-feeding, p. 273

Breast-feeding present in milk—manufacturer advises avoid; see also Pregnancy and Breast-feeding, p. 273

Side-effects nausea, abdominal pain; oedema; drowsiness (*rarely* encephalopathic symptoms including marked sedation, stupor, and confusion with non-specific slow wave EEG—reduce dose or withdraw), fatigue, excitation, agitation, dizziness, headache, nervousness, depression, aggression, paranoia, impaired concentration, impaired memory, tremor, paraesthesia, speech disorder, weight gain; visual field defects (see also under Cautions), blurred vision, nystagmus, diplopia; *less commonly* ataxia, psychosis, mania, and rash; occasional increase in seizure frequency (especially if myoclonic); *rarely* suicidal ideation and retinal disorders (including peripheral retinal neuropathy); *very rarely* hepatitis, optic neuritis and optic atrophy; *also reported* movement disorders in infantile spasms

Indication and dose

Adjunctive treatment of partial seizures with or without secondary generalisation not satisfactorily controlled with other antiepileptics
• By mouth

Neonate initially 15–20 mg/kg twice daily increased over 2–3 weeks to usual maintenance

dose 30–40 mg/kg twice daily; max. 75 mg/kg twice daily

Child 1 month–2 years initially 15–20 mg/kg twice daily increased over 2–3 weeks to usual maintenance dose 30–40 mg/kg twice daily; max. 75 mg/kg twice daily

Child 2–12 years initially 15–20 mg/kg (max. 250 mg) twice daily increased over 2–3 weeks to usual maintenance dose 30–40 mg/kg (max. 1.5 g) twice daily

Child 12–18 years initially 250 mg twice daily increased over 2–3 weeks to usual maintenance dose 1–1.5 g twice daily
Administration Tablets may be crushed and dispersed in liquid

• By rectum

Child 1 month–18 years dose as for oral therapy, see above
Administration dissolve contents of sachet in small amount of water and administer rectally

Infantile spasms as monotherapy
• By mouth

Neonate initially 15–25 mg/kg twice daily adjusted according to response over 7 days to usual maintenance dose 40–50 mg/kg twice daily; max. 75 mg/kg twice daily

Child 1 month–2 years initially 15–25 mg/kg twice daily adjusted according to response over 7 days to usual maintenance dose 40–50 mg/kg twice daily; max. 75 mg/kg twice daily

Sabril® (Sanofi-Aventis) [PoM]
Tablets, f/c, scored, vigabatrin 500 mg, net price 100-tab pack = £30.84. Label: 3, 8, counselling, driving (see notes above)

Powder, sugar-free, vigabatrin 500 mg/sachet. Net price 50-sachet pack = £17.08. Label: 3, 8, 13, counselling, driving (see notes above)

Note The contents of a sachet should be dissolved in water or a soft drink immediately before taking

Benzodiazepines

Clonazepam is occasionally used in tonic-clonic or partial seizures, but its sedative side-effects may be prominent. **Clobazam** may be used as adjunctive therapy in the treatment of epilepsy, but the effectiveness of these and other **benzodiazepines** may wane considerably after weeks or months of continuous therapy.

Hepatic impairment Benzodiazepines can precipitate coma if used in hepatic impairment. Start with smaller initial doses or reduce dose; avoid in severe impairment.

Renal impairment Children with renal impairment have increased cerebral sensitivity to benzodiazepines; start with small doses in severe impairment.

Pregnancy There is a risk of neonatal withdrawal symptoms when benzodiazepines are used during pregnancy. Avoid regular use and use only if there is a clear indication such as seizure control. High doses administered during late pregnancy or labour may cause neonatal hypothermia, hypotonia, and respiratory depression.

Breast-feeding Benzodiazepines are present in milk, and should be avoided if possible during breast-feeding.

CLOBAZAM

Cautions see Diazepam, section 4.8.2

Contra-indications see Diazepam, section 4.8.2

Hepatic impairment see notes above

Renal impairment see notes above

Pregnancy see notes above

Breast-feeding see notes above

Side-effects see Diazepam, section 4.8.2

Licensed use not licensed for use in children under 3 years

Indication and dose

Adjunctive therapy for epilepsy, monotherapy under specialist supervision for catamenial (menstruation) seizures (usually for 7–10 days each month, just before and during menstruation), cluster seizures

* By mouth

  Child 1 month–12 years initially 125 micrograms/kg twice daily increased every 5 days to usual maintenance dose of 250 micrograms/kg twice daily; max. 500 micrograms/kg twice daily, not exceeding 15 mg twice daily

  Child 12–18 years initially 10 mg twice daily increased every 5 days to usual maintenance dose of 10–15 mg twice daily; max. 30 mg twice daily

¹**Clobazam** (Non-proprietary) PoM JHS
Tablets, clobazam 10 mg. Net price 30-tab pack = £4.68. Label: 2 or 19, 8, counselling, driving (see notes above)
Brands include *Frisium®* JHS

Tablets, clobazam 5 mg available on a named patient basis
1. JHS except for epilepsy and endorsed 'SLS'

◢Extemporaneous formulations available see Extemporaneous Preparations, p. 8

CLONAZEPAM

Cautions see notes above; respiratory disease; spinal or cerebellar ataxia; myasthenia gravis (avoid if unstable); history of alcohol or drug abuse, depression or suicidal ideation; debilitated; avoid sudden withdrawal; acute porphyria (section 9.8.2); **interactions:** see p. 271 and Appendix 1 (anxiolytics and hypnotics)
Driving Drowsiness may affect performance of skilled tasks (e.g. driving); effects of alcohol enhanced

Contra-indications respiratory depression; acute pulmonary insufficiency; sleep apnoea syndrome

Hepatic impairment see notes above

Renal impairment see notes above

Pregnancy see notes above

Breast-feeding see notes above

Side-effects drowsiness, fatigue, dizziness, muscle hypotonia, coordination disturbances; also poor concentration, restlessness, confusion, amnesia, dependence, and withdrawal; salivary or bronchial hypersecretion in infants and small children; *rarely* gastro-intestinal symptoms, respiratory depression, headache, paradoxical effects including aggression and anxiety, sexual dysfunction, urinary incontinence, urticaria, pruritus, reversible hair loss, skin pigmentation changes; dysarthria, and visual disturbances on long-term treatment; blood disorders reported; **overdo-** sage: see Emergency Treatment of Poisoning, p. 41

Indication and dose

All forms of epilepsy

* By mouth

  Child 1 month–1 year initially 250 micrograms at night for 4 nights, increased over 2–4 weeks to usual maintenance dose of 0.5–1 mg at night (may be given in 3 divided doses if necessary)

  Child 1–5 years initially 250 micrograms at night for 4 nights, increased over 2–4 weeks to usual maintenance of 1–3 mg at night (may be given in 3 divided doses if necessary)

  Child 5–12 years initially 500 micrograms at night for 4 nights, increased over 2–4 weeks to usual maintenance dose of 3–6 mg at night (may be given in 3 divided doses if necessary)

  Child 12–18 years initially 1 mg at night for 4 nights, increased over 2–4 weeks to usual maintenance dose of 4–8 mg at night (may be given in 3–4 divided doses if necessary)

Note Clonazepam doses in BNFC may differ from those in product literature

Administration for administration *by mouth*, injection solution may be given orally

4 Central nervous system

◻ **CLONAZEPAM** (*continued*)

Rivotril® (Roche) PoM
Tablets, both scored, clonazepam 500 micrograms (beige), net price 100 = £3.77; 2 mg (white), 100 = £5.03. Label: 2, 8, counselling, driving (see notes above)

Injection, section 4.8.2

Liquid, clonazepam 0.5 mg/5 mL; 2 mg/5 mL; 2.5 mg/mL
Available from 'special-order' manufacturers or specialist importing companies, see p. 957

◢ Extemporaneous formulations available see Extemporaneous Preparations, p. 8

◢ **NITRAZEPAM**

Cautions avoid abrupt withdrawal; respiratory disease; acute porphyria (section 9.8.2); muscle weakness and myasthenia gravis; **interactions**: Appendix 1 (anxiolytics and hypnotics)

Contra-indications respiratory depression, acute pulmonary insufficiency, sleep apnoea syndrome; marked neuromuscular respiratory weakness including myasthenia gravis

Hepatic impairment see notes above

Renal impairment see notes above

Side-effects drowsiness, confusion, ataxia; see also under Diazepam (section 4.8.2); **overdosage**: see Emergency Treatment of Poisoning, p. 41

Licensed use not licensed for use in children

Indication and dose

Infantile spasms
• By mouth

  Child 1 month–2 years initially 125 micrograms/kg twice daily, adjusted according to response over 2–3 weeks to 250 micrograms/kg twice daily; max. 500 micrograms/kg (not exceeding 5 mg) twice daily; total daily dose may alternatively be given in 3 divided doses

Nitrazepam (Non-proprietary) PoM
Oral suspension, nitrazepam 2.5 mg/5 mL, net price 150 mL = £5.09. Label: 1, 8
Brands include *Somnite®* NHS

Other drugs

Acetazolamide (section 11.6), a carbonic anhydrase inhibitor, has a specific role in treating epilepsy associated with menstruation. It can also be used in conjunction with other antiepileptics for tonic-clonic or partial seizures.

Piracetam is used as adjunctive treatment for cortical myoclonus.

4.8.2 Drugs used in status epilepticus

Immediate measures to manage status epilepticus include positioning the child to avoid injury, supporting respiration including the provision of oxygen, maintaining blood pressure, and the correction of any hypoglycaemia. **Pyridoxine** (section 9.6.2) should be administered if the status epilepticus is caused by pyridoxine deficiency.

Convulsive status epilepticus should be treated urgently with intravenous **lorazepam**. Intravenous **diazepam** is effective but it is associated with a high risk of venous thrombophlebitis (reduced by using an emulsion formulation of diazepam injection). **Clonazepam** can also be used as an alternative.

Where facilities for resuscitation are not immediately available, **midazolam** can be given into the buccal cavity, or **diazepam** can be administered as a rectal solution; the buccal route may be more acceptable in children.

> **Important**
> If seizures recur or fail to respond 20 minutes after onset, phenytoin sodium, fosphenytoin, or phenobarbital sodium should be used; contact paediatric intensive care unit if seizures continue at 30 minutes after onset.
>
> If these measures fail to control seizures 40 minutes after onset, anaesthesia with thiopental (section 15.1.1) or midazolam (section 15.1.4) should be instituted with full intensive care support. Lidocaine infusion has also been used but requires specialist management.

Phenytoin sodium may be given by slow intravenous injection, with ECG monitoring, followed by the maintenance dosage if appropriate. Intramuscular use of phenytoin is not recommended (absorption is slow and erratic).

Alternatively, **fosphenytoin**, a pro-drug of phenytoin, can be given more rapidly and when given intravenously causes fewer injection-site reactions than phenytoin. Intravenous administration requires ECG monitoring. Although it can also be given intramuscularly, absorption is too slow by this route for treatment of status epilepticus. Doses of fosphenytoin should be expressed in terms of phenytoin sodium.

Paraldehyde given rectally causes little respiratory depression and is therefore useful where facilities for resuscitation are poor.

For **neonatal seizures**, see p. 274.

Non-convulsive status epilepticus   The urgency to treat non-convulsive status epilepticus depends upon the severity of the child's condition. If there is incomplete loss of awareness, oral antiepileptic therapy should be restarted or continued. Children who fail to respond to oral antiepileptic therapy or have complete lack of awareness can be treated in the same way as convulsive status epilepticus although anaesthesia is rarely needed.

CLONAZEPAM

Cautions see Clonazepam, section 4.8.1; facilities for reversing respiratory depression with mechanical ventilation must be at hand (but see also notes above)

Intravenous infusion Intravenous infusion of clonazepam is potentially hazardous (especially if prolonged), calling for close and constant observation and best carried out in specialist centres with intensive care facilities. Prolonged infusion may lead to accumulation and delay recovery

Contra-indications see Clonazepam, section 4.8.1; avoid injections containing benzyl alcohol in neonates (see under preparations below)

Hepatic impairment see Benzodiazepines, section 4.8.1

Renal impairment see Benzodiazepines, section 4.8.1

Pregnancy see Benzodiazepines, section 4.8.1

Breast-feeding see Benzodiazepines, section 4.8.1

Side-effects see Clonazepam, section 4.8.1; hypotension and apnoea

Indication and dose

Status epilepticus

- By intravenous injection over at least 2 minutes

  Neonate 100 micrograms/kg repeated after 24 hours if necessary (avoid unless there is no safer alternative)

  Child 1 month–12 years 50 micrograms/kg (max. 1 mg) repeated if necessary

  Child 12–18 years 1 mg repeated if necessary

- By intravenous infusion

  Child 1 month–12 years initially 50 micrograms/kg (max. 1 mg) *by intravenous injection* then *by intravenous infusion* 10 micrograms/kg/ hour adjusted according to response; max. 60 micrograms/kg/hour

  Child 12–18 years initially 1 mg *by intravenous injection* then *by intravenous infusion* 10 micrograms/kg/hour adjusted according to response; max. 60 micrograms/kg/hour

Other forms of epilepsy section 4.8.1

Administration for *intravenous injection*, dilute to a concentration of 500 micrograms/mL with Water for Injections

For *intravenous infusion*, dilute to a concentration of 12 micrograms/mL with Glucose 5% *or* Sodium Chloride 0.9%; incompatible with bicarbonate; adsorbed on PVC—glass infusion apparatus preferred (if PVC apparatus used, complete infusion within 2 hours)

Rivotril® (Roche) [PoM]
Injection, clonazepam 1 mg/mL in solvent, net price 1-mL amp (with 1 mL water for injections) = 61p
Excipients include benzyl alcohol (avoid in neonates unless there is no safer alternative available, see Excipients, p. 3), ethanol, propylene glycol

◢Oral preparations
Section 4.8.1

DIAZEPAM

Cautions respiratory disease, muscle weakness and myasthenia gravis, history of drug or alcohol abuse, marked personality disorder; avoid prolonged use (and abrupt withdrawal thereafter); when given parenterally, close observation required until full recovery from sedation; when given intravenously, facilities for reversing respiratory depression with mechanical ventilation must be at hand (but see also notes above); porphyria (section 9.8.2); **interactions:** Appendix 1 (anxiolytics and hypnotics)

Skilled tasks Drowsiness may affect performance of skilled tasks (e.g. driving); effects of alcohol enhanced

Contra-indications respiratory depression; marked neuromuscular respiratory weakness including unstable myasthenia gravis; acute pulmonary insufficiency; sleep apnoea syndrome; not for chronic psychosis; should not

be used alone in depression or in anxiety with depression; avoid injections containing benzyl alcohol in neonates (see under preparations below)

Hepatic impairment see Benzodiazepines, section 4.8.1

Renal impairment see Benzodiazepines, section 4.8.1

Pregnancy see Benzodiazepines, section 4.8.1

Breast-feeding see Benzodiazepines, section 4.8.1

Side-effects drowsiness and lightheadedness the next day; confusion and ataxia; amnesia; dependence; paradoxical increase in aggression (see also section 4.1); muscle weakness; *occasionally:* headache, vertigo, hypotension, salivation changes, gastro-intestinal disturbances, visual

4

Central nervous system

◁ **DIAZEPAM** (continued)

disturbances, dysarthria, tremor, changes in libido, incontinence, urinary retention; blood disorders and jaundice reported; skin reactions; on intravenous injection, pain, thrombophlebitis, and rarely apnoea; **overdosage**: see Emergency Treatment of Poisoning, p. 41

Licensed use Diazepam Rectubes® and Stesolid Rectal Tubes® not licensed for use in children under 1 year

Indication and dose

> Status epilepticus, febrile convulsions (section 4.8.3), convulsions caused by poisoning
> • By intravenous injection over 3–5 minutes
>
> **Neonate** 300–400 micrograms/kg repeated once after 10 minutes if necessary
>
> **Child 1 month–12 years** 300–400 micrograms/kg repeated once after 10 minutes if necessary
>
> **Child 12–18 years** 10–20 mg repeated once after 10 minutes if necessary
>
> • By rectum (as rectal solution)
>
> **Neonate** 1.25–2.5 mg repeated once after 10 minutes if necessary
>
> **Child 1 month–2 years** 5 mg repeated once after 10 minutes if necessary

> **Child 2–12 years** 5–10 mg repeated once after 10 minutes if necessary
>
> **Child 12–18 years** 10–20 mg repeated once after 10 minutes if necessary

> Muscle spasm section 10.2.2

> Peri-operative use section 15.1.4.1

Diazepam (Non-proprietary) ⓅⓄⓂ
Injection (solution), diazepam 5 mg/mL. Net price 2-mL amp = 45p
Excipients include benzyl alcohol (avoid in neonates, see Excipients, p. 3), ethanol, propylene glycol

Injection (emulsion), diazepam 5 mg/mL (0.5%). Net price 2-mL amp = 92p
Brands include Diazemuls®

Rectal tubes (= rectal solution), diazepam 2 mg/mL, net price 1.25-mL (2.5-mg) tube = 90p, 2.5-mL (5-mg) tube = £1.67; 4 mg/mL, 2.5-mL (10-mg) tube = £1.65
Brands include Diazepam Rectubes®, Stesolid®

◢ **Oral preparations**
Section 15.1.4.1

▰ FOSPHENYTOIN SODIUM

Note Fosphenytoin is a pro-drug of phenytoin

Cautions see Phenytoin Sodium; resuscitation facilities must be available; **interactions**: see p. 271 and Appendix 1 (phenytoin)

Contra-indications see Phenytoin Sodium

Hepatic impairment consider 10–25% reduction in dose or infusion rate (except initial dose for status epilepticus)

Renal impairment consider 10–25% reduction in dose or infusion rate (except initial dose for status epilepticus)

Pregnancy see Phenytoin (section 4.8.1)

Breast-feeding see Phenytoin (section 4.8.1)

Side-effects see Phenytoin Sodium

Important Intravenous infusion of fosphenytoin has been associated with severe cardiovascular reactions including asystole, ventricular fibrillation, and cardiac arrest. Hypotension, bradycardia, and heart block have also been reported. The following are recommended:

- monitor heart rate, blood pressure, and respiratory function for duration of infusion;
- observe patient for at least 30 minutes after infusion;
- if hypotension occurs, reduce infusion rate or discontinue;
- reduce dose or infusion rate in renal or hepatic impairment.

Indication and dose

> Expressed as **phenytoin sodium equivalent** (PE); fosphenytoin sodium 1.5 mg ≡ phenytoin sodium 1 mg

> Status epilepticus
> • By intravenous infusion (at a rate of 2–3 mg(PE)/kg/minute)
>
> **Child 5–18 years** initially 20 mg(PE)/kg, then (at a rate of 1–2 mg(PE)/kg/minute) 4–5 mg(PE)/kg; total daily dose may be given in 1–4 divided doses; adjusted according to response and trough plasma-phenytoin concentration

> Prophylaxis or treatment of seizures associated with neurosurgery or head injury
> • By intravenous infusion (at a rate of 1–2 mg(PE)/kg/minute)
>
> **Child 5–18 years** initially 10–15 mg(PE)/kg then 4–5 mg(PE)/kg daily; total daily dose may be given in 1–4 divided doses; adjusted according to response and trough plasma-phenytoin concentration

> Temporary substitution for oral phenytoin
> • By intravenous infusion (at a rate of 1–2 mg(PE)/kg/minute)
>
> **Child 5–18 years** same dose and dosing frequency as oral phenytoin therapy

Note Fosphenytoin sodium doses in BNFC may differ from those in product literature

Note Prescriptions for fosphenytoin sodium should state the dose in terms of phenytoin sodium equivalent (PE)

Administration for intermittent intravenous infusion, dilute to a concentration of 1.5–25 mg (PE)/mL with Glucose 5% or Sodium Chloride 0.9%

◁ **FOSPHENYTOIN SODIUM** (*continued*)

Pro-Epanutin® (Pfizer) (PoM)
  Injection, fosphenytoin sodium 75 mg/mL
  (equivalent to phenytoin sodium 50 mg/mL), net
  price 10-mL vial = £40.00
  Electrolytes phosphate 3.7 micromol/mg fosphenytoin sodium (phosphate 5.6 micromol/mg phenytoin sodium)

◢ LORAZEPAM

Cautions see Diazepam; facilities for reversing
respiratory depression with mechanical ventilation must be available

Contra-indications see Diazepam

Hepatic impairment see Benzodiazepines, section 4.8.1

Renal impairment see Benzodiazepines, section
4.8.1

Pregnancy see Benzodiazepines, section 4.8.1

Breast-feeding see Benzodiazepines, section
4.8.1

Side-effects see Diazepam; hypotension and
apnoea

Indication and dose

  Status epilepticus
  • By slow intravenous injection

    Neonate 100 micrograms/kg as a single dose,
    repeated once after 10 minutes if necessary

    Child 1 month–12 years 100 micrograms/kg
    (max. 4 mg) as a single dose, repeated once after
    10 minutes if necessary

    Child 12–18 years 4 mg as a single dose,
    repeated once after 10 minutes if necessary

Administration for *intravenous injection*, dilute with
an equal volume of Sodium Chloride 0.9% or
Water for Injections (for neonates, dilute injection
solution to a concentration of 100 micrograms/
mL)

◢**Preparations**
Section 15.1.4.1

◢ MIDAZOLAM

Cautions see Midazolam, section 15.1.4

Contra-indications see Midazolam, section 15.1.4

Hepatic impairment see Midazolam, section
15.1.4

Renal impairment see Midazolam, section 15.1.4

Pregnancy see Midazolam, section 15.1.4

Breast-feeding see Midazolam, section 15.1.4

Side-effects see Midazolam, section 15.1.4

Licensed use injection not licensed for use in
status epilepticus

Indication and dose

  Status epilepticus
  • By buccal administration

    Neonate 300 micrograms/kg, repeated once
    after 10 minutes if necessary

    Child 1–6 months 300 micrograms/kg (max.
    2.5 mg), repeated once after 10 minutes if
    necessary

    Child 6 months–1 year 2.5 mg, repeated once
    after 10 minutes if necessary

    Child 1–5 years 5 mg, repeated once after 10
    minutes if necessary

    Child 5–10 years 7.5 mg, repeated once after 10
    minutes if necessary

    Child 10–18 years 10 mg, repeated once after
    10 minutes if necessary

  • By intravenous administration

    Neonate initially *by intravenous injection* 150–
    200 micrograms/kg followed *by continuous
    intravenous infusion* of 60 micrograms/kg/hour
    (increased by 60 micrograms/kg/hour every 15
    minutes until seizure controlled); max.
    300 micrograms/kg/hour

    Child 1 month–18 years initially *by intravenous
    injection* 150–200 micrograms/kg followed *by
    continuous intravenous infusion* of 60 micro-
    grams/kg/hour (increased by 60 micrograms/
    kg/hour every 15 minutes until seizure con-
    trolled); max. 300 micrograms/kg/hour

Administration for *intravenous injection*, dilute with
Glucose 5% or Sodium Chloride 0.9%; rapid
intravenous injection (less than 2 minutes) may
cause seizure-like myoclonus in preterm neonate
For *buccal administration*, injection solution may
be given buccally or by mouth
Neonatal intensive care, dilute 15 mg/kg body-
weight to a final volume of 50 mL with infusion
fluid; an intravenous infusion rate of 0.1 mL/hour
provides a dose of 30 micrograms/kg/hour

◢**Preparations**
Section 15.1.4

◢ PARALDEHYDE

Cautions bronchopulmonary disease; **interactions:** Appendix 1 (paraldehyde)

Contra-indications gastric disorders; rectal
administration in colitis

Hepatic impairment use with caution

4 Central nervous system

◻ **PARALDEHYDE** (continued)

Pregnancy avoid unless essential—crosses placenta

Breast-feeding avoid unless essential—present in milk

Side-effects rashes; rectal irritation after enema

Licensed use not licensed for use in children as an enema

Indication and dose

Status epilepticus
- By rectum (doses expressed as undiluted paraldehyde)

  Neonate 0.4 mL/kg as a single dose

  Child 1 month–18 years 0.4 mL/kg (max. 10 mL) as a single dose

Administration for *rectal administration*, do not administer paraldehyde undiluted

Paraldehyde (Non-proprietary) [PoM]
Enema, 8–50%, available from 'special-order' manufacturers or specialist importing companies, see p. 957

▍**PHENOBARBITAL SODIUM**

Phenobarbitone sodium

Cautions see Phenobarbital, section 4.8.1

Hepatic impairment see Phenobarbital, section 4.8.1

Renal impairment see Phenobarbital, section 4.8.1

Pregnancy see Pregnancy and Breast-feeding, p. 273

Breast-feeding see Phenobarbital, section 4.8.1

Side-effects see Phenobarbital, section 4.8.1

Indication and dose

Status epilepticus
- By slow intravenous injection (no faster than 1 mg/kg/minute)

  Neonate initially 20 mg/kg then 2.5–5 mg/kg once or twice daily

  Child 1 month–12 years initially 20 mg/kg then 2.5–5 mg/kg once or twice daily

  Child 12–18 years initially 20 mg/kg (max. 1 g) then 300 mg twice daily

Other forms of epilepsy section 4.8.1

Note For therapeutic purposes phenobarbital and phenobarbital sodium may be considered equivalent in effect

Administration for *intravenous injection*, dilute to a concentration of 20 mg/mL with Water for Injections

Phenobarbital (Non-proprietary) [CD]
Injection, phenobarbital sodium 200 mg/mL, net price 1-mL amp = £2.00
Excipients include propylene glycol 90% (see Excipients, p. 3)
Note Must be diluted before intravenous administration (see Administration)

◢**Oral preparations**
Section 4.8.1

▍**PHENYTOIN SODIUM**

Cautions hypotension and heart failure; resuscitation facilities must be available; injection solutions alkaline (irritant to tissues); see also p. 282; interactions: see p. 271 and Appendix 1 (phenytoin)

Contra-indications sinus bradycardia, sino-atrial block, and second- and third-degree heart block; Stokes-Adams syndrome; acute porphyria (section 9.8.2)

Hepatic impairment see Phenytoin, section 4.8.1

Pregnancy see Phenytoin, section 4.8.1

Breast-feeding see Phenytoin, section 4.8.1

Side-effects intravenous injection may cause cardiovascular and CNS depression (particularly if injection too rapid) with arrhythmias, hypotension, and cardiovascular collapse; alterations in respiratory function (including respiratory arrest); injection-site reactions, see also p. 282

Indication and dose

Status epilepticus, acute symptomatic seizures associated with trauma or neurosurgery
- By slow intravenous injection or infusion (with blood-pressure and ECG monitoring)

  Neonate initially 18 mg/kg as a loading dose then 2.5–5 mg/kg twice daily

  Child 1 month–12 years initially 18 mg/kg as a loading dose then 2.5–5 mg/kg twice daily

  Child 12–18 years initially 18 mg/kg as a loading dose then up to 100 mg 3–4 times daily

- By intramuscular injection
  Not recommended (see notes above)

Other forms of epilepsy section 4.8.1

Note Phenytoin sodium doses in BNFC may differ from those in product literature

Administration before and after administration flush intravenous line with Sodium Chloride 0.9%.

For *intravenous injection*, give at rate not exceeding 1 mg/kg/minute (max. 50 mg/minute).

For *intravenous infusion*, dilute to a concentration not exceeding 10 mg/mL with Sodium Chloride 0.9% and give through an in-line filter (0.22–0.50 micron) at a rate not exceeding 1 mg/kg/minute (max. 50 mg/minute); complete administration within 1 hour of preparation

Phenytoin (Non-proprietary) [PoM]
Injection, phenytoin sodium 50 mg/mL with propylene glycol 40% and alcohol 10% in water for injections, net price 5-mL amp = £3.40

◌ **PHENYTOIN SODIUM** (*continued*)

Epanutin® Ready-Mixed Parenteral (Pfizer) (PoM)
Injection, phenytoin sodium 50 mg/mL with propylene glycol 40% and alcohol 10% in water for
injections. Net price 5-mL amp = £4.88

◢ **Oral preparations**
Section 4.8.1

4.8.3 Febrile convulsions

Brief febrile convulsions need no specific treatment; antipyretic medication e.g.
paracetamol (section 4.7.1) is commonly used to reduce fever and prevent
further convulsions but evidence to support this practice is lacking. *Prolonged
febrile convulsions* (those lasting 5 minutes or longer), *recurrent convulsions*, or
those occurring in a child at known risk must be treated more actively, as there is
the possibility of resulting brain damage. **Diazepam** (section 4.8.2) is the drug of
choice given either by slow intravenous injection or preferably rectally in solution,
repeated if necessary. The rectal solution is generally preferred as satisfactory
absorption is achieved within minutes and administration is much easier. Suppositories are not suitable because absorption is too slow.

Intermittent prophylaxis (i.e. the anticonvulsant administered at the onset of
fever) is possible in only a small proportion of children; rectal administration of
diazepam is the treatment of choice.

Long-term anticonvulsant prophylaxis for febrile convulsions is rarely indicated.
Anticonvulsant treatment needs to be considered only for children at risk from
prolonged or complex febrile convulsions, including those whose first seizure
occurred at under 14 months or who have neurological abnormalities or who have
had previous prolonged or focal convulsions.

4.9 Drugs used in dystonias and related disorders

4.9.1 Dopaminergic drugs used in dystonias
4.9.2 Antimuscarinic drugs used in dystonias
4.9.3 Drugs used in essential tremor, chorea, tics, and related disorders

Dystonias may result from conditions such as cerebral palsy or may be related to
a deficiency of the neurotransmitter dopamine as in Segawa syndrome.

4.9.1 Dopaminergic drugs used in dystonias

Levodopa, the amino-acid precursor of dopamine, acts by replenishing depleted
striatal dopamine. It is given with an extracerebral **dopa-decarboxylase inhibitor**
that reduces the peripheral conversion of levodopa to dopamine, thereby limiting
side-effects such as nausea, vomiting and cardiovascular effects; additionally,
effective brain-dopamine concentrations can be achieved with lower doses of
levodopa. The extracerebral dopa-decarboxylase inhibitor most commonly used
in children is carbidopa (in **co-careldopa**).

Levodopa therapy should be initiated at a low dose and increased in small steps;
the final dose should be as low as possible. Intervals between doses should be
chosen to suit the needs of the individual child.

In severe dystonias related to cerebral palsy, improvement can be expected within
2 weeks. Children with Segawa syndrome are particularly sensitive to levodopa;
they may even become symptom free on small doses. Levodopa also has a role in
treating metabolic disorders such as defects in tetrahydrobiopterin synthesis and
dihydrobiopterin reductase deficiency. For the use of tetrahydrobiopterin in
metabolic disorders see section 9.4.1.

Children may experience nausea within 2 hours of taking a dose; nausea and
vomiting with co-careldopa is rarely dose-limiting but domperidone (section 4.6)
may be useful in controlling these effects.

4

Central nervous system

In dystonic cerebral palsy treatment with larger doses of levodopa is associated with the development of potentially troublesome motor complications including response fluctuations and dyskinesias. Response fluctuations are characterised by large variations in motor performance, with normal function during the 'on' period, and weakness and restricted mobility during the 'off' period.

Sudden onset of sleep

Excessive daytime sleepiness and sudden onset of sleep can occur with co-careldopa.

Children starting treatment with these drugs, and their carers, should be warned of the possibility of these effects and of the need to exercise caution when performing skilled tasks e.g. driving or operating machinery.

Children who have suffered excessive sedation or sudden onset of sleep should refrain from performing skilled tasks until those effects have stopped recurring.

CO-CARELDOPA

A mixture of carbidopa and levodopa; the proportions are expressed in the form *x/y* where *x* and *y* are the strengths in milligrams of carbidopa and levodopa respectively

Cautions see also notes above; pulmonary disease, peptic ulceration, cardiovascular disease, diabetes mellitus, osteomalacia, susceptibility to angle-closure glaucoma, history of skin melanoma (risk of activation), psychiatric illness (avoid if severe); warn children and carers about excessive drowsiness (see notes above); in prolonged therapy, psychiatric, hepatic, haematological, renal, and cardiovascular surveillance is advisable; warn patients to resume normal activities gradually; avoid abrupt withdrawal; **interactions:** Appendix 1 (levodopa)

Pregnancy use with caution—toxicity in *animal* studies

Breast-feeding may suppress lactation; present in milk—avoid

Side-effects see also notes above; anorexia, nausea and vomiting, insomnia, agitation, postural hypotension (rarely labile hypertension), dizziness, tachycardia, arrhythmias, reddish discoloration of urine and other body fluids; *rarely* hypersensitivity; *very rarely* angle-closure glaucoma; abnormal involuntary movements and psychiatric symptoms which include hypomania and psychosis may be dose-limiting; depression, drowsiness, headache, flushing, sweating, gastrointestinal bleeding, peripheral neuropathy, taste disturbance, pruritus, rash, and liver enzyme changes also reported; syndrome resembling neuroleptic malignant syndrome reported on withdrawal

Licensed use not licensed for use in children

Indication and dose

Dopamine-sensitive dystonias including Segawa syndrome and dystonias related to cerebral palsy

• By mouth, expressed as levodopa

Child 3 months–18 years initially 250 micrograms/kg 2–3 times daily of a preparation containing 1:4 carbidopa:levodopa, increased according to response every 2–3 days to max. 1 mg/kg three times daily

Treatment of defects in tetrahydrobiopterin synthesis and dihydrobiopterin reductase deficiency

• By mouth, expressed as levodopa

Neonate initially 250–500 micrograms/kg 4 times daily of a preparation containing 1:4 carbidopa:levodopa, increased according to response every 4–5 days to maintenance dose of 2.5–3 mg/kg 4 times daily; at higher doses consider preparation containing 1:10 carbidopa:levodopa; review regularly (every 3–6 months)

Child 1 month–18 years initially 250–500 micrograms/kg 4 times daily of a preparation containing 1:4 carbidopa:levodopa, increased according to response every 4–5 days to maintenance dose of 2.5–3 mg/kg 4 times daily; at higher doses consider preparation containing 1:10 carbidopa:levodopa; review regularly (every 3–6 months in early childhood)

Sinemet® (MSD) PoM

Sinemet-62.5® tablets, yellow, scored, co-careldopa 12.5/50 (carbidopa 12.5 mg (as monohydrate), levodopa 50 mg), net price 90-tab pack = £6.28. Label: 14, counselling, driving, see notes above

Note 2 tablets *Sinemet-62.5®* ≡ 1 tablet *Sinemet Plus®*; *Sinemet-62.5®* previously known as *Sinemet LS®*

Sinemet-110® tablets, blue, scored, co-careldopa 10/100 (carbidopa 10 mg (as monohydrate), levodopa 100 mg), net price 90-tab pack = £6.57. Label: 14, counselling, driving, see notes above

Sinemet-Plus® tablets, yellow, scored, co-careldopa 25/100 (carbidopa 25 mg (as monohydrate), levodopa 100 mg), net price 90-tab pack = £9.66. Label: 14, counselling, driving, see notes above

Sinemet-275® tablets, blue, scored, co-careldopa 25/250 (carbidopa 25 mg (as monohydrate), levodopa 250 mg), net price 90-tab pack = £13.72. Label: 14, counselling, driving, see notes above

4.9.2 Antimuscarinic drugs used in dystonias

Antimuscarinic drugs help to control dystonias.

The antimuscarinic drugs **procyclidine** and **trihexyphenidyl** (benzhexol) reduce the symptoms of dystonias, including those induced by antipsychotic drugs; there is no justification for giving them routinely in the absence of dystonic symptoms. Tardive dyskinesia is not improved by antimuscarinic drugs and may be made worse.

No important differences exist between the antimuscarinic drugs, but some children tolerate one better than another.

Cautions Antimuscarinics should be used with caution in cardiovascular disease, hypertension, psychotic disorders, pyrexia, and in those susceptible to angle-closure glaucoma. Antimuscarinics should not be withdrawn abruptly in children receiving long-term treatment. Antimuscarinics are liable to abuse. **Interactions:** Appendix 1 (Antimuscarinics).

Skilled tasks May affect performance of skilled tasks (e.g. driving).

Contra-indications Antimuscarinics should be avoided in gastro-intestinal obstruction and myasthenia gravis.

Hepatic and renal impairment Procyclidine and trihexyphenidyl should be used with caution in children with hepatic or renal impairment.

Side-effects Side-effects of antimuscarinics include constipation, dry mouth, nausea, vomiting, tachycardia, dizziness, confusion, euphoria, hallucinations, impaired memory, anxiety, restlessness, urinary retention, blurred vision, and rash. Angle-closure glaucoma may occur very rarely.

◢ PROCYCLIDINE HYDROCHLORIDE

Cautions see notes above
Contra-indications see notes above
Hepatic impairment see notes above
Renal impairment see notes above
Pregnancy use only if potential benefit outweighs risk
Breast-feeding no information available
Side-effects see notes above
Licensed use not licensed for use in children

Indication and dose

> Dystonias
> • By mouth
>   Child 7–12 years 1.25 mg 3 times daily
>   Child 12–18 years 2.5 mg 3 times daily

> Acute dystonia
> • By intramuscular or intravenous injection
>   Child under 2 years 0.5–2 mg as a single dose
>   Child 2–10 years 2–5 mg as a single dose

> Child 10–18 years 5–10 mg (occasionally more than 10 mg)

Note Usually effective in 5–10 minutes but may need 30 minutes for relief

Procyclidine (Non-proprietary) ⓅoM
Tablets, procyclidine hydrochloride 5 mg, net price 28-tab pack = £3.22. Counselling, driving

Arpicolin® (Rosemont) ⓅoM
Syrup, sugar-free, procyclidine hydrochloride 2.5 mg/5 mL, net price 150 mL = £4.22; 5 mg/5 mL, 150 mL pack = £7.54. Counselling, driving

Kemadrin® (GSK) ⓅoM
Tablets, scored, procyclidine hydrochloride 5 mg, net price 100-tab pack = £4.72. Counselling, driving

Kemadrin® (Auden Mckenzie) ⓅoM
Injection, procyclidine hydrochloride 5 mg/mL, net price 2-mL amp = £1.49

◢ TRIHEXYPHENIDYL HYDROCHLORIDE
(Benzhexol hydrochloride)

Cautions see notes above
Contra-indications see notes above
Hepatic impairment see notes above
Renal impairment see notes above
Pregnancy use only if potential benefit outweighs risk
Breast-feeding avoid
Side-effects see notes above
Licensed use not licensed for use in children

Indication and dose

> Dystonia
> • By mouth
>   Child 3 months–18 years 1–2 mg daily in 1–2 divided doses, increased every 3–7 days by 1 mg daily; adjusted according to response and side-effects; max. 2 mg/kg daily

Trihexyphenidyl (Non-proprietary) ⓅoM
Tablets, trihexyphenidyl hydrochloride 2 mg, net price 84-tab pack = £24.27; 5 mg, 100-tab pack = £15.60. Counselling, before or after food, driving

4

Central nervous system

◁ **TRIHEXYPHENIDYL HYDROCHLORIDE** (*continued*)

Broflex® (Alliance) PoM
Syrup, pink, black currant, trihexyphenidyl hydro-
chloride 5 mg/5 mL, net price 200 mL = £7.44.
Counselling, driving

4.9.3 Drugs used in essential tremor, chorea, tics, and related disorders

Haloperidol may be useful in improving motor tics and symptoms of Tourette
syndrome and related choreas (see section 4.2.1). **Pimozide** (section 4.2.1) and
sulpiride (section 4.2.1) are also used in Tourette syndrome.

Propranolol or another beta-adrenoceptor blocking drug (section 2.4) may be
useful in treating essential tremor or tremor associated with anxiety or thyrotoxicosis.

BOTULINUM TOXIN TYPE A

Cautions neurological disorders; history of dysphagia or aspiration

Contra-indications generalised disorders of
muscle activity (e.g. myasthenia gravis)

Pregnancy avoid unless essential—toxicity in
animal studies

Breast-feeding avoid (or avoid unless essential)—
no information available

Side-effects increased electrophysiologic jitter in
some distant muscles; misplaced injections may
paralyse nearby muscle groups and excessive
doses may paralyse distant muscles; influenza-
like symptoms, *rarely* arrhythmias, myocardial
infarction, seizures, hypersensitivity reactions
including rash, pruritus and anaphylaxis, antibody formation (substantial deterioration in
response), and injection-site reactions; *very rarely*
exaggerated muscle weakness, dysphagia, and
aspiration
Specific side-effects in paediatric cerebral palsy Drowsiness, paraesthesia, urinary incontinence, myalgia

Indication and dose

In children over 2 years for dynamic equinus foot
deformity caused by spasticity in ambulant paediatric cerebral palsy for dose consult product literature (**important: information specific to each
individual preparation and not interchangeable**)

Botox® (Allergan) PoM
Injection, powder for reconstitution, botulinum
toxin type A complex, net price 50-unit vial =
£77.50; 100-unit vial = £138.20; 200-unit vial =
£276.40

Dysport® (Ipsen) PoM
Injection, powder for reconstitution, botulinum
type A toxin-haemagglutinin complex, net price
500-unit vial = £157.00

4.10 Drugs used in substance dependence

This section includes drugs used in the treatment of neonatal abstinence
syndrome and cigarette smoking.

Treatment of alcohol or opioid dependence in children requires specialist management. The UK health departments have produced guidance on the treatment
of drug misuse in the UK. *Drug Misuse and Dependence: UK Guidelines on Clinical
Management (2007)* is available at www.nta.nhs.uk/publications.

Neonatal abstinence syndrome   Neonatal abstinence syndrome occurs at birth
as a result of intra-uterine exposure to opioids or high-dose benzodiazepines.

Treatment is usually initiated if:

- feeding becomes a problem and tube feeding is required;
- there is profuse vomiting or watery diarrhoea;
- the baby remains very unsettled after two consecutive feeds despite gentle
swaddling and the use of a pacifier.

Treatment involves weaning the baby from the drug on which it is dependent.
Morphine or **methadone** (section 4.7.2) can be used in babies of mothers who
have been taking opioids. Morphine is widely used because the dose can be easily
adjusted, but methadone may provide smoother control of symptoms. Weaning
babies from opioids usually takes 7–10 days.

Weaning babies from benzodiazepines that have a long half-life is difficult to
manage; **chlorpromazine** (section 4.2.1) may be used in these situations but

excessive sedation may occur. For babies who are dependent on barbiturates, phenobarbital (section 4.8.1) may be tried, although it does not control gastro-intestinal symptoms.

Cigarette smoking

Smoking cessation interventions are a cost-effective way of reducing ill health and prolonging life. Smokers should be advised to stop and offered help if interested in doing so, with follow-up where appropriate. If possible, smokers should have access to smoking cessation services for behavioural support.

Therapy to aid smoking cessation is chosen according to the smoker's likely compliance, availability of counselling and support, previous experience of smoking-cessation aids, contra-indications and adverse effects of the products, and the smoker's preferences.

Nicotine replacement therapy is an effective aid to smoking cessation. Cigarette smoking should stop completely before starting nicotine replacement therapy. If complete smoking cessation is not possible some nicotine preparations are licensed for use as part of a programme to reduce smoking before stopping completely; the smoking cessation regimen can be followed during a quit attempt.

NICOTINE

Cautions severe or unstable cardiovascular disease (including hospitalisation for severe arrhythmias, recent myocardial infarction, or recent cerebrovascular accident)—initiate under medical supervision; uncontrolled hyperthyroidism; diabetes mellitus (monitor blood-glucose concentration closely when initiating treatment); phaeochromocytoma; *oral preparations*, oesophagitis, gastritis, peptic ulcers; *patches*, exercise may increase absorption and side-effects, skin disorders (patches should not be placed on broken skin); **interactions:** Appendix 1 (nicotine)

Note Most warnings under Cautions also apply to continuation of cigarette smoking

Hepatic impairment caution in moderate to severe impairment

Renal impairment caution in severe impairment

Pregnancy use only if smoking cessation without nicotine replacement therapy fails; intermittent therapy preferred but avoid liquorice-flavoured nicotine products

Breast-feeding present in milk; intermittent therapy preferred

Side-effects gastro-intestinal disturbances (including nausea, vomiting, dyspepsia); headache, dizziness; influenza-like symptoms; dry mouth; rash; *less frequently* palpitation; *rarely* atrial fibrillation; *with nasal spray*, sneezing, epistaxis, watering eyes, ear sensations; *with lozenges*, thirst, paraesthesia of mouth, gingival bleeding, taste disturbances; *with patches*, skin reactions (discontinue if severe)—vasculitis also reported, blood pressure changes; *with patches* or *lozenges*, sleep disturbances, nightmares, chest pain; *with gum* or *lozenges*, mouth ulceration, increased salivation; *with gum, lozenge, sublingual tablets,* or *inhalator*, hiccups, throat irritation

Indication and dose

See under preparations, below

Nicorette® (McNeil)
Tablets (sublingual) (*Nicorette Microtab®*), nicotine (as a cyclodextrin complex) 2 mg, net price starter pack of 2 × 15-tablet discs with dispenser = £4.46; refill pack of 7 × 15-tablet discs = £12.12. Label: 26

Note Also available in lemon flavour; also available as *NicAssist®*
Excipients lemon flavour includes aspartame (section 9.4.1)
Dose

Smoking cessation
● By sublingual administration

Child 12–18 years individuals smoking *20 cigarettes or less daily*, 2 mg each hour; for patients who fail to stop smoking or have significant withdrawal symptoms, consider increasing to 4 mg each hour; individuals smoking *more than 20 cigarettes daily*, 4 mg each hour. Max. 80 mg daily; treatment continued for up to 8 weeks followed by gradual reduction over 4 weeks; review treatment if abstinence not achieved within 3 months

Chewing gum, sugar-free, nicotine (as resin) 2 mg, net price pack of 30 = £3.04, pack of 105 = £8.89, pack of 210 = £14.82; 4 mg, pack of 30 = £3.99, pack of 105 = £10.84, pack of 210 = £18.24

Note Also available in mint, freshfruit, freshmint, and icy white flavours. Also available as *NicAssist®*
Note *Nicorette®* Combi patch + gum (containing *Invisi* patches 15 mg and *Icy White* gum 2 mg) also available
Dose

Smoking cessation
● By mouth

Child 12–18 years individuals *smoking 20 cigarettes or less daily* initially chew one 2-mg piece slowly (chew gum until taste becomes strong, then rest gum between cheek and gum, when taste fades start chewing again) for approx. 30 minutes when urge to smoke occurs; individuals smoking *more than 20 cigarettes daily* or needing more than 15 pieces of 2-mg gum daily should use the 4-mg gum; max. 15 pieces of 4-mg gum daily; treatment continued for up to 8 weeks followed by gradual reduction over 4 weeks; review treatment if abstinence not achieved within 3 months

◻ **NICOTINE (continued)**

Smoking reduction
- **By mouth**

Child 12–18 years chew one piece when urge to smoke occurs between smoking episodes (chew gum until taste becomes strong, then rest gum between cheek and gum, when taste fades start chewing again); reduce smoking within 6 weeks and attempt smoking cessation within 6 months; review treatment if abstinence not achieved within 9 months

Note Children under 18 years should consult a healthcare professional before starting smoking-reduction regimen

Patches, self-adhesive, beige, nicotine, '5 mg' patch (releasing approx. 5 mg/16 hours), net price 7 = £9.07; '10 mg' patch (releasing approx. 10 mg/16 hours), 7 = £9.07; '15 mg' patch (releasing approx. 15 mg/16 hours), 2 = £2.85, 7 = £9.07

Note Also available as NicAssist®

Dose

Smoking cessation
- **By transdermal route**

Child 12–18 years apply on waking to dry, non-hairy skin on hip, chest, or upper arm, removing after approx. 16 hours, usually when retiring to bed; site next patch on different area (avoid using same area on consecutive days); initially '15-mg' patch for 16 hours daily for 8 weeks then if abstinence achieved '10-mg' patch for 16 hours daily for 2 weeks then '5-mg' patch for 16 hours daily for 2 weeks; review treatment if abstinence not achieved within 3 months—further courses may be given if considered beneficial

Invisi patches, self-adhesive, beige, nicotine, '10 mg' patch (releasing approx. 10 mg/16 hours), net price 7 = £9.97; '15 mg' patch (releasing approx. 15 mg/16 hours), 7 = £9.97; '25 mg' patch (releasing approx. 25 mg/16 hours), 7 = £9.97

Note Nicorette® Combi patch + gum (containing Invisi patches 15 mg and Icy White gum 2 mg) also available

Dose

Smoking cessation
- **By transdermal route**

Child 12–18 years apply on waking to dry, non-hairy skin on hip, chest, or upper arm, removing after approx. 16 hours, usually when retiring to bed; site next patch on different area (avoid using same area on consecutive days); individuals smoking 10 or more cigarettes daily, initially '25-mg' patch for 16 hours daily for 8 weeks then if abstinence achieved '15-mg' patch for 16 hours daily for 2 weeks then '10-mg' patch for 16 hours daily for 2 weeks; individuals smoking less than 10 cigarettes daily, initially '15-mg' patch for 16 hours daily for 8 weeks then '10-mg' patch for 16 hours daily for 4 weeks; review treatment if abstinence not achieved within 3 months—further courses may be given if considered beneficial

Note Patients using the '25-mg' patch who experience excessive side-effects that do not resolve within a few days should change to the '15-mg' patch for the remainder of the initial 8-week course before switching to the '10-mg' patch for the final 4 weeks

Nasal spray, nicotine 500 micrograms/metered spray, net price 200-spray unit = £13.40

Dose

Smoking cessation
- **Intranasally**

Child 12–18 years apply 1 spray into each nostril as required to max. twice an hour for 16 hours daily (max. 64 sprays daily) for 8 weeks, then reduce gradually over next 4 weeks (reduce by half at end of first 2 weeks, stop altogether at end of next 2 weeks); review treatment if abstinence not achieved within 3 months

Inhalator (nicotine-impregnated plug for use in inhalator mouthpiece), nicotine 10 mg/cartridge, net price 6-cartridge (starter) pack = £4.46, 42-cartridge (refill) pack = £14.01

Note Also available as NicAssist®

Dose

Smoking cessation
- **By inhalation**

Child 12–18 years inhale when urge to smoke occurs; initially use between 6 and 12 cartridges daily for up to 8 weeks, then reduce gradually over 4 weeks (reduce by half over first 2 weeks, stop altogether at end of next 2 weeks); review treatment if abstinence not achieved within 3 months

Smoking reduction
- **By inhalation**

Child 12–18 years inhale when urge to smoke occurs between smoking episodes; reduce smoking within 6 weeks and attempt smoking cessation within 6 months; review treatment if abstinence not achieved within 9 months

Note Children under 18 years should consult a healthcare professional before starting smoking-reduction regimen

Nicotinell® (Novartis Consumer Health)

Chewing gum, sugar-free, nicotine 2 mg, net price pack of 12 = £1.71, pack of 24 = £3.01, pack of 96 = £8.26; 4 mg, pack of 12 = £1.70, pack of 24 = £3.30, pack of 96 = £10.26

Note Also available in fruit, liquorice, and mint flavours

Dose

Smoking cessation
- **By mouth**

Child 12–18 years individuals smoking 20 cigarettes or less daily, initially chew one 2-mg piece slowly (chew gum until taste becomes strong, then rest gum between cheek and gum, when taste fades start chewing again) for approx. 30 minutes when urge to smoke occurs; individuals smoking more than 20 cigarettes daily should use the 4-mg strength; max. 60 mg daily; withdraw gradually; review treatment if abstinence not achieved within 3 months

Nicotinell mint lozenge, sugar-free, nicotine (as bitartrate) 1 mg, net price pack of 12 = £1.71, pack of 36 = £4.27, pack of 96 = £9.12; 2 mg, net price pack of 12 = £1.99, pack of 36 = £4.95, pack of 96 = £10.60. Label: 24

Excipients include aspartame (section 9.4.1)

Dose

Smoking cessation
- **By mouth**

Child 12–18 years individuals smoking 30 cigarettes or less daily, initially suck one 1-mg lozenge every 1–2 hours when urge to smoke occurs; individuals smoking more than 30 cigarettes daily should use 2-mg strength; max. 30 mg daily; withdraw gradually; review treatment if abstinence not achieved within 3 months

TTS Patches, self-adhesive, all yellowish-ochre, nicotine, '10' patch (releasing approx. 7 mg/24 hours), net price 7 = £9.12; '20' patch (releasing approx. 14 mg/24 hours), net price 2 = £2.57, 7 = £9.40; '30' patch (releasing approx. 21 mg/24 hours), net price 2 = £2.85, 7 = £9.97, 21 = £24.51

Dose

Smoking cessation
- **By transdermal route**

Child 12–18 years apply to dry, non-hairy skin on trunk or upper arm, removing after 24 hours and siting

⌐ **NICOTINE** (*continued*)

replacement patch on a different area (avoid using the same area for several days); individuals smoking *less than 20 cigarettes daily*, initially '20' patch daily; individuals smoking *20 or more cigarettes daily*, initially '30' patch daily; withdraw gradually, reducing dose every 3–4 weeks; review treatment if abstinence not achieved within 3 months

NiQuitin® (GSK Consumer Healthcare)
Chewing gum, sugar-free, mint-flavour, nicotine 2 mg (white), net price pack of 12 = £1.71, pack of 24 = £2.85, pack of 96 = £8.55; 4 mg (yellow), pack of 12 = £1.71, pack of 24 = £2.85, pack of 96 = £8.55

Dose

Smoking cessation
● **By mouth**
Child 12–18 years initially chew 1 piece slowly (chew gum until taste becomes strong, then rest gum between cheek and gum, when taste fades start chewing again) for approx. 30 minutes, when urge to smoke occurs; max. 15 pieces daily; withdraw gradually; review treatment if abstinence not achieved within 3 months

Smoking reduction
● **By mouth**
Child 12–18 years chew 1 piece when urge to smoke occurs between smoking episodes (chew gum until taste becomes strong, then rest gum between cheek and gum, when taste fades start chewing again); reduce smoking within 6 weeks and attempt cessation within 6 months; review treatment if abstinence not achieved within 9 months
Note Children under 18 years should consult a healthcare professional before starting smoking-reduction regimen

Temporary abstinence
● **By mouth**
Child 12–18 years chew 1 piece when urge to smoke occurs between smoking episodes; max. 15 pieces daily; review treatment if unable to undertake permanent quit attempt within 6 months

Lozenges, sugar-free, nicotine (as polacrilex) 2 mg, net price pack of 36 = £5.12, pack of 72 = £9.97; 4 mg, pack of 36 = £5.12, pack of 72 = £9.97. Contains 0.65 mmol Na⁺/lozenge. Label: 24
Excipients include aspartame (section 9.4.1)

Note Also available as *Pre-Quit 4 mg Lozenges* and *Mini Mint Lozenges*

Dose

Smoking cessation
● **By mouth**
Child 12–18 years initially suck 1 lozenge every 1–2 hours when urge to smoke occurs (max. 15 lozenges

daily) for 6 weeks, then 1 lozenge every 2–4 hours for 3 weeks, then 1 lozenge every 4–8 hours for 3 weeks; withdraw gradually; review treatment if abstinence not achieved within 3 months

Smoking reduction
● **By mouth**
Child 12–18 years suck 1 lozenge when urge to smoke occurs between smoking episodes (max. 15 lozenges daily); reduce smoking within 6 weeks and attempt cessation within 6 months; review treatment if abstinence not achieved within 3 months
Note Children under 18 years should consult a healthcare professional before starting a smoking-reduction regimen

Temporary abstinence
● **By mouth**
Child 12–18 years suck 1 lozenge every 1–2 hours when urge to smoke occurs between smoking episodes (max. 15 lozenges daily); review treatment if unable to undertake permanent quit attempt within 6 months

Patches, self-adhesive, pink/beige, nicotine '7 mg' patch (releasing approx. 7 mg/24 hours), net price 7 = £9.97; '14 mg' patch (releasing approx. 14 mg/24 hours), 7 = £9.97; '21 mg' patch (releasing approx. 21 mg/24 hours), 7 = £9.97, 14 = £18.79

Note Also available as a clear patch

Dose

Smoking cessation
● **By transdermal route**
Child 12–18 years apply on waking to dry, non-hairy skin, removing after 24 hours and siting replacement patch on different area (avoid using same area for 7 days); individuals smoking *10 or more cigarettes daily*, initially '21-mg' patch daily for 6 weeks then '14-mg' patch daily for 2 weeks then '7-mg' patch daily for 2 weeks. Individuals smoking *less than 10 cigarettes daily*, initially '14-mg' patch daily for 6 weeks then '7-mg' patch daily for 2 weeks; review treatment if abstinence not achieved within 3 months

Note Patients using the '21-mg' patch who experience excessive side-effects, which do not resolve within a few days, should change to '14-mg' patch for the remainder of the initial 6 weeks before switching to the '7-mg' patch for the final 2 weeks

4 **Central nervous system**

4.11 **Drugs for dementia**

Classification not used in *BNF for Children*.

5 Infections

5 Infections

This chapter includes advice on the drug management of the following:
anthrax, p. 364
bacterial infections: table 1, summary of antibacterial treatment, p. 305
bacterial infections: table 2, summary of antibacterial prophylaxis, p. 310
Lyme disease, p. 319
MRSA infections, p. 317
oral infections, p. 304 and p. 309

Notifiable diseases

Doctors must notify the Proper Officer of the local authority (usually the consultant in communicable disease control) when attending a patient suspected of suffering from any of the diseases listed below; a form is available from the Proper Officer.

Anthrax	Measles	Rubella
Cholera	Meningitis	Scarlet fever
Diphtheria	Meningococcal septicaemia	Smallpox
Dysentery (amoebic or bacillary)	(without meningitis)	Tetanus
Encephalitis, acute	Mumps	Tuberculosis
Food poisoning	Ophthalmia neonatorum	Typhoid fever
Haemorrhagic fever (viral)	Paratyphoid fever	Typhus
Hepatitis, viral	Plague	Whooping cough
Leprosy	Poliomyelitis, acute	Yellow fever
Leptospirosis	Rabies	
Malaria	Relapsing fever	

Note It is good practice for doctors to also inform the consultant in communicable disease control of instances of other infections (e.g. psittacosis) where there could be a public health risk.

5.1 Antibacterial drugs

5.1.1 Penicillins

5.1.2 Cephalosporins, carbapenems, and other beta-lactams

5.1.3 Tetracyclines

5.1.4 Aminoglycosides

5.1.5 Macrolides

5.1.6 Clindamycin

5.1.7 Some other antibacterials

5.1.8 Sulphonamides and trimethoprim

5.1.9 Antituberculosis drugs

5.1.10 Antileprotic drugs

5.1.11 Metronidazole

5.1.12 Quinolones

5.1.13 Urinary-tract infections

Choice of a suitable drug   Before selecting an antibacterial the clinician must first consider two factors—the child and the known or likely causative organism. Factors related to the child which must be considered include history of allergy, renal and hepatic function, susceptibility to infection (i.e. whether immunocompromised), ability to tolerate drugs by mouth, severity of illness, ethnic origin, age and, if an adolescent female, whether pregnant, breast-feeding or taking an oral contraceptive.

The known or likely organism and its antibacterial sensitivity, in association with the above factors, will suggest one or more antibacterials, the final choice depending on the microbiological, pharmacological, and toxicological properties.

The principles involved in selection of an antibacterial must allow for a number of variables including age, changing renal and hepatic function, increasing bacterial resistance, and new information on side-effects. Duration of therapy, dosage, and route of administration depend on site, type and severity of infection and response.

Antibacterial policies   Local policies often limit the antibacterials that may be used to achieve reasonable economy consistent with adequate cover, and to reduce the development of resistant organisms. A policy may indicate a range of drugs for general use, and permit other drugs only on the advice of the microbiologist or paediatric infectious diseases specialist.

Before starting therapy   The following principles should be considered before starting:

- Viral infections should not be treated with antibacterials. However, antibacterials may be indicated for treatment of secondary bacterial infection (e.g. bacterial pneumonia secondary to influenza);

- Samples should be taken for culture and sensitivity testing whenever possible; 'blind' antibacterial prescribing for unexplained pyrexia usually leads to further difficulty in establishing the diagnosis;

5

Infections

- Knowledge of **prevalent organisms** and their current **sensitivity** is of great help in choosing an antibacterial before bacteriological confirmation is available. Generally, narrow-spectrum antibacterials are preferred to broad-spectrum antibacterials unless there is a clear clinical indication (e.g. life-threatening sepsis);

- The **dose** of an antibacterial varies according to a number of factors including age, weight, hepatic function, renal function, and severity of infection. The prescribing of the so-called 'standard' dose in serious infections may result in failure of treatment or even death of the patient; therefore it is important to prescribe a dose appropriate to the condition. An inadequate dose may also increase the likelihood of antibacterial resistance. On the other hand, for an antibacterial with a narrow margin between the toxic and therapeutic dose (e.g. an aminoglycoside) it is also important to avoid an excessive dose and the concentration of the drug in the plasma may need to be monitored;

- The **route** of administration of an antibacterial often depends on the severity of the infection. Life-threatening infections often require intravenous therapy. Antibacterials that are well absorbed may be given by mouth even for some serious infections. Parenteral administration is also appropriate when the oral route cannot be used (e.g. because of vomiting) or if absorption is inadequate (e.g. in neonates and young children). Whenever possible painful intramuscular injections should be avoided in children;

- **Duration** of therapy depends on the nature of the infection and the response to treatment. Courses should not be unduly prolonged because they encourage resistance, they may lead to side-effects and they are costly. However, in certain infections such as tuberculosis or osteomyelitis it may be necessary to treat for prolonged periods.

Oral bacterial infections   Antibacterial drugs should only be prescribed for the *treatment* of oral infections on the basis of defined need. They may be used in conjunction with (but not as an alternative to) other appropriate measures, such as providing drainage or extracting a tooth.

The 'blind' prescribing of an antibacterial for unexplained pyrexia, cervical lymphadenopathy, or facial swelling can lead to difficulty in establishing the diagnosis. A sample should always be taken for bacteriology in the case of severe oral infection.

Oral infections which may require antibacterial treatment include acute periapical or periodontal abscess, cellulitis, acutely created oral-antral communication (and acute sinusitis), severe pericoronitis, localised osteitis, acute necrotising ulcerative gingivitis, and destructive forms of chronic periodontal disease. Most of these infections are readily resolved by the early establishment of drainage and removal of the cause (typically an infected necrotic pulp). Antibacterials may be indicated if treatment has to be delayed and they are essential in immunocompromised patients or in those with conditions such as diabetes. Certain rarer infections including bacterial sialadenitis, osteomyelitis, actinomycosis, and infections involving fascial spaces such as Ludwig's angina, require antibiotics and specialist hospital care.

Antibacterial drugs may also be useful after dental surgery in some cases of spreading infection. Infection may spread to involve local lymph nodes, to fascial spaces (where it can cause airway obstruction), or into the bloodstream (where it can lead to cavernous sinus thrombosis and other serious complications). Extension of an infection can also lead to maxillary sinusitis; osteomyelitis is a complication, which usually arises when host resistance is reduced.

If the oral infection fails to respond to antibacterial treatment within 48 hours the antibacterial should be changed, preferably on the basis of bacteriological investigation. Failure to respond may also suggest an incorrect diagnosis, lack of essential additional measures (such as drainage), poor host resistance, or poor patient compliance.

Combination of a penicillin (or erythromycin) with metronidazole may sometimes be helpful for the treatment of severe or resistant oral infections.

See also **Penicillins** (section 5.1.1), **Cephalosporins** (section 5.1.2.1), **Tetracyclines** (section 5.1.3), **Macrolides** (section 5.1.5), **Clindamycin** (section 5.1.6), **Metronidazole** (section 5.1.11), **Fusidic acid** (section 13.10.1.2).

Superinfection   In general, broad-spectrum antibacterial drugs such as the cephalosporins are more likely to be associated with adverse reactions related to the selection of resistant organisms e.g. *fungal infections* or *antibiotic-associated colitis* (pseudomembranous colitis); other problems associated with superinfection include vaginitis and pruritus ani.

Therapy   Suggested treatment is shown in Table 1. When the pathogen has been isolated treatment may be changed to a more appropriate antibacterial if necessary. If no bacterium is cultured the antibacterial can be continued or stopped on clinical grounds. Infections for which prophylaxis is useful are listed in table 2.

Switching from parenteral to oral treatment   The ongoing parenteral administration of an antibacterial should be reviewed regularly. In older children it may be possible to switch to an oral antibacterial; in neonates and infants this should be done more cautiously because of the relatively high incidence of bacteraemia and the possibility of variable oral absorption.

Prophylaxis   Infections for which antibacterial prophylaxis is useful are listed in Table 2. In most situations, only a short course of prophylactic antibacterial is needed. Longer-term antibacterial prophylaxis is appropriate in specific indications such as vesico-ureteric reflux

Table 1. Summary of antibacterial therapy

> If treating a patient suspected of suffering from a notifiable disease, the consultant in communicable disease control should be informed (see p. 303)

Gastro-intestinal system

Gastro-enteritis
Antibacterial not usually indicated
  Frequently self-limiting and may not be bacterial

Campylobacter enteritis
Clarithromycin[1] *or* ciprofloxacin
  Frequently self-limiting; treat severe infection

Salmonella
Ciprofloxacin *or* cefotaxime
  Treat invasive or severe infection; treat less severe infection in those at risk of developing invasive infection (e.g. immunocompromised, haemoglobinopathy, or child under 6 months)

Shigellosis
Azithromycin [unlicensed indication] *or* ciprofloxacin
  Antibacterial not indicated for mild cases. Amoxicillin or trimethoprim may be used if organism sensitive

Typhoid fever
Ciprofloxacin *or* cefotaxime *or* ceftriaxone
  Chloramphenicol may be an alternative; infections from Indian subcontinent, Middle-East, and South-East Asia may be multiple-antibacterial-resistant and sensitivity should be tested—azithromycin [unlicensed indication] may be an option in disease caused by multiple-antibacterial-resistant organisms

***Clostridium difficile* infection**
Oral metronidazole *or* oral vancomycin
  Treat for 10–14 days. Use vancomycin for third or subsequent episode of infection, for severe infection, for infection not responding to metronidazole, or in patients intolerant of metronidazole. For infection not responding to vancomycin, or for life-threatening infection, or in patients with ileus, use oral vancomycin + i/v metronidazole.

Necrotising enterocolitis in neonates
Benzylpenicillin + gentamicin + metronidazole *or* amoxicillin[2] + gentamicin + metronidazole *or* amoxicillin[2] + cefotaxime + metronidazole

Peritonitis
A cephalosporin + metronidazole *or* amoxicillin + gentamicin + metronidazole *or* piperacillin with tazobactam alone

Peritoneal dialysis-associated peritonitis
Either vancomycin[3] + ceftazidime added to dialysis fluid *or* vancomycin added to dialysis fluid + ciprofloxacin by mouth
  Treat for 14 days or longer

1. Where clarithromycin is suggested azithromycin or erythromycin may be used.
2. Where amoxicillin is suggested ampicillin may be used.
3. Where vancomycin is suggested teicoplanin may be used.

Cardiovascular system

Endocarditis: initial 'blind' therapy

Flucloxacillin (*or* benzylpenicillin if symptoms less severe) + gentamicin
Substitute flucloxacillin (*or* benzylpenicillin) with vancomycin + rifampicin if cardiac prostheses present, or if penicillin-allergic, or if meticillin-resistant *Staphylococcus aureus* suspected

Endocarditis caused by staphylococci

Flucloxacillin (*or* vancomycin + rifampicin if penicillin-allergic or if meticillin-resistant *Staphylococcus aureus*)
Treat for at least 4 weeks; treat prosthetic valve endocarditis for at least 6 weeks and if using flucloxacillin add rifampicin for at least 2 weeks

Endocarditis caused by streptococci (e.g. viridans streptococci)

Benzylpenicillin (*or* vancomycin[1] if penicillin-allergic or highly penicillin-resistant) + gentamicin
Treat endocarditis caused by fully sensitive streptococci with benzylpenicillin or vancomycin alone for 4 weeks *or* (if a large vegetation, intracardial abscess, or infected emboli are absent) with benzylpenicillin + gentamicin for 2 weeks. Treat more resistant organisms for 4–6 weeks (stopping gentamicin after 2 weeks for organisms moderately sensitive to penicillin); if aminoglycoside cannot be used and if streptococci moderately sensitive to penicillin, treat with benzylpenicillin alone for 4 weeks. Treat prosthetic valve endocarditis for at least 6 weeks (stopping gentamicin after 2 weeks if organisms fully sensitive to penicillin)

Endocarditis caused by enterococci (e.g. *Enterococcus faecalis*)

Amoxicillin[2] (*or* vancomycin[1] if penicillin-allergic or penicillin-resistant) + gentamicin
Treat for at least 4 weeks (at least 6 weeks for prosthetic valve endocarditis); if gentamicin-resistant, substitute gentamicin with streptomycin

Endocarditis caused by haemophilus, actinobacillus, cardiobacterium, eikenella, and kingella species ('HACEK' organisms)

Amoxicillin[2] (*or* ceftriaxone if amoxicillin-resistant) + gentamicin
Treat for 4 weeks (6 weeks for prosthetic valve endocarditis); stop gentamicin after 2 weeks

Respiratory system

Haemophilus influenzae epiglottitis

Cefotaxime *or* ceftriaxone *or* chloramphenicol

Uncomplicated community-acquired pneumonia

Neonate and child under 6 months, treat as for severe community acquired pneumonia of unknown aetiology

Child 6 months–5 years, oral amoxicillin[2] *or* oral clarithromycin[3]

Child 5–18 years, oral clarithromycin[3] (*or* oral amoxicillin[2] if *Streptococcus pneumoniae* suspected)
Add flucloxacillin if staphylococci suspected, e.g. in influenza or measles; treat for 7 days (14–21 days for infections caused by staphylococci); pneumococci with decreased penicillin sensitivity being isolated but not yet common in UK; use clarithromycin[3] if atypical pathogens suspected (more common in children over 5 years) or if penicillin-allergic

Severe community-acquired pneumonia of unknown aetiology

Neonate, benzylpenicillin + gentamicin

Child 1 month–18 years, co-amoxiclav *or* cefuroxime (*or* benzylpenicillin if lobar or *Streptococcus pneumoniae* suspected)
Use clarithromycin[3] if atypical pathogens such as mycoplasma (more common in children over 5 years) or chlamydia suspected or if penicillin allergic; in pneumococcal infection add vancomycin to beta-lactam antibacterial if organism highly penicillin- and cephalosporin-resistant. Treat for 7–10 days (may extend treatment to 14–21 days in some cases e.g. if staphylococci or Gram-negative enteric bacilli suspected)

Pneumonia possibly caused by atypical pathogens

Clarithromycin[3]
A quinolone is an alternative in Legionella infection (if severe Legionella infection, for the first few days add clarithromycin[3] or rifampicin to the quinolone *or* add rifampicin to clarithromycin).
Doxycycline is an alternative for chlamydia and mycoplasma infections in children over 12 years.
Treat for 14 days (usually 7–10 days for Legionella)

---

1. Where vancomycin is suggested teicoplanin may be used.
2. Where amoxicillin is suggested ampicillin may be used.
3. Where clarithromycin is suggested azithromycin or erythromycin may be used.

Hospital-acquired pneumonia

Early-onset infection (less than 5 days after admission to hospital), treat as for severe community-acquired pneumonia of unknown aetiology; if life-threatening infection, or if recent history of antibacterial treatment, or if resistant organisms suspected, treat as for late-onset hospital-acquired pneumonia

Late-onset infection (more than 5 days after admission to hospital), an antipseudomonal penicillin (e.g. piperacillin with tazobactam) *or* another antipseudomonal beta-lactam

> Treat for 7 days (longer if pseudomonas confirmed); add vancomycin if MRSA suspected; add an aminoglycoside for severe illness caused by *Pseudomonas aeruginosa*

Cystic fibrosis

Staphylococcal lung infection in cystic fibrosis

Flucloxacillin (*or* clarithromycin[1] *or* clindamycin if penicillin-allergic)

> In severe exacerbation use flucloxacillin or a broad-spectrum cephalosporin (e.g. cefuroxime); substitute with vancomycin[2] if meticillin-resistant *Staphylococcus aureus* suspected, and if necessary, add either rifampicin or sodium fusidate

***Haemophilus influenzae* lung infection in cystic fibrosis**

Amoxicillin *or* a broad-spectrum cephalosporin

> In severe exacerbation use a third-generation cephalosporin (e.g. cefotaxime)

Pseudomonal lung infection in cystic fibrosis

Ciprofloxacin + *nebulised* colistin

> In severe exacerbation treat with a parenteral aminoglycoside + an antipseudomonal beta-lactam antibacterial, and continue nebulised antibacterial

Central nervous system

Meningitis: Initial empirical therapy

- Transfer patient urgently to hospital

- If bacterial meningitis and especially if *meningococcal disease* suspected, general practitioners should give benzylpenicillin (see p. 316 for dose) before urgent transfer to hospital; cefotaxime (section 5.1.2) may be an alternative in penicillin allergy; chloramphenicol may be used if history of immediate hypersensitivity reaction to penicillins or to cephalosporins

- Consider adjunctive treatment with dexamethasone (section 6.3.2) starting before or with first dose of antibacterial; avoid dexamethasone in septic shock, suspected meningococcal septicaemia, or if immunocompromised, or in meningitis following surgery

- In hospital, if aetiology unknown:
  Neonate and Child 1–3 months, cefotaxime + amoxicillin[3]
  Child 3 months–18 years, cefotaxime

Meningitis caused by group B streptococcus

Benzylpenicillin + gentamicin *or* cefotaxime alone

> Treat for 14 days

Meningitis caused by meningococci

Benzylpenicillin *or* cefotaxime

> Treat for 7 days; substitute chloramphenicol if history of immediate hypersensitivity reaction to penicillin or to cephalosporins. To eliminate nasopharyngeal carriage see Table 2, section 5.1.

Meningitis caused by pneumococci

Cefotaxime

> Treat for 10–14 days; substitute benzylpenicillin if organism penicillin-sensitive; if organism highly penicillin- and cephalosporin-resistant, add vancomycin and if necessary rifampicin. Consider adjunctive treatment with dexamethasone starting before or with first dose of antibacterial (but may reduce penetration of vancomycin into cerebrospinal fluid; section 6.3.2)

Meningitis caused by *Haemophilus influenzae*

Cefotaxime

> Treat for at least 10 days; substitute chloramphenicol if history of immediate hypersensitivity reaction to penicillin or to cephalosporins, or if organism resistant to cefotaxime. Consider adjunctive treatment with dexamethasone (section 6.3.2) starting before or with first dose of antibacterial. For *H. influenzae* type b give rifampicin for 4 days before hospital discharge (see Table 2, section 5.1)

Meningitis caused by Listeria

Amoxicillin[3] + gentamicin

> Treat for at least 14 days. Consider stopping gentamicin after one week

---

1. Where clarithromycin is suggested azithromycin or erythromycin may be used.
2. Where vancomycin is suggested teicoplanin may be used.
3. Where amoxicillin is suggested ampicillin may be used.

5

Infections

Urinary tract
Urinary-tract infection
Child under 3 months of age, i/v amoxicillin[1] + gentamicin *or* i/v cephalosporin alone

Child over 3 months of age with uncomplicated lower urinary-tract infection, trimethoprim *or* nitrofurantoin *or* oral cephalosporin (e.g. cefalexin) *or* amoxicillin[1]
Treat for 3 days. Re-assess child if unwell 24–48 hours after initial assessment. Use amoxicillin only if organism sensitive

Child over 3 months of age with acute pyelonephritis, a cephalosporin or co-amoxiclav
Treat for 7–10 days

Genital system
Syphilis
Neonatal congenital syphilis, benzylpenicillin
Treat for 10 days. Also consider treating neonates with suspected congenital syphilis whose mothers were treated inadequately for syphilis, or whose mothers were treated for syphilis in the 4 weeks before delivery, or whose mothers were treated with non-penicillin antibacterials for syphilis

Syphilis in child under 12 years, benzylpenicillin *or* procaine benzylpenicillin [unlicensed]
Treat for 10 days

Syphilis in child 12–18 years, benzathine benzylpenicillin [unlicensed] *or* doxycycline *or* erythromycin
Treat early syphilis (infection of less than 2 years) with benzathine benzylpenicillin as a single dose (repeat dose after 7 days for females in the third trimester of pregnancy) or with doxycycline or erythromycin for 14 days. Treat late latent syphilis (asymptomatic infection of more than 2 years) with doxycycline for 28 days or with benzathine benzylpenicillin once weekly for 2 weeks. Treat asymptomatic contacts of patients with infectious syphilis with doxycycline for 14 days. Contact tracing recommended

Uncomplicated gonorrhoea
Child under 12 years, ceftriaxone

Child 12–18 years, cefixime [unlicensed indication] *or* ciprofloxacin
Single dose treatment in uncomplicated infection. Choice depends on locality where infection acquired. Pharyngeal infection requires treatment with ceftriaxone. Use ciprofloxacin only if organism sensitive. Contact tracing recommended; remember chlamydia

Uncomplicated genital chlamydial infection, non-gonococcal urethritis and non-specific genital infection
Child under 12 years, erythromycin for 14 days

Child 12–18 years, single dose of azithromycin *or* doxycycline for 7 days
Contact tracing recommended

Pelvic inflammatory disease
Child 2–12 years, erythromycin + metronidazole + i/m ceftriaxone
Treat for 14 days (use i/m ceftriaxone as a single dose)

Child 12–18 years, doxycycline + metronidazole + i/m ceftriaxone
Treat for 14 days (use i/m ceftriaxone as a single dose). Contact tracing recommended. If severely ill, seek specialist advice

Blood
Septicaemia: Initial empirical therapy
Neonate less than 48 hours old, benzylpenicillin + gentamicin *or* amoxicillin[1] + cefotaxime

Neonate more than 48 hours old, flucloxacillin + gentamicin *or* amoxicillin[1] + cefotaxime

Child 1 month–18 years, community-acquired septicaemia, aminoglycoside + amoxicillin[1] *or* cefotaxime alone *or* ceftriaxone alone
Use aminoglycoside + broad spectrum antipseudomonal beta-lactam antibacterial if pseudomonas suspected; add metronidazole if anaerobic infection suspected; add flucloxacillin or vancomycin[2] if Gram-positive infection suspected

Child 1 month–18 years, hospital-acquired septicaemia, a broad-spectrum antipseudomonal beta-lactam antibacterial (e.g. piperacillin with tazobactam, *Timentin*®, ceftazidime, imipenem (with cilastatin as *Primaxin*®) or meropenem)
Add aminoglycoside if pseudomonas suspected, or if multiple-resistant organisms suspected, or if severe sepsis; add vancomycin[2] if meticillin-resistant *Staphylococcus aureus* suspected; add metronidazole to broad-spectrum cephalosporin if anaerobic infection suspected

1. Where amoxicillin is suggested ampicillin may be used.
2. Where vancomycin is suggested teicoplanin may be used.

Septicaemia related to vascular catheter

Vancomycin[1]

Add a broad-spectrum antipseudomonal beta-lactam if Gram-negative sepsis suspected, especially in the immunocompromised. Consider removing vascular catheter, particularly if infection caused by *Staphylococcus aureus*, pseudomonas, or candida

Meningococcal septicaemia

Benzylpenicillin *or* cefotaxime

If meningococcal disease suspected, general practitioners advised to give a single dose of benzyl-penicillin before urgent transfer to hospital (see under Benzylpenicillin, section 5.1.1.1); cefotaxime (section 5.1.2) may be an alternative in penicillin allergy; chloramphenicol may be used if history of immediate hypersensitivity to penicillin or to cephalosporins. To eliminate nasopharyngeal carriage give rifampicin or ciprofloxacin before hospital discharge (see Table 2, section 5.1)

Musculoskeletal system

Osteomyelitis

Flucloxacillin (*or* clindamycin if history of immediate hypersensitivity reaction to penicillin), (*or* vancomycin[1] if meticillin-resistant *Staphylococcus aureus*)

Consider adding fusidic acid or rifampicin for initial 2 weeks. Treat acute infection for 6 weeks. Seek specialist advice if chronic infection or prostheses present

Septic arthritis

Flucloxacillin (*or* clindamycin if history of immediate hypersensitivity reaction to penicillin), (*or* vancomycin[1] if meticillin-resistant staphylococci suspected), (*or* cefotaxime if gonococcal arthritis or Gram-negative infection suspected)

Treat for 4–6 weeks (longer if infection complicated; treat gonococcal infection for 2 weeks). Seek specialist advice if prostheses present

Eye

Purulent conjunctivitis

Neonate, neomycin eye drops

Child 1 month–18 years, chloramphenicol *or* gentamicin eye-drops

Congenital chlamydial conjunctivitis

Erythromycin (by mouth)

Treat for 14 days

Congenital gonococcal conjunctivitis

Cefotaxime *or* ceftriaxone

Single-dose treatment

Ear, nose, and oropharynx

Pericoronitis

Metronidazole *or* amoxicillin

Antibacterial required only in presence of systemic features of infection or of trismus or persistent swelling despite local treatment; treat for 3 days or until symptoms resolve

Acute necrotising ulcerative gingivitis

Metronidazole *or* amoxicillin

Antibacterial required only if systemic features of infection; treat for 3 days or until symptoms resolve

Periapical or periodontal abscess

Amoxicillin *or* metronidazole

Antibacterial required only in severe disease with cellulitis or if systemic features of infection; treat for 5 days

Periodontitis

Metronidazole *or* doxycycline

Antibacterial required for severe disease or disease unresponsive to local treatment; doxycycline is an option in children over 12 years

Throat infections

Phenoxymethylpenicillin (*or* clarithromycin[2] if penicillin-allergic)

Most throat infections are caused by viruses and many do not require antibacterial therapy. Consider antibacterial if history of valvular heart disease, if marked systemic upset, if peritonsillar cellulitis or abscess, or if at increased risk from acute infection (e.g. in immunosuppression, cystic fibrosis); prescribe antibacterial for beta-haemolytic streptococcal pharyngitis; treat for 10 days. **Avoid** amoxicillin if possibility of glandular fever, see section 5.1.1.3. Initial parenteral therapy (in severe infection) with benzylpenicillin, then oral therapy with phenoxymethylpenicillin *or* amoxicillin[3]

1. Where vancomycin is suggested teicoplanin may be used.
2. Where clarithromycin is suggested azithromycin or erythromycin may be used.
3. Where amoxicillin is suggested ampicillin may be used.

5
Infections

Sinusitis

Amoxicillin[1] *or* clarithromycin[2]

Antibacterial should usually be used only for persistent symptoms and purulent discharge lasting at least 7 days or if severe symptoms. Also consider antibacterial for those at high risk of serious complications (e.g. in immunosuppression, cystic fibrosis). Treat for 7 days. Consider oral co-amoxiclav if no improvement after 48 hours. Initial parenteral therapy with co-amoxiclav or cefuroxime may be required in severe infections

Otitis externa

Flucloxacillin (*or* clarithromycin[2] if penicillin-allergic)

Consider systemic antibacterial if spreading cellulitis or child systemically unwell. Use ciprofloxacin (or an aminoglycoside) if pseudomonas suspected, see section 12.1.1

Otitis media

Amoxicillin[1] (*or* clarithromycin[2] if penicillin-allergic)

Many infections caused by viruses. Most uncomplicated cases resolve without antibacterial treatment. In children without systemic features, antibacterial treatment may be started after 72 hours if no improvement. Consider earlier treatment if deterioration, if systemically unwell, if at high risk of serious complications (e.g. in immunosuppression, cystic fibrosis), if mastoiditis present, or in children under 2 years of age with bilateral otitis media. Treat for 5 days (longer if severely ill); consider co-amoxiclav if no improvement after 48 hours; initial parenteral therapy in severe infection with co-amoxiclav or cefuroxime

Skin

Impetigo

Topical fusidic acid (*or* mupirocin if meticillin-resistant *Staphylococcus aureus*); oral flucloxacillin *or* clarithromycin[2] if widespread

A topical antibacterial can be applied to small areas of the skin and treatment for 7 days usually adequate; max. duration of topical treatment 10 days; seek local microbiology advice before using topical treatment in hospital. Oral treatment for 7 days; add phenoxymethylpenicillin to flucloxacillin if streptococcal infection suspected

Erysipelas

Phenoxymethylpenicillin (or clarithromycin[2] if penicillin-allergic)

Add flucloxacillin to phenoxymethylpenicillin if staphylococcus suspected; substitute benzylpenicillin for phenoxymethylpenicillin if parenteral treatment required

Cellulitis

Benzylpenicillin + flucloxacillin (or clarithromycin[2] alone if penicillin-allergic)

Substitute phenoxymethylpenicillin for benzylpenicillin if oral treatment appropriate; discontinue flucloxacillin if streptococcal infection confirmed. Substitute treatment with broad-spectrum antibacterials if patients at risk from anaerobic or Gram-negative infections (e.g. use co-amoxiclav alone for facial infection, orbital infection, or infection caused by animal or human bites. Use ceftazidime + clindamycin in immunocompromised patients)

Staphylococcal scalded skin syndrome

Flucloxacillin (*or* clarithromycin[2] if penicillin-allergic)

Treat for 7–10 days

Animal and human bites

Co-amoxiclav alone (*or* clindamycin if penicillin-allergic)

Cleanse wound thoroughly; for tetanus-prone wound, give human tetanus immunoglobulin (with adsorbed diphtheria [low dose] and tetanus vaccine if necessary, according to immunisation history and risk of infection), see under Tetanus Vaccines, section 14.4; consider rabies prophylaxis (section 14.4) for bites from animals in endemic countries; assess risk of blood-borne viruses

Acne—see section 13.6

Paronychia or 'septic spots' in neonate

Flucloxacillin

Add aminoglycoside if systemically unwell

Surgical wound infection

Flucloxacillin *or* co-amoxiclav

Table 2. Summary of antibacterial prophylaxis

Prevention of recurrence of rheumatic fever

Phenoxymethylpenicillin by mouth

Child 1 month–6 years 125 mg twice daily

Child 6–18 years 250 mg twice daily

or

Erythromycin by mouth

Child 1 month–2 years 125 mg twice daily

Child 2–18 years 250 mg twice daily

1. Where amoxicillin is suggested ampicillin may be used.
2. Where clarithromycin is suggested azithromycin or erythromycin may be used.

Prevention of secondary case of invasive group A streptococcal infection[1]

Phenoxymethylpenicillin by mouth

Neonate 12.5 mg/kg (max. 62.5 mg) every 6 hours for 10 days

Child 1 month–1 year 62.5 mg every 6 hours for 10 days

Child 1–6 years 125 mg every 6 hours for 10 days

Child 6–12 years 250 mg every 6 hours for 10 days

Child 12–18 years 250–500 mg every 6 hours for 10 days

If child penicillin allergic,

either erythromycin by mouth

Child 1 month–2 years 125 mg every 6 hours for 10 days

Child 2–8 years 250 mg every 6 hours for 10 days

Child 8–18 years 250–500 mg every 6 hours for 10 days

or azithromycin by mouth [unlicensed indication]

Child 6 months–12 years 12 mg/kg (max. 500 mg) once daily for 5 days

Child 12–18 years 500 mg once daily for 5 days

Prevention of secondary case of meningococcal meningitis[2]

Rifampicin by mouth

Neonate 5 mg/kg every 12 hours for 2 days

Child 1 month–1 year 5 mg/kg every 12 hours for 2 days

Child 1–12 years 10 mg/kg (max. 600 mg) every 12 hours for 2 days

Child 12–18 years 600 mg every 12 hours for 2 days

or

Ciprofloxacin by mouth [unlicensed indication]

Child 2–5 years 125 mg as a single dose

Child 5–12 years 250 mg as a single dose

Child 12–18 years 500 mg as a single dose

or

Ceftriaxone by intramuscular injection [unlicensed indication] (preferred if pregnant)

Child 1 month–12 years 125 mg as a single dose

Child 12–18 years 250 mg as a single dose

Prevention of secondary case of Haemophilus influenzae type b disease[2]

Rifampicin by mouth

Child 1–3 months 10 mg/kg once daily for 4 days

Child 3 months–12 years 20 mg/kg (max. 600 mg) once daily for 4 days

Child 12–18 years 600 mg once daily for 4 days

Prevention of secondary case of diphtheria in non-immune patient

Erythromycin by mouth

Child 1 month–2 years 125 mg every 6 hours for 7 days

Child 2–8 years 250 mg every 6 hours for 7 days

Child 8–18 years 500 mg every 6 hours for 7 days

Treat for further 10 days if nasopharyngeal swabs positive after first 7 days' treatment

1. For details of those who should receive chemoprophylaxis contact a consultant in communicable disease control (or a consultant in infectious diseases or the local Health Protection Agency Laboratory)
2. For details of those who should receive chemoprophylaxis contact a consultant in communicable disease control (or a consultant in infectious diseases or the local Health Protection Agency laboratory). Unless there has been direct exposure of the mouth or nose to infectious droplets from a patient with meningococcal disease who has received less than 24 hours of antibacterial treatment, healthcare workers do not generally require chemoprophylaxis.

Prevention of secondary case of pertussis in non-immune patient or partially immune patient

Erythromycin[1] by mouth

Child 1 month–2 years 125 mg every 6 hours for 7 days

Child 2–8 years 250 mg every 6 hours for 7 days

Child 8–18 years 250–500 mg every 6 hours for 7 days

Note Pertussis vaccine inappropriate for outbreak since 3 injections required for protection

Prevention of pneumococcal infection in asplenia or in patients with sickle-cell disease

Phenoxymethylpenicillin by mouth

Child 1 month–6 years 125 mg every 12 hours

Child 6–12 years 250 mg every 12 hours

Child 12–18 years 500 mg every 12 hours

If cover also needed for *H. influenzae* in child give amoxicillin instead

Child 1 month–5 years 125 mg every 12 hours

Child 5–12 years 250 mg every 12 hours

Child 12–18 years 500 mg every 12 hours

Note Antibiotic prophylaxis is not fully reliable; for vaccines in asplenia see p. 736

Prevention of *Staphylococcus aureus* lung infection in cystic fibrosis

Flucloxacillin by mouth

Neonate 125 mg every 12 hours

Child 1 month–3 years 125 mg every 12 hours; recurrent infection, 50 mg/kg every 12 hours

Child 3–18 years recurrent infection, 50 mg/kg every 12 hours

Prevention of tuberculosis in susceptible close contacts or those who have become tuberculin positive[2]

Isoniazid for 6 months

Neonate 5 mg/kg daily

Child 1 month –12 years 5 mg/kg daily (max. 300 mg daily)

Child 12–18 years 300 mg daily

or isoniazid + rifampicin for 3 months

Child 1 month–12 years isoniazid 5 mg/kg daily (max. 300 mg daily) + rifampicin 10 mg/kg daily (max. 450 mg daily if body-weight less than 50 kg; max. 600 mg daily if body-weight over 50 kg)

Child 12–18 years isoniazid 300 mg daily + rifampicin 600 mg daily (rifampicin 450 mg daily if body-weight less than 50 kg)

or (if isoniazid-resistant tuberculosis) rifampicin for 6 months

Child 1 month–12 years 10 mg/kg daily (max. 450 mg daily if body-weight less than 50 kg; max. 600 mg daily if body-weight over 50 kg)

Child 12–18 years 600 mg daily (450 mg daily if body-weight less than 50 kg)

1. Where erythromycin is suggested another macrolide (e.g. azithromycin or clarithromycin) may be used.
2. For details of those who should receive chemoprophylaxis contact the lead clinician for local tuberculosis services (or a consultant in communicable disease control). See also section 5.1.9, for advice on immunocompromised patients and on prevention of tuberculosis

Prevention of gas-gangrene in high lower-limb amputations or following major trauma

i/v benzylpenicillin

Child 1 month–12 years 25 mg/kg (max. 600 mg) every 6 hours for 5 days

Child 12–18 years 300–600 mg every 6 hours for 5 days

or if penicillin-allergic i/v or oral metronidazole

Child 1 month–12 years 7.5 mg/kg (max. 500 mg) every 8 hours for 5 days

Child 12–18 years 400–500 mg every 8 hours for 5 days

Prevention of infection in gastro-intestinal procedures
Operations on stomach or oesophagus[1]

Single dose[2] of i/v gentamicin *or* i/v cefuroxime *or* i/v co-amoxiclav
Add i/v teicoplanin[3] if high risk of meticillin-resistant *Staphylococcus aureus*

Open biliary surgery[1]

Single dose[2] of i/v cefuroxime + i/v metronidazole[4] *or* i/v gentamicin + i/v metronidazole[4]
Add i/v teicoplanin[3] if high risk of meticillin-resistant *Staphylococcus aureus*

Resections of colon and rectum, and resections in inflammatory bowel disease, and appendicectomy[1]

Single dose[2] of i/v gentamicin + i/v metronidazole[4] *or* i/v cefuroxime + i/v metronidazole[4] *or* i/v co-amoxiclav alone
Add i/v teicoplanin[3] if high risk of meticillin-resistant *Staphylococcus aureus*

Endoscopic retrograde cholangiopancreatography[1]

Single dose of i/v gentamicin *or* oral or i/v ciprofloxacin
Prophylaxis recommended if pancreatic pseudocyst, immunocompromised, history of liver transplantation, or risk of incomplete biliary drainage

Percutaneous endoscopic gastrostomy or jejunostomy[1]

Single dose of i/v co-amoxiclav or i/v cefuroxime
Use single dose of i/v teicoplanin[3] if history of allergy to penicillins or cephalosporins, or if high risk of meticillin-resistant *Staphylococcus aureus*

Prevention of infection in orthopaedic surgery
Closed fractures[1]

Single dose[2] of i/v cefuroxime *or* i/v flucloxacillin
If history of allergy to penicillins or to cephalosporins or if high risk of meticillin-resistant *Staphylococcus aureus*, use single dose[2] of i/v teicoplanin[3]

Open fractures

i/v cefuroxime alone *or* i/v flucloxacillin + i/v gentamicin
If history of allergy to penicillins or to cephalosporins or if high risk of meticillin-resistant *Staphylococcus aureus*, use i/v teicoplanin[3] + i/v gentamicin. Use cefuroxime + metronidazole for complex open fractures with extensive soft tissue damage. Prophylaxis continued for 24 hours (longer if complex open fractures)

Prevention of infection in obstetric surgery
Termination of pregnancy

Single dose[2] of oral metronidazole
If genital chlamydial infection cannot be ruled out, give doxycycline (section 5.1.3) postoperatively

1. Intravenous antibacterial prophylaxis should be given up to 30 minutes before the procedure
2. Additional intra-operative or postoperative doses of antibacterial may be given for prolonged procedures or if there is major blood loss
3. Where teicoplanin is suggested vancomycin may be used
4. Metronidazole may alternatively be given by suppository but to allow adequate absorption, it should be given 2 hours before surgery

5 Infections

Prevention of endocarditis

> **NICE Guidance**
>
> Antimicrobial prophylaxis against infective endocarditis in children and adults undergoing interventional procedures (March 2008)
>
> Antibacterial prophylaxis and chlorhexidine mouthwash are **not** recommended for the prevention of endocarditis in patients undergoing dental procedures.
>
> Antibacterial prophylaxis is **not** recommended for the prevention of endocarditis in patients undergoing procedures of the:
>
> - upper and lower respiratory tract (including ear, nose, and throat procedures and bronchoscopy);
> - genito-urinary tract (including urological, gynaecological, and obstetric procedures);
> - upper and lower gastro-intestinal tract.
>
> While these procedures can cause bacteraemia, there is no clear association with the development of infective endocarditis. Prophylaxis may expose patients to the adverse effects of antimicrobials when the evidence of benefit has not been proven.
>
> Any infection in patients at risk of endocarditis[1] should be investigated promptly and treated appropriately to reduce the risk of endocarditis.
>
> If patients at risk of endocarditis[1] are undergoing a gastro-intestinal or genito-urinary tract procedure at a site where infection is suspected, they should receive appropriate antibacterial therapy that includes cover against organisms that cause endocarditis.
>
> Patients at risk of endocarditis[1] should be:
>
> - advised to maintain good oral hygiene;
> - told how to recognise signs of infective endocarditis, and advised when to seek expert advice.

> **Dermatological procedures**
>
> Advice of a Working Party of the British Society for Antimicrobial Chemotherapy is that patients who undergo dermatological procedures[2] do not require antibacterial prophylaxis against endocarditis.

Joint prostheses and dental treatment

> **Joint prostheses and dental treatment**
>
> Advice of a Working Party of the British Society for Antimicrobial Chemotherapy is that patients with prosthetic joint implants (including total hip replacements) do not require antibacterial prophylaxis for dental treatment. The Working Party considers that it is unacceptable to expose patients to the adverse effects of antibacterials when there is no evidence that such prophylaxis is of any benefit, but that those who develop any intercurrent infection require prompt treatment with antibacterials to which the infecting organisms are sensitive.
>
> The Working Party has commented that joint infections have rarely been shown to follow dental procedures and are even more rarely caused by oral streptococci.

---

1. Patients at risk of endocarditis include those with valve replacement, acquired valvular heart disease with stenosis or regurgitation, structural congenital heart disease (including surgically corrected or palliated structural conditions, but excluding isolated atrial septal defect, fully repaired ventricular septal defect, fully repaired patent ductus arteriosus, ure devices considered to be endothelialised), hypertrophic cardiomyopathy, or a previous episode of infective ditis.

itish Association of Dermatologists Therapy Guidelines and Audit Subcommittee advise that such ological procedures include skin biopsies and excision of moles or of malignant lesions

Infections

5

Immunosuppression and indwelling intraperitoneal catheters

> Immunosuppression and indwelling intraperitoneal catheters
> Advice of a Working Party of the British Society for Antimicrobial Che-
> motherapy is that patients who are immunosuppressed (including transplant
> patients) and patients with indwelling intraperitoneal catheters do not require
> antibacterial prophylaxis for dental treatment provided there is no other
> indication for prophylaxis.
> The Working Party has commented that there is little evidence that dental
> treatment is followed by infection in immunosuppressed and immunodeficient
> patients nor is there evidence that dental treatment is followed by infection in
> patients with indwelling intraperitoneal catheters.

5.1.1 Penicillins

5.1.1.1 Benzylpenicillin and phenoxymethylpenicillin
5.1.1.2 Penicillinase-resistant penicillins
5.1.1.3 Broad-spectrum penicillins
5.1.1.4 Antipseudomonal penicillins
5.1.1.5 Mecillinams

The penicillins are bactericidal and act by interfering with bacterial cell wall
synthesis. They diffuse well into body tissues and fluids, but penetration into the
cerebrospinal fluid is poor except when the meninges are inflamed. They are
excreted in the urine in therapeutic concentrations.

Hypersensitivity reactions   The most important side-effect of the penicillins is
hypersensitivity which causes rashes and anaphylaxis and can be fatal. Allergic
reactions to penicillins occur in 1–10% of exposed individuals; anaphylactic
reactions occur in fewer than 0.05% of treated patients. Individuals with a history
of anaphylaxis, urticaria, or rash immediately after penicillin administration are at
risk of immediate hypersensitivity to a penicillin; these individuals should not
receive a penicillin. Children who are allergic to one penicillin will be allergic to all
because the hypersensitivity is related to the basic penicillin structure. As patients
with a history of immediate hypersensitivity to penicillins may also react to the
cephalosporins and other beta-lactam antibiotics, they should not receive these
antibiotics; aztreonam may be less likely to cause hypersensitivity in penicillin-
sensitive patients and can be used with caution. If a penicillin (or another beta-
lactam antibiotic) is essential in a child with immediate hypersensitivity to penicillin then specialist advice should be sought on hypersensitivity testing or using a
beta-lactam antibiotic with a different structure to the penicillin that caused the
hypersensitivity (see also p. 326).

Individuals with a history of a minor rash (i.e. non-confluent, non-pruritic rash
restricted to a small area of the body) or a rash that occurs more than 72 hours
after penicillin administration are probably not allergic to penicillin and in these
individuals a penicillin should not be withheld unnecessarily for serious infections;
the possibility of an allergic reaction should, however, be borne in mind. Other
beta-lactam antibiotics (including cephalosporins) can be used in these patients.

Other side effects   A rare but serious toxic effect of the penicillins is encephalopathy due to cerebral irritation. This may result from excessively high doses or in
patients with severe renal failure. The penicillins should **not** be given by intrathecal injection because they can cause encephalopathy which may be fatal.

Another problem relating to high doses of penicillin, or normal doses given to
patients with renal failure, is the accumulation of electrolyte since most injectable
penicillins contain either sodium or potassium.

Diarrhoea frequently occurs during oral penicillin therapy. It is most common
with broad-spectrum penicillins, which can also cause antibiotic-associated colitis.

5

Infections

5.1.1.1 Benzylpenicillin and phenoxymethylpenicillin

Benzylpenicillin (Penicillin G) remains an important and useful antibiotic but is inactivated by bacterial beta-lactamases. It is effective for many streptococcal (including pneumococcal), gonococcal, and meningococcal infections and also for anthrax (section 5.1.12), diphtheria, gas-gangrene, leptospirosis, and treatment of Lyme disease (section 5.1.1.3) in children. It is also used in combination with gentamicin for the empirical treatment of sepsis in neonates less than 48 hours old. Pneumococci, meningococci, and gonococci which have decreased sensitivity to penicillin have been isolated; **benzylpenicillin is no longer the drug of first choice for pneumococcal meningitis**. Although benzylpenicillin is effective in the treatment of tetanus, metronidazole (section 5.1.11) is preferred. Benzylpenicillin is inactivated by gastric acid and absorption from the gastro-intestinal tract is low; therefore it must be given by injection.

Benzathine benzylpenicillin or **procaine benzylpenicillin** is used in the treatment of syphilis (see Table 1 section 5.1); both are available from 'special-order' manufacturers or specialist importing companies, see p. 957.

Phenoxymethylpenicillin (Penicillin V) has a similar antibacterial spectrum to benzylpenicillin, but is less active. It is gastric acid-stable, so is suitable for oral administration. It should not be used for serious infections because absorption can be unpredictable and plasma concentrations variable. It is indicated principally for respiratory-tract infections in children, for streptococcal tonsillitis, and for continuing treatment after one or more injections of benzylpenicillin when clinical response has begun. It should not be used for meningococcal or gonococcal infections. Phenoxymethylpenicillin is used for prophylaxis against streptococcal infections following rheumatic fever and against pneumococcal infections following splenectomy or in sickle cell disease.

Oral infections Phenoxymethylpenicillin is effective for dentoalveolar abscess.

BENZYLPENICILLIN SODIUM
(Penicillin G)

Cautions history of allergy; false-positive urinary glucose (if tested for reducing substances); **interactions:** Appendix 1 (penicillins)

Contra-indications penicillin hypersensitivity

Renal impairment neurotoxicity—high doses may cause convulsions. Estimated glomerular filtration rate 10–50 mL/minute/1.73 m², use normal dose every 8–12 hours; estimated glomerular filtration rate less than 10 mL/minute/ 1.73 m² use normal dose every 12 hours

Pregnancy not known to be harmful

Breast-feeding trace amounts in milk—not known to be harmful, but be alert for hypersensitivity in infant

Side-effects hypersensitivity reactions including urticaria, fever, joint pains, rashes, angioedema, anaphylaxis, serum sickness-like reactions; *rarely* CNS toxicity including convulsions (especially with high doses or in severe renal impairment), interstitial nephritis, haemolytic anaemia, leucopenia, thrombocytopenia and coagulation disorders; also reported diarrhoea (including antibiotic-associated colitis)

Indication and dose

Mild to moderate susceptible infections (including throat infections, otitis media, pneumonia, cellulitis, neonatal sepsis, Table 1, section 5.1)

• By intramuscular injection or by slow intravenous injection or infusion (intravenous route recommended in neonates and infants)

Neonate under 7 days 25 mg/kg every 12 hours; dose doubled in severe infection

Neonate 7–28 days 25 mg/kg every 8 hours; dose doubled in severe infection

Child 1 month–18 years 25 mg/kg every 6 hours; increased to 50 mg/kg every 4–6 hours (max. 2.4 g every 4 hours) in severe infection

Endocarditis (combined with another antibacterial if necessary, see Table 1, section 5.1)

• By slow intravenous injection or infusion

Child 1 month–18 years 25 mg/kg every 4 hours, increased if necessary to 50 mg/kg (max. 2.4 g) every 4 hours

Meningitis, meningococcal disease

• By slow intravenous injection or infusion

Neonate 75 mg/kg every 8 hours

Child 1 month–18 years 50 mg/kg every 4–6 hours (max. 2.4 g every 4 hours)

Important. If bacterial meningitis and especially if meningococcal disease is suspected, general practitioners are advised to give a single injection of benzylpenicillin by intravenous injection (or by intramuscular injection) before transferring the patient urgently to hospital. Suitable doses are: Infant under 1 year 300 mg; Child 1–9 years 600 mg, 10 years and over 1.2 g. In penicillin allergy, cefotaxime (section 5.1.2) may be an alternative; chloramphenicol may be used if there is a history of anaphylaxis to penicillins

Treatment or prevention of neonatal group B streptococcus infection

• By slow intravenous injection or infusion

Neonate under 7 days 50 mg/kg every 12 hours

Neonate 7–28 days 50 mg/kg every 8 hours

⌐ **BENZYLPENICILLIN SODIUM** (*continued*)

Prophylaxis in limb amputation Table 2, section 5.1

Safe practice Intrathecal injection of benzylpenicillin is **not** recommended

Administration Intravenous route recommended in neonates and infants. For *intravenous infusion*, dilute with Glucose 5% *or* Sodium Chloride 0.9%; give over 15–30 minutes. Longer administration time is particularly important when using doses of 50 mg/kg (or greater) to avoid CNS toxicity

Crystapen® (Genus) ℗ₒₘ
Injection, powder for reconstitution, benzylpenicillin sodium (unbuffered), net price 600-mg vial = 95p, 2-vial 'GP pack' = £2.64; 1.2-g vial = £1.89
Electrolytes Na⁺ 1.68 mmol/600-mg vial; 3.36 mmol/1.2-g vial

◤ PHENOXYMETHYLPENICILLIN

(Penicillin V)

Cautions see under Benzylpenicillin; **interactions**: Appendix 1 (penicillins)

Contra-indications see under Benzylpenicillin

Pregnancy not known to be harmful

Breast-feeding trace amounts in milk—not known to be harmful, but be alert for hypersensitivity in infant

Side-effects see under Benzylpenicillin

Indication and dose

Susceptible infections including oral infections, tonsillitis, otitis media, erysipelas, cellulitis

• By mouth

Child 1 month–1 year 62.5 mg 4 times daily; increased up to 12.5 mg/kg 4 times daily in severe infection

Child 1–6 years 125 mg 4 times daily; increased up to 12.5 mg/kg 4 times daily in severe infection

Child 6–12 years 250 mg 4 times daily; increased up to 12.5 mg/kg 4 times daily in severe infection

Child 12–18 years 500 mg 4 times daily; increased in severe infection up to 1 g 4 times daily

Prevention of pneumococcal infection in asplenia or sickle cell disease, see Table 2, section 5.1

Prevention of recurrence of rheumatic fever, see Table 2, section 5.1

Prevention of group A streptococcal infection, see Table 2, section 5.1

Phenoxymethylpenicillin (Non-proprietary) ℗ₒₘ
Tablets, phenoxymethylpenicillin (as potassium salt) 250 mg, net price 28-tab pack = £1.29. Label: 9, 23
Dental prescribing on NHS Phenoxymethylpenicillin Tablets may be prescribed

Oral solution, phenoxymethylpenicillin (as potassium salt) for reconstitution with water, net price 125 mg/5 mL, 100 mL = £1.90; 250 mg/5 mL, 100 mL = £2.59. Label: 9, 23
Dental prescribing on NHS Phenoxymethylpenicillin Oral Solution may be prescribed

5 | **Infections**

5.1.1.2 Penicillinase-resistant penicillins

Most staphylococci are now resistant to benzylpenicillin because they produce penicillinases. **Flucloxacillin**, however, is not inactivated by these enzymes and is thus effective in infections caused by penicillin-resistant staphylococci, which is the main indication for its use. Flucloxacillin is acid-stable and can, therefore, be given by mouth as well as by injection.

Flucloxacillin is well absorbed from the gut. For a warning on hepatic disorders see under Flucloxacillin.

MRSA Infection from *Staphylococcus aureus* strains resistant to meticillin [now discontinued] (meticillin-resistant *Staph. aureus*, MRSA) and to flucloxacillin can be difficult to manage. Treatment is guided by the sensitivity of the infecting strain.

Rifampicin (section 5.1.9) or **sodium fusidate** (section 5.1.7) should **not** be used alone because resistance may develop rapidly. **Clindamycin** alone or a combination of rifampicin and sodium fusidate can be used for *skin and soft-tissue infections* caused by MRSA; a **tetracycline** is an alternative in children over 12 years of age. A **glycopeptide** (e.g. vancomycin, section 5.1.7) can be used for severe skin and soft-tissue infections associated with MRSA. A combination of a glycopeptide and sodium fusidate *or* a glycopeptide and rifampicin can be considered for skin and soft-tissue infections that have failed to respond to a single antibacterial. **Linezolid** (section 5.1.7) should be reserved for skin and soft-tissue infections that have not responded to other antibacterials or for children who cannot tolerate other antibacterials.

A **glycopeptide** can be used for *pneumonia* associated with MRSA. **Linezolid** should be reserved for hospital-acquired pneumonia that has not responded to other antibacterials or for children who cannot tolerate other antibacterials.

Trimethoprim or **nitrofurantoin** can be used for *urinary-tract infections* caused by MRSA; a **tetracycline** is an alternative in children over 12 years of age. A **glycopeptide** can be used for urinary-tract infections that are severe or resistant to other antibacterials.

A **glycopeptide** can be used for *septicaemia* associated with MRSA.

For the management of endocarditis, osteomyelitis, or septic arthritis associated with MRSA, see Table 1, section 5.1.

Prophylaxis with vancomycin or teicoplanin (alone or in combination with another antibacterial active against other pathogens) is appropriate for patients undergoing surgery if:

- there is a history of MRSA colonisation or infection without documented eradication;
- there is a risk that the patient's MRSA carriage has recurred;
- the patient comes from an area with a high prevalence of MRSA.

It is important that hospitals have infection control guidelines to minimise MRSA transmission, including policies on isolation and treatment of MRSA carriers and on hand hygiene. For eradication of nasal carriage of MRSA, see section 12.2.3.

FLUCLOXACILLIN

Cautions see under Benzylpenicillin (section 5.1.1.1); risk of kernicterus in jaundiced neonates when high doses given parenterally; **interactions**: Appendix 1 (penicillins)

> **Hepatic disorders** Cholestatic jaundice and hepatitis may occur very rarely, up to several weeks after treatment with flucloxacillin has been stopped. Administration for more than 2 weeks and increasing age are risk factors. Healthcare professionals are reminded that:
> - flucloxacillin should not be used in patients with a history of hepatic dysfunction associated with flucloxacillin;
> - flucloxacillin should be used with caution in patients with hepatic impairment;
> - careful enquiry should be made about hypersensitivity reactions to beta-lactam antibacterials.

Contra-indications see under Benzylpenicillin (section 5.1.1.1)

Hepatic impairment see Cautions and Hepatic Disorders above

Renal impairment use normal dose every 8 hours if estimated glomerular filtration rate less than 10 mL/minute/1.73 m^2

Pregnancy not known to be harmful

Breast-feeding trace amounts in milk—not known to be harmful but be alert for hypersensitivity in infant

Side-effects see under Benzylpenicillin (section 5.1.1.1); also gastro-intestinal disturbances; *very rarely* hepatitis and cholestatic jaundice reported (see also Hepatic Disorders above)

Indication and dose

Infections due to beta-lactamase-producing staphylococci including otitis externa; adjunct in pneumonia, impetigo, cellulitis
- By mouth

Neonate under 7 days 25 mg/kg twice daily

Neonate 7–21 days 25 mg/kg 3 times daily

Neonate 21–28 days 25 mg/kg 4 times daily

Child 1 month–2 years 62.5–125 mg 4 times daily

Child 2–10 years 125–250 mg 4 times daily

Child 10–18 years 250–500 mg 4 times daily

- By intramuscular injection

Child 1 month–18 years 12.5–25 mg/kg every 6 hours (max. 500 mg every 6 hours)

- By slow intravenous injection or by intravenous infusion

Neonate under 7 days 25 mg/kg every 12 hours; may be doubled in severe infection

Neonate 7–21 days 25 mg/kg every 8 hours; may be doubled in severe infection

Neonate 21–28 days 25 mg/kg every 6 hours; may be doubled in severe infection

Child 1 month–18 years 12.5–25 mg/kg every 6 hours (max. 1 g every 6 hours); may be doubled in severe infection

Osteomyelitis (Table 1, section 5.1), cerebral abscess, staphylococcal meningitis
- By slow intravenous injection or by intravenous infusion

Neonate under 7 days 50–100 mg/kg every 12 hours

Neonate 7–21 days 50–100 mg/kg every 8 hours

Neonate 21–28 days 50–100 mg/kg every 6 hours

Child 1 month–18 years 50 mg/kg (max. 2 g) every 6 hours

◻ **FLUCLOXACILLIN** (*continued*)

Endocarditis (Table 1, section 5.1)
- **By slow intravenous injection or by intravenous infusion**

  Child 1 month–18 years 50 mg/kg (max. 2 g) every 6 hours

Prevention of staphylococcal lung infection in cystic fibrosis

  Table 2, section 5.1

Staphylococcal lung infection in cystic fibrosis
- **By mouth**

  Child 1 month–18 years 12.5–25 mg/kg (max. 1 g) 4 times daily; total daily dose may alternatively be given in 3 divided doses

Administration for *intermittent intravenous infusion*, dilute reconstituted solution in Glucose 5% *or* Sodium Chloride 0.9% and give over 30–60 minutes

Flucloxacillin (Non-proprietary) ▣ PoM
  Capsules, flucloxacillin (as sodium salt) 250 mg, net price 28 = £1.84; 500 mg, 28 = £2.50. Label: 9, 23
  Brands include *Floxapen*®, *Fluclomix*®, *Ladropen*®

  Oral solution (= elixir or syrup), flucloxacillin (as sodium salt) for reconstitution with water, 125 mg/5 mL, net price 100 mL = £3.67; 250 mg/5 mL, 100 mL = £26.70. Label: 9, 23
  Note Sugar-free versions are available and can be ordered by specifying 'sugar-free' on the prescription

  Injection, powder for reconstitution, flucloxacillin (as sodium salt). Net price 250-mg vial = £1.23; 500-mg vial = £2.45; 1-g vial = £4.90

5.1.1.3 Broad-spectrum penicillins

Ampicillin is active against certain Gram-positive and Gram-negative organisms but is inactivated by penicillinases including those produced by *Staphylococcus aureus* and by common Gram-negative bacilli such as *Escherichia coli*. Ampicillin is also active against *Listeria* spp. and enterococci. Almost all staphylococci, approx. 60% of *E. coli* strains and approx. 20% of *Haemophilus influenzae* strains are now resistant. The likelihood of resistance should therefore be considered before using ampicillin for the 'blind' treatment of infections; in particular, it should not be used for hospital patients without checking sensitivity.

Ampicillin can be given by mouth, but less than half the dose is absorbed and absorption is further decreased by the presence of food in the gut. Ampicillin is well excreted in the bile and urine.

Amoxicillin (amoxycillin) is a derivative of ampicillin and has a similar antibacterial spectrum. It is better absorbed than ampicillin when given by mouth, producing higher plasma and tissue concentrations; unlike ampicillin, absorption is not affected by the presence of food in the stomach.

Amoxicillin or ampicillin are principally indicated for the treatment of community-acquired pneumonia and middle ear infections, both of which may be due to *Streptococcus pneumoniae* and *H. influenzae*, and for urinary-tract infections (section 5.1.13). They are also used in the treatment of endocarditis and listerial meningitis. Amoxicillin may also be used for the treatment of Lyme disease [not licensed], see below.

Maculopapular rashes occur commonly with ampicillin (and amoxicillin) but are not usually related to true penicillin allergy. They often occur in children with glandular fever; broad-spectrum penicillins should not therefore be used for 'blind' treatment of a sore throat. Rashes are also common in children with acute or chronic lymphocytic leukaemia or in cytomegalovirus infection.

Co-amoxiclav consists of amoxicillin with the beta-lactamase inhibitor clavulanic acid. Clavulanic acid itself has no significant antibacterial activity but, by inactivating beta-lactamases, it makes the combination active against beta-lactamase-producing bacteria that are resistant to amoxicillin. These include resistant strains of *Staph. aureus*, *E. coli*, and *H. influenzae*, as well as many *Bacteroides* and *Klebsiella* spp. Co-amoxiclav should be reserved for infections likely, or known, to be caused by amoxicillin-resistant beta-lactamase-producing strains.

A combination of ampicillin with flucloxacillin (as co-fluampicil) is available to treat infections involving either streptococci or staphylococci (e.g. cellulitis).

Lyme disease Lyme disease should generally be treated by those experienced in its management. **Amoxicillin** [unlicensed indication], **cefuroxime axetil** or **doxycycline** are the antibacterials of choice for *early Lyme disease* or *Lyme arthritis* but doxycycline should only be used in children over 12 years of age. If these antibacterials are contra-indicated, a **macrolide** (e.g. erythromycin) can be used for early Lyme disease. Intravenous administration of **ceftriaxone**, **cefotaxime** (section 5.1.2.1), or **benzylpenicillin** (p. 316) is recommended for Lyme disease associated with cardiac or neurological complications. The duration of treatment is usually 2–4 weeks; Lyme arthritis may require further treatment.

Oral infections Amoxicillin or ampicillin are as effective as phenoxymethylpenicillin (section 5.1.1.1) but they are better absorbed; however, they may encourage emergence of resistant organisms.

Like phenoxymethylpenicillin, amoxicillin and ampicillin are ineffective against bacteria that produce beta-lactamases. Co-amoxiclav is active against beta-lactamase-producing bacteria that are resistant to amoxicillin. Co-amoxiclav may be used for severe dental infection with spreading cellulitis or dental infection not responding to first-line antibacterial treatment.

AMOXICILLIN
(Amoxycillin)

Cautions see under Ampicillin; maintain adequate hydration with high doses (particularly during parenteral therapy); **interactions**: Appendix 1 (penicillins)

Contra-indications see under Ampicillin

Renal impairment risk of crystalluria with high doses (particularly during parenteral therapy) in mild to moderate impairment; reduce dose in severe impairment; rashes more common and risk of crystalluria

Pregnancy not known to be harmful

Breast-feeding trace amounts in milk—not known to be harmful but be alert for hypersensitivity in infant

Side-effects see under Ampicillin

Indication and dose

Susceptible infections including urinary-tract infections, sinusitis, uncomplicated community-acquired pneumonia, oral infections (Table 1, section 5.1), *Haemophilus influenzae* infections, Lyme disease (see notes above), salmonellosis

• By mouth

Neonate under 7 days 30 mg/kg (max. 62.5 mg) twice daily; dose doubled in severe infection

Neonate 7–28 days 30 mg/kg (max. 62.5 mg) 3 times daily; dose doubled in severe infection

Child 1 month–1 year 62.5 mg 3 times daily; dose doubled in severe infection, community-acquired pneumonia, salmonellosis, or Lyme disease

Child 1–5 years 125 mg 3 times daily; dose doubled in severe infection, community-acquired pneumonia, salmonellosis, or Lyme disease

Child 5–18 years 250 mg 3 times daily; dose doubled in severe infection, community-acquired pneumonia, salmonellosis, or Lyme disease

• By intravenous injection or infusion

Neonate under 7 days 30 mg/kg every 12 hours; dose doubled in severe infection, community-acquired pneumonia, or salmonellosis

Neonate 7–28 days 30 mg/kg every 8 hours; dose doubled in severe infection, community-acquired pneumonia, or salmonellosis

Child 1 month–18 years 20–30 mg/kg (max. 500 mg) every 8 hours; dose doubled in severe infection (max. 4 g daily)

Otitis media
• By mouth

Child 1 month–18 years 40 mg/kg daily in 3 divided doses (max. 1.5 g daily in 3 divided doses)

Listerial meningitis (in combination with another antibacterial, Table 1, section 5.1), group B streptococcal infection, enterococcal endocarditis (in combination with another antibiotic)
• By intravenous infusion

Neonate under 7 days 50 mg/kg every 12 hours; dose may be doubled in meningitis

Neonate 7–28 days 50 mg/kg every 8 hours; dose may be doubled in meningitis

Child 1 month–18 years 50 mg/kg every 4–6 hours (max. 2 g every 4 hours)

Cystic fibrosis (treatment of asymptomatic *H. influenzae* carriage or mild exacerbations)
• By mouth

Child 1 month–1 year 125 mg 3 times daily

Child 1–7 years 250 mg 3 times daily

Child 7–18 years 500 mg 3 times daily

Helicobacter pylori eradication section 1.3

Administration Displacement value may be significant when reconstituting injection, consult local guidelines. Dilute intravenous injection to a concentration of 50 mg/mL (100 mg/mL for neonates). May be further diluted with Glucose 5% or Glucose 10% or Sodium chloride 0.9% or 0.45% for intravenous infusion. Give intravenous infusion over 30 minutes when using doses over 30 mg/kg

Amoxicillin (Non-proprietary) ⒫ⓞⓜ
Capsules, amoxicillin (as trihydrate) 250 mg, net price 21 = £1.22; 500 mg, 21 = £1.55. Label: 9
Brands include *Amix*®, *Amoram*®, *Amoxident*®, *Galenamox*®, *Rimoxallin*®
Dental prescribing on NHS Amoxicillin Capsules may be prescribed

◁ **AMOXICILLIN** (*continued*)

Oral suspension, amoxicillin (as trihydrate) for reconstitution with water, 125 mg/5 mL, net price 100 mL = £1.44; 250 mg/5 mL, 100 mL = £1.52. Label: 9
Note Sugar-free versions are available and can be ordered by specifying 'sugar-free' on the prescription
Brands include *Amoram*®, *Galenamox*®, *Rimoxallin*®
Dental prescribing on NHS Amoxicillin Oral Suspension may be prescribed

Sachets, sugar-free, amoxicillin (as trihydrate) 3 g/sachet, net price 2-sachet pack = £6.77, 14-sachet pack = £31.94. Label: 9, 13
Dental prescribing on NHS Amoxicillin Sachets may be prescribed as Amoxicillin Oral Powder

Injection, powder for reconstitution, amoxicillin (as sodium salt), net price 250-mg vial = 32p; 500-mg vial = 66p; 1-g vial = £1.16

Amoxil® (GSK) ℗ₒℳ
Capsules, both maroon/gold, amoxicillin (as trihydrate), 250 mg, net price 21-cap pack = £3.45; 500 mg, 21-cap pack = £6.91. Label: 9

Paediatric suspension, amoxicillin 125 mg (as trihydrate)/1.25 mL when reconstituted with water, net price 20 mL (peach- strawberry- and lemon-flavoured) = £3.25. Label: 9, counselling , use of pipette
Excipients include sucrose 600 mg/1.25 mL

Sachets SF, powder, sugar-free, amoxicillin (as trihydrate) 3 g/sachet, 2-sachet pack (peach- strawberry- and lemon-flavoured) = £2.99. Label: 9, 13

Injection, powder for reconstitution, amoxicillin (as sodium salt), net price 500-mg vial = 56p; 1-g vial = £1.12
Electrolytes Na⁺ 3.3 mmol/g

◢ **AMPICILLIN**

Cautions history of allergy; erythematous rashes common in glandular fever, cytomegalovirus infection, and acute or chronic lymphocytic leukaemia (see notes above); **interactions:** Appendix 1 (penicillins)

Contra-indications penicillin hypersensitivity

Renal impairment if estimated glomerular filtration rate less than $10 \, mL/minute/1.73 \, m^2$ reduce dose or frequency—rashes more common

Pregnancy not known to be harmful

Breast-feeding trace amounts in milk—not known to be harmful but be alert for hypersensitivity in infant

Side-effects nausea, vomiting, diarrhoea; rashes (discontinue treatment); rarely, antibiotic-associated colitis; see also under Benzylpenicillin (section 5.1.1.1)

Indication and dose

Susceptible infections including urinary-tract infections, otitis media, sinusitis, uncomplicated community-acquired pneumonia, oral infections (Table 1, section 5.1), *Haemophilus influenzae* infections, salmonellosis
• By mouth

Neonate under 7 days 30 mg/kg (max. 62.5 mg) twice daily; dose doubled in severe infection

Neonate 7–21 days 30 mg/kg (max. 62.5 mg) 3 times daily; dose doubled in severe infection

Neonate 21–28 days 30 mg/kg (max. 62.5 mg) 4 times daily; dose doubled in severe infection

Child 1 month–1 year 62.5 mg 4 times daily; dose doubled in severe infection, community-acquired pneumonia, or salmonellosis

Child 1–5 years 125 mg 4 times daily; dose doubled in severe infection, community-acquired pneumonia, or salmonellosis

Child 5–12 years 250 mg 4 times daily; dose doubled in severe infection, community-acquired pneumonia, or salmonellosis

Child 12–18 years 500 mg 4 times daily; dose doubled in severe infection

• By intravenous injection or infusion

Neonate under 7 days 30 mg/kg every 12 hours; dose doubled in severe infection, community-acquired pneumonia, or salmonellosis

Neonate 7–21 days 30 mg/kg every 8 hours; dose doubled in severe infection, community-acquired pneumonia, or salmonellosis

Neonate 21–28 days 30 mg/kg every 6 hours; dose doubled in severe infection, community-acquired pneumonia, or salmonellosis

Child 1 month–18 years 25 mg/kg (max. 1 g) every 6 hours; dose doubled in severe infection

Listerial meningitis, group B streptococcal infection, enterococcal endocarditis (in combination with another antibacterial, see Table 1, section 5.1)
• By intravenous infusion

Neonate under 7 days 50 mg/kg every 12 hours; dose doubled in meningitis

Neonate 7–21 days 50 mg/kg every 8 hours; dose doubled in meningitis

Neonate 21–28 days 50 mg/kg every 6 hours; dose doubled in meningitis

Child 1 month–18 years 50 mg/kg every 4–6 hours (max. 2 g every 4 hours)

Administration *Oral*: administer at least 30 minutes before food
Injection: displacement value may be significant when reconstituting injection, consult local guidelines. Dilute intravenous injection to a concentration of 50–100 mg/mL. May be further diluted with glucose 5% or 10% or sodium chloride 0.9% or 0.45% for infusion. Give over 30 minutes when using doses of greater than 50 mg/kg to avoid CNS toxicity including convulsions.

Ampicillin (Non-proprietary) ℗ₒℳ
Capsules, ampicillin 250 mg, net price 28 = £5.44; 500 mg, 28 = £26.09. Label: 9, 23
Brands include *Rimacillin*®
Dental prescribing on NHS Ampicillin Capsules may be prescribed

5

Infections

◻ **AMPICILLIN (continued)**

Oral suspension, ampicillin 125 mg/5 mL when reconstituted with water, net price 100 mL = £6.19; 250 mg/5 mL, 100 mL = £12.80. Label: 9, 23
Brands include *Rimacillin®*
Dental prescribing on NHS Ampicillin Oral Suspension may be prescribed

Injection, powder for reconstitution, ampicillin (as sodium salt), net price 500-mg vial = £7.83

Penbritin® (Chemidex) PoM
Capsules, both grey/red, ampicillin (as trihydrate) 250 mg, net price 28-cap pack = £2.10; 500 mg, 28-cap pack = £5.28. Label: 9, 23

Syrup, apricot- caramel- and peppermint-flavoured, ampicillin (as trihydrate) for reconstitution with water, 125 mg/5 mL, net price 100 mL = £3.78; 250 mg/5 mL, 100 mL = £7.39. Label: 9, 23
Excipients include sucrose 3.6 g/5 mL

◀**With flucloxacillin**
Co-fluampicil (Non-proprietary) PoM
Capsules, co-fluampicil 250/250 (flucloxacillin 250 mg as sodium salt, ampicillin 250 mg as trihydrate), net price 28-cap pack = £19.09. Label: 9, 22
Brands include *Flu-Amp®*

Magnapen® (Wockhardt) PoM
Syrup, co-fluampicil 125/125 (flucloxacillin 125 mg as magnesium salt, ampicillin 125 mg as trihydrate)/5 mL when reconstituted with water, net price 100 mL = £4.99. Label: 9, 22
Excipients include sucrose 3.14 g/5 mL

Injection 500 mg, powder for reconstitution, co-fluampicil 250/250 (flucloxacillin 250 mg as sodium salt, ampicillin 250 mg as sodium salt), net price per vial = £1.33
Electrolytes Na⁺ 1.3 mmol/vial

◣ CO-AMOXICLAV

A mixture of amoxicillin (as the trihydrate or as the sodium salt) and clavulanic acid (as potassium clavulanate); the proportions are expressed in the form *x*/*y* where *x* and *y* are the strengths in milligrams of amoxicillin and clavulanic acid respectively

Cautions see under Ampicillin and notes above; maintain adequate hydration with high doses (particularly during parenteral therapy); **interactions**: Appendix 1 (penicillins)
Cholestatic jaundice Cholestatic jaundice can occur either during or shortly after the use of co-amoxiclav. An epidemiological study has shown that the risk of acute liver toxicity was about 6 times greater with co-amoxiclav than with amoxicillin; these reactions have only rarely been reported in children. Jaundice is usually self-limiting and very rarely fatal. The duration of treatment should be appropriate to the indication and should not usually exceed 14 days

Contra-indications penicillin hypersensitivity, history of co-amoxiclav-associated or penicillin-associated jaundice or hepatic dysfunction

Hepatic impairment monitor liver function in liver disease. See also Cholestatic Jaundice above

Renal impairment *Co-amoxiclav 125/31 suspension, 250/62 suspension, 250/125 tablets, or 500/125 tablets*: use normal dose every 12 hours if estimated glomerular filtration rate 10–30 mL/minute/1.73 m². Use the normal dose recommended for mild or moderate infections every 12 hours if estimated glomerular filtration rate less than 10 mL/minute/1.73 m².

Co-amoxiclav 400/57 suspension: avoid if estimated glomerular filtration rate less than 30 mL/minute/1.73 m².

Co-amoxiclav injection: use normal initial dose and then use half normal dose every 12 hours if estimated glomerular filtration rate 10–30 mL/minute/1.73 m²; use normal initial dose and then use half normal dose every 24 hours if estimated glomerular filtration rate less than 10 mL/minute/1.73 m²

Pregnancy not known to be harmful

Breast-feeding trace amounts present in milk—not known to be harmful but be alert for hypersensitivity in the infant

Side-effects see under Ampicillin; hepatitis, cholestatic jaundice (see above); Stevens-Johnson syndrome, toxic epidermal necrolysis, exfoliative dermatitis, vasculitis reported; rarely prolongation of bleeding time, dizziness, headache, convulsions (particularly with high doses or in renal impairment); superficial staining of teeth with suspension, phlebitis at injection site

Indication and dose

Infections due to beta-lactamase-producing strains (where amoxicillin alone not appropriate) including respiratory-tract infections, genito-urinary and abdominal infections, cellulitis, animal bites

- **By mouth, expressed as co-amoxiclav (see also under Twice Daily Oral Preparations below)**

Neonate 0.25 mL/kg of *125/31* suspension 3 times daily

Child 1 month–1 year 0.25 mL/kg of *125/31* suspension 3 times daily; dose doubled in severe infection

Child 1–6 years 5 mL of *125/31* suspension 3 times daily *or* 0.25 mL/kg of *125/31* suspension 3 times daily; dose doubled in severe infection

Child 6–12 years 5 mL of *250/62* suspension 3 times daily *or* 0.15 mL/kg of *250/62* suspension 3 times daily; dose doubled in severe infection

Child 12–18 years one *250/125* strength tablet 3 times daily; increased in severe infections to one *500/125* strength tablet 3 times daily

- **By intravenous injection over 3–4 minutes or by intravenous infusion, expressed as co-amoxiclav**

Preterm neonate and neonate under 7 days 30 mg/kg every 12 hours

Neonate 7–28 days 30 mg/kg every 8 hours

Child 1–3 months 30 mg/kg every 8 hours

Child 3 months–12 years 30 mg/kg every 8 hours increased in more serious infections to 30 mg/kg every 6 hours

Child 12–18 years 1.2 g every 8 hours increased in more serious infections to 1.2 g every 6 hours

◻ **CO-AMOXICLAV (*continued*)**

Severe dental infection with spreading cellulitis or dental infection not responding to first-line antibacterial, see notes above
- **By mouth, expressed as co-amoxiclav**
  Child 12–18 years one *250/125* strength tablet every 8 hours for 5 days

Administration for *intermittent intravenous infusion* dilute reconstituted solution to a concentration of 10 mg/mL with Sodium Chloride 0.9% or Water for Injections; give over 30–40 minutes and complete infusion within 4 hours of reconstitution.

Co-amoxiclav (Non-proprietary) ⟨PoM⟩
Tablets, co-amoxiclav 250/125 (amoxicillin 250 mg as trihydrate, clavulanic acid 125 mg as potassium salt), net price 21-tab pack = £3.17. Label: 9
Dental prescribing on NHS Co-amoxiclav 250/125 Tablets may be prescribed

Tablets, co-amoxiclav 500/125 (amoxicillin 500 mg as trihydrate, clavulanic acid 125 mg as potassium salt), net price 21-tab pack = £6.30. Label: 9

Oral suspension, co-amoxiclav 125/31 (amoxicillin 125 mg as trihydrate, clavulanic acid 31.25 mg as potassium salt)/5 mL when reconstituted with water, net price 100 mL = £4.20. Label: 9
Dental prescribing on NHS Co-amoxiclav 125/31 Suspension may be prescribed

Oral suspension, co-amoxiclav 250/62 (amoxicillin 250 mg as trihydrate, clavulanic acid 62.5 mg as potassium salt)/5 mL when reconstituted with water, net price 100 mL = £6.29. Label: 9
Dental prescribing on NHS Co-amoxiclav 250/62 Suspension may be prescribed

Injection 500/100, powder for reconstitution, co-amoxiclav 500/100 (amoxicillin 500 mg as sodium salt, clavulanic acid 100 mg as potassium salt), net price per vial = £1.26

Injection 1000/200, powder for reconstitution, co-amoxiclav 1000/200 (amoxicillin 1 g as sodium salt, clavulanic acid 200 mg as potassium salt), net price per vial = £2.52

Augmentin® (GSK) ⟨PoM⟩
Tablets 375 mg, f/c, co-amoxiclav 250/125 (amoxicillin 250 mg as trihydrate, clavulanic acid 125 mg as potassium salt), net price 21-tab pack = £4.28. Label: 9

Tablets 625 mg, f/c, co-amoxiclav 500/125 (amoxicillin 500 mg as trihydrate, clavulanic acid 125 mg as potassium salt). Net price 21-tab pack = £8.16. Label: 9

Suspension '125/31 SF', sugar-free, co-amoxiclav 125/31 (amoxicillin 125 mg as trihydrate, clavulanic acid 31.25 mg as potassium salt)/5 mL when reconstituted with water. Net price 100 mL (raspberry- and orange-flavoured) = £4.08. Label: 9
Excipients include aspartame 12.5 mg/5 mL (section 9.4.1)

Suspension '250/62 SF', sugar-free, co-amoxiclav 250/62 (amoxicillin 250 mg as trihydrate, clavulanic acid 62.5 mg as potassium salt)/5 mL when reconstituted with water. Net price 100 mL (raspberry- and orange-flavoured) = £5.74. Label: 9
Excipients include aspartame 12.5 mg/5 mL (section 9.4.1)

Injection 600 mg, powder for reconstitution, co-amoxiclav 500/100 (amoxicillin 500 mg as sodium salt, clavulanic acid 100 mg as potassium salt). Net price per vial = £1.33
Electrolytes Na⁺ 1.35 mmol, K⁺ 0.5 mmol/600-mg vial

Injection 1.2 g, powder for reconstitution, co-amoxiclav 1000/200 (amoxicillin 1 g as sodium salt, clavulanic acid 200 mg as potassium salt). Net price per vial = £2.65
Electrolytes Na⁺ 2.7 mmol, K⁺ 1 mmol/1.2-g vial

◢ **Twice daily oral preparations**
Co-amoxiclav (Non-proprietary) ⟨PoM⟩
Suspension '400/57', co-amoxiclav 400/57 (amoxicillin 400 mg as trihydrate, clavulanic acid 57 mg as potassium salt)/5 mL when reconstituted with water. Net price 35 mL = £4.21, 70 mL = £5.91. Label: 9
Excipients may include aspartame (section 9.4.1)
Brands include *Augmentin-Duo®*
Dose

> **Child 2 months–2 years** 0.15 mL/kg twice daily, doubled in severe infection
>
> **Child 2–6 years (13–21 kg)** 2.5 mL twice daily, doubled in severe infection
>
> **Child 7–12 years (22–40 kg)** 5 mL twice daily, doubled in severe infections

5 **Infections**

5.1.1.4 **Antipseudomonal penicillins**

The carboxypenicillin, **ticarcillin**, is principally indicated for serious infections caused by *Pseudomonas aeruginosa* although it also has activity against certain other Gram-negative bacilli including *Proteus* spp. and *Bacteroides fragilis*.

Ticarcillin is now available only in combination with clavulanic acid (section 5.1.1.3); the combination (*Timentin®*) is active against beta-lactamase-producing bacteria resistant to ticarcillin.

The ureidopenicillin, **piperacillin**, is more active than ticarcillin against *Ps. aeruginosa*. Piperacillin is now only available in combination with the beta-lactamase inhibitor tazobactam.

These antipseudomonal penicillins may be used for the empirical treatment of septicaemia in immunocompromised children but otherwise should generally be reserved for serious infections resistant to other antibacterials. For pseudomonas septicaemias (especially in neutropenia or endocarditis) these antipseudomonal penicillins should be given with an aminoglycoside (e.g. gentamicin, section 5.1.4) since they have a synergistic effect.

Piperacillin with tazobactam is used in cystic fibrosis for the treatment of *Ps. aeruginosa* colonisation when ciprofloxacin and nebulised colistin have been ineffective; it can also be used in infective exacerbations, when it is combined with an aminoglycoside.

Owing to the sodium content of many of these antibiotics, high doses may lead to hypernatraemia.

PIPERACILLIN WITH TAZOBACTAM

Cautions see under Benzylpenicillin (section 5.1.1.1); **interactions:** Appendix 1 (penicillins)

Contra-indications see under Benzylpenicillin (section 5.1.1.1)

Renal impairment dose expressed as a combination of piperacillin and tazobactam (both as sodium salts). Child under 12 years 90 mg/kg (max. 4.5 g) every 8 hours if estimated glomerular filtration rate 20–40 mL/minute/1.73 m²; 90 mg/kg (max. 4.5 g) every 12 hours if estimated glomerular filtration rate less than 20 mL/minute/1.73 m². Child 12–18 years max. 4.5 g every 8 hours if estimated glomerular filtration rate 20–80 mL/minute/1.73 m²; max. 4.5 g every 12 hours if estimated glomerular filtration rate less than 20 mL/minute/1.73 m²

Pregnancy manufacturer advises use only if potential benefit outweighs risk

Breast-feeding present in milk—manufacturer advises use only if potential benefit outweighs risk

Side-effects see under Benzylpenicillin (section 5.1.1.1); also nausea, vomiting, diarrhoea; *less commonly* stomatitis, dyspepsia, constipation, jaundice, hypotension, headache, insomnia, and injection-site reactions; *rarely* abdominal pain, hepatitis, oedema, fatigue and eosinophilia; *very rarely* hypoglycaemia, hypokalaemia, pancytopenia, Stevens-Johnson syndrome, and toxic epidermal necrolysis

Licensed use not licensed for use in children under 12 years (except for children with neutropenia and complicated appendicitis)

Indication and dose

> Note Expressed as a combination of piperacillin and tazobactam (both as sodium salts) in a ratio of 8:1

> **Lower respiratory tract, urinary-tract, intra-abdominal and skin infections, and bacterial septicaemia**
> • By intravenous injection over 3–5 minutes or by intravenous infusion
>> Neonate 90 mg/kg every 8 hours

> Child 1 month–12 years 90 mg/kg every 6–8 hours; (max 4.5 g every 6 hours)
> Child 12–18 years 2.25–4.5 g every 6–8 hours, usually 4.5 g every 8 hours

> **Infections in children with neutropenia** in combination with an aminoglycoside
> • By intravenous injection over 3–5 minutes or by intravenous infusion
>> Child 1 month–18 years 90 mg/kg (max. 4.5 g) every 6 hours

> **Complicated appendicitis**
> • By intravenous injection over 3–5 minutes or by intravenous infusion
>> Child 2–12 years 112.5 mg/kg (max. 4.5 g) every 8 hours for 5–14 days

Administration displacement value may be significant when reconstituting injection, consult local guidelines. For *intravenous infusion*, dilute reconstituted solution to a concentration of 15–90 mg/mL with Glucose 5% *or* Sodium Chloride 0.9% (*or* Compound Sodium Lactate for *Tazocin*® brand only), *or* to a concentration of 90 mg/mL with Water for Injections; give over 20–30 minutes

Piperacillin with tazobactam (Non-proprietary) ⓅoM
Injection 2.25 g, powder for reconstitution, piperacillin 2 g (as sodium salt), tazobactam 250 mg (as sodium salt), net price 2.25-g vial = £7.16

Injection 4.5 g, powder for reconstitution, piperacillin 4 g (as sodium salt), tazobactam 500 mg (as sodium salt), net price 4.5-g vial = £14.21

Tazocin® (Wyeth) ⓅoM
Injection 2.25 g, powder for reconstitution, piperacillin 2 g (as sodium salt), tazobactam 250 mg (as sodium salt), net price 2.25-g vial = £7.65
Electrolytes Na⁺ 5.58 mmol/2.25-g vial

Injection 4.5 g, powder for reconstitution, piperacillin 4 g (as sodium salt), tazobactam 500 mg (as sodium salt), net price 4.5-g vial = £15.17
Electrolytes Na⁺ 11.16 mmol/4.5-g vial

TICARCILLIN WITH CLAVULANIC ACID

Cautions see under Benzylpenicillin (section 5.1.1.1); **interactions:** Appendix 1 (penicillins)
Cholestatic jaundice For a warning on cholestatic jaundice possibly associated with clavulanic acid, see under Co-amoxiclav

Contra-indications see under Benzylpenicillin (section 5.1.1.1)

Hepatic impairment manufacturer advises caution in severe impairment; also cholestatic jaundice, see under Co-amoxiclav

Renal impairment Neonate reduce dose if estimated glomerular filtration rate less than 60 mL/minute/1.73 m². Child 1 month–18 years use normal dose every 8 hours if estimated glomerular filtration rate 30–60 mL/minute/1.73 m²; use half normal dose every 8 hours if estimated glomerular filtration rate 10–30 mL/minute/1.73 m²; use half normal dose every 12 hours if estimated glomerular filtration rate less than 10 mL/minute/1.73 m²

Pregnancy not known to be harmful

◁ **TICARCILLIN WITH CLAVULANIC ACID (***continued***)**

Breast-feeding trace amounts present in milk—not known to be harmful, but be alert for hypersensitivity in the infant

Side-effects see under Benzylpenicillin (section 5.1.1.1); also nausea, vomiting, coagulation disorders, haemorrhagic cystitis (more frequent in children), injection-site reactions, Stevens-Johnson syndrome, toxic epidermal necrolysis, hypokalaemia, eosinophilia

Indication and dose

> Note Expressed as a combination of ticarcillin (as sodium salt) and clavulanic acid (as potassium salt) in a ratio of 15:1

> **Infections due to *Pseudomonas* and *Proteus* spp.** see notes above
> ● **By intravenous infusion**
>
> > **Preterm neonate body-weight under 2 kg** 80 mg/kg every 12 hours

> **Preterm neonate body-weight over 2 kg and neonate** 80 mg/kg every 8 hours, increased to every 6 hours in more severe infections

> **Child 1 month–18 years and body-weight under 40 kg** 80 mg/kg every 8 hours, increased to every 6 hours in more severe infections

> **Child under 18 years and body-weight over 40 kg** 3.2 g every 6–8 hours, increased to every 4 hours in more severe infections

Administration Displacement value may be important, consult local guidelines. For intermittent infusion, dilute reconstituted solution further to a concentration of 16–32 mg/mL with glucose 5% *or* to a concentration of 32 mg/mL with water for injections; infuse over 30–40 minutes.

Timentin® (GSK) [PoM]
Injection 3.2 g, powder for reconstitution, ticarcillin 3 g (as sodium salt), clavulanic acid 200 mg (as potassium salt). Net price per vial = £5.44
Electrolytes Na⁺ 16 mmol, K⁺ 1 mmol / 3.2-g vial

5.1.1.5 Mecillinams

Pivmecillinam has significant activity against many Gram-negative bacteria including *Escherichia coli*, klebsiella, enterobacter, and salmonellae. It is not active against *Pseudomonas aeruginosa* or enterococci. Pivmecillinam is hydrolysed to mecillinam, which is the active drug.

PIVMECILLINAM HYDROCHLORIDE

Cautions see under Benzylpenicillin (section 5.1.1.1); also liver and renal function tests required in long-term use; avoid in acute porphyria (section 9.8.2); **interactions**: Appendix 1 (penicillins)

Contra-indications see under Benzylpenicillin (section 5.1.1.1); also carnitine deficiency, oesophageal strictures, gastro-intestinal obstruction, infants under 3 months

Pregnancy not known to be harmful, but manufacturer advises avoid

Breast-feeding trace amounts in milk

Side-effects see under Benzylpenicillin (section 5.1.1.1); nausea, vomiting, dyspepsia; also reduced serum and total body carnitine (especially with long-term or repeated use)

Licensed use not licensed for use in children under 3 months

Indication and dose

> **Acute uncomplicated cystitis**
> ● **By mouth**
>
> > **Child body-weight over 40 kg** initially 400 mg then 200 mg every 8 hours for 3 days

> **Chronic or recurrent bacteriuria**
>
> > **Child body-weight over 40 kg** 400 mg every 6–8 hours

> **Urinary-tract infections**
>
> > **Child body-weight under 40 kg** 5–10 mg/kg every 6 hours; total daily dose may alternatively be given in 3 divided doses

> **Salmonellosis** not recommended therefore no dose stated

> Counselling Tablets should be swallowed whole with plenty of fluid during meals while sitting or standing

Selexid® (LEO) [PoM]
Tablets, f/c, pivmecillinam hydrochloride 200 mg, net price 10-tab pack = £4.50. Label: 9, 21, 27, counselling, posture (see Dose above)

5.1.2 Cephalosporins, carbapenems, and other beta-lactams

Antibiotics in this section include the **cephalosporins**, such as cefotaxime, ceftazidime, cefuroxime, cefalexin and cefradine, the **monobactam**, aztreonam, and the **carbapenems**, imipenem (a thienamycin derivative), meropenem, and ertapenem.

5

Infections

5.1.2.1 Cephalosporins

The cephalosporins are broad-spectrum antibacterials which are used for the treatment of septicaemia, pneumonia, meningitis, biliary-tract infections, peritonitis, and urinary-tract infections. The pharmacology of the cephalosporins is similar to that of the penicillins, excretion being principally renal. Cephalosporins penetrate the cerebrospinal fluid poorly unless the meninges are inflamed; cefotaxime and ceftriaxone are suitable cephalosporins for infections of the CNS (e.g meningitis).

The principal side-effect of the cephalosporins is hypersensitivity and about 0.5–6.5% of penicillin-sensitive patients will also be allergic to the cephalosporins. Patients with a history of immediate hypersensitivity to penicillin should not receive a cephalosporin. If a cephalosporin is essential in these patients because a suitable alternative antibacterial is not available, then cefixime, cefotaxime, ceftazidime, ceftriaxone, or cefuroxime can be used with caution; cefaclor, cefadroxil, cefalexin, and cefradine should be avoided.

Antibiotic-associated colitis may occur with the use of broad-spectrum cephalosporins, particularly second- and third-generation cephalosporins.

Cefradine (cephradine) has generally been replaced by the newer cephalosporins.

Cefuroxime is a 'second generation' cephalosporin that is less susceptible than the earlier cephalosporins to inactivation by beta-lactamases. It is, therefore, active against certain bacteria that are resistant to the other drugs and has greater activity against *Haemophilus influenzae* and *Neisseria gonorrhoeae*.

Cefotaxime, **ceftazidime** and **ceftriaxone** are 'third generation' cephalosporins with greater activity than the 'second generation' cephalosporins against certain Gram-negative bacteria. However, they are less active than cefuroxime against Gram-positive bacteria, most notably *Staphylococcus aureus*. Their broad antibacterial spectrum may encourage superinfection with resistant bacteria or fungi.

Ceftazidime has good activity against pseudomonas. It is also active against other Gram-negative bacteria.

Ceftriaxone has a longer half-life and therefore needs to be given only once daily. Indications include serious infections such as septicaemia, pneumonia, and meningitis. The calcium salt of ceftriaxone forms a precipitate in the gall bladder which may rarely cause symptoms but these usually resolve when the antibacterial is stopped. In neonates, ceftriaxone may displace bilirubin from plasmaalbumin and should be avoided in neonates with unconjugated hyperbilirubinaemia, hypoalbuminaemia, acidosis or impaired bilirubin binding.

Orally active cephalosporins   The orally active 'first generation' cephalosporins, **cefalexin** (cephalexin), **cefradine**, and **cefadroxil** and the 'second generation' cephalosporin, **cefaclor**, have a similar antimicrobial spectrum. They are useful for urinary-tract infections which do not respond to other drugs or which occur in pregnancy, respiratory-tract infections, otitis media, sinusitis, and skin and soft-tissue infections. Cefaclor has good activity against *H. influenzae*, but it is associated with protracted skin reactions especially in children. Cefadroxil has a long duration of action and can be given twice daily; it has poor activity against *H. influenzae*. **Cefuroxime axetil**, an ester of the 'second generation' cephalosporin cefuroxime, has the same antibacterial spectrum as the parent compound; it is poorly absorbed and needs to be given with food to maximise absorption.

Cefixime has a longer duration of action than the other cephalosporins that are active by mouth. It is presently only licensed for acute infections.

Cefpodoxime proxetil is more active than the other oral cephalosporins against respiratory bacterial pathogens and it is licensed for upper and lower respiratory-tract infections.

For treatment of Lyme disease, see section 5.1.1.3.

Oral infections   The cephalosporins offer little advantage over the penicillins in dental infections, often being less active against anaerobes. Infections due to oral streptococci (often termed viridans streptococci) which become resistant to penicillin are usually also resistant to cephalosporins. This is of importance in the case of children who have had rheumatic fever and are on long-term penicillin therapy. Cefalexin and cefradine have been used in the treatment of oral infections.

CEFACLOR

Cautions sensitivity to beta-lactam antibacterials (avoid if history of immediate hypersensitivity reaction, see also notes above and p. 315); false positive urinary glucose (if tested for reducing substances) and false positive Coombs' test; **interactions:** Appendix 1 (cephalosporins)

Contra-indications cephalosporin hypersensitivity

Renal impairment no dosage adjustment required, manufacturer advises caution

Pregnancy not known to be harmful

Breast-feeding present in milk in low concentration, considered compatible with breast-feeding

Side-effects diarrhoea and rarely antibiotic-associated colitis (CSM has warned both more likely with higher doses), nausea and vomiting, abdominal discomfort, headache; allergic reactions including rashes, pruritus, urticaria, serum sickness-like reactions with rashes, fever and arthralgia, and anaphylaxis; Stevens-Johnson syndrome, toxic epidermal necrolysis reported; disturbances in liver enzymes, transient hepatitis and cholestatic jaundice; other side-effects reported include eosinophilia and blood disorders (including thrombocytopenia, leucopenia, agranulocytosis, aplastic anaemia and haemolytic anaemia); reversible interstitial nephritis, hyperactivity, nervousness, sleep disturbances, hallucinations, confusion, hypertonia, and dizziness

Indication and dose

> **Infections due to sensitive Gram-positive and Gram-negative bacteria** but see notes above
> * By mouth
>
>> **Child 1 month–12 years** 20 mg/kg daily in 3 divided doses, doubled for severe infection (usual max. 1 g daily)
>>
>> *or*
>>
>> **Child 1 month–1 year** 62.5 mg 3 times daily; dose doubled for severe infections
>>
>> **Child 1–5 years** 125 mg 3 times daily; dose doubled for severe infections

> **Child 5–12 years** 250 mg 3 times daily; dose doubled for severe infections
>
> **Child 12–18 years** 250 mg 3 times daily; dose doubled for severe infections (max. 4 g daily)

> **Asymptomatic carriage of *Haemophilus influenzae* or mild exacerbations in cystic fibrosis**
> * By mouth
>
>> **Child 1 month–1 year** 125 mg every 8 hours
>>
>> **Child 1–7 years** 250 mg 3 times daily
>>
>> **Child 7–18 years** 500 mg 3 times daily

Cefaclor (Non-proprietary) ⟨PoM⟩

Capsules, cefaclor (as monohydrate) 250 mg, net price 21-cap pack = £4.31; 500 mg, 50-cap pack = £27.22. Label: 9
Brands include *Keftid*®

Suspension, cefaclor (as monohydrate) for reconstitution with water, 125 mg/5 mL, net price 100 mL = £5.16; 250 mg/5 mL, 100 mL = £10.32. Label: 9

Note Sugar-free versions are available and can be ordered by specifying 'sugar-free' on the prescription
Brands include *Keftid*®

Distaclor® (Flynn) ⟨PoM⟩

Capsules, cefaclor (as monohydrate) 500 mg (violet/grey), net price 21-cap pack = £18.19. Label: 9

Suspension, both pink, cefaclor (as monohydrate) for reconstitution with water, 125 mg/5 mL, net price 100 mL = £4.13; 250 mg/5 mL, 100 mL = £8.26. Label: 9

Distaclor MR® (Flynn) ⟨PoM⟩

Tablets, m/r, both blue, cefaclor (as monohydrate) 375 mg. Net price 14-tab pack = £8.31. Label: 9, 21, 25

Dose

> **Susceptible infections**
>> **Child 12–18 years** 375 mg every 12 hours with food, dose doubled for pneumonia

> **Lower urinary-tract infections**
>> **Child 12–18 years** 375 mg every 12 hours with food

CEFADROXIL

Cautions see under Cefaclor; **interactions:** Appendix 1 (cephalosporins)

Contra-indications see under Cefaclor

Renal impairment reduce dose if estimated glomerular filtration rate less than 50 mL/minute/1.73 m²

Pregnancy not known to be harmful

Breast-feeding present in milk in low concentrations

Side-effects see under Cefaclor

Indication and dose

> **Infections due to sensitive Gram-positive and Gram-negative bacteria** but see notes above
> * By mouth
>
>> **Child 1 month–1 year** 12.5 mg/kg twice daily
>>
>> **Child 1–6 years** 250 mg twice daily

> **Child 6–18 years**
>
>> **Body-weight under 40 kg** 500 mg twice daily;
>>
>> **Body-weight over 40 kg** 0.5–1 g twice daily (1 g once daily for skin, soft tissue and uncomplicated urinary-tract infections)

Cefadroxil (Non-proprietary) ⟨PoM⟩

Capsules, cefadroxil (as monohydrate) 500 mg, net price 20-cap pack = £2.81. Label: 9

Baxan® (Bristol-Myers Squibb) ⟨PoM⟩

Capsules, cefadroxil (as monohydrate) 500 mg, net price 20-cap pack = £5.05. Label: 9

Suspension, cefadroxil (as monohydrate) for reconstitution with water, 125 mg/5 mL, net price 60 mL = £1.57; 250 mg/5 mL, 60 mL = £3.11; 500 mg/5 mL, 60 mL = £4.66. Label: 9

5 Infections

CEFALEXIN
(Cephalexin)

Cautions see under Cefaclor; **interactions:** Appendix 1 (cephalosporins)

Contra-indications see under Cefaclor

Renal impairment reduce dose in moderate impairment

Pregnancy not known to be harmful

Breast-feeding present in milk in low concentrations, considered compatible with breast-feeding

Side-effects see under Cefaclor

Indication and dose

Infections due to sensitive Gram-positive and Gram-negative bacteria but see notes above
• By mouth

Neonate under 7 days 25 mg/kg (max. 125 mg) twice daily

Neonate 7–21 days 25 mg/kg (max. 125 mg) 3 times daily

Neonate 21–28 days 25 mg/kg (max. 125 mg) 4 times daily

Child 1 month–12 years 12.5 mg/kg twice daily; dose doubled in severe infection; max. 25 mg/kg 4 times daily (max. 1 g 4 times daily) or

Child 1 month–1 year 125 mg twice daily

Child 1–5 years 125 mg 3 times daily

Child 5–12 years 250 mg 3 times daily

Child 12–18 years 500 mg 2–3 times daily, increased to 1–1.5 g 3–4 times daily for severe infection

Prophylaxis of recurrent urinary-tract infection
• By mouth

Child 1 month–18 years 12.5 mg/kg at night (max. 125 mg at night)

Cefalexin (Non-proprietary) PoM
Capsules, cefalexin 250 mg, net price 28-cap pack = £2.01; 500 mg, 21-cap pack = £2.59. Label: 9

Dental prescribing on NHS Cefalexin Capsules may be prescribed

Tablets, cefalexin 250 mg, net price 28-tab pack = £2.34; 500 mg, 21-tab pack = £2.63. Label: 9

Dental prescribing on NHS Cefalexin Tablets may be prescribed

Oral suspension, cefalexin for reconstitution with water, 125 mg/5 mL, net price 100 mL = £1.97; 250 mg/5 mL, 100 mL = £2.23. Label: 9

Dental prescribing on NHS Cefalexin Oral Suspension may be prescribed

Ceporex® (Co-Pharma) PoM
Capsules, both caramel/grey, cefalexin 250 mg, net price 28-cap pack = £4.02; 500 mg, 28-cap pack = £7.85. Label: 9

Tablets, all pink, f/c, cefalexin 250 mg, net price 28-tab pack = £4.02; 500 mg, 28-tab pack = £7.85. Label: 9

Syrup, all orange, cefalexin for reconstitution with water, 125 mg/5 mL, net price 100 mL = £1.43; 250 mg/5 mL, 100 mL = £2.87; 500 mg/5 mL, 100 mL = £5.57. Label: 9

Keflex® (Flynn) PoM
Capsules, cefalexin 250 mg (green/white), net price 28-cap pack = £1.46; 500 mg (pale green/dark green), 21-cap pack = £1.98. Label: 9

Tablets, both peach, cefalexin 250 mg, net price 28-tab pack = £1.60; 500 mg (scored), 21-tab pack = £2.08. Label: 9

Suspension, cefalexin for reconstitution with water, 125 mg/5 mL, net price 100 mL = 84p; 250 mg/5 mL, 100 mL = £1.40. Label: 9

CEFIXIME

Cautions see under Cefaclor; **interactions:** Appendix 1 (cephalosporins)

Contra-indications see under Cefaclor

Renal impairment reduce dose if estimated glomerular filtration rate less than 20 mL/minute/1.73 m^2

Pregnancy not known to be harmful

Breast-feeding manufacturer advises avoid—no information available

Side-effects see under Cefaclor

Indication and dose

Acute infections due to sensitive Gram-positive and Gram-negative bacteria, but see notes above
• By mouth

Child 6 months–1 year 75 mg daily

Child 1–5 years 100 mg daily

Child 5–10 years 200 mg daily

Child 10–18 years 200–400 mg daily or 100–200 mg twice daily

Gonorrhoea [unlicensed indication, see also Table 1, section 5.1]
• By mouth

Child 12–18 years 400 mg as a single dose

Suprax® (Sanofi-Aventis) PoM
Tablets, f/c, scored, cefixime 200 mg. Net price 7-tab pack = £13.23. Label: 9

Paediatric oral suspension, cefixime 100 mg/5 mL when reconstituted with water, net price 50 mL (with double-ended spoon for measuring 3.75 mL or 5 mL since dilution not recommended) = £10.53, 100 mL = £18.91. Label: 9

CEFOTAXIME

Cautions see under Cefaclor; **interactions:** Appendix 1 (cephalosporins)

Contra-indications see under Cefaclor

Renal impairment usual initial dose, then use half normal dose if estimated glomerular filtration rate less than 5 mL/minute/1.73 m²

Pregnancy not known to be harmful

Breast-feeding present in milk in low concentration, considered compatible with breast-feeding

Side-effects see under Cefaclor; rarely arrhythmias following rapid injection reported

Indication and dose

Infections due to sensitive Gram-positive and Gram-negative bacteria, surgical prophylaxis, Haemophilus epiglottitis and meningitis (Table 1, section 5.1) see also notes above

• **By intramuscular or by intravenous injection or intravenous infusion**

Neonate under 7 days 25 mg/kg every 12 hours; dose doubled in severe infection and meningitis

Neonate 7–21 days 25 mg/kg every 8 hours; dose doubled in severe infection and meningitis

Neonate 21–28 days 25 mg/kg every 6–8 hours; dose doubled in severe infection and meningitis

Child 1 month–18 years 50 mg/kg every 8–12 hours; increase to every 6 hours in very severe infections and meningitis (max. 12 g daily)

Important. If bacterial meningitis and especially if meningococcal disease is suspected the patient should be transferred urgently to hospital. If benzylpenicillin cannot be given (e.g. because of an allergy), a single

dose of cefotaxime may be given (if available) before urgent transfer to hospital. Suitable doses of cefotaxime by intravenous injection (or by intramuscular injection) are Child under 12 years 50 mg/kg; Child over 12 years 1 g; chloramphenicol (section 5.1.7) may be used if there is a history of anaphylaxis to penicillins or cephalosporins

Congenital gonococcal conjunctivitis

• **By intramuscular injection**

Neonate 100 mg/kg as a single dose

Gonorrhoea

• **By intramuscular or by intravenous injection or intravenous infusion**

Child 12–18 years 500 mg as a single dose

Severe exacerbations of *Haemophilus influenzae* infection in cystic fibrosis

• **By intravenous injection or intravenous infusion**

Child 1 month–18 years 50 mg/kg every 6–8 hours (max. 12 g daily)

Administration Displacement value may be significant, consult local guidelines. For intermittent intravenous infusion dilute in glucose 5% *or* sodium chloride 0.9% *or* compound sodium lactate *or* water for injections; administer over 20–60 minutes; incompatible with alkaline solutions

Cefotaxime (Non-proprietary) PoM

Injection, powder for reconstitution, cefotaxime (as sodium salt), net price 500-mg vial = £2.14; 1-g vial = £4.31; 2-g vial = £8.57

CEFPODOXIME

Cautions see under Cefaclor; **interactions:** Appendix 1 (cephalosporins)

Contra-indications see under Cefaclor

Renal impairment increase dose interval to every 24 hours if estimated glomerular filtration rate 10–40 mL/minute/1.73 m². Increase dose interval to every 48 hours if estimated glomerular filtration rate less than 10 mL/minute/1.73 m²

Pregnancy not known to be harmful

Breast-feeding present in milk in low concentration

Side-effects see under Cefaclor

Indication and dose

Upper respiratory-tract infections (but in pharyngitis and tonsillitis reserved for infections which are recurrent, chronic, or resistant to other antibacterials), lower respiratory-tract infections (including bronchitis and pneumonia), skin and soft tissue infections, uncomplicated urinary-tract infections

• **By mouth**

Child 15 days–6 months 4 mg/kg twice daily

Child 6 months–2 years 40 mg twice daily

Child 3–8 years 80 mg twice daily

Child 9–12 years 100 mg twice daily

Child 12–18 years 100 mg twice daily (increased to 200 mg twice daily in sinusitis, skin and soft tissue infections, uncomplicated upper urinary tract infections and if necessary in lower respiratory tract infections)

Uncomplicated gonorrhoea

• **By mouth**

Child 12–18 years 200 mg as a single dose

Orelox® (Sanofi-Aventis) PoM

Tablets, f/c, cefpodoxime 100 mg (as proxetil), net price 10-tab pack = £9.78. Label: 5, 9, 21

Oral suspension, cefpodoxime (as proxetil) for reconstitution with water, 40 mg/5 mL, net price 100 mL = £11.50. Label: 5, 9, 21

Excipients include aspartame (section 9.4.1)

5

Infections

CEFRADINE

(Cephradine)

Cautions see under Cefaclor; **interactions:** Appendix 1 (cephalosporins)

Contra-indications see under Cefaclor

Renal impairment reduce dose if estimated glomerular filtration rate less than 20 mL/minute/1.73 m²

Pregnancy not known to be harmful

Breast-feeding present in milk in low concentrations

Side-effects see under Cefaclor

Licensed use not licensed for use in children for prevention of *Staphylococcus aureus* lung infection in cystic fibrosis

Indication and dose

Infections due to sensitive Gram-positive and Gram-negative bacteria but see notes above

• By mouth

Child 7–12 years 12.5–25 mg/kg twice daily (total daily dose may alternatively be given in 3–4 divided doses)

Child 12–18 years 0.5–1 g twice daily *or* 250–500 mg 4 times daily; up to 1 g 4 times daily in severe infections

Prevention of *Staphylococcus aureus* lung infection in cystic fibrosis

• By mouth

Child 7–18 years 2 g twice daily

Cefradine (Non-proprietary) [PoM]

Capsules, cefradine 250 mg, net price 20-cap pack = £4.04; 500 mg, 20-cap pack = £7.59. Label: 9
Brands include *Nicef*®

Dental prescribing on NHS Cefradine Capsules may be prescribed

CEFTAZIDIME

Cautions see under Cefaclor; **interactions:** Appendix 1 (cephalosporins)

Contra-indications see under Cefaclor

Renal impairment reduce dose if estimated glomerular filtration rate less than 50 mL/minute/1.73 m²

Pregnancy not known to be harmful

Breast-feeding present in milk in low concentration, considered compatible with breast-feeding

Side-effects see under Cefaclor

Licensed use nebulised route unlicensed

Indication and dose

Infections due to sensitive Gram-positive and Gram-negative bacteria but see notes above

• By intravenous injection or infusion

Neonate under 7 days 25 mg/kg every 24 hours; dose doubled in severe infection and meningitis

Neonate 7–21 days 25 mg/kg every 12 hours; dose doubled in severe infection and meningitis

Neonate 21–28 days 25 mg/kg every 8 hours; dose doubled in severe infection and meningitis

Child 1 month–18 years 25 mg/kg every 8 hours; dose doubled in severe infection, febrile neutropenia and meningitis (max. 6 g daily)

Pseudomonal lung infection in cystic fibrosis

• By intravenous injection or infusion or by deep intramuscular injection

Child 1 month–18 years 50 mg/kg every 8 hours (max. 9 g daily)

Chronic *Burkholderia cepacia* infection in cystic fibrosis

• By inhalation of nebulised solution

Child 1 month–18 years 1 g twice daily

Administration For parenteral administration, intravenous route recommended in children. Displacement value may be significant, consult local guidelines. For intermittent intravenous infusion dilute reconstituted solution further to a concentration of not more than 40 mg/mL in Glucose 5% or Glucose 10% or Sodium chloride 0.9% or Compound sodium lactate.

For nebulisation, dissolve dose in 3 mL of water for injection

Ceftazidime (Non-proprietary) [PoM]

Injection, powder for reconstitution, ceftazidime (as pentahydrate), with sodium carbonate, net price 1-g vial = £8.50; 2-g vial = £17.90

Fortum® (GSK) [PoM]

Injection, powder for reconstitution, ceftazidime (as pentahydrate), with sodium carbonate, net price 500-mg vial = £4.40; 1-g vial = £8.79; 2-g vial = £17.59; 3-g vial = £25.76
Electrolytes Na⁺ 2.3 mmol/g

Kefadim® (Flynn) [PoM]

Injection, powder for reconstitution, ceftazidime (as pentahydrate), with sodium carbonate, net price 1-g vial = £7.92; 2-g vial = £15.84
Electrolytes Na⁺ 2.3 mmol/g

CEFTRIAXONE

Cautions see under Cefaclor; neonates; may displace bilirubin from serum albumin, administer over 60 minutes in neonates (see also Contra-

indications); treatment longer than 14 days, renal failure, dehydration—risk of ceftriaxone precipi-

◻ **CEFTRIAXONE** (*continued*)

tation in gall bladder; **interactions:** Appendix 1 (cephalosporins)

Contra-indications see under Cefaclor; neonates less than 41 weeks postmenstrual age; neonates over 41 weeks postmenstrual age with jaundice, hypoalbuminaemia, or acidosis; concomitant treatment with intravenous calcium (including total parenteral nutrition containing calcium) in neonates over 41 weeks postmenstrual age—risk of precipitation in urine and lungs

Hepatic impairment if hepatic impairment is accompanied by severe renal impairment, reduce dose and monitor plasma concentration

Renal impairment max. 50 mg/kg daily (max. 2 g daily) in severe renal impairment; also monitor plasma concentration if hepatic impairment accompanied by severe renal impairment

Pregnancy not known to be harmful

Breast-feeding present in milk in low concentration, considered compatible with breast-feeding

Side-effects see under Cefaclor; calcium ceftriaxone precipitates in urine (particularly in very young, dehydrated or those who are immobilised) or in gall bladder—consider discontinuation if symptomatic; rarely prolongation of prothrombin time, pancreatitis

Licensed use not licensed for congenital gonococcal conjunctivitis or early syphilis; not licensed for use in children under 12 years of age for uncomplicated gonorrhoea or pelvic inflammatory disease

Indication and dose

Infections due to sensitive Gram-positive and Gram-negative bacteria
* By intravenous infusion over 60 minutes
  Neonate 20–50 mg/kg once daily

* By deep intramuscular injection, or by intravenous injection over 2–4 minutes, or by intravenous infusion
  Child 1 month–12 years
  Body-weight under 50 kg 50 mg/kg once daily; up to 80 mg/kg daily in severe infections and meningitis; doses of 50 mg/kg and over by intravenous infusion only
  Body-weight 50 kg and over dose as for child 12–18 years
  Child 12–18 years 1 g daily; 2–4 g daily in severe infections and meningitis; intramuscular doses over 1 g divided between more than one site; single intravenous doses above 1 g by intravenous infusion only

Congenital gonococcal conjunctivitis
* By intravenous infusion over 60 minutes or by deep intramuscular injection
  Neonate 25–50 mg/kg (max.125 mg) as a single dose

Uncomplicated gonorrhoea, pelvic inflammatory disease (Table 1, section 5.1)
* By deep intramuscular injection
  Child under 12 years
  Body-weight under 45 kg 125 mg as a single dose
  Body-weight over 45 kg 250 mg as a single dose
  Child 12–18 years 250 mg as a single dose

Early syphilis
* By deep intramuscular injection
  Child 12–18 years 500 mg daily for 10 days

Surgical prophylaxis
* By deep intramuscular injection or by intravenous injection over at least 2–4 minutes, or (for colorectal surgery) by intravenous infusion
  Child 12–18 years 1 g at induction; colorectal surgery, 2 g at induction; intramuscular doses over 1 g divided between more than one site

Prophylaxis of meningococcal meningitis Table 2, section 5.1

Administration Displacement value may be significant, consult local guidelines. For *intravenous infusion*, dilute reconstituted solution with Glucose 5% or 10% *or* Sodium Chloride 0.9%; give over at least 30 minutes (60 minutes in neonates). Not to be given simultaneously with parenteral nutrition or infusion fluids containing calcium, even by different infusion lines; may be infused sequentially with infusion fluids containing calcium if flush with sodium chloride 0.9% between infusions or give infusions by different infusion lines at different sites; see also Contra-indications above

For *intramuscular injection* ceftriaxone may be mixed with 1% Lidocaine Hydrochloride Injection to reduce pain at intramuscular injection site; final concentration 250–350 mg/mL.

Ceftriaxone (Non-proprietary) ▢PoM▢
Injection, powder for reconstitution, ceftriaxone (as sodium salt), net price 1-g vial = £10.17; 2-g vial = £20.36

Rocephin® (Roche) ▢PoM▢
Injection, powder for reconstitution, ceftriaxone (as sodium salt), net price 250-mg vial = £2.45; 1-g vial = £9.77; 2-g vial = £19.57
Electrolytes Na^+ 3.6 mmol/g

◼ **CEFUROXIME**

Cautions see under Cefaclor; **interactions:** Appendix 1 (cephalosporins)

Contra-indications see under Cefaclor

Renal impairment reduce parenteral dose if estimated glomerular filtration rate less than 20 mL/minute/1.73 m²

Pregnancy not known to be harmful

5 Infections

△ **CEFUROXIME** (*continued*)

Breast-feeding present in milk in low concentration

Side-effects see under Cefaclor

Licensed use not licensed for treatment of Lyme disease in children under 12 years

Indication and dose

Infections due to sensitive Gram-positive and Gram-negative bacteria
• By mouth (as cefuroxime axetil),

   Child 3 months–2 years 10 mg/kg (max. 125 mg) twice daily

   Child 2–12 years 15 mg/kg (max. 250 mg) twice daily

   Child 12–18 years 250 mg twice daily; dose doubled in severe lower respiratory-tract infections, or if pneumonia suspected; dose reduced to 125 mg twice daily in lower urinary-tract infection

• By intravenous injection or infusion or by intramuscular injection

   Neonate under 7 days 25 mg/kg every 12 hours; dose doubled in severe infection, intravenous route only

   Neonate 7–21 days 25 mg/kg every 8 hours; dose doubled in severe infection, intravenous route only

   Neonate 21–28 days 25 mg/kg every 6 hours; dose doubled in severe infection, intravenous route only

   Child 1 month–18 years 20 mg/kg (max. 750 mg) every 8 hours; increase to 50–60 mg/kg (max. 1.5 g) every 6–8 hours in severe infection and cystic fibrosis

Lyme disease (see also section 5.1.1.3)
• By mouth

   Child 3 months–12 years 15 mg/kg (max. 500 mg) twice daily for 14–21 days (for 28 days in Lyme arthritis)

   Child 12–18 years 500 mg twice daily for 14–21 days (for 28 days in Lyme arthritis)

Surgical prophylaxis
• By intravenous injection

   Child 1 month–18 years 50 mg/kg (max. 1.5 g) at induction, up to 3 further doses of 30 mg/kg (max. 750 mg) may be given by *intramuscular or intravenous injection* every 8 hours for high-risk procedures

Administration Single doses over 750 mg should be administered by the intravenous route only. Displacement value may be significant when reconstituting injection, consult local guidelines. For intermittent intravenous infusion, dilute reconstituted solution further in glucose 5% *or* sodium chloride 0.9%; give over 30 minutes.

Cefuroxime (Non-proprietary) ℗oM
   Tablets, cefuroxime (as axetil) 250 mg, net price 14-tab pack = £9.29. Label: 9, 21, 25

Zinacef® (GSK) ℗oM
   Injection, powder for reconstitution, cefuroxime (as sodium salt). Net price 250-mg vial = 94p; 750-mg vial = £2.34; 1.5-g vial = £4.70
   Electrolytes Na⁺ 1.8 mmol/750-mg vial

Zinnat® (GSK) ℗oM
   Tablets, both f/c, cefuroxime (as axetil) 125 mg, net price 14-tab pack = £4.65; 250 mg, 14-tab pack = £9.29. Label: 9, 21, 25

   Suspension, cefuroxime (as axetil) 125 mg/5 mL when reconstituted with water, net price 70 mL (tutti-frutti-flavoured) = £5.30. Label: 9, 21
   Excipients include aspartame (section 9.4.1), sucrose 3.1 g/ 5 mL

5.1.2.2 Carbapenems

The carbapenems are beta-lactam antibacterials with a broad-spectrum of activity which includes many Gram-positive and Gram-negative bacteria, and anaerobes; **imipenem** and **meropenem** have good activity against *Pseudomonas aeruginosa*. The carbapenems are not active against meticillin-resistant *Staphylococcus aureus* and *Enterococcus faecium*.

Imipenem and meropenem are used for the treatment of severe hospital-acquired infections and polymicrobial infections caused by multiple-antibacterial resistant organisms (including septicaemia, hospital-acquired pneumonia, intra-abdominal infections, skin and soft-tissue infections, and complicated urinary-tract infections).

Ertapenem is licensed for treating abdominal and gynaecological infections and for community-acquired pneumonia, but it is not active against atypical respiratory pathogens and it has limited activity against penicillin-resistant pneumococci. Unlike the other carbapenems, ertapenem is not active against *Pseudomonas* or against *Acinetobacter* spp.

Imipenem is partially inactivated in the kidney by enzymatic activity and is therefore administered in combination with **cilastatin**, a specific enzyme inhibitor, which blocks its renal metabolism. Meropenem and ertapenem are stable to the renal enzyme which inactivates imipenem and therefore can be given without cilastatin.

Side-effects of imipenem with cilastatin are similar to those of other beta-lactam antibiotics; neurotoxicity has been observed at very high dosage, in renal failure, or in patients with CNS disease. Meropenem has less seizure-inducing potential and can be used to treat central nervous system infection. Ertapenem has been associated with seizures uncommonly.

ERTAPENEM

Cautions hypersensitivity to beta-lactam antibacterials (avoid if history of immediate hypersensitivity reaction, see also p. 315); renal impairment, CNS disorders—risk of seizures; **interactions:** Appendix 1 (ertapenem)

Renal impairment risk of seizures; avoid if estimated glomerular filtration rate less than 30 mL/minute/1.73 m^2

Pregnancy manufacturer advises avoid unless potential benefit outweighs risk

Breast-feeding present in milk—manufacturer advises avoid

Side-effects diarrhoea, nausea, vomiting, headache, injection-site reactions, rash, pruritus, raised platelet count; *less commonly* dry mouth, taste disturbances, dyspepsia, abdominal pain, anorexia, constipation, melaena, antibiotic-associated colitis, bradycardia, hypotension, chest pain, oedema, pharyngeal discomfort, dyspnoea, dizziness, sleep disturbances, confusion, asthenia, seizures, raised glucose, petechiae; *rarely* dysphagia, cholecystitis, liver disorder (including jaundice), arrhythmia, increase in blood pressure, syncope, nasal congestion, cough, wheezing, anxiety, depression, agitation, tremor, pelvic peritonitis, renal impairment, muscle cramp, scleral disorder, blood disorders (including neutropenia, thrombocytopenia, haemorrhage), hypoglycaemia, electrolyte disturbances; also reported hallucinations and dyskinesia

Indication and dose

Abdominal infections, acute gynaecological infections, community-acquired pneumonia

• By intravenous infusion

Child 3 months–13 years 15 mg/kg every 12 hours (max. 1 g daily)

Child 13–18 years 1 g once daily

Administration reconstitute 1 g with 10 mL Water for Injections or Sodium Chloride 0.9%; for *intermittent intravenous infusion*, dilute requisite dose in Sodium Chloride 0.9% to a final concentration not exceeding 20 mg/mL; incompatible with glucose solutions

Invanz® (MSD) ▣
Intravenous infusion, powder for reconstitution, ertapenem (as sodium salt), net price 1-g vial = £31.65
Electrolytes Na$^+$ 6 mmol/1-g vial

IMIPENEM WITH CILASTATIN

Cautions CNS disorders (e.g. epilepsy); hypersensitivity to beta-lactam antibacterials (avoid if history of immediate hypersensitivity reaction, see also p. 315); **interactions:** Appendix 1 (imipenem with cilastatin)

Renal impairment reduce dose if estimated glomerular filtration rate less than 70 mL/minute/1.73 m^2; risk of CNS side-effects

Pregnancy manufacturer advises avoid unless potential benefit outweighs risk (toxicity in *animal* studies)

Breast-feeding present in milk but unlikely to be absorbed (however, manufacturer advises avoid)

Side-effects nausea, vomiting, diarrhoea (antibiotic-associated colitis reported), taste disturbances, tooth or tongue discoloration, hearing loss; blood disorders, positive Coombs' test; allergic reactions (with rash, pruritus, urticaria, Stevens-Johnson syndrome, fever, anaphylactic reactions, rarely toxic epidermal necrolysis, exfoliative dermatitis); myoclonic activity, convulsions, confusion and mental disturbances reported; slight increases in liver enzymes and bilirubin reported, rarely hepatitis; increases in serum creatinine and blood urea; red coloration of urine in children reported; local reactions: erythema, pain and induration, and thrombophlebitis

Licensed use not licensed for use in children under 3 months; not licensed for use in children with renal impairment

Indication and dose

Aerobic and anaerobic Gram-positive and Gram-negative infections, hospital-acquired septicaemia Table 1, section 5.1; not indicated for CNS infections

• By intravenous infusion
expressed in terms of imipenem

Neonate under 7 days 20 mg/kg every 12 hours

Neonate 7–21 days 20 mg/kg every 8 hours

Neonate 21–28 days 20 mg/kg every 6 hours

Child 1–3 months 20 mg/kg every 6 hours

Child 3 months–18 years

Body-weight under 40 kg 15 mg/kg (max. 500 mg) every 6 hours

Body-weight over 40 kg 250–500 mg every 6 hours; less sensitive organisms up to 12.5 mg/kg (max. 1 g) every 6 hours; total daily dose may alternatively be given in 3 divided doses

Cystic fibrosis

• By intravenous infusion

Child 1 month–18 years

Body-weight under 40 kg 22.5 mg/kg every 6 hours

Body-weight over 40 kg 1 g every 6–8 hours

Administration for intermittent intravenous infusion dilute to a concentration of 5 mg (as imi-

◁ **IMIPENEM WITH CILASTATIN** (*continued*)

penem)/mL in sodium chloride 0.9% *or* sodium chloride and glucose; give up to 500 mg over 20–30 minutes; give 1 g over 40–60 minutes

Primaxin® (MSD) [PoM]
Intravenous infusion, powder for reconstitution, imipenem (as monohydrate) 500 mg with cilastatin (as sodium salt) 500 mg, net price per vial = £12.00
Electrolytes Na⁺ 1.72 mmol/vial

■ MEROPENEM

Cautions hypersensitivity to beta-lactam antibacterials (avoid if history of immediate hypersensitivity reaction, see also p. 315); **interactions:** Appendix 1 (meropenem)

Hepatic impairment monitor transaminase and bilirubin concentrations

Renal impairment use normal dose every 12 hours if estimated glomerular filtration rate 26–50 mL/minute/1.73 m²; use half normal dose every 12 hours if estimated glomerular filtration rate 10–25 mL/minute/1.73 m²; use half normal dose every 24 hours if estimated glomerular filtration rate less than 10 mL/minute/1.73 m²

Pregnancy manufacturer advises use only if potential benefit outweighs risk—no information available

Breast-feeding unlikely to be absorbed (but manufacturer advises avoid unless potential benefit outweighs risk)

Side-effects nausea, vomiting, diarrhoea (antibiotic-associated colitis reported), abdominal pain, disturbances in liver function tests; headache; thrombocytaemia, positive Coombs' test; rash, pruritus, injection-site reactions; *less commonly* eosinophilia and thrombocytopenia; *rarely* convulsions; also reported paraesthesia, leucopenia, haemolytic anaemia, reduction in partial thromboplastin time, Stevens-Johnson syndrome, and toxic epidermal necrolysis

Licensed use not licensed for use in children for infection in neutropenia; not licensed for use in children under 3 months

Indication and dose

Aerobic and anaerobic Gram-positive and Gram-negative infections, hospital-acquired septicaemia Table 1, section 5.1

• By intravenous injection over 5 minutes or by intravenous infusion

Neonate under 7 days 20 mg/kg every 12 hours, dose doubled in severe infection

Neonate 7–28 days 20 mg/kg every 8 hours; dose doubled in severe infection

Child 1 month–12 years

Body-weight under 50 kg 10 mg/kg every 8 hours; dose doubled in hospital-acquired pneumonia, peritonitis, septicaemia and infections in neutropenic patients

Body-weight over 50 kg dose as for child 12–18 years

Child 12–18 years 500 mg every 8 hours; dose doubled in hospital-acquired pneumonia, peritonitis, septicaemia and infections in neutropenic patients

Meningitis

• By intravenous injection over 5 minutes or by intravenous infusion

Neonate under 7 days 40 mg/kg every 12 hours

Neonate 7–28 days 40 mg/kg every 8 hours

Child 1 month–12 years

Body-weight under 50 kg 40 mg/kg every 8 hours

Body-weight over 50 kg dose as for child 12–18 years

Child 12–18 years 2 g every 8 hours

Exacerbations of chronic lower respiratory-tract infections in cystic fibrosis

• By intravenous injection over 5 minutes or by intravenous infusion

Child 1 month–18 years 40 mg/kg every 8 hours (max. 2 g every 8 hours)

Administration Displacement value may be significant, consult local guidelines. For intermittent intravenous infusion dilute reconstituted solution further in glucose 5% *or* glucose 10% *or* sodium chloride 0.9% and give over 15–30 minutes

Meronem® (AstraZeneca) [PoM]
Injection, powder for reconstitution, meropenem (as trihydrate), net price 500-mg vial = £8.60; 1-g vial = £17.19
Electrolytes Na⁺ 3.9 mmol/g

5.1.2.3 Other beta-lactam antibiotics

Aztreonam is a monocyclic beta-lactam ('monobactam') antibiotic with an antibacterial spectrum limited to Gram-negative aerobic bacteria including *Pseudomonas aeruginosa*, *Neisseria meningitidis*, and *Haemophilus influenzae*; it should not be used alone for 'blind' treatment since it is not active against Gram-positive organisms. Aztreonam is also effective against *Neisseria gonorrhoeae* (but not against concurrent chlamydial infection). Side-effects are similar to those of the other beta-lactams although aztreonam may be less likely to cause hypersensitivity in penicillin-sensitive patients.

▲ AZTREONAM

Cautions hypersensitivity to beta-lactam antibiotics; **interactions**: Appendix 1 (aztreonam)

Contra-indications aztreonam hypersensitivity

Hepatic impairment experience limited, monitor liver function

Renal impairment usual initial dose, then half normal dose if estimated glomerular filtration rate 10–30 mL/minute/1.73 m²; usual initial dose, then one-quarter normal dose if estimated glomerular filtration rate less than 10 mL/minute/1.73 m²

Pregnancy manufacturer advises avoid—crosses placenta and no further information available

Breast-feeding present in milk in low concentration, considered compatible with breast-feeding

Side-effects nausea, vomiting, diarrhoea, abdominal cramps; mouth ulcers, altered taste; jaundice and hepatitis; flushing; hypersensitivity reactions; blood disorders (including thrombocytopenia and neutropenia); rashes, injection-site reactions; *rarely* hypotension, seizures, asthenia, confusion, dizziness, headache, halitosis, and breast tenderness; *very rarely* antibiotic-associated colitis, gastro-intestinal bleeding, and toxic epidermal necrolysis

Licensed use not licensed for use in children under 7 days

Indication and dose

Gram-negative infections including *Pseudomonas aeruginosa*, *Haemophilus influenzae*, and *Neisseria meningitidis*

• By intravenous injection over 3–5 minutes or by intravenous infusion

Neonate under 7 days 30 mg/kg every 12 hours

Neonate 7–28 days 30 mg/kg every 6–8 hours

Child 1 month–2 years 30 mg/kg every 6–8 hours

Child 2–12 years 30 mg/kg every 6–8 hours increased to 50 mg/kg every 6–8 hours in severe infection and cystic fibrosis (max. 2 g every 6 hours)

Child 12–18 years 1 g every 8 hours or 2 g every 12 hours; 2 g every 6–8 hours for severe infections (including systemic *Ps. aeruginosa* and lung infections in cystic fibrosis)

Administration Displacement value may be significant, consult local guidelines. For intermittent intravenous infusion, dilute reconstituted solution further in Glucose 5% *or* Sodium chloride 0.9% *or* Ringer's solution *or* Compound sodium lactate to a concentration of less than 20 mg/mL; to be given over 20–60 minutes

Azactam® (Squibb) PoM
Injection, powder for reconstitution, aztreonam. Net price 1-g vial = £9.59; 2-g vial = £19.20

5.1.3 Tetracyclines

The tetracyclines are broad-spectrum antibiotics whose value has decreased owing to increasing bacterial resistance. In children over 12 years of age they are useful for infections caused by chlamydia (trachoma, psittacosis, salpingitis, urethritis, and lymphogranuloma venereum), rickettsia (including Q-fever), brucella (doxycycline with either streptomycin or rifampicin), and the spirochaete, *Borrelia burgdorferi* (Lyme disease—see section 5.1.1.3). They are also used in respiratory and genital mycoplasma infections, in acne, in destructive (refractory) periodontal disease, in exacerbations of chronic respiratory diseases (because of their activity against *Haemophilus influenzae*), and for leptospirosis in penicillin hypersensitivity (as an alternative to erythromycin).

Microbiologically, there is little to choose between the various tetracyclines, the only exception being **minocycline** which has a broader spectrum; it is active against *Neisseria meningitidis* and has been used for meningococcal prophylaxis but is no longer recommended because of side-effects including dizziness and vertigo (see Table 2, section 5.1 for current recommendations). Compared to other tetracyclines, minocycline is associated with a greater risk of lupus-erythematosus-like syndrome. Minocycline sometimes causes irreversible pigmentation.

For the role of tetracyclines in the management of meticillin-resistant *Staphylococcus aureus* (MRSA) infections, see p. 317.

Oral infections In children over 12 years of age, tetracyclines can be effective against oral anaerobes but the development of resistance (especially by oral streptococci) has reduced their usefulness for the treatment of acute oral infections; they may still have a role in the treatment of destructive (refractory) forms of periodontal disease. Doxycycline has a longer duration of action than tetracycline or oxytetracycline and need only be given once daily; it is reported to be more active against anaerobes than some other tetracyclines.

For the use of doxycycline in the treatment of recurrent aphthous ulceration, oral herpes, or as an adjunct to gingival scaling and root planing for periodontitis, see section 12.3.1 and section 12.3.2.

Cautions Tetracyclines may increase muscle weakness in patients with myasthenia gravis, and exacerbate systemic lupus erythematosus. Antacids, and aluminium, calcium, iron, magnesium and zinc salts decrease the absorption of tetracyclines; milk also reduces the absorption of demeclocycline, oxytetracycline, and tetracycline. Other **interactions**: Appendix 1 (tetracyclines).

Contra-indications Deposition of tetracyclines in growing bone and teeth (by binding to calcium) causes staining and occasionally dental hypoplasia, and they should **not** be given to children under 12 years, or to pregnant or breast-feeding women. However, doxycycline may be used in children for treatment and post-exposure prophylaxis of anthrax when an alternative antibacterial cannot be given [unlicensed indication]. Tetracyclines should not be given to children with acute porphyria (section 9.8.2).

Hepatic impairment Tetracyclines should be avoided or used with caution in children with hepatic impairment. Tetracyclines should also be used with caution in those receiving potentially hepatotoxic drugs.

Renal impairment With the exception of **doxycycline** and **minocycline**, the tetracyclines may exacerbate renal failure and should **not** be given to children with renal impairment.

Pregnancy Tetracyclines should **not** be given to pregnant women; effects on skeletal development have been documented in the first trimester of pregnancy in *animal* studies. Administration during the second or third trimester may cause discoloration of the child's teeth, and maternal hepatotoxicity has been reported with large parenteral doses.

Breast-feeding Tetracyclines should **not** be given to women who are breast-feeding (although absorption and therefore discoloration of teeth in the infant is probably usually prevented by chelation with calcium in milk).

Side-effects Side-effects of the tetracyclines include nausea, vomiting, diarrhoea (antibiotic-associated colitis reported occasionally), dysphagia, and oesophageal irritation. Other rare side-effects include hepatotoxicity, pancreatitis, blood disorders, photosensitivity (particularly with demeclocycline), and hypersensitivity reactions (including rash, exfoliative dermatitis, Stevens-Johnson syndrome, urticaria, angioedema, anaphylaxis, pericarditis). Headache and visual disturbances may indicate benign intracranial hypertension (discontinue treatment); bulging fontanelles have been reported in infants.

▌TETRACYCLINE

Cautions see notes above

Contra-indications see notes above

Hepatic impairment see notes above; max. 1 g daily in divided doses

Renal impairment see notes above

Pregnancy see notes above

Breast-feeding see notes above

Side-effects see notes above; also acute renal failure, skin discoloration

Indication and dose

Susceptible infections see notes above

● By mouth

Child 12–18 years 250 mg 4 times daily, increased in severe infections to 500 mg 3–4 times daily

Acne section 13.6.2

Non-gonococcal urethritis

● By mouth

Child 12–18 years 500 mg 4 times daily for 7–14 days (21 days if failure or relapse after first course)

Tetracycline (Non-proprietary) PoM
Tablets, coated, tetracycline hydrochloride 250 mg, net price 28-tab pack = £9.10. Label: 7, 9, 23, counselling, posture

Dental prescribing on NHS Tetracycline Tablets may be prescribed

---

▌DEMECLOCYCLINE HYDROCHLORIDE

Cautions see notes above, but photosensitivity more common (avoid exposure to sunlight or sun lamps)

Contra-indications see notes above

Hepatic impairment see notes above; max. 1 g daily in divided doses

◻ **DEMECLOCYCLINE HYDROCHLORIDE** (*continued*)

Renal impairment see notes above
Pregnancy see notes above
Breast-feeding see notes above
Side-effects see notes above; also reversible nephrogenic diabetes insipidus, acute renal failure

Indication and dose

Susceptible infections see notes above
• By mouth
   Child 12–18 years 150 mg 4 times daily *or* 300 mg twice daily

Ledermycin® (Goldshield) ℗Ⓞℳ
Capsules, red, demeclocycline hydrochloride 150 mg, net price 28-cap pack = £16.02. Label: 7, 9, 11, 23

DOXYCYCLINE

Cautions see notes above; alcohol dependence; photosensitivity reported (avoid exposure to sunlight or sun lamps)
Contra-indications see notes above
Hepatic impairment see notes above
Renal impairment use with caution (avoid excessive doses)
Pregnancy see notes above
Breast-feeding see notes above
Side-effects see notes above; also anorexia, dry mouth, flushing, anxiety, and tinnitus
Licensed use not licensed for use in children under 12 years

Indication and dose

Susceptible infections see notes above
• By mouth
   Child 12–18 years 200 mg on first day, then 100 mg daily; severe infections (including refractory urinary-tract infections) 200 mg daily

Early syphilis
• By mouth
   Child 12–18 years 100 mg twice daily for 14 days

Late latent syphilis
• By mouth
   Child 12–18 years 100 mg twice daily for 28 days

Uncomplicated genital chlamydia, non-gonococcal urethritis, pelvic inflammatory disease Table 1, section 5.1
• By mouth
   Child 12–18 years 100 mg twice daily for 7 days (14 days in pelvic inflammatory disease)

Lyme disease (see also section 5.1.1.3)
• By mouth
   Child 12–18 years 100 mg twice daily for 10–14 days (for 28 days in Lyme arthritis)

Anthrax (treatment or post-exposure prophylaxis) see also section 5.1.12
• By mouth
   Child under 12 years (only if alternative antibacterial cannot be given) 2.5 mg/kg twice daily (max. 100 mg twice daily)
   Child 12–18 years 100 mg twice daily

Acne section 13.6.2

Adjunct to gingival scaling and root planing for periodontitis section 12.3.1

Counselling Capsules should be swallowed whole with plenty of fluid during meals while sitting or standing
Note Doxycycline doses in BNF for Children may differ from those in product literature

Doxycycline (Non-proprietary) ℗Ⓞℳ
Capsules, doxycycline (as hyclate) 50 mg, net price 28-cap pack = £2.02; 100 mg, 8-cap pack = £1.25. Label: 6, 9, 11, 27, counselling, posture
Brands include *Doxylar®*
Dental prescribing on NHS Doxycycline Capsules 100 mg may be prescribed

Vibramycin-D® (Pfizer) ℗Ⓞℳ
Dispersible tablets, yellow, scored, doxycycline 100 mg, net price 8-tab pack = £4.91. Label: 6, 9, 11, 13

LYMECYCLINE

Cautions see notes above
Contra-indications see notes above
Hepatic impairment see notes above
Renal impairment see notes above
Pregnancy see notes above
Breast-feeding see notes above
Side-effects see notes above

Indication and dose

Susceptible infections see notes above
• By mouth
   Child 12–18 years 408 mg twice daily, increased to 1.224–1.632 g daily in severe infections

Acne
• By mouth
   Child 12–18 years 408 mg daily for at least 8 weeks

◻ **LYMECYCLINE** (continued)

Tetralysal 300® (Galderma) PoM
Capsules, red/yellow, lymecycline 408 mg
(= tetracycline 300 mg). Net price 28-cap pack =
£7.77, 56-cap pack = £14.97. Label: 6, 9

MINOCYCLINE

Cautions see notes above; if treatment continued
for longer than 6 months, monitor every 3
months for hepatotoxicity, pigmentation and for
systemic lupus erythematosus—discontinue if
these develop or if pre-existing systemic lupus
erythematosus worsens

Contra-indications see notes above

Hepatic impairment see notes above

Renal impairment use with caution (avoid excessive doses)

Pregnancy see notes above

Breast-feeding see notes above

Side-effects see notes above; also dizziness and
vertigo (more common in women); *rarely* anorexia, tinnitus, impaired hearing, hyperaesthesia,
paraesthesia, acute renal failure, pigmentation
(sometimes irreversible), and alopecia; *very rarely*
systemic lupus erythematosus, discoloration of
conjunctiva, tears, and sweat

Indication and dose

Susceptible infections see notes above
● By mouth
    Child 12–18 years 100 mg twice daily

Acne section 13.6.2

Counselling Tablets or capsules should be swallowed
whole with plenty of fluid while sitting or standing

Minocycline (Non-proprietary) PoM
Capsules, minocycline (as hydrochloride) 50 mg,
net price 56-cap pack = £15.27; 100 mg, 28-cap
pack = £13.09. Label: 6, 9, counselling, posture
Brands include *Aknemin®*

Tablets, minocycline (as hydrochloride) 50 mg, net
price 28-tab pack = £4.09; 100 mg, 28-tab pack =
£7.87. Label: 6, 9, counselling, posture

◢Modified release

Acnamino® MR (Dexcel) PoM
Capsules, m/r, buff/brown (enclosing pink and
peach tablets), minocycline (as hydrochloride)
100 mg, net price 56-cap pack = £21.14. Label: 6, 25
Dose
    Acne
    ● By mouth
        Child 12–18 years 1 capsule daily

Minocin MR® (Meda) PoM
Capsules, m/r, orange/brown (enclosing yellow
and white pellets), minocycline (as hydrochloride)
100 mg. Net price 56-cap pack = £20.08. Label: 6,
25
Dose
    Acne
    ● By mouth
        Child 12–18 years 1 capsule daily

Sebomin MR® (Actavis) PoM
Capsules, m/r, orange, minocycline (as hydro-
chloride) 100 mg, net price 56-cap pack = £20.32.
Label: 6, 25
Dose
    Acne
    ● By mouth
        Child 12–18 years 1 capsule daily

OXYTETRACYCLINE

Cautions see notes above

Contra-indications see notes above

Hepatic impairment see notes above

Renal impairment see notes above

Pregnancy see notes above

Breast-feeding see notes above

Side-effects see notes above

Indication and dose

Susceptible infections see notes above
● By mouth
    Child 12–18 years 250–500 mg 4 times daily

Acne section 13.6.2

Oxytetracycline (Non-proprietary) PoM
Tablets, coated, oxytetracycline dihydrate 250 mg,
net price 28-tab pack = £1.42. Label: 7, 9, 23
Brands include *Oxymycin®*
Dental prescribing on NHS Oxtetracycline Tablets may be
prescribed

5.1.4 Aminoglycosides

These include amikacin, gentamicin, neomycin, streptomycin, and tobramycin.
All are bactericidal and active against some Gram-positive and many Gram-
negative organisms. Amikacin, gentamicin, and tobramycin are also active against
Pseudomonas aeruginosa; streptomycin is active against *Mycobacterium tuberculosis*
and is now almost entirely reserved for tuberculosis (section 5.1.9).

The aminoglycosides are not absorbed from the gut (although there is a risk of absorption in inflammatory bowel disease and liver failure) and must therefore be given by injection for systemic infections.

Most side-effects of this group of antibiotics are dose-related; therefore care must be taken with dosage and whenever possible treatment should not exceed 7 days. The important side-effects are ototoxicity, and nephrotoxicity; they occur most commonly in children with renal failure.

Aminoglycosides may impair neuromuscular transmission and should not be given to children with myasthenia gravis; large doses given during surgery have been responsible for a transient myasthenic syndrome in patients with normal neuromuscular function.

Aminoglycosides should preferably not be given with potentially ototoxic diuretics (e.g. furosemide (frusemide)); if concurrent use is unavoidable, administration of the aminoglycoside and of the diuretic should be separated by as long a period as practicable.

Renal impairment   Excretion of aminoglycosides is principally via the kidney and accumulation occurs in renal impairment. Ototoxicity and nephrotoxicity occur commonly in patients with renal failure. If there is impairment of renal function, the interval between doses must be increased; if the renal impairment is severe, the dose itself should be reduced as well. Serum-aminoglycoside concentrations **must** be monitored in patients with renal impairment, see Serum Concentrations below; renal, auditory, and vestibular function should also be monitored. A once-daily, high-dose regimen of an aminoglycoside should be avoided in children over 1 month of age with a creatinine clearance less than $20\,\text{mL/minute/}1.73\,\text{m}^2$.

Once daily dosage   *Once daily administration* of aminoglycosides is more convenient, provides adequate serum concentrations, and has largely superseded *multiple-daily dose regimens* (given in 2–3 divided doses during the 24 hours). Local guidelines on dosage and serum concentrations should be consulted. A once-daily, high-dose regimen of an aminoglycoside should be avoided in children with endocarditis or burns of more than 20% of the total body surface area, or in children over 1 month of age with a creatinine clearance of less than $20\,\text{mL/minute/}1.73\,\text{m}^2$. The *extended interval dose regimen* is used in neonates to reflect the changes in renal function that occur with increasing gestational and postnatal age (see Neonates below).

Serum concentrations   Serum concentration monitoring avoids both excessive and subtherapeutic concentrations thus preventing toxicity and ensuring efficacy. In children with normal renal function, aminoglycoside concentration should be measured initially after 3 or 4 doses of a multiple daily dose regimen; children with renal impairment may require earlier and more frequent measurement of aminoglycoside concentration.

Blood samples should be taken just before the next dose is administered ('trough' concentration). If the pre-dose ('trough') concentration is high, the interval between doses must be increased. For multiple daily dose regimens, blood samples should also be taken approximately 1 hour after intramuscular or intravenous administration ('peak' concentration). If the post-dose ('peak') concentration is high, the dose must be decreased.

Serum-aminoglycoside concentration should be measured in all children and **must** be determined in infants, in neonates, in obesity, and in cystic fibrosis, *or* if high doses are being given, *or* if there is renal impairment.

Cystic fibrosis   A higher dose of parenteral aminoglycoside is often required in children with cystic fibrosis because renal clearance of the aminoglycoside is increased. For the role of aminoglycosides in the treatment of pseudomonal lung infections in cystic fibrosis see Table 1, section 5.1. Nebulised tobramycin is used for chronic pseudomonal lung infection in cystic fibrosis; however, resistance may develop, and some children do not respond to treatment. Gentamicin can be used similarly [unlicensed use].

Endocarditis   Gentamicin is used in combination with other antibiotics for the treatment of bacterial endocarditis (Table 1, section 5.1). Serum-gentamicin concentration should be determined twice each week (more often in renal

5
Infections

impairment). **Streptomycin** may be used as an alternative in gentamicin-resistant enterococcal endocarditis.

Gentamicin is the aminoglycoside of choice in the UK and is used widely for the treatment of serious infections. It has a broad spectrum but is inactive against anaerobes and has poor activity against haemolytic streptococci and pneumococci. When used for the 'blind' therapy of undiagnosed serious infections it is usually given in conjunction with a penicillin or metronidazole (or both). Gentamicin is used together with another antibiotic for the treatment of endocarditis (see above and Table 1, section 5.1).

Loading and maintenance doses may be calculated on the basis of the patient's weight and renal function (e.g. using a nomogram); adjustments are then made according to serum-gentamicin concentrations. High doses are occasionally indicated for serious infections, especially in the neonate, children with cystic fibrosis or the immunocompromised patient; whenever possible treatment should not exceed 7 days.

Amikacin is more stable than gentamicin to enzyme inactivation. Amikacin is used in the treatment of serious infections caused by gentamicin-resistant Gram-negative bacilli.

Tobramycin has similar activity to gentamicin. It is slightly more active against *Ps. aeruginosa* but shows less activity against certain other Gram-negative bacteria. Tobramycin may be administered by nebuliser for the treatment of *Ps. aeruginosa* infection in cystic fibrosis (see Cystic Fibrosis, above).

Neomycin is too toxic for parenteral administration and can only be used for infections of the skin or mucous membranes or to reduce the bacterial population of the colon prior to bowel surgery or in hepatic failure. Oral administration may lead to malabsorption. Small amounts of neomycin may be absorbed from the gut in children with hepatic failure and, as these children may also be uraemic, cumulation may occur with resultant ototoxicity.

Neonates   As aminoglycosides are eliminated principally via the kidney, neonatal treatment must reflect the changes in glomerular filtration that occur with increasing gestational and postnatal age. In patients on single daily dose regimens it may become necessary to prolong the dose interval to more than 24 hours if the trough concentration is high.

Pregnancy   There is a risk of auditory or vestibular nerve damage when aminoglycosides are used in the second and third trimesters of pregnancy. The risk is greatest with streptomycin (section 5.1.9). The risk is probably very small with gentamicin and tobramycin, but their use should be avoided unless essential (if given, serum-aminoglycoside concentration monitoring is essential).

GENTAMICIN

Cautions neonates, infants (adjust dose and monitor renal, auditory and vestibular function together with serum gentamicin concentrations); avoid prolonged use; conditions characterised by muscular weakness; see also notes above; **interactions**: Appendix 1 (aminoglycosides)

Contra-indications myasthenia gravis

Renal impairment see notes above

Pregnancy see notes above

Side-effects vestibular and auditory damage, nephrotoxicity; rarely, hypomagnesaemia on prolonged therapy, antibiotic-associated colitis; also reported, nausea, vomiting, rash, blood disorders; see also notes above

Licensed use not licensed for nebulisation

Pharmacokinetics *Extended interval dose regimen in neonates*: pre-dose ('trough') concentration should be less than 2 mg/litre

Once daily dose regimen: pre-dose ('trough') concentration should be less than 1 mg/litre

Multiple daily dose regimen: one hour ('peak') serum concentration should be 5–10 mg/litre (3–5 mg/litre for endocarditis, 8–12 mg/litre in cystic fibrosis); pre-dose ('trough') concentration should be less than 2 mg/litre (less than 1 mg/litre for endocarditis)

Intrathecal/intraventricular injection: cerebrospinal fluid concentration should not exceed 10 mg/litre

Indication and dose

> To avoid excessive dosage in obese or severely oedematous children, use ideal weight for height to calculate parenteral dose and monitor serum-gentamicin concentration closely

Neonatal sepsis

- Extended interval dose regimen by slow intravenous injection or intravenous infusion

  Neonate less than 32 weeks postmenstrual age
  4–5 mg/kg every 36 hours

  Neonate 32 weeks and over postmenstrual age
  4–5 mg/kg every 24 hours

◻ **GENTAMICIN** (continued)

- **Multiple daily dose regimen by slow intravenous injection**

  Neonate less than 29 weeks postmenstrual age 2.5 mg/kg every 24 hours

  Neonate 29–35 weeks postmenstrual age 2.5 mg/kg every 18 hours

  Neonate over 35 weeks postmenstrual age 2.5 mg/kg every 12 hours

Septicaemia, meningitis and other CNS infections, biliary-tract infection, acute pyelonephritis, endocarditis (see notes above), pneumonia in hospital patients, adjunct in listerial meningitis (Table 1, section 5.1)

- **Once daily dose regimen (not for endocarditis or meningitis) by intravenous infusion**

  Child 1 month–18 years initially 7 mg/kg, then adjusted according to serum-gentamicin concentration

- **Multiple daily dose regimen by intramuscular or by slow intravenous injection over at least 3 minutes**

  Child 1 month–12 years 2.5 mg/kg every 8 hours

  Child 12–18 years 2 mg/kg every 8 hours

Pseudomonal lung infection in cystic fibrosis

- **Multiple daily dose regimen by slow intravenous injection over at least 3 minutes or by intravenous infusion**

  Child 1 month–18 years 3 mg/kg every 8 hours

- **By inhalation of nebulised solution**

  Child 1 month–2 years 40 mg twice daily

  Child 2–8 years 80 mg twice daily

  Child 8–18 years 160 mg twice daily

Bacterial ventriculitis and CNS infection (supplement to systemic therapy)

- **By intrathecal or intraventricular injection, seek specialist advice**

  Neonate seek specialist advice

Child 1 month–18 years 1 mg daily (increased if necessary to 5 mg daily)
Note only preservative-free, intrathecal preparation should be used

Eye section 11.3.1

Ear section 12.1.1

Note Local guidelines may vary

Administration for *intravenous infusion*, dilute in Glucose 5% or Sodium Chloride 0.9%; give over 30 minutes

For *nebulisation*, dilute preservative-free preparation in 3 mL sodium chloride 0.9%. Administer after physiotherapy and bronchodilators

For *intrathecal* or *intraventricular injection*, use preservative-free intrathecal preparations only

Gentamicin (Non-proprietary) ℗ℴℳ
Injection, gentamicin (as sulphate), net price 40 mg/mL, 1-mL amp = £1.40, 2-mL amp = £1.54, 2-mL vial = £1.48

Paediatric injection, gentamicin (as sulphate) 10 mg/mL, net price 2-mL vial = £1.80

Intrathecal injection, gentamicin (as sulphate) 5 mg/mL, net price 1-mL amp = 74p

Intravenous infusion, gentamicin (as sulphate) 1 mg/mL in sodium chloride intravenous infusion 0.9%, net price 80-mL (80 mg) bottle = £1.95; 3 mg/mL, 80-mL (240 mg) bottle = £5.95, 120-mL (360 mg) bottle = £8.45

Cidomycin® (Sanofi-Aventis) ℗ℴℳ
Injection, gentamicin (as sulphate) 40 mg/mL. Net price 2-mL amp or vial = £1.48

Genticin® (Amdipharm) ℗ℴℳ
Injection, gentamicin (as sulphate) 40 mg/mL. Net price 2-mL amp = £1.40

Isotonic Gentamicin Injection (Baxter) ℗ℴℳ
Intravenous infusion, gentamicin (as sulphate) 800 micrograms/mL in sodium chloride intravenous infusion 0.9%. Net price 100-mL (80-mg) *Viaflex*® bag = £1.61
Electrolytes Na⁺ 15.4 mmol/100-mL bag

▰ **AMIKACIN**

Cautions see under Gentamicin; interactions: Appendix 1 (aminoglycosides)
Contra-indications see under Gentamicin
Renal impairment see notes above
Pregnancy see notes above
Side-effects see under Gentamicin
Pharmacokinetics *Multiple dose regimen*: one-hour ('peak') serum concentration should not exceed 30 mg/litre; pre-dose ('trough') concentration should be less than 10 mg/litre
Once daily dose regimen: pre-dose ('trough') concentration should be less than 5 mg/litre
Licensed use dose for cystic fibrosis not licensed

Indication and dose

To avoid excessive dosage in obese or severely oedematous children, use ideal weight for height to calculate dose and monitor serum-amikacin concentration closely

Neonatal sepsis

- **Extended interval dose regimen by slow intravenous injection over 3–5 minutes or by intravenous infusion**

  Neonate 15 mg/kg every 24 hours

- **Multiple daily dose regimen by intramuscular or by slow intravenous injection or by infusion**

  Neonate loading dose of 10 mg/kg then 7.5 mg/kg every 12 hours

5
Infections

342 5.1.4 Aminoglycosides

◻ AMIKACIN *(continued)*

Serious Gram-negative infections resistant to gentamicin
• By slow intravenous injection over 3–5 minutes
Child 1 month–12 years 7.5 mg/kg every 12 hours

Child 12–18 years 7.5 mg/kg every 12 hours, increased to 7.5 mg/kg every 8 hours in severe infections, max. 500 mg every 8 hours for up to 10 days (max. cumulative dose 15 g)

Once daily dose regimen (not for endocarditis or meningitis)
• By intravenous injection or infusion
Child 1 month–18 years initially 15 mg/kg, then adjusted according to serum-amikacin concentration

Pseudomonal lung infection in cystic fibrosis
• Multiple daily dose regimen by slow intravenous injection or infusion
Child 1 month–18 years 10 mg/kg every 8 hours (max. 500 mg every 8 hours)

Note Local dosage guidelines may vary

Administration for *intravenous infusion*, dilute with Glucose 5% *or* Sodium Chloride 0.9%; give over 30 minutes

Amikacin (Non-proprietary) PoM
Injection, amikacin (as sulphate) 250 mg/mL. Net price 2-mL vial = £10.14
Electrolytes Na⁺ 0.56 mmol/500-mg vial

Amikin® (Bristol-Myers Squibb) PoM
Injection, amikacin (as sulphate) 50 mg/mL. Net price 2-mL vial = £2.11
Electrolytes Na⁺< 0.5 mmol/vial

▌ TOBRAMYCIN

Cautions see under Gentamicin; **interactions:** Appendix 1 (aminoglycosides)
Specific cautions for inhaled treatment Other inhaled drugs should be administered before tobramycin; monitor for bronchospasm with initial dose, measure peak flow before and after nebulisation—if bronchospasm occurs, repeat test using bronchodilator; monitor renal function before treatment and then annually; severe haemoptysis

Contra-indications see under Gentamicin
Renal impairment see notes above
Pregnancy see notes above
Side-effects see under Gentamicin; *on inhalation*, mouth ulcers, taste disturbances, voice alteration, cough, bronchospasm (see Cautions)
Pharmacokinetics *Intravenous extended interval dose regimen in neonates or multiple daily dose regimen:* one-hour ('peak') serum concentration should not exceed 10 mg/litre (8–12 mg/litre in cystic fibrosis); pre-dose ('trough') concentration should be less than 2 mg/litre
Once daily dose regimen: pre-dose ('trough') concentration should be less than 1 mg/litre

Indication and dose

To avoid excessive dosage in obese or severely oedematous children, use ideal weight for height to calculate parenteral dose and monitor serum-tobramycin concentration closely

Neonatal sepsis
• Extended interval dose regimen by intravenous injection over 3–5 minutes or by intravenous infusion
Neonate less than 32 weeks postmenstrual age 4–5 mg/kg every 36 hours
Neonate 32 weeks and over postmenstrual age 4–5 mg/kg every 24 hours

• Multiple daily dose regimen by intramuscular injection or by slow intravenous injection or by intravenous infusion
Neonate under 7 days 2 mg/kg every 12 hours
Neonate 7–28 days 2–2.5 mg/kg every 8 hours

Septicaemia, meningitis and other CNS infections, biliary-tract infection, acute pyelonephritis, pneumonia in hospital patients
• Multiple daily dose regimen by slow intravenous injection over 3–5 minutes
Child 1 month–12 years 2–2.5 mg/kg every 8 hours
Child 12–18 years 1 mg/kg every 8 hours; in severe infections up to 5 mg/kg daily in divided doses every 6–8 hours (reduced to 3 mg/kg daily as soon as clinically indicated)

• Once daily dose regimen by intravenous infusion
Child 1 month–18 years initially 7 mg/kg, then adjusted according to serum-tobramycin concentration

Pseudomonal lung infection in cystic fibrosis
• Multiple daily dose regimen by slow intravenous injection over 3–5 minutes
Child 1 month–18 years 8–10 mg/kg/daily in 3 divided doses

• Once daily dose regimen by intravenous infusion over 30 minutes
Child 1 month–18 years initially 10 mg/kg (max. 660 mg), then adjusted according to serum-tobramycin concentration

Chronic pulmonary *Pseudomonas aeruginosa* infection in patients with cystic fibrosis
• By inhalation of nebulised solution
Child 6–18 years 300 mg every 12 hours for 28 days, subsequent courses repeated after 28-day interval without tobramycin nebuliser solution

Note Local dosage guidelines may vary
Administration for *intravenous infusion*, dilute with Glucose 5% *or* Sodium Chloride 0.9%; give over 20–60 minutes

TOBRAMYCIN (continued)

Parenteral

Tobramycin (Non-proprietary) [PoM]
Injection, tobramycin (as sulphate) 40 mg/mL, net price 1-mL (40-mg) vial = £4.00, 2-mL (80-mg) vial = £4.16, 6-mL (240-mg) vial = £19.20

Inhalation

Bramitob® (Chiesi) [PoM]
Nebuliser solution, tobramycin 75 mg/mL, net price 56 x 4-mL (300-mg) unit = £1187.00

Tobi® (Novartis) [PoM]
Nebuliser solution, tobramycin 60 mg/mL, net price 56 × 5-mL (300-mg) unit = £1187.20

5.1.5 Macrolides

Erythromycin has an antibacterial spectrum that is similar but not identical to that of penicillin; it is thus an alternative in penicillin-allergic patients.

Indications for erythromycin include respiratory infections, whooping cough, legionnaires' disease, and campylobacter enteritis. It is active against many penicillin-resistant staphylococci but some are now also resistant to erythromycin; it has poor activity against *Haemophilus influenzae*. Erythromycin is also active against chlamydia and mycoplasmas.

Erythromycin causes nausea, vomiting, and diarrhoea in some children; in mild to moderate infections this can be avoided by giving a lower dose or the total dose in 4 divided doses but if a more serious infection, such as Legionella pneumonia, is suspected higher doses are needed.

Clarithromycin is an erythromycin derivative with slightly greater activity than the parent compound. Tissue concentrations are higher than with erythromycin. It is given twice daily.

Azithromycin is a macrolide with slightly less activity than erythromycin against Gram-positive bacteria but enhanced activity against some Gram-negative organisms including *H. influenzae*. Plasma concentrations are very low but tissue concentrations are much higher. It has a long tissue half-life and once daily dosage is recommended. Azithromycin is also used in the treatment of trachoma [unlicensed indication] (section 11.3.1).

For the role of erythromycin, azithromycin, and clarithromycin in the treatment of Lyme disease, see section 5.1.1.3.

Azithromycin and clarithromycin cause fewer gastro-intestinal side-effects than erythromycin.

Spiramycin is also a macrolide (section 5.4.7).

Oral infections   Erythromycin is an alternative for oral infections in penicillin-allergic patients or where a beta-lactamase producing organism is involved. However, many organisms are now resistant to erythromycin or rapidly develop resistance; its use should therefore be limited to short courses. Metronidazole (section 5.1.11) may be preferred as an alternative to a penicillin.

ERYTHROMYCIN

Cautions neonate under 2 weeks (risk of hypertrophic pyloric stenosis); predisposition to QT interval prolongation (including electrolyte disturbances, concomitant use of drugs that prolong QT interval); acute porphyria (section 9.8.2); **interactions:** Appendix 1 (macrolides)

Hepatic impairment may cause idiosyncratic hepatotoxicity

Renal impairment reduce dose in severe renal impairment (ototoxicity)

Pregnancy not known to be harmful

Breast-feeding only small amounts in milk—not known to be harmful

Side-effects nausea, vomiting, abdominal discomfort, diarrhoea (antibiotic-associated colitis reported); less frequently urticaria, rashes and other allergic reactions; reversible hearing loss reported after large doses; cholestatic jaundice, pancreatitis, cardiac effects (including chest pain and arrhythmias), myasthenia-like syndrome, Stevens-Johnson syndrome, and toxic epidermal necrolysis also reported

Indication and dose

Susceptible infections in patients with penicillin hypersensitivity, oral infections (see notes above), campylobacter enteritis, respiratory-tract infections (including legionnaires' disease), skin infections, chlamydial ophthalmia

• **By mouth**

Neonate 12.5 mg/kg every 6 hours

Child 1 month–2 years 125 mg 4 times daily; dose doubled in severe infections

Child 2–8 years 250 mg 4 times daily; dose doubled in severe infections

5 Infections

◻ **ERYTHROMYCIN (continued)**

Child 8–18 years 250–500 mg 4 times daily; dose doubled in severe infections
Note Total daily dose may be given in two divided doses

- **By intermittent intravenous infusion**

  Neonate 10–12.5 mg/kg every 6 hours

  Child 1 month–18 years 12.5 mg/kg (max. 1 g) every 6 hours

- **By continuous intravenous infusion**

  Child 1 month–18 years 50 mg/kg daily (max. 4 g daily); mild infections (oral treatment not possible) 25 mg/kg daily

Early syphilis
- **By mouth**

  Child 12–18 years 500 mg 4 times daily for 14 days

Uncomplicated genital chlamydia, non-gono-coccal urethritis
- **By mouth**

  Child 12–18 years 500 mg twice daily for 14 days

Lyme disease (see also section 5.1.1.3)
- **By mouth**

  Child 1 month–18 years 12.5 mg/kg (max. 500 mg) 4 times daily for 14–21 days

Prophylaxis against pneumococcal infection
- **By mouth**

  Child 1 month–2 years 125 mg twice daily

  Child 2–8 years 250 mg twice daily

  Child 8–18 years 500 mg twice daily

Gastric stasis section 1.2

Acne vulgaris section 13.6

Diphtheria, whooping cough prophylaxis Table 2, section 5.1

Prevention of group A streptococcal infection Table 2, section 5.1

Administration Dilute reconstituted solution further in glucose 5% (neutralised with Sodium bicarbonate) or sodium chloride 0.9% to a concentration of 1 mg/mL for continuous infusion

and 1–5 mg/mL for intermittent infusion; give intermittent infusion over 20–60 minutes
Concentration of up to 10 mg/mL may be used in fluid-restriction if administered via a central venous catheter

Erythromycin (Non-proprietary) ⁅PoM⁆
Capsules, enclosing e/c microgranules, erythromycin 250 mg, net price 28-cap pack = £5.95. Label: 5, 9, 25
Brands include *Tiloryth*®

Tablets, e/c, erythromycin 250 mg, net price 28 = £1.97. Label: 5, 9, 25

Dental prescribing on NHS Erythromycin Tablets e/c may be prescribed

Erythromycin Ethyl Succinate (Non-proprietary) ⁅PoM⁆
Oral suspension, erythromycin (as ethyl succinate) for reconstitution with water 125 mg/5 mL, net price 100 mL = £1.79; 250 mg/5 mL, 100 mL = £2.38; 500 mg/5 mL, 100 mL = £3.90. Label: 9

Note Sugar-free versions are available and can be ordered by specifying 'sugar-free' on the prescription
Brands include *Primacine*®
Dental prescribing on NHS Erythromycin Ethyl Succinate Oral Suspension may be prescribed

Erythromycin Lactobionate (Non-proprietary) ⁅PoM⁆
Intravenous infusion, powder for reconstitution, erythromycin (as lactobionate), net price 1-g vial = £9.98

Erymax® (Cephalon) ⁅PoM⁆
Capsules, opaque orange/clear orange, enclosing orange and white e/c pellets, erythromycin 250 mg, net price 28-cap pack = £5.72, 112-cap pack = £22.87. Label: 5, 9, 25

Erythrocin® (Abbott) ⁅PoM⁆
Tablets, both f/c, erythromycin (as stearate), 250 mg, net price 100–tab pack = £18.20; 500 mg, 100–tab pack = £36.40. Label: 9
Dental prescribing on NHS May be prescribed as Erythromycin Stearate Tablets

Erythroped® (Abbott) ⁅PoM⁆
Suspension SF, sugar-free, banana-flavoured, erythromycin (as ethyl succinate) for reconstitution with water, 125 mg/5 mL (*Suspension PI SF*), net price 140 mL = £3.06; 250 mg/5 mL, 140 mL = £5.95; 500 mg/5 mL (*Suspension SF Forte*), 140 mL = £10.56. Label: 9

Erythroped A® (Abbott) ⁅PoM⁆
Tablets, yellow, f/c, erythromycin 500 mg (as ethyl succinate). Net price 28-tab pack = £10.78. Label: 9
Dental prescribing on NHS May be prescribed as Erythromycin Ethyl Succinate Tablets

---

AZITHROMYCIN

Cautions see under Erythromycin; **interactions:** Appendix 1 (macrolides)

Hepatic impairment manufacturer advises avoid in severe liver disease—no information available

Pregnancy manufacturer advises use only if adequate alternatives not available

Breast-feeding present in milk; use only if no suitable alternative

Side-effects see under Erythromycin; also anorexia, dyspepsia, flatulence, dizziness, headache, drowsiness, convulsions, arthralgia, and disturbances in taste and smell; *rarely* constipation, hepatitis, hepatic failure, syncope, insomnia, agitation, anxiety, asthenia, paraesthesia, hyperactivity, thrombocytopenia, haemolytic anaemia, insterstitial nephritis, acute renal failure, photosensitivity, tooth and tongue discoloration

◻ **AZITHROMYCIN** (*continued*)

Licensed use not licensed for typhoid fever, Lyme disease, or prophylaxis of group A streptococcal infection

Indication and dose

Respiratory-tract infections, otitis media, skin and soft-tissue infections
- **By mouth**

  Child over 6 months 10 mg/kg once daily (max. 500 mg once daily) for 3 days
  or

  Body-weight 15–25 kg 200 mg once daily for 3 days

  Body-weight 26–35 kg 300 mg once daily for 3 days

  Body-weight 36–45 kg 400 mg once daily for 3 days

  Body-weight over 45 kg 500 mg once daily for 3 days

Infection in cystic fibrosis
- **By mouth**

  Child 6 months–18 years 10 mg/kg once daily (max. 500 mg once daily) for 3 days; course repeated after 1 week, then repeat as necessary

Chronic *Pseudomonas aeruginosa* infection in cystic fibrosis
- **By mouth**

  Child 6–18 years

  Body-weight 25–40 kg 250 mg 3 times a week

  Body-weight over 40 kg 500 mg 3 times a week

Uncomplicated genital chlamydial infections and non-gonococcal urethritis
- **By mouth**

  Child 12–18 years 1 g as a single dose

Lyme disease (see also section 5.1.1.3), mild to moderate typhoid due to multiple-antibacterial resistant organisms
- **By mouth**

  Child 6 months–18 years 10 mg/kg once daily (max. 500 mg) for 7–10 days (for 7 days in typhoid)

Prevention of group A streptococcal infection
Table 2, section 5.1

Azithromycin (Non-proprietary) ⓅⓄⓂ
Capsules, azithromycin (as dihydrate) 250 mg, net price 4-cap pack = £8.85, 6-cap pack = £13.27. Label: 5, 9, 23

[1]Tablets, azithromycin (as monohydrate hemi-ethanolate) 250 mg, net price 4-tab pack = £8.81; 500 mg, 3-tab pack = £7.15. Label: 5, 9
1. Azithromycin tablets can be sold to the public for the treatment of confirmed, asymptomatic *Chlamydia trachomatis* genital infection in those over 16 years of age, and for the epidemiological treatment of their sexual partners, subject to max. single dose of 1 g, max. daily dose 1 g, and a pack size of 1 g

Zithromax® (Pfizer) ⓅⓄⓂ
Capsules, azithromycin (as dihydrate) 250 mg, net price 4-cap pack = £7.16, 6-cap pack = £10.74. Label: 5, 9, 23

Oral suspension, cherry/banana-flavoured, azithromycin (as dihydrate) 200 mg/5 mL when reconstituted with water. Net price 15-mL pack = £4.06, 22.5-mL pack = £6.10, 30-mL pack = £11.04. Label: 5, 9

Dental prescribing on NHS May be prescribed as Azithromycin Oral Suspension 200 mg/5 mL

◼ **CLARITHROMYCIN**

Cautions see under Erythromycin; **interactions:** Appendix 1 (macrolides)

Hepatic impairment hepatic dysfunction including jaundice reported

Renal impairment use half normal dose if estimated glomerular filtration rate less than 30 mL/minute/1.73 m^2; avoid *Klaricid XL®* if estimated glomerular filtration rate less than 30 mL/minute/1.73 m^2

Pregnancy manufacturer advises avoid unless potential benefit outweighs risk

Breast-feeding manufacturer advises avoid unless potential benefit outweighs risk—present in milk

Side-effects see under Erythromycin; also dyspepsia, tooth and tongue discoloration, smell and taste disturbances, stomatitis, glossitis, and headache; *less commonly* hepatitis, arthralgia, and myalgia; *rarely* tinnitus; *very rarely* pancreatitis, dizziness, insomnia, nightmares, anxiety, confusion, psychosis, paraesthesia, convulsions, hypoglycaemia, renal failure, leucopenia, and thrombocytopenia; on intravenous infusion, local tenderness, phlebitis

Licensed use intravenous route not licensed for use in children

Indication and dose

Respiratory-tract infections, mild to moderate skin and soft tissue infections, otitis media
- **By mouth**

  Neonate 7.5 mg/kg twice daily

  Child 1 month–12 years

  Body-weight under 8 kg 7.5 mg/kg twice daily

  Body-weight 8–11 kg 62.5 mg twice daily

  Body-weight 12–19 kg 125 mg twice daily

  Body-weight 20–29 kg 187.5 mg twice daily

  Body-weight 30–40 kg 250 mg twice daily

  Child 12–18 years 250 mg twice daily for 7 days, increased if necessary in severe infections to 500 mg every 12 hours for up to 14 days

5

Infections

5 Infections

□ **CLARITHROMYCIN** *(continued)*

• By intravenous infusion into large proximal vein

Child 1 month–12 years 7.5 mg/kg every 12 hours

Child 12–18 years 500 mg every 12 hours

Lyme disease (see also section 5.1.1.3)
• By mouth

Child 1 month–12 years 7.5 mg/kg (max. 500 mg) twice daily for 14–21 days

Child 12–18 years 500 mg twice daily for 14–21 days

Helicobacter pylori **eradication** section 1.3

Administration for intermittent intravenous infusion dilute reconstituted solution further in Glucose 5% *or* Sodium chloride 0.9% to a concentration of 2 mg/mL; give into large proximal vein over 60 minutes

Clarithromycin (Non-proprietary) PoM
Tablets, clarithromycin 250 mg, net price 14-tab pack = £3.34; 500 mg, 14-tab pack = £5.45. Label: 9

Klaricid® (Abbott) PoM
Tablets, both yellow, f/c, clarithromycin 250 mg, net price 14-tab pack = £7.14; 500 mg, 14-tab pack = £11.53, 20-tab pack = £16.47. Label: 9

Paediatric suspension, clarithromycin for reconstitution with water 125 mg/5 mL, net price 70 mL = £5.36, 100 mL = £9.23; 250 mg/5 mL, 70 mL = £10.72. Label: 9

Granules, clarithromycin 250 mg/sachet, net price 14-sachet pack = £11.68. Label: 9, 13

Intravenous infusion, powder for reconstitution, clarithromycin. Net price 500-mg vial = £9.45
Electrolytes Na$^+$< 0.5 mmol/500-mg vial

Klaricid XL® (Abbott) PoM
Tablets, m/r, yellow, clarithromycin 500 mg, net price 7-tab pack = £6.46, 14-tab pack = £12.71. Label: 9, 21, 25

Dose
• By mouth

Child 12–18 years 500 mg once daily (doubled in severe infections) for 7–14 days

5.1.6 Clindamycin

Clindamycin is active against Gram-positive cocci, including streptococci and penicillin-resistant staphylococci, and also against many anaerobes, especially *Bacteroides fragilis*. It is well concentrated in bone and excreted in bile and urine.

Clindamycin is recommended for staphylococcal joint and bone infections such as osteomyelitis, and intra-abdominal sepsis; it is an alternative to macrolides for erysipelas or cellulitis in penicillin-allergic patients. It is also used in combination with other antibacterials for cellulitis in immunocompromised children. Clindamycin can also be used for infections associated with meticillin-resistant *Staphylococcus aureus* (MRSA) in bone and joint infections, and skin and soft-tissue infections.

Clindamycin has been associated with antibiotic-associated colitis (section 1.5), which may be fatal. Although it can occur with most antibacterials, antibiotic-associated colitis occurs more frequently with clindamycin. Children should therefore discontinue treatment immediately if diarrhoea develops.

Oral infections Clindamycin should not be used routinely for the treatment of oral infections because it may be no more effective than penicillins against anaerobes and there may be cross-resistance with erythromycin-resistant bacteria. Clindamycin can be used for the treatment of dentoalveolar abscess that has not responded to penicillin or to metronidazole.

CLINDAMYCIN

Cautions discontinue immediately if diarrhoea or colitis develops; monitor liver and renal function on prolonged therapy and in neonates and infants; avoid rapid intravenous administration; avoid in acute porphyria (section 9.8.2); **interactions:** Appendix 1 (clindamycin)

Contra-indications diarrhoeal states; avoid injections containing benzyl alcohol in neonates (see under preparations below)

Pregnancy not known to be harmful

Breast-feeding amount probably too small to be harmful; bloody diarrhoea reported in 1 infant

Side-effects diarrhoea (discontinue treatment), abdominal discomfort, oesophagitis, oesophageal ulcers, taste disturbances, nausea, vomiting, antibiotic-associated colitis; jaundice; leucopenia, eosinophilia, and thrombocytopenia reported; polyarthritis reported; rash, pruritus, urticaria, anaphylactoid reactions, Stevens-Johnson syndrome, toxic epidermal necrolysis, exfoliative and vesiculobullous dermatitis reported; pain, induration, and abscess after intramuscular injection; thrombophlebitis after intravenous injection

◁ **CLINDAMYCIN (continued)**

Indication and dose

Staphylococcal bone and joint infections, peritonitis see notes above
* **By mouth**

  Neonate under 14 days 3–6 mg/kg 3 times daily

  Neonate 14–28 days 3–6 mg/kg 4 times daily

  Child 1 month–12 years 3–6 mg/kg 4 times daily (body-weight under 10 kg, minimum dose 37.5 mg 3 times daily)

  Child 12–18 years 150–300 mg 4 times daily; in severe infections 450 mg 4 times daily

* **By deep intramuscular injection or by intravenous infusion**

  Child 1 month–12 years 3.75–6.25 mg/kg 4 times daily; increased up to 10 mg/kg 4 times daily in severe infections; total daily dose may alternatively be given in 3 divided doses

  Child 12–18 years 150–675 mg 4 times daily; total daily dose may alternatively be given in 2–3 divided doses; in life-threatening infection up to 1.2 g 4 times daily; single doses above 600 mg by intravenous infusion only; single doses by intravenous infusion not to exceed 1.2 g

Staphylococcal lung infection in cystic fibrosis
* **By mouth**

  Child 1 month–18 years 5–7 mg/kg (max. 600 mg) 4 times daily

Treatment of falciparum malaria, see p. 401

Administration for *intravenous infusion*, dilute to a concentration of not more than 18 mg/mL with Glucose 5% *or* Sodium Chloride 0.9%; give over 10–60 minutes at a max. rate of 20 mg/kg/hour

Clindamycin (Non-proprietary) [PoM]
Capsules, clindamycin (as hydrochloride) 150 mg, net price 24-cap pack = £18.03. Label: 9, 27, counselling, see above (diarrhoea)
Dental prescribing on NHS Clindamycin Capsules may be prescribed

Liquid, 75 mg/5 mL available from 'special-order' manufacturers or specialist importing companies, see p. 957

Dalacin C® (Pharmacia) [PoM]
Capsules, clindamycin (as hydrochloride) 75 mg (green/white), net price 24-cap pack = £7.45; 150 mg, (white), 24-cap pack = £13.72. Label: 9, 27, counselling, see above (diarrhoea)
Dental prescribing on NHS May be prescribed as Clindamycin Capsules

Injection, clindamycin (as phosphate) 150 mg/mL, net price 2-mL amp = £6.20; 4-mL amp = £12.35
Excipients include benzyl alcohol (avoid in neonates, see Excipients, p. 3)

5.1.7 Some other antibacterials

Antibacterials discussed in this section include chloramphenicol, fusidic acid, glycopeptide antibiotics (vancomycin and teicoplanin), linezolid, and the polymyxin, colistin.

Chloramphenicol

Chloramphenicol is a potent broad-spectrum antibiotic; however, it is associated with serious haematological side-effects when given systemically and should therefore be reserved for the treatment of life-threatening infections, particularly those caused by *Haemophilus influenzae*, and also for typhoid fever. Chloramphenicol is also used in cystic fibrosis for the treatment of respiratory *Burkholderia cepacia* infection resistant to other antibacterials.

Grey baby syndrome may follow excessive doses in neonates with immature hepatic metabolism; monitoring of plasma concentrations is recommended.

Chloramphenicol eye drops (section 11.3.1) and chloramphenicol ear drops (section 12.1.1) are also available.

CHLORAMPHENICOL

Cautions avoid repeated courses and prolonged treatment; blood counts required before and periodically during treatment; monitor plasma-chloramphenicol concentration in neonates (see below); **interactions:** Appendix 1 (chloramphenicol)

Contra-indications acute porphyria (section 9.8.2)

Hepatic impairment avoid if possible—increased risk of bone-marrow depression; reduce dose and monitor plasma-chloramphenicol concentration

Renal impairment avoid in severe impairment unless no alternative; dose-related depression of haematopoiesis

Pregnancy manufacturer advises avoid; neonatal grey-baby syndrome if used in third trimester

Breast-feeding manufacturer advises avoid; use another antibiotic; may cause bone-marrow toxicity in infant; concentration in milk usually insufficient to cause 'grey-baby syndrome'

Side-effects blood disorders including reversible and irreversible aplastic anaemia (with reports of resulting leukaemia), peripheral neuritis, optic

☐ CHLORAMPHENICOL (continued)

neuritis, headache, depression, urticaria, erythema multiforme, nausea, vomiting, diarrhoea, stomatitis, glossitis, dry mouth; nocturnal haemoglobinuria reported; grey syndrome (abdominal distension, pallid cyanosis, circulatory collapse) may follow excessive doses in neonates with immature hepatic metabolism (see Pharmacokinetics below)

Pharmacokinetics plasma concentration monitoring required in neonates and preferred in those under 4 years of age, and in hepatic impairment; recommended peak plasma concentration (approx. 1 hour after end of intravenous injection or infusion or 2 hours after oral administration) 15–25 mg/litre; pre-dose ('trough') concentration should not exceed 15 mg/litre

Indication and dose

See notes above

• **By intravenous injection**

Neonate up to 14 days 12.5 mg/kg twice daily

Neonate 14–28 days 12.5 mg/kg 2–4 times daily
Note Check dosage carefully; overdosage can be fatal (see also pharmacokinetics above)

• **By mouth or by intravenous injection or infusion**

Child 1 month–18 years 12.5 mg/kg every 6 hours; dose may be doubled in severe infections such as septicaemia, meningitis and epiglottitis providing plasma-chloramphenicol concentrations are measured and high doses reduced as soon as indicated

Administration Displacement value may be significant for injection, consult local guidelines. For intermittent intravenous infusion, dilute reconstituted solution further in glucose 5% *or* sodium chloride 0.9%

Chloramphenicol (Non-proprietary) ⓅⓞⓂ
Capsules, chloramphenicol 250 mg. Net price 60 = £377.00

◢Extemporaneous formulations available see Extemporaneous Preparations, p. 8

Kemicetine® (Pharmacia) ⓅⓞⓂ
Injection, powder for reconstitution, chloramphenicol (as sodium succinate). Net price 1-g vial = £1.39
Electrolytes Na⁺ 3.14 mmol/g

Fusidic acid

Fusidic acid and its salts are narrow-spectrum antibiotics. The only indication for their use is in infections caused by penicillin-resistant staphylococci, especially osteomyelitis, as they are well concentrated in bone; they are also used for staphylococcal endocarditis. A second antistaphylococcal antibiotic is usually required to prevent emergence of resistance during treatment.

◤ SODIUM FUSIDATE

Cautions monitor liver function with high doses or on prolonged therapy; elimination may be reduced in hepatic impairment or biliary disease or biliary obstruction; **interactions:** Appendix 1 (fusidic acid)

Hepatic impairment impaired biliary excretion, avoid or reduce dose; possibly increased risk of hepatotoxicity, monitor liver function

Pregnancy not known to be harmful; manufacturer advises use only if potential benefit outweighs risk

Breast-feeding present in milk; manufacturer advises caution

Side-effects nausea, vomiting, reversible jaundice, especially after high dosage or rapid infusion (withdraw therapy if persistent); rarely hypersensitivity reactions, acute renal failure (usually with jaundice), blood disorders

Indication and dose

Penicillin-resistant staphylococcal infection including osteomyelitis, staphylococcal endocarditis in combination with other antibacterials see under Preparations, below

Sodium fusidate (LEO) ⓅⓞⓂ
Intravenous infusion, powder for reconstitution, sodium fusidate 500 mg (= fusidic acid 480 mg),

with buffer, net price per vial (with diluent) = £70.04
Electrolytes Na⁺ 3.1 mmol/vial when reconstituted with buffer

Dose

As sodium fusidate
• **By intravenous infusion**

Neonate 10 mg/kg every 12 hours

Child 1 month–18 years 6–7 mg/kg (max. 500 mg) every 8 hours

Administration reconstitute with buffer solution provided; further dilute to 1 mg/mL with Sodium chloride 0.9% *or* Glucose 5% intravenous infusion (but see below); infuse over at least 6 hours via a superficial vein or 2 hours via a central venous line; incompatible in solution of pH less than 7.4

Fucidin® (LEO) ⓅⓞⓂ
Tablets, f/c, sodium fusidate 250 mg, net price 10-tab pack = £6.02. Label: 9

Dose

As sodium fusidate
• **By mouth**
Child 12–18 years 500 mg every 8 hours, dose doubled for severe infections

Skin infection as sodium fusidate
• **By mouth**
Child 12–18 years 250 mg every 12 hours for 5–10 days

◁ SODIUM FUSIDATE (continued)

Suspension, off-white, banana- and orange-flavoured, fusidic acid 250 mg/5 mL, net price 50 mL = £6.73. Label: 9, 21

Dose

As fusidic acid
- By mouth

Neonate 15 mg/kg 3 times daily

Child 1 month–1 year 15 mg/kg 3 times daily

Child 1–5 years 250 mg 3 times daily

Child 5–12 years 500 mg 3 times daily

Child 12–18 years 750 mg 3 times daily

Note Fusidic acid is incompletely absorbed and doses recommended for suspension are proportionately higher than those for sodium fusidate tablets

Vancomycin and teicoplanin

The glycopeptide antibiotics vancomycin and teicoplanin have bactericidal activity against aerobic and anaerobic Gram-positive bacteria including multi-resistant *Staphylococci*. However, there are reports of *Staphylococcus aureus* with reduced susceptibility to glycopeptides. There are increasing reports of glycopeptide-resistant *Enterococci*.

Vancomycin is used *by the intravenous route* in the prophylaxis and treatment of serious infections caused by Gram-positive cocci. Vancomycin is principally excreted via the kidney and dose reduction is necessary in renal impairment.

Penetration in to cerebrospinal fluid is poor; vancomycin may be administered by the intrathecal or intraventricular route for treatment of meningitis [unlicensed]. Vancomycin (added to dialysis fluid) is also used in the treatment of peritonitis associated with peritoneal dialysis [unlicensed route] (Table 1 section 5.1).

Vancomycin given *by mouth* for 10–14 days is effective in the treatment of *Clostridium difficile* infection (see also section 1.5); low doses are considered adequate (higher dose may be considered if the infection fails to respond or if it is life-threatening). Vancomycin is also used by mouth in prophylaxis of neonatal necrotising enterocolitis. Vancomycin should **not** be given by mouth for systemic infections since it is not significantly absorbed.

Teicoplanin is similar to vancomycin but has a significantly longer duration of action allowing once-daily administration. Plasma concentration monitoring is not usually necessary, but may help optimise therapy. Unlike vancomycin, teicoplanin can be given by intramuscular as well as by intravenous injection; it is not given by mouth.

VANCOMYCIN

Cautions avoid rapid infusion (risk of anaphylactoid reactions, see Side-effects); rotate infusion sites; avoid if history of deafness; all patients require plasma-vancomycin measurement (after 3 or 4 doses if renal function normal, earlier if renal impairment), blood counts, urinalysis, and renal function tests; monitor auditory function in renal impairment; teicoplanin sensitivity; systemic absorption may follow oral administration especially in inflammatory bowel disorders or following multiple doses; **interactions**: Appendix 1 (vancomycin)

Renal impairment reduce dose—monitor plasma-vancomycin concentration and renal function regularly; see also Cautions above

Pregnancy manufacturer advises use only if potential benefit outweighs risk—plasma-vancomycin concentration monitoring essential to reduce risk of fetal toxicity

Breast-feeding present in milk—significant absorption following oral administration unlikely

Side-effects after parenteral administration: nephrotoxicity including renal failure and interstitial nephritis; ototoxicity (discontinue if tinnitus occurs); blood disorders including neutropenia (usually after 1 week or high cumulative dose), rarely agranulocytosis and thrombocytopenia; nausea; chills; fever; eosinophilia, anaphylaxis, rashes (including exfoliative dermatitis, Stevens-Johnson syndrome, toxic epidermal necrolysis, and vasculitis); phlebitis (irritant to tissue); on rapid infusion, severe hypotension (including shock and cardiac arrest), wheezing, dyspnoea, urticaria, pruritus, flushing of the upper body ('red man' syndrome), pain and muscle spasm of back and chest

Pharmacokinetics plasma concentration monitoring required; pre-dose ('trough') concentration should be 10–15 mg/litre (15–20 mg/litre for less sensitive strains of meticillin-resistant *Staphylococcus aureus*)

Licensed use not licensed for intraventricular use

Indication and dose

Infections due to Gram-positive bacteria including osteomyelitis, septicaemia and soft-tissue infections see notes above

- By intravenous infusion

Neonate less than 29 weeks postmenstrual age 15 mg/kg every 24 hours, adjusted according to plasma concentration

5 Infections

5 Infections

◯ **VANCOMYCIN** *(continued)*

Neonate 29–35 weeks postmenstrual age
15 mg/kg every 12 hours, adjusted according to plasma concentration

Neonate over 35 weeks postmenstrual age
15 mg/kg every 8 hours, adjusted according to plasma concentration

Child 1 month–18 years 15 mg/kg every 8 hours (maximum daily dose 2 g), adjusted according to plasma concentration

Clostridium difficile infection (see also notes above)
● **By mouth**

Child 1 month–5 years 5 mg/kg 4 times daily for 10–14 days (increased up to 10 mg/kg 4 times daily if infection fails to respond or is life-threatening)

Child 5–12 years 62.5 mg 4 times daily for 10–14 days (increased up to 250 mg 4 times daily if infection fails to respond or is life-threatening)

Child 12–18 years 125 mg 4 times daily for 10–14 days (increased up to 500 mg 4 times daily if infection fails to respond or is life-threatening)

Prophylaxis of necrotising enterocolitis in neonates
● **By mouth**

Neonate 15 mg/kg 3 times daily

CNS infection e.g. ventriculitis
● **By intraventricular administration, seek specialist advice**

Neonate 10 mg once every 24 hours

Child 1 month–18 years 10 mg once every 24 hours
Note for all children reduce to 5 mg daily if ventricular size reduced or increase to 15–20 mg once daily if ventricular size increased. Adjust dose according to CSF concentration after 3-4 days; aim for pre-dose ('trough') concentration less than 10 mg/litre. If CSF not draining freely reduce dose frequency to once every 2–3 days

Peritonitis associated with peritoneal dialysis
Add to each bag of dialysis fluid to achieve a concentration of 20–25 mg/litre

Note Vancomycin doses in BNF for Children may differ from those in product literature

Administration Displacement value may be significant, consult product literature and local guidelines. For intermittent intravenous infusion, the reconstituted preparation should be further diluted in sodium chloride 0.9% *or* glucose 5% to a concentration of up to 5 mg/mL; give over at least 60 minutes (rate not to exceed 10 mg/minute for doses over 500 mg); use continuous infusion only if intermittent not available (limited evidence); 10 mg/mL can be used if infused via a central venous line over at least 1 hour

Injection may be given orally; flavouring syrups may be added to the solution at the time of administration

Safe Practice For intraventricular administration, seek specialist advice

Vancomycin (Non-proprietary) PoM
Capsules, vancomycin (as hydrochloride) 125 mg, net price 28-cap pack = £132.47; 250 mg, 28-cap pack = £132.47. Label: 9

Injection, powder for reconstitution, vancomycin (as hydrochloride), for use as an infusion, net price 500-mg vial = £7.25; 1-g vial = £14.50

Note Can be used to prepare solution for oral administration

Vancocin® (Flynn) PoM
Matrigel capsules, vancomycin (as hydrochloride) 125 mg, net price 28-cap pack = £88.31. Label: 9

Injection, powder for reconstitution, vancomycin (as hydrochloride), for use as an infusion, net price 500-mg vial = £8.05; 1-g vial = £16.11

Note Can be used to prepare solution for oral administration

▲ **TEICOPLANIN**

Cautions vancomycin sensitivity; blood counts and liver and kidney function tests required—monitor renal and auditory function on prolonged administration during renal impairment or if other nephrotoxic or neurotoxic drugs given; monitor plasma-teicoplanin concentration if severe sepsis or burns, deep-seated staphylococcal infection (including bone and joint infection), endocarditis, renal impairment, and in intravenous drug abusers; **interactions:** Appendix 1 (teicoplanin)

Renal impairment reduce dose on day 4: use half normal dose if estimated glomerular filtration rate 40–60 mL/minute/1.73 m^2 and use one-third normal dose if estimated glomerular filtration rate less than 40 mL/minute/1.73 m^2; see also Cautions above

Pregnancy manufacturer advises use only if potential benefit outweighs risk

Breast-feeding no information available

Side-effects nausea, vomiting, diarrhoea; rash, pruritus, fever, bronchospasm, rigors, urticaria, angioedema, anaphylaxis; dizziness, headache; blood disorders including eosinophilia, leucopenia, neutropenia, and thrombocytopenia; disturbances in liver enzymes, transient increase of serum creatinine, renal failure; tinnitus, mild hearing loss, and vestibular disorders also reported; rarely exfoliative dermatitis, Stevens-Johnson syndrome, toxic epidermal necrolysis; local reactions include erythema, pain, thrombophlebitis, injection site abscess and rarely flushing with infusion

Pharmacokinetics plasma-teicoplanin concentration is not measured routinely because there is no clear relationship between plasma-teicoplanin concentration and toxicity. However, the plasma-teicoplanin concentration can be used to opti-

◁ **TEICOPLANIN** (*continued*)

mise treatment in some patients (see Cautions). Pre-dose ('trough') concentration should be greater than 10 mg/litre (greater than 15–20 mg/litre in endocarditis) but less than 60 mg/litre

Indication and dose

Potentially serious Gram-positive infections including endocarditis, and serious infections due to Staphylococcus aureus

• **By intravenous injection or intravenous infusion over 30 minutes**

Neonate initially 16 mg/kg for one dose followed 24 hours later by 8 mg/kg once daily (intravenous infusion only)

Child 1 month–18 years in moderate infections initially 10 mg/kg (max. 400 mg) every 12 hours for 3 doses, then 6 mg/kg (max. 200 mg) once daily; in severe infections or in neutropenia initially 10 mg/kg (max. 400 mg) every 12 hours for 3 doses then 10 mg/kg (max. 400 mg) once daily; after first 3 doses, subsequent doses can be given by intramuscular injection if necessary although intravenous route preferable for children

Administration For intermittent intravenous infusion, dilute reconstituted solution further in sodium chloride 0.9% *or* glucose 5% *or* compound sodium lactate intravenous infusion; give over 30 minutes. Intermittent intravenous infusion preferred in neonates

Targocid® (Sanofi-Aventis) PoM
Injection, powder for reconstitution, teicoplanin, net price 200-mg vial (with diluent) = £3.57; 400-mg vial (with diluent) = £6.10
Electrolytes Na$^+$< 0.5 mmol/200- and 400-mg vial

Linezolid

Linezolid, an oxazolidinone antibacterial, is active against Gram-positive bacteria including meticillin-resistant *Staphylococcus aureus* (MRSA), and glycopeptide-resistant enterococci. Resistance to linezolid can develop with prolonged treatment or if the dose is less than that recommended. Linezolid should be reserved for infections caused by Gram-positive bacteria when the organisms are resistant to other antibacterials or when patients cannot tolerate other antibacterials. Linezolid is **not** active against common Gram-negative organisms; it must be given in combination with other antibacterials for mixed infections that also involve Gram-negative organisms. There is limited information on use in children and expert advice should be sought. A higher incidence of blood disorders and optic neuropathy have been reported in patients receiving linezolid for more than the maximum recommended duration of 28 days.

LINEZOLID

Cautions monitor full blood count (including platelet count) weekly (see also Blood Disorders below); unless close observation and blood-pressure monitoring possible, avoid in uncontrolled hypertension, phaeochromocytoma, carcinoid tumour, thyrotoxicosis, bipolar depression, schizophrenia, or acute confusional states; **interactions:** Appendix 1 (MAOIs)

Blood disorders Haematopoietic disorders (including thrombocytopenia, anaemia, leucopenia, and pancytopenia) have been reported in patients receiving linezolid. It is recommended that full blood counts are monitored weekly. Close monitoring is recommended in patients who:

• receive treatment for more than 10–14 days;
• have pre-existing myelosuppression;
• are receiving drugs that may have adverse effects on haemoglobin, blood counts, or platelet function;
• have severe renal impairment.

If significant myelosuppression occurs, treatment should be stopped unless it is considered essential, in which case intensive monitoring of blood counts and appropriate management should be implemented.

CHM advice (optic neuropathy) Severe optic neuropathy may occur rarely, particularly if linezolid is used for longer than 28 days. The CHM recommends that:

• patients should be warned to report symptoms of visual impairment (including blurred vision, visual field defect, changes in visual acuity and colour vision) immediately;
• patients experiencing new visual symptoms (regardless of treatment duration) should be evaluated promptly, and referred to an ophthalmologist if necessary;
• visual function should be monitored regularly if treatment is required for longer than 28 days.

Monoamine oxidase inhibition Linezolid is a reversible, non-selective monoamine oxidase inhibitor (MAOI). Patients should avoid consuming large amounts of tyramine-rich foods (such as mature cheese, yeast extracts, undistilled alcoholic beverages, and fermented soya bean products). In addition, linezolid should not be given with another MAOI or within 2 weeks of stopping another MAOI. Unless close observation and blood-pressure monitoring is possible, avoid in those receiving SSRIs, 5HT$_1$ agonists ('triptans'), tricyclic antidepressants, sympathomimetics, dopaminergics, buspirone, pethidine and possibly other opioid analgesics. For other interactions see Appendix 1 (MAOIs)

Contra-indications see Monoamine Oxidase Inhibition above

Hepatic impairment no dose adjustment necessary but in severe hepatic impairment use only if potential benefit outweighs risk

Renal impairment no dose adjustment necessary but metabolites may accumulate if estimated

5

Infections

⌂ LINEZOLID (continued)

glomerular filtration rate less than 30 mL/minute/1.73 m²; see also Blood Disorders above

Pregnancy manufacturer advises use only if potential benefit outweighs risk—no information available

Breast-feeding manufacturer advises avoid—present in milk in *animal* studies

Side-effects diarrhoea (antibiotic-associated colitis reported), nausea, vomiting, taste disturbances, headache; *less commonly* thirst, dry mouth, glossitis, stomatitis, tongue discoloration, abdominal pain, dyspepsia, gastritis, constipation, pancreatitis, hypertension, fever, fatigue, dizziness, insomnia, hypoaesthesia, paraesthesia, tinnitus, polyuria, anaemia, leucopenia, thrombocytopenia, eosinophilia, electrolyte disturbances, blurred vision, rash, pruritus, diaphoresis, and injection-site reactions; *very rarely* renal failure, pancytopenia and Stevens-Johnson syndrome; also reported tooth discoloration, convulsions, lactic acidosis; peripheral and optic neuropathy reported on prolonged therapy (see also CHM Advice above)

Licensed use not licensed for use in children

Indication and dose

Pneumonia, complicated skin and soft-tissue infections caused by Gram-positive bacteria (initiated under expert supervision)

- By mouth or by intravenous infusion over 30–120 minutes

  Neonate under 7 days 10 mg/kg every 12 hours, increase to every 8 hours if poor response

  Neonate over 7 days 10 mg/kg every 8 hours

  Child 1 month–12 years 10 mg/kg (max. 600 mg) every 8 hours

  Child 12–18 years 600 mg every 12 hours

Zyvox® (Pharmacia) ▼ PoM
Tablets, f/c, linezolid 600 mg, net price 10-tab pack = £445.00. Label: 9, 10, patient information leaflet

Suspension, yellow, linezolid 100 mg/5 mL when reconstituted with water, net price 150 mL (orange-flavoured) = £222.50. Label: 9, 10 patient information leaflet
Excipients include aspartame 20 mg/5 mL (section 9.4.1)

Intravenous infusion, linezolid 2 mg/mL, net price 300-mL *Excel®* bag = £44.50
Excipients include Na⁺ 5 mmol/300-mL bag, glucose 13.71 g/300-mL bag

Polymyxins

The polymyxin antibiotic, **colistin**, is active against Gram-negative organisms including *Pseudomonas aeruginosa*, *Acinetobacter baumanii*, and *Klebsiella pneumoniae*. It is **not** absorbed by mouth and is given by injection for a systemic effect. Intravenous administration of colistin should be reserved for Gram-negative infections resistant to other antibacterials; its major adverse effects are dose-related neurotoxicity and nephrotoxicity.

Colistin is used by mouth in bowel sterilisation regimens in neutropenic patients (usually with nystatin); it is **not** recommended for gastro-intestinal infections. It is also given by inhalation of a nebulised solution as an adjunct to standard antibacterial therapy in patients with cystic fibrosis.

Both colistin and polymyxin B are included in some preparations for topical application.

COLISTIN

Cautions acute porphyria (section 9.8.2); risk of bronchospasm on inhalation—may be prevented or treated with a selective beta₂ agonist; **interactions**: Appendix 1 (polymyxins)

Contra-indications myasthenia gravis

Renal impairment monitor plasma-colistin concentration during parenteral treatment. Reduce parenteral dose in moderate to severe impairment

Pregnancy avoid—possible risk of fetal toxicity especially in second and third trimesters

Breast-feeding present in milk but poorly absorbed from gut; manufacturers advise avoid (or use only if potential benefit outweighs risk)

Side-effects neurotoxicity reported especially with excessive doses (including apnoea, perioral and peripheral paraesthesia, vertigo; rarely vasomotor instability, slurred speech, confusion, psychosis, visual disturbances); nephrotoxicity; hypersensitivity reactions including rash; injection-site reactions; inhalation may cause sore throat, sore mouth, cough, bronchospasm

Pharmacokinetics see notes above; plasma concentration monitoring required for intravenous treatment in renal impairment and cystic fibrosis; recommended 'peak' plasma-colistin concentration (approx. 30 minutes after intravenous injection or infusion) 10–15 mg/litre (125–200 units/mL); colistin sulphate may be absorbed from the gastro-intestinal tract in infants under 6 months old

Indication and dose

Pseudomonas aeruginosa infection in cystic fibrosis

- By slow intravenous injection into a totally implantable venous access device, or by intravenous infusion (but see notes above)

  Child 1 month–18 years

  Body-weight under 60 kg 16 666–25 000 units/kg every 8 hours

◻ **COLISTIN (continued)**

Body-weight over 60 kg 1–2 million units every 8 hours

• **By inhalation of nebulised solution**

Child 1 month–2 years 500 000–1 million units twice daily

Child 2–18 years 1–2 million units twice daily

Administration For *intravenous infusion*, dilute to a concentration of 40 000 units/mL with Sodium Chloride 0.9%; give over 30 minutes

For *slow intravenous injection* into a totally implantable venous access device, dilute to a concentration of 90 000 units/mL for child under 12 years (200 000 units/mL for child over 12 years)

For *nebulisation* administer required dose in 2–4 mL of sodium chloride 0.9% (or water for injections). Colistin must not be mixed with tobramycin as they are chemically unstable

together; it may be mixed with gentamicin if used immediately

Colomycin® (Forest) PoM
Injection, powder for reconstitution, colistimethate sodium (colistin sulphomethate sodium). Net price 1 million-unit vial = £1.68; 2 million-unit vial = £3.09
Electrolytes (before reconstitution) Na⁺< 0.5 mmol/1 million-unit and 2 million-unit vial
Note *Colomycin®* Injection (dissolved in physiological saline) may be used for nebulisation

Promixin® (Profile) PoM
Powder for nebuliser solution, colistimethate sodium (colistin sulphomethate sodium), net price 1 million-unit vial = £4.60.

Injection, powder for reconstitution, colistimethate sodium (colistin sulphomethate sodium), net price 1 million unit-vial = £2.30
Electrolytes (before reconstitution) Na⁺< 0.5 mmol/1 million-unit vial

5.1.8 Sulphonamides and trimethoprim

The importance of the sulphonamides has decreased as a result of increasing bacterial resistance and their replacement by antibacterials which are generally more active and less toxic.

Sulfamethoxazole (sulphamethoxazole) and trimethoprim are used in combination (as **co-trimoxazole**) because of their synergistic activity. However, co-trimoxazole is associated with rare but serious side-effects e.g. Stevens-Johnson syndrome and blood dyscrasias, notably bone marrow depression and agranulocytosis (see CSM recommendations below). Co-trimoxazole should be avoided in children less than 6 weeks of age (except for treatment and prophylaxis of *pneumocystis pneumonia*) because of the risk of kernicterus. There is a risk of haemolytic anaemia if used in children with glucose-6-phosphate dehydrogenase (G6PD) deficiency (section 9.1.5).

> **Restrictions on the use of co-trimoxazole**
> Co-trimoxazole should be limited to the role of drug of choice in *Pneumocystis jirovecii* (*Pneumocystis carinii*) pneumonia; it is also indicated for *toxoplasmosis* and *nocardiasis*. It should now only be considered for use in *acute exacerbations of chronic bronchitis* and *infections of the urinary tract* when there is good bacteriological evidence of sensitivity to co-trimoxazole and good reason to prefer this combination to a single antibacterial; similarly it should only be used in *acute otitis media in children* when there is good reason to prefer it.

Trimethoprim can be used alone for urinary- and respiratory-tract infections and for shigellosis and invasive salmonella infections. Trimethoprim has side-effects similar to co-trimoxazole but they are less severe and occur less frequently.

For *topical preparations* of sulphonamides used in the treatment of burns see section 13.10.1.1.

CO-TRIMOXAZOLE

A mixture of trimethoprim and sulfamethoxazole in the proportions of 1 part to 5 parts
Cautions maintain adequate fluid intake; avoid in blood disorders (unless under specialist supervision); monitor blood counts on prolonged treatment; discontinue immediately if blood disorders or rash develop; predisposition to folate deficiency; asthma; G6PD deficiency (section 9.1.5); avoid in infants under 6 weeks (except for treatment or prophylaxis of pneumocystis pneumonia); **interactions**: Appendix 1 (trimethoprim, sulfamethoxazole)

Contra-indications acute porphyria (section 9.8.2)

Hepatic impairment manufacturer advises avoid in severe liver disease

Renal impairment use half normal dose if estimated glomerular filtration rate 15–30 mL/minute/1.73 m²; avoid if estimated glomerular filtration rate less than 15 mL/minute/1.73 m² and if plasma-sulfamethoxazole concentration cannot be monitored

◻ CO-TRIMOXAZOLE (continued)

Pregnancy teratogenic risk in first trimester (trimethoprim a folate antagonist). Neonatal haemolysis and methaemoglobinaemia in third trimester; fear of increased risk of kernicterus in neonates appears to be unfounded

Breast-feeding small risk of kernicterus in jaundiced infants and of haemolysis in G6PD-deficient infants (due to sulfamethoxazole)

Side-effects nausea, diarrhoea; headache, hyperkalaemia; rash (very rarely including Stevens-Johnson syndrome, toxic epidermal necrolysis, photosensitivity)—discontinue immediately; less commonly vomiting; very rarely glossitis, stomatitis, anorexia, liver damage (including jaundice and hepatic necrosis), pancreatitis, antibiotic-associated colitis, myocarditis, cough and shortness of breath, pulmonary infiltrates, aseptic meningitis, depression, convulsions, peripheral neuropathy, ataxia, tinnitus, vertigo, hallucinations, hypoglycaemia, blood disorders (including leucopenia, thrombocytopenia, megaloblastic anaemia, eosinophilia), hyponatraemia, renal disorders including interstitial nephritis, arthralgia, myalgia, vasculitis, systemic lupus erythematosus, and uveitis; rhabdomyolysis reported in HIV-infected patients

Pharmacokinetics plasma concentration monitoring may be required with high doses or during moderate to severe renal impairment; seek expert advice

Licensed use not licensed for use in children under 6 weeks

Indication and dose

Treatment of susceptible infections (but see notes above) dose expressed as co-trimoxazole
- By mouth
  Child 6 weeks–12 years 24 mg/kg twice daily or
  Child 6 weeks–6 months 120 mg twice daily
  Child 6 months–6 years 240 mg twice daily
  Child 6–12 years 480 mg twice daily
  Child 12–18 years 960 mg twice daily
- By intravenous infusion
  Child 6 weeks–18 years 18 mg/kg every 12 hours; increased in severe infection to 27 mg/kg (max. 1.44 g) every 12 hours

Treatment of Pneumocystis jirovecii (P. carinii) infections (undertaken where facilities for appropriate monitoring available—consult microbiologist and product literature)
- By mouth or by intravenous infusion
  Child 1 month–18 years 60 mg/kg every 12 hours for 14 days; total daily dose may alternatively be given in 3–4 divided doses
  Note oral route preferred

Prophylaxis of Pneumocystis jirovecii (P. carinii) infections
- By mouth
  Child 1 month–18 years 450 mg/m^2 (max 960 mg) twice daily for three days of the week (either consecutively or on alternate days)
  Note dose regimens may vary, consult local guidelines

Note 480 mg of co-trimoxazole consists of sulfamethoxazole 400 mg and trimethoprim 80 mg

Administration for intermittent intravenous infusion may be further diluted in glucose 5% and 10% or sodium chloride 0.9% or Ringer's intravenous solution. Dilute contents of 1 ampoule (5 mL) to 125 mL, 2 ampoules (10 mL) to 250 mL or 3 ampoules (15 mL) to 500 mL; suggested duration of infusion 60–90 minutes (but may be adjusted according to fluid requirements); if fluid restriction necessary, 1 ampoule (5 mL) may be diluted with 75 mL glucose 5% and the required dose infused over max. 60 minutes; check container for haze or precipitant during administration. In severe fluid restriction may be given undiluted via a central venous line

Co-trimoxazole (Non-proprietary) ⒫ℴ𝔐
Tablets, co-trimoxazole 480 mg, net price 28-tab pack = £13.12; 960 mg, 100 = £23.46. Label: 9
Brands include Fectrim®, Fectrim® Forte

Paediatric oral suspension, co-trimoxazole 240 mg/5 mL, net price 100 mL = £1.12. Label: 9

Oral suspension, co-trimoxazole 480 mg/5 mL. Net price 100 mL = £4.41. Label: 9

Septrin® (GSK) ⒫ℴ𝔐
Tablets, co-trimoxazole 480 mg, net price 100-tab pack = £15.52. Label: 9

Forte tablets, scored, co-trimoxazole 960 mg, net price 100-tab pack = £23.46. Label: 9

Adult suspension, co-trimoxazole 480 mg/5 mL, net price 100 mL (vanilla-flavoured) = £4.41. Label: 9

Paediatric suspension, sugar-free, co-trimoxazole 240 mg/5 mL. Net price 100 mL (banana- and vanilla-flavoured) = £2.45. Label: 9

Intravenous infusion, co-trimoxazole 96 mg/mL. To be diluted before use. Net price 5-mL amp = £1.78
Electrolytes Na$^+$ 1.7 mmol/5 mL
Excipients include alcohol 13.2%, propylene glycol, sulphites

---

▶ TRIMETHOPRIM

Cautions predisposition to folate deficiency; manufacturer recommends blood counts on long-term therapy (but evidence of practical value unsatisfactory); neonates (specialist supervision required); acute porphyria (section 9.8.2); **interactions:** Appendix 1 (trimethoprim)

Blood disorders On long-term treatment, patients and their carers should be told how to recognise signs of blood

◁ **TRIMETHOPRIM** (*continued*)

disorders and advised to seek immediate medical attention if symptoms such as fever, sore throat, rash, mouth ulcers, purpura, bruising or bleeding develop

Contra-indications blood dyscrasias

Renal impairment use half normal dose after 3 days if estimated glomerular filtration rate 15–30 mL/minute/1.73 m²; use half normal dose if estimated glomerular filtration rate less than 15 mL/minute/1.73 m² (monitor plasma-tri-methoprim concentration if estimated glomerular filtration rate less than 10 mL/minute/1.73 m²)

Pregnancy teratogenic risk in first trimester (folate antagonist); manufacturers advise avoid

Breast-feeding present in milk—short-term use not known to be harmful

Side-effects gastro-intestinal disturbances including nausea and vomiting, pruritus, rashes, hyperkalaemia, depression of haematopoiesis; rarely erythema multiforme, toxic epidermal necrolysis, photosensitivity and other allergic reactions including angioedema and anaphylaxis; aseptic meningitis reported

Licensed use not licensed for use in children under 6 weeks

Indication and dose

Urinary-tract infections; respiratory-tract infections
• By mouth

Neonate initially 3 mg/kg as a single dose then 1–2 mg/kg twice daily

Child 1 month–12 years 4 mg/kg (max. 200 mg) twice daily

or

Child 6 weeks–6 months 25 mg twice daily

Child 6 months–6 years 50 mg twice daily

Child 6–12 years 100 mg twice daily

Child 12–18 years 200 mg twice daily

Prophylaxis of urinary-tract infection
• By mouth

Neonate 2 mg/kg at night

Child 1 month–12 years 2 mg/kg (max. 100 mg) at night

Child 12–18 years 100 mg at night

Pneumocystis pneumonia see , p. 417

Trimethoprim (Non-proprietary) ⓅⓄⓂ
Tablets, trimethoprim 100 mg, net price 28 = 99p; 200 mg, 14-tab pack = 95p. Label: 9
Brands include *Trimopan*®

Suspension, trimethoprim 50 mg/5 mL, net price 100 mL = £2.62. Label: 9

5.1.9 Antituberculosis drugs

Tuberculosis is treated in two phases—an *initial phase* using 4 drugs and a *continuation phase* using two drugs in fully sensitive cases. Treatment requires specialised knowledge, particularly where the disease involves resistant organisms or non-respiratory organs.

The regimens given below are recommended for the treatment of tuberculosis in the UK; variations occur in other countries. Either the unsupervised regimen or the supervised regimen described below should be used; the two regimens should **not** be used concurrently. Compliance with therapy is a major determinant of its success. Treatment needs to be carefully monitored in families in whom concordance may be problematic.

Initial phase The concurrent use of 4 drugs during the initial phase is designed to reduce the bacterial population as rapidly as possible and to prevent the emergence of drug-resistant bacteria. The drugs are best given as combination preparations, provided the respective dose of each drug is appropriate, unless the child is unable to swallow the tablets or one of the components cannot be given because of resistance or intolerance. The treatment of choice for the initial phase is the daily use of isoniazid, rifampicin, pyrazinamide and ethambutol. However, care is needed in young children receiving ethambutol because of the difficulty in testing eyesight and in obtaining reports of visual symptoms (see below). Treatment should be started without waiting for culture results if clinical features or histology results are consistent with tuberculosis; treatment should be continued even if initial culture results are negative. The initial phase drugs should be continued for 2 months. Where a positive culture for *M. tuberculosis* has been obtained, but susceptibility results are not available after 2 months, treatment with rifampicin, isoniazid, pyrazinamide and ethambutol should be continued until full susceptibility is confirmed, even if this is for longer than 2 months.

Streptomycin is rarely used in the UK although it may be used in the initial phase of treatment if resistance to isoniazid has been established before therapy is commenced and ethambutol is contra-indicated.

5 Infections

Continuation phase   After the initial phase, treatment is continued for a further 4 months with isoniazid and rifampicin (preferably given as a combination preparation). Longer treatment is necessary for meningitis, direct spinal cord involvement, and for resistant organisms which may also require modification of the regimen.

Unsupervised treatment   The following regimen should be used for those who are likely to take antituberculous drugs reliably **without supervision**. Children and families who are unlikely to comply with daily administration of antituberculous drugs should be treated with the regimen described under Supervised Treatment.

Recommended dosage for standard unsupervised 6-month treatment

Isoniazid (for 2-month initial and 4-month continuation phases)
Child 1 month–18 years 10 mg/kg (max. 300 mg) once daily

Rifampicin (for 2-month initial and 4–month continuation phase)
Child 1 month–18 years 10 mg/kg once daily (max. 450 mg if body-weight under 50 kg; if body-weight 50 kg and over max. 600 mg)

Pyrazinamide (for 2-month initial phase only)
Child 1 month–18 years 35 mg/kg once daily (max. 1.5 g if body-weight under 50 kg; if body-weight 50 kg and over max. 2 g)

Ethambutol (for 2-month initial phase only)
Child 1 month–18 years 15 mg/kg once daily

Note In general, doses should be rounded up to facilitate administration of suitable volumes of liquid or an appropriate strength of tablet. The exception is ethambutol due to the risk of toxicity. Doses may also need to be recalculated to allow for weight gain in younger children.
The fixed-dose combination preparations (*Rifater®, Rifinah®*) are unlicensed for use in children. Consideration may be given to use of these preparations in older children, provided the respective dose of each drug is appropriate for the weight of the child.

Pregnancy   The standard regimen (above) may be used during pregnancy. Streptomycin should not be given in pregnancy.

Breast-feeding   The standard regimen (above) may be used during breast-feeding.

Neonates   Congenital tuberculosis is acquired from maternal extrapulmonary sites at birth, particularly the genital tract; if infection is suspected, the baby will require treatment with isoniazid 10 mg/kg once daily, rifampicin 10 mg/kg once daily, pyrazinamide 35 mg/kg once daily, and ethambutol 15 mg/kg once daily. Isoniazid, rifampicin, pyrazinamide, and ethambutol are used for 2 months during the initial phase of treatment. After the initial phase, treatment is continued for a further 4 months with isoniazid and rifampicin.

Supervised treatment   Drug administration needs to be **fully supervised** (directly observed therapy, DOT) in children or families who cannot comply reliably with the treatment regimen. These patients are given isoniazid, rifampicin, pyrazinamide and ethambutol (or streptomycin) 3 times a week under supervision for the first 2 months followed by isoniazid and rifampicin 3 times a week for a further 4 months.

Recommended dosage for intermittent supervised 6-month treatment

Isoniazid (for 2-month initial and 4-month continuation phases)
Child 1 month–18 years, 15 mg/kg (max. 900 mg) 3 times a week

Rifampicin (for 2-month initial and 4-month continuation phases)
Child 1 month–18 years, 15 mg/kg (max. 900 mg) 3 times a week

Pyrazinamide (for 2-month initial phase only)
Child 1 month–18 years, 50 mg/kg (max. 2 g 3 times a week if body-weight under 50 kg; max. 2.5 g 3 times a week if body-weight 50 kg and over)

Ethambutol (for 2-month initial phase only)
Child 1 month–18 years, 30 mg/kg 3 times a week

Note In general, doses should be rounded up to facilitate administration of suitable volumes of liquid or an appropriate strength of tablet. The exception is ethambutol due to the risk of toxicity. Doses may also need to be recalculated to allow for weight gain in younger children.
The fixed-dose combination preparations (*Rifater®, Rifinah®*) are unlicensed for use in children. Consideration may be given to use of these preparations in older children, provided the respective dose of each drug is appropriate for the weight of the child.

Immunocompromised patients   Multi-resistant *Mycobacterium tuberculosis* may be present in immunocompromised children. The organism should always be cultured to confirm its type and drug sensitivity. Confirmed *M. tuberculosis* infection sensitive to first-line drugs should be treated with a standard 6-month regimen; after completing treatment, children should be closely monitored. The regimen may need to be modified if infection is caused by resistant organisms, and specialist advice is needed.

Specialist advice should be sought about tuberculosis treatment or chemoprophylaxis in a HIV-positive individual; care is required in choosing the regimen and in avoiding potentially hazardous interactions. Starting antiretroviral treatment in the first 2 months of antituberculosis treatment increases the risk of immune reconstitution syndrome.

Infection may also be caused by other mycobacteria e.g. *M. avium* complex in which case specialist advice on management is needed.

Corticosteroids   A corticosteroid should be given (in addition to antituberculosis therapy) for meningeal or pericardial tuberculosis.

Prevention of tuberculosis   Chemoprophylaxis may be required in children who are close contacts of a case of smear-positive pulmonary tuberculosis and who are severely immunosuppressed (including congenital immunodeficiencies, cytotoxic or immunosuppressive therapy) and in those who have evidence of latent tuberculosis and require treatment with immunosuppressants; expert advice should be sought.

Chemoprophylaxis involves use of either isoniazid alone for 6 months or of isoniazid and rifampicin for 3 months (see Table 2, section 5.1).

For prevention of tuberculosis in susceptible close contacts or those who have become tuberculin-positive, see Table 2, section 5.1. For advice on immunisation against tuberculosis and tuberculin testing, see section 14.4.

Monitoring   Since isoniazid, rifampicin and pyrazinamide are associated with liver toxicity, *hepatic function* should be checked before treatment with these drugs. Those with pre-existing liver disease should have frequent checks particularly in the first 2 months. If there is no evidence of liver disease (and pre-treatment liver function is normal), further checks are only necessary if the patient develops fever, malaise, vomiting, jaundice or unexplained deterioration during treatment. In view of the need to comply fully with antituberculous treatment on the one hand and to guard against serious liver damage on the other, children and their carers should be informed carefully how to recognise signs of liver disorders and advised to discontinue treatment and seek **immediate** medical attention should symptoms of liver disease occur.

Renal function should be checked before treatment with antituberculous drugs and appropriate dosage adjustments made. Streptomycin or ethambutol should preferably be avoided in patients with renal impairment, but if used, the dose should be reduced and the plasma-drug concentration monitored.

Visual acuity should be tested before ethambutol is used (see below).

> Major causes of treatment failure are incorrect prescribing by the physician and inadequate compliance by the child or their carer. Monthly tablet counts and urine examination (rifampicin imparts an orange-red coloration) may be useful indicators of compliance with treatment. Avoid both excessive and inadequate dosage. Treatment should be supervised by a specialist paediatrician.

Isoniazid is cheap and highly effective. Like rifampicin it should always be included in any antituberculous regimen unless there is a specific contra-indication. Its only common side-effect is peripheral neuropathy which is more likely to occur where there are pre-existing risk factors such as diabetes, chronic renal failure, malnutrition and HIV infection. In these circumstances, and in breast-fed infants treated with isoniazid, pyridoxine (section 9.6.2) should be given prophylactically from the start of treatment. Other side-effects such as hepatitis (important: see Monitoring above) and psychosis are rare.

Rifampicin, a rifamycin, is a key component of any antituberculous regimen. Like isoniazid it should always be included unless there is a specific contra-indication.

During the first two months ('initial phase') of rifampicin administration transient disturbance of liver function with elevated serum transaminases is common but generally does not require interruption of treatment. Occasionally more serious liver toxicity requires a change of treatment particularly in those with pre-existing liver disease (important: see Monitoring above).

On intermittent treatment six toxicity syndromes have been recognised—influenza-like, abdominal, and respiratory symptoms, shock, renal failure, and thrombocytopenic purpura—and can occur in 20 to 30% of patients.

Rifampicin induces hepatic enzymes which accelerate the metabolism of several drugs including oestrogens, corticosteroids, phenytoin, sulphonylureas, and anticoagulants; **interactions:** Appendix 1 (rifamycins). **Important:** the effectiveness of hormonal contraceptives is reduced and alternative family planning advice should be offered (section 7.3.1).

Rifabutin is indicated in adults for *prophylaxis* against *M. avium* complex infections in patients with a low CD4 count; it is also licensed in adults for the *treatment* of non-tuberculous mycobacterial disease and pulmonary tuberculosis. There is limited experience in children. As with rifampicin it induces hepatic enzymes and the effectiveness of hormonal contraceptives is reduced requiring alternative family planning methods.

Pyrazinamide is a bactericidal drug only active against intracellular dividing forms of *Mycobacterium tuberculosis*; it exerts its main effect only in the first two or three months. It is particularly useful in tuberculous meningitis because of good meningeal penetration. It is not active against *M. bovis*. Serious liver toxicity may occasionally occur (important: see Monitoring above).

Ethambutol is included in a treatment regimen if isoniazid resistance is suspected; it can be omitted if the risk of resistance is low.

Side-effects of ethambutol are largely confined to visual disturbances in the form of loss of acuity, colour blindness, and restriction of visual fields. These toxic effects are more common where excessive dosage is used or if the child's renal function is impaired. The earliest features of ocular toxicity are subjective and children and their carers should be advised to discontinue therapy immediately if deterioration in vision develops and promptly seek further advice. Early discontinuation of the drug is almost always followed by recovery of eyesight. Those who cannot understand warnings about visual side-effects should, if possible, be given an alternative drug. In particular, ethambutol should be used with caution in children until they are at least 5 years old and capable of reporting symptomatic visual changes accurately.

Where possible visual acuity should be tested by Snellen chart before treatment with ethambutol.

Streptomycin is now rarely used in the UK except for resistant organisms. Plasma-drug concentration should be measured in patients with impaired renal function in whom streptomycin must be used with great care. Side-effects increase after a cumulative dose of 100 g, which should only be exceeded in exceptional circumstances.

Drug-resistant tuberculosis should be treated by a specialist paediatrician with experience in such cases, and where appropriate facilities for infection-control exist. Second-line drugs available for infections caused by resistant organisms, or when first-line drugs cause unacceptable side-effects, include amikacin, capreomycin, cycloserine, newer macrolides (e.g. azithromycin and clarithromycin), quinolones (e.g. moxifloxacin) and protionamide (prothionamide; no longer on UK market). Availability of suitable formulations may limit choice in children.

CYCLOSERINE

Cautions monitor haematological, renal, and hepatic function; **interactions:** Appendix 1 (cycloserine)

Contra-indications epilepsy, depression, severe anxiety, psychotic states, alcohol dependence, acute porphyria (section 9.8.2)

Renal impairment reduce dose and monitor blood-cycloserine concentration; avoid in severe impairment

Pregnancy manufacturer advises use only if potential benefit outweighs risk—crosses the placenta

Breast-feeding present in milk—amount too small to be harmful

Side-effects mainly neurological, including headache, dizziness, vertigo, drowsiness, tremor, convulsions, confusion, psychosis, depression (discontinue or reduce dose if symptoms of CNS

◻ **CYCLOSERINE** (*continued*)

toxicity); rashes, allergic dermatitis (discontinue or reduce dose); megaloblastic anaemia; changes in liver function tests; heart failure at high doses reported

Pharmacokinetics blood concentration should not exceed a peak concentration of 30 mg/litre (measured 3–4 hours after the dose); penetrates CNS

Licensed use licensed for use in children (age range not specified by manufacturer)

Indication and dose

Tuberculosis resistant to first-line drugs, used in combination with other drugs
• By mouth
    Child 2–12 years initially 5 mg/kg (max. 250 mg) twice daily, adjusted according to blood

concentration and response up to 10 mg/kg (max. 500 mg) twice daily

Child 12–18 years initially 250 mg twice daily for 2 weeks adjusted according to blood concentration and response to max. 500 mg twice daily

Cycloserine (King) [PoM]
Capsules, red/grey cycloserine 250 mg, net price 100-cap pack = £303.45. Label: 2, 8

ETHAMBUTOL HYDROCHLORIDE

Cautions test visual acuity before treatment and warn patients to report visual changes—see notes above; young children (see notes above)—routine ophthalmological monitoring recommended

Contra-indications optic neuritis, poor vision

Renal impairment reduce dose; if creatinine clearance less than 30 mL/minute/1.73 m^2, monitor plasma-ethambutol concentration; risk of optic nerve damage

Pregnancy not known to be harmful; see notes above

Breast-feeding amount too small to be harmful

Side-effects optic neuritis, red/green colour blindness, peripheral neuritis, rarely rash, pruritus, urticaria, thrombocytopenia

Pharmacokinetics 'peak' concentration (2–2.5 hours after dose) should be 2–6 mg/litre (7–

22 micromol/litre); 'trough' (pre-dose) concentration should be less than 1 mg/litre (4 micromol/litre); for advice on laboratory assay of ethambutol contact the Poisons Unit at New Cross Hospital (Tel (020) 7771 5360)

Indication and dose

Tuberculosis, used in combination with other drugs see notes above

Ethambutol (Non-proprietary) [PoM]
Tablets, ethambutol hydrochloride 100 mg (yellow), net price 56-tab pack = £11.51; 400 mg (grey), 56-tab pack = £42.74. Label: 8

◢ Extemporaneous formulations available see Extemporaneous Preparations, p. 8

ISONIAZID

Cautions slow acetylator status (increased risk of side-effects); epilepsy; history of psychosis; alcohol dependence, malnutrition, diabetes mellitus, HIV infection (risk of peripheral neuritis); acute porphyria (section 9.8.2); **interactions:** Appendix 1 (isoniazid)

Hepatic disorders Children and their carers should be told how to recognise signs of liver disorder, and advised to discontinue treatment and seek immediate medical attention if symptoms such as persistent nausea, vomiting, malaise or jaundice develop

Contra-indications drug-induced liver disease

Hepatic impairment use with caution; monitor liver function regularly and particularly frequently in the first 2 months; see also Hepatic Disorders above

Renal impairment reduce dose if estimated glomerular filtration rate less than 10 mL/minute/1.73 m^2; risk of peripheral neuropathy

Pregnancy not known to be harmful; see notes above

Breast-feeding monitor infant for possible toxicity; theoretical risk of convulsions and neuropathy; prophylactic pyridoxine advisable in mother and infant

Side-effects nausea, vomiting, constipation, dry mouth; peripheral neuritis with high doses (pyridoxine prophylaxis, see notes above), optic neuritis, convulsions, psychotic episodes, vertigo; hypersensitivity reactions including fever, Stevens-Johnson syndrome, purpura; blood disorders including agranulocytosis, haemolytic anaemia, aplastic anaemia; hepatitis; pancreatitis; interstitial pneumonitis; systemic lupus erythematosus-like syndrome, pellagra, hyperreflexia, difficulty with micturition, hyperglycaemia, and gynaecomastia reported; hearing loss and tinnitus (in children with end-stage renal impairment)

Indication and dose

Tuberculosis, used in combination with other drugs see notes above

Isoniazid (Non-proprietary) [PoM]
Tablets, isoniazid 50 mg, net price 56-tab pack = £9.72; 100 mg, 28-tab pack = £9.80. Label: 8, 22

Injection, isoniazid 25 mg/mL, net price 2-mL amp = £11.04

◢ Extemporaneous formulations available see Extemporaneous Preparations, p. 8

5

Infections

PYRAZINAMIDE

Cautions diabetes; **interactions**: Appendix 1 (pyrazinamide)

Hepatic disorders Children and their carers should be told how to recognise signs of liver disorder, and advised to discontinue treatment and seek immediate medical attention if symptoms such as persistent nausea, vomiting, malaise or jaundice develop

Contra-indications acute porphyria (section 9.8.2)

Hepatic impairment monitor hepatic function—idiosyncratic hepatotoxicity more common; avoid in severe hepatic impairment; see also Hepatic Disorders above

Pregnancy manufacturer advises use only if potential benefit outweighs risk; see also notes above

Breast-feeding amount too small to be harmful

Side-effects hepatotoxicity including fever, anorexia, hepatomegaly, splenomegaly, jaundice, liver failure; nausea, vomiting, dysuria, arthralgia, sideroblastic anaemia, thrombocytopenia, rash and occasionally photosensitivity

Licensed use not licensed

Indication and dose

Tuberculosis in combination with other drugs
see notes above

Pyrazinamide (Non-proprietary) [PoM]
Tablets, scored, pyrazinamide 500 mg. Label: 8
Available from 'special-order' manufacturers or specialist importing companies, see p. 957

◢Extemporaneous formulations available see Extemporaneous Preparations, p. 8

RIFABUTIN

Cautions see under Rifampicin; acute porphyria (section 9.8.2)

Hepatic impairment reduce dose in severe impairment

Renal impairment use half normal dose if estimated glomerular filtration rate less than 30 mL/minute/1.73 m²

Pregnancy manufacturer advises avoid—no information available

Breast-feeding manufacturer advises avoid—no information available

Side-effects nausea, vomiting; leucopenia, thrombocytopenia, anaemia, rarely haemolysis; raised liver enzymes, jaundice, rarely hepatitis; uveitis following high doses or administration with drugs which raise plasma concentration—see also **interactions**: Appendix 1 (rifamycins); arthralgia, myalgia, influenza-like syndrome, dyspnoea; also hypersensitivity reactions including fever, rash, eosinophilia, bronchospasm, shock; skin, urine, saliva and other body secretions coloured orange-red; asymptomatic corneal opacities reported with long-term use

Licensed use not licensed for use in children

Indication and dose

Prophylaxis of *Mycobacterium avium* complex infections in immunosuppressed patients with low CD4 count (see product literature) Also see notes above
• By mouth
  Child 1–12 years 5 mg/kg (max. 300 mg) once daily
  Child 12–18 years 300 mg once daily

Treatment of non-tuberculous mycobacterial disease, in combination with other drugs
• By mouth
  Child 1month–12 years 5 mg/kg once daily for up to 6 months after cultures negative
  Child 12–18 years 450–600 mg once daily for up to 6 months after cultures negative

Treatment of pulmonary tuberculosis, in combination with other drugs
• By mouth
  Child 12–18years 150–450 mg once daily for at least 6 months

Mycobutin® (Pharmacia) [PoM]
Capsules, red-brown, rifabutin 150 mg. Net price 30-cap pack = £90.38. Label: 8, 14, counselling, lenses, see under Rifampicin

◢Extemporaneous formulations available see Extemporaneous Preparations, p. 8

RIFAMPICIN

Cautions liver function tests and blood counts in hepatic disorders, and on prolonged therapy, see also below; acute porphyria (section 9.8.2); **important**: advise those on hormonal contraceptives to use additional means (see also section 7.3.1); discolours soft contact lenses; see also

notes above; **interactions**: Appendix 1 (rifamycins)

Note If treatment interrupted re-introduce with low dosage and increase gradually; discontinue permanently if serious side-effects develop

Hepatic disorders Children and their carers should be told how to recognise signs of liver disorder, and advised to discontinue treatment and seek immediate medical attention if symptoms such as persistent nausea, vomiting, malaise or jaundice develop

Contra-indications jaundice

◁ **RIFAMPICIN (continued)**

Hepatic impairment impaired elimination; monitor liver function; avoid or do not exceed 8 mg/kg daily; see also Cautions above

Pregnancy manufacturers advise very high doses teratogenic in *animal* studies in first trimester; risk of neonatal bleeding may be increased in third trimester; see also notes above

Breast-feeding amount too small to be harmful

Side-effects gastro-intestinal symptoms including anorexia, nausea, vomiting, diarrhoea (antibiotic-associated colitis reported); headache, drowsiness; those occurring mainly on intermittent therapy include influenza-like symptoms (with chills, fever, dizziness, bone pain), respiratory symptoms (including shortness of breath), collapse and shock, haemolytic anaemia, disseminated intravascular coagulation and acute renal failure, thrombocytopenic purpura; alterations of liver function, jaundice; flushing, urticaria, and rashes; other side-effects reported include oedema, psychoses, adrenal insufficiency, muscular weakness and myopathy, exfoliative dermatitis, toxic epidermal necrolysis, Stevens-Johnson syndrome, pemphigoid reactions, leucopenia, eosinophilia, menstrual disturbances; urine, saliva, and other body secretions coloured orange-red; thrombophlebitis reported if infusion used for prolonged period

Licensed use not licensed for use in children for pruritus due to cholestasis

Indication and dose

> **Tuberculosis, in combination with other drugs**
> see notes above

> **Prophylaxis of meningococcal meningitis and *Haemophilus influenzae* (type b) infection** Table 2, section 5.1

> **Brucellosis, legionnaires disease, serious staphylococcal infections, in combination with other antibacterials**
> • **By mouth or by intravenous infusion**
>
> > **Neonates** 5–10 mg/kg twice daily
> >
> > **Child 1 month–1 year** 5–10 mg/kg twice daily
> >
> > **Child 1–18 years** 10 mg/kg (max. 600 mg) twice daily

> **Pruritus due to cholestasis**
> • **By mouth**
>
> > **Child 1 month–18 years** 5–10 mg/kg (max. 600 mg) once daily

Administration Displacement value may be significant, consult local reconstitution guidelines; reconstitute with solvent provided. May be further diluted with glucose 5% or sodium chloride 0.9% to a final concentration of 1.2 mg/mL. Infuse over 2–3 hours.

Rifampicin (Non-proprietary) ℗ℴ℧

Capsules, rifampicin 150 mg, net price 100 = £18.81; 300 mg, 100 = £41.74. Label: 8, 14, 22, counselling, see contact lenses above

Rifadin® (Sanofi-Aventis) ℗ℴ℧

Capsules, rifampicin 150 mg (blue/red), net price 100-cap pack = £18.32; 300 mg (red), 100-cap pack = £36.63. Label: 8, 14, 22, counselling, see contact lenses above

Syrup, red, rifampicin 100 mg/5 mL (raspberry-flavoured). Net price 120 mL = £3.56. Label: 8, 14, 22, counselling, see contact lenses above
Excipients include sucrose

Intravenous infusion, powder for reconstitution, rifampicin. Net price 600-mg vial (with solvent) = £7.67
Electrolytes Na⁺ < 0.5 mmol/vial

Rimactane® (Sandoz) ℗ℴ℧

Capsules, rifampicin 150 mg (red), net price 60-cap pack = £11.35; 300 mg (red/brown), 60-cap pack = £22.69. Label: 8, 14, 22, counselling, see contact lenses above

◀ **Combined preparations**
See notes above

Rifater® (Sanofi-Aventis) ℗ℴ℧

Tablets, pink, s/c, rifampicin 120 mg, isoniazid 50 mg, pyrazinamide 300 mg. Net price 100-tab pack = £21.95. Label: 8, 14, 22, counselling, see contact lenses above

Rifinah 150® (Sanofi-Aventis) ℗ℴ℧

Tablets, pink, s/c, rifampicin 150 mg, isoniazid 100 mg, net price 84-tab pack = £15.91. Label: 8, 14, 22, counselling, see contact lenses above
Note Some stock packaged as *Rifinah* 100/150 mg

Rifinah 300® (Sanofi-Aventis) ℗ℴ℧

Tablets, orange, s/c, rifampicin 300 mg, isoniazid 150 mg, net price 56-tab pack = £21.02. Label: 8, 14, 22, counselling, see contact lenses above
Note Some stock packaged as *Rifinah* 150/300 mg

5

Infections

▰ **STREPTOMYCIN**

Cautions see under Aminoglycosides, section 5.1.4; measure plasma-concentration in renal impairment; **interactions:** Appendix 1 (aminoglycosides)

Contra-indications see under Aminoglycosides, section 5.1.4

Renal impairment see under Aminoglycosides, section 5.1.4

Pregnancy see under Aminoglycosides, section 5.1.4

Side-effects see under Aminoglycosides, section 5.1.4; also hypersensitivity reactions, paraesthesia of mouth

Pharmacokinetics one-hour ('peak') concentration should be 15–40 mg/litre; pre-dose ('trough') concentration should be less than 5 mg/litre (less than 1 mg/litre in renal impairment)

◻ **STREPTOMYCIN** (*continued*)

Licensed use not licensed for use in children

Indication and dose

Tuberculosis, resistant to other treatment, in combination with other drugs
- By deep intramuscular injection

    Child 1 month–18 years 15 mg/kg (max. 1 g) once daily

Adjunct to doxycycline in brucellosis, expert advice essential
- By deep intramuscular injection

    Child 1 month–18 years 5–10 mg/kg every 6 hours; total daily dose may alternatively be given in 2–3 divided doses

Streptomycin Sulphate (Non-proprietary) PoM
Injection, powder for reconstitution, streptomycin (as sulphate), net price 1-g vial = £8.25
Available as an unlicensed preparation from UCB Pharma

5.1.10 Antileprotic drugs

Classification not used in *BNF for Children*.

5.1.11 Metronidazole

Metronidazole is an antimicrobial drug with high activity against anaerobic bacteria and protozoa. It is also used for surgical and gynaecological sepsis in which its activity against colonic anaerobes, especially *Bacteroides fragilis*, is important. Metronidazole by mouth is effective for the treatment of *Clostridium difficile* infection (see also section 1.5); it can be given by intravenous infusion if oral treatment is inappropriate. Metronidazole is well absorbed orally and the intravenous route is normally reserved for severe infections. Metronidazole by the rectal route is an effective alternative to the intravenous route when oral administration is not possible. Intravenous metronidazole is used for the treatment of established cases of tetanus; diazepam (section 10.2.2) and tetanus immunoglobulin (section 14.5.2) are also used.

Topical metronidazole (section 13.10.1.2) reduces the odour produced by anaerobic bacteria in fungating tumours; it is also used in the management of rosacea (section 13.6).

Oral infections Metronidazole is an alternative to a penicillin for the treatment of many oral infections where the patient is allergic to penicillin or the infection is due to beta-lactamase-producing anaerobes (Table 1, section 5.1). It is the drug of first choice for the treatment of acute necrotising ulcerative gingivitis (Vincent's infection) and pericoronitis; suitable alternatives are amoxicillin (section 5.1.1.3) and erythromycin (section 5.1.5). For these purposes treatment with metronidazole for 3 days is sufficient, but the duration of treatment may need to be longer in pericoronitis. Tinidazole is licensed for the treatment of acute ulcerative gingivitis.

◢ METRONIDAZOLE

Cautions disulfiram-like reaction with alcohol, clinical and laboratory monitoring advised if treatment exceeds 10 days; **interactions:** Appendix 1 (metronidazole)

Hepatic impairment in severe liver disease reduce total daily dose to one-third, and give once daily; use with caution in hepatic encephalopathy

Pregnancy manufacturer advises avoidance of high-dose regimens; use only if potential benefit outweighs risk

Breast-feeding significant amount in milk; manufacturer advises avoid large single doses though otherwise compatible; may give milk a bitter taste

Side-effects gastro-intestinal disturbances (including nausea and vomiting), taste disturbances, furred tongue, oral mucositis, anorexia; *very rarely* hepatitis, jaundice, pancreatitis, drowsiness, dizziness, headache, ataxia, psychotic disorders, darkening of urine, thrombocytopenia, pancytopenia, myalgia, arthralgia, visual disturbances, rash, pruritus, and erythema multiforme; on prolonged or intensive therapy peripheral neuropathy, transient epileptiform seizures, and leucopenia

Licensed use not licensed for use in neonates or children under 1 year

Indication and dose

Protozoal infections section 5.4.2

Anaerobic infections (usually treated for 7 days and for 10–14 days in *Clostridium difficile* infection)
- By mouth

    Child 1 month–12 years 7.5 mg/kg (max. 400 mg) every 8 hours

    Child 12–18 years 400 mg every 8 hours

◻ **METRONIDAZOLE** (*continued*)

- **By rectum**

  Child 1 month–1 year 125 mg 3 times daily for 3 days, then twice daily thereafter

  Child 1–5 years 250 mg 3 times daily for 3 days, then twice daily thereafter

  Child 5–12 years 500 mg 3 times daily, for 3 days, then twice daily thereafter

  Child 12–18 years 1 g 3 times daily for 3 days, then twice daily thereafter

- **By intravenous infusion over 20–30 minutes**

  Neonate 15 mg/kg as a single loading dose, followed after 24 hours by 7.5 mg/kg every 12 hours thereafter

  Child 1 month–18 years 7.5 mg/kg (max. 500 mg) every 8 hours

Pelvic inflammatory disease (see also Table 1, section 5.1)

- **By mouth**

  Child 12–18 years 400 mg twice daily for 14 days

Acute ulcerative gingivitis and other acute dental infections

- **By mouth**

  Child 1–3 years 50 mg every 8 hours

  Child 3–7 years 100 mg every 12 hours

  Child 7–10 years 100 mg every 8 hours

  Child 10–18 years 200 mg every 8 hours

Helicobacter pylori eradication section 1.3

Surgical prophylaxis

- **By mouth or by intravenous infusion**

  Child 1 month–12 years 7.5 mg/kg 2 hours before surgery; up to 3 further doses of 7.5 mg/kg may be given every 8 hours for high-risk procedures

  Child 12–18 years 400–500 mg 2 hours before surgery; up to 3 further doses of 400–500 mg may be given every 8 hours for high-risk procedures

- **By rectum**

  Child 5–10 years 500 mg 2 hours before surgery; up to 3 further doses of 500 mg may be given every 8 hours for high-risk procedures

  Child 10–18 years 1 g 2 hours before surgery; up to 3 further doses of 1 g may be given every 8 hours for high-risk procedures

Note Metronidazole doses in BNF for Children may differ from those in product literature

Metronidazole (Non-proprietary) ℗ℴ𝕄
Tablets, metronidazole 200 mg, net price 21-tab pack = £1.09; 400 mg, 21-tab pack = £1.21. Label: 4, 9, 21, 25, 27
Brands include *Vaginyl*®
Dental prescribing on NHS Metronidazole Tablets may be prescribed

Tablets, metronidazole 500 mg, net price 21-tab pack = £28.43. Label: 4, 9, 21, 25, 27
Dental prescribing on NHS Metronidazole Tablets may be prescribed

Suspension, metronidazole (as benzoate) 200 mg/ 5 mL. Net price 100 mL = £7.94. Label: 4, 9
Brands include *Norzol*®
Dental prescribing on NHS Metronidazole Oral Suspension may be prescribed

Intravenous infusion, metronidazole 5 mg/mL. Net price 20-mL amp = £1.56, 100-mL container = £3.41

Flagyl® (Winthrop) ℗ℴ𝕄
Tablets, both f/c, ivory, metronidazole 200 mg, net price 21-tab pack = £4.49; 400 mg, 14-tab pack = £6.34. Label: 4, 9, 21, 25, 27
Suppositories, metronidazole 500 mg, net price 10 = £15.18; 1 g, 10 = £23.06. Label: 4, 9

Flagyl S® (Winthrop) ℗ℴ𝕄
Suspension, orange- and lemon-flavoured, metronidazole (as benzoate) 200 mg/5 mL. Net price 100 mL = £11.18. Label: 4, 9

Metrolyl® (Sandoz) ℗ℴ𝕄
Intravenous infusion, metronidazole 5 mg/mL, net price 100-mL Steriflex® bag = £1.22
Electrolytes Na⁺ 14.53 mmol/100-mL bag

Suppositories, metronidazole 500 mg, net price 10 = £12.34; 1 g, 10 = £18.34. Label: 4, 9

5.1.12 Quinolones

Nalidixic acid is effective in uncomplicated urinary-tract infections.

Ciprofloxacin is active against both Gram-positive and Gram-negative bacteria. It is particularly active against Gram-negative bacteria, including salmonella, shigella, campylobacter, neisseria, and pseudomonas. Ciprofloxacin has only moderate activity against Gram-positive bacteria such as *Streptococcus pneumoniae* and *Enterococcus faecalis*; it should not be used for pneumococcal pneumonia. It is active against chlamydia and some mycobacteria. Most anaerobic organisms are not susceptible. Ciprofloxacin is licensed in children over 1 year of age for pseudomonal infections in cystic fibrosis, for complicated urinary-tract infections, and for treatment and prophylaxis of inhalation anthrax. When the benefits of treatment outweigh the risks, ciprofloxacin is licensed in children over 1 year of age for severe infections of the respiratory tract and of the gastro-intestinal system (including typhoid fever). It is also used in the treatment of septicaemia caused by multi-resistant organisms (usually hospital acquired) and gonorrhoea

5

Infections

(although resistance is increasing). Ciprofloxacin is also used in the prophylaxis of meningococcal disease.

Many staphylococci are resistant to quinolones and their use should be avoided in MRSA infections.

Ofloxacin eye drops are used in ophthalmic infections (section 11.3.1).

There is much less experience of the other quinolones in children; expert advice should be sought.

Anthrax *Inhalation* or *gastro-intestinal anthrax* should be treated initially with either **ciprofloxacin** or, in children over 12 years, **doxycycline** [unlicensed indication] (section 5.1.3) combined with one or two other antibacterials (such as amoxicillin, benzylpenicillin, chloramphenicol, clarithromycin, clindamycin, imipenem with cilastatin, rifampicin [unlicensed indication], and vancomycin). When the condition improves and the sensitivity of the *Bacillus anthracis* strain is known, treatment may be switched to a single antibacterial. Treatment should continue for 60 days because germination may be delayed.

Cutaneous anthrax should be treated with either ciprofloxacin [unlicensed indication] or doxycycline [unlicensed indication] (section 5.1.3) for 7 days. Treatment may be switched to amoxicillin (section 5.1.1.3) if the infecting strain is susceptible. Treatment may need to be extended to 60 days if exposure is due to aerosol. A combination of antibacterials for 14 days is recommended for cutaneous anthrax with systemic features, extensive oedema, or lesions of the head or neck.

Ciprofloxacin or doxycycline may be given for *post-exposure prophylaxis*. If exposure is confirmed, antibacterial prophylaxis should continue for 60 days. Antibacterial prophylaxis may be switched to amoxicillin after 10–14 days if the strain of *B. anthracis* is susceptible. Vaccination against anthrax (section 14.4) may allow the duration of antibacterial prophylaxis to be shortened.

Cautions Quinolones should be used with caution in children with a history of epilepsy or conditions that predispose to seizures, in G6PD deficiency (section 9.1.5), myasthenia gravis (risk of exacerbation). Exposure to excessive sunlight should be avoided (discontinue if photosensitivity occurs). The CSM has warned that quinolones may induce **convulsions** in patients with or without a history of convulsions; taking NSAIDs at the same time may also induce them. Other **interactions**: Appendix 1 (quinolones).

Quinolones cause arthropathy in the weight-bearing joints of immature *animals* and are therefore generally not recommended in children and growing adolescents. However, the significance of this effect in humans is uncertain and in some specific circumstances short-term use of a quinolone in children is justified. **Nalidixic acid** is used for resistant urinary-tract infections in children over 3 months of age.

> **Tendon damage**
> Tendon damage (including rupture) has been reported rarely in patients receiving quinolones. Tendon rupture may occur within 48 hours of starting treatment; cases have also been reported several months after stopping a quinolone. Healthcare professionals are reminded that:
> - quinolones are contra-indicated in patients with a history of tendon disorders related to quinolone use;
> - the risk of tendon damage is increased by the concomitant use of corticosteroids;
> - if tendinitis is suspected, the quinolone should be discontinued immediately.

Contra-indications Quinolone hypersensitivity.

Pregnancy Quinolones should be avoided in pregnancy because they have been shown to cause arthropathy in *animal* studies; safer alternatives are available.

Side-effects Side-effects of the quinolones include nausea, vomiting, dyspepsia, abdominal pain, diarrhoea (rarely antibiotic-associated colitis), headache, dizziness, rash (very rarely Stevens-Johnson syndrome and toxic epidermal necrolysis). Less frequent side-effects include anorexia, sleep disturbances, asthenia, confusion, anxiety, depression, hallucinations, tremor, blood disorders (including eosinophilia, leucopenia, thrombocytopenia), arthralgia, myalgia, disturbances in vision and taste. Other side-effects reported rarely or very rarely include hepatic dysfunction (including jaundice and hepatitis), hypotension, vasculitis, dyspnoea, convulsions, psychoses, paraesthesia, renal failure, interstitial nephritis, tendon inflammation and damage (see also Tendon Damage above), photosensitivity, disturbances in hearing and smell. The drug should be **discontinued** if psychiatric, neurological or hypersensitivity reactions (including severe rash) occur.

CIPROFLOXACIN

Cautions see notes above; avoid excessive alkalinity of urine and ensure adequate fluid intake (risk of crystalluria); **interactions:** Appendix 1 (quinolones)

Skilled tasks May impair performance of skilled tasks (e.g. driving)

Contra-indications see notes above

Renal impairment reduce dose if estimated glomerular filtration rate less than 30 mL/minute/1.73 m^2—consult product literature

Pregnancy see notes above

Breast-feeding amount probably too small to be harmful but manufacturer advises avoid

Side-effects see notes above; also flatulence, pain and phlebitis at injection site; *rarely* dysphagia, pancreatitis, chest pain, tachycardia, syncope, oedema, hot flushes, abnormal dreams, sweating, hyperglycaemia, and erythema nodosum; *very rarely* movement disorders, tinnitus, vasculitis, and tenosynovitis

Licensed use licensed for use in children over 1 year for complicated urinary-tract infections, for pseudomonal lower respiratory-tract infections in cystic fibrosis, for prophylaxis and treatment of inhalational anthrax; licensed for use in children over 1 year for other infections where the benefit is considered to outweigh the potential risks; not licensed for use in children for gastro-intestinal anthrax; not licensed for use in children for prophylaxis of meningococcal meningitis; not licensed for use in children under 1 year of age

Indication and dose

Complicated urinary-tract infections
● By mouth
Neonate 10 mg/kg twice daily
Child 1 month–18 years 10 mg/kg twice daily; dose doubled in severe infection (max. 750 mg twice daily)

● By intravenous infusion over 60 minutes
Neonate 6 mg/kg every 12 hours
Child 1 month–18 years 6 mg/kg every 8 hours; increased to 10 mg/kg every 8 hours in severe infection (max. 400 mg every 8 hours)

Severe respiratory-tract infections, gastro-intestinal infections; see notes above
● By mouth
Neonate 15 mg/kg twice daily
Child 1 month–18 years 20 mg/kg (max. 750 mg) twice daily

● By intravenous infusion over 60 minutes
Neonate 10 mg/kg every 12 hours

Child 1 month–18 years 10 mg/kg (max. 400 mg) every 8 hours

Pseudomonal lower respiratory-tract infection in cystic fibrosis
● By mouth
Child 1 month–18 years 20 mg/kg (max. 750 mg) twice daily

● By intravenous infusion over 60 minutes
Child 1 month–18 years 10 mg/kg (max. 400 mg) every 8 hours

Gonorrhoea
● By mouth
Child 12–18 years 500 mg as a single dose

Anthrax (treatment and post-exposure prophylaxis, see notes above)
● By mouth
Child 1 month–18 years 15 mg/kg (max. 500 mg) twice daily

● By intravenous infusion over 60 minutes
Child 1 month–18 years 10 mg/kg (max. 400 mg) every 12 hours

Eye infections section 11.3.1

Prophylaxis of meningococcal meningitis Table 2, section 5.1

Ciprofloxacin (Non-proprietary) ℗oM
Tablets, ciprofloxacin (as hydrochloride) 100 mg, net price 6-tab pack = £1.26; 250 mg, 10-tab pack = £1.09, 20-tab pack = £1.23; 500 mg, 10-tab pack = £1.18, 20-tab pack = £1.40; 750 mg, 10-tab pack = £5.52. Label: 7, 9, 25, counselling, driving

Intravenous infusion, ciprofloxacin (as lactate) 2 mg/mL, net price 50-mL bottle = £8.00, 100-mL bottle = £15.00, 200-mL bottle = £22.00

Ciproxin® (Bayer Schering) ℗oM
Tablets, all f/c, ciprofloxacin (as hydrochloride) 250 mg (scored), net price 10-tab pack = £7.21, 20-tab pack = £14.42; 500 mg (scored), 10-tab pack = £13.65, 20-tab pack = £27.29; 750 mg, 10-tab pack = £19.22. Label: 7, 9, 25, counselling, driving

Suspension, strawberry-flavoured, ciprofloxacin for reconstitution with diluent provided, 250 mg/5 mL, net price 100 mL = £16.50. Label: 7, 9, 25, counselling, driving

Intravenous infusion, ciprofloxacin (as lactate) 2 mg/mL, in sodium chloride 0.9%, net price 50-mL bottle = £8.31, 100-mL bottle = £16.23, 200-mL bottle = £24.70
Electrolytes Na+ 15.4 mmol/100-mL bottle

5 Infections

■ NALIDIXIC ACID

Cautions see notes above; avoid in acute porphyria (section 9.8.2); false positive urinary glucose (if tested for reducing substances); monitor blood counts, renal and liver function if treatment exceeds 2 weeks; **interactions:** Appendix 1 (quinolones)

Contra-indications see notes above

Hepatic impairment manufacturer advises caution in liver disease

Renal impairment use with caution; avoid if estimated glomerular filtration rate less than 20 mL/minute/1.73 m²

Pregnancy see notes above

Breast-feeding risk to infant very small but one case of haemolytic anaemia reported

Side-effects see notes above; also reported toxic psychosis, increased intracranial pressure, cranial nerve palsy, metabolic acidosis

Licensed use not licensed for use in children under 3 months of age

Indication and dose

> **Urinary tract infection resistant to other antibiotics**
> - By mouth
>
>   **Child 3 months–12 years** 12.5 mg/kg 4 times daily for 7 days, reduced to 7.5 mg/kg 4 times daily in prolonged therapy or 15 mg/kg twice daily for prophylaxis
>
>   **Child 12–18 years** 900 mg 4 times daily for 7 days, reduced in chronic infections to 600 mg 4 times daily

Nalidixic acid (Rosemont) [PoM]
Suspension, pink, nalidixic acid 300 mg/5 mL, net price 150 mL (raspberry- and strawberry-flavoured) = £11.42. Label: 9, 11
Excipients include sucrose 450 mg/5 mL

5.1.13 Urinary-tract infections

Urinary-tract infection is more common in adolescent girls than in boys; when it occurs in adolescent boys there is frequently an underlying abnormality of the renal tract. Recurrent episodes of infection are an indication for radiological investigation especially in children in whom untreated pyelonephritis may lead to permanent kidney damage.

Escherichia coli is the most common cause of urinary-tract infection; *Staphylococcus saprophyticus* is also common in sexually active young women. Less common causes include Proteus and Klebsiella spp. *Pseudomonas aeruginosa* infections usually occur in the hospital setting and may be associated with functional or anatomical abnormalities of the renal tract. *Staphylococcus epidermidis* and *Enterococcus faecalis* infection may complicate catheterisation or instrumentation.

> Whenever possible a specimen of urine should be collected for culture and sensitivity testing before starting antibacterial therapy. The antibacterial chosen should reflect current local bacterial sensitivity to antibacterials.

Urinary-tract infections in children require prompt antibacterial treatment to minimise the risk of renal scarring. Uncomplicated 'lower' urinary-tract infections in *children over 3 months* of age can be treated with trimethoprim, nitrofurantoin, a first generation cephalosporin, or amoxicillin for 3 days; children should be reassessed if they continue to be unwell 24–48 hours after the initial assessment.

Acute pyelonephritis in children over 3 months of age can be treated with a first generation cephalosporin or co-amoxiclav for 7–10 days. If the patient is severely ill, then the infection is best treated initially by intravenous injection of a broad-spectrum antibacterial such as cefotaxime or co-amoxiclav; gentamicin is an alternative.

Children under 3 months of age should be transferred to hospital and treated initially with intravenous antibacterials such as ampicillin with gentamicin, or cefotaxime alone, until the infection responds; full doses of oral antibacterials are then given for a further period.

Resistant infections Widespread bacterial resistance, especially to amoxicillin, ampicillin, and trimethoprim has increased the importance of urine culture before therapy. Alternatives for resistant organisms include co-amoxiclav (amoxicillin with clavulanic acid), an oral cephalosporin, pivmecillinam, or a quinolone.

Antibacterial prophylaxis Recurrent episodes of infection are an indication for imaging tests. *Antibacterial prophylaxis* with low doses of trimethoprim or nitrofurantoin may be considered for children with recurrent infection, significant urinary-tract anomalies, or significant kidney damage. Nitrofurantoin is contra-indicated in children under 3 months of age because of the theoretical possibility of haemolytic anaemia.

Pregnancy Urinary-tract infection in *pregnancy* may be asymptomatic and requires prompt treatment to prevent progression to acute pyelonephritis. Penicillins and cephalosporins are suitable for treating urinary-tract infection during pregnancy. Nitrofurantoin may also be used but it should be avoided at term. Sulphonamides, quinolones, and tetracyclines should be avoided during pregnancy; trimethoprim should also preferably be avoided particularly in the first trimester.

Renal impairment In *renal failure* antibacterials normally excreted by the kidney accumulate with resultant toxicity unless the dose is reduced. This applies especially to the aminoglycosides which should be used with great caution; tetracyclines, methamine, and nitrofurantoin should be avoided altogether.

NITROFURANTOIN

Cautions anaemia; diabetes mellitus; electrolyte imbalance; vitamin B and folate deficiency; pulmonary disease; on long-term therapy, monitor liver function and monitor for pulmonary symptoms (discontinue if deterioration in lung function); susceptibility to peripheral neuropathy; false positive urinary glucose (if tested for reducing substances); urine may be coloured yellow or brown; **interactions:** Appendix 1 (nitrofurantoin)

Contra-indications infants less than 3 months old, G6PD deficiency (section 9.1.5), acute porphyria (section 9.8.2)

Hepatic impairment use with caution; cholestatic jaundice and chronic active hepatitis reported

Renal impairment avoid if estimated glomerular filtration rate less than 60 mL/minute/1.73 m^2; risk of peripheral neuropathy; ineffective because of inadequate urine concentrations

Pregnancy avoid at term—may produce neonatal haemolysis

Breast-feeding avoid; only small amounts in milk but enough to produce haemolysis in G6PD-deficient infants (section 9.1.5)

Side-effects anorexia, nausea, vomiting, and diarrhoea; acute and chronic pulmonary reactions (pulmonary fibrosis reported; possible association with lupus erythematosus-like syndrome); peripheral neuropathy; also reported, hypersensitivity reactions (including angio-edema, anaphylaxis, sialadenitis, urticaria, rash and pruritus); rarely, cholestatic jaundice, hepatitis, exfoliative dermatitis, erythema multiforme, pancreatitis, arthralgia, blood disorders (including agranulocytosis, thrombocytopenia, and aplastic anaemia), benign intracranial hypertension, and transient alopecia

Indication and dose

Acute uncomplicated urinary-tract infection
● By mouth
    Child 3 months–12 years 750 micrograms/kg 4 times daily for 3–7 days

Child 12–18 years 50 mg 4 times daily for 3–7 days; increased to 100 mg 4 times daily in severe chronic recurrent infections

Prophylaxis of urinary-tract infection (but see Cautions)
● By mouth
    Child 3 months–12 years 1 mg/kg at night
    Child 12–18 years 50–100 mg at night

Nitrofurantoin (Non-proprietary) ℗ℴ𝓜
Tablets, nitrofurantoin 50 mg, net price 28-tab pack = £1.84; 100 mg, 28-tab pack = £4.67 Label: 9, 14, 21

Oral suspension, nitrofurantoin 25 mg/5 mL, net price 300 mL = £65.00. Label: 9, 14, 21

Furadantin® (Goldshield) ℗ℴ𝓜
Tablets, all yellow, scored, nitrofurantoin 50 mg, net price 100-tab pack = £9.79; 100 mg, 100-tab pack = £18.11. Label: 9, 14, 21

Macrobid® (Goldshield) ℗ℴ𝓜
Capsules, m/r, blue/yellow, nitrofurantoin 100 mg (as nitrofurantoin macrocrystals and nitrofurantoin monohydrate). Net price 14-cap pack = £4.89. Label: 9, 14, 21, 25

Dose
Uncomplicated urinary-tract infection
    Child 12–18 years 1 capsule twice daily with food

Genito-urinary surgical prophylaxis
    Child 12–18 years 1 capsule twice daily on day of procedure and for 3 days after

Macrodantin® (Goldshield) ℗ℴ𝓜
Capsules, yellow/white, nitrofurantoin 50 mg (as macrocrystals), net price 30-cap pack = £2.49; 100 mg (yellow/white), 20 = £3.21. Label: 9, 14, 21

5.2 Antifungal drugs

Treatment of fungal infections

The systemic treatment of common fungal infections is outlined below; specialist treatment is required in most forms of systemic or disseminated fungal infections.

For local treatment of fungal infections, see section 7.2.2 (genital), section 7.4.4 (bladder), section 11.3.2 (eye), section 12.1.1 (ear), section 12.3.2 (oropharynx), and section 13.10.2 (skin).

Aspergillosis Aspergillosis most commonly affects the respiratory tract but in severely immunocompromised patients, invasive forms can affect the heart, brain, and skin. **Amphotericin** (liposomal formulation preferred if toxicity or renal impairment are concerns) or **voriconazole** can be used to treat aspergillosis. **Itraconazole** is an alternative for refractory infection or for patients who cannot tolerate amphotericin. Itraconazole is also used as an adjunct in the treatment of allergic bronchopulmonary aspergillosis. **Caspofungin** is licensed in children for invasive aspergillosis unresponsive to amphotericin or to itraconazole, or in children who cannot tolerate amphotericin or itraconazole.

Candidiasis Many superficial candidal infections, including infections of the skin (section 13.10.2), are treated locally. Systemic antifungal treatment is required in widespread or intractable infection. Vaginal candidiasis can be treated with locally acting antifungals (section 7.2.2); alternatively, fluconazole can be given by mouth.

Oropharyngeal candidiasis generally responds to topical therapy (section 12.3.2). Fluconazole is given by mouth for unresponsive infections; it is reliably absorbed and is effective. Itraconazole can be used for fluconazole-resistant infections. Topical therapy may not be adequate in immunocompromised children and an oral triazole antifungal is preferred.

For *deep and disseminated candidiasis*, either **amphotericin** by intravenous infusion or an **echinocandin** (e.g. caspofungin) can be used. **Fluconazole** is an alternative for *Candida albicans* infection in clinically stable children who have not received an azole antifungal recently. **Voriconazole** can be used for infections caused by fluconazole-resistant *Candida* spp. when oral therapy is required, or when the infection has not responded to amphotericin or an echinocandin, or in children intolerant of amphotericin or an echinocandin. In refractory cases, **flucytosine** can be used with intravenous amphotericin.

Cryptococcosis Cryptococcosis is uncommon but infection in the immunocompromised, especially HIV-infected children, can be life-threatening; cryptococcal meningitis is the most common form of fungal meningitis. The treatment of choice in cryptococcal meningitis is **amphotericin** by intravenous infusion with **flucytosine** by intravenous infusion for 2 weeks, followed by **fluconazole** by mouth for 8 weeks or until cultures are negative. In cryptococcosis, fluconazole is sometimes given alone as an alternative in AIDS patients with mild localised infection or in those who cannot tolerate amphotericin. Following successful treatment, fluconazole can be used for prophylaxis against relapse until immunity recovers.

Histoplasmosis Histoplasmosis is rare in temperate climates; it can be life-threatening, particularly in HIV-infected children. **Itraconazole** can be used for the treatment of immunocompetent children with indolent non-meningeal infection, including chronic pulmonary histoplasmosis. **Amphotericin** by intravenous infusion is preferred in children with fulminant or severe infections. Following successful treatment, itraconazole can be used for prophylaxis against relapse.

Skin and nail infections Mild localised fungal infections of the skin (including tinea corporis, tinea cruris, and tinea pedis) respond to topical therapy (section 13.10.2). Systemic therapy is appropriate if topical therapy fails, if many areas are affected, or if the site of infection is difficult to treat such as in infections of the nails (onychomycosis) and of the scalp (tinea capitis).

Oral imidazole or triazole antifungals (particularly **itraconazole**) and **terbinafine** are used more frequently than griseofulvin because they have a broader spectrum of activity and require a shorter duration of treatment.

Tinea capitis is treated systemically; additional topical application of an antifungal (section 13.10.2) may reduce transmission. **Griseofulvin** is used for tinea capitis; it is effective against infections caused by *Trichophyton tonsurans* and *Microsporum spp.* Terbinafine is used for tinea capitis caused by *T. tonsurans* [unlicensed indication]; fluconazole is an alternative [unlicensed indication]. The role of terbinafine in the management of *Microsporum* infections is uncertain.

Pityriasis versicolor (section 13.10.2) may be treated with **itraconazole** by mouth if topical therapy is ineffective; **fluconazole** by mouth is an alternative. Oral **terbinafine** is **not** effective for pityriasis versicolor.

Antifungal treatment may not be necessary in asymptomatic children with tinea infection of the nails. If treatment is necessary, a systemic antifungal is more effective than topical therapy. **Terbinafine** and **itraconazole** have largely replaced griseofulvin for the systemic treatment of *onychomycosis*, particularly of the toenail; they should be used under specialist advice. Although terbinafine is not licensed for use in children, it is considered to be the drug of choice for onychomycosis. Itraconazole can be administered as intermittent 'pulse' therapy. For the role of topical antifungals in the treatment of onychomycosis, see section 13.10.2

Immunocompromised children   Immunocompromised children are at particular risk of fungal infections and may receive antifungal drugs prophylactically; oral triazole antifungals are the drugs of choice for prophylaxis. **Fluconazole** is more reliably absorbed than **itraconazole**, but fluconazole is not effective against *Aspergillus* spp. Itraconazole is preferred in patients at risk of invasive aspergillosis. **Micafungin** can be used for prophylaxis of candidiasis in patients undergoing haematopoietic stem cell transplantation when fluconazole or itraconazole cannot be used.

Amphotericin by intravenous infusion or **caspofungin** is used for the empirical *treatment* of serious fungal infections in immunocompromised children.

Drugs used in fungal infections

Polyene antifungals   The polyene antifungals include amphotericin and nystatin; neither drug is absorbed when given by mouth. They are used for oral, oropharyngeal, and perioral infections by local application in the mouth (section 12.3.2).

Amphotericin by intravenous infusion is used for the treatment of systemic fungal infections and is active against most fungi and yeasts. It is highly protein bound and penetrates poorly into body fluids and tissues. When given parenterally amphotericin is toxic and side-effects are common. Lipid formulations of amphotericin (*Abelcet®* and *AmBisome®*) are significantly less toxic and are recommended when the conventional formulation of amphotericin is contraindicated because of toxicity, especially nephrotoxicity, or when response to conventional amphotericin is inadequate; lipid formulations are more expensive.

Nystatin is used principally for *Candida albicans* infections of the skin (section 13.10.2) and mucous membranes, including intestinal candidiasis.

Imidazole antifungals   The imidazole antifungals include clotrimazole, econazole, sulconazole, and tioconazole. They are used for the local treatment of vaginal candidiasis (section 7.2.2) and for dermatophyte infections (section 13.10.2).

Ketoconazole is better absorbed by mouth than other imidazoles. It has been associated with fatal hepatotoxicity; the CSM has advised that prescribers should weigh the potential benefits of ketoconazole treatment against the risk of liver damage and should carefully monitor patients both clinically and biochemically. It should not be used by mouth for superficial fungal infections.

Miconazole (section 12.3.2) can be used locally for oral infections; it is also effective in intestinal infections. Systemic absorption may follow use of miconazole oral gel and may result in significant drug interactions.

Triazole antifungals   **Fluconazole** is very well absorbed after oral administration. It also achieves good penetration into the cerebrospinal fluid to treat fungal meningitis.

Itraconazole is active against a wide range of dermatophytes. There is limited information available on use in children. Itraconazole capsules require an acid environment in the stomach for optimal absorption.

Itraconazole has been associated with liver damage and should be avoided or used with caution in children with liver disease; fluconazole is less frequently associated with hepatotoxicity.

Voriconazole is a broad-spectrum antifungal drug which is licensed in adults for the treatment of life-threatening infections.

Echinocandin antifungals The echinocandin antifungals (e.g. **caspofungin**) are only active against *Aspergillus* spp. and *Candida* spp; however **micafungin** is not used for the treatment of aspergillosis.

Other antifungals Flucytosine is used with amphotericin in a synergistic combination. Bone marrow depression can occur which limits its use, particularly in children with AIDS; weekly blood counts are necessary during prolonged therapy. Resistance to flucytosine can develop during therapy and sensitivity testing is essential before and during treatment.

Griseofulvin is effective for widespread or intractable dermatophyte infections but has been superseded by newer antifungals, particularly for nail infections. Griseofulvin is used in the treatment of tinea capitis. It is the drug of choice for trichophyton infections in children. Duration of therapy is dependent on the site of the infection and may extend to a number of months.

Terbinafine is the drug of choice for fungal nail infections and is also used for ringworm infections where oral treatment is considered appropriate.

▲ AMPHOTERICIN
(Amphotericin B)

Cautions when given parenterally, toxicity common (close supervision necessary and close observation required for at least 30 minutes after test dose; see Anaphylaxis below); hepatic and renal function tests, blood counts and plasma electrolyte (including plasma-potassium and magnesium concentration) monitoring required; corticosteroids (avoid except to control reactions); avoid rapid infusion (risk of arrhythmias); **interactions:** Appendix 1 (amphotericin)

Anaphylaxis The CSM has advised that anaphylaxis occurs rarely with any intravenous amphotericin product and a test dose is advisable before the first infusion; the patient should be carefully observed for at least 30 minutes after the test dose. Prophylactic antipyretics or hydrocortisone should only be used in patients who have previously experienced acute adverse reactions (in whom continued treatment with amphotericin is essential)

Renal impairment use only if no alternative; nephrotoxicity may be reduced with use of lipid formulation

Pregnancy not known to be harmful, but manufacturers advise avoid unless potential benefit outweighs risk

Breast-feeding no information available

Side-effects when given parenterally, anorexia, nausea and vomiting, diarrhoea, epigastric pain; febrile reactions, headache, muscle and joint pain; anaemia; disturbances in renal function (including hypokalaemia and hypomagnesaemia) and renal toxicity; also cardiovascular toxicity (including arrhythmias, blood pressure changes), blood disorders, neurological disorders (including hearing loss, diplopia, convulsions, peripheral neuropathy, encephalopathy), abnormal liver function (discontinue treatment), rash, anaphylactoid reactions (see Anaphylaxis, above); pain and thrombophlebitis at injection site

Licensed use intravenous conventional formulation amphotericin (*Fungizone*®) is licensed for use in children (age range not specified by manufacturer); *Ambisome*® not licensed for use in children under 1 month

Indication and dose

Systemic fungal infections
- **By intravenous infusion**
  see preparations
  Note Different preparations of intravenous amphotericin vary in their pharmacodynamics, pharmacokinetics, dosage, and administration; these preparations should **not** be considered interchangeable. To avoid confusion, prescribers should specify the brand to be dispensed.

Fungizone® (Squibb) ℗ₒM
Intravenous infusion, powder for reconstitution, amphotericin (as sodium deoxycholate complex), net price 50-mg vial = £3.96
Electrolytes Na⁺ < 0.5 mmol/vial

Dose

Systemic fungal infection
- **By intravenous infusion**

  Neonate 1 mg/kg once daily (initial test dose of 100 micrograms/kg included as part of first dose); after 7 days, may be reduced to 1 mg/kg on alternate days

  Child 1 month–18 years initial test dose of 100 micrograms/kg (max. 1 mg) included as part of first dose of 250 micrograms/kg daily; increased over 2–4 days, if tolerated, to 1 mg/kg daily; in severe infection max. 1.5 mg/kg daily or on alternate days
  Note prolonged treatment usually necessary; if interrupted for longer than 7 days, recommence at 250 micrograms/kg daily and increase gradually

  Administration For *intravenous infusion*, reconstitute each vial with 10 mL Water for Injections and shake immediately to produce a 5 mg/mL colloidal solution; dilute further in Glucose 5% to a concentration of 100 micrograms/mL (in fluid-restricted children, up to 400 micrograms/mL given via a central line); pH of glucose solution must not be below 4.2 (check each container—consult product literature for details of buffer); infuse over 4–6 hours, or if tolerated over a minimum of 2 hours (initial test dose given over 20–30 minutes); begin infusion immediately after dilution and protect from light; incompatible with Sodium Chloride solutions—flush existing intravenous line with Glucose 5% or use separate line; an in-line filter (pore size no less than 1 micron) may be used

▲ Lipid formulations

Abelcet® (Cephalon) ℗ₒM
Intravenous infusion, amphotericin 5 mg/mL as lipid complex with L-α-dimyristoylphosphatidyl-

◻ **AMPHOTERICIN (continued)**

choline and L-α-dimyristoylphosphatidylglycerol, net price 20-mL vial = £82.13 (hosp. only)

Dose

> Severe invasive candidiasis; severe systemic fungal infections in children not responding to conventional amphotericin or to other antifungal drugs or where toxicity or renal impairment precludes conventional amphotericin, including invasive aspergillosis, cryptococcal meningitis and disseminated cryptococcosis in children with HIV
> - **By intravenous infusion**
>   **Child 1 month–18 years** initial test dose of 100 micrograms/kg (max. 1 mg) then 5 mg/kg once daily

Administration for *intravenous infusion*, allow suspension to reach room temperature, shake gently to ensure no yellow settlement, withdraw requisite dose (using 17–19 gauge needle) into one or more 20-mL syringes; replace needle on syringe with a 5-micron filter needle provided (fresh needle for each syringe) and dilute in Glucose 5% to a concentration of 2 mg/mL; preferably give *via* an infusion pump at a rate of 2.5 mg/kg/hour (initial test dose given over 15 minutes); an in-line filter (pore size no less than 15 micron) may be used; do not use sodium chloride or other electrolyte solutions—flush existing intravenous line with Glucose 5% or use separate line

AmBisome® (Gilead) ℞

Intravenous infusion, powder for reconstitution, amphotericin 50 mg encapsulated in liposomes, net price 50-mg vial = £96.69
Electrolytes Na⁺< 0.5 mmol/vial
Excipients include sucrose 900 mg/vial

Dose

> Severe systemic or deep mycoses where toxicity (particularly nephrotoxicity) precludes use of conventional amphotericin
> - **By intravenous infusion**
>   **Neonate** 1 mg/kg once daily (initial test dose of 100 micrograms/kg included as part of first dose);

increased if necessary to 3 mg/kg once daily; max. 5 mg/kg once daily

Child 1 month–18 years initial test dose 100 micrograms/kg (max. 1 mg) then 1 mg/kg once daily, increased if necessary to 3 mg/kg once daily; max. 5 mg/kg once daily

> Suspected or proven infection in febrile neutropenic patients unresponsive to broad-spectrum antibacterials
> - **By intravenous infusion**
>   **Child 1 month–18 years** initial test dose 100 micrograms/kg (max. 1 mg) then 3 mg/kg once daily until afebrile for 3 consecutive days; max. period of treatment 42 days; max. 5 mg/kg once daily

> Visceral leishmaniasis see section 5.4.5 and product literature

Administration for *intravenous infusion*, reconstitute each vial with 12 mL Water for Injections and shake vigorously to produce a preparation containing 4 mg/mL; withdraw requisite dose from vial and introduce into Glucose 5% through the 5-micron filter provided, to produce a final concentration of 0.2–2 mg/mL; infuse over 30–60 minutes (initial test dose given over 10 minutes); incompatible with sodium chloride solutions—flush existing intravenous line with Glucose 5% or use separate line

▰ **CASPOFUNGIN**

Cautions interactions: Appendix 1 (caspofungin)
Hepatic impairment usual initial dose, then use 70% of normal maintenance dose in moderate impairment; no information available for severe impairment
Pregnancy manufacturer advises avoid unless essential—toxicity in *animal* studies
Breast-feeding present in milk in *animal* studies—manufacturer advises avoid
Side-effects nausea, diarrhoea, vomiting; tachycardia, hypotension, flushing; dyspnoea; headache; hypokalaemia, hypomagnesaemia; arthralgia; rash, pruritus, sweating, injection-site reactions; *less commonly* abdominal pain, dyspepsia, dysphagia, dry mouth, taste disturbances, anorexia, constipation, flatulence, cholestasis, hepatic dysfunction, ascites, palpitation, arrhythmia, chest pain, heart failure, thrombophlebitis, hypertension, bronchospasm, cough, dizziness, fatigue, paraesthesia, hypoaesthesia, sleep disturbances, tremor, anxiety, disorientation, hyperglycaemia, renal failure, hypocalcaemia, metabolic acidosis, anaemia, thrombocytopenia, leucopenia, myalgia, muscular weakness, blurred vision, and erythema multiforme; also reported, acute respiratory distress syndrome, anaphylaxis, and hypercalcaemia

Indication and dose

> Invasive aspergillosis either unresponsive to amphotericin or itraconazole or in patients intolerant of amphotericin or itraconazole; invasive candidiasis (see notes above); empirical treatment of systemic fungal infections in patients with neutropenia
> - **By intravenous infusion**
>   **Neonate** 25 mg/m² once daily
>   **Child 1 month–3 months** 25 mg/m² once daily
>   **Child 3 months–1 year** 50 mg/m² once daily
>   **Child 1–18 years** 70 mg/m² (max. 70 mg) on first day then 50 mg/m² (max. 70 mg) once daily; increased to 70 mg/m² (max. 70 mg) daily if lower dose tolerated but inadequate response

Administration for *intravenous infusion*, allow vial to reach room temperature; initially reconstitute 50 mg with 10.5 mL Water for Injections to produce a 5.2 mg/mL solution, or reconstitute 70 mg with 10.5 mL Water for Injections to produce a 7.2 mg/mL solution; mix gently to dissolve; dilute requisite dose to a final concentration not exceeding 500 micrograms/mL with Sodium Chloride 0.9%; give over 60 minutes; incompatible with glucose solutions

◁ **CASPOFUNGIN** (*continued*)

Cancidas® (MSD) ▼ PoM
Intravenous infusion, powder for reconstitution, caspofungin (as acetate), net price 50-mg vial = £327.67; 70-mg vial = £416.78

FLUCONAZOLE

Cautions concomitant use with hepatotoxic drugs, monitor liver function with high doses or extended courses—discontinue if signs or symptoms of hepatic disease (risk of hepatic necrosis); susceptibility to QT interval prolongation; **interactions**: Appendix 1 (antifungals, triazole)

Contra-indications acute porphyria (section 9.8.2)

Hepatic impairment toxicity with related drugs

Renal impairment usual initial dose then halve subsequent doses if estimated glomerular filtration rate less than 50 mL/minute/1.73m²

Pregnancy manufacturer advises avoid—multiple congenital abnormalities reported with long-term high doses

Breast-feeding present in milk but amount probably too small to be harmful

Side-effects nausea, abdominal discomfort, diarrhoea, flatulence, headache, rash (discontinue treatment or monitor closely if infection invasive or systemic); less frequently dyspepsia, vomiting, taste disturbance, hepatic disorders, angioedema, anaphylaxis, dizziness, seizures, alopecia, pruritus, toxic epidermal necrolysis, Stevens-Johnson syndrome (severe cutaneous reactions more likely in AIDS patients), hyperlipidaemia, leucopenia, thrombocytopenia, and hypokalaemia reported

Licensed use not licensed for tinea infections in children, or for vaginal candidiasis in girls under 16 years, or for prevention of relapse of cryptococcal meningitis after completion of primary therapy in children with AIDS

Indication and dose

Mucosal candidiasis (except genital)
- By mouth or by intravenous infusion
  Neonate under 2 weeks 3–6 mg/kg on first day then 3 mg/kg every 72 hours

  Neonate 2–4 weeks 3–6 mg/kg on first day then 3 mg/kg every 48 hours

  Child 1 month–12 years 3–6 mg/kg on first day then 3 mg/kg (max. 100 mg) daily for 7–14 days in oropharyngeal candidiasis (max. 14 days except in severely immunocompromised patients); for 14–30 days in other mucosal infections (e.g. oesophagitis, candiduria, non-invasive bronchopulmonary infections)

  Child 12–18 years 50 mg daily (100 mg daily in unusually difficult infections) given for 7–14 days in oropharyngeal candidiasis (max. 14 days except in severely immunocompromised patients); for 14–30 days in other mucosal infections (e.g. oesophagitis, candiduria, non-invasive bronchopulmonary infections)

Vaginal candidiasis (see also Recurrent Vulvovaginal Candidiasis, section 7.2.2)
- By mouth
  Child under 16 years (post-puberty) a single dose of 150 mg

  Child 16–18 years a single dose of 150 mg

Candidal balanitis
- By mouth
  Child 16–18 years a single dose of 150 mg

Tinea pedis, corporis, cruris, pityriasis versicolor, and dermal candidiasis
- By mouth
  Child 1 month–18 years 3 mg/kg (max. 50 mg) daily for 2–4 weeks (for up to 6 weeks in tinea pedis); max. duration of treatment 6 weeks

Tinea capitis caused by *Trichophyton spp.*
- By mouth
  Child 1–18 years 6 mg/kg (max. 300 mg) daily for 2–4 weeks

Invasive candidal infections (including candidaemia and disseminated candidiasis) and cryptococcal infections (including meningitis)
- By mouth or by intravenous infusion
  Neonate under 2 weeks 6–12 mg/kg every 72 hours, treatment continued according to response (at least 8 weeks for cryptococcal meningitis)

  Neonate 2–4 weeks 6–12 mg/kg every 48 hours, treatment continued according to response (at least 8 weeks for cryptococcal meningitis)

  Child 1 month–18 years 6–12 mg/kg (max. 800 mg) daily, treatment continued according to response (at least 8 weeks for cryptococcal meningitis)

Prevention of relapse of cryptococcal meningitis in AIDS patients after completion of primary therapy
- By mouth or by intravenous infusion
  Child 1 month–18 years 6 mg/kg (max. 200 mg) daily

Prevention of fungal infections in immunocompromised patients
- By mouth or by intravenous infusion
  Neonate under 2 weeks according to extent and duration of neutropenia, 3–12 mg/kg every 72 hours

  Neonate 2–4 weeks according to extent and duration of neutropenia, 3–12 mg/kg every 48 hours

▱ FLUCONAZOLE (*continued*)

Child 1 month–18 years according to extent and duration of neutropenia, 3–12 mg/kg (max. 400 mg) daily; 12 mg/kg (max. 400 mg) daily if high risk of systemic infections e.g. following bone-marrow transplantation; commence treatment before anticipated onset of neutropenia and continue for 7 days after neutrophil count in desirable range

Administration for *intravenous infusion*, give over 10–30 minutes; do not exceed an infusion rate of 5–10 mL/minute

Fluconazole (Non-proprietary) ℞
  [1]Capsules, fluconazole 50 mg, net price 7-cap pack = £1.20; 150 mg, single-capsule pack = £1.04; 200 mg, 7-cap pack = £4.46. Label: 9, (50 and 200 mg)
  Dental prescribing on NHS Fluconazole Capsules 50 mg may be prescribed

Intravenous infusion, fluconazole 2 mg/mL, net price 25-mL bottle = £7.31; 100-mL bottle = £29.27

Diflucan® (Pfizer) ℞
  [1]Capsules, fluconazole 50 mg (blue/white), net price 7-cap pack = £16.61; 150 mg (blue), single-capsule pack = £7.12; 200 mg (purple/white), 7-cap pack = £66.42. Label: 9, (50 and 200 mg)

Oral suspension, orange-flavoured, fluconazole for reconstitution with water, 50 mg/5 mL, net price 35 mL = £16.61; 200 mg/5 mL, 35 mL = £66.42. Label: 9
  Dental prescribing on NHS May be prescribed as Fluconazole Oral Suspension 50 mg/5 mL

Intravenous infusion, fluconazole 2 mg/mL in sodium chloride intravenous infusion 0.9%, net price 25-mL bottle = £7.32; 100-mL bottle = £29.28
Electrolytes Na⁺ 15 mmol/100-mL bottle

▰ FLUCYTOSINE

Cautions blood disorders; liver- and kidney-function tests and blood counts required (weekly in blood disorders); **interactions:** Appendix 1 (flucytosine)

Renal impairment liver- and kidney-function tests and blood counts required weekly; use normal dose every 12 hours if estimated glomerular filtration rate 20–40 mL/minute/1.73 m²; use normal dose every 24 hours if estimated glomerular filtration rate 10–20 mL/minute/1.73 m²; use initial normal dose if estimated glomerular filtration rate less than 10 mL/minute/1.73 m² and then adjust dose according to plasma-flucytosine concentration

Pregnancy teratogenic in *animal* studies; manufacturer advises use only if potential benefit outweighs risk

Breast-feeding manufacturer advises avoid

Side-effects nausea, vomiting, diarrhoea, rashes; less frequently cardiotoxicity, confusion, hallucinations, convulsions, headache, sedation, vertigo, alterations in liver function tests (hepatitis and hepatic necrosis reported), and toxic epidermal necrolysis; blood disorders including thrombocytopenia, leucopenia, and aplastic anaemia reported

Pharmacokinetics for plasma-concentration monitoring blood should be taken shortly before starting the next infusion. Plasma concentration for optimum response 25–50 mg/litre (200–400 micromol/litre)—should not be allowed to exceed 80 mg/litre (620 micromol/litre)

Licensed use tablets not licensed

Indication and dose

Systemic yeast and fungal infections, adjunct to amphotericin in severe systemic candidiasis and in other severe or long-standing infections
  • By *intravenous infusion* or *by mouth*

  Neonate 50 mg/kg every 12 hours

  Child 1 month–18 years 50 mg/kg every 6 hours; extremely sensitive organisms, 25–37.5 mg/kg every 6 hours may be sufficient; treatment continued usually for not more than 7 days

Cryptococcal meningitis (adjunct to amphotericin, see Cryptococcosis, p. 368)
  • By *intravenous infusion* or *by mouth*

  Neonate 50 mg/kg every 12 hours

  Child 1 month–18 years 25 mg/kg every 6 hours for 2 weeks

Administration for *intravenous infusion*, give over 20–40 minutes through a giving set with a 15-micron filter

Ancotil® (Meda) ℞
  Intravenous infusion, flucytosine 10 mg/mL. Net price 250-mL infusion bottle = £30.33 (hosp. only)
  Electrolytes Na⁺ 34.5 mmol/250-mL bottle

Note Flucytosine tablets may be available from 'special-order' manufacturers or specialist importing companies, see p. 957

◣Extemporaneous formulations available see Extemporaneous Preparations, p. 8

▰ GRISEOFULVIN

Cautions interactions: Appendix 1 (griseofulvin)
  Skilled tasks May impair performance of skilled tasks; effects of alcohol enhanced

Contra-indications systemic lupus erythematosus (risk of exacerbation); acute porphyria (section 9.8.2)

Hepatic impairment avoid in severe liver disease

Pregnancy avoid (fetotoxicity and teratogenicity in *animals*); effective contraception required during and for at least 1 month after administration (**important**: effectiveness of oral contraceptives reduced, see also p. 486); also males should avoid

---

1. Capsules can be sold to the public for vaginal candidiasis and associated candidal balanitis in those aged 16–18 years, in a container or packaging containing not more than 150 mg and labelled to show a max. dose of 150 mg

5

Infections

◁ GRISEOFULVIN (*continued*)

fathering a child during and for at least 6 months after treatment

Breast-feeding avoid—no information available

Side-effects nausea, vomiting, diarrhoea; headache; less frequently hepatotoxicity, dizziness, confusion, fatigue, sleep disturbances, impaired co-ordination, peripheral neuropathy, leucopenia, systemic lupus erythematosus, rash (including rarely erythema multiforme, toxic epidermal necrolysis), and photosensitivity

Licensed use tablets licensed for use in children (age range not specified by manufacturer); suspension not licensed

Indication and dose

Dermatophyte infections where topical therapy has failed or is inappropriate
• By mouth
    Child 1 month–12 years 10 mg/kg (max. 500 mg) once daily or in divided doses; in severe infection dose may be doubled, reducing when response occurs

Child 12–18 years 500 mg once daily or in divided doses; in severe infection dose may be doubled, reducing when response occurs

Tinea capitis caused by *Trichophyton tonsurans*
• By mouth
    Child 1 month–12 years 15–20 mg/kg (max. 1 g) once daily or in divided doses

    Child 12–18 years 1 g once daily or in divided doses

Griseofulvin (Non-proprietary) PoM
Tablets, griseofulvin 125 mg, net price 100 = £33.80; 500 mg, 100 = £87.60. Label: 9, 21, counselling, skilled tasks

Suspension, griseofulvin 125 mg/5 mL. Label: 9, 21, counselling, skilled tasks
Available via specialist importing companies

■ **ITRACONAZOLE**

Cautions absorption reduced in AIDS and neutropenia (monitor plasma-itraconazole concentration and increase dose if necessary); susceptibility to congestive heart failure (see also Heart Failure, below); **interactions**: Appendix 1 (antifungals, triazole)

Hepatotoxicity Potentially life-threatening hepatotoxicity reported very rarely—discontinue if signs of hepatitis develop. Avoid or use with caution if history of hepatotoxicity with other drugs or in active liver disease. Monitor liver function if treatment continues for longer than one month, if receiving other hepatotoxic drugs, if history of hepatotoxicity with other drugs, or in hepatic impairment

Counselling Children or their carers should be told how to recognise signs of liver disorder and advised to seek prompt medical attention if symptoms such as anorexia, nausea, vomiting, fatigue, abdominal pain or dark urine develop

Heart failure Following reports of heart failure, caution is advised when prescribing itraconazole to patients at high risk of heart failure. Those at risk include:
• patients receiving high doses and longer treatment courses;
• those with cardiac disease;
• patients receiving treatment with negative inotropic drugs, e.g. calcium channel blockers.
Itraconazole should be avoided in patients with ventricular dysfunction or a history of heart failure unless the infection is serious.

Contra-indications acute porphyria (section 9.8.2)

Hepatic impairment use only if potential benefit outweighs risk of hepatotoxicity (see Hepatotoxicity above); dose reduction may be necessary

Renal impairment risk of congestive heart failure; bioavailability of oral formulations possibly reduced; use intravenous infusion with caution if estimated glomerular filtration rate 30–80 mL/minute/1.73 m² (monitor renal function); avoid intravenous infusion if estimated glomerular filtration rate less than 30 mL/minute/1.73 m²

Pregnancy manufacturer advises use only in life-threatening situations (toxicity at high doses in

animal studies); ensure effective contraception during treatment and until the next menstrual period following end of treatment

Breast-feeding small amounts present in milk—may accumulate; manufacturer advises avoid

Side-effects nausea, abdominal pain; rash; *less commonly* vomiting, dyspepsia, taste disturbances, flatulence, diarrhoea, constipation, oedema, headache, dizziness, paraesthesia (discontinue treatment if neuropathy), menstrual disorder, and alopecia; *rarely* hypoaesthesia, urinary frequency, leucopenia, visual disturbances, and tinnitus; also reported, heart failure (see Cautions above), hypertriglyceridaemia, hepatitis (see Hepatotoxicity above), erectile dysfunction, thrombocytopenia, hypokalaemia, myalgia, arthralgia, photosensitivity, toxic epidermal necrolysis, and Stevens-Johnson Syndrome; *with intravenous injection* hypertension and hyperglycaemia

Licensed use *Sporanox*® capsules and *Sporanox*® *Pulse* are not licensed for use in children under 12 years; *Sporanox*® liquid and *Sporanox*® infusion are not licensed for use in children (age range not specified by manufacturer)

Indication and dose

Oropharyngeal candidiasis
• By mouth
    Child 1 month–12 years 3–5 mg/kg once daily; max. 100 mg daily (200 mg daily in AIDS or neutropenia) for 15 days

    Child 12–18 years 100 mg once daily (200 mg once daily in AIDS or neutropenia) for 15 days

Pityriasis versicolor
• By mouth
    Child 1 month–12 years 3–5 mg/kg (max. 200 mg) once daily for 7 days

    Child 12–18 years 200 mg once daily for 7 days

◻ **ITRACONAZOLE** (*continued*)

Tinea corporis and tinea cruris
- **By mouth**

    Child 1 month–12 years 3–5 mg/kg (max. 100 mg) once daily for 15 days

    Child 12–18 years *either* 100 mg once daily for 15 days *or* 200 mg once daily for 7 days

Tinea pedis and tinea manuum
- **By mouth**

    Child 1 month–12 years 3–5 mg/kg (max. 100 mg) once daily for 30 days

    Child 12–18 years *either* 100 mg once daily for 30 days *or* 200 mg twice daily for 7 days

Onychomycosis
- **By mouth**

    Child 1–12 years course ('pulse') of 5 mg/kg (max. 200 mg) daily for 7 days; subsequent courses repeated after 21 day intervals; fingernails 2 courses, toenails 3 courses

    Child 12–18 years *either* 200 mg once daily for 3 months *or* course ('pulse') of 200 mg twice daily for 7 days, subsequent courses repeated after 21-day intervals; fingernails 2 courses, toenails 3 courses

Systemic aspergillosis, candidiasis and cryptococcosis including cryptococcal meningitis where other antifungal drugs inappropriate or ineffective (limited information available)
- **By mouth**

    Child 1 month–18 years 5 mg/kg (max. 200 mg) once daily; increased in invasive or disseminated disease and in cryptococcal meningitis to 5 mg/kg (max. 200 mg) twice daily

- **By intravenous infusion**

    Child 1 month–18 years 2.5 mg/kg (max. 200 mg) every 12 hours for 2 days, then 2.5 mg/kg (max. 200 mg) once daily for max. 12 days

Histoplasmosis
- **By mouth**

    Child 1 month–18 years 5 mg/kg (max. 200 mg) 1–2 times daily

Maintenance in AIDS patients to prevent relapse of underlying fungal infection and prophylaxis in neutropenia when standard therapy inappropriate
- **By mouth**

    Child 1 month–18 years 5 mg/kg (max. 200 mg) once daily, increased to 5 mg/kg (max. 200 mg) twice daily if low plasma-itraconazole concentration (see Cautions)

Prophylaxis of deep fungal infections (when standard therapy inappropriate) in patients with haematological malignancy or undergoing bone-marrow transplantation who are expected to become neutropenic
- **By mouth (liquid preparation only)**

    Child 1 month–18 years 2.5 mg/kg twice daily starting before transplantation or before chemotherapy (taking care to avoid interaction with cytotoxic drugs) and continued until neutrophil count recovers

Administration For *intravenous infusion*, dilute 250 mg with 50 mL Sodium Chloride 0.9% and give requisite dose through an in-line filter (0.2 micron) over 60 minutes

Itraconazole (Non-proprietary) [PoM]
Capsules, enclosing coated beads, itraconazole 100 mg, net price 15-cap pack = £9.31. Label: 5, 9, 21, 25, counselling, hepatotoxicity

Sporanox® (Janssen-Cilag) [PoM]
Capsules, blue/pink, enclosing coated beads, itraconazole 100 mg, net price 4-cap pack = £3.75; 15-cap pack = £14.05; 28-cap pack (*Sporanox®-Pulse*) = £26.24; 60-cap pack = £56.21. Label: 5, 9, 21, 25, counselling, hepatotoxicity

Oral liquid, sugar-free, cherry-flavoured, itraconazole 10 mg/mL, net price 150 mL (with 10-mL measuring cup) = £46.72. Label: 9, 23, counselling, administration, hepatotoxicity

Counselling Do not take with food; swish around mouth and swallow, do not rinse afterwards

Concentrate for intravenous infusion, itraconazole 10 mg/mL. For dilution before use. Net price 25-mL amp (with infusion bag and filter) = £63.84
Excipients include propylene glycol

▮ **KETOCONAZOLE** ◁

Cautions predisposition to adrenocortical insufficiency; **interactions:** Appendix 1 (antifungals, imidazole)

Hepatotoxicity Potentially life-threatening hepatotoxicity reported very rarely; risk of hepatotoxicity greater if given for longer than 10 days. Monitor liver function before treatment, then on weeks 2 and 4 of treatment, then every month. Avoid or use with caution if abnormal liver function tests (avoid in active liver disease) or if history of hepatotoxicity with other drugs. For CSM advice see p. 369

Counselling Children and their carers should be told how to recognise signs of liver disorder and advised to seek prompt medical attention if symptoms such as anorexia, nausea, vomiting, fatigue, abdominal pain, jaundice, or dark urine develop

Contra-indications acute porphyria (section 9.8.2)

Hepatic impairment avoid (see also Hepatotoxicity above)

Pregnancy manufacturer advises avoid unless potential benefit outweighs risk (teratogenicity in *animal* studies)

Breast-feeding manufacturer advises avoid

Side-effects nausea, vomiting, abdominal pain; pruritus; *less commonly* diarrhoea, headache, dizziness, drowsiness, and rash; also reported fatal liver damage (see Hepatotoxicity above), dyspepsia, raised intracranial pressure, paraesthesia, adrenocortical insufficiency, erectile dysfunction, menstrual disorders, azoospermia (with high doses), gynaecomastia, thrombocytopenia, photophobia, photosensitivity, and alopecia

5 **Infections**

◻ **KETOCONAZOLE** (*continued*)

Indication and dose

Dermatophytoses and *Malassezia* folliculitis *either* resistant to fluconazole, terbinafine, or itraconazole *or* in patients intolerant of these antifungals; chronic mucocutaneous, cutaneous, and oropharyngeal candidiasis *either* resistant to fluconazole or itraconazole *or* in patients intolerant of these antifungals; see also CSM recommendations, p. 369

- By mouth

  Child body-weight 15–30 kg 100 mg once daily

  Child body-weight over 30 kg 200 mg once daily, increased if response inadequate to 400 mg once daily

  Note Treatment continued until symptoms have cleared and cultures negative, but see Cautions (max. duration of treatment 4 weeks for *Malassezia* infection)

Nizoral® (Janssen-Cilag) PoM ⬛
Tablets, scored, ketoconazole 200 mg. Net price 30-tab pack = £14.02. Label: 5, 9, 21, Counselling, hepatotoxicity

◢Extemporaneous formulations available see Extemporaneous Preparations, p. 8

◢ MICAFUNGIN

Cautions monitor renal function; **interactions**: Appendix 1 (micafungin)

Hepatotoxicity Potentially life-threatening hepatotoxicity reported. Monitor liver function—discontinue if significant and persistent abnormalities in liver function tests develop. Use with caution in hepatic impairment (avoid if severe) or if receiving other hepatotoxic drugs. Risk of hepatic side-effects greater in children under 1 year of age

Hepatic impairment use with caution in mild to moderate impairment; avoid in severe impairment; see also Hepatotoxicity above

Renal impairment use with caution; deterioration in renal function

Pregnancy manufacturer advises avoid unless essential—toxicity in *animal* studies

Breast-feeding manufacturer advises use only if potential benefit outweighs risk—present in milk in *animal* studies

Side-effects nausea, vomiting, diarrhoea, abdominal pain, hepatomegaly; blood pressure changes, tachycardia; headache, fever; hypokalaemia, hypomagnesaemia, hypocalcaemia, leucopenia, anaemia, thrombocytopenia, renal failure; rash, phlebitis; *less commonly* dyspepsia, constipation, hepatitis and cholestasis (see also Hepatotoxicity above), taste disturbances, anorexia, palpitation, bradycardia, flushing, dyspnoea, sleep disturbances, anxiety, confusion, dizziness, tremor, pancytopenia, eosinophilia, hyponatraemia, hyperkalaemia, hypophosphataemia, hyperhidrosis, and pruritus; *rarely* haemolytic anaemia

Indication and dose

Invasive candidiasis

- By intravenous infusion

  Neonate 2 mg/kg once daily (increased to 4 mg/kg daily if inadequate response) for at least 14 days

  Child 1 month–18 years, body-weight under 40 kg 2 mg/kg once daily (increased to 4 mg/kg daily if inadequate response) for at least 14 days

  Child 1 month–18 years, body-weight over 40 kg 100 mg once daily (increased to 200 mg daily if inadequate response) for at least 14 days

Oesophageal candidiasis

- By intravenous infusion

  Child 16–18 years, body-weight under 40 kg 3 mg/kg once daily

  Child 16–18 years, body-weight over 40 kg 150 mg once daily

Prophylaxis of candidiasis in children undergoing bone-marrow transplantation or who are expected to become neutropenic for over 10 days

- By intravenous infusion

  Neonate 1 mg/kg once daily; continue for at least 7 days after neutrophil count in desirable range

  Child 1 month–18 years, body-weight under 40 kg 1 mg/kg once daily; continue for at least 7 days after neutrophil count in desirable range

  Child 1 month–18 years, body-weight over 40 kg 50 mg once daily; continue for at least 7 days after neutrophil count in desirable range

Administration for *intravenous infusion* reconstitute each vial with 5 mL Glucose 5% *or* Sodium Chloride 0.9%; gently rotate vial, without shaking, to dissolve; dilute requisite dose to a concentration of 0.5–2 mg/mL with Glucose 5% *or* Sodium Chloride 0.9%; protect infusion from light; give over 60 minutes

Mycamine® (Astellas) ▼ PoM
Intravenous infusion, powder for reconstitution, micafungin (as sodium), net price 50-mg vial = £196.08; 100-mg vial = £341.00

◢ NYSTATIN

Pregnancy no information available, but absorption from gastro-intestinal tract negligible

Breast-feeding no information available, but absorption from gastro-intestinal tract negligible

Side-effects nausea, vomiting, diarrhoea at high doses; oral irritation and sensitisation; rash (including urticaria) and rarely Stevens-Johnson syndrome reported

◻ NYSTATIN (*continued*)

Licensed use suspension not licensed for treatment of intestinal candidiasis in neonates; suspension licensed for prophylaxis in neonates as once daily dose

Indication and dose

Treatment of intestinal candidiasis

• **By mouth**

Neonate 100 000 units 4 times daily after feeds

Child 1 month–12 years 100 000 units 4 times daily; immunocompromised children may require higher doses (e.g. 500 000 units 4 times daily)

Child 12–18 years 500 000 units 4 times daily; doubled in severe infection

---

Oral infection section 12.3.2

Skin infection section 13.10.2

Nystan® (Squibb) [PoM]
Suspension, yellow, nystatin 100 000 units/mL, net price 30 mL with pipette = £1.91. Label: 9, counselling, use of pipette
Excipients include alcohol

▌TERBINAFINE

Cautions psoriasis (risk of exacerbation); auto-immmune disease (risk of lupus-erythematosus-like effect) **interactions:** Appendix 1 (terbinafine)

Hepatic impairment manufacturer advises avoid—elimination reduced

Renal impairment use half normal dose if estimated glomerular filtration rate less than 50 mL/minute/1.73 m^2

Pregnancy manufacturer advises use only if benefit outweighs risk—no information available

Breast-feeding avoid—present in milk

Side-effects abdominal discomfort, anorexia, nausea, diarrhoea; headache; rash and urticaria occasionally with arthralgia or myalgia; *less commonly* taste disturbance; *rarely* liver toxicity (including jaundice, cholestasis and hepatitis)—discontinue treatment, angioedema, dizziness, malaise, paraesthesia, hypoaesthesia, photosensitivity, serious skin reactions (including Stevens-Johnson syndrome and toxic epidermal necrolysis)—discontinue treatment if progressive skin rash; *very rarely* psychiatric disturbances, blood disorders (including incidence of leucopenia higher and thrombocytopenia), lupus erythematosus-like effect, and exacerbation of psoriasis

Licensed use not licensed for use in children

Indication and dose

Dermatophyte infections of the nails, ringworm infections (including tinea pedis, cruris, corporis, and capitis) where oral therapy appropriate (due to site, severity or extent)

• **By mouth**

Child over 1 year; body-weight 10–20 kg 62.5 mg once daily

Child body-weight 20–40 kg 125 mg once daily

Child body-weight over 40 kg 250 mg once daily

Note treatment usually for 4 weeks in tinea capitis, 2–6 weeks in tinea pedis, 2–4 weeks in tinea cruris, 4 weeks in tinea corporis, 6 weeks–3 months in nail infections (occasionally longer in toenail infections)

Fungal skin infections section 13.10.2

Terbinafine (Non-proprietary) [PoM]
Tablets, terbinafine (as hydrochloride) 250 mg, net price 14-tab pack = £2.70, 28-tab pack = £3.22. Label: 9

Lamisil® (Novartis) [PoM]
Tablets, off-white, scored, terbinafine (as hydrochloride) 250 mg, net price 14-tab pack = £23.16, 28-tab pack = £44.66. Label: 9

▌VORICONAZOLE

Cautions electrolyte disturbances, cardiomyopathy, bradycardia, symptomatic arrhythmias, history of QT interval prolongation, concomitant use with other drugs that prolong QT interval; avoid exposure to sunlight; patients at risk of pancreatitis; monitor liver function before treatment and during treatment; haematological malignancy (increased risk of hepatic reactions); monitor renal function; **interactions:** Appendix 1 (antifungals, triazole)

Contra-indications acute porphyria (section 9.8.2)

Hepatic impairment in mild to moderate hepatic cirrhosis use usual initial dose then halve subsequent doses; no information available for severe hepatic cirrhosis—manufacturer advises use only if potential benefit outweighs risk

Renal impairment excipient in intravenous infusion solution may accumulate if estimated glom-

erular filtration rate less than 50 mL/minute/1.73 m^2—manufacturer advises use intravenous infusion only if potential benefit outweighs risk and monitor renal function; alternatively, use tablets or oral suspension (no dose adjustment required)

Pregnancy toxicity in *animal* studies—manufacturer advises avoid unless potential benefit outweighs risk; effective contraception required during treatment

Breast-feeding manufacturer advises avoid—no information available

Side-effects gastro-intestinal disturbances (including nausea, vomiting, abdominal pain, diarrhoea), jaundice; oedema, hypotension, chest pain; respiratory distress syndrome, sinusitis; headache, dizziness, asthenia, anxiety, depression, confusion, agitation, hallucinations, paraesthesia, tremor; influenza-like symptoms; hypo-

◻ **VORICONAZOLE** (*continued*)

glycaemia; haematuria; blood disorders (including anaemia, thrombocytopenia, leucopenia, pancytopenia), acute renal failure, hypokalaemia; visual disturbances including altered perception, blurred vision, and photophobia; rash, pruritus, photosensitivity, alopecia, cheilitis; injection-site reactions; *less commonly* cholecystitis, pancreatitis, hepatitis, constipation, arrhythmias (including QT interval prolongation), syncope, raised serum cholesterol, hypersensitivity reactions (including flushing), ataxia, nystagmus, hypoaesthesia, adrenocortical insufficiency, arthritis, blepharitis, optic neuritis, scleritis, glossitis, gingivitis, psoriasis, and Stevens-Johnson syndrome; *rarely* pseudomembranous colitis, convulsions, sleep disturbances, tinnitus, hearing disturbances, extrapyramidal effects, hypertonia, hypothyroidism, hyperthyroidism, discoid lupus erythematosus, toxic epidermal necrolysis, retinal haemorrhage, optic atrophy, and taste disturbances

Indication and dose

> Invasive aspergillosis; serious infections caused by *Scedosporium* spp., *Fusarium* spp., or invasive fluconazole-resistant *Candida* spp. (including *C. krusei*)
>
> • By mouth
>
> **Child 2–12 years** (oral suspension recommended) 200 mg every 12 hours
>
> **Child 12–18 years, body-weight under 40 kg** 200 mg every 12 hours for 2 doses then 100 mg every 12 hours, increased if necessary to 150 mg every 12 hours

> **Child 12–18 years, body-weight over 40 kg** 400 mg every 12 hours for 2 doses then 200 mg every 12 hours, increased if necessary to 300 mg every 12 hours
>
> • By intravenous infusion
>
> **Child 2–12 years** 7 mg/kg every 12 hours (reduced to 4 mg/kg every 12 hours if not tolerated) for max. 6 months
>
> **Child 12–18 years** 6 mg/kg every 12 hours for 2 doses, then 4 mg/kg every 12 hours (reduced to 3 mg/kg every 12 hours if not tolerated) for max. 6 months

Administration For *intravenous infusion*, reconstitute each 200 mg with 19 mL Water for Injections to produce a 10 mg/mL solution; dilute dose to concentration of 0.5–5 mg/mL with Glucose 5% *or* Sodium Chloride 0.9% and give at a rate not exceeding 3 mg/kg/hour

Vfend® (Pfizer) PoM
Tablets, f/c, voriconazole 50 mg, net price 28-tablet pack = £275.68; 200 mg, 28-tab pack = £1102.74. Label: 9, 11, 23

Oral suspension, voriconazole 200 mg/5 mL when reconstituted with water, net price 75 mL (orange-flavoured) = £551.37. Label: 9, 11, 23

Intravenous infusion, powder for reconstitution, voriconazole, net price 200-mg vial = £77.14
Excipients include sulphobutylether beta cyclodextrin sodium (risk of accumulation in renal impairment)
Electrolytes Na⁺ 9.47 mmol/vial

5.3 Antiviral drugs

5.3.1 HIV infection
5.3.2 Herpesvirus infections
5.3.3 Viral hepatitis
5.3.4 Influenza
5.3.5 Respiratory syncytial virus

The majority of virus infections resolve spontaneously in immunocompetent subjects. A number of specific treatments for viral infections are available, particularly for the immunocompromised. This section includes notes on herpes simplex and varicella-zoster, human immunodeficiency virus, cytomegalovirus, respiratory syncytial virus, viral hepatitis and influenza.

5.3.1 HIV infection

There is no cure for infection caused by the human immunodeficiency virus (HIV) but a number of drugs slow or halt disease progression. Drugs for HIV infection (antiretrovirals) may be associated with serious side-effects. Although antiretrovirals increase life expectancy considerably and decrease the risk of complications associated with premature ageing, mortality and morbidity remain slightly higher than in uninfected individuals.

The natural progression of HIV disease is different in children compared to adults; drug treatment should only be undertaken by specialists within a formal paediatric HIV clinical network. Guidelines and dose regimens are under constant review and for this reason specific dose recommendations have not been included in *BNF for Children*.

Further information on the management of children with HIV can be obtained from the Children's HIV Association (CHIVA) www.chiva.org.uk; and further information on antiretroviral use and toxicity can be obtained from the Paediatric European Network for Treatment of AIDS (PENTA) website www.pentatrials.org.

Principles of treatment   Treatment is aimed at suppressing viral replication for as long as possible; it should be started before the immune system is irreversibly damaged. The need for early drug treatment should, however, be balanced against the risk of toxicity. Commitment to treatment and strict adherence over many years are required; the regimen chosen should take into account convenience and the child's tolerance of treatment. The development of drug resistance is reduced by using a combination of drugs; such combinations should have synergistic or additive activity while ensuring that their toxicity is not additive. It is recommended that viral sensitivity to antiretroviral drugs is established before starting treatment or before switching drugs if the infection is not responding.

Initiation of treatment   Treatment is started in all HIV infected children under 1 year of age regardless of clinical and immunological parameters. In children over 1 year of age, treatment is based on the child's age, CD4 cell count, viral load, and symptoms. The choice of antiviral treatment for children should take into account the method and frequency of administration, risk of side-effects, compatibility of drugs with food, palatability, and the appropriateness of the formulation. Initiating treatment with a combination of drugs ('highly active antiretroviral therapy' which includes 2 nucleoside reverse transcriptase inhibitors with *either* a non-nucleoside reverse transcriptase inhibitor *or* a boosted protease inhibitor) is recommended. The metabolism of many antiretrovirals varies in young children; it may therefore be necessary to adjust the dose according to the plasma-drug concentration. Children who require treatment for both HIV and chronic hepatitis B should receive antivirals that are active against both diseases (section 5.3.3).

Switching therapy   Deterioration of the condition (including clinical, virological changes, and CD4 cell changes) may require a complete change of therapy. The choice of an alternative regimen depends on factors such as the response to previous treatment, tolerance, and the possibility of cross-resistance.

Pregnancy   Treatment of HIV infection in pregnancy aims to minimise the viral load and disease progression in the mother and reduce the risk of toxicity to the fetus (but the teratogenic potential of most antiretroviral drugs is unknown). Combination antiretroviral therapy represents optimal treatment but all options require **careful assessment** by a specialist. Combination antiretroviral therapy may be associated with a greater risk of preterm delivery. Consideration also needs to be given to preventing transmission of the infection to the neonate (see below).

Prevention of transmission to neonate   Zidovudine given in the perinatal period to the mother and the neonate reduces transmission to the baby. However, optimal treatment of the mother's HIV infection with combination treatment maximises the chance of preventing transmission. Local protocols and national guidelines (www.bhiva.org) should be consulted for recommendations on treatment during pregnancy and the perinatal period.

Breast-feeding   Breast-feeding by HIV-positive mothers may cause HIV infection in the infant and should be avoided.

Post-exposure prophylaxis   Children exposed to HIV infection through needle-stick injury or by another route should be sent to an accident and emergency department for post-exposure prophylaxis [unlicensed indication]. Antiretrovirals for prophylaxis are chosen on the basis of efficacy and potential for toxicity.

Drugs used for HIV infection   Zidovudine, a nucleoside reverse transcriptase inhibitor (or 'nucleoside analogue'), was the first anti-HIV drug to be introduced. Other nucleoside reverse transcriptase inhibitors include **abacavir**, **didanosine**, **emtricitabine**, **lamivudine**, **stavudine**, and **tenofovir**.

The protease inhibitors include **atazanavir**, **darunavir**, **fosamprenavir** (a pro-drug of amprenavir), **indinavir**, **lopinavir**, **nelfinavir**, **ritonavir**, **saquinavir**, and **tipranavir**. Ritonavir in low doses boosts the activity of atazanavir, darunavir, fosamprenavir, indinavir, lopinavir, saquinavir, and tipranavir increasing the persistence of plasma concentrations of these drugs; at such a low dose, ritonavir has no intrinsic antiviral activity. A combination of lopinavir with low-dose ritonavir is available for use in children over 2 years. The protease inhibitors are metabolised by cytochrome P450 enzyme systems and therefore have a significant potential for drug interactions. Protease inhibitors are associated with lipodystrophy and metabolic effects (see below).

The non-nucleoside reverse transcriptase inhibitors **efavirenz**, **etravirine**, and **nevirapine** are active against the subtype HIV-1 but not HIV-2, a subtype that is rare in the UK. These drugs may interact with a number of drugs metabolised in the liver. Nevirapine is associated with a high incidence of rash (including Stevens-Johnson syndrome) and fatal hepatitis. Rash is also associated with efavirenz and etravirine but it is usually milder. Psychiatric or CNS disturbances are common with efavirenz. CNS disturbances are often self-limiting and can be reduced by taking the dose at bedtime (especially in the first 2–4 weeks of treatment). Efavirenz has also been associated with an increased plasma cholesterol concentration. Etravirine is used in regimens containing a boosted protease inhibitor for HIV infection resistant to other non-nucleoside reverse transcriptase inhibitors and protease inhibitors.

Enfuvirtide, which inhibits the fusion of HIV to the host cell, is licensed for managing infection that has failed to respond to a regimen of other antiretroviral drugs. Enfuvirtide should be combined with other potentially active antiretroviral drugs; it is given by subcutaneous injection.

Maraviroc is an antagonist of the CCR5 chemokine receptor. It is used in patients exclusively infected with CCR5–tropic HIV.

Raltegravir is an inhibitor of HIV integrase. It is used for the treatment of HIV infection resistant to multiple antiretrovirals.

Immune reconstitution syndrome   Improvement in immune function as a result of antiretroviral treatment may provoke a marked inflammatory reaction against residual opportunistic organisms.

Lipodystrophy syndrome   Metabolic effects associated with antiretroviral treatment include *fat redistribution*, *insulin resistance*, and *dyslipidaemia*; collectively these have been termed *lipodystrophy syndrome*. Children should be encouraged to lead a healthy lifestyle that reduces their long-term cardiovascular risk. Plasma lipids and blood glucose should be measured before starting antiretroviral therapy, after 3–6 months of treatment, and then at least annually. Insulin resistance and hyperglycaemia occur only rarely in children.

Fat redistribution (with loss of subcutaneous fat, increased abdominal fat, 'buffalo hump' and breast enlargement) is associated with regimens containing protease inhibitors and nucleoside reverse transcriptase inhibitors. Stavudine, and to a lesser extent zidovudine, are associated with a higher risk of lipoatrophy and should be used only if alternative regimens are not suitable.

Dyslipidaemia is associated with antiretroviral treatment, particularly with protease inhibitors; in children, hypercholesterolaemia appears to be more common than hypertriglyceridaemia. Protease inhibitors and nucleoside reverse transcriptase inhibitors are associated with insulin resistance and hyperglycaemia but they occur rarely in children. Of the protease inhibitors, atazanavir and darunavir are less likely to cause dyslipidaemia, while saquinavir and atazanavir are less likely to impair glucose tolerance.

Osteonecrosis   Osteonecrosis has been reported in children with advanced HIV disease or following long-term exposure to combination antiretroviral therapy.

Nucleoside reverse transcriptase inhibitors

Cautions

Lactic acidosis   Life-threatening lactic acidosis associated with hepatomegaly and hepatic steatosis has been reported with nucleoside reverse transcriptase inhibitors. They should be used with caution in children with hepatomegaly, hepatitis (especially hepatitis C treated with interferon alfa and ribavirin), liver-enzyme abnormalities and with other risk factors for liver disease and hepatic steatosis. Treatment with the nucleoside reverse transcriptase inhibitor should be **discontinued** in case of symptomatic hyperlactataemia, lactic acidosis, progressive hepatomegaly or rapid deterioration of liver function. Stavudine, especially with didanosine, is associated with a higher risk of lactic acidosis and should be used only if alternative regimens are not suitable.

Hepatic impairment Nucleoside reverse transcriptase inhibitors should be used with caution in children with hepatic impairment (greater risk of hepatic side-effects, see also Lactic Acidosis above). However, some nucleoside reverse transcriptase inhibitors are used in children who also have chronic hepatitis B.

Pregnancy See p. 379

Breast-feeding See p. 379

Side-effects Side-effects of the nucleoside reverse transcriptase inhibitors include gastro-intestinal disturbances (such as nausea, vomiting, abdominal pain, flatulence and diarrhoea), anorexia, pancreatitis, liver damage (see also Lactic Acidosis, above), dyspnoea, cough, headache, insomnia, dizziness, fatigue, blood disorders (including anaemia, neutropenia, and thrombocytopenia), myalgia, arthralgia, rash, urticaria, and fever. See notes above for Lipodystrophy Syndrome (p. 380) and Osteonecrosis (p. 380).

ABACUR
ABACAVIR

Cautions see notes above; also test for HLA-B*5701 allele before treatment (or if re-starting treatment and HLA-B*5701 status not known)—increased risk of hypersensitivity reaction in presence of HLA-B*5701 allele; **interactions:** Appendix 1 (abacavir)

Hypersensitivity reactions Life-threatening hypersensitivity reactions reported—characterised by fever or rash and possibly nausea, vomiting, diarrhoea, abdominal pain, dyspnoea, cough, lethargy, malaise, headache, and myalgia; less frequently mouth ulceration, oedema, hypotension, sore throat, acute respiratory distress syndrome, anaphylaxis, paraesthesia, arthralgia, conjunctivitis, lymphadenopathy, lymphocytopenia and renal failure; rarely myolysis; laboratory abnormalities may include raised liver function tests (see Lactic Acidosis above) and creatine kinase; symptoms usually appear in the first 6 weeks, but may occur at any time; monitor for symptoms every 2 weeks for 2 months; discontinue immediately if any symptom of hypersensitivity develops and do not rechallenge (risk of more severe hypersensitivity reaction); discontinue if hypersensitivity cannot be ruled out, even when other diagnoses possible—if rechallenge necessary it must be carried out in hospital setting; if abacavir is stopped for any reason other than hypersensitivity, exclude hypersensitivity reaction as the cause and rechallenge only if medical assistance is readily available; care needed with concomitant use of drugs which cause skin toxicity

Counselling Children and carers should be told the importance of regular dosing (intermittent therapy may increase the risk of sensitisation), how to recognise signs of hypersensitivity, and advised to seek immediate medical attention if symptoms develop or before re-starting treatment; children or their carers should be advised to keep Alert Card with them at all times

Hepatic impairment see notes above; also avoid in moderate impairment unless essential; avoid in severe impairment

Renal impairment manufacturer advises avoid in end-stage renal disease; avoid *Kivexa®* and *Trizivir®* if estimated glomerular filtration rate less than 50 mL/minute/1.73 m^2

Pregnancy manufacturer advises avoid (toxicity in *animal* studies); see also Pregnancy, p. 379

Breast-feeding see p. 379

Side-effects see notes above; also hypersensitivity reactions (see above); *very rarely* Stevens-Johnson syndrome and toxic epidermal necrolysis; rash and gastro-intestinal disturbances more common in children

Licensed use *Ziagen®* not licensed for use in children under 3 months; *Kivexa®* not licensed for use in children under 12 years; *Trizivir®* not licensed for use in children

Indication and dose

HIV infection in combination with other antiretroviral drugs

For dose, consult Guidelines (see notes above)

Ziagen® (ViiV) �PoM
Tablets, yellow, f/c, scored, abacavir (as sulphate) 300 mg, net price 60-tab pack = £221.81. Counselling, hypersensitivity reactions

Oral solution, sugar-free, banana and strawberry flavoured, abacavir (as sulphate) 20 mg/mL, net price 240-mL = £59.15. Counselling, hypersensitivity reactions
Excipients include propylene glycol

◢ **With lamivudine**
For cautions, contra-indications and side-effects see under individual drugs

Kivexa® (ViiV) PoM
Tablets, orange, f/c, abacavir (as sulphate) 600 mg, lamivudine 300 mg, net price 30-tab pack = £373.94. Counselling, hypersensitivity reactions

◢ **With lamivudine and zidovudine**
Note use only if child is stabilised (for 6–8 weeks) on the individual components in the same proportions. For cautions, contra-indications and side-effects see under individual drugs

Trizivir® (ViiV) PoM
Tablets, blue-green, f/c, abacavir (as sulphate) 300 mg, lamivudine 150 mg, zidovudine 300 mg, net price 60-tab pack = £540.40. Counselling, hypersensitivity reactions

DIDANOSINE
(ddI, DDI)

Cautions see notes above; also history of pancreatitis (preferably avoid, otherwise extreme caution, see also below); peripheral neuropathy or hyperuricaemia (see under Side-effects); ophthalmological examination (including visual acuity, colour vision, and dilated fundus examination) recommended annually or if visual

◯ **DIDANOSINE** (*continued*)

changes occur; **interactions:** Appendix 1 (didanosine)

Pancreatitis If symptoms of pancreatitis develop or if serum lipase is raised and pancreatitis is confirmed, discontinue treatment. Whenever possible avoid concomitant treatment with other drugs known to cause pancreatic toxicity (e.g. intravenous pentamidine isetionate); monitor closely if concomitant therapy unavoidable. Since significant elevations of triglycerides cause pancreatitis monitor closely if triglycerides elevated

Hepatic impairment see notes above

Renal impairment reduce dose if estimated glomerular filtration rate less than 60 mL/minute/1.73 m²; consult product literature

Pregnancy manufacturer advises use only if potential benefit outweighs risk

Breast-feeding see p. 379

Side-effects see notes above; also pancreatitis (less common in children, see also under cautions), liver failure, anaphylactic reactions, peripheral neuropathy (switch to another antiretroviral if peripheral neuropathy develops), diabetes mellitus, hypoglycaemia, acute renal failure, rhabdomyolysis, dry eyes, retinal and optic nerve changes, dry mouth, parotid gland enlargement, sialadenitis, alopecia, hyperuricaemia (suspend if raised significantly)

Licensed use tablets not licensed for use in children under 3 months; EC capsules not licensed for use in children under 6 years

Indication and dose

HIV infection in combination with other antiretroviral drugs

For dose, consult Guidelines (see notes above)

Videx® (Bristol-Myers Squibb) (PoM)
Tablets, with calcium and magnesium antacids, didanosine 25 mg, net price 60-tab pack = £25.56. Label: 23, counselling, administration, see below
Excipients include aspartame equivalent to phenylalanine 36.5 mg per tablet (section 9.4.1)

Note Antacids in formulation may affect absorption of other drugs—see **interactions:** Appendix 1 (antacids)

Administration to ensure sufficient antacid, each dose to be taken as at least 2 tablets (child under 1 year 1 tablet) chewed thoroughly, crushed or dispersed in water; clear apple juice may be added for flavouring; tablets to be taken 2 hours after lopinavir with ritonavir capsules and oral solution or atazanavir with ritonavir

Videx® EC capsules, enclosing e/c granules, didanosine 125 mg, net price 30-cap pack = £49.16; 200 mg, 30-cap pack = £78.65; 250 mg, 30-cap pack = £98.31; 400 mg, 30-cap pack = £157.30. Label: 25, counselling, administration, see below

Administration capsules should be swallowed whole and taken at least 2 hours before or 2 hours after food

---

▮ **EMTRICITABINE**

Cautions see notes above; also on discontinuation, monitor patients with hepatitis B (risk of exacerbation of hepatitis); **interactions:** Appendix 1 (emtricitabine)

Hepatic impairment see notes above and Cautions above

Renal impairment reduce dose or increase dosage interval if estimated glomerular filtration rate less than 50 mL/minute/1.73 m²; consult product literature

Pregnancy manufacturer advises use only if essential—no information available

Breast-feeding see p. 379

Side-effects see notes above; also abnormal dreams, pruritus, and hyperpigmentation

Licensed use not licensed for use in children under 4 months

Indication and dose

HIV infection in combination with other antiretroviral drugs

For dose, consult Guidelines (see notes above)

Emtriva® (Gilead) (PoM)
Capsules, white/blue, emtricitabine 200 mg, net price 30-cap pack = £163.50

Oral solution, orange, emtricitabine 10 mg/mL, net price 170-mL pack (candy-flavoured) = £46.50
Electrolytes Na⁺ 460 micromol/mL

Note 240 mg oral solution ≡ 200 mg capsule; where appropriate the capsule may be used instead of the oral solution

◢ **With tenofovir**
See under Tenofovir

◢ **With efavirenz and tenofovir**
See under Tenofovir

▮ **LAMIVUDINE**
(3TC)

Cautions see notes above; **interactions:** Appendix 1 (lamivudine)

Chronic hepatitis B Recurrent hepatitis in patients with chronic hepatitis B may occur on discontinuation of lamivudine. When treating chronic hepatitis B with lamivudine, monitor liver function tests every 3 months, and viral and serological markers of hepatitis B every 3–6 months, more frequently in patients with advanced liver disease or following transplantation (monitoring to continue after discontinuation)—consult product literature

Hepatic impairment see notes above and Cautions above

Renal impairment reduce dose if estimated glomerular filtration rate less than 50 mL/minute/1.73 m²; consult product literature

Pregnancy see p. 379

Breast-feeding see p. 379

Side-effects see notes above; also peripheral neuropathy, muscle disorders including rhabdomyolysis, nasal symptoms, alopecia

Licensed use *Epivir®* not licensed for use in children under 3 months; *Zeffix®* not licensed for use in children

◻ **LAMIVUDINE** *(continued)*

Indication and dose

See preparations, below

Epivir® (ViiV) ꜰᴏᴹ
Tablets, f/c, lamivudine 150 mg (scored, white), net price 60-tab pack = £152.14; 300 mg (grey), 30-tab pack = £167.21

Oral solution, banana- and strawberry-flavoured, lamivudine 50 mg/5 mL, net price 240-mL pack = £41.41
Excipients include sucrose 1 g/5 mL

Dose

HIV infection in combination with other antiretroviral drugs

For dose, consult Guidelines (see notes above)

Zeffix® (ViiV) ꜰᴏᴹ
Tablets, brown, f/c, lamivudine 100 mg, net price 28-tab pack = £78.09

Oral solution, banana and strawberry flavoured, lamivudine 25 mg/5 mL, net price 240-mL pack = £22.79
Excipients include propylene glycol, sucrose 1 g/5 mL

Dose

Chronic hepatitis B infection with *either* compensated liver disease (with evidence of viral replication and histology of active liver inflammation or fibrosis), *or* decompensated liver disease

• By mouth
  Child 2–12 years 3 mg/kg (max. 100 mg) once daily
  Child 12–18 years 100 mg once daily
  Note Children receiving lamivudine for concomitant HIV infection should continue to receive lamivudine in a dose appropriate for HIV infection

◀**With abacavir**
See under Abacavir

◀**With zidovudine**
See under Zidovudine

◀**With abacavir and zidovudine**
See under Abacavir

▰ **STAVUDINE**

(d4T)

Cautions see notes above; also history of peripheral neuropathy (see under Side-effects); history of pancreatitis or concomitant use with other drugs associated with pancreatitis; **interactions:** Appendix 1 (stavudine)

Hepatic impairment see notes above

Renal impairment reduce dose to 50% if estimated glomerular filtration rate 25–50 mL/minute/1.73 m²; reduce dose to 25% if estimated glomerular filtration rate less than 25 mL/minute/1.73 m²

Pregnancy manufacturer advises use only if potential benefit outweighs risk

Breast-feeding see p. 379

Side-effects see notes above; also peripheral neuropathy (switch to another antiretroviral if peripheral neuropathy develops), abnormal dreams, cognitive dysfunction, drowsiness, depression, pruritus; *less commonly* anxiety, gynaecomastia

Licensed use capsules not licensed for use in children under 3 months

Indication and dose

HIV infection in combination with other antiretroviral drugs

For dose, consult Guidelines (see notes above)

Zerit® (Bristol-Myers Squibb) ꜰᴏᴹ
Capsules, stavudine 20 mg (brown), net price 56-cap pack = £142.28; 30 mg (light orange/dark orange), 56-cap pack = £149.20; 40 mg (dark orange), 56-cap pack = £153.70 (all hosp. only)

Oral solution, cherry-flavoured, stavudine for reconstitution with water, 1 mg/mL, net price 200 mL = £23.40

▰ **TENOFOVIR DISOPROXIL**

Cautions see notes above; also test renal function and serum phosphate before treatment, then every 4 weeks (more frequently if at increased risk of renal impairment) for 1 year and then every 3 months, interrupt treatment if renal function deteriorates or serum phosphate decreases; concomitant or recent use of nephrotoxic drugs; on discontinuation, monitor patients with hepatitis B (risk of exacerbation of hepatitis); **interactions:** Appendix 1 (tenofovir)

Hepatic impairment see notes above and Cautions above

Renal impairment increase dose interval if estimated glomerular filtration rate less than 50 mL/minute/1.73 m²; avoid *Atripla®* if estimated glomerular filtration rate less than 50 mL/minute/1.73 m²; avoid *Truvada®* if estimated glom-erular filtration rate less than 30 mL/minute/1.73 m²

Pregnancy manufacturer advises use only if potential benefit outweighs risk—no information available

Breast-feeding see p. 379

Side-effects see notes above; also hypophosphataemia; *rarely* renal failure; also reported nephrogenic diabetes insipidus, reduced bone density, hypokalaemia, myopathy, and rhabdomyolysis

Licensed use not licensed for use in children

Indication and dose

HIV infection in combination with other antiretroviral drugs

For dose, consult Guidelines (see notes above)

◻ **TENOFOVIR DISOPROXIL (continued)**

Viread® (Gilead) ▼ PoM
Tablets, f/c, blue, tenofovir disoproxil (as fumarate) 245 mg, net price 30-tab pack = £255.00. Label: 21, counselling, administration

Counselling Children with swallowing difficulties may disperse tablet in half a glass of water, orange juice, or grape juice (but bitter taste)

◢**With emtricitabine**
For **cautions**, **contra-indications**, and **side-effects** see under individual drugs

Truvada® (Gilead) PoM
Tablets, blue, f/c, tenofovir disoproxil (as fumarate) 245 mg, emtricitabine 200 mg, net price 30-tab

pack = £418.50. Label: 21, Counselling, administration

Children with swallowing difficulties may disperse tablet in half a glass of water, orange juice, or grape juice (but bitter taste)

◢**With efavirenz and emtricitabine**
For **cautions**, **contra-indications**, and **side-effects** see under individual drugs

Atripla® (Gilead) PoM
Tablets, pink, f/c, efavirenz 600 mg, emtricitabine 200 mg, tenofovir disoproxil (as fumarate) 245 mg, net price 30-tab pack = £626.90. Label: 23, 25

▰ **ZIDOVUDINE**

(Azidothymidine, AZT)
Note The abbreviation AZT which is sometimes used for zidovudine has also been used for another drug

Cautions see notes above; also haematological toxicity particularly with high dose and advanced disease—monitor full blood count after 4 weeks of treatment, then every 3 months; vitamin B₁₂ deficiency (increased risk of neutropenia); if anaemia or myelosuppression occur, reduce dose or interrupt treatment according to product literature, or consider other treatment; **interactions**: Appendix 1 (zidovudine)

Contra-indications abnormally low neutrophil count or haemoglobin concentration (consult product literature); neonates with hyperbilirubinaemia requiring treatment other than phototherapy, or with raised transaminase (consult product literature); acute porphyria (section 9.8.2)

Hepatic impairment see notes above; also accumulation may occur

Renal impairment reduce dose if estimated glomerular filtration rate less than 10 mL/minute/1.73 m²; consult product literature

Pregnancy limited information available; manufacturer advises use only if clearly indicated; see also p. 379

Breast-feeding see p. 379

Side-effects see notes above; also anaemia (may require transfusion), taste disturbance, chest pain, influenza-like symptoms, paraesthesia, neuropathy, convulsions, dizziness, drowsiness, anxiety, depression, loss of mental acuity, myopathy, gynaecomastia, urinary frequency, sweating, pruritus, pigmentation of nails, skin and oral mucosa

Licensed use *Combivir®* is not licensed for use in children with body-weight under 14 kg

Indication and dose

> HIV infection in combination with other antiretroviral drugs; prevention of maternal-fetal HIV transmission
>
> For dose, consult Guidelines (see notes above including Prevention of Transmission to Neonate)

Administration for *intermittent intravenous infusion*, dilute to a concentration of 2 mg/mL or 4 mg/mL with Glucose 5% and give over 1 hour.
For administration *by mouth*, *Combivir®* tablets may be crushed and mixed with semi-solid food or liquid just before administration

Retrovir® (ViiV) PoM
Capsules, zidovudine 100 mg (white/blue band), net price 100-cap pack = £110.98; 250 mg (blue/white/dark blue band), 40-cap pack = £110.98

Oral solution, sugar-free, strawberry-flavoured, zidovudine 50 mg/5 mL, net price 200-mL pack with 10-mL oral syringe = £22.20

Injection, zidovudine 10 mg/mL. For dilution and use as an intravenous infusion. Net price 20-mL vial = £11.14

◢**With lamivudine**
For **cautions**, **contra-indications**, and **side-effects** see under individual drugs

Combivir® (ViiV) PoM
Tablets, f/c, zidovudine 300 mg, lamivudine 150 mg, net price 60-tab pack = £318.60

◢**With abacavir and lamivudine**
See under Abacavir

▰ **Protease inhibitors**

Cautions Protease inhibitors should be used with caution in diabetes (see also Lipodystrophy Syndrome, p. 380). Caution is also needed in children with haemophilia who may be at increased risk of bleeding.

Contra-indications Protease inhibitors should not be given to patients with acute porphyria (but see section 9.8.2).

Hepatic impairment Protease inhibitors should be used with caution in children with chronic hepatitis B or C (increased risk of hepatic side-effects).

Pregnancy See p. 379

Breast-feeding See p. 379

Side-effects Side-effects of the protease inhibitors include gastro-intestinal disturbances (including diarrhoea, nausea, vomiting, abdominal pain, flatulence), anorexia, hepatic dysfunction, pancreatitis; blood disorders including anaemia, neutropenia, and thrombocytopenia; sleep disturbances, fatigue, headache, dizziness, paraesthesia, myalgia, myositis, rhabdomyolysis; taste disturbances; rash, pruritus, Stevens-Johnson syndrome, hypersensitivity reactions including anaphylaxis; see also Lipodystrophy Syndrome (p. 380) and Osteonecrosis (p. 380).

ATAZANAVIR

Cautions see notes above; concomitant use with drugs that prolong PR interval; cardiac conduction disorders; predisposition to QT interval prolongation (including electrolyte disturbances, concomitant use of drugs that prolong QT interval); **interactions:** Appendix 1 (atazanavir)

Contra-indications see notes above

Hepatic impairment see notes above; also use with caution in mild impairment; avoid in moderate to severe impairment

Pregnancy manufacturer advises use only if potential benefit outweighs risk; theoretical risk of hyperbilirubinaemia in neonate if used at term

Breast-feeding see p. 379

Side-effects see notes above; also mouth ulcers, dry mouth, hypertension, syncope, chest pain, dyspnoea, peripheral neuropathy, abnormal dreams, amnesia, disorientation, depression, anxiety, weight changes, increased appetite, gynaecomastia, nephrolithiasis, urinary frequency, haematuria, proteinuria, arthralgia, and alopecia; *rarely* hepatosplenomegaly, oedema, palpitation, and abnormal gait; also reported cholelithiasis, cholecystitis, and torsade de pointes

Licensed use not licensed for use in children

Indication and dose

HIV infection in combination with other antiretroviral drugs

    For dose, consult Guidelines (see notes above)

Reyataz® (Bristol-Myers Squibb) [PoM]
Capsules, atazanavir (as sulphate) 150 mg (dark blue/light blue), net price 60-cap pack = £303.38; 200 mg (dark blue), 60-cap pack = £303.38; 300 mg (red/blue), 30-cap pack = £303.38. Label: 5, 21

DARUNAVIR

Cautions see notes above; also sulphonamide sensitivity; **interactions:** Appendix 1 (darunavir)

Contra-indications see notes above

Hepatic impairment see notes above; also manufacturer advises caution in mild to moderate impairment; avoid in severe impairment—no information available

Pregnancy manufacturer advises use only if potential benefit outweighs risk—no information available

Breast-feeding see p. 379

Side-effects see notes above; also haematemesis, myocardial infarction, chest pain, QT interval prolongation, syncope, bradycardia, tachycardia, palpitation, hypertension, flushing, peripheral oedema, dyspnoea, cough, peripheral neuropathy, anxiety, confusion, memory impairment, depression, abnormal dreams, convulsions, increased appetite, weight changes, pyrexia, hypothyroidism, osteoporosis, gynaecomastia, erectile dysfunction, reduced libido, dysuria, polyuria, nephrolithiasis, renal failure, arthralgia, visual disturbances, dry eyes, conjunctival hyperaemia, rhinorrhoea, throat irritation, dry mouth, stomatitis, nail discoloration, acne, seborrhoeic dermatitis, eczema, increased sweating, and alopecia

Licensed use not licensed for use in children not previously treated with antiretroviral therapy; not licensed for use in children under 6 years and body-weight under 20 kg, previously treated with antiretroviral therapy

Indication and dose

In combination with other antiretroviral drugs, for HIV infection resistant to other protease inhibitors in children previously treated with antiretrovirals

    For dose, consult Guidelines (see notes above)

Prezista® (Janssen-Cilag) ▼ [PoM]
Tablets, f/c, darunavir (as ethanolate) 75 mg (white), net price 480-tab pack = £446.70; 150 mg (white), 240-tab pack = £446.70; 400 mg (light orange), 60-tab pack = £297.80; 600 mg (orange), 60-tab pack = £446.70. Label: 21

FOSAMPRENAVIR

Note Fosamprenavir is a pro-drug of amprenavir

Cautions see notes above; **interactions:** Appendix 1 (fosamprenavir)

Rash Rash may occur, usually in the second week of therapy; discontinue permanently if severe rash with systemic or allergic symptoms or, mucosal involvement; if rash mild or moderate, may continue without interruption—usually resolves within 2 weeks and may respond to antihistamines

Contra-indications see notes above

◻ **FOSAMPRENAVIR** *(continued)*

Hepatic impairment see notes above; also manufacturer advises caution in mild impairment; reduce dose in moderate to severe impairment

Pregnancy toxicity in *animal* studies; manufacturer advises use only if potential benefit outweighs risk

Breast-feeding see p. 379

Side-effects see notes above; also reported, rash including rarely Stevens-Johnson syndrome (see also Rash above)

Licensed use not licensed for use in children under 6 years and body-weight under 25 kg

Indication and dose

HIV infection in combination with other antiretroviral drugs

For dose, consult Guidelines (see notes above)

Note 700 mg fosamprenavir is equivalent to approx. 600 mg amprenavir

Telzir® (ViiV) [PoM]

Tablets, f/c, pink, fosamprenavir (as calcium) 700 mg, net price 60-tab pack = £274.92

Oral suspension, fosamprenavir (as calcium) 50 mg/mL, net price 225-mL pack (grape-bubble-gum-and peppermint-flavoured) (with 10-mL oral syringe) = £73.31. Counselling, administration
Excipients include propylene glycol

Administration In children, oral suspension should be taken with food

▌INDINAVIR

Cautions see notes above; ensure adequate hydration (risk of nephrolithiasis); children at risk of nephrolithiasis (monitor for nephrolithiasis); **interactions**: Appendix 1 (indinavir)

Contra-indications see notes above; also contra-indicated in neonates (risk of hyperbilirubinaemia)

Hepatic impairment see notes above; also increased risk of nephrolithiasis; reduce dose in mild to moderate impairment; not studied in severe impairment

Renal impairment use with caution; monitor for nephrolithiasis

Pregnancy toxicity in *animal* studies, manufacturer advises use only if potential benefit outweighs risk; theoretical risk of hyperbilirubinaemia and renal stones in neonate if used at term

Breast-feeding see p. 379

Side-effects see notes above; also reported, dry mouth, hypoaesthesia, dry skin, hyperpigmentation, alopecia, paronychia, interstitial nephritis (with medullary calcification and cortical atrophy in asymptomatic severe leucocyturia), nephro-lithiasis (may require interruption or discontinuation), dysuria, haematuria, crystalluria, proteinuria, pyuria, pyelonephritis; haemolytic anaemia

Licensed use not licensed for use in children under 4 years

Indication and dose

HIV infection in combination with nucleoside reverse transcriptase inhibitors

For dose, consult Guidelines (see notes above)

Crixivan® (MSD) [PoM]

Capsules, indinavir (as sulphate), 200 mg, net price 360-cap pack = £226.28; 400 mg, 180-cap pack = £226.28. Label: 27, counselling, administration

Counselling Administer 1 hour before or 2 hours after a meal; may be administered with a low-fat light meal (may be mixed with apple sauce); in combination with didanosine tablets, allow 1 hour between each drug (antacids in didanosine tablets reduce absorption of indinavir); in combination with low-dose ritonavir, give with food
Note Dispense in original container (contains desiccant)

▌LOPINAVIR WITH RITONAVIR

Cautions see notes above; concomitant use with drugs that prolong QT or PR interval; cardiac conduction disorders, structural heart disease; pancreatitis (see below); **interactions**: Appendix 1 (lopinavir, ritonavir)
Pancreatitis Signs and symptoms suggestive of pancreatitis (including raised serum lipase) should be evaluated—discontinue if pancreatitis diagnosed

Contra-indications see notes above

Hepatic impairment see notes above; also avoid oral solution—high propylene glycol content; manufacturer advises avoid tablets in severe impairment

Renal impairment avoid oral solution due to high propylene glycol content

Pregnancy avoid oral solution due to high propylene glycol content; manufacturer advises use tablets only if potential benefit outweighs risk (toxicity in *animal* studies)

Breast-feeding see p. 379

Side-effects see notes and Cautions above; also electrolyte disturbances; *less commonly* dysphagia, appetite changes, weight changes, cholecystitis, hypertension, myocardial infarction, palpitation, thrombophlebitis, vasculitis, chest pain, oedema, dyspnoea, cough, agitation, anxiety, amnesia, ataxia, hypertonia, confusion, depression, abnormal dreams, extrapyramidal effects, neuropathy, influenza-like syndrome, Cushing's syndrome, hypothyroidism, menorrhagia, amenorrhoea, sexual dysfunction, breast enlargement, dehydration, nephritis, hypercalciuria, lactic acidosis, arthralgia, hyperuricaemia, abnormal vision, otitis media, tinnitus, dry mouth, sialadenitis, mouth ulceration, periodontitis, acne, alopecia, dry skin, sweating, skin discoloration, nail disorders; *rarely* prolonged PR interval

Licensed use not licensed for use in children under 2 years

◁ **LOPINAVIR WITH RITONAVIR** (*continued*)

Indication and dose

HIV infection in combination with other antiretroviral drugs

For dose, consult Guidelines (see notes above)

Kaletra® (Abbott) [PoM]
Tablets, pale yellow, f/c, lopinavir 100 mg, ritonavir 25 mg, net price 60-tab pack = £76.85. Label: 25

Tablets, yellow, f/c, lopinavir 200 mg, ritonavir 50 mg, net price 120-tab pack = £307.39. Label: 25

Oral solution, lopinavir 400 mg, ritonavir 100 mg/5 mL, net price 5 × 60-mL packs = £307.39. Label: 21
Excipients include propylene glycol 153 mg/mL (see Excipients, p. 3), alcohol 42%

Counselling Oral solution tastes bitter

NELFINAVIR

Cautions see notes above; **interactions:** Appendix 1 (nelfinavir)

Contra-indications see notes above

Hepatic impairment see notes above; also manufacturer advises caution

Renal impairment manufacturer advises caution

Pregnancy manufacturer advises use only if potential benefit outweighs risk—no information available

Breast-feeding see p. 379

Side-effects see notes above; also reported, fever

Licensed use not licensed for use in children under 3 years

Indication and dose

HIV infection in combination with other antiretroviral drugs

For dose, consult Guidelines (see notes above)

Viracept® (Roche) [PoM]
Tablets, blue, f/c, nelfinavir (as mesilate) 250 mg, net price 300-tab pack = £262.51. Label: 21

RITONAVIR

Cautions see notes above; concomitant use with drugs that prolong PR interval; cardiac conduction disorders, structural heart disease; pancreatitis (see below); **interactions:** Appendix 1 (ritonavir)

Pancreatitis Signs and symptoms suggestive of pancreatitis (including raised serum lipase) should be evaluated—discontinue if pancreatitis diagnosed

Contra-indications see notes above

Hepatic impairment see notes above; also avoid in decompensated liver disease; in severe impairment without decompensation, use 'booster' doses with caution (avoid treatment doses)

Pregnancy manufacturer advises use only if potential benefit outweighs risk—toxicity in *animal* studies

Breast-feeding see p. 379

Side-effects see notes and Cautions above; also diarrhoea (may impair absorption—close monitoring required), vasodilatation, cough, throat irritation, anxiety, perioral and peripheral paraesthesia, hyperaesthesia, fever, decreased blood-thyroxine concentration, electrolyte disturbances, raised uric acid, dry mouth, mouth ulcers, and sweating; *less commonly* increased prothrombin time and dehydration; syncope,

postural hypotension, seizures, menorrhagia, and renal failure also reported

Licensed use not licensed for use in children under 2 years

Indication and dose

HIV infection in combination with other antiretroviral drugs; low doses used to increase effect of some protease inhibitors

For dose, consult Guidelines (see notes above)

Norvir® (Abbott) [PoM]
Capsules, ritonavir 100 mg, net price 84-cap pack = £94.35. Label 21
Excipients include alcohol 12%

Oral solution, sugar-free, ritonavir 400 mg/5 mL, net price 5 × 90-mL packs (with measuring cup) = £403.20. Label: 21, counselling, administration
Excipients include alcohol, propylene glycol

Counselling Oral solution contains 43% alcohol; bitter taste can be masked by mixing with chocolate milk; do not mix with water, measuring cup must be dry
Administration of ritonavir and didanosine should be separated by at least 2 hours

◀**With lopinavir**
See under Lopinavir with ritonavir

SAQUINAVIR

Cautions see notes above; concomitant use of garlic (avoid garlic capsules—reduces plasma-saquinavir concentration); **interactions:** Appendix 1 (saquinavir)

Contra-indications see notes above

Hepatic impairment see notes above; also manufacturer advises caution in moderate impairment; avoid in severe impairment

Renal impairment use with caution if estimated glomerular filtration rate less than 30 mL/minute/1.73 m²

Pregnancy manufacturer advises use only if potential benefit outweighs risk

Breast-feeding see p. 379

Side-effects see notes above; also dyspnoea, increased appetite, peripheral neuropathy, convulsions, changes in libido, renal impairment, dry mouth, and alopecia

Licensed use not licensed for use in children under 16 years

◁ **SAQUINAVIR** (*continued*)

Indication and dose

> HIV infection in combination with other antiretroviral drugs
>
> For dose, consult Guidelines (see notes above)

Invirase® (Roche) PoM

Capsules, brown/green, saquinavir (as mesilate) 200 mg, net price 270-cap pack = £230.70. Label: 21

Tablets, orange, f/c, saquinavir (as mesilate) 500 mg, net price 120-tab pack = £256.33. Label: 21

TIPRANAVIR

Cautions see notes above; also patients at risk of increased bleeding from trauma, surgery, or other pathological conditions; concomitant use of drugs that increase risk of bleeding; **interactions:** Appendix 1 (tipranavir)

Hepatotoxicity Potentially life-threatening hepatotoxicity reported; monitor liver function before treatment then every 2 weeks for 1 month, then every 3 months. Discontinue if signs or symptoms of hepatitis develop or if liver-function abnormality develops (consult product literature)

Contra-indications see notes above

Hepatic impairment see notes above; also manufacturer advises caution in mild impairment; avoid in moderate or severe impairment—no information available

Pregnancy manufacturer advises use only if potential benefit outweighs risk—toxicity in *animal* studies

Breast-feeding see p. 379

Side-effects see notes above; also dyspnoea, anorexia, peripheral neuropathy, influenza-like symptoms, renal impairment, and photosensitivity; *rarely* dehydration

Licensed use capsules not licensed for use in children under 12 years; oral solution not licensed for use in children under 2 years or in children over 12 years

Indication and dose

> HIV infection resistant to other protease inhibitors, in combination with other antiretroviral drugs in children previously treated with antiretrovirals
>
> For dose, consult Guidelines (see notes above)

Aptivus® (Boehringer Ingelheim) ▼ PoM

Capsules, pink, tipranavir 250 mg, net price 120-cap pack = £441.00. Label: 5, 21
Excipients include ethanol 100 mg per capsule

Oral solution, toffee-and mint-flavoured, tipranavir 100 mg/mL, net price 95-mL pack = £129.65. Label: 5, 21, counselling, crystallisation
Excipients include vitamin E 78 mg/mL

Note The bioavailability of *Aptivus®* oral solution is higher than that of the capsules; the oral solution is **not** interchangeable with the capsules on a milligram-for-milligram basis

Counselling Children and carers should be told to observe the oral solution for crystallisation; the bottle should be replaced if more than a thin layer of crystals form (doses should continue to be taken at the normal time until the bottle is replaced)

Non-nucleoside reverse transcriptase inhibitors

EFAVIRENZ

Cautions history of mental illness or seizures; **interactions:** Appendix 1 (efavirenz)

Rash Rash, usually in the first 2 weeks, is the most common side-effect; discontinue if severe rash with blistering, desquamation, mucosal involvement or fever; if rash mild or moderate, may continue without interruption—usually resolves within 1 month

Psychiatric disorders Children or their carers should be advised to seek immediate medical attention if symptoms such as severe depression, psychosis or suicidal ideation occur

Contra-indications acute porphyria (but see section 9.8.2)

Hepatic impairment in mild to moderate liver disease, monitor for dose-related side-effects (e.g. CNS effects) and liver function; avoid in severe impairment; greater risk of hepatic side-effects in chronic hepatitis B or C

Renal impairment manufacturer advises caution in severe renal failure—no information available

Pregnancy manufacturer advises avoid (effective contraception required during treatment and for 12 weeks after treatment); use efavirenz only if no alternative available

Breast-feeding see p. 379

Side-effects rash including Stevens-Johnson syndrome (see Rash above); abdominal pain, diarrhoea, nausea, vomiting; anxiety, depression, sleep disturbances, abnormal dreams, dizziness, headache, fatigue, impaired concentration (administration at bedtime especially in first 2–4 weeks reduces CNS effects); pruritus; *less commonly* pancreatitis, hepatitis, psychosis, mania, suicidal ideation, amnesia, ataxia, convulsions, and blurred vision; also reported hepatic failure, flushing, raised serum cholesterol (see Lipodystrophy syndrome, p. 380), tremor, gynaecomastia, tinnitus, photosensitivity; see also Osteonecrosis, p. 380

Licensed use capsules and oral solution not licensed for use in children under 3 years and body-weight under 13 kg; tablets not licensed for use in children with body-weight under 40 kg

Indication and dose

> HIV infection in combination with other antiretroviral drugs
>
> For dose, consult Guidelines (see notes above)

Sustiva® (Bristol-Myers Squibb) PoM

Capsules, efavirenz 50 mg (yellow/white), net price 30-cap pack = £16.73; 100 mg (white), 30-cap

◻ **EFAVIRENZ (continued)**

pack = £33.41; 200 mg (yellow), 90-cap pack = £200.27. Label: 23

Administration Capsules may be opened and contents added to food (contents have a peppery taste) [unlicensed use]

Tablets, f/c, yellow, efavirenz 600 mg, net price 30-tab pack = £200.27. Label: 23

Oral solution, sugar-free, strawberry and mint fla-vour, efavirenz 30 mg/mL, net price 180-mL pack = £53.84

Note The bioavailability of *Sustiva*® oral solution is lower than that of the capsules and tablets; the oral solution is **not** interchangeable with either capsules or tablets on a milligram-for-milligram basis

◢**With emtricitabine and tenofovir**
See under Tenofovir

▮ **ETRAVIRINE**

Cautions interactions: Appendix 1 (etravirine)

Hypersensitivity reactions Rash, usually in the second week, is the most common side-effect and appears more frequently in females. Life-threatening hypersensitivity reactions reported usually during week 3–6 of treatment and characterised by rash, eosinophilia, and systemic symptoms (including fever, general malaise, myalgia, arthralgia, blistering, oral lesions, conjunctivitis, and hepatitis). Discontinue permanently if hypersensitivity reaction or severe rash develop. If rash mild or moderate (without signs of hypersensitivity reaction), may continue without interruption— usually resolves within 2 weeks

Counselling Children and carers should be told how to recognise hypersensitivity reactions and advised to seek immediate medical attention if hypersensitivity reaction or severe rash develop

Contra-indications acute porphyria (but see section 9.8.2)

Hepatic impairment use with caution in moderate impairment; avoid in severe impairment—no information available; greater risk of hepatic side-effects in chronic hepatitis B or C

Pregnancy manufacturer advises use only if potential benefit outweighs risk

Breast-feeding see p. 379

Side-effects rash (including Stevens-Johnson syndrome rarely and toxic epidermal necrolysis very rarely; see also Hypersensitivity Reactions above); gastro-oesophageal reflux, nausea, abdominal pain, flatulence, gastritis; hyper-tension; peripheral neuropathy; diabetes, hyper-lipidaemia (see also Lipodystrophy Syndrome, p. 380); renal failure; anaemia; *less commonly* pancreatitis, haematemesis, hepatitis, chest pain, bronchospasm, drowsiness, malaise, gynaeco-mastia, blurred vision, dry mouth, and sweating; also reported, haemorrhagic stroke; see also Osteonecrosis, p. 380

Licensed use not licensed for use in children

Indication and dose

> **In combination with other antiretroviral drugs (including a boosted protease inhibitor) for HIV infection resistant to other non-nucleoside reverse transcriptase inhibitors and protease inhibitors**
>
> For dose, consult Guidelines (see notes above)

Administration for children with swallowing diffi-culties, tablets may be dispersed in a glass of water just before administration

Intelence® (Janssen-Cilag) ▼ PoM
Tablets, etravirine 100 mg, net price 120-tab pack = £307.35. Label: 21
counselling, rash, and hypersensitivity reactions
Note Dispense in original container (contains desiccant)

▮ **NEVIRAPINE**

Cautions chronic hepatitis B or C, high CD4 cell count, and females (all at greater risk of hepatic side-effects); **interactions:** Appendix 1 (nevira-pine)

Hepatic disease Potentially life-threatening hepatotoxi-city including fatal fulminant hepatitis reported usually in first 6 weeks; close monitoring required during first 18 weeks; monitor liver function before treatment then every 2 weeks for 2 months then after 1 month and then regularly; discontinue permanently if abnormalities in liver function tests accompanied by hypersensitivity reaction (rash, fever, arthralgia, myalgia, lymphadenopa-thy, hepatitis, renal impairment, eosinophilia, granulocy-topenia); suspend if severe abnormalities in liver function tests but no hypersensitivity reaction—discontinue per-manently if significant liver function abnormalities recur; monitor patient closely if mild to moderate abnormalities in liver function tests with no hypersensitivity reaction

Rash Rash, usually in first 6 weeks, is most common side-effect; incidence reduced if introduced at low dose and dose increased gradually; monitor closely for skin reac-tions during first 18 weeks; discontinue permanently if severe rash or if rash accompanied by blistering, oral lesions, conjunctivitis, facial oedema, general malaise or hypersensitivity reactions; if rash mild or moderate may continue without interruption but dose should not be increased until rash resolves

Counselling Children and carers should be told how to recognise hypersensitivity reactions and advised to discontinue treatment and seek immediate medical attention if severe skin reaction, hypersensitivity reactions or symptoms of hepatitis develop

Contra-indications acute porphyria (but see sec-tion 9.8.2); post-exposure prophylaxis

Hepatic impairment manufacturer advises cau-tion in moderate impairment; avoid in severe impairment; see also Hepatic Disease, above

Pregnancy although manufacturers advise avoid, may be appropriate to use if clearly indicated; see also p. 379

Breast-feeding see p. 379

Side-effects rash including Stevens-Johnson syndrome and rarely, toxic epidermal necrolysis (see also Cautions above); nausea, hepatitis (see also Hepatic Disease above), headache; *less com-monly* vomiting, abdominal pain, fatigue, fever, and myalgia; *rarely* diarrhoea, angioedema, anaphylaxis, hypersensitivity reactions (may involve hepatic reactions and rash, see Hepatic Disease above), arthralgia, anaemia, and granu-locytopenia; *very rarely* neuropsychiatric reac-tions; see also Osteonecrosis, p. 380

5

Infections

△ **NEVIRAPINE** (*continued*)

Licensed use tablets, not licensed for use in children weighing less than 50 kg or with body surface area less than 1.25 m²

Indication and dose

HIV infection in combination with other antiretroviral drugs

For dose, consult Guidelines (see notes above)

Note Dose titration should not exceed 28 days; alternative treatment should be considered. Dose titration should be repeated if treatment interrupted for more than 7 days

Viramune® (Boehringer Ingelheim) ▼[PoM]
Tablets, nevirapine 200 mg, net price 14-tab pack = £39.67, 60-tab pack = £170.00. Counselling, hypersensitivity reactions

Suspension, nevirapine 50 mg/5 mL, net price 240-mL pack = £50.40. Counselling, hypersensitivity reactions

---

Other antiretrovirals

ENFUVIRTIDE

Cautions
Hypersensitivity reactions Hypersensitivity reactions including rash, fever, nausea, vomiting, chills, rigors, low blood pressure, respiratory distress, glomerulonephritis, and raised liver enzymes reported; discontinue immediately if any signs or symptoms of systemic hypersensitivity develop and do not rechallenge
Counselling Children and carers should be told how to recognise signs of hypersensitivity, and advised to discontinue treatment and seek prompt medical attention if symptoms develop
Hepatic impairment manufacturer advises caution—no information available; chronic hepatitis B or C (possibly greater risk of hepatic side-effects)
Pregnancy manufacturer advises use only if potential benefit outweighs risk
Breast-feeding see p. 379
Side-effects injection-site reactions; pancreatitis, gastro-oesophageal reflux disease, anorexia, weight loss; hypertriglyceridaemia; peripheral neuropathy, asthenia, tremor, anxiety, nightmares, irritability, impaired concentration, vertigo; pneumonia, sinusitis, influenza-like illness; diabetes mellitus; haematuria; renal calculi,

lymphadenopathy; myalgia; conjunctivitis; dry skin, acne, erythema, skin papilloma; *less commonly* hypersensitivity reactions (see Cautions); see also Osteonecrosis, p. 380

Licensed use not licensed for use in children under 6 years

Indication and dose

HIV infection in combination with other antiretroviral drugs for resistant infection or for children intolerant to other antiretroviral regimens

For dose, consult Guidelines (see notes above)

Administration for *subcutaneous injection*, reconstitute with 1.1 mL Water for Injections and allow to stand (for up to 45 minutes) to dissolve; do **not** shake or invert vial

Fuzeon® (Roche) [PoM]
Injection, powder for reconstitution, enfuvirtide 108 mg (= enfuvirtide 90 mg/mL when reconstituted with 1.1 mL Water for Injections), net price 108-mg vial = £18.39 (with solvent, syringe, and alcohol swabs). Counselling, hypersensitivity reactions

MARAVIROC

Cautions cardiovascular disease; chronic hepatitis B or C; **interactions:** Appendix 1 (maraviroc)
Hepatic impairment use with caution
Renal impairment if estimated glomerular filtration rate less than 80 mL/minute/1.73 m², consult product literature
Pregnancy manufacturer advises use only if potential benefit outweighs risk—toxicity in *animal* studies
Breast-feeding see p. 379
Side-effects nausea, vomiting, abdominal pain, dyspepsia, constipation, diarrhoea; cough; dizziness, paraesthesia, asthenia, sleep disturbances, headache, weight loss; muscle spasms, back pain; taste disturbances; rash, pruritus; *less commonly* pancreatitis, hepatic cirrhosis, rectal bleeding, myocardial infarction, myocardial ischaemia,

bronchospasm, seizures, hallucinations, loss of consciousness, polyneuropathy, pancytopenia, neutropenia, lymphadenopathy, renal failure, polyuria, and myositis; see also Osteonecrosis, p. 380

Licensed use not licensed for use in children

Indication and dose

CCR5–tropic HIV infection in combination with other antiretroviral drugs in children previously treated with antiretrovirals

For dose, consult Guidelines (see notes above)

Celsentri® (Pfizer) ▼[PoM]
Tablets, blue, f/c, maraviroc 150 mg, net price 60-tab pack = £551.10; 300 mg, 60-tab pack = £551.10

RALTEGRAVIR

Cautions risk factors for myopathy or rhabdomyolysis; **interactions:** Appendix 1 (raltegravir)

Hepatic impairment chronic hepatitis B or C (greater risk of hepatic side-effects); use with

◁ **RALTEGRAVIR (continued)**

caution in severe impairment—no information available

Pregnancy manufacturer advises avoid—toxicity in *animal* studies

Breast-feeding see p. 379

Side-effects diarrhoea, nausea, vomiting, abdominal pain, flatulence; hypertriglyceridaemia; dizziness, headache, insomnia, abnormal dreams, asthenia; rash (Stevens-Johnson syndrome reported); *less commonly* gastritis, hepatitis, pancreatitis, dry mouth, gastro-oesophageal reflux, taste disturbances, pain on swallowing, peptic ulcer, constipation, rectal bleeding, lipodystrophy (see Lipodystrophy Syndrome, p. 380), palpitation, ventricular extrasystoles, bradycardia, hypertension, flushing, chest pain, oedema, dysphonia, epistaxis, nasal congestion, drowsiness, anxiety, appetite changes, confusion, impaired memory and attention, depression, pyrexia, chills, carpal tunnel syndrome, tremor, peripheral neuropathy, erectile dysfunction, gynaecomastia, menopausal symptoms, renal failure, nocturia, polydipsia, anaemia, neutropenia, arthralgia, myalgia, visual disturbances, tinnitus, acne, pruritus, hyperhidrosis, dry skin, skin papilloma, and alopecia; *also reported* suicidal ideation; see also Osteonecrosis, p. 380

Licensed use not licensed for use in children under 16 years

Indication and dose

> In combination with other antiretroviral drugs for HIV infection resistant to multiple antiretrovirals
>
> For dose, consult Guidelines (see notes above)

Isentress® (MSD) ▼ [PoM]

Tablets, pink, f/c, raltegravir (as potassium salt) 400 mg, net price 60-tab pack = £647.29. Label: 25

5.3.2 Herpesvirus infections

5.3.2.1 Herpes simplex and varicella–zoster infection
5.3.2.2 Cytomegalovirus infection

5.3.2.1 Herpes simplex and varicella–zoster infection

The two most important herpesvirus pathogens are herpes simplex virus (herpesvirus hominis) and varicella–zoster virus.

Herpes simplex infections Herpes infection of the mouth and lips and in the eye is generally associated with herpes simplex virus serotype 1 (HSV-1); other areas of the skin may also be infected, especially in immunodeficiency. Genital infection is most often associated with HSV-2 and also HSV-1. Treatment of herpes simplex infection should start as early as possible and usually within 5 days of the appearance of the infection.

In individuals with good immune function, mild infection of the eye (ocular herpes, section 11.3.3) and of the lips (herpes labialis or cold sores, section 13.10.3) is treated with a topical antiviral drug. Primary herpetic gingivostomatitis is managed by changes to diet and with analgesics (section 12.3.2). Severe infection, neonatal herpes infection or infection in immunocompromised individuals requires treatment with a systemic antiviral drug. Primary or recurrent genital herpes simplex infection is treated with an antiviral drug given by mouth. Persistance of a lesion or recurrence in an immunocompromised child may signal the development of resistance.

Specialist advice should be sought for systemic treatment of herpes simplex infection in pregnancy.

Varicella–zoster infections Regardless of immune function and the use of any immunoglobulins, neonates with *chickenpox* should be treated with a parenteral antiviral to reduce the risk of severe disease. Oral therapy is not recommended as absorption is variable.

Chickenpox in otherwise healthy children between 1 month and 12 years is usually mild and antiviral treatment is not usually required. Chickenpox is more severe in adolescents than in children; antiviral treatment started within 24 hours of the onset of rash may reduce the duration and severity of symptoms in otherwise healthy adolescents. Antiviral treatment is generally recommended in immunocompromised patients and those at special risk (e.g. because of severe cardiovascular or respiratory disease or chronic skin disorder); in such cases, an antiviral is given for 10 days with at least 7 days of parenteral treatment.

In pregnancy severe chickenpox may cause complications, especially varicella pneumonia. Specialist advice should be sought for the treatment of chickenpox during pregnancy.

Neonates and children who have been exposed to chickenpox and are at special risk of complications may require prophylaxis with varicella-zoster immunoglobulin (see under Disease-specific Immunoglobulins, section 14.5.2). Prophylactic intravenous aciclovir should be considered for neonates whose mothers develop chickenpox 4 days before to 2 days after delivery.

In *herpes zoster* (shingles) systemic antiviral treatment can reduce the severity and duration of pain, reduce complications, and reduce viral shedding. Treatment with the antiviral should be started within 72 hours of the onset of rash and is usually continued for 7–10 days. Immunocompromised patients at high risk of disseminated or severe infection should be treated with a parenteral antiviral drug. Chronic pain which persists after the rash has healed (postherpetic neuralgia) requires specific management (section 4.7.3).

Choice Aciclovir is active against herpesviruses but does not eradicate them. Uses of aciclovir include systemic treatment of varicella–zoster and the systemic and topical treatment of herpes simplex infections of the skin (section 13.10.3) and mucous membranes (section 7.2.2). It is used by mouth for severe herpetic stomatitis (see also p. 665). Aciclovir eye ointment (section 11.3.3) is used for herpes simplex infections of the eye; it is combined with systemic treatment for ophthalmic zoster.

Famciclovir, a prodrug of penciclovir, is similar to aciclovir and is licensed in adults for use in herpes zoster and genital herpes; there is limited information available on use in children. Penciclovir itself is used as a cream for herpes simplex labialis (section 13.10.3).

Valaciclovir is an ester of aciclovir, licensed in adults for herpes zoster and herpes simplex infections of the skin and mucous membranes (including genital herpes); it is also licensed in children over 12 years for preventing cytomegalovirus disease following renal transplantation. Valaciclovir may be used for the treatment of mild herpes zoster in immunocompromised children over 12 years; treatment should be initiated under specialist supervision. Valaciclovir once daily may reduce the risk of transmitting genital herpes to heterosexual partners—specialist advice should be sought.

ACICLOVIR
(Acyclovir)

Cautions maintain adequate hydration (especially with infusion or high doses, or during renal impairment); **interactions:** Appendix 1 (aciclovir)

Renal impairment see Cautions above; also risk of neurological reactions increased; use normal *intravenous* dose every 12 hours if estimated glomerular filtration rate 25–50 mL/minute/1.73 m² (every 24 hours if estimated glomerular filtration rate 10–25 mL/minute/1.73 m²); consult product literature for intravenous dose if estimated glomerular filtration rate less than 10 mL/minute/1.73 m². For *herpes zoster*, use normal oral dose every 8 hours if estimated glomerular filtration rate 10–25 mL/minute/1.73 m² (every 12 hours if estimated glomerular filtration rate less than 10 mL/minute/1.73 m²). For *herpes simplex*, use normal oral dose every 12 hours if estimated glomerular filtration rate less than 10 mL/minute/1.73 m²

Pregnancy not known to be harmful—manufacturers advise use only when potential benefit outweighs risk

Breast-feeding significant amount in milk after systemic administration; not known to be harmful but manufacturers advise caution

Side-effects nausea, vomiting, abdominal pain, diarrhoea, headache, fatigue, rash, urticaria, pruritus, photosensitivity; *very rarely* hepatitis, jaundice, dyspnoea, neurological reactions (including dizziness, confusion, hallucinations, convulsions, ataxia, dysarthria, and drowsiness), acute renal failure, anaemia, thrombocytopenia, and leucopenia; on *intravenous infusion*, severe local inflammation (sometimes leading to ulceration), and *very rarely* agitation, tremors, psychosis and fever

Licensed use tablets and suspension not licensed for treatment of herpes zoster in children (age range not specified by manufacturer); intravenous infusion not licensed for herpes zoster in children under 18 years; tablets and suspension not licensed for attenuation of chickenpox (if varicella-zoster immunoglobulin not indicated) in children under 18 years

Indication and dose

Herpes simplex treatment

• By mouth

Child 1 month–2 years 100 mg 5 times daily, usually for 5 days (longer if new lesions appear during treatment or if healing incomplete); dose doubled if immunocompromised or if absorption impaired

Child 2–18 years 200 mg 5 times daily, usually for 5 days (longer if new lesions appear during treatment or if healing incomplete); dose doubled if immunocompromised or if absorption impaired

• By intravenous infusion

Neonate 20 mg/kg every 8 hours for 14 days (21 days if CNS involvement)

◁ ACICLOVIR (continued)

Child 1–3 months 20 mg/kg every 8 hours for 14 days (21 days if CNS involvement)

Child 3 months–12 years 250 mg/m^2 every 8 hours usually for 5 days, dose doubled if CNS involvement (given for up to 21 days) or if immunosuppressed

Child 12–18 years 5 mg/kg every 8 hours usually for 5 days, dose doubled if CNS involvement (given for up to 21 days) or if immuno-suppressed
Note To avoid excessive dose in obese patients parenteral dose should be calculated on the basis of ideal weight for height

Herpes simplex prophylaxis in the immuno-compromised
• By mouth
Child 1 month–2 years 100–200 mg 4 times daily

Child 2–18 years 200–400 mg 4 times daily

Chickenpox and herpes zoster infection
• By mouth
Child 1 month–2 years 200 mg 4 times daily for 5 days

Child 2–6 years 400 mg 4 times daily for 5 days

Child 6–12 years 800 mg 4 times daily for 5 days

Child 12–18 years 800 mg 5 times daily for 7 days

• By intravenous infusion
Neonate 10–20 mg/kg every 8 hours for at least 7 days

Child 1–3 months 10–20 mg/kg every 8 hours for at least 7 days

Child 3 months–12 years 250 mg/m^2 every 8 hours usually for 5 days, dose doubled if immunocompromised

Child 12–18 years 5 mg/kg every 8 hours usually for 5 days, dose doubled if immuno-compromised
Note To avoid excessive dose in obese patients parenteral dose should be calculated on the basis of ideal weight for height

Prophylaxis of chickenpox after delivery (see notes above)
• By intravenous infusion
Neonate 10 mg/kg every 8 hours; continued until serological tests confirm absence of virus

Attenuation of chickenpox if varicella–zoster immunoglobulin not indicated
• By mouth
Child 1 month–18 years 10 mg/kg 4 times daily for 7 days starting 1 week after exposure

Herpesvirus skin infections section 13.10.3

Herpesvirus eye infections section 11.3.3

Administration for *intravenous infusion*, reconstitute to 25 mg/mL with Water for Injections or Sodium Chloride 0.9% then dilute to concentration of 5 mg/mL with Sodium Chloride 0.9% or Sodium Chloride and Glucose or Compound Sodium Lactate and give over 1 hour; alternatively, may be administered in a concentration of 25 mg/mL using a suitable infusion pump and central venous access and given over 1 hour

Aciclovir (Non-proprietary) PoM
Tablets, aciclovir 200 mg, net price 25-tab pack = £4.01; 400 mg, 56-tab pack = £9.28; 800 mg, 35-tab pack = £11.42. Label: 9
Brands include *Virovir*®
Dental prescribing on NHS Aciclovir Tablets 200 mg or 800 mg may be prescribed

Dispersible tablets, aciclovir 200 mg, net price 25-tab pack = £2.26; 400 mg, 56-tab pack = £6.88; 800 mg, 35-tab pack = £6.29. Label: 9

Suspension, aciclovir 200 mg/5 mL, net price 125 mL = £34.55; 400 mg/5 mL, 100 mL = £37.54. Label: 9
Dental prescribing on NHS Aciclovir Oral Suspension 200 mg/5 mL may be prescribed

Intravenous infusion, powder for reconstitution, aciclovir (as sodium salt), net price 250-mg vial = £9.13; 500-mg vial = £20.22
Electrolytes Na$^+$ 1.1 mmol/250-mg vial

Intravenous infusion, aciclovir (as sodium salt), 25 mg/mL, net price 10-mL (250-mg) vial = £10.37; 20-mL (500-mg) vial = £19.21; 40-mL (1-g) vial = £40.44
Electrolytes Na$^+$ 1.16 mmol/250-mg vial

Zovirax® (GSK) PoM
Tablets, all dispersible, f/c, aciclovir 200 mg, net price 25-tab pack = £18.07; 800 mg (scored, *Shingles Treatment Pack*), 35-tab pack = £67.13. Label: 9

Suspension, both off-white, sugar-free, aciclovir 200 mg/5 mL (banana-flavoured), net price 125 mL = £29.53; 400 mg/5 mL (*Double Strength Suspension*, orange-flavoured), 100 mL = £33.01. Label: 9

Intravenous infusion, powder for reconstitution, aciclovir (as sodium salt), net price 250-mg vial = £9.75; 500-mg vial = £18.07
Electrolytes Na$^+$ 1.1 mmol/250-mg vial

▌VALACICLOVIR

Note Valaciclovir is a pro-drug of aciclovir
Cautions see under Aciclovir
Hepatic impairment manufacturer advises caution with high doses used for preventing cytomegalovirus disease—no information available in children
Renal impairment maintain adequate hydration; for *herpes zoster*, 1 g every 12 hours if estimated

glomerular filtration rate 15–30 mL/minute/1.73 m^2 (every 24 hours if estimated glomerular filtration rate less than 15 mL/minute/1.73 m^2); for *treatment of herpes simplex*, 500 mg every 24 hours if estimated glomerular filtration rate less than 15 mL/minute/1.73 m^2; for *suppression of herpes simplex*, 250 mg (500 mg in immunocompromised) every 24 hours if estimated glomerular

VALACICLOVIR (continued)

filtration rate less than 15 mL/minute/1.73 m²; reduce dose according to estimated glomerular filtration rate for *cytomegalovirus prophylaxis* following renal transplantation (consult product literature)

Pregnancy see under Aciclovir

Breast-feeding see under Aciclovir

Side-effects see under Aciclovir but neurological reactions more frequent with high doses

Licensed use not licensed for use in children except for CMV prophylaxis in children over 12 years

Indication and dose

Herpes zoster in immunocompromised
• By mouth
Child 12–18 years 1 g 3 times daily for 7 days

Treatment of herpes simplex
• By mouth
Child 12–18 years first episode, 500 mg twice

daily for 5 days (longer if new lesions appear during treatment or if healing incomplete); recurrent infection, 500 mg twice daily for 5 days

Suppression of herpes simplex
• By mouth
Child 12–18 years 500 mg daily in 1–2 divided doses (in immunocompromised or HIV-positive patients, 500 mg twice daily)

Prevention of cytomegalovirus disease following renal transplantation (preferably starting within 72 hours of transplantation)
• By mouth
Child 12–18 years 2 g 4 times daily usually for 90 days

Valtrex® (GSK) PoM
Tablets, f/c, valaciclovir (as hydrochloride) 250 mg, net price 60-tab pack = £130.87; 500 mg, 10-tab pack = £21.86, 42-tab pack = £91.61. Label: 9

5.3.2.2 Cytomegalovirus infection

Recommendations for the optimum maintenance therapy of cytomegalovirus (CMV) infections and the duration of treatment are subject to rapid change.

Ganciclovir is related to aciclovir but it is more active against cytomegalovirus; it is also much more toxic than aciclovir and should therefore be prescribed under specialist supervision and only when the potential benefit outweighs the risks. Ganciclovir is administered by intravenous infusion for the *initial treatment* of CMV infection. The use of ganciclovir may also be considered for symptomatic congenital CMV infection. Ganciclovir causes profound myelosuppression when given with zidovudine; the two should not normally be given together particularly during initial ganciclovir therapy. The likelihood of ganciclovir resistance increases in patients with a high viral load or in those who receive the drug over a long duration; cross-resistance to cidofovir is common.

Valaciclovir (section 5.3.2.1) is licensed for use in children over 12 years for prevention of cytomegalovirus disease following renal transplantation.

Foscarnet is also active against cytomegalovirus; it is toxic and can cause renal impairment.

Cidofovir is given in combination with probenecid for CMV retinitis in AIDS patients when ganciclovir and foscarnet are contra-indicated. Cidofovir is nephrotoxic. There is limited information on its use in children.

For local treatment of CMV retinitis, see section 11.3.3.

GANCICLOVIR

Cautions close monitoring of full blood count (severe deterioration may require correction and possibly treatment interruption); history of cytopenia; potential carcinogen and teratogen; radiotherapy; ensure adequate hydration during intravenous administration; vesicant—infuse into vein with adequate flow preferably using plastic cannula; possible risk of long-term carcinogenic or reproductive toxicity; **interactions:** Appendix 1 (ganciclovir)

Contra-indications hypersensitivity to valganciclovir, ganciclovir, aciclovir, or valaciclovir;

abnormally low haemoglobin, neutrophil, or platelet counts (consult product literature)

Renal impairment reduce dose if estimated glomerular filtration rate less than 70 mL/minute/1.73 m²; consult product literature

Pregnancy avoid—teratogenic risk; ensure effective contraception during treatment and barrier contraception for males during and for at least 90 days after treatment

Breast-feeding avoid—no information available

Side-effects diarrhoea, nausea, vomiting, dyspepsia, abdominal pain, constipation, flatulence, dysphagia, taste disturbance, hepatic dysfunc-

△ **GANCICLOVIR (continued)**

tion; dyspnoea, chest pain, cough; headache, insomnia, convulsions, dizziness, peripheral neuropathy, depression, anxiety, confusion, abnormal thinking, fatigue, weight loss, anorexia; infection, pyrexia, night sweats; anaemia, leucopenia, thrombocytopenia, pancytopenia, renal impairment; myalgia, arthralgia; macular oedema, retinal detachment, vitreous floaters, eye pain; ear pain; dermatitis, pruritus; injection-site reactions; *less commonly* mouth ulcers, pancreatitis, arrhythmias, hypotension, anaphylactic reactions, psychosis, tremor, male infertility, haematuria, disturbances in hearing and vision, and alopecia

Licensed use not licensed for use in children

Indication and dose

Life-threatening or sight-threatening cytomegalovirus infections in immunocompromised patients only; prevention of cytomegalovirus disease during immunosuppressive therapy following organ transplantation

• By intravenous infusion

Child 1 month–18 years initially (induction) 5 mg/kg every 12 hours for 14–21 days for treatment or for 7–14 days for prevention; maintenance (for patients at risk of relapse of

retinitis), 6 mg/kg daily on 5 days per week *or* 5 mg/kg daily until adequate recovery of immunity; if retinitis progresses initial induction treatment may be repeated

Congenital cytomegalovirus infection of the CNS

• By intravenous infusion

Neonate 6 mg/kg every 12 hours for 6 weeks

Local treatment of CMV retinitis section 11.3.3

Administration for *intravenous infusion*, reconstitute with Water for Injections (500 mg/10 mL) then dilute to a concentration of not more than 10 mg/mL with Glucose 5% *or* Sodium Chloride 0.9% and give over 1 hour

Cymevene® (Roche) [PoM]
Intravenous infusion, powder for reconstitution, ganciclovir (as sodium salt). Net price 500-mg vial = £30.37
Electrolytes Na⁺ 2 mmol/500-mg vial

Caution in handling Ganciclovir is toxic and personnel should be adequately protected during handling and administration; if solution comes into contact with skin or mucosa, wash off immediately with soap and water

◼ FOSCARNET SODIUM

Cautions monitor electrolytes, particularly calcium and magnesium; monitor serum creatinine every second day during induction and every week during maintenance; ensure adequate hydration; avoid rapid infusion; **interactions:** Appendix 1 (foscarnet)

Renal impairment reduce dose; consult product literature

Pregnancy avoid

Breast-feeding avoid—present in milk in *animal* studies

Side-effects nausea, vomiting, diarrhoea (occasionally constipation and dyspepsia), abdominal pain, anorexia; changes in blood pressure and ECG; headache, fatigue, mood disturbances (including psychosis), asthenia, paraesthesia, convulsions, tremor, dizziness, and other neurological disorders; rash; impairment of renal function including acute renal failure; hypocalcaemia (sometimes symptomatic) and other electrolyte disturbances; abnormal liver function tests; decreased haemoglobin concentration, leucopenia, granulocytopenia, thrombocytopenia; thrombophlebitis if given undiluted by peripheral vein; genital irritation and ulceration (due to high concentrations excreted in urine); isolated reports of pancreatitis

Licensed use not licensed for use in children

Indication and dose

CMV disease

• By intravenous infusion

Child 1 month–18 years induction 60 mg/kg every 8 hours for 2–3 weeks then maintenance 60 mg/kg daily, increased to 90–120 mg/kg if tolerated; if disease progresses on maintenance dose, repeat induction regimen

Mucocutaneous herpes simplex infection

• By intravenous infusion

Child 1 month–18 years 40 mg/kg every 8 hours for 2–3 weeks or until lesions heal

Administration for *intravenous infusion*, give undiluted solution via a central venous catheter; alternatively dilute to a concentration of 12 mg/mL with Glucose 5% *or* Sodium Chloride 0.9% for administration via a peripheral vein; give over at least 1 hour (give doses greater than 60 mg/kg over 2 hours)

Foscavir® (AstraZeneca) [PoM]
Intravenous infusion, foscarnet sodium hexahydrate 24 mg/mL, net price 250-mL bottle = £34.49

5.3.3 Viral hepatitis

Treatment for viral hepatitis should be initiated by a specialist in hepatology or infectious diseases. The management of uncomplicated acute viral hepatitis is largely symptomatic. Hepatitis B and hepatitis C viruses are major causes of chronic hepatitis. For details on immunisation against hepatitis A and B infections, see section 14.4 (active immunisation) and section 14.5 (passive immunisation).

Chronic hepatitis B Interferon alfa (section 8.2.4), **peginterferon alfa-2a**, **lamivudine** (section 5.3.1), **adefovir dipivoxil**, **entecavir**, and **tenofovir diso-proxil** have a role in the treatment of chronic hepatitis B in adults, but their role in children has not been well established. Specialist supervision is required for the management of chronic hepatitis B.

Tenofovir, or a combination of tenofovir with either emtricitabine or lamivudine, may be used with other antiretrovirals, as part of 'highly active antiretroviral therapy' (section 5.3.1) in children who require treatment for both HIV and chronic hepatitis B. If children infected with both HIV and chronic hepatitis B only require treatment for chronic hepatitis B, they should receive antivirals that are not active against HIV. Management of these children should be co-ordinated between HIV and hepatology specialists.

Chronic hepatitis C Treatment should be considered for children with moderate or severe liver disease. Specialist supervision is required and the regimen is chosen according to the genotype of the infecting virus and the viral load. A combination of **ribavirin** (section 5.3.5) with either **interferon alfa** (section 8.2.4) or **peginterferon alfa-2b** is licensed for use in children over 3 years with chronic hepatitis C. A combination of peginterferon alfa (BNF Section 8.2.4) and ribavirin is preferred.

5.3.4 Influenza

For advice on immunisation against influenza, see section 14.4.

Oseltamivir and **zanamivir** reduce replication of influenza A and B viruses by inhibiting viral neuraminidase. They are most effective for the treatment of influenza if started within a few hours of the onset of symptoms; oseltamivir is licensed for use within 48 hours of the first symptoms while zanamivir is licensed for use within 36 hours of the first symptoms. In otherwise healthy individuals they reduce the duration of symptoms by about 1–1.5 days. For further information on the treatment of influenza, see NICE guidance, p. 397.

Oseltamivir and zanamivir are licensed for post-exposure prophylaxis of influenza when influenza is circulating in the community. Oseltamivir should be given within 48 hours of exposure to influenza while zanamivir should be given within 36 hours of exposure to influenza (see also NICE guidance, p. 397). Oseltamivir and zanamivir are also licensed for use in exceptional circumstances (e.g. when vaccination does not cover the infecting strain) to prevent influenza in an epidemic.

Oseltamivir in children under 1 year of age Data on the use of oseltamivir in children under 1 year of age is limited. Furthermore, oseltamivir may be ineffective in neonates because they may not be able to metabolise oseltamivir to its active form. In exceptional circumstances, oseltamivir can be used (under specialist supervision) for the treatment or post-exposure prophylaxis of influenza in children under 1 year of age. The Department of Health has advised (May 2009) that during a pandemic, treatment with oseltamivir can be overseen by healthcare professionals experienced in assessing children.

Amantadine is licensed for prophylaxis and treatment of influenza A in children over 10 years of age, but it is no longer recommended (see NICE guidance, p. 397).

Information on pandemic influenza, avian influenza, and swine influenza can be found at www.dh.gov.uk/pandemicflu and at www.hpa.org.uk.

Pregnancy and breast-feeding Although safety data are limited, either oseltamivir or zanamivir can be used in women who are pregnant or breast-feeding when the potential benefit outweighs the risk (e.g. during a pandemic). Zanamivir is the preferred drug during pregnancy; however, oseltamivir is recommended during severe infection or when zanamivir cannot be used. Oseltamivir is the preferred drug in women who are breast-feeding.

NICE guidance

Oseltamivir, zanamivir, and amantadine for prophylaxis and treatment of influenza (September 2008 and February 2009)

The drugs described here are not a substitute for vaccination, which remains the most effective way of preventing illness from influenza.

- Amantadine is **not** recommended for prophylaxis or treatment of influenza.
- Oseltamivir or zanamivir are **not** recommended for seasonal prophylaxis against influenza.
- When influenza is circulating in the community[1], either oseltamivir or zanamivir is recommended (in accordance with UK licensing) for post-exposure prophylaxis in at-risk children who are not effectively protected by influenza vaccine, and who have been in close contact with someone suffering from influenza-like illness in the same household or residential setting. Oseltamivir should be given within 48 hours of exposure to influenza while zanamivir should be given within 36 hours of exposure to influenza.
- When influenza is circulating in the community[1], oseltamivir or zanamivir is recommended (in accordance with UK licensing) for the treatment of influenza in at-risk children who can start treatment within 48 hours (within 36 hours for zanamivir) of the onset of symptoms.
- During local outbreaks of influenza-like illness, when there is a high level of certainty that influenza is present, either oseltamivir or zanamivir may be used for post-exposure prophylaxis or treatment in at-risk children (regardless of influenza vaccination) living in long-term residential or nursing homes.

At-risk children are those who have one or more of the following conditions:

- chronic respiratory disease (including asthma);
- chronic heart disease;
- chronic renal disease;
- chronic liver disease;
- chronic neurological disease;
- immunosuppression;
- diabetes mellitus.

This guidance does not cover the circumstances of a pandemic, an impending pandemic, or a widespread epidemic of a new strain of influenza to which there is little or no immunity in the community.

◢ OSELTAMIVIR

Renal impairment reduce dose by 50% if estimated glomerular filtration rate 10–30 mL/minute/1.73 m²; avoid if estimated glomerular filtration rate less than 10 mL/minute/1.73 m²

Pregnancy use only if potential benefit outweighs risk (e.g. during a pandemic); see also p. 396

Breast-feeding amount probably too small to be harmful; use only if potential benefit outweighs risk; (e.g. during a pandemic); see also p. 396

Side-effects nausea, vomiting, abdominal pain, diarrhoea; headache; conjunctivitis; *less commonly* eczema; also reported hepatitis, gastrointestinal bleeding, arrhythmias, neuropsychiatric disorders, visual disturbances, Stevens-Johnson syndrome, and toxic epidermal necrolysis

Licensed use not licensed for use in children under 1 year unless there is a pandemic

Indication and dose

Prevention of influenza

- **By mouth**

  Child under 1 month (see notes above) 2 mg/kg once daily for 10 days for post-exposure prophylaxis

  Child 1–3 months (see notes above) 2.5 mg/kg once daily for 10 days for post-exposure prophylaxis

  Child 3 months–1 year (see notes above) 3 mg/kg once daily for 10 days for post-exposure prophylaxis

  Child 1–13 years

  Body-weight under 15 kg 30 mg once daily for 10 days for post-exposure prophylaxis; for up to 6 weeks during an epidemic

  Body-weight 15–23 kg 45 mg once daily for 10 days for post-exposure prophylaxis; for up to 6 weeks during an epidemic

---

1. National surveillance schemes, including those run by the Health Protection Agency, should be used to indicate when influenza is circulating in the community.

5

Infections

◻ **OSELTAMIVIR (continued)**

Body-weight 23–40 kg 60 mg once daily for 10 days for post-exposure prophylaxis; for up to 6 weeks during an epidemic

Body-weight over 40 kg 75 mg once daily for 10 days for post-exposure prophylaxis; for up to 6 weeks during an epidemic

Child 13–18 years 75 mg once daily for 10 days for post-exposure prophylaxis; for up to 6 weeks during an epidemic

Treatment of influenza
• By mouth
Child under 1 month (see notes above) 2 mg/kg twice daily for 5 days

Child 1–3 months (see notes above) 2.5 mg/kg twice daily for 5 days

Child 3 months–1 year (see notes above) 3 mg/kg twice daily for 5 days

Child 1–13 years

Body-weight under 15 kg 30 mg twice daily for 5 days

Body-weight 15–23 kg 45 mg twice daily for 5 days

Body-weight 23–40 kg 60 mg twice daily for 5 days

Body-weight over 40 kg 75 mg twice daily for 5 days

Child 13–18 years 75 mg twice daily for 5 days

Administration if suspension not available, capsules can be opened and the contents mixed with a small amount of sweetened food, such as sugar water or chocolate syrup, just before administration

¹**Tamiflu®** (Roche) ▼ PoM
Capsules, oseltamivir (as phosphate) 30 mg (yellow), net price 10-cap pack = £7.86; 45 mg (grey), 10-cap pack = £15.72; 75 mg (grey-yellow), 10-cap pack = £15.72. Label: 9

Suspension, sugar-free, tutti-frutti-flavoured, oseltamivir (as phosphate) for reconstitution with water, 60 mg/5 mL, net price 75 mL = £15.72. Label: 9
Excipients include sorbitol 1.7 g/5 mL
Note Solutions prepared by 'Special Order' manufacturers may be a different concentration
1. ᴺᴴˢ except for the treatment and prophylaxis of influenza as indicated in the notes above and NICE guidance; endorse prescription 'SLS'

ZANAMIVIR

Cautions asthma and chronic pulmonary disease (risk of bronchospasm—short-acting bronchodilator should be available; avoid in severe asthma unless close monitoring possible and appropriate facilities available to treat bronchospasm); uncontrolled chronic illness; other inhaled drugs should be administered before zanamivir

Pregnancy use only if potential benefit outweighs risk (e.g. during a pandemic); see also p. 396

Breast-feeding amount probably too small to be harmful; use only if potential benefit outweighs risk (e.g. during a pandemic); see also p. 396

Side-effects very rarely bronchospasm, respiratory impairment, angioedema, urticaria, and rash; also reported neuropsychiatric disorders

Indication and dose

Post-exposure prophylaxis of influenza
• By inhalation of powder
Child 5–18 years 10 mg once daily for 10 days

Prevention of influenza during an epidemic
• By inhalation of powder
Child 5–18 years 10 mg once daily for up to 28 days

Treatment of influenza
• By inhalation of powder
Child 5–18 years 10 mg twice daily for 5 days

¹**Relenza®** (GSK) PoM
Dry powder for inhalation disks containing 4 blisters of zanamivir 5 mg/blister, net price 5 disks with *Diskhaler®* device = £16.36
1. ᴺᴴˢ except for the treatment and prophylaxis of influenza as indicated in the notes above and NICE guidance; endorse prescription 'SLS'

5.3.5 Respiratory syncytial virus

Ribavirin (tribavirin) inhibits a wide range of DNA and RNA viruses. It is licensed for administration by inhalation for the treatment of severe bronchiolitis caused by the respiratory syncytial virus (RSV) in infants, especially when they have other serious diseases. However, there is no evidence that ribavirin produces clinically relevant benefit in RSV bronchiolitis. Ribavirin is given by mouth with peginterferon alfa or interferon alfa for the treatment of chronic hepatitis C infection (see Viral Hepatitis, section 5.3.3). Ribavirin is also effective in Lassa fever and has also been used parenterally in the treatment of life-threatening RSV, parainfluenza virus, and adenovirus infections in immunocompromised children [unlicensed indications].

Palivizumab is a monoclonal antibody licensed for preventing serious lower respiratory-tract disease caused by respiratory syncytial virus in children at high risk of the disease; it should be prescribed under specialist supervision and on the basis of the likelihood of hospitalisation. Palivizumab should be considered for children under 6 months with haemodynamically significant left-to-right shunt congenital heart disease or who have pulmonary hypertension. It should also be considered for children under 2 years *either* with chronic lung disease who are using oxygen at home (or have been on prolonged oxygen treatment) *or* with severe congenital immunodeficiency. Palivizumab may also be used for the first 6–12 months of life in a child born at under 35 weeks gestation, if the child is considered by the specialist to be at special risk of hospitalisation. It is licensed for monthly use during the RSV season; the first dose should be administered before the start of the RSV season.

PALIVIZUMAB

Cautions moderate to severe acute infection or febrile illness; thrombocytopenia; serum-palivizumab concentration may be reduced after cardiac surgery

Contra-indications hypersensitivity to humanised monoclonal antibodies

Side-effects fever, injection-site reactions, nervousness; *less commonly* diarrhoea, vomiting, constipation, haemorrhage, rhinitis, cough, wheeze, pain, drowsiness, asthenia, hyperkinesia, leucopenia, and rash; also reported, apnoea, hypersensitivity reactions (including anaphylaxis), convulsions and thrombocytopenia

Licensed use not licensed in children with congenital immunodeficiency or in children born at 35 weeks gestation or less and older than 6 months (licensed in children under 6 months)

Indication and dose

> Prevention of serious disease caused by respiratory syncytial virus infection (see notes above)
>
> • By intramuscular injection (preferably in anterolateral thigh)
>
> **Neonate** 15 mg/kg once a month during season of RSV risk
>
> **Child 1 month–2 years** 15 mg/kg once a month during season of RSV risk (child undergoing cardiac bypass surgery, 15 mg/kg as soon as stable after surgery, then once a month during season of risk); injection volume over 1 mL should be divided between 2 or more sites

Synagis® (Abbott) ▼ PoM
Injection, powder for reconstitution, palivizumab, net price 50-mg vial = £360.40; 100-mg vial = £663.11

RIBAVIRIN

(Tribavirin)

Cautions

Specific cautions for inhaled treatment Maintain standard supportive respiratory and fluid management therapy; monitor electrolytes closely; monitor equipment for precipitation; pregnant women (and those planning pregnancy) should avoid exposure to aerosol

Specific cautions for systemic treatment Exclude pregnancy before treatment in females of childbearing age; effective contraception essential during treatment and for 4 months after treatment in females and for 7 months after treatment in males of childbearing age; routine monthly pregnancy tests recommended; condoms must be used if partner of male patient is pregnant (ribavirin excreted in semen); cardiac disease (assessment including ECG recommended before and during treatment—discontinue if deterioration); determine full blood count, platelets, electrolytes, serum creatinine, liver function tests and uric acid before starting treatment and then on weeks 2 and 4 of treatment, then as indicated clinically—adjust dose if adverse reactions or laboratory abnormalities develop (consult product literature); eye examination recommended before oral treatment; eye examination also recommended during oral treatment if pre-existing ophthalmological disorder or if decrease in vision reported—discontinue treatment if ophthalmological disorder deteriorates or if new ophthalmological disorder develops; test thyroid function before treatment and then every 3 months

Interactions: Appendix 1 (ribavirin)

Contra-indications

Specific contra-indications for systemic treatment Severe cardiac disease, including unstable or uncontrolled cardiac disease in previous 6 months; haemoglobinopathies; severe debilitating medical conditions; severe hepatic dysfunction or decompensated cirrhosis; autoimmune disease (including autoimmune hepatitis); history of severe psychiatric condition

Hepatic impairment no dosage adjustment required; use oral ribavirin with caution in severe hepatic dysfunction or decompensated cirrhosis

Renal impairment plasma-ribavirin concentration increased; manufacturer advises avoid oral ribavirin if estimated glomerular filtration rate less than 50 mL/minute/1.73 m^2; manufacturer advises use intravenous preparation with caution if estimated glomerular filtration rate less than 30 mL/minute/1.73 m^2

Pregnancy avoid; teratogenicity in *animal* studies; see also Cautions above

Breast-feeding avoid—no information available

Side-effects

Specific side-effects for inhaled treatment Worsening respiration, bacterial pneumonia, and pneumothorax reported; rarely non-specific anaemia and haemolysis

Specific side-effects for systemic treatment Haemolytic anaemia (anaemia may be improved by epoetin); also (in combination with peginterferon alfa or interferon alfa) nausea, vomiting, dyspepsia, abdominal pain, peptic ulcer, flatulence, diarrhoea, constipation, colitis, pancreatitis, growth retardation (including decrease in height and weight), appetite changes, weight loss, pulmonary embolism, chest pain, tachycardia, palpitation, syncope, cerebrovascular disease, peripheral oedema, changes in blood pressure, flushing, Raynaud's disease, hypertriglyceridaemia, dyspnoea, cough, interstitial pneumonitis, sleep disturbances, abnormal dreams, asthenia, impaired concentration and memory, psychoses, anxiety, depression, suicidal ideation, dizziness, hyperkinesia, tremor, hypertonia, seizures, ataxia, dysphonia, peripheral neuropathy, influenza-like symptoms, headache, hyperglycaemia, thyroid disorders, menstrual disturbances, virilism, testicular pain, micturition disorders, leucopenia, thrombocytopenia, aplastic anaemia, lymphadenopathy, hypocalcaemia, renal failure, hyperuricaemia, myalgia, arthralgia, systemic lupus erythematosus, vasculitis, sarcoidosis, eye changes (including blurred vision and retinopathy), rhinitis, tinnitus, hearing impairment, dry mouth, stomatitis, glossitis, taste disturbance, pharyngitis, gingivitis, tooth disorders, rash (including very rarely Stevens-Johnson syndrome and toxic epidermal necro-

◁ **RIBAVIRIN (continued)**

lysis), pruritus, urticaria, photosensitivity, psoriasis, alopecia, dry skin, skin discoloration, increased sweating

Licensed use inhalation licensed for use in children (age range not specified by manufacturer);
intravenous preparation not licensed

Indication and dose

Bronchiolitis
* **By aerosol inhalation or nebulisation (via small
particle aerosol generator)**

  Child 1 month–2 years inhale solution containing 20 mg/mL for 12–18 hours for at least 3
  days; max. 7 days

Life-threatening RSV, parainfluenza virus, and
adenovirus infection in immunocompromised
children (seek expert advice)
* **By intravenous infusion over 15 minutes**

  Child 1 month–18 years 33 mg/kg as a single
  dose, then 16 mg/kg every 6 hours for 4 days,
  then 8 mg/kg every 8 hours for 3 days

Chronic hepatitis C (in combination with interferon alfa or peginterferon alfa) in previously
untreated children without liver decompensation
* **By mouth**

  Child over 3 years; body-weight under 47 kg
  15 mg/kg daily in 2 divided doses

Child body-weight 47–50 kg 200 mg in the
morning and 400 mg in the evening

Child body-weight 50–65 kg 400 mg twice daily

Child body-weight 65–86 kg 400 mg in the
morning and 600 mg in the evening

Child body-weight 86–105 kg 600 mg twice
daily

Child body-weight over 105 kg 600 mg in the
morning and 800 mg in the evening

Rebetol® (Schering-Plough) PoM
Capsules, ribavirin 200 mg, net price 84-cap pack =
£163.80, 140-cap pack = £273.00, 168-cap pack =
£327.60. Label: 21

Oral solution, ribavirin 200 mg/5 mL, net price
100 mL (bubble-gum-flavoured) = £68.38. Label: 21

Virazole® (Meda) PoM
Inhalation◢ ribavirin 6 g for reconstitution with
300 mL water for injections. Net price 3 × 6-g vials
= £349.00

Intravenous infusion, 100 mg/mL, 10-mL amp
Available on a named-patient basis from Valeant

5.4 Antiprotozoal drugs

Advice on specific problems available from:

Advice for healthcare professionals

HPA (Health Protection Agency) Malaria Reference Laboratory www.hpa.org.uk/infections/topics_az/malaria	(020) 7636 3924 (prophylaxis only)
National Travel Health Network and Centre	0845 602 6712
Travel Medicine Team, Health Protection, Scotland (registered users of Travax only) www.travax.nhs.uk (for registered users of the NHS Travax website only)	(0141) 300 1100 (weekdays 2–4 p.m. only)
Birmingham	(0121) 424 0357
Liverpool	(0151) 705 3100
London	0845 155 5000 (treatment)
Oxford	(01865) 225 430

Advice for travellers

Hospital for Tropical Diseases, Travel Healthline www.fitfortravel.nhs.uk	020 7950 7799
WHO advice on international travel and health www.who.int/ith	
National Travel Health Network and Centre (NaTHNaC) www.nathnac.org/travel/index.htm	

Infections 5

5.4.1 Antimalarials

Recommendations on the prophylaxis and treatment of malaria reflect guidelines agreed by UK malaria specialists. Choice will depend on the age of the child (see below).

The centres listed above should be consulted for advice on special problems.

Treatment of malaria

If the infective species is **not known**, or if the infection is **mixed**, initial treatment should be as for *falciparum malaria* with quinine, *Malarone*® (proguanil with atovaquone), or *Riamet*® (artemether with lumefantrine). Falciparum malaria can progress rapidly in unprotected children and antimalarial treatment should be considered in those with features of severe malaria and possible exposure, even if the initial blood tests for the organism are negative.

Falciparum malaria (treatment)

Falciparum malaria (malignant malaria) is caused by *Plasmodium falciparum*. In most parts of the world *P. falciparum* is now resistant to chloroquine which should not therefore be given for treatment.

Quinine, *Malarone*® (proguanil with atovaquone), or *Riamet*® (artemether with lumefantrine) can be given *by mouth* if the child can swallow and retain tablets and there are no serious manifestations (e.g. impaired consciousness); quinine should be given *by intravenous infusion* (see below) if the child is seriously ill or unable to take tablets. **Mefloquine** is now rarely used for treatment because of concerns about resistance.

Oral. **Quinine** is well tolerated by children although the salts are bitter.

> The dosage regimen for quinine *by mouth* is:
> 10 mg/kg (of quinine salt[1]; max. 600 mg) every 8 hours for 7 days
> *together with or followed by*
> *either* **clindamycin** 7–13 mg/kg (max. 450 mg) every 8 hours for 7 days [unlicensed indication]
> *or*, in children over 12 years, **doxycycline** 200 mg once daily for 7 days

If the parasite is likely to be sensitive, **pyrimethamine** with **sulfadoxine** as a single dose [unlicensed] may be given (instead of either clindamycin or doxycycline) together with or after a course of quinine.

> The dose regimen for pyrimethamine with sulfadoxine by mouth is:
> Child up to 4 years and body-weight over 5 kg pyrimethamine 12.5 mg with sulfadoxine 250 mg as a single dose
>
> Child 5–6 years pyrimethamine 25 mg with sulfadoxine 500 mg as a single dose
>
> Child 7–9 years pyrimethamine 37.5 mg with sulfadoxine 750 mg as a single dose
>
> Child 10–14 years pyrimethamine 50 mg with sulfadoxine 1 g as a single dose
>
> Child 14–18 years pyrimethamine 75 mg with sulfadoxine 1.5 g as a single dose

Alternatively, *Malarone*®, or *Riamet*® may be given instead of quinine. It is not necessary to give clindamycin, doxycycline, or pyrimethamine with sulfadoxine after *Malarone*® or *Riamet*® treatment.

> The dose regimen for *Malarone*® *by mouth* is:
> Child body-weight 5–8 kg, 2 'paediatric' tablets once daily for 3 days
>
> Child body-weight 9–10 kg, 3 'paediatric' tablets once daily for 3 days
>
> Child body-weight 11–20 kg, 1 'standard' tablet once daily for 3 days
>
> Child body-weight 21–30 kg, 2 'standard' tablets once daily for 3 days
>
> Child body-weight 31–40 kg, 3 'standard' tablets once daily for 3 days
>
> Child body-weight over 40 kg, 4 'standard' tablets once daily for 3 days

5 Infections

---

1. Valid for quinine hydrochloride, dihydrochloride, and sulphate; not valid for quinine bisulphate which contains a correspondingly smaller amount of quinine.

402 5.4.1 Antimalarials

BNFC 2010–2011

The dose regimen for *Riamet®* *by mouth* is:

Child body-weight 5–15 kg 1 tablet initially, followed by 5 further doses of 1 tablet each given at 8, 24, 36, 48, and 60 hours (total 6 tablets over 60 hours)

Child body-weight 15–25 kg 2 tablets initially, followed by 5 further doses of 2 tablets each given at 8, 24, 36, 48, and 60 hours (total 12 tablets over 60 hours)

Child body-weight 25–35 kg 3 tablets initially, followed by 5 further doses of 3 tablets each given at 8, 24, 36, 48, and 60 hours (total 18 tablets over 60 hours)

Child 12–18 years and body-weight over 35 kg, 4 tablets initially followed by 5 further doses of 4 tablets each given at 8, 24, 36, 48, and 60 hours (total 24 tablets over 60 hours)

Parenteral. If the child is seriously ill or unable to swallow tablets, **quinine** should be given *by intravenous infusion*. The dose regimen for quinine *by intravenous infusion* is calculated on a mg/kg basis:

Neonates and children, loading dose[1,2] of 20 mg/kg (up to maximum 1.4 g) of quinine salt[3] infused over 4 hours *then 8 hours after the start of the loading dose*, maintenance dose of 10 mg/kg[4] (up to maximum 700 mg) of quinine salt[3] infused over 4 hours every 8 hours (until child can swallow tablets to complete the 7-day course *together with or followed by either* clindamycin or doxycycline as above).

Specialist advice should be sought in difficult cases (e.g. very high parasite count, deterioration on optimal doses of quinine, infection acquired in quinine-resistant areas of south-east Asia) because intravenous **artesunate** may be available for 'named-patient' use.

Pregnancy   Falciparum malaria is particularly dangerous in pregnancy, especially in the last trimester. The treatment doses of oral and intravenous quinine given above (including the loading dose) can safely be given in pregnancy. Clindamycin [unlicensed indication] should be given for 7 days with or after quinine. Doxycycline should be avoided in pregnancy (affects teeth and skeletal development in fetus); pyrimethamine with sulfadoxine, *Malarone®*, and *Riamet®* are also best avoided until more information is available.

Benign malarias (treatment)

Benign malaria is usually caused by *Plasmodium vivax* and less commonly by *P. ovale* and *P. malariae.* **Chloroquine**[5] is the drug of choice for the treatment of benign malarias (but chloroquine-resistant *P. vivax* infection has been reported from Indonesia, New Guinea and some adjacent islands).

Chloroquine alone is adequate for *P. malariae* infections but in the case of *P. vivax* and *P. ovale*, a *radical cure* (to destroy parasites in the liver and thus prevent relapses) is required. This is achieved with **primaquine**[6] given after the chloroquine.

The dosage regimen of chloroquine *by mouth* for benign malaria in children is:

initial dose of 10 mg/kg of base (max. 620 mg) *then*

a single dose of 5 mg/kg of base (max. 310 mg) after 6–8 hours *then*

a single dose of 5 mg/kg of base (max. 310 mg) daily for 2 days

For a *radical cure*, **primaquine**[6] [unlicensed] is then given to children over 6 months of age; specialist advice should be sought for children under 6 months of age. Primaquine is given in a dose of 250 micrograms/kg (max. 15 mg) daily for 14 days in *P. ovale* infection or 500 micrograms/kg (max. 30 mg) daily for 14 days in *P. vivax* infection.

---

1. In intensive care units the loading dose can alternatively be given as quinine salt[3] 7 mg/kg infused over 30 minutes followed immediately by 10 mg/kg over 4 hours then (after 8 hours) maintenance dose as described.
2. **Important:** the loading dose of 20 mg/kg should **not** be used if the patient has received quinine or mefloquine during the previous 12 hours
3. Valid for quinine hydrochloride, dihydrochloride, and sulphate; not valid for quinine bisulphate which contains a correspondingly smaller amount of quinine.
4. Maintenance dose should be reduced to 5–7 mg/kg of quinine salt[3] in children with severe renal impairment, severe hepatic impairment, or if parenteral treatment is required for more than 48 hours.
5. For the treatment of chloroquine-resistant benign malaria *Malarone®* [unlicensed indication], quinine, or *Riamet®* [unlicensed indication] can be used; as with chloroquine, primaquine should be given for radical cure.
6. Before starting primaquine, blood should be tested for glucose-6-phosphate dehydrogenase (G6PD) activity since the drug can cause haemolysis in G6PD-deficient patients. Specialist advice should be obtained in G6PD deficiency. In mild G6PD deficiency, primaquine in a dose of 750 micrograms/kg (max. 45 mg) once a week for 8 weeks, has been found useful and without undue harmful effects.

Parenteral   If the child is unable to take oral therapy, quinine can be given by *intravenous infusion*. The dose is 10 mg/kg[1] (max. 700 mg) of quinine salt[2] infused over 4 hours every 8 hours, changed to oral chloroquine as soon as the child's condition permits.

Pregnancy   Treatment doses of chloroquine can be given for benign malaria. In the case of *P. vivax* or *P. ovale*, however, the radical cure with primaquine should be **postponed** until the pregnancy is over; instead chloroquine should be continued at a dose of 10 mg/kg (max. 310 mg) each week during the pregnancy.

Prophylaxis against malaria

The recommendations on prophylaxis reflect guidelines agreed by UK malaria specialists; the advice is aimed at residents of the UK who travel to endemic areas. The choice of drug for a particular child should take into account:

- risk of exposure to malaria;
- extent of drug resistance;
- efficacy of the recommended drugs;
- side-effects of the drugs;
- patient-related factors (e.g. age, pregnancy, renal or hepatic impairment, compliance with prophylactic regimen).

Prophylactic doses are based on guidelines agreed by UK malaria experts and may differ from advice in product literature. **Weight is a better guide than age.** If in doubt obtain advice from specialist centre, see p. 400.

Protection against bites   Prophylaxis is not absolute, and breakthrough infection can occur with any of the drugs recommended. Personal protection against being bitten is very important. Mosquito nets impregnated with permethrin provide the most effective barrier protection against insects (infants should sleep with a mosquito net stretched over the cot or baby carrier); mats and vaporised insecticides are also useful. Diethyltoluamide (DEET) 20–50% in lotions, sprays, or roll-on formulations is safe and effective when applied to the skin of adults and children over 2 months of age. It can also be used during pregnancy and breast-feeding. The duration of protection varies according to the concentration of DEET and is longest for DEET 50%. Long sleeves and trousers worn after dusk also provide protection.

Length of prophylaxis   In order to determine tolerance and to establish habit, prophylaxis should generally be started one week (preferably 2–3 weeks in the case of mefloquine) before travel into an endemic area (or if not possible at earliest opportunity up to 1 or 2 days before travel); *Malarone®* or doxycycline prophylaxis should be started 1–2 days before travel. Prophylaxis should be continued for **4 weeks after leaving** (except for *Malarone®* prophylaxis which should be stopped 1 week after leaving).

In those requiring long-term prophylaxis, chloroquine and proguanil may be used for periods of over 5 years. Mefloquine is licensed for use up to 1 year (although it has been used for up to 3 years without undue problems). Doxycycline can be used for up to 2 years. *Malarone®* is licensed for use for up to 28 days but can be used for up to 1 year (and possibly longer) with caution. Specialist advice should be sought for long-term prophylaxis.

Return from malarial region   It is important to be aware that **any illness** that occurs within 1 year and **especially within 3 months of return might be malaria** even if all recommended precautions against malaria were taken. Travellers and carers of children should be **warned** of this and told that if they develop any illness **particularly within 3 months** of their return they should go **immediately** to a doctor and specifically mention their exposure to malaria.

Epilepsy   Both chloroquine and mefloquine are unsuitable for malaria prophylaxis in children with a history of epilepsy. In areas *without chloroquine resistance*, proguanil alone is recommended; in areas *with chloroquine resistance*, doxycycline or *Malarone®* may be considered. The metabolism of doxycycline may be influenced by antiepileptics (see **interactions**: Appendix 1 (tetracyclines)).

1. Maintenance dose should be reduced to 5–7 mg/kg of quinine salt[2] in children with severe renal impairment, severe hepatic impairment, or if parenteral treatment is required for more than 48 hours.
2. Valid for quinine hydrochloride, dihydrochloride, and sulphate; not valid for quinine bisulphate which contains a correspondingly smaller amount of quinine.

5

Infections

Asplenia Asplenic children (or those with severe splenic dysfunction) are at particular risk of severe malaria. If travel to malarious areas is unavoidable, rigorous precautions are required against contracting the disease.

Renal impairment Avoidance (or dosage reduction) of proguanil is recommended since it is excreted by the kidneys. *Malarone*® should not be used for prophylaxis in children with estimated glomerular filtration rate less than 30 mL/minute/1.73 m². Chloroquine is only partially excreted by the kidneys and reduction of the dose for prophylaxis is not required except in severe impairment. Mefloquine is considered to be appropriate to use in renal impairment and does not require dosage reduction. Doxycycline is also considered to be appropriate.

Pregnancy Travel to malarious areas should be avoided during pregnancy; if travel is unavoidable, effective prophylaxis must be used. Chloroquine and proguanil can be given in the usual doses during pregnancy, but these drugs are not appropriate for most areas because their effectiveness has declined, particularly in sub-saharan Africa; in the case of proguanil, folic acid 5 mg daily should be given. The centres listed on p. 400 should be consulted for advice on prophylaxis in chloroquine-resistant areas. Although the manufacturer advises that mefloquine should not be used during pregnancy, particularly in the first trimester, unless the potential benefit outweighs the risk, studies of mefloquine in pregnancy (including use in the first trimester) indicate that it can be considered for travel to chloroquine-resistant areas. Doxycycline is contra-indicated during pregnancy. *Malarone*® should be avoided during pregnancy unless there is no suitable alternative.

Breast-feeding Prophylaxis is required in **breast-fed infants**; although antimalarials are present in milk, the amounts are too variable to give reliable protection.

Specific recommendations

Where a journey requires two regimens, the regimen for the higher risk area should be used for the whole journey. Those travelling to remote or little-visited areas may require expert advice.

Risk may vary in different parts of a country—check under all risk levels

Important Settled immigrants and their carers (or long-term visitors) to the UK may be unaware that they will have **lost some of their immunity** and also that the areas where they previously lived **may now be malarious**

North Africa, the Middle East, and Central Asia

Very low risk Risk *very low* in Algeria, Egypt (but *low risk* in El Faiyum, see below), Georgia (south-east, July–October), Kyrgystan (but *low risk* in south-west, see below), Libya, rural Morocco, most tourist areas of Turkey (but *low risk* in Adana and border with Syria, see below), Uzbekistan (extreme south-east only):

chemoprophylaxis not recommended but avoid mosquito bites and consider malaria if fever presents

Low risk Risk *low* in Armenia (June–October), Azerbaijan (southern border areas, June–September), Egypt (El Faiyum only, June–October), Iran (northern border with Azerbaijan, May–October; *variable risk* in rural south-east provinces; see below), rural north Iraq (May–November), Kyrgystan (south-west, May–October), north border of Syria (May–October), Turkey (plain around Adana and east of there, border with Syria, March–November), Turkmenistan (south-east only, June–October):

preferably

chloroquine *or* (if chloroquine not appropriate) proguanil hydrochloride

Variable risk   Risk *variable* and *chloroquine resistance present* in Afghanistan (below 2000 m, May–November), Iran (rural south-east provinces, March–November, see also *Low Risk* above), Oman (remote rural areas only), Saudi Arabia (south-west and rural areas of western region; no risk in Mecca, Medina, Jeddah, or high-altitude areas of Asir Province), Tajikistan (June–October), Yemen (no risk in Sana'a):

> chloroquine + proguanil hydrochloride *or* (if chloroquine + proguanil not appropriate and child over 12 years) doxycycline

Sub-Saharan Africa

No chemoprophylaxis recommended for Cape Verde (some risk on São Tiago) and Mauritius (but avoid mosquito bites and consider malaria if fever presents)

Very high risk   Risk *very high* (or *locally very high*) and *chloroquine resistance very widespread* in Angola, Benin, Botswana (northern half, November–June), Burkina Faso, Burundi, Cameroon, Central African Republic, Chad, Comoros, Congo, Democratic Republic of the Congo (formerly Zaïre), Djibouti, Equatorial Guinea, Eritrea, Ethiopia (below 2000 m; no risk in Addis Ababa), Gabon, Gambia, Ghana, Guinea, Guinea-Bissau, Ivory Coast, Kenya, Liberia, Madagascar, Malawi, Mali, Mauritania (all year in south; July–October in north), Mozambique, Namibia (all year along Kavango and Kunene rivers; November–June in northern third), Niger, Nigeria, Principe, Rwanda, São Tomé, Senegal, Sierra Leone, Somalia, South Africa (low-altitude areas of Mpumalanga and Limpopo Provinces, Kruger National Park, and north-east KwaZulu-Natal as far south as Jozini), Sudan, Swaziland, Tanzania, Togo, Uganda, Zambia, Zimbabwe (all year in Zambezi valley; November–June in other areas below 1200 m; risk negligible in Harare and Bulawayo):

> mefloquine *or* doxycycline (if child over 12) *or Malarone*®

Note In Zimbabwe and neighbouring countries, pyrimethamine with dapsone (also known as *Deltaprim*®) prophylaxis is used by local residents (sometimes with chloroquine—this regimen is not recommended).

South Asia

Low risk   Risk *low* in Bangladesh (but *high risk* in Chittagong Hill Tracts, see below), India (Kerala [southern states], Tamil Nadu, Karnataka, Southern Andhra Pradesh [including Hyderabad], Mumbai, Rajasthan [including Jaipur], Uttar Pradesh [including Agra], Haryana, Uttaranchal, Himachal Pradesh, Jammu, Kashmir, Punjab, Delhi; *variable risk* in other areas, see below; *high risk* in Assam), Sri Lanka (but *variable risk* north of Vavuniya, see below):

> chemoprophylaxis not recommended but avoid mosquito bites and consider malaria if fever present

Variable risk   Risk *variable* and *chloroquine resistance usually moderate* in southern districts of Bhutan, India (*low risk* in some areas, see above; *high risk* in Assam, see below), Nepal (below 1500 m, especially Terai districts; no risk in Kathmandu), Pakistan (below 2000 m), Sri Lanka (north of Vavuniya; *low risk* in other areas, see above):

> chloroquine + proguanil hydrochloride *or* (if chloroquine + proguanil not appropriate) mefloquine *or* doxycycline *or Malarone*®

High risk   Risk *high* and *chloroquine resistance high* in Bangladesh (only in Chittagong Hill Tracts; *low risk* in other areas, see above), India (Assam only; see also *Low Risk* and *Variable Risk* above):

> mefloquine *or* doxycycline (if child over 12) *or Malarone*® *or* (if mefloquine, doxycycline, or *Malarone*® not appropriate) chloroquine + proguanil hydrochloride

5

Infections

Infections

5

South-East Asia

Very low risk   Risk *very low* in Bali, Brunei, Cambodia (Angkor Wat and Siem Reap, but no risk in Phnom Penh; *substantial risk* in other areas, see below; *great risk* in western provinces, see below), main tourist areas of China (but *substantial risk* in Yunnan and Hainan, see below; *chloroquine prophylaxis* appropriate for other remote areas), Hong Kong, Korea (both North and South), Malaysia (both East and West including Cameron Highlands, but *substantial risk* in Sabah [except Kota Kinabalu], and *variable risk* in deep forests, see below), Singapore, Thailand (**important**: regional risk exists, see under *Great Risk*, below), Vietnam (cities, coast between Ho Chi Minh and Hanoi, and Mekong River until close to Cambodian border; *substantial risk* in other areas, see below):

> chemoprophylaxis not recommended but avoid mosquito bites and consider malaria if fever presents

Variable risk   Risk *variable* and *some chloroquine resistance* in Indonesia (very low risk in Bali, and cities but *substantial risk* in Irian Jaya [West Papua] and Lombok, see below), rural Philippines below 600 m (no risk in cities, Cebu, Bohol, and Catanduanes), deep forests of peninsular Malaysia and Sarawak (but *substantial risk* in Sabah, see below):

> chloroquine + proguanil hydrochloride *or* (if chloroquine + proguanil not appropriate) mefloquine *or* doxycycline *or Malarone®*

Substantial risk   Risk *substantial* and *drug resistance common* in Cambodia (no risk or *very low risk* in some areas, see above; *great risk* in western provinces, see below), China (Yunnan and Hainan; *chloroquine prophylaxis* appropriate for other remote areas; see also *Very Low Risk* above), East Timor, Irian Jaya [West Papua], Laos (no risk in Vientiane), Lombok, Malaysia (Sabah; see also *Very Low Risk* and *Variable Risk* above), Myanmar (formerly Burma; see also *Great Risk* below), Vietnam (*very low risk* in some areas, see above):

> mefloquine *or* doxycycline (if child over 12) *or Malarone®*

Great risk and drug resistance present   Risk *great and widespread chloroquine and mefloquine resistance present* in western provinces of Cambodia (see also *Very Low Risk* and *Substantial Risk* above), borders of Thailand with Cambodia, Laos and Myanmar (*very low risk* in Chang Rai and Kwai Bridge, see above), Myanmar (eastern Shan State):

> doxycycline (if child over 12) *or Malarone®*

Oceania

Risk   Risk *high* and *chloroquine resistance high* in Papua New Guinea (below 1800 m), Solomon Islands, Vanuatu:

> doxycycline (if child over 12) *or* mefloquine *or Malarone®*

Central and South America and the Caribbean

Very low risk   Risk *very low* in Jamaica:

> chemoprophylaxis not recommended but avoid mosquito bites and consider malaria if fever presents

Variable to low risk   Risk *variable to low* in Argentina (rural areas along northern borders only), rural Belize (except Belize district), Costa Rica (Limon Province except Puerto Limon and northern canton of Pococci), Dominican Republic, El Salvador (Santa Ana province in west), Guatemala (below 1500 m), Haiti, Honduras, Mexico (states of Oaxaca and Chiapas), Nicaragua, Panama (west of

Panama Canal but *variable to high risk* east of Panama Canal, see below), rural Paraguay:

> chloroquine *or* (if chloroquine not appropriate) proguanil hydrochloride

Variable to high risk   Risk *variable to high and chloroquine resistance present* in rural areas of Bolivia (below 2500 m; see below for Amazon basin area), Ecuador (below 1500 m; no malaria in Galapagos Islands and Guayaquil; see below for Esmeraldas Province), Panama (east of Panama Canal), Peru (rural areas east of the Andes and west of the Amazon basin area below 1500 m; see below for Amazon basin area), Venezuela (north of Orinoco river; *high risk* south of and including Orinoco river and Amazon basin area, see below; Caracas free of malaria):

> chloroquine + proguanil hydrochloride *or* (if chloroquine + proguanil not appropriate) mefloquine *or* doxycycline (if child over 12) *or Malarone®*

High risk   Risk *high* and *marked chloroquine resistance* in Bolivia (Amazon basin area; see also *variable to high risk* above), Brazil (throughout 'Legal Amazon' area which includes the Amazon basin area, Mato Grosso and Maranhao only; elsewhere *very low risk*—no chemoprophylaxis), Colombia (most areas below 800 m), Ecuador (Esmeraldas Province; *variable to high risk* in other areas, see above), French Guiana, all interior regions of Guyana, Peru (Amazon basin area; see also *variable to high risk* above), Suriname (except Paramaribo and coast), Venezuela (Amazon basin area, areas south of and including Orinoco river; see also *variable to high risk* above):

> mefloquine *or* doxycycline (if child over 12) *or Malarone®*

Standby treatment [unlicensed]

> Children and their carers visiting remote, malarious areas for prolonged periods should carry standby treatment if they are likely to be more than 24 hours away from medical care. Self-medication should be **avoided** if medical help is accessible.
>
> In order to avoid excessive self-medication, the traveller should be provided with **written instructions** that urgent medical attention should be sought if fever (38°C or more) develops 7 days (or more) after arriving in a malarious area and that self-treatment is indicated if medical help is not available within 24 hours of fever onset.
>
> In view of the continuing emergence of resistant strains and of the different regimens required for different areas expert advice should be sought on the best treatment course for an individual traveller. A drug used for chemoprophylaxis should not be considered for standby treatment for the same traveller.

5

Infections

Artemether with lumefantrine

Artemether with lumefantrine is licensed for the *treatment of acute uncomplicated falciparum malaria*.

ARTEMETHER WITH LUMEFANTRINE

Cautions electrolyte disturbances, concomitant use with other drugs known to cause QT-interval prolongation; monitor patients unable to take food (greater risk of recrudescence); **interactions:** Appendix 1 (artemether with lumefantrine) Skilled tasks Dizziness may affect performance of skilled tasks

Contra-indications history of arrhythmias, of clinically relevant bradycardia, and of congestive heart failure accompanied by reduced left ventricular ejection fraction; family history of sudden death or of congenital QT interval prolongation

Hepatic impairment manufacturer advises caution in severe impairment—monitor ECG and plasma potassium concentration

Renal impairment manufacturer advises caution in severe impairment—monitor ECG and plasma potassium concentration

◻ **ARTEMETHER WITH LUMEFANTRINE (*continued*)**

Pregnancy toxicity in *animal* studies with arte-mether; manufacturer advises use only if potential benefit outweighs risk

Breast-feeding manufacturer advises avoid breast-feeding for at least 1 week after last dose; present in milk in *animal* studies

Side-effects abdominal pain, anorexia, diarrhoea, vomiting, nausea; palpitation, prolonged QT interval; cough; headache, dizziness, sleep disturbances, asthenia, paraesthesia; arthralgia, myalgia; pruritus, rash; *less commonly* ataxia, hypoaesthesia, clonus

Indication and dose

Treatment of acute uncomplicated falciparum malaria see p. 401

Treatment of benign malaria see p. 402

Administration tablets may be crushed just before administration

Riamet® (Novartis) ▼ [PoM]
Tablets, yellow, artemether 20 mg, lumefantrine 120 mg, net price 24-tab pack = £22.50. Label: 21, counselling, skilled tasks

Chloroquine

Chloroquine is used for the *prophylaxis of malaria* in areas of the world where the *risk of chloroquine-resistant falciparum malaria is still low*. It is also used with proguanil when chloroquine-resistant falciparum malaria is present but this regimen may not give optimal protection (see specific recommendations by country, p. 404).

Chloroquine is **no longer recommended** for the *treatment of falciparum malaria* owing to widespread resistance, nor is it recommended if the infective species is *not known* or if the infection is *mixed*; in these cases treatment should be with quinine, *Malarone®*, or *Riamet®* (for details, see p. 401). It is still recommended for the *treatment of benign malarias* (for details, see p. 402).

CHLOROQUINE

Cautions may exacerbate psoriasis, neurological disorders (avoid for prophylaxis if history of epilepsy, see notes above), may aggravate myasthenia gravis, severe gastro-intestinal disorders, G6PD deficiency (see section 9.1.5); ophthalmic examination with long-term therapy; avoid concurrent therapy with hepatotoxic drugs—other **interactions**: Appendix 1 (chloroquine and hydroxychloroquine)

Hepatic impairment use with caution in moderate to severe impairment

Renal impairment manufacturers advise caution; see also Prophylaxis Against Malaria, p. 404

Pregnancy benefit of prophylaxis and treatment in malaria outweighs risk; see also Benign Malarias (treatment), p. 403 and Prophylaxis Against Malaria, p. 404

Breast-feeding amount in milk probably too small to be harmful; see also Prophylaxis Against Malaria, p. 404

Side-effects gastro-intestinal disturbances, headache; also hypotension, convulsions, visual disturbances, depigmentation or loss of hair, skin reactions (rashes, pruritus); rarely, bone-marrow suppression, hypersensitivity reactions such as urticaria and angioedema; other side-effects (not usually associated with malaria prophylaxis or treatment), see under Antimalarials, section 10.1.3; very toxic in **overdosage**—immediate advice from poisons centres essential (see also p. 41)

Indication and dose

Prophylaxis of malaria
- By mouth
  Dose (expressed as chloroquine base) preferably started 1 week before entering endemic area and continued for 4 weeks after leaving (see notes above)

  Child up to 12 weeks, body-weight under 6 kg
  37.5 mg once weekly

  Child 12 weeks–1 year, body-weight 6–10 kg
  75 mg once weekly

  Child 1–4 years, body-weight 10–16 kg
  112.5 mg once weekly

  Child 4–8 years, body-weight 16–25 kg 150 mg once weekly (or 155 mg once weekly if tablets used)

  Child 8–13 years, body-weight 25–45 kg
  225 mg once weekly (or 232.5 mg once weekly if tablets used)

  Child over 13 years, body-weight over 45 kg
  310 mg once weekly
  Counselling Warn travellers about **importance** of avoiding mosquito bites, **importance** of taking prophylaxis regularly, and **importance** of immediate visit to doctor if ill within 1 year and **especially** within 3 months of return. For details, see notes above

Treatment of benign malaria see p. 402

Note Chloroquine doses in BNFC may differ from those in product literature

◁ **CHLOROQUINE (continued)**

[1]**Avloclor®** (AstraZeneca) `PoM`
Tablets, scored, chloroquine phosphate 250 mg
(≡ chloroquine base 155 mg). Net price 20-tab
pack = £1.22. Label: 5, counselling, prophylaxis, see
above

[1]**Malarivon®** (Wallace Mfg) `PoM`
Syrup, chloroquine phosphate 80 mg/5 mL (≡
chloroquine base 50 mg/5 mL), net price 75 mL =
£8.75. Label: 5, counselling, prophylaxis, see above

[1]**Nivaquine®** (Sanofi-Aventis) `PoM`
Syrup, golden, chloroquine sulphate 68 mg/5 mL
(≡ chloroquine base 50 mg/5 mL), net price

100 mL = £4.60. Label: 5, counselling, prophylaxis,
see above

◀**With proguanil**
For cautions and side-effects of proguanil see Proguanil; for dose see Chloroquine and Proguanil

[1]**Paludrine/Avloclor®** (AstraZeneca)
Tablets, travel pack of 14 tablets of chloroquine
phosphate 250 mg (≡ chloroquine base 155 mg)
and 98 tablets of proguanil hydrochloride 100 mg,
net price 112-tab pack = £8.79. Label: 5, 21, counselling, prophylaxis, see above

---

Mefloquine

Mefloquine is used for the *prophylaxis of malaria* in areas of the world where there is a *high risk of chloroquine-resistant falciparum malaria* (for details, see specific recommendations by country, p. 404).

Mefloquine is now rarely used for the *treatment of falciparum malaria* because of increased resistance. It is rarely used for the treatment of benign malarias because better tolerated alternatives are available. Mefloquine should not be used for treatment if it has been used for prophylaxis.

◢ MEFLOQUINE

Cautions cardiac conduction disorders; epilepsy
(avoid for prophylaxis); not recommended in
infants under 3 months (5 kg); **interactions:**
Appendix 1 (mefloquine)
Skilled tasks Dizziness or a disturbed sense of balance
may affect performance of skilled tasks; effects may
persist for up to 3 weeks

Contra-indications hypersensitivity to quinine;
avoid for prophylaxis if history of psychiatric
disorders (including depression) or convulsions

Hepatic impairment avoid for chemoprophylaxis
in severe liver disease

Pregnancy manufacturer advises adequate
contraception during prophylaxis and for 3
months after stopping (teratogenicity in *animal*
studies), but see also p. 404

Breast-feeding present in milk but risk to infant
minimal; see also, p. 404

Side-effects nausea, vomiting, dyspepsia, abdominal pain, diarrhoea; headache, dizziness, sleep
disturbances; *less frequently* anorexia, bradycardia, fatigue, abnormal dreams, fever, tinnitus,
and neuropsychiatric reactions (including sensory and motor neuropathies, tremor, ataxia,
anxiety, depression, panic attacks, agitation, hallucinations, psychosis, convulsions); *rarely* suicidal ideation; *very rarely* pneumonitis; also
reported, circulatory disorders (including hypotension and hypertension), chest pain, tachycardia, palpitation, cardiac conduction disorders,
oedema, dyspnoea, encephalopathy, leucopenia,
leucocytosis, thrombocytopenia, muscle weakness, myalgia, arthralgia, visual disturbances,

vestibular disorders, rash (including Stevens-Johnson syndrome), pruritus, and alopecia

Licensed use not licensed for use in children
under 5 kg body-weight and under 3 months

Indication and dose

Prophylaxis of malaria preferably started 2½
weeks before entering endemic area and continued for 4 weeks after leaving (see notes above)
• By mouth
  Child body-weight 5–16 kg 62.5 mg once
  weekly
  Child body-weight 16–25 kg 125 mg once
  weekly
  Child body-weight 25–45 kg 187.5 mg once
  weekly
  Child body-weight over 45 kg 250 mg once
  weekly
  Long-term chemoprophylaxis Mefloquine prophylaxis
  can be taken for up to 1 year
  Counselling Inform travellers and carers of children
  travelling about adverse reactions of mefloquine and,
  if they occur, to seek medical advice on alternative
  antimalarials before the next dose is due. Also warn
  travellers and carers of children travelling about
  importance of avoiding mosquito bites, **importance**
  of taking prophylaxis regularly, and **importance** of
  immediate visit to doctor if ill within 1 year and
  especially within 3 months of return. For details, see
  notes above
  Note Mefloquine doses in BNFC may differ from those
  in product literature

Administration Tablet may be crushed and mixed
with food such as jam or honey just before
administration

---

1. Can be sold to the public provided it is licensed and labelled for the prophylaxis of malaria. Drugs for malaria prophylaxis not prescribable on the NHS; health authorities may investigate circumstances under which antimalarials are prescribed

◻ **MEFLOQUINE (continued)**

[1]**Lariam**® (Roche) [PoM]
Tablets, scored, mefloquine (as hydrochloride)
250 mg. Net price 8-tab pack = £14.53. Label: 21,

25, 27, counselling, skilled tasks, prophylaxis, see above

Primaquine

Primaquine is used to eliminate the liver stages of *P. vivax* or *P. ovale following chloroquine treatment* (for details, see p. 402).

PRIMAQUINE

Cautions G6PD deficiency (test blood, see under Benign Malarias (treatment), p. 402); systemic diseases associated with granulocytopenia (e.g. juvenile idiopathic arthritis, lupus erythematosus); **interactions**: Appendix 1 (primaquine)

Pregnancy risk of neonatal haemolysis and methaemoglobinaemia in third trimester; see also, p. 403

Breast-feeding no information available; theoretical risk of haemolysis in G6PD-deficient infants

Side-effects nausea, vomiting, anorexia, abdominal pain; *less commonly* methaemoglobinaemia, haemolytic anaemia especially in G6PD deficiency, leucopenia

Licensed use not licensed

Indication and dose

> Adjunct in the treatment of *Plasmodium vivax* and *P. ovale* malaria (eradication of liver stages) for dose see Benign Malarias, p. 402

Primaquine (Non-proprietary)
Tablets, primaquine (as phosphate) 7.5 mg or 15 mg
Available from 'special-order' manufacturers or specialist importing companies, see p. 957

Proguanil

Proguanil is used (usually *with chloroquine*, but occasionally *alone*) for the *prophylaxis of malaria*, (for details, see specific recommendations by country, p. 404).

Proguanil used alone is not suitable for the *treatment of malaria*; however, *Malarone*® (a combination of atovaquone with proguanil) is licensed for the treatment of acute uncomplicated falciparum malaria.

Malarone® is also used for the *prophylaxis of falciparum malaria* in areas of widespread mefloquine or chloroquine resistance. *Malarone*® is also used as an alternative to mefloquine or doxycycline. *Malarone*® is particularly suitable for short trips to highly chloroquine-resistant areas because it needs to be taken only for 7 days after leaving an endemic area.

PROGUANIL HYDROCHLORIDE

Cautions interactions: Appendix 1 (proguanil)

Renal impairment (see notes under Prophylaxis against malaria). Use half normal dose if estimated glomerular filtration rate 20–60 mL/minute/1.73 m². Use one-quarter normal dose on alternate days if estimated glomerular filtration rate 10–20 mL/minute/1.73 m². Use one-quarter normal dose once weekly if estimated glomerular filtration rate less than 10 mL/minute/1.73 m²; increased risk of haematological toxicity.

Pregnancy benefit of prophylaxis in malaria outweighs risk; adequate folate supplements should be given to mother; see also p. 404

Breast-feeding amount in milk probably too small to be harmful when used for malaria prophylaxis; see also p. 404

Side-effects mild gastric intolerance, diarrhoea, and constipation; occasionally mouth ulcers and stomatitis; *very rarely* cholestasis, vasculitis, skin reactions and hair loss

Indication and dose

> Prophylaxis of malaria preferably started 1 week before entering endemic area and continued for 4 weeks after leaving (see notes above)
> - By mouth
>   Child up to 12 weeks, body-weight under 6 kg 25 mg once daily
>   Child 12 weeks–1 year, body-weight 6–10 kg 50 mg once daily
>   Child 1–4 years, body-weight 10–16 kg 75 mg once daily
>   Child 4–8 years, body-weight 16–25 kg 100 mg once daily
>   Child 8–13 years, body-weight 25–45 kg 150 mg once daily
>   Child over 13 years, body-weight over 45 kg 200 mg once daily
> **Counselling** Warn travellers and carers of children travelling about **importance** of avoiding mosquito bites, **importance** of taking prophylaxis regularly, and **importance** of immediate visit to doctor if ill within

---

1. Drugs for malaria prophylaxis not prescribable on the NHS; health authorities may investigate circumstances under which antimalarials prescribed

◁ PROGUANIL HYDROCHLORIDE (*continued*)

1 year and **especially** within 3 months of return. For details, see notes above
Note Proguanil doses in BNFC may differ from those in product literature

Administration Tablets may be crushed and mixed with food such as milk, jam or honey just before administration

[1] **Paludrine®** (AstraZeneca)
Tablets, scored, proguanil hydrochloride 100 mg. Net price 98-tab pack = £7.43. Label: 21, counselling, prophylaxis, see above

◢**With chloroquine**
See under Chloroquine

■ PROGUANIL HYDROCHLORIDE WITH ATOVAQUONE

Cautions diarrhoea or vomiting (reduced absorption of atovaquone); efficacy not evaluated in cerebral or complicated malaria (including hyperparasitaemia, pulmonary oedema or renal failure); **interactions**: see Appendix 1 (proguanil, atovaquone)

Renal impairment avoid for malaria prophylaxis and, if possible, for treatment if estimated glomerular filtration rate less than 30 mL/minute/ 1.73 m^2

Pregnancy manufacturer advises avoid unless essential

Breast-feeding use only if no suitable alternative available; see also Breast-feeding, p. 404

Side-effects abdominal pain, nausea, vomiting, diarrhoea; cough; headache, dizziness, insomnia, abnormal dreams, depression, anorexia, fever; rash, pruritus; *less frequently* stomatitis, palpitation, anxiety, blood disorders, hyponatraemia, and hair loss; also reported hepatitis, cholestasis, tachycardia, hallucinations, seizures, vasculitis, mouth ulcers, and Stevens-Johnson syndrome

Indication and dose

See preparations

Counselling Warn travellers about **importance** of avoiding mosquito bites, **importance** of taking prophylaxis regularly, and **importance** of immediate visit to doctor if ill within 1 year and **especially** within 3 months of return. For details, see notes above

[2] **Malarone®** (GSK) PoM
Tablets ('standard'), pink, f/c, proguanil hydrochloride 100 mg, atovaquone 250 mg. Net price 12-tab pack = £25.21. Label: 21, counselling, prophylaxis, see above

Dose
Prophylaxis of malaria started 1–2 days before entering endemic area and continued for 1 week after leaving
• By mouth
  Child body-weight over 40 kg 1 tablet daily

Treatment of malaria
• By mouth
  Child body-weight 11–21 kg 1 tablet daily for 3 days
  Child body-weight 21–31 kg 2 tablets once daily for 3 days
  Child body-weight 31–40 kg 3 tablets once daily for 3 days
  Child body-weight over 40 kg 4 tablets once daily for 3 days

[2] **Malarone® Paediatric** (GSK) PoM
Paediatric tablets, pink, f/c proguanil hydrochloride 25 mg, atovaquone 62.5 mg, net price 12-tab pack = £6.26. Label: 21, counselling, prophylaxis, see above

Dose
Prophylaxis of malaria started 1–2 days before entering endemic area and continued for 1 week after leaving
• By mouth
  Child body-weight 11–21 kg 1 tablet once daily
  Child body-weight 21–31 kg 2 tablets once daily
  Child body-weight 31–40 kg 3 tablets once daily
  Child body-weight over 40 kg use *Malarone®* ('standard') tablets, see above

Treatment of malaria
• By mouth
  Child body-weight 5–9 kg 2 tablets once daily for 3 days
  Child body-weight 9–11 kg 3 tablets once daily for 3 days
  Child body-weight 11 kg and over use *Malarone®* ('standard') tablets, see above

Administration tablets may be crushed and mixed with food or milky drink just before administration

5 Infections

Pyrimethamine

Pyrimethamine should not be used alone, but is used with sulfadoxine.

Pyrimethamine with sulfadoxine is not recommended for the *prophylaxis of malaria*, but can be used in the treatment of *falciparum malaria* with (or following) *quinine*.

---

1. Can be sold to the public provided it is licensed and labelled for the prophylaxis of malaria. Drugs for malaria prophylaxis not prescribable on the NHS; health authorities may investigate circumstances under which antimalarials are prescribed
2. Drugs for malaria prophylaxis not prescribable on the NHS; health authorities may investigate circumstances under which antimalarials prescribed

PYRIMETHAMINE WITH SULFADOXINE

Cautions see under Pyrimethamine (section 5.4.7) and under Co-trimoxazole (section 5.1.8); not recommended for prophylaxis (severe side-effects on long-term use); **interactions**: Appendix 1 (pyrimethamine, sulphonamides)

Contra-indications see under Pyrimethamine (section 5.4.7) and under Co-trimoxazole (section 5.1.8); sulphonamide allergy

Pregnancy possible teratogenic risk in *first trimester* as pyrimethamine is a folate antagonist; in *third trimester*—risk of neonatal haemolysis and methaemoglobinaemia; fear of increased risk of neonatal kernicterus appears unfounded; see also p. 402

Breast-feeding small risk of neonatal kernicterus in jaundiced infants; risk of haemolysis in G6PD-deficient child due to sulfadoxine

Side-effects see under Pyrimethamine (section 5.4.7) and under Co-trimoxazole (section 5.1.8); pulmonary infiltrates (e.g. eosinophilic or allergic alveolitis) reported—discontinue if cough or shortness of breath

Licensed use not licensed for use in children of body-weight under 5 kg

Indication and dose

Adjunct to quinine in treatment of *Plasmodium falciparum* malaria see p. 401

Prophylaxis not recommended by UK malaria experts

Pyrimethamine with sulfadoxine (Non-proprietary) PoM

Tablets, scored, pyrimethamine 25 mg, sulfadoxine 500 mg, net price 3-tab pack = 74p

Note Also known as *Fansidar®*

Available from 'special-order' manufacturers or specialist importing companies, see p. 957

Quinine

Quinine is not suitable for the *prophylaxis of malaria*.

Quinine is used for the *treatment of falciparum malaria* or if the infective species is *not known* or if the infection is *mixed* (for details see p. 401).

QUININE

Cautions cardiac disease (including atrial fibrillation, conduction defects, heart block)—monitor ECG during parenteral treatment; monitor blood glucose and electrolyte concentration during parenteral treatment; G6PD deficiency (see section 9.1.5); **interactions**: Appendix 1 (quinine)

Contra-indications haemoglobinuria, myasthenia gravis, optic neuritis, tinnitus

Hepatic impairment for treatment of malaria in severe impairment, reduce parenteral maintenance dose to 5–7 mg/kg of quinine salt

Renal impairment for treatment of malaria in severe impairment, reduce parenteral maintenance dose to 5–7 mg/kg of quinine salt

Pregnancy risk of teratogenesis with high doses in *first trimester*, but in malaria benefit of treatment outweighs risk, see also p. 402

Breast-feeding present in milk but not known to be harmful

Side-effects cinchonism, including tinnitus, headache, hot and flushed skin, nausea, abdominal pain, rashes, visual disturbances (including temporary blindness), confusion; cardiovascular effects (see Cautions); hypersensitivity reactions including angioedema; hypoglycaemia (especially after parenteral administration); blood disorders (including thrombocytopenia and intravascular coagulation); acute renal failure; photosensitivity; very toxic in **overdosage**—immediate advice from poisons centres essential (see also p. 41)

Licensed use injection not licensed

Indication and dose

Treatment of malaria see p. 401

Note Quinine (anhydrous base) 100 mg ≡ quinine bisulphate 169 mg ≡ quinine dihydrochloride 122 mg ≡ quinine hydrochloride 122 mg ≡ quinine sulphate 121 mg. Quinine bisulphate 300-mg tablets are available but provide less quinine than 300 mg of the dihydrochloride, hydrochloride, or sulphate

Administration for *intravenous infusion*, dilute to a concentration of 2 mg/mL (max. 30 mg/mL in fluid restriction) with Glucose 5% *or* Sodium Chloride 0.9% and give over 4 hours

Quinine Sulphate (Non-proprietary) PoM

Tablets, coated, quinine sulphate 200 mg, net price 28-tab pack = £2.63; 300 mg, 28-tab pack = £2.43

Quinine Dihydrochloride (Non-proprietary) PoM

Injection, quinine dihydrochloride 300 mg/mL. For dilution and use as an infusion. 1- and 2-mL amps

Available from 'special-order' manufacturers or specialist importing companies, see p. 957

Note Intravenous injection of quinine is so hazardous that it has been superseded by infusion

Tetracyclines

Doxycycline (section 5.1.3) is used in children over 12 years for the *prophylaxis of malaria* in areas of *widespread mefloquine or chloroquine resistance*. Doxycycline is also used as an alternative to mefloquine or *Malarone®* (for details, see specific recommendations by country, p. 404).

Doxycycline is also used as an *adjunct to quinine in the treatment of falciparum malaria* (for details see p. 401).

DOXYCYCLINE

Cautions section 5.1.3
Contra-indications section 5.1.3
Hepatic impairment section 5.1.3
Renal impairment section 5.1.3
Pregnancy section 5.1.3
Breast-feeding section 5.1.3
Side-effects section 5.1.3
Licensed use not licensed for use in children under 12 years

Indication and dose

Prophylaxis of malaria preferably started 1–2 days before entering endemic area and continued for 4 weeks after leaving (see notes above)
• By mouth
  Child over 12 years 100 mg once daily

Treatment of falciparum malaria see p. 401

◢Preparations
Section 5.1.3

5.4.2 Amoebicides

Metronidazole is the drug of choice for *acute invasive amoebic dysentery* since it is very effective against vegetative forms of *Entamoeba histolytica* which can cause ulceration of the large intestine. **Tinidazole** is also effective. Metronidazole and tinidazole are also active against amoebae which may have migrated to the liver. Treatment with metronidazole (or tinidazole) is followed by a 10-day course of diloxanide furoate.

Diloxanide furoate is the drug of choice for asymptomatic patients with *E. histolytica* cysts in the faeces; metronidazole and tinidazole are relatively ineffective. Diloxanide furoate is relatively free from toxic effects and the usual course is of 10 days, given alone for chronic infections or following metronidazole or tinidazole treatment.

For *amoebic abscesses* of the liver **metronidazole** is effective; tinidazole is an alternative. Aspiration of the abscess is indicated where it is suspected that it may rupture or where there is no improvement after 72 hours of metronidazole; the aspiration may need to be repeated. Aspiration aids penetration of metronidazole and, for abscesses with large volume of pus, if carried out in conjunction with drug therapy, may reduce the period of disability.

Diloxanide furoate is not effective against hepatic amoebiasis, but a 10-day course should be given at the completion of metronidazole or tinidazole treatment to destroy any amoebae in the gut.

DILOXANIDE FUROATE

Pregnancy manufacturer advises avoid—no information available
Breast-feeding manufacturer advises avoid
Side-effects flatulence, vomiting, urticaria, pruritus
Licensed use not licensed for use in children under 25 kg body-weight
Indication and dose

Chronic amoebiasis and as adjunct to metronidazole or tinidazole in acute amoebiasis
• By mouth
  Child 1 month–12 years 6.6 mg/kg 3 times daily for 10 days

  Child 12–18 years 500 mg 3 times daily for 10 days

Diloxanide (Sovereign) [PoM]
Tablets, diloxanide furoate 500 mg, net price 30-tab pack = £42.95. Label: 9

◢Extemporaneous formulations available see Extemporaneous Preparations, p. 8

METRONIDAZOLE

Cautions section 5.1.11
Hepatic impairment section 5.1.11
Pregnancy section 5.1.11
Breast-feeding section 5.1.11
Side-effects section 5.1.11
Indication and dose
Anaerobic infections section 5.1.11

◁ **METRONIDAZOLE** *(continued)*

Invasive intestinal amoebiasis, extra-intestinal amoebiasis (including liver abscess)
- By mouth

Child 1–3 years 200 mg 3 times daily for 5 days in intestinal infection (for 5–10 days in extra-intestinal infection)

Child 3–7 years 200 mg 4 times daily for 5 days in intestinal infection (for 5–10 days in extra-intestinal infection)

Child 7–10 years 400 mg 3 times daily for 5 days in intestinal infection (for 5–10 days in extra-intestinal infection)

Child 10–18 years 800 mg 3 times daily for 5 days in intestinal infection (for 5–10 days in extra-intestinal infection)

Urogenital trichomoniasis
- By mouth

Child 1–3 years 50 mg 3 times daily for 7 days

Child 3–7 years 100 mg twice daily for 7 days

Child 7–10 years 100 mg 3 times daily for 7 days

Child 10–18 years 200 mg 3 times daily for 7 days *or* 400–500 mg twice daily for 5–7 days, *or* 2 g as a single dose

Giardiasis
- By mouth

Child 1–3 years 500 mg once daily for 3 days

Child 3–7 years 600–800 mg once daily for 3 days

Child 7–10 years 1 g once daily for 3 days

Child 10–18 years 2 g once daily for 3 days *or* 400 mg 3 times daily for 5 days *or* 500 mg twice daily for 7–10 days

◀**Preparations**
Section 5.1.11

■ **TINIDAZOLE**

Cautions see under Metronidazole (section 5.1.11); avoid in acute porphyria (section 9.8.2); **interactions:** Appendix 1 (tinidazole)

Pregnancy manufacturer advises avoid in first trimester

Breast-feeding present in milk—manufacturer advises avoid breast-feeding during and for 3 days after stopping treatment

Side-effects see under Metronidazole (section 5.1.11)

Licensed use licensed for use in children (age range not specified by manufacturer)

Indication and dose

Intestinal amoebiasis
- By mouth

Child 1 month–12 years 50–60 mg/kg (max. 2 g) once daily for 3 days

Child 12–18 years 2 g once daily for 2–3 days

Amoebic involvement of liver
- By mouth

Child 1 month–12 years 50–60 mg/kg (max. 2 g) once daily for 5 days

Child 12–18 years 1.5–2 g once daily for 3–6 days

Urogenital trichomoniasis and giardiasis
- By mouth

Child 1 month–12 years single dose of 50–75 mg/kg (max. 2 g) (repeated once if necessary)

Child 12–18 years single dose of 2 g (repeated once if necessary)

Fasigyn® (Pfizer) ᴾᵒᴹ
Tablets, f/c, tinidazole 500 mg, net price 16-tab pack = £11.04. Label: 4, 9, 21, 25

5.4.3 Trichomonacides

Metronidazole (section 5.4.2) is the treatment of choice for *Trichomonas vaginalis* infection. Contact tracing is recommended and sexual contacts should be treated simultaneously. If metronidazole is ineffective, **tinidazole** (section 5.4.2) may be tried.

5.4.4 Antigiardial drugs

Metronidazole (section 5.4.2) is the treatment of choice for *Giardia lamblia* infections. **Tinidazole** (section 5.4.2) may be used as an alternative to metronidazole.

5.4.5 Leishmaniacides

Cutaneous leishmaniasis frequently heals spontaneously but if skin lesions are extensive or unsightly, treatment is indicated, as it is in visceral leishmaniasis (kala-azar). Leishmaniasis should be treated under specialist supervision.

Sodium stibogluconate, an organic pentavalent antimony compound, is the treatment of choice for visceral leishmaniasis. The dose is 20 mg/kg daily (max. 850 mg) for at least 20 days by intramuscular or intravenous injection; the dosage varies with different geographical regions and expert advice should be obtained. Skin lesions can also be treated with sodium stibogluconate.

Amphotericin is used with or after an antimony compound for visceral leishmaniasis unresponsive to the antimonial alone; side-effects may be reduced by using liposomal amphotericin (*AmBisome*®—section 5.2) at a dose of 1–3 mg/kg daily for 10–21 days to a cumulative dose of 21–30 mg/kg *or* at a dose of 3 mg/kg for 5 consecutive days followed by a single dose of 3 mg/kg 6 days later. *Abelcet*®, a lipid formulation of amphotericin is also likely to be effective but less information is available.

Pentamidine isetionate (pentamidine isethionate) (section 5.4.8) has been used in antimony-resistant visceral leishmaniasis, but although the initial response is often good, the relapse rate is high; it is associated with serious side-effects. Other treatments include paromomycin [unlicensed], available from 'special-order' manufacturers or specialist importing companies, see p. 957

SODIUM STIBOGLUCONATE

Cautions intravenous injections must be given slowly over 5 minutes (to reduce risk of local thrombosis) and stopped if coughing or substernal pain; mucocutaneous disease (see below); monitor ECG before and during treatment; heart disease (withdraw if conduction disturbances occur); treat intercurrent infection (e.g. pneumonia)

Mucocutaneous disease Successful treatment of mucocutaneous leishmaniasis may induce severe inflammation around the lesions (may be life-threatening if pharyngeal or tracheal involvement)—may require corticosteroid

Hepatic impairment use with caution

Renal impairment avoid in significant impairment

Pregnancy manufacturer advises use only if potential benefit outweighs risk

Breast-feeding amount probably too small to be harmful

Side-effects anorexia, nausea, vomiting, abdominal pain; ECG changes; coughing (see Cautions); headache, lethargy, arthralgia, myalgia; *rarely* jaundice, flushing, bleeding from nose or gum, substernal pain (see Cautions), vertigo, fever, sweating, and rash; also reported pancreatitis and anaphylaxis; pain and thrombosis on intravenous administration, intramuscular injection also painful

Licensed use licensed for use in children (age range not specified by manufacturer)

Indication and dose

Leishmaniasis for dose, see notes above

Administration injection should be filtered immediately before administration using a filter of 5 microns or less; see also Cautions above

Pentostam® (GSK) ▒PoM▒
Injection, sodium stibogluconate equivalent to pentavalent antimony 100 mg/mL. Net price 100-mL bottle = £66.43

5.4.6 Trypanocides

The prophylaxis and treatment of trypanosomiasis is difficult and differs according to the strain of organism. Expert advice should therefore be obtained.

5.4.7 Drugs for toxoplasmosis

Most infections caused by *Toxoplasma gondii* are self-limiting, and treatment is not necessary. Exceptions are children with eye involvement (toxoplasma choroidoretinitis), and those who are immunosuppressed. Toxoplasmic encephalitis is a common complication of AIDS. The treatment of choice is a combination of **pyrimethamine** and **sulfadiazine** (sulphadiazine), given for several weeks (expert advice **essential**). Pyrimethamine is a folate antagonist, and adverse reactions to this combination are relatively common (folinic acid supplements (see p. 509) and weekly blood counts needed). Alternative regimens use combinations of pyrimethamine with clindamycin or clarithromycin or azithromycin. Long-term secondary prophylaxis is required after treatment of toxoplasmosis

5 Infections

in immunocompromised patients; prophylaxis should continue until immunity recovers.

If toxoplasmosis is acquired in pregnancy, transplacental infection may lead to severe disease in the fetus; specialist advice should be sought on management. Spiramycin may reduce the risk of transmission of maternal infection to the fetus. When there is evidence of placental or fetal infection, pyrimethamine may be given with sulfadiazine and folinic acid after the first trimester.

In neonates without signs of toxoplasmosis, but born to mothers known to have become infected, spiramycin is given while awaiting laboratory results. If toxoplasmosis is confirmed in the infant, pyrimethamine and sulfadiazine are given for 12 months, together with folinic acid.

PYRIMETHAMINE

Cautions blood counts required with prolonged treatment; history of seizures—avoid large loading doses; **interactions**: Appendix 1 (pyrimethamine)

Hepatic impairment manufacturer advises caution

Renal impairment manufacturer advises caution

Pregnancy theoretical teratogenic risk in first trimester (folate antagonist); adequate folate supplement should be given to mother

Breast-feeding present in milk—avoid breast-feeding during toxoplasmosis treatment; avoid other folate antagonists

Side-effects depression of haematopoiesis with high doses, rashes, insomnia

Licensed use not licensed for use in children under 5 years

Indication and dose

Toxoplasmosis in pregnancy (in combination with sulfadiazine and folinic acid (section 8.1)), see notes above

• By mouth

  Child 12–18 years 50 mg once daily until delivery

Congenital toxoplasmosis (in combination with sulfadiazine and folinic acid (section 8.1)),

• By mouth

  Neonate 1 mg/kg twice daily for 2 days, *then* 1 mg/kg once daily for 6 months, *then* 1 mg/kg 3 times a week for 6 months

Malaria no dose stated because not recommended alone

Daraprim® (GSK) [PoM]
Tablets, scored, pyrimethamine 25 mg. Net price 30-tab pack = £2.60

Extemporaneous formulations available see Extemporaneous Preparations, p. 8

SPIRAMYCIN

Cautions cardiac disease, arrhythmias (including predisposition to QT interval prolongation)

Contra-indications sensitivity to other macrolides

Hepatic impairment use with caution

Breast-feeding present in breast milk

Side-effects gastro-intestinal disturbances including nausea, vomiting, diarrhoea; dizziness, headache; rash; hepatotoxicity; *rarely*, prolongation of QT interval, thrombocytopenia and vasculitis

Licensed use not licensed

Indication and dose

Toxoplasmosis in pregnancy see notes above

• By mouth

  Child 12–18 years 1.5 g twice daily until delivery

Chemoprophylaxis of congenital toxoplasmosis

• By mouth

  Neonate 50 mg/kg twice daily

Spiramycin (Non-proprietary)
Tablets, spiramycin 750 000 units (250 mg); 1.5 million units (500 mg); 3 million units (1 g)

Syrup, spiramycin 75 000 units/mL (25 mg/mL)

Note 3000 units ≡ 1 mg spiramycin
Available from 'special-order' manufacturers or specialist importing companies, see p. 957

SULFADIAZINE

Cautions see under Co-trimoxazole, section 5.1.8

Contra-indications see under Co-trimoxazole, section 5.1.8

Renal impairment use with caution; avoid in severe impairment; high risk of crystalluria

⌀ SULFADIAZINE (*continued*)

Pregnancy risk of neonatal haemolysis and methaemoglobinaemia in third trimester; fear of increased risk of kernicterus in neonates appears to be unfounded

Breast-feeding small risk of kernicterus in jaundiced infants and of haemolysis in G6PD-deficient infants

Side-effects see under Co-trimoxazole, section 5.1.8

Licensed use not licensed for use in toxoplasmosis

Indication and dose

Toxoplasmosis in pregnancy (in combination with pyrimethamine and folinic acid (section 8.1)), see notes above
• By mouth
   Child 12–18 years 1 g 3 times daily until delivery

Congenital toxoplasmosis (in combination with pyrimethamine and folinic acid (section 8.1))
• By mouth
   Neonate 50 mg/kg twice daily for 12 months

Sulfadiazine (Non-proprietary) ℗ₒₘ
Tablets, sulfadiazine 500 mg, net price 56-tab pack = £37.50. Label: 9, 27

◢Extemporaneous formulations available see Extemporaneous Preparations, p. 8

5.4.8 Drugs for pneumocystis pneumonia

Pneumonia caused by *Pneumocystis jirovecii* (*Pneumocystis carinii*) occurs in immunosuppressed children; it is a common cause of pneumonia in AIDS. Pneumocystis pneumonia should generally be treated by those experienced in its management. Blood gas measurement is used to assess disease severity.

Treatment

Mild to moderate disease Co-trimoxazole (section 5.1.8) in high dosage is the drug of choice for the treatment of mild to moderate pneumocystis pneumonia.

A combination of **dapsone** with **trimethoprim** 5 mg/kg every 6–8 hours (section 5.1.8) is given by mouth for the treatment of mild to moderate disease [unlicensed indication] in children who cannot tolerate co-trimoxazole.

A combination of **clindamycin** (section 5.1.6) and **primaquine** (section 5.4.1) may be used in the treatment of mild to moderate disease [unlicensed indication]; this combination is associated with considerable toxicity.

Severe disease Co-trimoxazole (section 5.1.8) in high dosage, given by mouth or by intravenous infusion, is the drug of choice for the treatment of severe pneumocystis pneumonia. **Pentamidine isetionate** given by intravenous infusion is an alternative for children who cannot tolerate co-trimoxazole, or who have not responded to it. Pentamidine isetionate is a potentially toxic drug that can cause severe hypotension during or immediately after infusion.

Corticosteroid treatment can be lifesaving in those with severe pneumocystis pneumonia (see Adjunctive Therapy below).

Adjunctive therapy In moderate to severe pneumocystis infections associated with HIV infection, prednisolone (section 6.3.2) is given by mouth in a dose of 2 mg/kg (max. 80 mg daily) for 5 days (alternatively, hydrocortisone may be given parenterally); the dose is then reduced over the next 16 days and then stopped. Corticosteroid treatment should ideally be started at the same time as the anti-pneumocystis therapy and certainly no later than 24–72 hours afterwards. The corticosteroid should be withdrawn before anti-pneumocystis treatment is complete.

Prophylaxis

Prophylaxis against pneumocystis pneumonia should be given to all children with a history of the infection. Prophylaxis against pneumocystis pneumonia should also be considered for severely immunocompromised children. Prophylaxis should continue until immunity recovers sufficiently. It should not be discontinued if the child has oral candidiasis, continues to lose weight, or is receiving cytotoxic therapy or long-term immunosuppressant therapy.

Co-trimoxazole (section 5.1.8) by mouth is the drug of choice for prophylaxis against pneumocystis pneumonia. Co-trimoxazole may be used in infants born to mothers with a high risk of transmission of infection.

Inhaled **pentamidine isetionate** is better tolerated than parenteral pentamidine. Intermittent inhalation of pentamidine isetionate is used for prophylaxis against pneumocystis pneumonia in children unable to tolerate co-trimoxazole. It is effective but children may be prone to extrapulmonary infection. Alternatively, **dapsone** can be used.

DAPSONE

Cautions cardiac or pulmonary disease; anaemia (treat severe anaemia before starting); susceptibility to haemolysis including G6PD deficiency (section 9.1.5); avoid in acute porphyria (section 9.8.2); **interactions:** Appendix 1 (dapsone)

Blood disorders On long-term treatment, children and their carers should be told how to recognise signs of blood disorders and advised to seek immediate medical attention if symptoms such as fever, sore throat, rash, mouth ulcers, purpura, bruising or bleeding develop

Pregnancy neonatal haemolysis and methaemoglobinaemia reported in third trimester; folic acid 5 mg daily should be given to mother throughout pregnancy

Breast-feeding haemolytic anaemia; although significant amount in milk, risk to infant very small unless infant is G6PD deficient

Side-effects haemolysis, methaemoglobinaemia, neuropathy, allergic dermatitis (rarely including toxic epidermal necrolysis and Stevens-Johnson syndrome), anorexia, nausea, vomiting, tachycardia, headache, insomnia, psychosis, hepatitis, agranulocytosis; dapsone syndrome (rash with fever and eosinophilia)—discontinue immediately (may progress to exfoliative dermatitis, hepatitis, hypoalbuminaemia, psychosis and death)

Licensed use not licensed for treatment of *P. jirovecii* pneumonia; monotherapy not licensed for children for prophylaxis of *P. jirovecii* pneumonia

Indication and dose

Treatment of *Pneumocystis jirovecii* (*P. carinii*) pneumonia (in combination with trimethoprim)
• By mouth

Child 1 month–12 years 2 mg/kg (max. 100 mg) once daily

Child 13–18 years 100 mg once daily

Prophylaxis of *Pneumocystis jirovecii* (*P. carinii*) pneumonia
• By mouth

Child 1 month–18 years 2 mg/kg (max. 100 mg) once daily

Dapsone (Non-proprietary) PoM
Tablets, dapsone 50 mg, net price 28-tab pack = £24.54; 100 mg 28-tab pack = £35.81. Label: 8

PENTAMIDINE ISETIONATE

Cautions risk of severe hypotension following administration (establish baseline blood pressure and administer with child lying down; monitor blood pressure closely during administration, and at regular intervals, until treatment concluded); hypokalaemia, hypomagnesaemia, coronary heart disease, bradycardia, history of ventricular arrhythmias, concomitant use with other drugs known to prolong Q-T interval; hypertension or hypotension; hyperglycaemia or hypoglycaemia; leucopenia, thrombocytopenia, or anaemia; carry out laboratory monitoring according to product literature; care required to protect personnel during handling and administration; **interactions:** Appendix 1 (pentamidine isetionate)

Hepatic impairment use with caution

Renal impairment reduce intravenous dose for pneumocystis pneumonia if estimated glomerular filtration rate less than 10 mL/minute/1.73 m²; consult product literature

Pregnancy manufacturer advises avoid unless essential

Breast-feeding manufacturer advises avoid unless essential

Side-effects severe reactions, sometimes fatal, due to hypotension, hypoglycaemia, pancreatitis, and arrhythmias; also leucopenia, thrombocytopenia, acute renal failure, hypocalcaemia; also reported: azotaemia, abnormal liver-function tests, anaemia, hyperkalaemia, nausea and vomiting, dizziness, syncope, flushing, hyperglycaemia, rash, and taste disturbances; Stevens-Johnson syndrome reported; on inhalation, bronchoconstriction (may be prevented by prior use of bronchodilators), cough and shortness of breath; discomfort, pain, induration, abscess formation, and muscle necrosis at injection site

Licensed use *nebuliser solution* not licensed for use in children; nebuliser solution not licensed for primary prevention of pneumocystis pneumonia

Indication and dose

Treatment of *Pneumocystis jirovecii* (*P. carinii*) pneumonia
• By intravenous infusion

Child 1 month–18 years 4 mg/kg once daily for at least 14 days

Prophylaxis of *Pneumocystis jirovecii* (*P. carinii*) pneumonia
• By inhalation of nebulised solution (using suitable equipment—consult product literature)

Child 5–18 years 300 mg every 4 weeks *or* 150 mg every 2 weeks

◁ **PENTAMIDINE ISETIONATE** (*continued*)

Visceral leishmaniasis (kala-azar, section 5.4.5)
- **By deep intramuscular injection**

  Child 1–18 years 3–4 mg/kg on alternate days to max. total of 10 injections; course may be repeated if necessary

Cutaneous leishmaniasis
- **By deep intramuscular injection**

  Child 1–18 years 3–4 mg/kg once or twice weekly until condition resolves (but see also section 5.4.5)

Trypanosomiasis
- **By deep intramuscular injection or intravenous infusion**

  Child 1–18 years 4 mg/kg daily or on alternate days to total of 7–10 injections

Administration Direct intravenous injection should be avoided whenever possible and **never** given rapidly; intramuscular injections should be deep and preferably given into the buttock.

For *intravenous infusion*, reconstitute 300 mg with 3–5 mL Water for Injections (displacement value may be significant), then dilute required dose with 50–250 mL Glucose 5% *or* Sodium Chloride 0.9%; give over at least 60 minutes

Pentacarinat® (Sanofi-Aventis) PoM

Injection, powder for reconstitution, pentamidine isetionate, net price 300-mg vial = £30.45

Nebuliser solution, pentamidine isetionate, net price 300-mg bottle = £32.15

Caution in handling Pentamidine isetionate is toxic and personnel should be adequately protected during handling and administration—consult product literature

5.5 Anthelmintics

5.5.1 Drugs for threadworms
5.5.2 Ascaricides
5.5.3 Drugs for tapeworm infections
5.5.4 Drugs for hookworms
5.5.5 Schistosomicides
5.5.6 Filaricides
5.5.7 Drugs for cutaneous larva migrans
5.5.8 Drugs for strongyloidiasis

Advice on prophylaxis and treatment of helminth infections is available from the following specialist centres:

Birmingham	(0121) 424 0357
Scottish Centre for Infection and Environmental Health (registered users of Travax only)	(0141) 300 1100 (weekdays 2–4 p.m. only)
Liverpool	(0151) 708 9393
London	(020) 7387 9300 (treatment advice only)

5.5.1 Drugs for threadworms

(pinworms, *Enterobius vermicularis*)

Anthelmintics are effective in threadworm infections, but their use needs to be combined with hygiene measures to break the cycle of auto-infection. All members of the family require treatment.

Adult threadworms do not live for longer than 6 weeks and for development of fresh worms, ova must be swallowed and exposed to the action of digestive juices in the upper intestinal tract. Direct multiplication of worms does not take place in the large bowel. Adult female worms lay ova on the perianal skin which causes pruritus; scratching the area then leads to ova being transmitted on fingers to the mouth, often via food eaten with unwashed hands. Washing hands and scrubbing nails before each meal and after each visit to the toilet is essential. A bath taken immediately after rising will remove ova laid during the night.

Mebendazole is the drug of choice for treating threadworm infection in children over 6 months. It is given as a single dose; as reinfection is very common, a second dose may be given after 2 weeks.

Piperazine is available in combination with sennosides as a single-dose preparation.

5

Infections

MEBENDAZOLE

Cautions interactions: Appendix 1 (mebendazole)

Note The patient information leaflet in the *Vermox*® pack includes the statement that it is not suitable for women known to be pregnant or for children under 2 years

Pregnancy manufacturer advises avoid—toxicity in *animal* studies

Breast-feeding amount present in milk too small to be harmful but manufacturer advises avoid

Side-effects *very rarely* abdominal pain, diarrhoea; convulsions (in infants) and rash (including Stevens-Johnson syndrome and toxic epidermal necrolysis) reported

Licensed use not licensed for use in children under 2 years

Indication and dose

Threadworms
• By mouth
Child 6 months—18 years 100 mg as a single dose; if reinfection occurs second dose may be needed after 2 weeks

Whipworms, hookworms (section 5.5.4)
• By mouth
Child 1—18 years 100 mg twice daily for 3 days

Roundworms (section 5.5.2)
• By mouth
Child 1—2 years 100 mg twice daily for 3 days
Child 2—18 years 100 mg twice daily for 3 days *or* 500 mg as a single dose

¹**Mebendazole** (Non-proprietary) (PoM)
Tablets, chewable, mebendazole 100 mg
1. Mebendazole tablets can be sold to the public if supplied for oral use in the treatment of enterobiasis in children over 2 years provided its container or package is labelled to show a max. single dose of 100 mg and it is supplied in a container or package containing not more than 800 mg

Vermox® (Janssen-Cilag) (PoM)
Tablets, orange, scored, chewable, mebendazole 100 mg. Net price 6-tab pack = £1.36
Suspension, mebendazole 100 mg/5 mL. Net price 30 mL = £1.59

PIPERAZINE

Cautions epilepsy

Note Packs on sale to the general public carry a warning to avoid in epilepsy, liver or kidney disease, and to seek medical advice during pregnancy

Hepatic impairment manufacturer advises avoid

Renal impairment use with caution; avoid in severe renal impairment; risk of neurotoxicity

Pregnancy not known to be harmful but manufacturer advises avoid in first trimester

Breast-feeding present in milk—manufacturer advises avoid breast-feeding for 8 hours after dose (express and discard milk during this time)

Side-effects nausea, vomiting, colic, diarrhoea, allergic reactions including urticaria, bronchospasm, and rare reports of arthralgia, fever, Stevens-Johnson syndrome and angioedema; rarely dizziness, muscular inco-ordination ('worm wobble'); drowsiness, nystagmus, vertigo, blurred vision, confusion and clonic contractions in children with neurological or renal abnormalities

Indication and dose
See under preparation, below

◢With sennosides
For cautions, contra-indications, side-effects of senna see section 1.6.2

Pripsen® (Thornton & Ross)
Oral powder, piperazine phosphate 4 g, total sennosides (calculated as sennoside B) 15.3 mg/sachet. Net price two-dose sachet pack = £1.73. Label: 13

Dose
(Stirred into milk or water)

Threadworms
• By mouth
Child 3 months–1 year 1 level 2.5-mL spoonful as a single dose in the morning, repeated after 14 days
Child 1–6 years 1 level 5-mL spoonful as a single dose in the morning, repeated after 14 days
Child 6–18 years content of 1 sachet as a single dose (in the morning), repeated after 14 days

Roundworms first dose as for threadworms; repeat at monthly intervals for up to 3 months if reinfection risk

5.5.2 Ascaricides
(common roundworm infections)

Mebendazole (section 5.5.1) is effective against *Ascaris lumbricoides* and is generally considered to be the drug of choice.

Levamisole [unlicensed] (available from 'special-order' manufacturers or specialist importing companies, see p. 957) is an alternative when mebendazole cannot be used. It is very well tolerated; mild nausea or vomiting has been reported in about 1% of treated patients.

Piperazine may be given in a single dose, see Piperazine, above.

▲ LEVAMISOLE

Cautions epilepsy; juvenile idiopathic arthritis; Sjögren's syndrome

Contra-indications blood disorders

Hepatic impairment use with caution—dose adjustment may be necessary

Pregnancy embryotoxic in *animal* studies, avoid if possible

Breast-feeding no information available

Side-effects nausea, vomiting, diarrhoea; dizziness, headache; on *prolonged treatment* taste disturbances, insomnia, convulsions, influenza-like syndrome, blood disorders, vasculitis, arthralgia, myalgia, rash

Licensed use not licensed

Indication and dose

> **Roundworm** (*Ascaris lumbricoides*)
> * By mouth
> > **Child 1 month–18 years** 2.5–3 mg/kg (max. 150 mg) as a single dose

> **Hookworm**
> * By mouth
> > **Child 1 month–18 years** 2.5 mg/kg (max. 150 mg) as a single dose repeated after 7 days if severe

> **Nephrotic syndrome (specialist supervision section 6.3.2)**
> * By mouth
> > **Child 1month–18 years** 2.5 mg/kg (max. 150 mg) on alternate days

Levamisole (Non-proprietary) PoM
Tablets, levamisole (as hydrochloride) 50 mg
Label: 4
Available from 'special-order' manufacturers or specialist importing companies, see p. 957

5.5.3 Drugs for tapeworm infections

Taenicides

Niclosamide [unlicensed] (available from 'special-order' manufacturers or specialist importing companies, see p. 957) is the most widely used drug for tapeworm infections and side-effects are limited to occasional gastro-intestinal upset, lightheadedness, and pruritus; it is not effective against larval worms. Fears of developing cysticercosis in *Taenia solium* infections have proved unfounded. All the same, an antiemetic can be given before treatment and a laxative can be given 2 hours after niclosamide.

Praziquantel [unlicensed] is available from Merck Serono (*Cysticide*®); it is as effective as niclosamide and is given to children over 4 years of age as a single dose of 5–10 mg/kg after a light breakfast (*or* as a single dose of 25 mg/kg for *Hymenolepis nana*).

Hydatid disease

Cysts caused by *Echinococcus granulosus* grow slowly and asymptomatic children do not always require treatment. Surgical treatment remains the method of choice in many situations. **Albendazole** [unlicensed] (available from 'special-order' manufacturers or specialist importing companies, see p. 957 is used in conjunction with surgery to reduce the risk of recurrence or as primary treatment in inoperable cases. Albendazole is given to children over 2 years of age in a dose of 7.5 mg/kg twice daily (max. 400 mg twice daily) for 28 days followed by 14-day break and then repeated for up to 2–3 cycles. Alveolar echinococcosis due to *E. multilocularis* is usually fatal if untreated. Surgical removal with albendazole cover is the treatment of choice, but where effective surgery is impossible, repeated cycles of albendazole (for a year or more) may help. Careful monitoring of liver function is particularly important during drug treatment.

5.5.4 Drugs for hookworms

(ancylostomiasis, necatoriasis)

Hookworms live in the upper small intestine and draw blood from the point of their attachment to their host. An iron-deficiency anaemia may occur and, if present, effective treatment of the infection requires not only expulsion of the worms but treatment of the anaemia.

Mebendazole (section 5.5.1) has a useful broad-spectrum activity, and is effective against hookworms. **Albendazole** [unlicensed] (available from 'special-order' manufacturers or specialist importing companies, see p. 957) given as a single dose of 400 mg in children over 2 years, is an alternative. **Levamisole** is also effective (section 5.5.2).

5 Infections

5.5.5 Schistosomicides
(bilharziasis)

Adult *Schistosoma haematobium* worms live in the genito-urinary veins and adult *S. mansoni* in those of the colon and mesentery. *S. japonicum* is more widely distributed in veins of the alimentary tract and portal system.

Praziquantel [unlicensed] is available from Merck Serono (*Cysticide*®) and is effective against all human schistosomes. In children over 4 years the dose is 20 mg/kg followed after 4–6 hours by a further dose of 20 mg/kg (20 mg/kg 3 times daily for one day for *S. japonicum* infections). No serious adverse effects have been reported. Of all the available schistosomicides, it has the most attractive combination of effectiveness, broad-spectrum activity, and low toxicity.

5.5.6 Filaricides

Diethylcarbamazine [unlicensed] (available from 'special-order' manufacturers or specialist importing companies, see p. 957) is effective against microfilariae and adult worms of *Loa loa*, *Wuchereria bancrofti*, and *Brugia malayi*. To minimise reactions, treatment in children over 1 month is commenced with a dose of diethylcarbamazine citrate 1 mg/kg in divided doses on the first day and increased gradually over 3 days to 6 mg/kg daily (3 mg/kg daily if child under 10 years) in divided doses; length of treatment varies according to infection type, and usually gives a radical cure for these infections. Close medical supervision is necessary particularly in the early phase of treatment. In heavy infections there may be a febrile reaction, and in heavy *Loa loa* infection there is a small risk of encephalopathy. In such cases treatment must be given under careful in-patient supervision and stopped at the first sign of cerebral involvement (and specialist advice sought).

Ivermectin [unlicensed] (available from 'special-order' manufacturers or specialist importing companies, see p. 957) is very effective in *onchocerciasis* and it is now the drug of choice. In children over 5 years, a single dose of 150 micrograms/kg by mouth produces a prolonged reduction in microfilarial levels. Retreatment at intervals of 6 to 12 months depending on symptoms must be given until the adult worms die out. Reactions are usually slight and most commonly take the form of temporary aggravation of itching and rash. Diethylcarbamazine or suramin should no longer be used for onchocerciasis because of their toxicity.

5.5.7 Drugs for cutaneous larva migrans
(creeping eruption)

Dog and cat hookworm larvae may enter human skin where they produce slowly extending itching tracks usually on the foot. Single tracks can be treated with topical tiabendazole (no commercial preparation available). Multiple infections respond to **ivermectin**, **albendazole** or **tiabendazole** (thiabendazole) by mouth (all unlicensed and available from 'special-order' manufacturers or specialist importing companies, see p. 957).

5.5.8 Drugs for strongyloidiasis

Adult forms of *Strongyloides stercoralis* live in the gut and produce larvae which penetrate the gut wall and invade the tissues, setting up a cycle of auto-infection. **Ivermectin** [unlicensed] in a dose of 200 micrograms/kg daily for 2 days is the treatment of choice for chronic *Strongyloides* infection in children over 5 years. **Albendazole** [unlicensed] is an alternative in children over 2 years given in a dose of 400 mg twice daily for 3 days, repeated after 3 weeks if necessary.

Both of these drugs are available from 'special-order' manufacturers or specialist importing companies, see p. 957.

6 Endocrine system

> This chapter includes advice on the drug management of the following:
> Adrenal suppression during illness, trauma or surgery, p. 452
> Serious infections in patients taking corticosteroids, p. 453
> Nephrotic syndrome, p. 452
> Delayed puberty, p. 460
> Precocious puberty, p. 464
> Diabetes insipidus, p. 471

For hormonal contraception, see section 7.3.

6.1 Drugs used in diabetes

6.1.1 Insulins
6.1.2 Oral antidiabetic drugs
6.1.3 Diabetic ketoacidosis
6.1.4 Treatment of hypoglycaemia
6.1.5 Treatment of diabetic nephropathy and neuropathy
6.1.6 Diagnostic and monitoring devices for diabetes mellitus

Diabetes mellitus occurs because of a lack of insulin or resistance to its action. It is diagnosed by measuring fasting or random blood-glucose concentration (and occasionally by oral glucose tolerance test). Although there are many subtypes, the two principle classes of diabetes are type 1 diabetes and type 2 diabetes.

Type 1 diabetes, (formerly referred to as insulin-dependent diabetes mellitus (IDDM)), is due to a deficiency of insulin following autoimmune destruction of pancreatic beta cells and is the most common form of diabetes in children. Children with type 1 diabetes require administration of insulin.

Type 2 diabetes, (formerly referred to as non-insulin-dependent diabetes mellitus (NIDDM)), is rare in children but the incidence is increasing, particularly in adolescents, as obesity increases. It results from reduced secretion of insulin or from peripheral resistance to the action of insulin, or from a combination of both. Although children may be controlled on diet alone, many require oral antidiabetic drugs or insulin to maintain satisfactory control. There is limited information available on the use of oral anti-diabetic drugs in children (see section 6.1.2). In overweight individuals, type 2 diabetes may be prevented by losing weight and increasing physical activity.

Genetic defects of beta-cell function (formerly referred to as maturity-onset diabetes of the young (MODY)), describes a number of rare disease states, characterised by onset of mild hyperglycaemia, generally before 25 years of age. A sulphonylurea such as gliclazide (p. 437) may be effective in these patients.

Treatment of diabetes   Treatment should be aimed at alleviating symptoms and minimising the risk of long-term complications (see below).

Diabetes is a strong risk factor for cardiovascular disease later in life. Other risk factors for cardiovascular disease (smoking, hypertension, obesity and hyperlipidaemia) should be addressed. The use of an ACE inhibitor (section 2.5.5.1) and of a lipid-regulating drug (section 2.12) can be beneficial in children with diabetes and a high cardiovascular disease risk. For reference to the use of an ACE inhibitor in the management of diabetic nephropathy, see section 6.1.5.

Prevention of diabetic complications   Although rare, retinopathy, neuropathy and nephropathy can occur in children with diabetes. Screening for complications should begin 5 years after diagnosis of diabetes or from 12 years of age. Optimal glycaemic control in both type 1 diabetes and type 2 diabetes reduces, in the long term, the risk of microvascular complications including retinopathy, development of proteinuria and to some extent neuropathy.

A measure of the total glycosylated (or glycated) haemoglobin (HbA_1) or a specific fraction (HbA_{1c}) provides a good indication of long-term glycaemic control. Overall it is ideal to aim for an HbA_{1c} concentration of 48–59 mmol/mol (6.5–7.5%) or less (reference range 20–42 mmol/mol *or* 4–6%), but this cannot always be achieved and for those using insulin there is a significantly increased risk of disabling hypoglycaemia.

Measurement of HbA_{1c}

HbA_{1c} values currently expressed as a percentage, are aligned to the assay used in the Diabetes Control and Complications Trial (DCCT). A new standard, specific for HbA_{1c}, has been created by the International Federation of Clinical Chemistry and Laboratory Medicine (IFCC), which expresses HbA_{1c} values in *mmol of glycosylated haemoglobin per mol of haemoglobin*. UK laboratories now express results in both IFCC-standardised units (mmol/mol) and DCCT-aligned units (%). From 1 June 2011, results will only be reported in IFCC-standardised units.

Equivalent values

IFCC-HbA_{1c} (mmol/mol)	DCCT-HbA_{1c} (%)
42	6.0
48	6.5
53	7.0
59	7.5
64	8.0
75	9.0

Laboratory measurement of serum-fructosamine concentration is technically simpler and cheaper than the measurement of HbA_{1c} and can be used to assess control over short periods of time, particularly when HbA_{1c} monitoring is invalid (e.g. disturbed erythrocyte turnover or abnormal haemoglobin type).

Tight control of blood pressure in hypertensive children with type 2 diabetes may reduce mortality significantly and protects visual acuity (by reducing considerably the risks of maculopathy and retinal photocoagulation) (see also section 2.5).

Driving   Information on the requirements for driving vehicles by individuals receiving treatment for diabetes is available in the BNF (section 6.1) or from the DVLA at www.dvla.gov.uk/medical.aspx.

6.1.1 Insulins

Insulin is a polypeptide hormone that plays a key role in the regulation of carbohydrate, fat, and protein metabolism. There are differences in the amino-acid sequence of animal insulins, human insulins, and the human insulin analogues. Human sequence insulin may be produced semisynthetically by enzymatic modification of porcine insulin (emp) or biosynthetically by recombinant DNA technology using bacteria (crb, prb) or yeast (pyr).

Immunological resistance to insulin action is uncommon. Preparations of human sequence insulin should theoretically be less immunogenic than other insulin preparations, but no real advantage has been shown in trials.

Insulin is inactivated by gastro-intestinal enzymes, and must therefore be given by injection; the subcutaneous route is ideal in most circumstances. Insulin is usually injected into the thighs, buttocks, or abdomen; absorption from a limb site can be increased if the limb is used in strenuous exercise after the injection. Generally, subcutaneous insulin injections cause few problems; lipodystrophy may occur and is a factor in poor glycaemic control. Lipodystrophy can be minimised by using different injection sites in rotation. Local allergic reactions are rare.

Insulin should be given to all children with type 1 diabetes; it may also be needed to treat type 2 diabetes either when other methods cannot control the condition or during periods of acute illness or peri-operatively. Insulin is required in all instances of ketoacidosis (section 6.1.3), which can develop rapidly in children.

Management of diabetes with insulin   The aim of treatment is to achieve the best possible control of blood-glucose concentration without making the child or carer obsessional and to avoid disabling hypoglycaemia; close co-operation is needed between the child or carer and the medical team to achieve good control and thereby reduce the risk of complications.

Insulin preparations can be divided into 3 types:

- those of **short** duration which have a relatively rapid onset of action, namely soluble insulin and the rapid-acting insulin analogues, insulin aspart, insulin glulisine, and insulin lispro (section 6.1.1.1);
- those with an **intermediate** action, e.g. isophane insulin (section 6.1.1.2); and
- those whose action is slower in onset and lasts for **long** periods, e.g. protamine zinc insulin, insulin detemir, and insulin glargine (section 6.1.1.2)

The duration of the action of a particular type of insulin can vary from one child to another, and needs to be assessed individually.

Mixtures of insulin preparations may be required and appropriate combinations have to be determined for the individual child. Treatment should be started with several doses of short-acting insulin (soluble insulin or a rapid-acting insulin analogue) given throughout the day with a longer-acting insulin given once or twice daily. Alternatively, for those who have difficulty with, or prefer not to use, multiple daily injection regimens or in whom such regimens fail to achieve adequate glycaemic control, a mixture of premixed short- and intermediate-acting insulins (most commonly in a proportion of 30% soluble insulin and 70% isophane insulin) can be given twice daily. The dose of short-acting or rapid-acting insulin (or the proportion of the short-acting soluble insulin component in premixed insulin) can be increased in those with excessive postprandial hyperglycaemia. The dose of insulin is increased gradually according to the child's individual requirements, taking care to avoid troublesome hypoglycaemia.

6

Endocrine system

Initiation of insulin may be followed by a partial remission phase or 'honeymoon period' when lower doses of insulin are required than are subsequently necessary to maintain glycaemic control.

Examples of insulin regimens

- Multiple injection regimen: short-acting insulin or rapid-acting insulin analogue, before meals
  With intermediate-acting or long-acting insulin, once or twice daily;

- Short-acting insulin or rapid-acting insulin analogue mixed with intermediate-acting insulin, twice daily (before breakfast and the main evening meal);

- Short-acting insulin or rapid-acting insulin analogue mixed with intermediate-acting insulin, before breakfast
  With short-acting or rapid-acting insulin analogue alone, before afternoon snack or the main evening meal, and intermediate-acting insulin or long-acting insulin, at bedtime;

- Continuous subcutaneous insulin infusion (see below).

Insulin requirements   Most prepubertal children require around 0.6–0.8 units/kg/day of insulin after the initial temporary remission phase. Unless the child has a very sedentary life-style, a requirement for higher doses may indicate poor compliance, poor absorption of insulin from the injection site (e.g. because of lipohypertrophic sites), or the beginning of puberty. During puberty up to 1.5–2 units/kg/day of insulin may be required, especially during growth spurts. Around 1 year after menarche or after the growth spurt in boys, the dose may need to be adjusted to avoid excessive weight gain. Insulin requirements can be *increased* by infection, stress, and accidental or surgical trauma. Insulin requirements can be *reduced* in very active individuals, in those with certain endocrine disorders (e.g. Addison's disease, hypopituitarism), or in coeliac disease. Insulin requirements should be assessed frequently in all these circumstances.

Hepatic impairment   Insulin requirements may be decreased in patients with hepatic impairment.

Renal impairment   Insulin requirements may fall in patients with renal impairment and therefore dose reduction may be necessary. The compensatory response to hypoglycaemia is impaired in renal impairment.

Pregnancy and breast-feeding   During pregnancy and breast-feeding, insulin requirements may alter and doses should be assessed frequently by an experienced diabetes physician. The dose of insulin generally needs to be increased in the second and third trimesters of pregnancy. The short-acting insulin analogues, insulin aspart and insulin lispro, are not known to be harmful, and may be used during pregnancy and breast-feeding. The safety of long-acting insulin analogues in pregnancy has not been established, therefore isophane insulin is recommended where longer-acting insulins are needed.

Insulin administration   Insulin is generally given by *subcutaneous injection* 30 minutes before a meal, except for rapid-acting insulins, which should be given immediately before, with, or even immediately after a meal (section 6.1.1.1); the injection site should be rotated to prevent lipodystrophy. Injection devices ('pens') (section 6.1.1.3), which hold the insulin in a cartridge and meter the required dose, are convenient to use. Insulin syringes (for use with needles) are less popular with children and carers, but may be required for insulins not available in cartridge form.

For intensive insulin regimens multiple subcutaneous injections (3 or more times daily) are usually recommended.

Short-acting insulins (soluble insulin, insulin aspart, insulin glulisine, and insulin lispro) can also be given by *continuous subcutaneous infusion* using a portable infusion pump. This device delivers a continuous basal insulin infusion and patient-activated bolus doses at meal times. This technique is appropriate only for children who suffer recurrent hypoglycaemia or marked morning rise in blood-glucose concentration despite optimised multiple-injection regimens. Children on subcutaneous insulin infusion must be highly motivated, able to monitor their blood-glucose concentration or have it monitored by a carer, and have expert training, advice, and supervision from an experienced healthcare team.

NICE guidance

Continuous subcutaneous insulin infusion for the treatment of diabetes mellitus (type 1) (July 2008)

Continuous subcutaneous insulin infusion is recommended as an option in children over 12 years with type 1 diabetes:

- who suffer repeated or unpredictable hypoglycaemia, whilst attempting to achieve optimal glycaemic control with multiple-injection regimens, **or**

- whose glycaemic control remains inadequate (HbA$_{1c}$ over 8.5%) despite optimised multiple-injection regimens (including the use of long-acting insulin analogues where appropriate).

Continuous subcutaneous insulin infusion is also recommended as an option for children under 12 years with type 1 diabetes for whom multiple-injection regimens are considered impractical or inappropriate. Children on insulin pumps should undergo a trial of multiple-injection therapy between the ages of 12 and 18 years.

Soluble insulin by the *intravenous route* is reserved for urgent treatment e.g in diabetic ketoacidosis, and for fine control in serious illness and in the peri-operative period (see under Diabetes and Surgery, below).

Monitoring   All carers and children need to be trained to monitor blood-glucose concentrations (section 6.1.6). Since blood-glucose concentration varies substantially throughout the day, 'normoglycaemia' cannot always be achieved throughout a 24-hour period without causing damaging hypoglycaemia. It is therefore best to recommend that children should maintain a blood-glucose concentration of between 4 and 10 mmol/litre for most of the time (4–8 mmol/litre before meals and less than 10 mmol/litre after meals), while accepting that on occasions, for brief periods, it will be above these values; efforts should be made to prevent the blood-glucose concentration from falling below 4 mmol/litre. Children using multiple injection regimens should understand how to adjust their insulin dose according to their carbohydrate intake. With fixed-dose insulin regimens, the carbohydrate intake needs to be regulated, and should be distributed throughout the day to match the insulin regimen. The intake of energy and of simple and complex carbohydrates should be adequate to allow normal growth and development but obesity must be avoided.

Hypoglycaemia   Hypoglycaemia is a potential problem for all children using insulin, and they and their carers should be given careful instruction on how to avoid it.

Very tight control of diabetes lowers the blood-glucose concentration needed to trigger hypoglycaemic symptoms; an increase in the frequency of hypoglycaemic episodes may reduce the warning symptoms experienced by the child. Loss of warning of hypoglycaemia among insulin-treated children can be a serious hazard, especially for cyclists and drivers.

To restore the warning signs, episodes of hypoglycaemia must be minimised; this involves appropriate adjustment of insulin type, dose, and frequency, together with suitable timing and quantity of meals and snacks.

Diabetes and surgery   Children with type 1 diabetes should undergo surgery in centres with facilities for, and expertise in, the care of children with diabetes. Detailed local protocols should be available to all healthcare professionals involved in the treatment of these children.

Children with type 1 diabetes who require surgery:

- should be admitted to hospital for general anaesthesia;

- should receive insulin, even if they are fasting, to avoid ketoacidosis;

- should receive glucose infusion when fasting before an anaesthetic to prevent hypoglycaemia;

- should have careful monitoring of blood-glucose concentration because surgery may cause hyperglycaemia.

Elective surgery   Surgery in children with diabetes is best scheduled early on the list, preferably in the morning. If glycaemic control is poor it is advisable to admit

6

Endocrine system

the child well in advance of surgery. On the *evening before surgery*, blood-glucose should be measured frequently, especially before meals and snacks and at bedtime; urine should be tested for ketones. The usual evening or bedtime insulin and bedtime snack should be given. Ketosis or severe hypoglycaemia require correction, preferably by overnight intravenous infusion (section 6.1.3 and section 6.1.4), and the surgery may need to be postponed.

For *minor procedures that require fasting*, a slight modification of the usual regimen may be all that is necessary e.g. for early morning procedures delay insulin and food until immediately after the procedure.

For *other types of elective surgery*, consult local treatment protocols.

Emergency surgery Intravenous fluids and an insulin infusion should be started immediately (see Intravenous Fluids and Continuous Insulin Infusion, below). If ketoacidosis is present the recommendations for diabetic ketoacidosis should be followed (section 6.1.3).

Intravenous fluids and continuous insulin infusion Blood-glucose and plasma-electrolyte concentrations must be measured frequently in a child receiving intravenous support. Intravenous infusion should be continued until after the child starts to eat and drink. The following infusions should be used and adjusted according to the child's fluid and electrolyte requirements:

- Constant infusion of sodium chloride 0.45% and glucose 5% intravenous infusion together with potassium chloride 20 mmol/litre (provided that plasma-potassium concentration is not raised) at a rate determined by factors such as volume depletion and age; the amount of potassium chloride infused is adjusted according to plasma electrolyte measurements;

- Constant infusion of soluble insulin 1 unit/mL in sodium chloride 0.9% intravenous infusion initially at a rate of 0.025 units/kg/hour (up to 0.05 units/kg/hour if the child is unwell), then adjusted according to blood-glucose concentration (frequent monitoring necessary) in line with locally agreed protocols and the child's volume depletion and age;

- Blood-glucose concentration should be maintained between 5 and 10 mmol/litre. If the glucose concentration falls below 5 mmol/litre, glucose 10% intravenous infusion may be required; conversely, if the glucose concentration persistently exceeds 14 mmol/litre, sodium chloride 0.9% intravenous infusion should be substituted;

- The insulin infusion may be stopped temporarily for 10–15 minutes if blood-glucose concentration falls below 4 mmol/litre.

The usual subcutaneous insulin regimen should be started before the first meal (but the dose may need to be 10–20% higher than usual if the child is still bedbound or unwell) and the intravenous insulin infusion stopped 1 hour later. If glycaemic control is not adequately achieved, additional insulin can be given in the following ways:

- additional doses of soluble insulin at any of the 4 injection times (before meals or bedtime) *or*

- temporary addition of intravenous insulin infusion to subcutaneous regimen *or*

- complete reversion to intravenous insulin infusion (particularly if the child is unwell).

Neonatal diabetes Neonatal diabetes is a rare condition that presents with acidosis, dehydration, hyperglycaemia, and rarely ketosis; it responds to continuous insulin infusion. When the neonate is stable, treatment can be switched to subcutaneous insulin given once or twice a day. Treatment is normally required for 4–6 weeks in transient forms, but may be required permanently in some cases.

Neonatal hyperglycaemia Newborn babies are relatively intolerant of glucose, especially in the first week of life and if premature. If intravenous glucose is necessary e.g. for total parenteral nutrition, infuse at a lower rate for 6–12 hours and the glucose intolerance should resolve. Insulin is not needed for such transient glucose intolerance, but may be needed if blood-glucose concentration is persistently high.

6.1.1.1 **Short-acting insulins**

Soluble insulin is a short-acting form of insulin. For maintenance regimens it is usual to inject it 15 to 30 minutes before meals.

Soluble insulin is the most appropriate form of insulin for use in diabetic emergencies and at the time of surgery. It can be given intravenously and intramuscularly, as well as subcutaneously.

When injected subcutaneously, soluble insulin has a rapid onset of action (30 to 60 minutes), a peak action between 2 and 4 hours, and a duration of action of up to 8 hours.

When injected intravenously, soluble insulin has a very short half-life of only about 5 minutes and its effect disappears within 30 minutes.

The rapid-acting human insulin analogues, **insulin aspart**, **insulin glulisine**, and **insulin lispro**, have a faster onset (10–20 minutes) and shorter duration of action (2–5 hours) than soluble insulin; as a result, compared with soluble insulin, fasting and preprandial blood-glucose concentrations are a little higher, postprandial blood-glucose concentration is a little lower, and hypoglycaemia occurs slightly less frequently. These rapid-acting insulins are ideal for prandial dosing in a multiple injection regimen in combination with a long-acting insulin once or twice daily. Insulin aspart, insulin glulisine, and insulin lispro can be administered by subcutaneous infusion (see Insulin Administration, above). Insulin aspart and insulin lispro can also be administered intravenously and can be used as alternatives to soluble insulin for diabetic emergencies and at the time of surgery.

INSULIN

(Insulin Injection; Neutral Insulin; Soluble Insulin)

A sterile solution of insulin (i.e. bovine or porcine) or of human insulin; pH 6.6–8.0

Cautions section 6.1.1; **interactions**: Appendix 1 (antidiabetics)

Hepatic impairment section 6.1.1

Renal impairment section 6.1.1

Pregnancy section 6.1.1

Breast-feeding section 6.1.1

Side-effects see notes above; transient oedema; local reactions and fat hypertrophy at injection site; rarely hypersensitivity reactions including urticaria, rash; overdose causes hypoglycaemia

Indication and dose

Hyperglycaemia, surgery in children with diabetes

● **By intravenous infusion**

Neonate 0.02–0.125 units/kg/hour, adjusted according to blood-glucose concentration, see also notes above

Child 1 month–18 years 0.025–0.1 units/kg/hour, adjusted according to blood-glucose concentration, see also notes above

Diabetes mellitus

● **By subcutaneous injection**

According to requirements (see notes above)
Note Rotate injection site to reduce local reactions and fat hypertrophy

Administration For *intravenous infusion*, dilute to a concentration of 1 unit/mL with Sodium Chloride 0.9% and mix thoroughly; insulin may be adsorbed by plastics, flush giving set with 5 mL of infusion fluid containing insulin.

Neonatal intensive care, dilute 5 units to a final volume of 50 mL with infusion fluid; an intravenous infusion rate of 0.1 mL/kg/hour provides a dose of 0.01 units/kg/hour

◢**Highly purified animal**

Counselling Show container to child or carer and confirm the expected version is dispensed

Hypurin® Bovine Neutral (Wockhardt) PoM
Injection, soluble insulin (bovine, highly purified) 100 units/mL. Net price 10-mL vial = £18.48; cartridges (for *Autopen® Classic*) 5 × 3 mL = £27.72

Hypurin® Porcine Neutral (Wockhardt) PoM
Injection, soluble insulin (porcine, highly purified) 100 units/mL. Net price 10-mL vial = £16.80; cartridges (for *Autopen® Classic*) 5 × 3 mL = £25.20

◢**Human sequence**

Counselling Show container to child or carer and confirm the expected version is dispensed

Actrapid® (Novo Nordisk) PoM
Injection, soluble insulin (human, pyr) 100 units/mL. Net price 10-mL vial = £7.48

Note Not recommended for use in subcutaneous insulin infusion pumps—may precipitate in catheter or needle

Humulin S® (Lilly) PoM
Injection, soluble insulin (human, prb) 100 units/mL. Net price 10-mL vial = £15.68; 5 × 3-mL cartridge (for *Autopen® Classic* or *HumaPen®*) = £26.71

Insuman® Rapid (Sanofi-Aventis) PoM
Injection, soluble insulin (human, crb) 100 units/mL, net price 5 × 3-mL cartridge (for *OptiPen® Pro 1*) = £22.52; 5 × 3-mL *Insuman® Rapid OptiSet®* prefilled disposable injection devices (range 2–40 units, allowing 2-unit dosage adjustment) = £26.81

Note Not recommended for use in subcutaneous insulin infusion pumps

◢**Mixed preparations**

See Biphasic Isophane Insulin (section 6.1.1.2)

6 Endocrine system

INSULIN ASPART

(Recombinant human insulin analogue)

Cautions section 6.1.1; **interactions:** Appendix 1 (antidiabetics)

Hepatic impairment section 6.1.1

Renal impairment section 6.1.1

Pregnancy section 6.1.1

Breast-feeding section 6.1.1

Side-effects see under Insulin

Licensed use not licensed for use in children under 2 years

Indication and dose

Diabetes mellitus

- By subcutaneous injection
  Immediately before meals or when necessary shortly after meals, according to requirements

- By subcutaneous infusion, intravenous injection or intravenous infusion
  According to requirements

Administration for *intravenous infusion*, dilute to a concentration of 0.05–1 unit/mL with Glucose 5% or Sodium Chloride 0.9% and mix thoroughly; insulin may be adsorbed by plastics, flush giving set with 5 mL of infusion fluid containing insulin.

NovoRapid® (Novo Nordisk) (PoM)
Injection, insulin aspart (recombinant human insulin analogue) 100 units/mL, net price 10-mL vial = £16.60; *Penfill®* cartridge (for *Innovo®* and *NovoPen®* devices) 5 × 3-mL = £29.14; 5 × 3-mL *FlexPen®* prefilled disposable injection devices (range 1–60 units, allowing 1-unit dosage adjustment) = £32.00

Counselling Show container to child or carer and confirm the expected version is dispensed

INSULIN GLULISINE

(Recombinant human insulin analogue)

Cautions section 6.1.1; **interactions:** Appendix 1 (antidiabetics)

Hepatic impairment section 6.1.1

Renal impairment section 6.1.1

Pregnancy section 6.1.1

Breast-feeding section 6.1.1

Side-effects see under Insulin

Licensed use not licensed for children under 6 years

Indication and dose

Diabetes mellitus

- By subcutaneous injection
  Immediately before meals or when necessary shortly after meals, according to requirements

- By subcutaneous infusion
  According to requirements

Apidra® (Sanofi-Aventis) (PoM)
Injection, insulin glulisine (recombinant human insulin analogue) 100 units/mL, net price 10-mL vial = £16.60; 5 × 3-mL cartridge (for *OptiPen® Pro 1* and *Autopen® 24*) = £28.30; 5 × 3-mL *OptiClik®* cartridge (for *OptiClik® Pen* (NHS)) = £30.27; 5 × 3-mL *Apidra® Optiset®* prefilled disposable injection devices (range 2–40 units, allowing 2-unit dosage adjustment) = £28.30; 5 × 3-mL *Apidra® SoloStar®* prefilled disposable injection devices (range 1–80 units, allowing 1-unit dosage adjustment) = £25.00

Counselling Show container to patient and confirm that patient is expecting the version dispensed

Note The *Scottish Medicines Consortium* (p. 4) has advised (October 2008) that *Apidra®* is accepted for restricted use within NHS Scotland for the treatment of children over 6 years with diabetes mellitus in whom the use of a short-acting insulin analogue is appropriate

INSULIN LISPRO

(Recombinant human insulin analogue)

Cautions section 6.1.1; children under 12 years (use only if benefit likely compared to soluble insulin); **interactions:** Appendix 1 (antidiabetics)

Hepatic impairment section 6.1.1

Renal impairment section 6.1.1

Pregnancy section 6.1.1

Breast-feeding section 6.1.1

Side-effects see under Insulin

Indication and dose

Diabetes mellitus

- By subcutaneous injection
  Shortly before meals or when necessary shortly after meals, according to requirements

- By subcutaneous infusion, or intravenous injection, or intravenous infusion
  According to requirements

Administration For *intravenous infusion*, dilute to a concentration of 0.1–1 unit/mL with Glucose 5% or Sodium Chloride 0.9% and mix thoroughly; insulin may be adsorbed by plastics, flush giving set with 5 mL of infusion fluid containing insulin.

Humalog® (Lilly) (PoM)
Injection, insulin lispro (recombinant human insulin analogue) 100 units/mL. Net price 10-mL vial = £16.61; 5 × 3-mL cartridge (for *Autopen® Classic* or *HumaPen®*) = £28.31; 5 × 3-mL *Humalog®-Pen* prefilled disposable injection devices (range 1–60 units, allowing 1-unit dosage adjustment) = £29.46; 5 × 3-mL *Humalog® KwikPen* prefilled disposable injection devices (range 1–60 units, allowing 1-unit dosage adjustment) = £29.46

Counselling Show container to child or carer and confirm the expected version is dispensed

6.1.1.2 **Intermediate- and long-acting insulins**

When given by subcutaneous injection, intermediate- and long-acting insulins have an onset of action of approximately 1–2 hours, a maximal effect at 4–12 hours, and a duration of 16–35 hours. Some are given twice daily in conjunction with short-acting (soluble) insulin, and others are given once daily. Soluble insulin can be mixed with intermediate and long-acting insulins (except insulin detemir and insulin glargine), essentially retaining the properties of the two components, although there may be some blunting of the initial effect of the soluble insulin component (especially on mixing with protamine zinc insulin, see below).

Close monitoring of blood glucose is essential when introducing a change to the insulin regimen; the total daily dose as well as any concomitant treatment may need to be adjusted.

Isophane insulin is a suspension of insulin with protamine; it is of particular value for initiation of twice-daily insulin regimens. Isophane can be mixed with soluble insulin before injection but ready-mixed preparations may be more appropriate (**biphasic isophane insulin**, **biphasic insulin aspart**, or **biphasic insulin lispro**).

Insulin zinc suspension (30% amorphous, 70% crystalline) has a more prolonged duration of action.

Protamine zinc insulin is usually given once daily with short-acting (soluble) insulin. It has the drawback of binding with the soluble insulin when mixed in the same syringe and is now rarely used.

Insulin detemir and **insulin glargine** are long-acting human insulin analogues with a prolonged duration of action; insulin detemir is given once or twice daily and insulin glargine is given once daily. These long-acting insulins are ideal for once or twice daily dosing in a multiple injection regimen in combination with a short-acting insulin before meals.

NICE (May 2009) has recommended that, if insulin is required in patients with type 2 diabetes, insulin detemir or insulin glargine may be considered for those:

- who require assistance with injecting insulin *or*

- whose lifestyle is significantly restricted by recurrent symptomatic hypoglycaemia *or*

- who would otherwise need twice-daily basal insulin injections in combination with oral antidiabetic drugs *or*

- who cannot use the device needed to inject isophane insulin.

INSULIN DETEMIR

(Recombinant human insulin analogue—long-acting)

Cautions section 6.1.1; **interactions**: Appendix 1 (antidiabetics)

Hepatic impairment section 6.1.1

Renal impairment section 6.1.1

Pregnancy section 6.1.1

Breast-feeding section 6.1.1

Side-effects see under Insulin (section 6.1.1.1)

Licensed use not licensed for use in children under 6 years

Indication and dose

Diabetes mellitus

- By subcutaneous injection

  Child over 6 years according to requirements

Levemir® (Novo Nordisk) ⓅⓄⓂ

Injection, insulin detemir (recombinant human insulin analogue) 100 units/mL, net price 5 × 3-mL cartridge (for *NovoPen®* devices) = £42.00; 5 × 3-mL *FlexPen®* prefilled disposable injection device (range 1–60 units, allowing 1-unit dosage adjustment) = £42.00; 5 × 3-mL *Levemir InnoLet®* prefilled disposable injection devices (range 1–50 units, allowing 1-unit dosage adjustment) = £44.85

Counselling Show container to child or carer and confirm the expected version is dispensed

INSULIN GLARGINE

(Recombinant human insulin analogue—long acting)

Cautions section 6.1.1; **interactions**: Appendix 1 (antidiabetics)

Hepatic impairment section 6.1.1

Renal impairment section 6.1.1

Pregnancy section 6.1.1

Breast-feeding section 6.1.1

Side-effects see under Insulin (section 6.1.1.1)

Licensed use not licensed for use in children under 6 years

6

Endocrine system

◁ **INSULIN GLARGINE (continued)**

Indication and dose

Diabetes mellitus
• By subcutaneous injection
  According to requirements

Lantus® (Sanofi-Aventis) [PoM]
Injection, insulin glargine (recombinant human insulin analogue) 100 units/mL, net price 10-mL vial = £26.00; 5 × 3-mL cartridge (for *OptiPen® Pro 1* and *Autopen® 24*) = £39.00; 5 × 3-mL *OptiClik®* cartridge (for *OptiClik® Pen* [NHS]) = £40.36; 5 × 3-mL *Lantus® OptiSet®* prefilled disposable injection devices (range 2–40 units, allowing 2-unit dosage adjustment) = £39.00; 5 × 3-mL *Lantus® SoloStar®* prefilled disposable injection devices (range 1–80 units, allowing 1-unit dosage adjustment) = £40.36

Note The *Scottish Medicines Consortium* (p. 4) has advised (October 2002) that insulin glargine is accepted for restricted use within NHS Scotland for the treatment of type 1 diabetes:

• in those who are at risk of or experience unacceptable frequency or severity of nocturnal hypoglycaemia on attempting to achieve better hypoglycaemic control during treatment with other insulins

• as a once daily insulin therapy for patients who require a carer to administer their insulin.

It is **not** recommended for routine use in patients with type 2 diabetes unless they suffer from recurrent episodes of hypoglycaemia or require assistance with their insulin injections.

Counselling Show container to child or carer and confirm the expected version is dispensed

---

▣ INSULIN ZINC SUSPENSION

(Insulin Zinc Suspension (Mixed)—long acting)
A sterile neutral suspension of bovine insulin or of human insulin in the form of a complex obtained by the addition of a suitable zinc salt; consists of rhombohedral crystals (10–40 microns) and of particles of no uniform shape (not exceeding 2 microns)

Cautions section 6.1.1; **interactions:** Appendix 1 (antidiabetics)

Hepatic impairment section 6.1.1

Renal impairment section 6.1.1

Pregnancy section 6.1.1

Breast-feeding section 6.1.1

Side-effects see under Insulin (section 6.1.1.1)

Indication and dose

Diabetes mellitus
• By subcutaneous injection
  According to requirements

◢**Highly purified animal**

Hypurin® Bovine Lente (Wockhardt) [PoM]
Injection, insulin zinc suspension (bovine, highly purified) 100 units/mL. Net price 10-mL vial = £18.48

Counselling Show container to child or carer and confirm the expected version is dispensed

---

▣ ISOPHANE INSULIN

(Isophane Insulin Injection; Isophane Protamine Insulin Injection; Isophane Insulin (NPH)—intermediate acting)
A sterile suspension of bovine or porcine insulin or of human insulin in the form of a complex obtained by the addition of protamine sulphate or another suitable protamine

Cautions section 6.1.1; **interactions:** Appendix 1 (antidiabetics)

Hepatic impairment section 6.1.1

Renal impairment section 6.1.1

Pregnancy section 6.1.1

Breast-feeding section 6.1.1

Side-effects see under Insulin (section 6.1.1.1); protamine may cause allergic reactions

Indication and dose

Diabetes mellitus
• By subcutaneous injection
  According to requirements

◢**Highly purified animal**

Counselling Show container to child or carer and confirm the expected version is dispensed

Hypurin® Bovine Isophane (Wockhardt) [PoM]
Injection, isophane insulin (bovine, highly purified) 100 units/mL. Net price 10-mL vial = £18.48; cartridges (for *Autopen® Classic*) 5 × 3 mL = £27.72

Hypurin® Porcine Isophane (Wockhardt) [PoM]
Injection, isophane insulin (porcine, highly purified) 100 units/mL. Net price 10-mL vial = £16.80; cartridges (for *Autopen® Classic*) 5 × 3 mL = £25.20

◢**Human sequence**

Counselling Show container to child or carer and confirm the expected version is dispensed

Insulatard® (Novo Nordisk) [PoM]
Injection, isophane insulin (human, pyr) 100 units/mL. Net price 10-mL vial = £7.48; *Insulatard Penfill®* cartridge (for *Innovo®*, or *Novopen®* devices) 5 × 3 mL = £19.08; 5 × 3-mL *Insulatard InnoLet®* prefilled disposable injection devices (range 1–50 units, allowing 1-unit dosage adjustment) = £20.40

Humulin I® (Lilly) [PoM]
Injection, isophane insulin (human, prb) 100 units/mL. Net price 10-mL vial = £15.68; 5 × 3-mL cartridge (for *Autopen® Classic* or *HumaPen®*) = £26.71; 5 × 3-mL *Humulin I-Pen®* prefilled disposable injection devices (range 1–60 units, allowing 1-unit dosage adjustment) = £28.44

Insuman® Basal (Sanofi-Aventis) [PoM]
Injection, isophane insulin (human, crb) 100 units/mL, net price 5-mL vial = £5.61; 5 × 3-mL cartridge (for *OptiPen® Pro 1*) = £22.52; 5 × 3-mL *Insuman® Basal OptiSet®* prefilled disposable injection devices (range 2–40 units, allowing 2-unit dosage adjustment) = £26.81

◢**Mixed preparations**

See Biphasic Isophane Insulin (p. 434)

▲ PROTAMINE ZINC INSULIN

(Protamine Zinc Insulin Injection—long acting)
A sterile suspension of insulin in the form of a complex obtained by the addition of a suitable protamine and zinc chloride; this preparation was included in BP 1980 but is not included in BP 1988

Cautions section 6.1.1; see also notes above; **interactions:** Appendix 1 (antidiabetics)

Hepatic impairment section 6.1.1

Renal impairment section 6.1.1

Pregnancy section 6.1.1

Breast-feeding section 6.1.1

Side-effects see under Insulin (section 6.1.1.1); protamine may cause allergic reactions

Indication and dose

Diabetes mellitus
- By subcutaneous injection
  According to requirements

Hypurin® Bovine Protamine Zinc (Wockhardt) ⓅⓄⓂ
Injection, protamine zinc insulin (bovine, highly purified) 100 units/mL. Net price 10-mL vial = £18.48

Counselling Show container to child or carer and confirm the expected version is dispensed

---

▰ Biphasic insulins

Biphasic insulins are pre-mixed insulin preparations containing various combinations of short-acting (soluble) or rapid-acting (analogue) insulin and an intermediate-acting insulin.

The percentage of short-acting insulin varies from 10% to 50%. These preparations should be administered by subcutaneous injection up to 15 minutes before or soon after a meal.

▲ BIPHASIC INSULIN ASPART

(Intermediate-acting insulin)

Cautions section 6.1.1; **interactions:** Appendix 1 (antidiabetics)

Hepatic impairment section 6.1.1

Renal impairment section 6.1.1

Pregnancy section 6.1.1

Breast-feeding section 6.1.1

Side-effects see under Insulin (section 6.1.1.1); protamine may cause allergic reactions

Indication and dose

Diabetes mellitus
- By subcutaneous injection
  Up to 10 minutes before or soon after a meal, according to requirements

NovoMix® 30 (Novo Nordisk) ⓅⓄⓂ
Injection, biphasic insulin aspart (recombinant human insulin analogue), 30% insulin aspart, 70% insulin aspart protamine, 100 units/mL, net price 5 × 3-mL *Penfill®* cartridges (for *Innovo®* and *NovoPen®* devices) = £29.43; 5 × 3-mL *FlexPen®* prefilled disposable injection devices (range 1–60 units, allowing 1-unit dosage adjustment) = £32.00

Counselling Show container to child or carer and confirm the expected version is dispensed; the proportions of the two components should be checked **carefully** (the order in which the proportions are stated may not be the same in other countries)

▲ BIPHASIC INSULIN LISPRO

(Intermediate-acting insulin)

Cautions see section 6.1.1 and Insulin Lispro; **interactions:** Appendix 1 (antidiabetics)

Hepatic impairment section 6.1.1

Renal impairment section 6.1.1

Pregnancy section 6.1.1

Breast-feeding section 6.1.1

Side-effects see under Insulin (section 6.1.1.1); protamine may cause allergic reactions

Indication and dose

Diabetes mellitus
- By subcutaneous injection
  Up to 15 minutes before or soon after a meal, according to requirements

Humalog® Mix25 (Lilly) ⓅⓄⓂ
Injection, biphasic insulin lispro (recombinant human insulin analogue), 25% insulin lispro, 75% insulin lispro protamine, 100 units/mL, net price 5 × 3-mL cartridge (for *Autopen® Classic* or *HumaPen®*) = £29.46; 5 × 3-mL prefilled disposable injection devices (range 1–60 units, allowing 1-unit dosage adjustment) = £30.98; 5 × 3-mL *Humalog®*
Mix25 KwikPen prefilled disposable injection devices (range 1–60 units allowing 1-unit dosage adjustment) = £30.98

Counselling Show container to child or carer and confirm the expected version is dispensed; the proportions of the two components should be checked **carefully** (the order in which the proportions are stated may not be the same in other countries)

Humalog® Mix50 (Lilly) ⓅⓄⓂ
Injection, biphasic insulin lispro (recombinant human insulin analogue), 50% insulin lispro, 50% insulin lispro protamine, 100 units/mL, net price 5 × 3-mL cartridge (for *Autopen® Classic* or *HumaPen®*) = £29.46; 5 × 3-mL prefilled disposable injection devices (range 1–60 units, allowing 1-unit dosage adjustment) = £29.46; 5 × 3-mL *Humalog® Mix50 KwikPen* prefilled disposable injection devices (range 1–60 units, allowing 1-unit dosage adjustment) = £30.98

Counselling Show container to child or carer and confirm the expected version is dispensed; the proportions of the two components should be checked **carefully** (the order in which the proportions are stated may not be the same in other countries)

6

Endocrine system

BIPHASIC ISOPHANE INSULIN

(Biphasic Isophane Insulin Injection—intermediate acting)

A sterile buffered suspension of either porcine or human insulin complexed with protamine sulphate (or another suitable protamine) in a solution of insulin of the same species

Cautions section 6.1.1; **interactions:** Appendix 1 (antidiabetics)

Hepatic impairment section 6.1.1

Renal impairment section 6.1.1

Pregnancy section 6.1.1

Breast-feeding section 6.1.1

Side-effects see under Insulin (section 6.1.1.1); protamine may cause allergic reactions

Indication and dose

Diabetes mellitus
• By subcutaneous injection
According to requirements

◢Highly purified animal

Counselling Show container to child or carer and confirm the expected version is dispensed; the proportions of the two components should be checked **carefully** (the order in which the proportions are stated may not be the same in other countries)

Hypurin® Porcine 30/70 Mix (Wockhardt) PoM
Injection, biphasic isophane insulin (porcine, highly purified), 30% soluble, 70% isophane, 100 units/mL. Net price 10-mL vial = £16.80; cartridges (for *Autopen® Classic*) 5 × 3 mL = £25.20

◢Human sequence

Counselling Show container to child or carer and confirm the expected version is dispensed; the proportions of the two components should be checked **carefully** (the order in which the proportions are stated may not be the same in other countries)

Mixtard® 30 (Novo Nordisk) PoM
Injection, biphasic isophane insulin (human, pyr),
30% soluble, 70% isophane, 100 units/mL. Net price 10-mL vial = £7.48; *Mixtard 30 Penfill®* cartridge (for *Innovo® or Novopen®* devices) 5 × 3 mL = £19.08; 5 × 3-mL *Mixtard 30 InnoLet®* prefilled disposable injection devices (range 1–50 units allowing 1-unit dosage adjustment) = £19.87

Humulin M3® (Lilly) PoM
Injection, biphasic isophane insulin (human, prb), 30% soluble, 70% isophane, 100 units/mL. Net price 10-mL vial = £15.68; 5 × 3-mL cartridge (for *Autopen® Classic* or *HumaPen®*) = £26.71

Insuman® Comb 15 (Sanofi-Aventis) PoM
Injection, biphasic isophane insulin (human, crb), 15% soluble, 85% isophane, 100 units/mL, net price 5 × 3-mL *Insuman® Comb 15 OptiSet®* prefilled disposable injection devices (range 2–40 units, allowing 2-unit dosage adjustment) = £26.81

Insuman® Comb 25 (Sanofi-Aventis) PoM
Injection, biphasic isophane insulin (human, crb), 25% soluble, 75% isophane, 100 units/mL, net price 5-mL vial = £5.61; 5 × 3-mL cartridge (for *OptiPen® Pro 1*) = £22.52; 5 × 3-mL *Insuman® Comb 25 OptiSet®* prefilled disposable injection devices (range 2–40 units, allowing 2-unit dosage adjustment) = £26.81

Insuman® Comb 50 (Sanofi-Aventis) PoM
Injection, biphasic isophane insulin (human, crb), 50% soluble, 50% isophane, 100 units/mL, net price; 5 × 3-mL cartridge (for *OptiPen® Pro 1*) = £22.52; 5 × 3-mL *Insuman® Comb 50 OptiSet®* prefilled disposable injection devices (range 2–40 units, allowing 2-unit dosage adjustment) = £26.81

6.1.1.3 Hypodermic equipment

Carers and children should be advised on the safe disposal of lancets, single-use syringes, and needles. Suitable arrangements for the safe disposal of contaminated waste must be made before these products are prescribed for patients who are carriers of infectious diseases.

◢Injection devices

Autopen® (Owen Mumford)
Injection device; *Autopen® 24* (for use with Sanofi-Aventis 3-mL insulin cartridges), allowing 1-unit dosage adjustment, max. 21 units (single-unit version) *or* 2 unit dosage adjustment, max. 42 units (2 unit version), net price (both) = £15.55; *Autopen® Classic* (for use with Lilly and Wockhardt 3-mL insulin cartridges), allowing 1-unit dosage adjustment, max. 21 units (single-unit version) *or* 2 unit dosage adjustment, max. 42 units (2-unit version), net price (all) = £15.79

HumaPen® Luxura (Lilly)
Injection device, for use with *Humulin®* and *Humalog®* 3-mL cartridges; allowing 1-unit dosage adjustment, max. 60 units, net price = £26.36

HumaPen® Luxura HD (Lilly)
Injection device, for use with *Humulin®* and *Humalog®* 3-mL cartridges; allowing 0.5-unit dosage adjustment, max. 30 units, net price = £26.36

NovoPen® (Novo Nordisk)
Injection device; for use with *Penfill®* insulin cartridges; *NovoPen® Junior* (for 3-mL cartridges), allowing 0.5-unit dosage adjustment, max. 35 units, net price = £24.79;

NovoPen® 3 Demi (for 3-mL cartridges), allowing 0.5-unit dosage adjustment, max. 35 units, net price = £25.21; *NovoPen® 4* (for 3-mL cartridges), allowing 1-unit dosage adjustment, max. 60 units, net price = £26.56

OptiClik® (Sanofi-Aventis)
Injection device, for use with *Lantus OptiClik®* insulin cartridges, allowing 1-unit dosage adjustment, max. 80 units, net price = £20.13

OptiPen® Pro 1 (Sanofi-Aventis)
Injection device, for use with *Insuman®* insulin cartridges; allowing 1-unit dosage adjustment, max. 60 units, net price = £22.00

SQ-PEN® (Medical House)
Needle-free insulin delivery device for use with any 10-mL vial *or* any 3-mL cartridge of insulin, allowing 1-unit dosage adjustment, max. 50 units, net price *starter pack* (*SQ-PEN®* device, 1 practice nozzle, 1 nozzle, 1 3-mL adaptor, 1 10-mL adaptor) = £147.83, *3-month consumables pack* for 10-mL adaptor (7 nozzles, 5 × 10-mL insulin vial adaptors) = £18.08, for 3-mL adaptor (7 nozzles, 15 × 3-mL insulin cartridge adaptors) = £30.82; *vial adaptor pack* (6 insulin vial adaptors) = £7.66, *cartridge adaptor pack* (6 insulin cartridge adaptors) = £7.66; *nozzle pack* (6 nozzles) = £10.03

◢Lancets

Lancets—sterile, single use (Drug Tariff)

BD Micro-Fine®+ 100 = £3.16, 200 = £6.13; *Cleanlet Fine*®
100 = £3.19, 200 = £6.13; [1] *Finepoint*® 100 = £3.51;
[1] *FreeStyle*® 200 = £6.94; [1] *GlucoMen*® Fine 100 = £3.55,
200 = £6.88; *Hypoguard Supreme*® 100 = £2.75; [1] *Microlet*®
(formerly *Ascensia Microlet*®) 100 = £3.76, 200 = £7.17;
[1] *Milward Steri-Let*®, 23 gauge, 100 = £3.00, 200 = £5.70,
28 gauge, 100 = £3.00, 200 = £5.70; [1] *Monolet*® 100 =
£3.28, 200 = £6.24; *Monolet*® *Extra* 100 = £3.28; *MPD Ultra
Thin*®, 100 = £3.30, 200 = £6.50; *Multiclix*® 204 = £9.20;
[1] *One Touch UltraSoft*® 100 = £3.58; [2] *Softclix*® 200 = £7.35;
[2] *Softclix XL*® 50 = £1.84; *Thin Lancets*, 200 = £7.08; [1] *Unilet
ComforTouch*® 100 = £3.60, 200 = £6.83; [1] *Unilet General
Purpose Superlite*® 100 = £3.67, 200 = £6.96; *Unistik 3
Comfort*®, 28-gauge, 100 = £6.24, 200 = £12.20; *Unistik 3
Extra*®, 21-gauge, 100 = £6.24, 200 = £12.20; *Unistik 3
Normal*®, 23-gauge, 100 = £6.24, 200 = £12.20; *Universal*®,
200 = £6.37; *Vitrex Soft*®, 23-gauge, 100 = £3.00, 200 =
£5.70; *Vitrex Gentle*® 28-gauge, 100 = £3.19, 200 = £6.13;
WaveSense Ultra-Thin® 28-gauge, 200 = £6.90, 33-gauge,
200 = £6.90

Compatible finger-pricking devices (unless indicated
otherwise, see footnotes), all 〔NHS〕: *B-D Optimus*®,
Glucolet®, *Monojector*®, *Penlet II*®, *Soft Touch*®

1. 〔NHS〕 *Autolet*® and 〔NHS〕 *Autolet Impression*® are also
   compatible finger-pricking devices
2. Use 〔NHS〕 *Softclix*® finger-pricking device

◢Needles

Hypodermic Needle, Sterile single use (Drug Tariff)

For use with reusable glass syringe, sizes 0.5 mm (25G),
0.45 mm (26G), 0.4 mm (27G). Net price 100-needle pack
= £2.70

Brands include *Microlance*®, *Monoject*®

Needles for Prefilled and Reusable Pen Injectors (Drug
Tariff)

Screw on, needle length 6.1 mm or less, net price 100-
needle pack = £12.53; 6.2–9.9 mm, 100-needle pack =
£8.89; 10 mm or more, 100-needle pack = £8.89

Brands include *BD Micro-Fine*®+, *Comfort Point*®,
NovoFine®, *Novofine Autocover*®, *Unifine*® *Pentips*

Snap on, needle length 6.1 mm or less, net price 100-
needle pack = £12.02; 6.2–9.9 mm, 100-needle pack =
£8.52; 10 mm or more, 100-needle pack = £8.52

Brands include *Penfine*®

◢Syringes

Hypodermic Syringe (Drug Tariff)

Calibrated glass with Luer taper conical fitting, for use
with U100 insulin. Net price 0.5 mL and 1 mL = £9.08

Brands include *Abcare*®

Pre-Set U100 Insulin Syringe (Drug Tariff)

Calibrated glass with Luer taper conical fitting, supplied
with dosage chart and strong box, for blind patients. Net
price 1 mL = £21.99

U100 Insulin Syringe with Needle (Drug Tariff)

Disposable with fixed or separate needle for single use or
single patient-use, colour coded orange. Needle length
8 mm, diameters 0.33 mm (29G), 0.3 mm (30G), net price
10 (with needle), 0.3 mL = £1.36, 0.5 mL = £1.31; needle
length 12 mm, diameters 0.45 mm (26G), 0.4 mm (27G),
0.36 mm (28G), 0.33 mm (29G), net price 10 (with needle),
0.3 mL = £1.45; 0.5 mL = £1.41; 1 mL = £1.42

Brands include *BD Micro-Fine*®+, *Clinipak*®, *Insupak*®,
Monoject® *Ultra*, *Omnikan*®, *Plastipak*®

◢Accessories

Needle Clipping (Chopping) Device (Drug Tariff)

Consisting of a clipper to remove needle from its hub and
container from which cut-off needles cannot be retrieved;
designed to hold 1200 needles, not suitable for use with
lancets. Net price = £1.33

Brands include *BD Safe-Clip*®

Sharpsguard (Drug Tariff)

Net price 1-litre sharpsbin = 85p

6.1.2 Oral antidiabetic drugs

6.1.2.1 Sulphonylureas
6.1.2.2 Biguanides
6.1.2.3 Other antidiabetic drugs

Oral antidiabetic drugs are used for the treatment of type 2 diabetes mellitus.
They should be prescribed only if the child fails to respond adequately to
restriction of energy and carbohydrate intake and an increase in physical activity.
They should be used to augment the effect of diet and exercise, and not to replace
them.

In children, type 2 diabetes does not usually occur until adolescence and
information on the use of oral antidiabetic drugs in children is limited. Treatment
with oral antidiabetic drugs should be initiated under specialist supervision **only**;
the initial dose should be at the lower end of the adult dose range and then
adjusted according to response.

Metformin (section 6.1.2.2) is the oral antidiabetic drug of choice because there is
most experience with this drug in children. If dietary changes and metformin do
not control the diabetes adequately, either a sulphonylurea (section 6.1.2.1) or
insulin (section 6.1.1) can be added.

Alternatively, oral therapy may be substituted with insulin.

When insulin is added to oral therapy, it is generally given at bedtime as isophane
or long-acting insulin, and when insulin replaces an oral regimen it may be given
as twice-daily injections of a biphasic insulin (or isophane insulin mixed with
soluble insulin), or a multiple injection regimen. Weight gain and hypoglycaemia
may be complications of insulin therapy but weight gain can be reduced if the
insulin is given in combination with metformin.

6

Endocrine system

Pregnancy and breast-feeding During pregnancy, women with *pre-existing diabetes* can be treated with metformin [unlicensed use], either alone or in combination with insulin (section 6.1.1). Metformin can be continued, or glibenclamide resumed, during breast-feeding for those with pre-existing diabetes. Women with *gestational diabetes* may be treated, with or without concomitant insulin (section 6.1.1), with glibenclamide from 11 weeks gestation (after organogenesis) [unlicensed use] or with metformin [unlicensed use]. Women with gestational diabetes should discontinue hypoglycaemic treatment after giving birth.

Other oral hypoglycaemic drugs are contra-indicated in pregnancy and breast-feeding.

6.1.2.1 Sulphonylureas

The sulphonylureas are not the first choice oral antidiabetics in children. They act mainly by augmenting insulin secretion and consequently are effective only when some residual pancreatic beta-cell activity is present; during long-term administration they also have an extrapancreatic action. All can cause hypoglycaemia but this is uncommon and usually indicates excessive dosage. Sulphonylurea-induced hypoglycaemia can persist for many hours and must always be treated in hospital.

Sulphonylureas are considered for children in whom metformin is contra-indicated or not tolerated. Several sulphonylureas are available but experience in children is limited; choice is determined by side-effects and the duration of action as well as the child's age and renal function. Glibenclamide, a long-acting sulphonylurea, is associated with a greater risk of hypoglycaemia and for this reason is generally avoided in children. Shorter-acting alternatives, such as **tolbutamide**, may be preferred.

Insulin therapy should be instituted temporarily during intercurrent illness (such as coma, infection, and trauma). Sulphonylureas should be omitted on the morning of surgery; insulin is often required because of the ensuing hyperglycaemia in these circumstances.

Sulphonylureas can be useful in the management of certain forms of diabetes that result from genetic defects of beta-cell function; there is most experience with gliclazide.

Cautions Sulphonylureas encourage weight gain and should be prescribed only if poor control and symptoms persist despite adequate attempts at dieting; metformin (section 6.1.2.2) is considered the drug of choice in children.

Contra-indications Sulphonylureas should be avoided where possible in acute porphyria (section 9.8.2). Sulphonylureas are contra-indicated in the presence of ketoacidosis.

Hepatic impairment Sulphonylureas should be avoided or a reduced dose should be used in severe hepatic impairment, because there is an increased risk of hypoglycaemia. Jaundice may occur.

Renal impairment Sulphonylureas should be used with care in those with mild to moderate renal impairment, because of the hazard of hypoglycaemia; they should be avoided where possible in severe renal impairment. If necessary, the short-acting drug tolbutamide can be used in renal impairment, as can gliclazide which is principally metabolised in the liver, but careful monitoring of blood-glucose concentration is essential; care is required to use the lowest dose that adequately controls blood glucose.

Pregnancy The use of sulphonylureas in pregnancy should generally be avoided because of the risk of neonatal hypoglycaemia; however, glibenclamide can be used during the second and third trimesters of pregnancy in women with gestational diabetes, see section 6.1.2.

Breast-feeding The use of sulphonylureas (except glibenclamide [unlicensed use], see section 6.1.2) in breast-feeding should be avoided because there is a theoretical possibility of hypoglycaemia in the infant.

Side-effects   Side-effects of sulphonylureas are generally mild and infrequent and include gastro-intestinal disturbances such as nausea, vomiting, diarrhoea and constipation.

Sulphonylureas can occasionally cause a disturbance in liver function, which rarely leads to cholestatic jaundice, hepatitis, and hepatic failure. Hypersensitivity reactions can occur, usually in the first 6–8 weeks of therapy. They consist mainly of allergic skin reactions which progress rarely to erythema multiforme or exfoliative dermatitis, fever, and jaundice; photosensitivity has rarely been reported with glipizide. Blood disorders are also rare but include leucopenia, thrombocytopenia, agranulocytosis, pancytopenia, haemolytic anaemia, and aplastic anaemia.

GLIBENCLAMIDE

Cautions   see notes above; **interactions:** Appendix 1 (antidiabetics)
Contra-indications   see notes above
Hepatic impairment   see notes above
Renal impairment   see notes above
Pregnancy   see notes above
Breast-feeding   see notes above
Side-effects   see notes above
Licensed use   not licensed for use in children

Indication and dose

Type 2 diabetes mellitus, maturity-onset diabetes of the young (specialist management only, see notes above)
- By mouth
  Child 12–18 years initially 2.5 mg daily with or immediately after breakfast, adjusted according to response, max. 15 mg daily

Glibenclamide (Non-proprietary) ▣ᴾᵒᴹ
Tablets, glibenclamide 2.5 mg, net price 28-tab pack = 93p; 5 mg, 28-tab pack = 93p

GLICLAZIDE

Cautions   see notes above; **interactions:** Appendix 1 (antidiabetics)
Contra-indications   see notes above
Hepatic impairment   see notes above
Renal impairment   see notes above
Pregnancy   see notes above
Breast-feeding   see notes above
Side-effects   see notes above
Licensed use   not licensed for use in children

Indication and dose

Type 2 diabetes mellitus, maturity-onset diabetes of the young (specialist management only, see notes above)
- By mouth
  Child 12–18 years initially 20 mg once daily with breakfast, adjusted according to response; up to 160 mg as a single dose; max. 160 mg twice daily

Gliclazide (Non-proprietary) ▣ᴾᵒᴹ
Tablets, scored, gliclazide 80 mg, net price 28-tab pack = £1.11, 60-tab pack = £1.45
Brands include *DIAGLYK*®

Diamicron® (Servier) ▣ᴾᵒᴹ
Tablets, scored, gliclazide 80 mg, net price 60-tab pack = £4.38

TOLBUTAMIDE

Cautions   see notes above; **interactions:** Appendix 1 (antidiabetics)
Contra-indications   see notes above
Hepatic impairment   see notes above
Renal impairment   see notes above
Pregnancy   see notes above
Breast-feeding   see notes above
Side-effects   see notes above; also headache, tinnitus
Licensed use   not licensed for use in children

Indication and dose

Type 2 diabetes mellitus (see notes above), specialist management only
- By mouth
  Child 12–18 years 0.5–1.5 g (max. 2 g) daily in divided doses with or immediately after meals *or* as a single dose with or immediately after breakfast

Tolbutamide (Non-proprietary) ▣ᴾᵒᴹ
Tablets, tolbutamide 500 mg. Net price 28-tab pack = £1.55

◄ Extemporaneous formulations available see Extemporaneous Preparations, p. 8

6.1.2.2 Biguanides

Metformin, the only available biguanide, has a different mode of action from the sulphonylureas, and is not interchangeable with them. It exerts its effect mainly by decreasing gluconeogenesis and by increasing peripheral utilisation of glucose; since it acts only in the presence of endogenous insulin it is effective only if there are some residual functioning pancreatic islet cells.

Metformin is the drug of first choice in children with type 2 diabetes, in whom strict dieting has failed to control diabetes. When the combination of strict diet and metformin treatment fails, other options to be considered under specialist management only, include:

- combining with insulin (section 6.1.1) but weight gain and hypoglycaemia can be problems (weight gain minimised if insulin given at night);
- combining with a sulphonylurea (section 6.1.2.1) (reports of increased hazard with this combination remain unconfirmed).

Insulin treatment is almost always required in medical and surgical emergencies; insulin should also be substituted before elective surgery (omit metformin on the morning of surgery and give insulin if required).

Hypoglycaemia does not usually occur with metformin; other advantages are the lower incidence of weight gain and lower plasma-insulin concentration. It does not exert a hypoglycaemic action in non-diabetic subjects unless given in over-dose.

Gastro-intestinal side-effects are initially common with metformin, and may persist in some children, particularly when high doses are given. A slow increase in dose may improve tolerability.

Very rarely, metformin can provoke lactic acidosis which is most likely to occur in children with renal impairment, see Lactic Acidosis below.

METFORMIN HYDROCHLORIDE

Cautions see notes above; determine renal function before treatment and once or twice annually during treatment; **interactions**: Appendix 1 (antidiabetics)

Lactic acidosis Use with caution in renal impairment—increased risk of lactic acidosis; avoid in significant renal impairment. Withdraw or interrupt treatment in those at risk of tissue hypoxia or sudden deterioration in renal function, such as those with dehydration, severe infection, shock, sepsis, acute heart failure, respiratory failure, or hepatic impairment

Contra-indications ketoacidosis, use of iodine-containing X-ray contrast media (do not restart metformin until renal function returns to normal) and use of general anaesthesia (suspend metformin on the morning of surgery and restart when renal function returns to normal)

Hepatic impairment withdraw if tissue hypoxia likely

Renal impairment see under Cautions

Pregnancy used in pregnancy for both pre-existing and gestational diabetes—see also Pregnancy and Breast-feeding, p. 436

Breast-feeding may be used during breast–feeding—see also Pregnancy and Breast-feeding, p. 436

Side-effects anorexia, nausea, vomiting, diarrhoea (usually transient), abdominal pain, taste disturbance; *rarely* lactic acidosis (withdraw treatment), decreased vitamin-B_{12} absorption, erythema, pruritus and urticaria; hepatitis also reported

Licensed use not licensed for use in children under 10 years

Indication and dose

Diabetes mellitus (see notes above) specialist supervision **only**

- By mouth

  Child 8–10 years initially 200 mg once daily adjusted according to response at intervals of at least 1 week; max. 2 g daily in 2–3 divided doses

  Child 10–18 years initially 500 mg once daily adjusted according to response at intervals of at least 1 week; max. 2 g daily in 2–3 divided doses

Metformin (Non-proprietary) ⟨PoM⟩
Tablets, coated, metformin hydrochloride 500 mg, net price 28-tab pack = 98p, 84-tab pack= £1.46; 850 mg, 56-tab pack = £1.33. Label: 21

Oral solution, sugar-free, metformin hydrochloride 500 mg/5 mL, net price 100 mL = £56.16. Label: 21
Brands include *Metsol®*

Glucophage® (Merck Serono) ⟨PoM⟩
Tablets, f/c, metformin hydrochloride 500 mg, net price 84-tab pack = £2.88; 850 mg, 56-tab pack = £3.20. Label: 21

Oral powder, sugar-free, metformin hydrochloride 500 mg/sachet, net price 30-sachet pack = £3.29, 60-sachet pack = £6.58; 1 g/sachet, 30-sachet pack = £6.58, 60-sachet pack = £13.16. Label: 13, 21, counselling, administration
Excipients include aspartame (section 9.4.1)

Counselling The contents of each sachet should be mixed with 150 mL of water and taken immediately

6.1.2.3 **Other antidiabetic drugs**

There is little experience of the use of **acarbose** in children. It has been used in older children; therapy should be initiated by an appropriate expert.

The use of nateglinide in combination with a sulphonylurea is generally reserved for the management of some subtypes of diabetes resulting from genetic defects of beta-cell function or other syndromes of diabetes and requires specialist management.

6.1.3 **Diabetic ketoacidosis**

The management of diabetic ketoacidosis involves the replacement of fluid and electrolytes and the administration of insulin. Guidelines for the Management of Diabetic Ketoacidosis, published by the British Society of Paediatric Endocrinology and Diabetes[1], should be followed. Clinically well children with mild ketoacidosis who are dehydrated up to 5% usually respond to oral rehydration and subcutaneous insulin. For those who do not respond, or are clinically unwell, or are dehydrated by more than 5%, insulin and replacement fluids are best given by intravenous infusion.

- To restore circulating volume for children in *shock*, give 10 mL/kg **sodium chloride 0.9%** as a rapid infusion, repeat as necessary up to a maximum of 30 mL/kg.

- Further fluid should be given by intravenous infusion at a rate that replaces deficit and provides maintenance over 48 hours; initially use **sodium chloride 0.9%**, changing to **sodium chloride 0.45%** and **glucose 5%** after 12 hours if response is adequate and plasma-sodium concentration is stable.

- Include **potassium chloride** in the fluids unless anuria is suspected, adjust according to plasma-potassium concentration.

- Insulin infusion is necessary to switch off ketogenesis and reverse acidosis; it should not be started until at least 1 hour after the start of intravenous rehydration fluids.

- **Soluble insulin** should be diluted (and **mixed thoroughly**) with **sodium chloride 0.9%** intravenous infusion to a concentration of 1 unit/mL and infused at a rate of 0.1 units/kg/hour.

- **Sodium bicarbonate** infusion (1.26% or 2.74%) is rarely necessary and is used only in cases of extreme acidosis (blood pH less than 6.9) and shock, since the acid-base disturbance is normally corrected by treatment with insulin.

- Once blood glucose falls to 14 mmol/litre, **glucose intravenous infusion 5%** *or* **10%** should be added to the fluids.

- The insulin infusion rate can be reduced to no less than 0.05 units/kg/hour when blood-glucose concentration has fallen to 14 mmol/litre *and* blood pH is greater than 7.3 *and* a glucose infusion has been started (see above); it is continued until the child is ready to take food by mouth. Subcutaneous insulin can then be started.

- The insulin infusion should not be stopped until 1 hour after starting subcutaneous soluble or long-acting insulin, or 10 minutes after starting subcutaneous insulin aspart, or insulin glulisine, or insulin lispro.

Hyperosmolar hyperglycaemic state or hyperosmolar hyperglycaemic nonketotic coma occurs rarely in children. Treatment is similar to that of diabetic ketoacidosis, although lower rates of insulin infusion and slower rehydration may be required.

6.1.4 **Treatment of hypoglycaemia**

Prompt treatment of hypoglycaemia in children from any cause is essential as severe hypoglycaemia may cause subsequent neurological damage. Hyperinsulinism, fatty acid oxidation disorders and glycogen storage disease are less common causes of acute hypoglycaemia in children.

Initially glucose 10–20 g is given by mouth either in liquid form or as granulated sugar or sugar lumps. Approximately 10 g of glucose is available from 2 teaspoons of sugar, 3 sugar lumps, *Glucogel*® (formerly known as *Hypostop*® *Gel*, glucose 10 g/25 g tube, available from BBI Healthcare), *Dextrogel*® (glucose 10 g/25 g

6

Endocrine system

---

1. Available at www.bsped.org.uk

tube, available from M & A Pharmachem), and non-diet versions of *Lucozade®* *Energy Original* 55 mL, *Coca-Cola®* 100 mL, and *Ribena® Blackcurrant* 18 mL (to be diluted). If necessary this can be repeated in 10–15 minutes. After initial treatment, a snack providing sustained availability of carbohydrate (e.g. a sandwich, fruit, milk, or biscuits) or the next meal, if it is due, can prevent blood-glucose concentration from falling again.

Hypoglycaemia which causes unconsciousness or seizures is an emergency. **Glucagon**, a polypeptide hormone produced by the alpha cells of the islets of Langerhans, increases blood-glucose concentration by mobilising glycogen stored in the liver. In hypoglycaemia, if sugar cannot be given by mouth, glucagon can be given by injection. Carbohydrates should be given as soon as possible to restore liver glycogen; glucagon is not appropriate for chronic hypoglycaemia. Glucagon can be issued to parents or carers of insulin-treated children for emergency use in hypoglycaemic attacks. It is often advisable to prescribe it on an 'if necessary' basis for hospitalised insulin-treated children, so that it can be given rapidly by the nurses during a hypoglycaemic emergency. If not effective in 10 minutes intravenous glucose should be given.

Alternatively, 5 mL/kg of glucose intravenous infusion 10% (500 mg/kg of glucose) (section 9.2.2) can be given intravenously into a large vein through a large-gauge needle; care is required since this concentration is irritant especially if extravasation occurs. Glucose intravenous infusion 50% is **not** recommended, as it is very viscous and hypertonic. Close monitoring is necessary, particularly in the case of an overdose with a long-acting insulin because further administration of glucose may be required. Children whose hypoglycaemia is caused by an oral antidiabetic drug should be transferred to hospital because the hypoglycaemic effects of these drugs can persist for many hours.

Glucagon is not effective in the treatment of hypoglycaemia due to fatty acid oxidation or glycogen storage disorders.

Neonatal hypoglycaemia Neonatal hypoglycaemia at birth is treated with **glucose intravenous infusion 10%** given at a rate of 5 mL/kg/hour. An initial dose of 2.5 mL/kg over 5 minutes may be required if hypoglycaemia is severe enough to cause loss of consciousness or seizures. Mild asymptomatic persistent hypoglycaemia may respond to a single dose of **glucagon**. Glucagon has also been used in the short-term management of endogenous hyperinsulinism.

GLUCAGON

Cautions see notes above, insulinoma, glucagonoma; ineffective in chronic hypoglycaemia, starvation, and adrenal insufficiency; delayed hypoglycaemia when used as a diagnostic test—deaths reported (ensure a meal is eaten before discharge)

Contra-indications phaeochromocytoma

Side-effects nausea, vomiting, diarrhoea, hypokalaemia, rarely hypersensitivity reactions

Licensed use unlicensed for growth hormone test and hyperinsulinism

Indication and dose

Hypoglycaemia associated with diabetes
• By subcutaneous, intramuscular, or intravenous injection

Neonate 20 micrograms/kg

Child 1 month–2 years 500 micrograms

Child 2–18 years, body-weight less than 25 kg 500 micrograms; body-weight over 25 kg 1 mg

Endogenous hyperinsulinism
• By intramuscular or intravenous injection

Neonate 200 micrograms/kg (max. 1 mg) as a single dose

Child 1 month–2 years 1 mg as a single dose

• By continuous intravenous infusion

Neonate 1–18 micrograms/kg/hour, adjusted according to response (max. 50 micrograms/kg/hour)

Child 1 month–2 years 1–10 micrograms/kg/hour, increased if necessary
Administration Do not add to infusion fluids containing calcium—precipitation may occur

Diagnosis of growth hormone secretion specialist centre only (section 6.5.1)
• By intramuscular injection

Child 1 month–18 years 100 micrograms/kg (max. 1 mg) as a single dose; dose may vary, consult local guidelines

Beta-blocker poisoning, see p. 41

Note 1 unit of glucagon = 1 mg of glucagon

[1]**GlucaGen® HypoKit** (Novo Nordisk) PoM
Injection, powder for reconstitution, glucagon (rys) as hydrochloride with lactose, net price 1-mg vial with prefilled syringe containing water for injection = £11.52
1. PoM restriction does not apply where administration is for saving life in emergency

Chronic hypoglycaemia

Diazoxide is useful in the management of chronic hypoglycaemia due to excessive insulin secretion, either from a tumour involving the islets of Langerhans or from persisting hyperinsulinaemic hypoglycaemia of infancy (nesidioblastosis, see also glucagon above). Diazoxide has no place in the management of acute hypoglycaemia. **Chlorothiazide** 3–5 mg/kg twice daily (section 2.2.1) reduces diazoxide-induced sodium and water retention and has the added benefit of potentiating the glycaemic effect of diazoxide.

If diazoxide and chlorothiazide fail to suppress excessive glucose requirements in chronic hypoglycaemia then **octreotide** or **nifedipine** (section 2.6.2) can be added. Octreotide suppresses secretion of growth hormone, but growth is unlikely to be affected in the long term.

DIAZOXIDE

Cautions ischaemic heart disease; monitor blood pressure, during prolonged use monitor white cell and platelet count, and regularly assess growth, bone, and psychological development; avoid the intravenous route if possible; extravasation can cause tissue necrosis and single doses of 300 mg have been associated with angina and cerebral and myocardial infarction; **interactions:** Appendix 1 (diazoxide)

Contra-indications see section 2.5.1

Renal impairment increased sensitivity to hypotensive and hyperglycaemic effect; dose reduction may be required

Pregnancy prolonged use in second or third trimesters may produce alopecia and impaired glucose tolerance in neonate; inhibits uterine activity

Side-effects anorexia, nausea, vomiting, hyperuricaemia, sodium and water retention, hyperglycaemia, hypotension, oedema, tachycardia, arrhythmias, extrapyramidal effects; hypertrichosis on prolonged treatment

Licensed use chronic intractable hypoglycaemia (for use in hypertensive crisis see section 2.5.1)

Indication and dose

> **Chronic intractable hypoglycaemia**
> • By mouth or by intravenous injection
>
> > **Neonate** initially 5 mg/kg twice daily to establish response, adjust dose according to response; usual maintenance dose 1.5–3 mg/kg 2–3 times daily; up to 7 mg/kg 3 times daily may be required in some cases, higher doses unlikely to be beneficial
>
> > **Child 1 month–18 years** initially 1.7 mg/kg 3 times daily then adjusted according to response; usual maintenance dose 1.5–3 mg/kg 2–3 times daily; up to 5 mg/kg 3 times daily may be required in some cases, higher doses unlikely to be beneficial

Eudemine® (UCB Pharma) [PoM]
Tablets, diazoxide 50 mg, net price 100 = £44.64

Injection, see section 2.5.1

◢ Extemporaneous formulations available see Extemporaneous Preparations, p. 8

OCTREOTIDE

Cautions avoid abrupt withdrawal of short-acting octreotide—see Side-effects below; in insulinoma (risk of increased depth and duration of hypoglycaemia—monitor closely when initiating treatment and changing doses); diabetes mellitus (antidiabetic requirements may be reduced); monitor thyroid function on long-term therapy; **interactions:** Appendix 1 (octreotide)

Pregnancy possible effect on fetal growth, avoid unless benefit outweighs risk; effective contraception required during treatment

Breast-feeding avoid unless essential—present in milk in *animal* studies

Side-effects anorexia, nausea, vomiting, abdominal pain, bloating, flatulence, diarrhoea, constipation, and steatorrhoea (administer between meals or at bedtime to reduce gastro-intestinal side-effects); bradycardia, dyspnoea, headache, dizziness; postprandial glucose tolerance may be impaired, rarely persistent hyperglycaemia with chronic administration; hypoglycaemia has also been reported; reduced gall bladder motility and bile flow; gallstones reported after long-term treatment; abrupt withdrawal of subcutaneous

octreotide is associated with biliary colic and pancreatitis; rash, alopecia; pain and irritation at injection site—sites should be rotated; *rarely* pancreatitis shortly after administration; hepatitis also reported

Licensed use not licensed in children

Indication and dose

> **Persistent hyperinsulinaemic hypoglycaemia unresponsive to diazoxide and glucose**
> • By subcutaneous injection
>
> > **Neonate** initially 2–5 micrograms/kg every 6–8 hours, adjusted according to response; up to 7 micrograms/kg every 4 hours may rarely be required
>
> > **Child 1 month–18 years** initially 1–2 micrograms/kg every 4–6 hours, dose adjusted according to response; up to 7 micrograms/kg every 4 hours may rarely be required

> **Bleeding from oesophageal or gastric varices**
> • By continuous intravenous infusion
>
> > **Child 1 month–18 years** 1 microgram/kg/hour, higher doses may be required initially; when no

6

Endocrine system

OCTREOTIDE (continued)

active bleeding reduce dose over 24 hours; usual max. 50 micrograms/hour

Administration for *intravenous infusion*, dilute with Sodium Chloride 0.9% to a concentration of 10–50%

Sandostatin® (Novartis) PoM
Injection, octreotide (as acetate) 50 micrograms/mL, net price 1-mL amp = £3.72; 100 micrograms/mL, 1-mL amp = £6.53; 200 micrograms/mL 5-mL vial = £69.66; 500 micrograms/mL, 1-mL amp = £33.87

6.1.5 Treatment of diabetic nephropathy and neuropathy

Diabetic nephropathy

Regular review of diabetic children over 12 years of age should include an annual test for microalbuminuria (the earliest sign of nephropathy). If reagent strip tests (*Micral-Test II®* NHS or *Microbumintest®* NHS) are used and prove positive, the result should be confirmed by laboratory analysis of a urine sample. Microalbuminuria can occur transiently during puberty; if it persists (at least 3 positive tests) treatment with an ACE inhibitor (section 2.5.5.1) or an angiotensin-II receptor antagonist (section 2.5.5.2) under specialist guidance should be considered; to minimise the risk of renal deterioration, blood pressure should be carefully controlled (section 2.5).

ACE inhibitors can potentiate the hypoglycaemic effect of insulin and oral anti-diabetic drugs; this effect is more likely during the first weeks of combined treatment and in children with renal impairment.

For the treatment of hypertension in diabetes, see section 2.5.

Diabetic neuropathy

Clinical neuropathy is rare in children whose diabetes is well controlled.

6.1.6 Diagnostic and monitoring devices for diabetes mellitus

Blood monitoring

Blood **glucose** monitoring using a meter gives a direct measure of the glucose concentration at the time of the test and can detect hypoglycaemia as well as hyperglycaemia. Carers and children should be properly trained in the use of blood glucose monitoring systems and the appropriate action to take on the results obtained. Inadequate understanding of the normal fluctuations in blood glucose can lead to confusion and inappropriate action.

Children using multiple injection regimens should understand how to adjust their insulin dose according to their carbohydrate intake. With fixed-dose insulin regimens, the carbohydrate intake needs to be regulated, and should be distributed throughout the day to match the insulin regimen.

Note In the UK blood-glucose concentration is expressed in mmol/litre and Diabetes UK advises that these units should be used for self-monitoring of blood glucose. In other European countries units of mg/100 mL (or mg/dL) are commonly used.
It is advisable to check that the meter is pre-set in the correct units.

If the blood glucose level is high or if the child is unwell, blood **ketones** should be measured according to local guidelines in order to detect diabetic ketoacidosis (section 6.1.3). Children and their carers should be trained in the use of blood ketone monitoring systems and to take appropriate action on the results obtained, including when to seek medical attention.

Urinalysis

Tests for glucose range from reagent strips specific to glucose to reagent tablets which detect all reducing sugars. *Clinitest®* is rarely used now; *Clinistix®* is suitable for screening purposes only. It is rarely necessary for children to test themselves for ketones unless they become unwell—see also Blood Monitoring, above.

Microalbuminuria can be detected with *Micral-Test II®* NHS or *Microbumintest®* NHS but this should be followed by confirmation in the laboratory, since false positive results are common.

Endocrine system

6

Meters and test strips

Meter (all JHS)	Type of monitoring	Meter retail price	Compatible test strips	Test strip net price	Sensitivity range (mmol/litre)	Manufacturer
Accu-Chek® Active[1]	Blood glucose		Active®	50-strip pack = £14.76	0.6–33.3	Roche Diagnostics
Accu-Chek® Advantage[1]	Blood glucose		Advantage Plus®	50-strip pack = £14.76	0.6–33.3	Roche Diagnostics
Accu-Chek® Aviva	Blood glucose	£14.94	Aviva®	50-strip pack = £14.49	0.6–33.3	Roche Diagnostics
Accu-Chek® Compact[1]	Blood glucose		Compact®	3 × 17-strip pack = £14.88	0.6–33.3	Roche Diagnostics
Accu-Chek® Compact Plus	Blood glucose	£14.94	Compact®	3 × 17-strip pack = £14.88	0.6–33.3	Roche Diagnostics
Accutrend®[1]	Blood glucose		BM-Accutest®	50-strip pack = £14.31	1.1–33.3	Roche Diagnostics
Ascensia Breeze®[1]	Blood glucose		Ascensia® Autodisc	5 × 10-disc pack = £14.62	0.6–33.3	Bayer Diabetes Care
Ascensia Esprit® 2[1]	Blood glucose		Ascensia® Autodisc	5 × 10-disc pack = £14.62	0.6–33.3	Bayer Diabetes Care
Breeze 2®	Blood glucose	£14.34	Breeze 2®	5 × 10-disc pack = £14.34	0.6–33.3	Bayer Diabetes Care
Contour®	Blood glucose	£10.80	Contour® Formerly Ascensia® Microfill	50-strip pack = £14.74	0.6–33.3	Bayer Diabetes Care
FreeStyle®[1]	Blood glucose		FreeStyle®	50-strip pack = £14.62	1.1–27.8	Abbott
FreeStyle Freedom®[1]	Blood glucose		FreeStyle®	50-strip pack = £14.62	1.1–27.8	Abbott
FreeStyle Freedom Lite®	Blood glucose	£11.49	FreeStyle Lite®	50-strip pack = £14.62	1.1–27.8	Abbott
FreeStyle Lite®	Blood glucose	£14.94	FreeStyle Lite®	50-strip pack = £14.62	1.1–27.8	Abbott
FreeStyle Mini®[1]	Blood glucose		FreeStyle®	50-strip pack = £14.62	1.1–27.8	Abbott
GlucoMen® Glycó[1]	Blood glucose		GlucoMen®	50-strip pack = £13.67	1.1–33.3	Menarini Diagnostics
GlucoMen® LX	Blood glucose	£14.94	GlucoMen® LX	50-strip pack = £14.33	1.1–33.3	Menarini Diagnostics
GlucoMen® PC[1]	Blood glucose		GlucoMen®	50-strip pack = £13.67	1.1–33.3	Menarini Diagnostics
GlucoMen® Visio	Blood glucose	£10.34	GlucoMen® Visio Sensor	50-strip pack = £14.53	1.1–33.3	Menarini Diagnostics
Glucotrend®[1]	Blood glucose		Active®	50-strip pack = £14.76	0.6–33.3	Roche Diagnostics
Hypoguard® Supreme Extra	Blood glucose	£45.00	Hypoguard® Supreme	50-strip pack = £12.00	2.2–27.7	Hypoguard
Hypoguard® Supreme Plus	Blood glucose	£35.00	Hypoguard® Supreme	50-strip pack = £12.00	2.2–27.7	Hypoguard
MediSense® Precision QID[1]	Blood glucose		MediSense G2®	50-strip pack = £13.67	1.1–33.3	Abbott
One Touch® II[1]	Blood glucose		One Touch®	50-strip pack = £14.37	1.1–33.3	LifeScan
One Touch® Basic[1]	Blood glucose		One Touch®	50-strip pack = £14.37	1.1–33.3	LifeScan

6 Endocrine system

1. Meter no longer available

Meter (all ʰˢ)	Type of monitoring	Meter retail price	Compatible test strips	Test strip net price	Sensitivity range (mmol/ litre)	Manufacturer
One Touch® Profile[1]	Blood glucose		One Touch®	50-strip pack = £14.37	1.1–33.3	LifeScan
One Touch Ultra®[1]	Blood glucose		One Touch Ultra®	50-strip pack = £14.53	1.1–33.3	LifeScan
One Touch Ultra 2®	Blood glucose	£25.98	One Touch Ultra®	50-strip pack = £14.53	1.1–33.3	LifeScan
One Touch UltraEasy®	Blood glucose	£25.98	One Touch Ultra®	50-strip pack = £14.53	1.1–33.3	LifeScan
One Touch UltraSmart®[2]	Blood glucose		One Touch Ultra®	50-strip pack = £14.53	1.1–33.3	LifeScan
One Touch® Vita[2]	Blood glucose		One Touch® Vita	50-strip pack = £14.53	1.1–33.3	LifeScan
Optium®[1]	Blood ketones		Optium® β-ketone	10-strip pack = £19.55	0–8.0	Abbott
Optium Xceed®	Blood glucose	£17.24	Optium Plus® Formerly Medisense® Optium Plus	50-strip pack = £14.53	1.1–27.8	Abbott
	Blood ketones		Optium® β-ketone	10-strip pack = £19.55	0–8.0	Abbott
PocketScan®[1]	Blood glucose		PocketScan®	50-strip pack = £14.19	1.1–33.3	LifeScan
Prestige®	Blood glucose	£8.62	Prestige®	50-strip pack = £14.51	1.4–33.3	Home Diagnostics
TRUEone®	Blood glucose	n/a	All-in-one test strips and meter	50-strip pack with meter = £14.36	1.1–33.3	Home Diagnostics
TRUEresult®[2]	Blood glucose	£11.74	TRUEresult®	50-strip pack = £14.36	1.1–33.3	Home Diagnostics
TRUEresult twist®[2]	Blood glucose	£11.74	TRUEresult®	50-strip pack = £14.36	1.1–33.3	Home Diagnostics
TRUEtrack®	Blood glucose	£8.62	TRUEtrack®	50-strip pack = £14.25	1.1–33.3	Home Diagnostics
WaveSense Jazz®	Blood glucose	£24.99	WaveSense Jazz®	50-strip pack = £14.45	1.1–33.3	WaveSense

1. Meter no longer available
2. Free of charge from diabetes healthcare professionals

◢ Glucose

Clinistix® (Bayer Diabetes Care)
Reagent strips, for detection of glucose in urine. Net price 50-strip pack = £3.27

Clinitest® (Bayer Diabetes Care)
Reagent tablets, for detection of glucose and other reducing substances in urine. Net price 36-tab pack = £2.00

Diabur-Test 5000® (Roche Diagnostics)
Reagent strips, for detection of glucose in urine. Net price 50-strip pack = £2.85

Diastix® (Bayer Diabetes Care)
Reagent strips, for detection of glucose in urine. Net price 50-strip pack = £2.78

Medi-Test® Glucose (BHR)
Reagent strips, for detection of glucose in urine. Net price 50-strip pack = £2.30

◢ Ketones

Ketostix® (Bayer Diabetes Care)
Reagent strips, for detection of ketones in urine. Net price 50-strip pack = £2.95

Ketur Test® (Roche Diagnostics)
Reagent strips, for detection of ketones in urine. Net price 50-strip pack = £2.74

◢ Protein

Albustix® (Siemens)
Reagent strips, for detection of protein in urine. Net price 50-strip pack = £4.10

Medi-Test® Protein 2 (BHR)
Reagent strips, for detection of protein in urine. Net price 50-strip pack = £3.22

◢ Other reagent strips available for urinalysis include:

Combur-3 Test® ʰˢ (glucose and protein—Roche Diagnostics), Clinitek Microalbumin® ʰˢ (albumin and creatinine—Siemens), Ketodiastix® ʰˢ (glucose and ketones—Bayer Diagnostics), Medi-Test Combi 2® ʰˢ (glucose and protein—BHR), Micral-Test II® ʰˢ (albumin—Roche Diagnostics), Microalbustix® ʰˢ (albumin and creatinine—Siemens), Microbumintest® ʰˢ (albumin—Bayer Diagnostics), Uristix® ʰˢ (glucose and protein—Siemens)

Endocrine system

6

Oral glucose tolerance test

The oral glucose tolerance test is used mainly for diagnosis of impaired glucose tolerance; it is not recommended or necessary for routine diagnostic use when severe symptoms of hyperglycaemia are present. However, it is used for the investigation of insulin resistance, glycogen storage disease, and excessive growth hormone secretion. In children who have less severe symptoms and blood-glucose concentrations that do not establish or exclude diabetes (e.g. impaired fasting glycaemia), an oral glucose tolerance test may be required. A dose of 1.75 g/kg (max. 75 g) of anhydrous glucose is used. It is also used to establish the presence of gestational diabetes; this generally involves giving anhydrous glucose 75 g (equivalent to Glucose BP 82.5 g) by mouth to the fasting patient, and measuring blood-glucose concentration at intervals. The appropriate amount of glucose should be given with 200–300 mL fluid. Alternatively anhydrous glucose 75 g can be given as 113 mL *Polycal*® (Nutricia Clinical) with extra fluid to administer a total volume of 200–300 mL.

6.2 Thyroid and antithyroid drugs

6.2.1 Thyroid hormones
6.2.2 Antithyroid drugs

6.2.1 Thyroid hormones

Thyroid hormones are used in hypothyroidism (juvenile myxoedema), and also in diffuse non-toxic goitre, congenital or neonatal hypothyroidism, and Hashimoto's thyroiditis (lymphadenoid goitre). Neonatal hypothyroidism requires prompt treatment to facilitate normal development.

Levothyroxine sodium (thyroxine sodium) is the treatment of choice for *maintenance* therapy.

Doses for congenital hypothyroidism and juvenile myxoedema should be titrated according to clinical response, growth assessment, and measurement of plasma thyroxine and thyroid-stimulating hormone concentrations. In congenital hypothyroidism higher initial doses may normalise metabolism more quickly, with associated beneficial effects on mental development.

Liothyronine sodium has a similar action to levothyroxine but is more rapidly metabolised and has a more rapid effect; 20–25 micrograms is equivalent to approximately 100 micrograms of levothyroxine. Its effects develop after a few hours and disappear within 24 to 48 hours of discontinuing treatment. It may be used in *severe hypothyroid states* when a rapid response is desired.

Liothyronine by intravenous injection is the treatment of choice in *hypothyroid coma*. Adjunctive therapy includes intravenous fluids, hydrocortisone, and treatment of infection; assisted ventilation is often required.

LEVOTHYROXINE SODIUM
(Thyroxine sodium)

Cautions panhypopituitarism or predisposition to adrenal insufficiency (initiate corticosteroid therapy before starting levothyroxine); cardiac disorders (monitor ECG; start at low dose and carefully titrate); long-standing hypothyroidism, diabetes insipidus, diabetes mellitus (dose of antidiabetic drugs including insulin may need to be increased); **interactions:** Appendix 1 (thyroid hormones)

Pregnancy monitor maternal serum-thyrotrophin concentration—levothyroxine may cross the placenta and excessive maternal concentration can be detrimental to fetus

Breast-feeding amount too small to affect tests for neonatal hypothyroidism

Side-effects usually at excessive dosage include diarrhoea, vomiting; anginal pain, arrhythmias, palpitation, tachycardia, benign intracranial hypertension; tremor, restlessness, excitability, insomnia, headache, flushing, sweating, fever, heat intolerance, weight loss, nervousness; craniosynostosis and premature closure of epiphyses; menstrual irregularities; eosinophilia, liver dysfunction; muscle cramps, muscular weakness; transient hair loss; hypersensitivity reactions including rash, pruritus and oedema also reported

446 6.2.2 Antithyroid drugs

◁ **LEVOTHYROXINE SODIUM** (*continued*)

Indication and dose

Hypothyroidism

Note Levothyroxine equivalent to 100 micrograms/m²/day can be used as a guide to the requirements in children

• **By mouth**

Neonate initially 10–15 micrograms/kg once daily (max. 50 micrograms daily), adjusted in steps of 5 micrograms/kg every 2 weeks or as necessary; usual maintenance dose 20–50 micrograms daily

Child 1 month–2 years initially 5 micrograms/kg once daily (max. 50 micrograms daily) adjusted in steps of 10–25 micrograms daily every 2–4 weeks until metabolism normalised; usual maintenance dose 25–75 micrograms daily

Child 2–12 years initially 50 micrograms once daily adjusted in steps of 25 micrograms da-

ily every 2–4 weeks until metabolism normalised; usual maintenance dose 75–100 micrograms daily

Child 12–18 years initially 50 micrograms once daily adjusted in steps of 25–50 micrograms daily every 3–4 weeks until metabolism normalised; usual maintenance dose 100–200 micrograms daily

Levothyroxine (Non-proprietary) ℗
Tablets, levothyroxine sodium 25 micrograms, net price 28-tab pack = £2.15; 50 micrograms, 28-tab pack = £1.10; 100 micrograms, 28-tab pack = £1.09
Brands include *Eltroxin*®

Oral solution, levothyroxine sodium 25 micrograms/5 mL, net price 100 mL = £42.75; 50 micrograms/5 mL, 100 mL = £44.90; 100 micrograms/5 mL, 100 mL = £52.75
Brands include *Evotrox*® (sugar-free)

▌LIOTHYRONINE SODIUM
(ʟ-Tri-iodothyronine sodium)

Cautions severe and prolonged hypothyroidism (initiate corticosteroid therapy in adrenal insufficiency); cardiac disorders (monitor ECG; start at low dose and carefully titrate); diabetes insipidus, diabetes mellitus (dose of antidiabetic drugs including insulin may need to be increased); **interactions:** Appendix 1 (thyroid hormones)

Pregnancy does not cross the placenta in significant amounts; monitor maternal thyroid function tests—dosage adjustment may be necessary

Breast-feeding amount too small to affect tests for neonatal hypothyroidism

Side-effects usually at excessive dosage include diarrhoea; anginal pain, arrhythmias, palpitation, tachycardia; restlessness, excitability, headache, flushing, sweating, weight loss; muscle cramps, muscle weakness

Licensed use unlicensed for use in children

Indication and dose
See also notes above

Hypothyroidism
• **By mouth**
Child 12–18 years initially 10–20 micrograms daily gradually increased to 60 micrograms daily in 2–3 divided doses

• **By slow intravenous injection**
(replacement for oral levothyroxine)

Convert **daily** levothyroxine dose to liothyronine (see below) and give in 2–3 divided doses, adjusted according to response
Note 2 micrograms liothyronine equivalent to approx. 8 micrograms levothyroxine

Hypothyroid coma
• **By slow intravenous injection**
Child 12–18 years 5–20 micrograms repeated every 12 hours or up to every 4 hours if necessary; *alternatively* initially 50 micrograms then 25 micrograms every 8 hours reducing to 25 micrograms twice daily

Liothyronine sodium (Goldshield) ℗
Tablets, scored, liothyronine sodium 20 micrograms, net price 28-tab pack = £23.77

Triiodothyronine (Goldshield) ℗
Injection, powder for reconstitution, liothyronine sodium (with dextran). Net price 20-microgram amp = £37.92

6.2.2 Antithyroid drugs

Antithyroid drugs are used for hyperthyroidism either to prepare children for thyroidectomy or for long-term management. In the UK carbimazole is the most commonly used drug. Propylthiouracil can be used in those who suffer sensitivity reactions to carbimazole as sensitivity is not necessarily displayed to both drugs. Both drugs act primarily by interfering with the synthesis of thyroid hormones.

Treatment in children should be undertaken by a specialist.

CSM warning (neutropenia and agranulocytosis)

Doctors are reminded of the importance of recognising bone marrow suppression induced by carbimazole and the need to stop treatment promptly.

1. Children and their carers should be asked to report symptoms and signs suggestive of infection, especially sore throat.
2. A white blood cell count should be performed if there is any clinical evidence of infection.
3. Carbimazole should be stopped promptly if there is clinical or laboratory evidence of neutropenia.

Carbimazole or **propylthiouracil** are initially given in large doses to block thyroid function. This dose is continued until the child becomes euthyroid, usually after 4 to 8 weeks, and is then gradually reduced to a maintenance dose of 30–60% of the initial dose. Alternatively high-dose treatment is continued in combination with levothyroxine replacement (*blocking-replacement regimen*); this is particularly useful when dose adjustment proves difficult or relapse is a problem. Treatment is usually continued for 12 to 24 months. The blocking-replacement regimen is **not** suitable during pregnancy. Hypothyroidism should be avoided particularly during pregnancy as it can cause fetal goitre.

When substituting, carbimazole 1 mg is considered equivalent to propylthiouracil 10 mg but the dose may need adjusting according to response.

Rashes and pruritus are common with carbimazole but they can be treated with antihistamines without discontinuing therapy; alternatively propylthiouracil can be substituted. If a child on carbimazole develops a sore throat it should be reported immediately because of the rare complication of agranulocytosis (see CSM warning, above).

Iodine has been used as an adjunct to antithyroid drugs for 10 to 14 days before partial thyroidectomy; however, there is little evidence of a beneficial effect. Iodine should not be used for long-term treatment because its antithyroid action tends to diminish.

Radioactive sodium iodide (^{131}I) solution is used increasingly for the treatment of thyrotoxicosis at all ages, particularly where medical therapy or compliance is a problem, in patients with cardiac disease, and in patients who relapse after thyroidectomy.

Propranolol (section 2.4) is useful for rapid relief of thyrotoxic symptoms and can be used in conjunction with antithyroid drugs or as an adjunct to radioactive iodine. Beta-blockers are also useful in neonatal thyrotoxicosis and in supraventricular arrhythmias due to hyperthyroidism. Propranolol has been used in conjunction with iodine to prepare mildly thyrotoxic patients for surgery but it is preferable to make the patient euthyroid with carbimazole. Laboratory tests of thyroid function are not altered by beta-blockers. Most experience in treating thyrotoxicosis has been gained with propranolol but **atenolol** (section 2.4) is also used.

Thyrotoxic crisis ('thyroid storm') requires emergency treatment with intravenous administration of fluids, propranolol and hydrocortisone as sodium succinate, as well as oral iodine solution and carbimazole or propylthiouracil which may need to be administered by nasogastric tube.

Neonatal hyperthyroidism is treated with carbimazole or propylthiouracil, usually for 8 to 12 weeks. In severe symptomatic disease iodine may be needed to block the thyroid and propranolol required to treat peripheral symptoms.

Pregnancy and breast-feeding Radioactive iodine therapy is contra-indicated during pregnancy. Propylthiouracil and carbimazole can be given but the blocking-replacement regimen (see above) is **not** suitable. Rarely, carbimazole has been associated with congenital defects, including aplasia cutis of the neonate—use carbimazole in pregnancy only if propylthiouracil is not suitable. Both propylthiouracil and carbimazole cross the placenta and in high doses can cause fetal goitre and hypothyroidism—the lowest dose that will control the hyperthyroid state should be used (requirements in Graves' disease tend to fall during pregnancy).

Carbimazole and propylthiouracil are present in breast milk but this does not preclude breast-feeding as long as neonatal development is closely monitored and the lowest effective dose is used.

6 Endocrine system

CARBIMAZOLE

Hepatic impairment use with caution in mild to moderate impairment; avoid in severe hepatic impairment

Pregnancy see notes above

Breast-feeding amount in milk may be sufficient to affect neonatal thyroid function therefore lowest effective dose should be used; see notes above

Side-effects nausea, mild gastro-intestinal disturbances, taste disturbance, hepatic disorders (including hepatitis and jaundice), headache, fever, malaise; rash, pruritus, arthralgia; *rarely* myopathy, alopecia, bone marrow suppression (including pancytopenia and agranulocytosis, see **CSM warning** above), hypersensitivity reactions

Indication and dose

Hyperthyroidism (including Graves' disease), thyrotoxic crisis, thyrotoxicosis

• By mouth

   Neonate initially 250 micrograms/kg 3 times daily until euthyroid then adjust as necessary (see notes above); higher initial doses (up to 1 mg/kg daily) are occasionally required, particularly in thyrotoxic crisis

   Child 1 month–12 years initially 250 micrograms/kg (max. 10 mg) 3 times daily until euthyroid then adjusted as necessary (see notes above); higher initial doses occasionally required, particularly in thyrotoxic crisis

   Child 12–18 years initially 10 mg 3 times daily until euthyroid then adjusted as necessary (see notes above); higher initial doses occasionally required, particularly in thyrotoxic crisis
   Counselling Warn child and carers to tell doctor immediately if sore throat, mouth ulcers, bruising, fever, malaise, or non-specific illness develops

Carbimazole (Non-proprietary) PoM
   Tablets, carbimazole 5 mg, net price 100-tab pack = £4.53; 20 mg, 100-tab pack = £16.83. Counselling, blood disorder symptoms

Neo-Mercazole® (Amdipharm) PoM
   Tablets, both pink, carbimazole 5 mg, net price 100-tab pack = £3.85; 20 mg, 100-tab pack = £11.44. Counselling, blood disorder symptoms
Administration tablets may be crushed in water and used immediately

◢Extemporaneous formulations available see Extemporaneous Preparations, p. 8

IODINE AND IODIDE

Cautions not for long-term treatment

Pregnancy neonatal goitre and hypothyroidism; see also notes above

Breast-feeding stop breast-feeding; danger of neonatal hypothyroidism or goitre; appears to be concentrated in milk; see also notes above

Side-effects hypersensitivity reactions including coryza-like symptoms, headache, lacrimation, conjunctivitis, pain in salivary glands, laryngitis, bronchitis, rashes; on prolonged treatment depression, insomnia, impotence; goitre in infants of mothers taking iodides

Indication and dose
   See under preparation

Aqueous Iodine Oral Solution
   Oral solution, iodine 5%, potassium iodide 10% in purified water, freshly boiled and cooled, total

   iodine 130 mg/mL, net price 500 mL = £5.95. Label: 27

Dose
   Neonatal thyrotoxicosis
   • By mouth
      Neonate 0.05–0.1 mL 3 times daily

   Thyrotoxicosis (pre-operative)
   • By mouth
      Neonate 0.1–0.3 mL 3 times daily
      Child 1 month–18 years 0.1–0.3 mL 3 times daily

   Thyrotoxic crisis
   • By mouth
      Child 1 month–1 year 0.2–0.3 mL 3 times daily
Administration Dilute well with milk or water

PROPYLTHIOURACIL

Hepatic impairment reduce dose

Renal impairment estimated glomerular filtration rate 10–50 mL/minute/1.73 m^2, use 75% of normal dose; estimated glomerular filtration rate less than 10 mL/minute/1.73 m^2, use 50% of normal dose

Pregnancy see notes above

Breast-feeding monitor infant's thyroid status but amount in milk probably too small to affect infant; high doses may affect neonatal thyroid function; see also notes above

Side-effects see under Carbimazole; leucopenia; rarely cutaneous vasculitis, thrombocytopenia, aplastic anaemia, hypoprothrombinaemia, hepatitis, encephalopathy, hepatic necrosis

(sometimes fatal), nephritis, lupus erythematous-like syndromes

Licensed use not licensed for use in children under 6 years of age

Indication and dose

Hyperthyroidism (including Graves' disease), thyrotoxic crisis, thyrotoxicosis

• By mouth

   Neonate initially 2.5–5 mg/kg twice daily until euthyroid then adjusted as necessary (see notes above); higher doses occasionally required, particularly in thyrotoxic crisis

   Child 1 month–1 year initially 2.5 mg/kg 3 times daily until euthyroid then adjusted as

◻ **PROPYLTHIOURACIL** (*continued*)

necessary (see notes above); higher doses occasionally required, particularly in thyrotoxic crisis

Child 1–5 years initially 25 mg 3 times daily until euthyroid then adjusted as necessary (see notes above); higher doses occasionally required, particularly in thyrotoxic crisis

Child 5–12 years initially 50 mg 3 times daily until euthyroid then adjusted as necessary (see notes above); higher doses occasionally required, particularly in thyrotoxic crisis

Child 12–18 years initially 100 mg 3 times daily administered until euthyroid then adjusted as necessary (see notes above); higher doses occasionally required, particularly in thyrotoxic crisis

Propylthiouracil (Non-proprietary) PoM
Tablets, propylthiouracil 50 mg. Net price 56-tab pack = £36.25

◢Extemporaneous formulations available see Extemporaneous Preparations, p. 8

◢ PROPRANOLOL HYDROCHLORIDE

Cautions see section 2.4
Contra-indications see section 2.4
Hepatic impairment section 2.4
Renal impairment section 2.4
Pregnancy section 2.4
Breast-feeding section 2.4
Side-effects see section 2.4
Licensed use see section 2.4

Indication and dose

Hyperthyroidism with autonomic symptoms, thyrotoxicosis, thyrotoxic crisis
• By mouth

Neonate initially 250–500 micrograms/kg every 6–8 hours, adjusted according to response

Child 1 month–18 years initially 250–500 micrograms/kg every 8 hours, then adjusted according to response; doses up to 1 mg/kg every 8 hours occasionally required, max. 40 mg every 8 hours

• By intravenous injection over 10 minutes

Neonate initially 20–50 micrograms/kg every 6–8 hours, adjusted according to response

Child 1 month–18 years initially 25–50 micrograms/kg (max. 5 mg) every 6–8 hours, adjusted according to response

◢Preparations
See section 2.4

6.3 Corticosteroids

6.3.1 Replacement therapy
6.3.2 Glucocorticoid therapy

6.3.1 Replacement therapy

The adrenal cortex normally secretes hydrocortisone (cortisol) which has glucocorticoid activity and weak mineralocorticoid activity. It also secretes the mineralocorticoid aldosterone.

In deficiency states, physiological replacement is best achieved with a combination of **hydrocortisone** (section 6.3.2) and the mineralocorticoid **fludrocortisone**; hydrocortisone alone does not usually provide sufficient mineralocorticoid activity for complete replacement.

In *Addison's disease* or following adrenalectomy, **hydrocortisone** by mouth is usually required. This is given in 2–3 divided doses, the larger in the morning and the smaller in the evening, mimicking the normal diurnal rhythm of cortisol secretion. The optimum daily dose is determined on the basis of clinical response. Glucocorticoid therapy is supplemented by fludrocortisone.

In *acute adrenocortical insufficiency*, **hydrocortisone** is given intravenously (preferably as sodium succinate) every 6 to 8 hours in sodium chloride intravenous infusion 0.9%.

In *hypopituitarism*, glucocorticoids should be given as in adrenocortical insufficiency, but since production of aldosterone is also regulated by the renin-angiotensin system a mineralocorticoid is not usually required. Additional replacement therapy with levothyroxine (section 6.2.1) and sex hormones (section 6.4) should be given as indicated by the pattern of hormone deficiency.

6

Endocrine system

In *congenital adrenal hyperplasia*, the pituitary gland increases production of corticotropin to compensate for reduced formation of cortisol; this results in excessive adrenal androgen production. Treatment is aimed at suppressing corticotropin using hydrocortisone (section 6.3.2). Careful and continual dose titration is required to avoid growth retardation and toxicity; for this reason potent, synthetic glucocorticoids such as dexamethasone are usually reserved for use in adolescents. The dose is adjusted according to clinical response and measurement of adrenal androgens and 17-hydroxyprogesterone. Salt-losing forms of congenital adrenal hyperplasia (where there is a lack of aldosterone production) require mineralocorticoid replacement. Mineralocorticoid replacement may also be beneficial even when salt-losing symptoms are not evident.

FLUDROCORTISONE ACETATE

Cautions section 6.3.2; **interactions:** Appendix 1 (corticosteroids)

Contra-indications section 6.3.2

Hepatic impairment see section 6.3.2

Renal impairment see section 6.3.2

Pregnancy see section 6.3.2

Breast-feeding see section 6.3.2

Side-effects section 6.3.2

Indication and dose

Mineralocorticoid replacement in adrenocortical insufficiency
• By mouth

Neonate initially 100 micrograms once daily, adjusted according to response; usual range 50–300 micrograms daily

Child 1 month–18 years initially 50–100 micrograms once daily; maintenance 50–300 micrograms once daily, adjusted according to response

Florinef® (Squibb) PoM

Tablets, scored, fludrocortisone acetate 100 micrograms. Net price 100-tab pack = £5.15. Label: 10, steroid card

▲ Extemporaneous formulations available see Extemporaneous Preparations, p. 8

Note Bioavailability uncertain, tablets may result in more reliable absorption and may be dispersed in water

6.3.2 Glucocorticoid therapy

In comparing the relative potencies of corticosteroids in terms of their anti-inflammatory (glucocorticoid) effects it should be borne in mind that high glucocorticoid activity in itself is of no advantage unless it is accompanied by relatively low mineralocorticoid activity (see Disadvantages of Corticosteroids below). The mineralocorticoid activity of **fludrocortisone** (section 6.3.1) is so high that its anti-inflammatory activity is of no clinical relevance. The table below shows equivalent anti-inflammatory doses.

Equivalent anti-inflammatory doses of corticosteroids
This table takes no account of mineralocorticoid effects, nor does it take account of variations in duration of action
Prednisolone 1 mg ≡ Betamethasone 150 micrograms
≡ Cortisone acetate 5 mg
≡ Deflazacort 1.2 mg
≡ Dexamethasone 150 micrograms
≡ Hydrocortisone 4 mg
≡ Methylprednisolone 800 micrograms
≡ Triamcinolone 800 micrograms

The relatively high mineralocorticoid activity of **cortisone** and **hydrocortisone**, and the resulting fluid retention, make them unsuitable for disease suppression on a long-term basis. However, they can be used for adrenal replacement therapy (section 6.3.1); hydrocortisone is preferred because cortisone requires conversion in the liver to hydrocortisone. Hydrocortisone is used on a short-term basis by intravenous injection for the emergency management of some conditions. The relatively moderate anti-inflammatory potency of hydrocortisone also makes it a useful topical corticosteroid for the management of inflammatory skin conditions because side-effects (both topical and systemic) are less marked (section 13.4); cortisone is not active topically.

Prednisolone has predominantly glucocorticoid activity and is the corticosteroid most commonly used by mouth for long-term disease suppression.

Betamethasone and **dexamethasone** have very high glucocorticoid activity in conjunction with insignificant mineralocorticoid activity. This makes them particularly suitable for high-dose therapy in conditions where fluid retention would be a disadvantage.

Betamethasone and dexamethasone also have a long duration of action and this, coupled with their lack of mineralocorticoid action makes them particularly suitable for conditions which require suppression of corticotropin (corticotrophin) secretion. Some esters of betamethasone and of **beclometasone** (beclomethasone) exert a considerably more marked topical effect (e.g. on the skin or the lungs) than when given by mouth; use is made of this to obtain topical effects whilst minimising systemic side-effects (e.g. for skin applications and asthma inhalations).

Deflazacort has a high glucocorticoid activity; it is derived from prednisolone.

Use of corticosteroids

Dosages of corticosteroids vary widely in different diseases and in different children. If the use of a corticosteroid can save or prolong life, as in exfoliative dermatitis, pemphigus, acute leukaemia or acute transplant rejection, high doses may need to be given, because the complications of therapy are likely to be less serious than the effects of the disease itself.

When long-term corticosteroid therapy is used in some chronic diseases, the adverse effects of treatment may become greater than the disabilities caused by the disease. To minimise side-effects the maintenance dose should be kept as low as possible.

When potentially less harmful measures are ineffective corticosteroids are used topically for the treatment of inflammatory conditions of the skin (section 13.4). Corticosteroids should be avoided or used only under specialist supervision in psoriasis (section 13.5).

Corticosteroids are used both topically (by rectum) and systemically (by mouth or intravenously) in the management of ulcerative colitis and Crohn's disease (section 1.5 and section 1.7.2).

Use can be made of the mineralocorticoid activity of fludrocortisone to treat postural hypotension in autonomic neuropathy.

High-dose corticosteroids should be avoided for the management of septic shock. However, low-dose hydrocortisone can be used in septic shock (section 2.7.1) that is resistant to volume expansion and catecholamines, and is accompanied by suspected or proven adrenal insufficiency.

The suppressive action of glucocorticoids on the hypothalamic-pituitary-adrenal axis is greatest and most prolonged when they are given at night. In most adults a single dose of 1 mg of dexamethasone at night is sufficient to inhibit corticotropin secretion for 24 hours. This is the basis of the 'overnight dexamethasone suppression test' for diagnosing Cushing's syndrome.

Betamethasone and dexamethasone are also appropriate for conditions where water retention would be a disadvantage.

A corticosteroid can be used in the management of raised intracranial pressure or cerebral oedema that occurs as a result of malignancy (see also p. 28); high doses of betamethasone or dexamethasone are generally used. However, a corticosteroid should **not** be used for the management of head injury or stroke because it is unlikely to be of benefit and may even be harmful.

In acute hypersensitivity reactions such as angioedema of the upper respiratory tract and anaphylactic shock, corticosteroids are indicated as an adjunct to emergency treatment with adrenaline (epinephrine) (section 3.4.3). In such cases hydrocortisone (as sodium succinate) by intravenous injection may be required.

In the management of asthma, corticosteroids are preferably used by inhalation (section 3.2) but systemic therapy along with bronchodilators is required for the emergency treatment of severe acute asthma (section 3.1.1).

Dexamethasone should not be used routinely for the prophylaxis and treatment of chronic lung disease in neonates because of an association with adverse neurological effects.

Corticosteroids may be useful in conditions such as auto-immune hepatitis, rheumatoid arthritis, and sarcoidosis; they may also lead to remissions of acquired haemolytic anaemia (section 9.1.3) and thrombocytopenic purpura (section 9.1.4).

High doses of a corticosteroid (usually prednisolone) are used in the treatment of *glomerular kidney disease*, including *nephrotic syndrome*. The condition frequently recurs; a corticosteroid given in high doses and for prolonged periods may delay relapse but the higher incidence of adverse effects limits the overall benefit. Those who suffer frequent relapses may be treated with prednisolone given in a low dose (daily or on alternate days) for 3–6 months; the dose should be adjusted to minimise effects on growth and development. Other drugs used in the treatment of glomerular kidney disease include levamisole (section 5.5.2), cyclophosphamide and chlorambucil (section 8.1.1), and ciclosporin (section 8.2.2). *Congenital nephrotic syndrome* may be resistant to corticosteroids and immunosuppressants; indometacin (section 10.1.1) and an ACE inhibitor such as captopril (section 2.5.5.1) have been used.

Corticosteroids can improve the prognosis of serious conditions such as systemic lupus erythematosus and polyarteritis nodosa; the effects of the disease process may be suppressed and symptoms relieved, but the underlying condition is not cured, although it may ultimately remit. It is usual to begin therapy in these conditions at fairly high dose and then to reduce the dose to the lowest commensurate with disease control.

For other references to the use of corticosteroids see Prescribing in Palliative Care (p. 26), section 8.2.2 (immunosuppression), section 10.1.2 (rheumatic diseases), section 11.4 (eye), section 12.1.1 (otitis externa), section 12.2.1 (allergic rhinitis), and section 12.3.1 (aphthous ulcers).

Administration

Whenever possible *local treatment* with creams, intra-articular injections, inhalations, eye-drops, or enemas should be used in preference to *systemic treatment*. The suppressive action of a corticosteroid on cortisol secretion is least when it is given as a single dose in the morning. In an attempt to reduce pituitary-adrenal suppression further, the total dose for two days can sometimes be taken as a single dose on alternate days; alternate-day administration has not been very successful in the management of asthma (section 3.2). Pituitary-adrenal suppression can also be reduced by means of intermittent therapy with short courses. In some conditions it may be possible to reduce the dose of corticosteroid by adding a small dose of an immunosuppressive drug (section 8.2.1).

Cautions and contra-indications of corticosteroids

Adrenal suppression

During prolonged therapy with corticosteroids, adrenal atrophy develops and can persist for years after stopping. Abrupt withdrawal after a prolonged period can lead to acute adrenal insufficiency, hypotension, or death (see Withdrawal of Corticosteroids, below). Withdrawal can also be associated with fever, myalgia, arthralgia, rhinitis, conjunctivitis, painful itchy skin nodules, and weight loss.

To compensate for a diminished adrenocortical response caused by prolonged corticosteroid treatment, any significant intercurrent illness, trauma, or surgical procedure requires a temporary increase in corticosteroid dose, or if already stopped, a temporary re-introduction of corticosteroid treatment. To avoid a precipitous fall in blood pressure during anaesthesia or in the immediate postoperative period, anaesthetists **must** know whether a patient is taking or has been taking a corticosteroid. A regimen for corticosteroid replacement may be necessary before and after surgery.

Children on long-term corticosteroid treatment should carry a Steroid Treatment Card (see p. 455) which gives guidance on minimising risk and provides details of prescriber, drug, dosage and duration of treatment.

Infections

Prolonged courses of corticosteroids increase susceptibility to infections and severity of infections; clinical presentation of infections may also be atypical. Serious infections, e.g. *septicaemia* and *tuberculosis*, may reach an advanced stage before being recognised, and *amoebiasis* or *strongyloidiasis* may be activated or exacerbated (exclude before initiating a corticosteroid in those at risk or with suggestive symptoms). Fungal or viral *ocular infections* may also be exacerbated (see also section 11.4.1).

Chickenpox   Unless they have had chickenpox, children receiving oral or parenteral corticosteroids for purposes other than replacement should be regarded as being *at risk of severe chickenpox* (see Steroid Treatment Card). Manifestations of fulminant illness include pneumonia, hepatitis and disseminated intravascular coagulation; rash is not necessarily a prominent feature.

Passive immunisation with varicella–zoster immunoglobulin (section 14.5.2) is needed for exposed non-immune children receiving systemic corticosteroids or for those who have used them within the previous 3 months. Confirmed chickenpox warrants specialist care and urgent treatment (section 5.3.2.1). Corticosteroids should not be stopped and dosage may need to be increased.

Topical, inhaled or rectal corticosteroids are less likely to be associated with an increased risk of severe chickenpox.

Measles   Children taking corticosteroids, and their carers, should be advised to take particular care to avoid exposure to measles and to seek urgent medical advice if exposure occurs. Prophylaxis with intramuscular normal immunoglobulin (section 14.5.1) may be needed.

Withdrawal of corticosteroids

The magnitude and speed of dose reduction in corticosteroid withdrawal should be determined on a case-by-case basis, taking into consideration the underlying condition that is being treated, and individual patient factors such as the likelihood of relapse and the duration of corticosteroid treatment. *Gradual* withdrawal of systemic corticosteroids should be considered in those whose disease is unlikely to relapse and have:

- recently received repeated courses (particularly if taken for longer than 3 weeks);
- taken a short course within 1 year of stopping long-term therapy;
- other possible causes of adrenal suppression;
- received more than 40 mg daily prednisolone (or equivalent) *or* 2 mg/kg daily for 1 week or 1 mg/kg daily for 1 month;
- been given repeat doses in the evening;
- received more than 3 weeks' treatment.

Systemic corticosteroids may be stopped abruptly in those whose disease is unlikely to relapse *and* who have received treatment for 3 weeks or less *and* who are not included in the patient groups described above.

During corticosteroid withdrawal the dose may be reduced rapidly down to physiological doses (equivalent to prednisolone 5 mg/m^2 daily) and then reduced more slowly. Assessment of the disease may be needed during withdrawal to ensure that relapse does not occur.

Psychiatric reactions

Systemic corticosteroids, particularly in high doses, are linked to psychiatric reactions including euphoria, nightmares, insomnia, irritability, mood lability, suicidal thoughts, psychotic reactions, and behavioural disturbances. A serious paranoid state or depression with risk of suicide can be induced, particularly in children with a history of mental disorder. These reactions frequently subside on reducing the dose or discontinuing the corticosteroid but they may also require specific management. Children and their carers should be advised to seek medical advice if psychiatric symptoms (especially depression and suicidal thoughts) occur and they should also be alert to the rare possibility of such reactions during withdrawal of corticosteroid treatment.

Systemic corticosteroids should be prescribed with care in those predisposed to psychiatric reactions, including those who have previously suffered corticosteroid-induced psychosis, or who have a personal or family history of psychiatric disorders.

Advice to children and carers

A patient information leaflet should be supplied to every patient when a systemic corticosteroid is prescribed. Children and carers should especially be advised of the following (for details, see Infections, Adrenal Suppression, and Psychiatric Reactions above and Withdrawal of Corticosteroids below):

- **Immunosupression** Prolonged courses of corticosteroids can increase susceptibility to infection and serious infections can go unrecognised. Unless already immune, children are at risk of severe **chickenpox** and should avoid close contact with people who have chickenpox or shingles. Similarly, precautions should also be taken against contracting **measles**;

- **Adrenal suppression** If the corticosteroid is given for longer than 3 weeks, treatment must not be stopped abruptly. Adrenal suppression can last for a year or more after stopping treatment and the child or carer must mention the course of corticosteroid when receiving treatment for any illness or injury;

- **Mood and behaviour changes** Corticosteroid treatment, especially with high doses, can alter mood and behaviour early in treatment—the child can become confused, irritable and suffer from delusion and suicidal thoughts. These effects can also occur when corticosteroid treatment is being withdrawn. Medical advice should be sought if worrying psychological changes occur;

- **Other serious effects** Serious gastro-intestinal, musculoskeletal, and ophthalmic effects which require medical help can also occur; for details see Side-effects of Corticosteroids, p. 456.

Steroid treatment cards (see p. 455) should be issued where appropriate. Doctors and pharmacists can obtain supplies of the card from:

England and Wales

3M Security Printing and Systems Limited
Gorse Street, Chadderton
Oldham, OL9 9QH
Tel: (0161) 683 2189
Fax: (0161) 683 2188
nhsforms@spsl.uk.com

Scotland

R.R. Donnelley Global Document Solutions
20–22 South Gyle Crescent
Edinburgh, EH12 9EB
Tel: (0131) 334 1229
Fax: (0131) 334 5946
ian.fruish@rrd.com

Northern Ireland

Pharmaceutical Directorate
Business Services Organisation
2 Franklin Street
Belfast, BT2 8DQ
Tel: (028) 9053 5652

Other cautions and contra-indications

Other cautions include: growth restriction—possibly irreversible, frequent monitoring required if history of tuberculosis (or X-ray changes), hypertension, congestive heart failure, diabetes mellitus including family history, osteoporosis, susceptibility to angle-closure glaucoma (including family history), ocular herpes simplex—

risk of corneal perforation, severe affective disorders (particularly if history of steroid-induced psychosis—see also Psychiatric Reactions above), epilepsy, peptic ulcer, hypothyroidism, history of steroid myopathy, ulcerative colitis, diverticulitis, recent intestinal anastomoses, thromboembolic disorders, myasthenia gravis; **interactions:** Appendix 1 (corticosteroids)

Other contra-indications include: systemic infection (unless specific therapy given); avoid live virus vaccines in those receiving immunosuppressive doses (serum antibody response diminished)

Hepatic impairment

When corticosteroids are administered orally or parenterally, the plasma-drug concentration may be increased in children with hepatic impairment. Corticosteroids should be used with caution in hepatic impairment and the child should be monitored closely.

Renal impairment

Oral and parenteral preparations of corticosteroids should be used with caution in children with renal impairment.

STEROID TREATMENT CARD

I am a patient on STEROID treatment which must not be stopped suddenly

- If you have been taking this medicine for more than three weeks, the dose should be reduced gradually when you stop taking steroids unless your doctor says otherwise.

- Read the patient information leaflet given with the medicine.

- Always carry this card with you and show it to anyone who treats you (for example a doctor, nurse, pharmacist or dentist). For one year after you stop the treatment, you must mention that you have taken steroids.

- If you become ill, or if you come into contact with anyone who has an infectious disease, consult your doctor promptly. If you have never had chickenpox, you should avoid close contact with people who have chickenpox or shingles. If you do come into contact with chickenpox, see your doctor urgently.

- Make sure that the information on the card is kept up to date.

6

Endocrine system

Pregnancy and breast-feeding

The benefit of treatment with corticosteroids during pregnancy and breast-feeding outweighs the risk; pregnant women with fluid retention should be monitored closely. Corticosteroid cover will be required during labour.

Following a review of the data on the safety of systemic corticosteroids used in pregnancy and breast-feeding the CSM (May 1998) concluded:

- corticosteroids vary in their ability to cross the placenta; betamethasone and dexamethasone cross the placenta readily while 88% of prednisolone is inactivated as it crosses the placenta;

- there is no convincing evidence that systemic corticosteroids increase the incidence of congenital abnormalities such as cleft palate or lip;

- when administration is prolonged or repeated during pregnancy, systemic corticosteroids increase the risk of intra-uterine growth restriction; there is no evidence of intra-uterine growth restriction following short-term treatment (e.g. prophylactic treatment for neonatal respiratory distress syndrome);

- any adrenal suppression in the neonate following prenatal exposure usually resolves spontaneously after birth and is rarely clinically important;

- prednisolone appears in small amounts in breast milk but maternal doses of up to 40 mg daily are unlikely to cause systemic effects in the infant; infants should be monitored for adrenal suppression if the mothers are taking a higher dose.

Side-effects of corticosteroids

Overdosage or prolonged use can exaggerate some of the normal physiological actions of corticosteroids leading to mineralocorticoid and glucocorticoid side-effects.

Corticosteroids suppress growth and can affect the development of puberty. It is important to use the lowest effective dose; alternate-day regimens may be appropriate and limit growth reduction. For the effect of corticosteroids given in pregnancy, see Pregnancy and Breast-feeding, above.

Mineralocorticoid side-effects include hypertension, sodium and water retention, and potassium, and calcium loss. They are most marked with fludrocortisone, but are significant with cortisone, hydrocortisone, corticotropin, and tetracosactide (tetracosactrin). Mineralocorticoid actions are negligible with the high potency glucocorticoids, betamethasone and dexamethasone, and occur only slightly with methylprednisolone, prednisolone, and triamcinolone.

Glucocorticoid side-effects include diabetes and osteoporosis (section 6.6); in addition high doses are associated with avascular necrosis of the femoral head. Muscle wasting (proximal myopathy) can also occur. Corticosteroid therapy is also weakly linked with peptic ulceration (the potential advantage of soluble or enteric-coated preparations to reduce the risk is speculative only). See also Psychiatric Reactions, p. 453.

High doses of corticosteroids can cause Cushing's syndrome, with moon face, striae, and acne; it is usually reversible on withdrawal of treatment, but this must always be gradually tapered to avoid symptoms of acute adrenal insufficiency (**important**: see also Adrenal Suppression, p. 452).

Side-effects can be minimised by using the lowest effective dose for the minimum period possible.

Other side effects include: *gastro-intestinal effects*: dyspepsia, abdominal distension, acute pancreatitis, oesophageal ulceration and candidiasis; *musculoskeletal effects*: muscle weakness, vertebral and long bone fractures, tendon rupture; *endocrine effects*: menstrual irregularities and amenorrhoea, hirsutism, weight gain, negative nitrogen and calcium balance, increased appetite; increased susceptibility to and severity of infection, reactivation of dormant tuberculosis; *neuropsychiatric effects*: psychological dependence, insomnia, increased intracranial pressure with papilloedema (usually after withdrawal), aggravation of schizophrenia, aggravation of epilepsy; *ophthalmic effects*: papilloedema, posterior subcapsular cataracts, corneal or scleral thinning and exacerbation of ophthalmic viral or fungal disease, increased intra-ocular pressure, exophthalmos, *very rarely* angle-closure glaucoma; *also* impaired healing, petechiae, ecchymoses, facial erythema, suppression of skin test reactions, urticaria, hyperhidrosis, skin atrophy, bruising, telangiectasia, myocardial rupture following recent myocardial infarction, congestive heart failure, leucocytosis, hyperglycaemia, hypersensitivity reactions (including anaphylaxis), thromboembolism, nausea, malaise, hiccups, headache, vertigo.

For other references to the side-effects of corticosteroids see section 1.5 (gastro-intestinal system), section 3.2 (asthma), section 11.4 (eye) and section 13.4 (skin).

BETAMETHASONE

Cautions see notes above
Contra-indications see notes above
Hepatic impairment see notes above
Renal impairment see notes above
Pregnancy see notes above; transient effect on fetal movements and heart rate
Breast-feeding see notes above
Side-effects see notes above
Licensed use *Betnesol*® tablets not licensed for use as mouthwash

Indication and dose

Suppression of inflammatory and allergic disorders; congenital adrenal hyperplasia; see also notes above

• By slow intravenous injection or by intravenous infusion

Child 1 month–1 year initially 1 mg repeated up to 4 times in 24 hours according to response

Child 1–6 years initially 2 mg repeated up to 4 times in 24 hours according to response

Child 6–12 years initially 4 mg repeated up to 4 times in 24 hours according to response

Child 12–18 years initially 4–20 mg repeated up to 4 times in 24 hours according to response

Eye section 11.4.1

Ear section 12.1.1

Nose section 12.2.1

Mouth section 12.3.1

Administration For *intravenous infusion*, dilute with Glucose 5% or Sodium Chloride 0.9%

Betnesol® (UCB Pharma) [PoM]
Injection, betamethasone 4 mg (as sodium phosphate) /mL. Net price 1-mL amp = £1.17. Label: 10, steroid card

DEFLAZACORT

Cautions see notes above
Contra-indications see notes above
Hepatic impairment see notes above
Renal impairment see notes above
Pregnancy see notes above
Breast-feeding see notes above
Side-effects see notes above

Indication and dose

Inflammatory and allergic disorders

• By mouth

Child 1 month–12 years 0.25–1.5 mg/kg once daily or on alternate days; up to 2.4 mg/kg (max. 120 mg) daily has been used in emergency situations

Child 12–18 years 3–18 mg once daily or on alternate days; up to 2.4 mg/kg (max. 120 mg) daily has been used in emergency situations

Nephrotic syndrome
• By mouth

Child 1 month–18 years initially 1.5 mg/kg once daily (max. 120 mg) reduced to lowest effective dose for maintenance

Calcort® (Sanofi-Aventis) [PoM]
Tablets, deflazacort 6 mg, net price 60-tab pack = £15.82. Label: 5, 10, steroid card

DEXAMETHASONE

Cautions see notes above
Contra-indications see notes above
Hepatic impairment see notes above
Renal impairment see notes above
Pregnancy see notes above
Breast-feeding see notes above
Side-effects see notes above; also perineal irritation may follow intravenous administration of the phosphate ester
Licensed use not licensed for use in bacterial meningitis

Note Dexamethasone 1 mg ≡ dexamethasone phosphate 1.2 mg ≡ dexamethasone sodium phosphate 1.3 mg

Indication and dose

Inflammatory and allergic disorders

• By mouth (as dexamethasone)

Child 1 month–18 years 10–100 micrograms/kg daily in 1–2 divided doses, adjusted according to response; up to 300 micrograms/kg daily may be required in emergency situations

• By intramuscular injection or slow intravenous injection or infusion (as dexamethasone phosphate)

Child 1 month–12 years 100–400 micrograms/kg daily in 1–2 divided doses; max. 24 mg daily

Child 12–18 years initially 0.5–24 mg daily

◻ **DEXAMETHASONE** (*continued*)

Life-threatening cerebral oedema
- **By intravenous injection (as dexamethasone phosphate)**

Child under 35 kg body-weight initially 20 mg, then 4 mg every 3 hours for 3 days, then 4 mg every 6 hours for 1 day, then 2 mg every 6 hours for 4 days, then decrease by 1 mg daily

Child over 35 kg body-weight initially 25 mg, then 4 mg every 2 hours for 3 days, then 4 mg every 4 hours for 1 day, then 4 mg every 6 hours for 4 days, then decrease by 2 mg daily

Bacterial meningitis (see section 5.1)
- **By slow intravenous injection (as dexamethasone phosphate)**

Child 2 months–18 years 150 micrograms/kg every 6 hours for 4 days starting before or with first dose of antibacterial

Physiological replacement
- **By mouth or by slow intravenous injection (as dexamethasone)**

Child 1 month–18 years 250–500 micrograms/m² every 12 hours, adjusted according to response

Croup section 3.1

Nausea and vomiting with chemotherapy section 8.1

Rheumatic disease section 10.1.2

Eye section 11.4.1

Administration for administration *by mouth* tablets may be dispersed in water or injection solution given by mouth

For *intravenous infusion* dilute with Glucose 5% or Sodium Chloride 0.9%; give over 15–20 minutes

Dexamethasone (Non-proprietary) PoM
Tablets, dexamethasone 500 micrograms, net price 28-tab pack = £29.50; 2 mg, 50-tab pack = £6.88, 100-tab pack = £13.08. Label: 10, steroid card, 21

Oral solution, sugar-free, dexamethasone (as dexamethasone sodium phosphate) 2 mg/5 mL, net price 150-mL = £42.30. Label: 10, steroid card, 21
Brands include *Dexsol®*

Injection, dexamethasone phosphate (as dexamethasone sodium phosphate) 4 mg/mL, net price 1-mL amp = £1.00, 2-mL vial = £1.98; 24 mg/mL, 5-mL vial = £16.66. Label: 10, steroid card

Injection, dexamethasone (as dexamethasone sodium phosphate) 4 mg/mL, net price 1-mL amp = 91p, 2-mL vial = £1.27. Label: 10, steroid card

HYDROCORTISONE

Cautions see notes above
Contra-indications see notes above
Hepatic impairment see notes above
Renal impairment see notes above
Pregnancy see notes above
Breast-feeding see notes above
Side-effects see notes above; also phosphate ester associated with paraesthesia and pain (particularly in the perineal region)

Indication and dose

Congenital adrenal hyperplasia see also section 6.3.1
- **By mouth**

Neonate 6–7 mg/m² every 8 hours, adjusted according to response

Child 1 month–18 years 5–6.5 mg/m² every 8 hours, adjusted according to response; usual maintenance 4–5 mg/m² every 8 hours but higher doses may be needed

Acute adrenocortical insufficiency (*Addisonian crisis*) see also notes above and section 6.3.1
- **By slow intravenous administration**

Neonate initially 10 mg as a slow intravenous injection then 100 mg/m² daily as a continuous infusion or in divided doses every 6–8 hours; adjusted according to response; when stable reduce over 4–5 days to oral maintenance dose

Child 1 month–12 years initially 2–4 mg/kg as a slow intravenous injection or infusion then 2–4 mg/kg every 6 hours; adjusted according to response; when stable reduce over 4–5 days to oral maintenance dose

Child 12–18 years 100 mg every 6 to 8 hours by slow intravenous injection or infusion

Adrenal hypoplasia, Addison's disease, chronic maintenance or replacement therapy
- **By mouth**

Neonate usual dose 4–5 mg/m² every 8 hours; higher doses may be needed

Child 1 month–18 years usual dose 4–5 mg/m² every 8 hours; higher doses may be needed
Note larger doses given in the morning and smaller doses in the evening

Inflammatory bowel disease—induction of remission see also section 1.5.2
- **By intravenous injection**

Child 2–18 years 2.5 mg/kg (max. 100 mg) every 6 hours

- **By continuous intravenous infusion**

Child 2–18 years 10 mg/kg daily (max. 400 mg daily)

Acute hypersensitivity reactions, angioedema see also section 3.4.3
- **By intramuscular or intravenous injection**

Child under 6 months initially 25 mg 3 times daily, adjusted according to response

Child 6 months–6 years initially 50 mg 3 times daily, adjusted according to response

Endocrine system

6

�𝄐 **HYDROCORTISONE** *(continued)*

Child 6–12 years initially 100 mg 3 times daily, adjusted according to response

Child 12–18 years initially 200 mg 3 times daily, adjusted according to response

Hypotension resistant to inotropic treatment and volume replacement (limited evidence)
● By intravenous injection

Neonate initially 2.5 mg/kg repeated if necessary after 4 hours, then 2.5 mg/kg every 6 hours for 48 hours or until blood pressure recovers, then dose reduced gradually over at least 48 hours

Child 1 month–18 years 1 mg/kg (max. 100 mg) every 6 hours

Severe acute asthma p. 172

Eye section 11.4.1

Haemorrhoids section 1.7.2

Rheumatic disease section 10.1.2

Shock section 2.7.1

Skin section 13.4

Administration for *intravenous administration*, dilute with Glucose 5% or Sodium Chloride 0.9%; for *intermittent infusion* give over 20–30 minutes.

For administration *by mouth*, injection solution may be swallowed [unlicensed use] but consider phosphate content; alternatively *Corlan*® pellets (section 12.3.1) may be swallowed [unlicensed use]—pellets should not be cut as may not provide appropriate dose

Hydrocortisone® (Non-proprietary) [PoM]
Tablets, scored, hydrocortisone 10 mg, net price 30-tab pack = £40.00; 20 mg, 30-tab pack = £42.00. Label: 10, steroid card, 21

¹**Efcortesol**® (Sovereign) [PoM] ◢
Injection, hydrocortisone 100 mg (as sodium phosphate)/mL, net price 1-mL amp = £1.08, 5-mL amp = £4.89. Label: 10, steroid card
Note Paraesthesia and pain (particularly in the perineal region) may follow intravenous injection of the phosphate ester
1. [PoM] restriction does not apply where administration is for saving life in emergency

¹**Solu-Cortef**® (Pharmacia) [PoM]
Injection, powder for reconstitution, hydrocortisone (as sodium succinate). Net price 100-mg vial = 92p, 100-mg vial with 2-mL amp water for injections = £1.16. Label: 10, steroid card
1. [PoM] restriction does not apply where administration is for saving life in emergency

◢ Extemporaneous formulations available see Extemporaneous Preparations, p. 8

◣ METHYLPREDNISOLONE

Cautions see notes above; rapid intravenous administration of large doses associated with cardiovascular collapse
Contra-indications see notes above
Hepatic impairment see notes above
Renal impairment see notes above
Pregnancy see notes above
Breast-feeding see notes above
Side-effects see notes above

Indication and dose
Inflammatory and allergic disorders
● By mouth, slow intravenous injection or by intravenous infusion
Child 1 month–18 years 0.5–1.7 mg/kg daily in 2–4 divided doses depending on condition and response

Treatment of graft rejection reactions
● By intravenous injection
Child 1 month–18 years 10–20 mg/kg or 400–600 mg/m² (max. 1 g) once daily for 3 days

Severe erythema multiforme (Stevens-Johnson syndrome), lupus nephritis, systemic onset juvenile idiopathic arthritis
● By intravenous injection
Child 1 month–18 years 10–30 mg/kg (max. 1 g) once daily or on alternate days for up to 3 doses

Immunosuppression section 8.2.2

Rheumatic disease section 10.1.2

Skin section 13.4

Administration intravenous injection given over 30 minutes; for intravenous infusion may be diluted with sodium chloride intravenous infusion 0.9% or 0.45%, or glucose intravenous infusion 5% or 10%

Medrone® (Pharmacia) [PoM]
Tablets, scored, methylprednisolone 2 mg (pink), net price 30-tab pack = £3.88; 4 mg, 30-tab pack = £6.19; 16 mg, 30-tab pack = £17.17; 100 mg (blue), 20-tab pack = £48.32. Label: 10, steroid card, 21

Solu-Medrone® (Pharmacia) [PoM]
Injection, powder for reconstitution, methylprednisolone (as sodium succinate) (all with solvent). Net price 40-mg vial = £1.58; 125-mg vial =

◻ **METHYLPREDNISOLONE** (*continued*)

£4.75; 500-mg vial = £9.60; 1-g vial = £17.30; 2-g vial = £32.86. Label: 10, steroid card

◢Intramuscular depot
Depo-Medrone® (Pharmacia) [PoM]
Injection (aqueous suspension), methylprednisolone acetate 40 mg/mL. Net price 1-mL vial =

£2.87; 2-mL vial = £5.15; 3-mL vial = £7.47. Label: 10, steroid card

Dose
• By deep intramuscular injection into gluteal muscle
Seek specialist advice

◢ PREDNISOLONE

Cautions see notes above; also Duchenne's muscular dystrophy (possible transient rhabdomyolysis and myoglobinuria following strenuous physical activity)

Contra-indications see notes above

Hepatic impairment see notes above

Renal impairment see notes above

Pregnancy see notes above

Breast-feeding see notes above

Side-effects see notes above

Indication and dose

Autoimmune inflammatory disorders (including juvenile idiopathic arthritis, connective tissue disorders and systemic lupus erythematosus)
• By mouth
Child 1 month–18 years initially 1–2 mg/kg once daily (usual max. 60 mg daily), then reduced after a few days if appropriate

Autoimmune hepatitis
• By mouth
Child 1 month–18 years initially 2 mg/kg once daily (max. 40 mg daily) then reduced to minimum effective dose

Corticosteroid replacement therapy
• By mouth
Child 12–18 years 5 mg/m² daily in 1–2 divided doses adjusted according to response

Infantile spasms
• By mouth
Child 1 month–2 years initially 10 mg 4 times daily for 14 days (if seizures not controlled after 7 days increase to 20 mg 3 times daily for 7 days); reduce dose gradually over 15 days until stopped (patients taking 40 mg daily, reduce dose in steps of 10 mg every 5 days, then stop; patients taking 60 mg daily, reduce dose to 40 mg daily for 5 days, then 20 mg daily for 5 days, then 10 mg daily for 5 days, then stop)

Idiopathic thrombocytopenic purpura
• By mouth
Child 1–10 years 1–2 mg/kg daily for max. 14 days *or* 4 mg/kg daily for max. 4 days

Nephrotic syndrome
• By mouth
Child 1 month–18 years initially 60 mg/m² once daily (max. 80 mg daily) for 4–6 weeks until proteinuria ceases then 40 mg/m² on alternate days for 4–6 weeks, then withdraw by reducing dose gradually; prevention of relapse 0.5–1 mg/kg once daily or on alternate days for 3–6 months

Asthma see p. 186

Ear section 12.1.1

Eye section 11.4.1

Immunosuppression section 8.2.2

Inflammatory bowel disease section 1.5.2

Pneumocystis pneumonia section 5.4.8

Rheumatic disease section 10.1.2

Prednisolone (Non-proprietary) [PoM]
Tablets, prednisolone 1 mg, net price 28-tab pack = £1.02; 5 mg, 28-tab pack = £1.09; 25 mg, 56-tab pack = £25.00. Label: 10, steroid card, 21

Tablets, both e/c, prednisolone 2.5 mg (brown), net price 30-tab pack = £4.67; 5 mg (red), 30-tab pack = £4.73. Label: 5, 10, steroid card, 25
Brands include *Deltacortril®*

Soluble tablets, prednisolone 5 mg (as sodium phosphate), net price 30-tab pack = £7.45. Label: 10, steroid card, 13, 21

6.4 Sex hormones

6.4.1 Female sex hormones
6.4.2 Male sex hormones and antagonists
6.4.3 Anabolic steroids

Sex hormone replacement therapy is indicated in children for the treatment of gonadotrophin deficiency, gonadal disorders, or delayed puberty that interferes with quality of life. Indications include constitutional delay in puberty, congenital or acquired hypogonadotrophic hypogonadism, hypergonadotrophic hypogonad-

6 Endocrine system

ism (Turner's syndrome, Klinefelter's syndrome), endocrine disorders (Cushing's syndrome or hyperprolactinaemia), and chronic illnesses, such as cystic fibrosis or sickle-cell disease, that may affect the onset of puberty.

Replacement therapy is generally started at the appropriate age for the development of puberty and should be managed by a paediatric endocrinologist. Patients with constitutional delay, chronic illness, or eating disorders may need only small doses of hormone supplements for 4 to 6 months to induce puberty and endogenous sex hormone production, which is then sustained. Patients with organic causes of hormone deficiency will require life-long replacement, adjusted to allow normal development.

Inadequate treatment may lead to poor bone mineralisation, resulting in fractures and osteoporosis.

6.4.1 Female sex hormones

6.4.1.1 Oestrogens
6.4.1.2 Progestogens

6.4.1.1 Oestrogens

Oestrogens are necessary for the development of female secondary sexual characteristics. If onset of puberty is delayed because of organic pathology, puberty can be induced with ethinylestradiol in increasing doses, guided by breast staging and uterine scans. Cyclical progestogen replacement is added after 12–18 months of oestrogen treatment (see section 6.4.1.2). Once the adult dosage of oestrogen has been reached (20 micrograms ethinylestradiol daily), it may be more convenient to provide replacement either as a low-dose oestrogen containing oral contraceptive formulation [unlicensed indication] (see section 7.3.1) or as a combined oestrogen and progestogen hormone replacement therapy preparation [unlicensed indication] (see BNF section 6.4.1.1). There is limited experience in the use of transdermal patches or gels in children; compliance and skin irritation are sometimes a problem.

Ethinylestradiol is occasionally used, under **specialist supervision**, for the management of hereditary haemorrhagic telangiectasia (but evidence of benefit is limited), for the prevention of tall stature, and in tests of growth hormone secretion (see below). Side-effects include nausea and fluid retention.

Topical oestrogen creams are used in the treatment of labial adhesions (see section 7.2.1)

▲ ETHINYLESTRADIOL

(Ethinyloestradiol)

Cautions see Combined Hormonal Contraceptives (section 7.3.1); **interactions**: Appendix 1 (Oestrogens)

Contra-indications cardiovascular disease (sodium retention with oedema), personal or family history of thromboembolism, acute porphyria; see also Combined Hormonal Contraceptives (section 7.3.1)

Hepatic impairment avoid in liver disease including disorders of hepatic excretion (e.g. Dubin-Johnson or Rotor syndromes), infective hepatitis (until liver function returns to normal), and jaundice

Pregnancy avoid

Breast-feeding avoid

Side-effects nausea, vomiting, headache, breast tenderness, changes in body weight, fluid retention, depression, chorea, skin reactions, chloasma, hypertension, may irritate contact lenses, impairment of liver function, hepatic tumours, rarely photosensitivity; see also Combined Hormonal Contraceptives (section 7.3.1)

Licensed use unlicensed for use in children

Indication and dose

See notes above

Induction of sexual maturation in girls
• By mouth
Initially 2 micrograms daily, increasing every 6 months to 5 micrograms, then to 10 micrograms, and then to 20 micrograms daily
Note after 12–18 months of treatment give progestogen for 7 days of each 28-day cycle

Maintenance of sexual maturation in girls
• By mouth
20 micrograms daily with cyclical progestogen for 7 days of each 28-day cycle

Prevention of tall stature in girls
• By mouth
Girls 2–12 years 20–50 micrograms daily

6 Endocrine system

◁ **ETHINYLESTRADIOL** (*continued*)

Pituitary priming before growth hormone secretion test in girls
- By mouth

  Girls with bone age above 10 years 100 micrograms daily for 3 days before test

Ethinylestradiol (Non-proprietary) ⒫ₒₘ
Tablets, ethinylestradiol (unlicensed) 10 micrograms, net price 21-tab pack = £25.01; 50 micrograms, 21-tab pack = £34.10; 1 mg, 28-tab pack = £46.75

Note 2 microgram tablets available from 'special-order' manufacturers or specialist-importing companies, see p. 957

6.4.1.2 Progestogens

There are two main groups of progestogen, *progesterone and its analogues* (dydrogesterone and medroxyprogesterone) and *testosterone analogues* (norethisterone and norgestrel). The newer progestogens (desogestrel, norgestimate, and gestodene) are all derivatives of norgestrel; levonorgestrel is the active isomer of norgestrel and has twice its potency. Progesterone and its analogues are less androgenic than the testosterone derivatives and neither progesterone nor dydrogesterone causes virilisation.

In delayed puberty cyclical progestogen is added after 12–18 months of oestrogen therapy (section 6.4.1.1) to establish a menstrual cycle; usually levonorgestrel 30 micrograms or norethisterone 5 mg daily are used for the last 7 days of each 28 day cycle.

Norethisterone is also used to postpone menstruation during a cycle; treatment is started 3 days before the expected onset of menstruation.

NORETHISTERONE

Cautions conditions that may worsen with fluid retention e.g. epilepsy, hypertension, migraine, asthma, cardiac dysfunction; susceptibility to thromboembolism (particular caution with high dose); history of depression; diabetes (monitor closely); **interactions**: Appendix 1 (progestogens)

Contra-indications history of liver tumours, severe liver impairment; severe arterial disease, undiagnosed vaginal bleeding; acute porphyria (section 9.8.2); history during pregnancy of idiopathic jaundice, severe pruritus, or pemphigoid gestationis

Hepatic impairment caution; avoid if severe

Renal impairment use with caution

Pregnancy avoid

Breast-feeding higher doses may suppress lactation and alter milk composition; use lowest effective dose

Side-effects menstrual disturbances, premenstrual-like syndrome (including bloating, fluid retention, breast tenderness), weight gain, nausea, headache, dizziness, insomnia, drowsiness, depression; skin reactions (including urticaria, pruritus, rash, and acne), hirsutism and alopecia; jaundice and anaphylactoid reactions also reported

Licensed use not licensed for use in children

Indication and dose

See notes above

Induction and maintenance of sexual maturation in females (combined with an oestrogen after 12–24 months oestrogen therapy)
- By mouth
  5 mg once daily for the last 7 days of a 28-day cycle

Postponement of menstruation
- By mouth
  5 mg 3 times daily, starting 3 days before expected onset of menstruation

Norethisterone (Non-proprietary) ⒫ₒₘ
Tablets, norethisterone 5 mg, net price 30-tab pack = £2.62

Primolut N® (Bayer Schering) ⒫ₒₘ
Tablets, norethisterone 5 mg. Net price 30-tab pack = £1.93

Utovlan® (Pharmacia) ⒫ₒₘ
Tablets, norethisterone 5 mg, net price 30-tab pack = £1.40, 90-tab pack = £4.21

6.4.2 Male sex hormones and antagonists

Androgens cause masculinisation; they are used as replacement therapy in androgen deficiency, in delayed puberty, and in those who are hypogonadal due to either pituitary or testicular disease.

When given to patients with hypopituitarism androgens can lead to normal sexual development and potency but not to fertility. If fertility is desired, the usual treatment is with gonadotrophins or pulsatile gonadotrophin-releasing hormone (section 6.5.1) which stimulates spermatogenesis as well as androgen production.

Intramuscular depot preparations of **testosterone esters** are preferred for replacement therapy. Testosterone enantate or propionate or alternatively *Sustanon®*, which consists of a mixture of testosterone esters and has a longer duration of action, can be used. For induction of puberty, depot testosterone injections are given monthly and the doses increased every 6 to 12 months according to response. Single ester testosterone injections may need to be given more frequently. Testosterone enantate is unlicensed in children. Implants of testosterone can be used for hypogonadism; the implants are replaced every 4 to 5 months.

Oral **testosterone undecanoate** is used for induction of puberty. An alternative approach that promotes growth rather than sexual maturation uses oral oxandrolone (section 6.4.3).

Chorionic gonadotrophin (section 6.5.1) has also been used in delayed puberty in the male to stimulate endogenous testosterone production, but has little advantage over testosterone.

Caution should be used when androgens or chorionic gonadotrophin are used in treating boys with delayed puberty since the fusion of epiphyses is hastened and may result in short stature.

Testosterone patches and topical gel are also available but experience of their use in children under 15 years is limited. Topical testosterone is applied to the penis in the treatment of microphallus; an extemporaneously prepared cream should be used because the alcohol in proprietary gel formulations causes irritation.

◢ TESTOSTERONE AND ESTERS

Cautions cardiac impairment, hypertension, epilepsy, migraine, diabetes mellitus, skeletal metastases (risk of hypercalcaemia); **interactions**: Appendix 1 (testosterone)

Contra-indications history of primary liver tumours, hypercalcaemia, nephrosis

Hepatic impairment avoid if possible—fluid retention and dose-related toxicity

Renal impairment use with caution—potential for fluid retention

Pregnancy avoid; causes masculinisation of female fetus

Breast-feeding avoid; may cause masculinisation in the female infant or precocious development in the male infant; high doses suppress lactation

Side-effects headache, depression, gastro-intestinal bleeding, nausea, cholestatic jaundice, changes in libido, gynaecomastia, polycythaemia, anxiety, asthenia, paraesthesia, hypertension, electrolyte disturbances including sodium retention with oedema and hypercalcaemia, weight gain; increased bone growth; androgenic effects such as hirsutism, male-pattern baldness, seborrhoea, acne, pruritus; excessive frequency and duration of penile erection, precocious sexual development and premature closure of epiphyses in pre-pubertal males, suppression of spermatogenesis in males and virilism in females; *rarely* liver tumours; sleep apnoea also reported; *with patches and gel*, local irritation and allergic reactions

Licensed use *Sustanon®* and *Viromone®* licensed for use in children; *Andropatch®* licensed for use in children over 15 years

Indication and dose

See also under preparations; specialist use only

Induction and maintenance of sexual maturation in males

• By mouth (as testosterone undecanoate)

Child over 12 years 40 mg on alternate days increasing according to response up to 120 mg daily

• By deep intramuscular injection of testosterone enantate or propionate

Child over 12 years 25–50 mg/m^2 every month increasing dose every 6–12 months according to response

• Patch

Child over 15 years apply to clean, dry, unbroken skin on back, abdomen, upper arms or thighs, removing after 24 hours and siting replacement patch on a different area (with an interval of 7 days before using the same site); initially apply patches equivalent to testosterone 5 mg/24 hours (2.5 mg/24 hours in non-virilised patients) at night (approx. 10 p.m.), then adjust to 2.5–7.5 mg every 24 hours according to plasma-testosterone concentration

Treatment of microphallus

• Topically

Apply 3 times daily for 3 weeks
Note Use only specially manufactured preparation (see notes above)

◢**Oral**

Restandol® Testocaps (Organon) [PoM]
Capsules, orange, testosterone undecanoate 40 mg in oily solution. Net price 30-cap pack = £8.72; 60-cap pack = £17.44. Label: 21, 25

◢**Intramuscular**

Testosterone Enantate (Non-proprietary) [PoM]
Injection (oily), testosterone enantate 250 mg/mL.
Net price 1-mL amp = £12.11

6

Endocrine system

◁ **TESTOSTERONE AND ESTERS** (*continued*)

Sustanon 250® (Organon) [PoM]
   Injection (oily), testosterone propionate 30 mg,
   testosterone phenylpropionate 60 mg, testosterone
   isocaproate 60 mg, and testosterone decanoate
   100 mg/mL, net price 1-mL amp = £2.50
   Excipients include arachis (peanut) oil, benzyl alcohol (see
   Excipients p. 3)

Viromone® (Nordic) [PoM]
   Injection, testosterone propionate 50 mg/mL, net
   price 2-mL amp = £4.50

◢ **Implant**
Testosterone (Organon) [PoM]
   Implant, testosterone 100 mg, net price = £7.40;
   200 mg = £13.79

Dose
   Maintenance of sexual maturation in males
      Child over 16 years 100–600 mg; 600 mg usually
      maintains plasma-testosterone concentration within
      the normal range for 4–5 months

◢ **Cream**
Testosterone
   Cream, testosterone 5% (other strengths available)
   Available from 'special-order' manufacturers or specialist
   importing companies, see p. 957

◢ **Transdermal preparations**
Andropatch® (GSK) [PoM]
   Patches, self-adhesive, releasing testosterone
   approx. 2.5 mg/24 hours, net price 60-patch pack =
   £47.19; releasing testosterone approx. 5 mg/
   24 hours, net price 30-patch pack = £47.19. Counselling, administration

---

Anti-androgens and precocious puberty

The gonadorelin stimulation test (section 6.5.1) is used to distinguish between
gonadotrophin-dependent (central) precocious puberty and *gonadotrophin-indepen-
dent precocious puberty*. Treatment requires specialist management.

Gonadorelin analogues, used in the management of gonadotrophin-dependent
precocious puberty, delay development of secondary sexual characteristics and
growth velocity.

Testolactone and **cyproterone** are used in the management of gonadotrophin-
independent precocious puberty, resulting from McCune-Albright syndrome,
familial male precocious puberty (testotoxicosis), hormone-secreting tumours,
and ovarian and testicular disorders. Testolactone inhibits the aromatisation of
testosterone, the rate limiting step in oestrogen synthesis. Cyproterone is a
progestogen with anti-androgen properties.

Spironolactone (section 2.2.3) is sometimes used in combination with testolactone because it has some androgen receptor blocking properties.

High blood concentration of sex hormones may activate release of gonadotrophin
releasing hormone, leading to development of secondary, central gonadotrophin-
dependent precocious puberty. This may require the addition of gonadorelin
analogues to prevent progression of pubertal development and skeletal maturation.

CYPROTERONE ACETATE

Cautions blood counts initially and throughout
   treatment; monitor adrenocortical function regularly; diabetes mellitus (see also Contra-indications)
   Skilled tasks Fatigue and lassitude may impair performance of skilled tasks (e.g. driving)

Contra-indications hepatic disease, severe diabetes (with vascular changes); sickle-cell anaemia, malignant or wasting disease, meningioma
   or history of meningioma, severe depression,
   history of thromboembolic disorders

Hepatic impairment monitor hepatic function
   regularly—dose-related toxicity, see Side-effects
   below

Side-effects fatigue and lassitude, breathlessness,
   weight changes, reduced sebum production (may
   clear acne), changes in hair pattern, gynaecomastia (rarely leading to galactorrhoea and
   benign breast nodules); rarely hypersensitivity

reactions, rash and osteoporosis; inhibition of
   spermatogenesis (see notes above); hepatotoxicity reported (including jaundice, hepatitis and
   hepatic failure)
   Hepatotoxicity Direct hepatic toxicity including jaundice,
   hepatitis and hepatic failure have been reported (usually
   after several months) with cyproterone acetate 200–
   300 mg daily. Liver function tests should be performed
   before treatment and whenever symptoms suggestive of
   hepatotoxicity occur—if confirmed cyproterone should
   normally be withdrawn unless the hepatotoxicity can be
   explained by another cause such as metastatic disease (in
   which case cyproterone should be continued only if the
   perceived benefit exceeds the risk)

Licensed use unlicensed for use in children

◻ **CYPROTERONE ACETATE** (*continued*)

Indication and dose

> Gonadotrophin-independent precocious
> puberty) (specialist use only; see also notes
> above)
> • **By mouth**
>   Initially 25 mg twice daily, adjusted according to
>   response

Cyproterone Acetate (Non-proprietary) PoM
Tablets, cyproterone acetate 50 mg, net price 56-
tab pack = £31.54. Label: 21, counselling, driving
Note 10 mg tablets available from 'special-order' manufacturers or specialist-importing companies, see p. 957

Androcur® (Bayer Schering) PoM
Tablets, scored, cyproterone acetate 50 mg, net
price 56-tab pack = £24.88. Label: 21, counselling,
driving

TESTOLACTONE

Cautions interactions: Appendix 1 (testolactone)
Pregnancy avoid
Breast-feeding no information available
Side-effects nausea, vomiting, anorexia, diarrhoea; hypertension; peripheral neuropathy;
weight changes; changes in hair pattern; rarely
hypersensitivity reactions, rash

Indication and dose

> Gonadotrophin-independent precocious
> puberty (specialist use only; see also notes above)
> • **By mouth**
>   5 mg/kg 3–4 times daily; up to 10 mg/kg 4 times
>   daily may be required

Testolactone PoM
Tablets, testolactone 50 mg
Available from 'special-order' manufacturers or specialist
importing companies, see p. 957

GOSERELIN

Cautions monitor bone mineral density
Contra-indications undiagnosed vaginal bleeding
Pregnancy avoid
Breast-feeding avoid
Side-effects changes in blood pressure, headache, mood changes including depression,
hypersensitivity reactions including urticaria,
pruritus, rash, asthma and anaphylaxis; changes
in scalp and body hair, weight changes, withdrawal bleeding, ovarian cysts (may require
withdrawal), breast swelling and tenderness
(males and females), visual disturbances,
paraesthesia, local reactions at injection site
Licensed use not licensed for use in children

Indication and dose

> Gonadotrophin-dependent precocious puberty
>   see notes above; for doses, see under prepara-
>   tions below
>   Note Injections may be required more frequently in
>   some cases

Administration Rotate injection site to prevent
atrophy and nodule formation

Novgos® (Genus) PoM
Implant, goserelin (as acetate) 3.6 mg in prefilled
syringe, net price = £67.30
Dose
> • **Implant, by subcutaneous injection into anterior
>   abdominal wall**
>   3.6 mg every 28 days

Zoladex® (AstraZeneca) PoM
Implant, goserelin (as acetate) 3.6 mg in *Safe-Sys-
tem*® syringe applicator, net price each = £84.14
Dose
> • **Implant, by subcutaneous injection into anterior
>   abdominal wall**
>   3.6 mg every 28 days

Zoladex® **LA** (AstraZeneca) PoM
Implant, goserelin (as acetate) 10.8 mg in *Safe-
System*® syringe applicator, net price each =
£267.48
Dose
> • **Implant, by subcutaneous injection into anterior
>   abdominal wall**
>   10.8 mg every 12 weeks

LEUPRORELIN ACETATE

Cautions see Goserelin
Contra-indications see Goserelin
Pregnancy avoid—teratogenic in *animal* studies
Breast-feeding avoid
Side-effects see Goserelin
Licensed use not licensed for use in children

Indication and dose

> Gonadotrophin-dependent precocious puberty
>   see notes above; for doses, see under prepara-
>   tions below
>   Note Injections may be required more frequently in
>   some cases

Administration Rotate injection site to prevent
atrophy and nodule formation

6

Endocrine system

◁ **LEUPRORELIN ACETATE** (*continued*)

Prostap® SR (Wyeth) PoM

Injection (microsphere powder for reconstitution), leuprorelin acetate, net price 3.75-mg vial with 1-mL vehicle-filled syringe = £75.24

Dose

• By subcutaneous or by intramuscular injection

    3.75 mg every four weeks (half this dose is sometimes used in children with body-weight under 20 kg)

Prostap® 3 (Wyeth) PoM

Injection (microsphere powder for reconstitution), leuprorelin acetate, net price 11.25-mg vial with 2-mL vehicle-filled syringe = £225.72

Dose

• By subcutaneous or by intramuscular injection

    11.25 mg every 12 weeks

▌ TRIPTORELIN

Cautions see Goserelin

Contra-indications see Goserelin

Pregnancy avoid

Breast-feeding avoid

Side-effects see Goserelin; also gastro-intestinal disturbances; asthenia; arthralgia

Indication and dose

> Gonadotrophin-dependent precocious puberty
>
>   see notes above; for doses see under preparations below

Administration rotate injection site to prevent atrophy and nodule formation

Decapeptyl® SR (Ipsen) PoM

Injection, (powder for suspension), m/r, triptorelin (as acetate), net price 11.25-mg vial (with diluent) = £207.00

Dose

• By intramuscular injection

    11.25 mg every 3 months

    Note Each vial includes an overage to allow accurate administration of 11.25 mg dose

Gonapeptyl® Depot (Ferring) PoM

Injection (powder for suspension), triptorelin (as acetate), net price 3.75-mg prefilled syringe (with prefilled syringe of vehicle) = £81.69

Dose

• By subcutaneous or by intramuscular injection

    Body-weight under 20 kg initially 1.875 mg on days 0, 14, and 28, then 1.875 mg every 4 weeks

    Body-weight 20–30 kg initially 2.5 mg on days 0, 14, and 28, then 2.5 mg every 4 weeks

    Body-weight over 30 kg initially 3.75 mg on days 0, 14, and 28, then 3.75 mg every 4 weeks; discontinue when bone maturation consistent with age over 12 years in girls and over 13 years in boys

    Note may be given every 3 weeks if necessary

▌ 6.4.3 Anabolic steroids

Anabolic steroids have some androgenic activity but in girls they cause less virilisation than androgens. They are used in the treatment of some *aplastic anaemias* (section 9.1.3). Oxandrolone is used to stimulate late pre-pubertal growth prior to induction of sexual maturation in boys with short stature and in girls with Turner's syndrome; specialist management is required.

▌ OXANDROLONE

Cautions see Testosterone (section 6.4.2); interactions: Appendix 1 (oxandrolone)

Contra-indications see Testosterone (section 6.4.2)

Hepatic impairment see Testosterone (section 6.4.2)

Renal impairment see Testosterone (section 6.4.2)

Pregnancy see Testosterone (section 6.4.2)

Breast-feeding see Testosterone (section 6.4.2)

Side-effects see Testosterone (section 6.4.2)

Indication and dose

> Stimulation of late pre-pubertal growth in boys with short stature
>
> • By mouth
>
>   Boys 10–18 years (or appropriate age) 1.25–2.5 mg daily for 3–6 months

> Stimulation of late pre-pubertal growth in girls with Turner's syndrome
>
> • By mouth
>
>   Girls in combination with growth hormone 0.625–2.5 mg daily

Oxandrolone

Tablets, oxandrolone 2.5 mg

Available from 'special-order' manufacturers or specialist importing companies, see p. 957

Endocrine system

6

6.5 Hypothalamic and pituitary hormones

6.5.1 Hypothalamic and anterior pituitary hormones including growth hormone
6.5.2 Posterior pituitary hormones and antagonists

Use of preparations in these sections requires detailed prior investigation of the patient and *should be reserved for specialist centres.*

6.5.1 Hypothalamic and anterior pituitary hormones including growth hormone

Anterior pituitary hormones

Corticotrophins

Tetracosactide (tetracosactrin), an analogue of corticotropin (adrenocorticotrophic hormone, ACTH), is used to test adrenocortical function; failure of plasma-cortisol concentration to rise after administration of tetracosactide indicates adrenocortical insufficiency. A low-dose test is considered by some clinicians to be more sensitive when used to confirm established, partial adrenal suppression.

Tetracosactide should be used with caution in patients with allergic disorders e.g. asthma and should be given only if no other ACTH preparations have been given previously. Tetracosactide depot injection (*Synacthen Depot®*) is also used in the treatment of infantile spasms (see Infantile spasms, section 4.8.1) but it is contraindicated in neonates because of the presence of benzyl alcohol in the injection. Corticotropin-releasing factor, corticorelin, (also known as corticotropin-releasing hormone, CRH) is used to test anterior pituitary function and secretion of corticotropin.

TETRACOSACTIDE
(Tetracosactrin)

Cautions as for corticosteroids, section 6.3.2; **important:** risk of anaphylaxis (medical supervision; consult product literature); **interactions:** Appendix 1 (corticosteroids)

Contra-indications as for corticosteroids, section 6.3.2; avoid injections containing benzyl alcohol in neonates (see under preparations)

Hepatic impairment see section 6.3.2

Renal impairment see section 6.3.2

Pregnancy avoid (but may be used diagnostically if essential)

Breast-feeding avoid (but may be used diagnostically if essential)

Side-effects as for corticosteroids, section 6.3.2

Licensed use not licensed for low-dose test for adrenocortical insufficiency or treatment of infantile spasms

Indication and dose

See notes above and under preparations below

Synacthen® (Alliance) PoM
Injection, tetracosactide 250 micrograms (as acetate)/mL. Net price 1-mL amp = £2.70

Dose

Diagnosis of adrenocortical insufficiency (30-minute test)
• By intramuscular or intravenous injection
Standard-dose test 145 micrograms/m² (max. 250 micrograms) as a single dose

Low-dose test 300 nanograms/m² as a single dose
Administration may be diluted in sodium chloride 0.9% to 250 nanograms/mL

Synacthen Depot® (Alliance) PoM
Injection (aqueous suspension), tetracosactide acetate 1 mg/mL, with zinc phosphate complex. Net price 1-mL amp = £3.87
Excipients include benzyl alcohol (avoid in neonates, see Excipients p. 3)

Dose

Infantile spasms
• By intramuscular injection
Child 1 month–2 years initially 500 micrograms on alternate days, adjusted according to response

CORTICORELIN
(Corticotrophin-releasing hormone, CRH)

Pregnancy avoid
Breast-feeding avoid

Side-effects flushing of face, neck and upper body, hypotension, mild sensation of taste or smell

Endocrine system

◁ **CORTICORELIN (continued)**

Licensed use not licensed

Indication and dose

Test of anterior pituitary function
• By intravenous injection over 30 seconds

    Child 1 month–18 years 1 microgram/kg (max. 100 micrograms) as a single dose

CRH Ferring® (Shire) [PoM]
Injection, corticorelin 100 micrograms

Gonadotrophins

Gonadotrophins are occasionally used in the treatment of hypogonadotrophic hypogonadism and associated oligospermia. There is no justification for their use in primary gonadal failure.

Chorionic gonadotrophin is used in the investigation of testicular function in suspected primary hypogonadism and incomplete masculinisation. It has also been used in delayed puberty in boys to stimulate endogenous testosterone production, but it has little advantage over testosterone (section 6.4.2).

CHORIONIC GONADOTROPHIN

(Human Chorionic Gonadotrophin; HCG)
A preparation of a glycoprotein fraction secreted by the placenta and obtained from the urine of pregnant women having the action of the pituitary luteinising hormone

Cautions cardiac impairment, asthma, epilepsy, migraine; prepubertal boys (risk of premature epiphyseal closure or precocious puberty)

Contra-indications androgen-dependent tumours

Renal impairment use with caution

Side-effects oedema (reduce dose), headache, tiredness, mood changes, gynaecomastia, local reactions

Licensed use unlicensed in children for test of testicular function

Indication and dose

Test of testicular function
• By intramuscular injection
  Short stimulation test:

    Child 1 month–18 years 1500–2000 units once daily for 3 days

  Prolonged stimulation test:

    Child 1 month–18 years 1500–2000 units twice weekly for 3 weeks

Hypogonadotrophic hypogonadism
• By intramuscular injection

    Child 1 month–18 years 1000–2000 units twice weekly, adjusted to response

Undescended testes
• By intramuscular injection

    Child 7–18 years initially 500 units 3 times weekly (1000 units twice weekly if over 17 years); adjusted to response; up to 4000 units 3 times weekly may be required; continue for 1–2 months after testicular descent

Choragon® (Ferring) [PoM]
Injection, powder for reconstitution, chorionic gonadotrophin. Net price 5000-unit amp (with solvent) = £3.26. For intramuscular injection

Pregnyl® (Organon) [PoM]
Injection, powder for reconstitution, chorionic gonadotrophin. Net price 1500-unit amp = £2.16; 5000-unit amp = £3.21 (both with solvent). For subcutaneous or intramuscular injection

---

Growth hormone

Growth hormone is used to treat proven deficiency of the hormone, Prader-Willi syndrome, Turner's syndrome, growth disturbance in children born small for gestational age, and chronic renal insufficiency (see NICE guidance below). Growth hormone is also used in Noonan syndrome and idiopathic short stature [unlicensed indications] under specialist management. Treatment should be initiated and monitored by a paediatrician with expertise in managing growth-hormone disorders; treatment can be continued under a shared-care protocol by a general practitioner.

Growth hormone of human origin (HGH; somatotrophin) has been replaced by a growth hormone of human sequence, **somatropin**, produced using recombinant DNA technology.

> **NICE guidance**
>
> Somatropin in children with growth failure (May 2002)
> Treatment with somatropin is recommended for children with:
>
> - proven growth-hormone deficiency;
> - Turner's syndrome;
> - Prader-Willi syndrome;
> - chronic renal insufficiency before puberty.
>
> Treatment should be discontinued if the response is poor (i.e. an increase in growth velocity of less than 50% from baseline) in the first year of therapy.
>
> In children with chronic renal insufficiency, treatment should be stopped after renal transplantation and not restarted for at least a year

Mecasermin, a human insulin-like growth factor-I (rhIGF-I), is licensed to treat growth failure in children with severe primary insulin-like growth factor-I deficiency (section 6.7.4).

SOMATROPIN

(Synthetic Human Growth Hormone)

Cautions diabetes mellitus (adjustment of antidiabetic therapy may be necessary), papilloedema (see under Side-effects), relative deficiencies of other pituitary hormones (notably hypothyroidism—manufacturers recommend periodic thyroid function tests but limited evidence of clinical value), history of malignant disease, disorders of the epiphysis of the hip (monitor for limping), resolved intracranial hypertension (monitor closely), initiation of treatment close to puberty not recommended in child born small for gestational age; Silver-Russell syndrome; rotate subcutaneous injection sites to prevent lipoatrophy; **interactions**: Appendix 1 (somatropin)

Contra-indications evidence of tumour activity (complete antitumour therapy and ensure intracranial lesions inactive before starting); not to be used after renal transplantation or for growth promotion in children with closed epiphyses (or near closure in Prader-Willi syndrome); severe obesity or severe respiratory syndrome in Prader-Willi syndrome

Pregnancy interrupt treatment if pregnancy occurs

Breast-feeding absorption from milk unlikely

Side-effects headache, funduscopy for papilloedema recommended if severe or recurrent headache, visual problems, nausea and vomiting occur—if papilloedema confirmed consider benign intracranial hypertension (rare cases reported); fluid retention (peripheral oedema), arthralgia, myalgia, carpal tunnel syndrome, paraesthesia, antibody formation, hypothyroidism, insulin resistance, hyperglycaemia, hypoglycaemia, reactions at injection site; leukaemia in children with growth hormone deficiency also reported

Licensed use not licensed for use in Noonan syndrome

Indication and dose

> **Gonadal dysgenesis (Turner's syndrome)**
> - By subcutaneous injection
>   45–50 micrograms/kg daily or 1.4 mg/m² daily

> **Deficiency of growth hormone**
> - By subcutaneous or intramuscular injection
>   23–39 micrograms/kg daily or 0.7–1 mg/m² daily

> **Prader-Willi syndrome**
> - By subcutaneous injection
>   **Children with growth velocity greater than 1 cm/year** in combination with energy-restricted diet, 35 micrograms/kg daily or 1 mg/m² daily; max. 2.7 mg daily

> **Chronic renal insufficiency (renal function decreased to less than 50%)**
> - By subcutaneous injection
>   45–50 micrograms/kg daily or 1.4 mg/m² daily (higher doses may be needed) adjusted if necessary after 6 months

> **Growth disturbance in children born small for gestational age whose growth has not caught up by 4 years of age or later; Noonan syndrome**
> - By subcutaneous injection
>   35 micrograms/kg daily or 1 mg/m² daily

Genotropin® (Pharmacia) ℗oM

Injection, two-compartment cartridge containing powder for reconstitution, somatropin (rbe) and diluent, net price 5.3-mg (16-unit) cartridge = £122.87, 12-mg (36-unit) cartridge = £278.20. For use with *Genotropin® Pen* ⟨JHS⟩ device (available free of charge from clinics). For subcutaneous injection

MiniQuick injection, two-compartment single-dose syringe containing powder for reconstitution, somatropin (rbe) and diluent, net price 0.2-mg (0.6-unit) syringe = £4.64; 0.4-mg (1.2-unit) syringe = £9.27; 0.6-mg (1.8-unit) syringe = £13.91; 0.8-mg (2.4-unit) syringe = £18.55; 1-mg (3-unit) syringe = £23.18; 1.2-mg (3.6-unit) syringe = £27.82; 1.4-mg (4.2-unit) syringe = £32.46; 1.6-mg (4.8-unit) syringe = £37.09; 1.8-mg (5.4-unit) syringe = £41.73; 2-mg (6-unit) syringe = £46.37. For subcutaneous injection

Humatrope® (Lilly) ℗oM

Injection, powder for reconstitution, somatropin (rbe), net price 6-mg (18-unit) cartridge = £108.00;

6

Endocrine system

◻ SOMATROPIN (continued)

12-mg (36-unit) cartridge = £216.00; 24-mg (72-unit) cartridge = £432.00; all supplied with diluent. For subcutaneous or intramuscular injection; cartridges for subcutaneous injection

Norditropin® (Novo Nordisk) PoM

SimpleXx injection, somatropin (epr) 3.3 mg (10 units)/mL, net price 1.5-mL (5-mg, 15-unit) cartridge = £106.95; 6.7 mg (20 units)/mL, 1.5-mL (10-mg, 30-unit) cartridge = £213.90; 10 mg (30 units)/mL, 1.5-mL (15-mg, 45-unit) cartridge = £320.85. For use with appropriate *NordiPen®* device (available free of charge from clinics). For subcutaneous injection

NutropinAq® (Ipsen) PoM

Injection, somatropin (rbe), net price 10 mg (30 units) 2-mL cartridge = £207.00. For use with *NutropinAq®* Pen ⟨NHS⟩ device (available free of charge from clinics). For subcutaneous injection

Omnitrope® (Sandoz) ▼ PoM

Injection, somatropin (rbe) 3.3 mg (10 units)/mL, net price 1.5 mL (5-mg, 15-unit) cartridge = £91.33; 6.7 mg (20 units)/mL, 1.5 mL (10-mg, 30-unit) cartridge = £182.66. For use with *Omnitrope Pen 5®* ⟨NHS⟩ and *Omnitrope Pen 10®* ⟨NHS⟩ devices respectively (available free of charge from clinics). For subcutaneous injection

Excipients include benzyl alcohol (in 5-mg cartridge) (avoid in neonates, see Excipients, p. 3)

Note Biosimilar medicine, see p. 2

Saizen® (Merck Serono) PoM

Injection, powder for reconstitution, somatropin (rmc), net price 1.33-mg (4-unit) vial (with diluent) = £29.28; 3.33-mg (10-unit) vial (with diluent) = £73.20. For subcutaneous or intramuscular injection

Excipients include benzyl alcohol (avoid in neonates, see Excipients, p. 3)

Click.easy®, powder for reconstitution, somatropin (rmc), net price 8-mg (24-unit) vial (in *Click.easy®* device with diluent) = £185.44. For use with *One.click®* ⟨NHS⟩ autoinjector device or *Cool.Click®* ⟨NHS⟩ needle-free device (both available free of charge from clinics). For subcutaneous injection

Zomacton® (Ferring) PoM

Injection, powder for reconstitution, somatropin (rbe), net price 4-mg (12-unit) vial (with diluent) = £79.69. For use with *ZomaJet 2 Vision®* ⟨NHS⟩ needle-free device (available free of charge from clinics) or with needles and syringes; 10 mg (30-unit) vial (with diluent) = £199.23, for use with *ZomaJet Vision X®* ⟨NHS⟩ needle-free device (available free of charge from clinics) or with needles and syringes. For subcutaneous injection

Excipients include benzyl alcohol (in 4-mg vial) (avoid in neonates, see Excipients, p. 3)

Hypothalamic hormones

Gonadorelin when injected intravenously in post-pubertal girls leads to a rapid rise in plasma concentrations of both luteinising hormone (LH) and follicle-stimulating hormone (FSH). It has not proved to be very helpful, however, in distinguishing hypothalamic from pituitary lesions. It is used in the assessment of delayed or precocious puberty.

Protirelin is a hypothalamic releasing hormone which stimulates the release of thyrotrophin from the pituitary. It is indicated for the diagnosis of mild hyper-thyroidism or hypothyroidism, but its use has been superseded by immunoassays for thyroid-stimulating hormone. Together with other tests protirelin may also be used to confirm hypopituitarism and hypothalamic disease in children with marginally lowered thyrotrophin.

Other growth hormone stimulation tests involve the use of insulin, glucagon, arginine, and clonidine [all unlicensed uses]. The tests should be carried out in specialist centres.

◼ GONADORELIN

(Gonadotrophin-releasing hormone; GnRH; LH–RH)

Cautions pituitary adenoma

Pregnancy avoid

Breast-feeding avoid

Side-effects rarely nausea, headache, abdominal pain, increased menstrual bleeding; rarely, hypersensitivity reaction on repeated administration of large doses; irritation at injection site

Licensed use not licensed for use in children under 1 year

Indication and dose

> Assessment of anterior pituitary function; assessment of delayed puberty
> * By subcutaneous or intravenous injection
>   **Child 1–18 years** 2.5 micrograms/kg (max. 100 micrograms) as a single dose

HRF® (Intrapharm) PoM

Injection, powder for reconstitution, gonadorelin. Net price 100-microgram vial (with diluent) = £13.72 (hosp. only)

Excipients include benzyl alcohol (avoid in neonates, see Excipients p. 3)

PROTIRELIN

(Thyrotrophin-releasing hormone; TRH)

Cautions severe hypopituitarism, myocardial ischaemia, bronchial asthma and obstructive airways disease

Pregnancy use with caution as limited information available

Breast-feeding breast enlargement and leakage of milk reported

Side-effects after rapid intravenous administration desire to micturate, flushing, dizziness, nausea, abnormal taste; transient increase in pulse rate and blood pressure; rarely bronchospasm

Indication and dose

Assessment of thyroid function and thyroid stimulating hormone reserve
- By intravenous injection

    Neonate 1 microgram/kg as a single dose; dose may vary—consult local protocol

    Child 1 month–18 years 1 microgram/kg (max. 200 micrograms) as a single dose; dose may vary—consult local protocol

Diagnosis of hypopituitarism and hypothalamic disease
- By intravenous injection

    Neonate 7 micrograms/kg as a single dose (unlicensed dose); dose may vary—consult local protocol

    Child 1 month–18 years 7 micrograms/kg (max. 200 micrograms) as a single dose (unlicensed dose); dose may vary—consult local protocol

Protirelin (Non-proprietary) ꜰᴏᴍ
Injection, protirelin 100 micrograms/mL. Net price 2-mL amp = £15.15

6.5.2 Posterior pituitary hormones and antagonists

Posterior pituitary hormones

Diabetes insipidus   Diabetes insipidus is caused by either a deficiency of antidiuretic hormone (ADH, vasopressin) secretion (cranial, neurogenic, or pituitary diabetes insipidus) or by failure of the renal tubules to react to secreted antidiuretic hormone (nephrogenic diabetes insipidus).

Vasopressin (antidiuretic hormone, ADH) is used in the treatment of *pituitary diabetes insipidus* as is its analogue **desmopressin**. Dosage is tailored to produce a regular diuresis every 24 hours to avoid water intoxication. Treatment may be required permanently or for a limited period only in diabetes insipidus following trauma or pituitary surgery.

Desmopressin is more potent and has a longer duration of action than vasopressin; unlike vasopressin it has no vasoconstrictor effect. It is given by mouth or intranasally for maintenance therapy, and by injection in the postoperative period or in unconscious patients. Desmopressin is also used in the differential diagnosis of diabetes insipidus; following an intramuscular or intranasal dose, restoration of the ability to concentrate urine after water deprivation confirms a diagnosis of pituitary diabetes insipidus. Failure to respond suggests nephrogenic diabetes insipidus. Fluid input must be managed carefully to avoid hyponatraemia; this test is not usually recommended in young children.

In *nephrogenic* and *partial pituitary diabetes insipidus* benefit may be gained from the paradoxical antidiuretic effect of thiazides (section 2.2.1) e.g. chlorothiazide 10–20 mg/kg (max. 500 mg) twice daily.

Other uses   Desmopressin is also used to boost factor VIII concentration in mild to moderate haemophilia and in von Willebrand's disease; it is also used to test fibrinolytic response. For a comment on use of desmopressin in nocturnal enuresis see section 7.4.2.

Vasopressin infusion is used to control variceal bleeding in portal hypertension, before introducing more definitive treatment. **Terlipressin**, a derivative of vasopressin, and octreotide are used similarly but experience in children is limited.

DESMOPRESSIN

Cautions see under Vasopressin; less pressor activity, but still considerable caution in cardiovascular disease and in hypertension (not indicated for nocturnal enuresis or nocturia in these circumstances); also considerable caution in cystic fibrosis; in nocturia and nocturnal enuresis limit fluid intake from 1 hour before dose until 8 hours afterwards; in nocturia periodic blood pressure and weight checks needed to monitor for fluid overload; **interactions:** Appendix 1 (desmopressin)

6 Endocrine system

◻ **DESMOPRESSIN** (*continued*)

For cautions specifically relating to the use of desmopressin in nocturnal enuresis see section 7.4.2

Hyponatraemic convulsions The CSM has advised that patients being treated for primary nocturnal enuresis should be warned to avoid fluid overload (including during swimming) and to stop taking desmopressin during an episode of vomiting or diarrhoea (until fluid balance normal). The risk of hyponatraemic convulsions can also be minimised by keeping to the recommended starting doses and by avoiding concomitant use of drugs which increase secretion of vasopressin (e.g. tricyclic antidepressants)

Contra-indications cardiac insufficiency and other conditions treated with diuretics; psychogenic polydipsia and polydipsia in alcohol dependence

Renal impairment use with caution; antidiuretic effect may be reduced

Pregnancy small oxytocic effect in third trimester; increased risk of pre-eclampsia

Breast-feeding amount too small to be harmful

Side-effects fluid retention, and hyponatraemia (in more serious cases with convulsions) on administration without restricting fluid intake; stomach pain, headache, nausea, vomiting, allergic reactions, and emotional disturbance in children also reported; epistaxis, nasal congestion, rhinitis with nasal spray

Licensed use not licensed for assessment of antidiuretic hormone secretion

Indication and dose

Assessment of antidiuretic hormone secretion (congenital deficiency suspected) (specialist use only)
• Intranasally
    Child 1 month–2 years initially 100–500 nanograms as a single dose

Assessment of antidiuretic hormone secretion (congenital deficiency not suspected) (specialist use only)
• Intranasally
    Child 1 month–2 years 1–5 micrograms as a single dose

Test for suspected diabetes insipidus (water deprivation test)
• Intranasally
    Neonate not recommended, use trial of treatment

    Child 1 month–2 years 5–10 micrograms as a single dose; not usually recommended, see notes above

    Child 2–12 years 10–20 micrograms as a single dose, see notes above

    Child 12–18 years 20 micrograms as a single dose, see notes above

• By subcutaneous or intramuscular injection
    Neonate not recommended, use trial of treatment

    Child 1 month–2 years 400 nanograms as a single dose; not usually recommended, see notes above

    Child 2–12 years 0.5–1 microgram as a single dose, see notes above

    Child 12–18 years 1–2 micrograms as a single dose, see notes above

Diabetes insipidus, treatment
• By mouth
(as desmopressin acetate)

    Neonate initially 1–4 micrograms 2–3 times daily, adjusted according to response

    Child 1 month–2 years initially 10 micrograms 2–3 times daily, adjusted according to response (range 30-150 micrograms daily)

    Child 2–12 years initially 50 micrograms 2–3 times daily, adjusted according to response (range 100-800 micrograms daily)

    Child 12–18 years initially 100 micrograms 2–3 times daily, adjusted according to response (range 0.2–1.2 mg daily)

• Sublingually
(as desmopressin base)

    Child 2–18 years initially 60 micrograms 3 times daily, adjusted according to response (range 40–240 micrograms 3 times daily)

• Intranasally
(as desmopressin acetate)

    Neonate initially 100–500 nanograms, adjusted according to response (range 1.25–10 micrograms daily in 1–2 divided doses)

    Child 1 month–2 years initially 2.5–5 micrograms 1–2 times daily, adjusted according to response

    Child 2–12 years initially 5–20 micrograms 1–2 times daily, adjusted according to response

    Child 12–18 years initially 10–20 micrograms 1–2 times daily, adjusted according to response

• By subcutaneous or intramuscular injection

    Neonate initially 100 nanograms once daily, adjusted according to response (intramuscular route only)

    Child 1 month–12 years initially 400 nanograms once daily, adjusted according to response

    Child 12–18 years initially 1–4 micrograms once daily, adjusted according to response

Primary nocturnal enuresis
• By mouth
(as desmopressin acetate)

    Child 5–18 years (preferably over 7 years) 200 micrograms at bedtime, increased to 400 micrograms at bedtime only if lower dose not effective (**important:** see also Cautions), reassess after 3 months by withdrawing treatment for at least 1 week

• Sublingually
(as desmopressin base)

    Child 5–18 years (preferably over 7 years) 120 micrograms at bedtime, increased to 240 micrograms at bedtime only if lower dose

◻ **DESMOPRESSIN** (*continued*)

not effective (**important:** see also Cautions); reassess after 3 months by withdrawing treatment for at least 1 week

Fibrinolytic response testing

- **By intravenous injection over 20 minutes or by subcutaneous injection**

  Child 2–18 years 300 nanograms/kg as a single dose; blood sampled after 20 minutes for fibrinolytic activity

Mild to moderate haemophilia and von Willebrand's disease

- **By intravenous infusion over 20 minutes or by subcutaneous injection**

  Child 1 month–18 years 300 nanograms/kg as a single dose immediately before surgery or after trauma; may be repeated at intervals of 12 hours if no tachycardia

- **Intranasally**

  Child 1–18 years 4 micrograms/kg as a single dose, for pre-operative use give 2 hours before procedure

Renal function testing

- **Intranasally**

  Child 1 month–1 year 10 micrograms (empty bladder at time of administration and restrict fluid intake to 50% at next 2 feeds to avoid fluid overload)

  Child 1–15 years 20 micrograms (empty bladder at time of administration and restrict fluid intake to 500 mL from 1 hour before until 8 hours after administration to avoid fluid overload)

  Child 15–18 years 40 micrograms (empty bladder at time of administration and restrict fluid intake to 500 mL from 1 hour before until 8 hours after administration to avoid fluid overload)

- **By subcutaneous or intramuscular injection**

  Child 1 month–1 year 400 nanograms (empty bladder at time of administration and restrict fluid intake to 50% at next 2 feeds to avoid fluid overload)

  Child 1–18 years 2 micrograms (empty bladder at time of administration and restrict fluid intake to 500 mL from 1 hour before until 8 hours after administration to avoid fluid overload)

Desmopressin acetate (Non-proprietary) PoM
Nasal spray, desmopressin acetate 10 micrograms/ metered spray, net price 6-mL unit (60 metered sprays) = £34.51. Counselling, fluid intake, see above
Brands include *Presinex*®
Note Children requiring dose of less than 10 micrograms should be given *DDAVP*® intranasal solution

DDAVP® (Ferring) ▼ PoM
Tablets, both scored, desmopressin acetate 100 micrograms, net price 90-tab pack = £44.12; 200 micrograms, 90-tab pack = £88.23. Counselling, fluid intake, see above

Note Tablets may be crushed

Oral lyophilisates, (*DDAVP*® *Melt*), desmopressin (as acetate) 60 micrograms, net price 100-tab pack = £50.53; 120 micrograms, 100-tab pack = £101.07; 240 micrograms, 100-tab pack = £202.14. Label: 26, counselling, fluid intake, see notes above

Intranasal solution, desmopressin acetate 100 micrograms/mL. Net price 2.5-mL dropper bottle and catheter = £9.72. Counselling, fluid intake, see above
Administration May be diluted with sodium chloride 0.9% to a concentration of 10 micrograms/mL

Injection, desmopressin acetate 4 micrograms/mL. Net price 1-mL amp = £1.10
Administration May be administered orally [unlicensed]; for intravenous infusion, to be diluted to a concentration not less than 1 microgram/mL as adheres to surfaces if very dilute; for higher doses used in mild to moderate haemophilia and von Willebrand's disease may be diluted with 30–50 mL sodium chloride 0.9% intravenous infusion

Desmotabs® (Ferring) PoM
Tablets, scored, desmopressin acetate 200 micrograms, net price 30-tab pack = £29.43. Counselling, fluid intake, see above

Note tablets may be crushed

Desmomelt® (Ferring) ▼ PoM
Oral lyophilisates, desmopressin (as acetate) 120 micrograms, net price 30-tab pack = £30.34; 240 micrograms, 30-tab pack = £60.68. Label: 26, counselling, fluid intake, see above

Desmospray® (Ferring) PoM
Nasal spray, desmopressin acetate 10 micrograms/ metered spray. Net price 6-mL unit (60 metered sprays) = £25.02. Counselling, fluid intake, see above
Note Children requiring dose of less than 10 micrograms should be given *DDAVP*® intranasal solution

Low dose Desmospray® PoM
Nasal spray, desmopressin acetate 2.5 micrograms/metered spray
Available from Ferring on a named-patient basis

Octim® (Ferring) PoM
Nasal spray, desmopressin acetate 150 micrograms/metered spray, net price 2.5-mL unit (25 metered sprays) = £576.60. Counselling, fluid intake, see above

Injection, desmopressin acetate 15 micrograms/ mL, net price 1-mL amp = £19.22
Administration for *intravenous infusion* dilute with 50 mL of Sodium Chloride 0.9% and give over 20 minutes

6

Endocrine system

�▰ TERLIPRESSIN

Cautions see under Vasopressin

Contra-indications see under Vasopressin

Pregnancy avoid

Breast-feeding no information available

Side-effects see under Vasopressin, but effects milder

◻ **TERLIPRESSIN** *(continued)*

Licensed use unlicensed for use in children

Indication and dose

> Adjunct in acute massive haemorrhage of gas-
> tro-intestinal tract or oesophageal varices
> (specialist use only)
>
> • By intravenous injection
>
> **Child 12–18 years** initially 2 mg then 1–2 mg
> every 4–6 hours until bleeding is controlled;
> max. duration of treatment 72 hours

Glypressin® (Ferring) [PoM]

Injection, terlipressin, powder for reconstitution,
net price 1-mg vial with 5 mL diluent = £18.47

Injection, terlipressin 0.12 mg/mL, solution for
injection, net price 1-mg (8.5 mL) vial = £19.39

◢ **VASOPRESSIN**

Cautions heart failure, hypertension, asthma, epilepsy, migraine or other conditions which might
be aggravated by water retention; avoid fluid
overload

Contra-indications vascular disease (especially
disease of coronary arteries) unless extreme
caution, chronic nephritis (until reasonable blood
nitrogen concentrations attained)

Renal impairment see Contra-indications

Pregnancy oxytocic effect in third trimester

Breast-feeding not known to be harmful

Side-effects fluid retention, pallor, tremor,
sweating, vertigo, headache, nausea, vomiting,
belching, abdominal cramps, desire to defaecate,
hypersensitivity reactions (including anaphylaxis), constriction of coronary arteries (may
cause anginal attacks and myocardial ischaemia),
peripheral ischaemia and rarely gangrene

Licensed use not licensed for use in children

Indication and dose

> Adjunct in acute massive haemorrhage of gas-
> tro-intestinal tract or oesophageal varices
> (specialist use only)
>
> • By continuous intravenous infusion (may also
> be infused directly into the superior mesenteric
> artery)
>
> **Child 1 month–18 years** initially 0.3 units/kg
> (max. 20 units) over 20–30 minutes *then*
> 0.3 units/kg/hour, adjusted according to
> response (max. 1 unit/kg/hour); if bleeding
> stops, continue at same dose for 12 hours, then
> withdraw gradually over 24–48 hours; max.
> duration of treatment 72 hours

Administration for *intravenous infusion* dilute with
Glucose 5% or Sodium Chloride 0.9% to a concentration of 0.2–1 unit/mL

◢Synthetic vasopressin

Pitressin® (Goldshield) [PoM]

Injection, argipressin (synthetic vasopressin)
20 units/mL. Net price 1-mL amp = £17.14 (hosp.
only)

6.6 Drugs affecting bone metabolism

6.6.1 Calcitonin
6.6.2 Bisphosphonates

The two main disorders of bone metabolism that occur in children are rickets and
osteoporosis. The two most common forms of rickets are Vitamin D deficiency
rickets (section 9.6.4) and hypophosphataemic rickets (section 9.5.2). See also
calcium (section 9.5.1.1).

Osteoporosis

Osteoporosis in children may be primary (e.g. *osteogenesis imperfecta* and *idiopathic juvenile osteoporosis*), or secondary (e.g. due to inflammatory disorders,
immobilisation, or corticosteroids); specialist management is required.

Corticosteroid-induced osteoporosis To reduce the risk of osteoporosis doses
of oral corticosteroids should be as low as possible and courses of treatment as
short as possible.

6.6.1 Calcitonin

Calcitonin is involved with parathyroid hormone in the regulation of bone turnover and hence in the maintenance of calcium balance and homeostasis. **Calcitonin (salmon)** (salcatonin, synthetic or recombinant salmon calcitonin) is used
to lower the plasma-calcium concentration in some patients with hypercalcaemia
(notably when associated with malignant disease).

CALCITONIN (SALMON)/SALCATONIN

Cautions history of allergy (skin test advised); heart failure; children—use for short periods only and monitor bone growth

Contra-indications hypocalcaemia

Renal impairment use with caution

Pregnancy avoid unless essential, toxicity in *animal* studies

Breast-feeding avoid unless essential, may inhibit lactation

Side-effects nausea, vomiting, diarrhoea, abdominal pain, flushing, dizziness, headache, taste disturbances; musculoskeletal pain; with nasal spray nose and throat irritation, rhinitis, sinusitis and epistaxis; *less commonly* diuresis, oedema, cough, visual disturbances, injection-site reactions, rash, hypersensitivity reactions including pruritus

Licensed use not licensed in children

Indication and dose

Hypercalcaemia (experience limited in children) (specialist use only)

- By subcutaneous or intramuscular injection

  Child 1 month–18 years 2.5–5 units/kg every 12 hours, max. 400 units every 6–8 hours,

adjusted according to response (no additional benefit with over 8 units/kg every 6 hours)

- By slow intravenous infusion

  Child 1 month–18 years 5–10 units/kg over at least 6 hours

Osteoporosis (specialist use only)

Refer for specialist advice, experience very limited

Administration for *intravenous infusion*, dilute injection solution (e.g. 400 units in 500 mL) with Sodium Chloride 0.9% and give over at least 6 hours; glass or hard plastic containers should not be used; some loss of potency on dilution and administration—use diluted solution without delay

Miacalcic® (Novartis) [PoM]
Nasal spray ▼, calcitonin (salmon) 200 units/metered spray, net price 2-mL unit (approx. 14 metered sprays) = £20.99

Injection, calcitonin (salmon) 50 units/mL, net price 1-mL amp = £4.27; 100 units/mL, 1-mL amp = £8.55; 200 units/mL, 2-mL vial = £30.75

6.6.2 Bisphosphonates

Bisphosphonates are adsorbed on to hydroxyapatite crystals in bone, slowing both their rate of growth and dissolution, and therefore reducing the rate of bone turnover.

A bisphosphonate such as **disodium pamidronate** is used in the management of severe forms of *osteogenesis imperfecta* and other causes of osteoporosis in children to reduce the number of fractures; the long-term effects of bisphosphonates in children have not been established. Single doses of biphosphonates are also used to manage hypercalaemia (section 9.5.1.2). Treatment should be initiated under specialist advice **only**.

> **MHRA/CHM advice (October 2007 and November 2009)**
> The risk of osteonecrosis of the jaw is substantially greater for patients receiving intravenous bisphosphonates in the treatment of cancer than for patients receiving oral bisphosphonates for osteoporosis or Paget's disease.
>
> Risk factors for developing osteonecrosis of the jaw that should be considered are: potency of bisphosphonate (highest for zoledronate), route of administration, cumulative dose, duration and type of malignant disease, concomitant treatment, smoking, comorbid conditions, and history of dental disease.
>
> All patients receiving bisphosphonates for cancer should have a dental check-up (and any necessary remedial work should be performed) before bisphosphonate treatment. However, urgent bisphosphonate treatment should not be delayed, and a dental check-up should be carried out as soon as possible in these patients. All other patients who are prescribed bisphosphonates should have a dental examination only if they have poor dental health.
>
> During bisphosphonate treatment patients should maintain good oral hygiene, receive routine dental check-ups, and report any oral symptoms.

ALENDRONIC ACID

Cautions upper gastro-intestinal disorders (dysphagia, symptomatic oesophageal disease, gastritis, duodenitis, or ulcers—see also under Contra-indications and Side-effects); history (within 1 year) of ulcers, active gastro-intestinal bleeding, or surgery of the upper gastro-intestinal tract; correct disturbances of calcium and mineral metabolism (e.g. vitamin-D deficiency, hypocalcaemia) before starting and monitor serum-calcium concentration during treatment; consider

6

Endocrine system

◁ **ALENDRONIC ACID (continued)**

dental check-up before initiating bisphosphonate (risk of osteonecrosis of the jaw, see MHRA/CHM advice, p. 475); exclude other causes of osteoporosis; atypical stress fractures reported (discontinue unless benefits of continued treatment clearly outweigh risks); **interactions:** Appendix 1 (bisphosphonates)

Contra-indications abnormalities of oesophagus and other factors which delay emptying (e.g. stricture or achalasia), hypocalcaemia,

Renal impairment avoid if estimated glomerular filtration rate is less than 35 mL/minute/1.73 m^2

Pregnancy avoid

Breast-feeding no information available

Side-effects oesophageal reactions (see below), abdominal pain and distension, dyspepsia, regurgitation, melaena, diarrhoea or constipation, flatulence, musculoskeletal pain, headache; *rarely* rash, pruritus, erythema, photosensitivity, uveitis, scleritis, transient decrease in serum phosphate; nausea, vomiting, gastritis, peptic ulceration, hypersensitivity reactions (including urticaria and angioedema), and atypical stress fractures with long term use also reported; myalgia, malaise, and fever at initiation of treatment; *very rarely* severe skin reactions (including

Stevens-Johnson syndrome), osteonecrosis of the jaw (see MHRA/CHM advice, p. 475)

Oesophageal reactions Severe oesophageal reactions (oesophagitis, oesophageal ulcers, oesophageal stricture and oesophageal erosions) have been reported; patients should be advised to stop taking the tablets and to seek medical attention if they develop symptoms of oesophageal irritation such as dysphagia, new or worsening heartburn, pain on swallowing or retrosternal pain

Licensed use not licensed for use in children

Indication and dose

See notes above, specialist use only

Counselling Swallow the tablets whole with a full glass of water on an empty stomach at least 30 minutes before breakfast (and any other oral medication); stand or sit upright for at least 30 minutes and do not lie down until after eating breakfast. Do not take the tablets at bedtime or before rising.

Fosamax® (MSD) (PoM)
Tablets, alendronic acid (as sodium alendronate) 10 mg, 28-tab pack = £23.12. Counselling, administration

Fosamax® Once Weekly (MSD) (PoM)
Tablets, alendronic acid (as sodium alendronate) 70 mg, net price 4-tab pack = £22.80. Counselling, administration

▌ DISODIUM PAMIDRONATE

Disodium pamidronate was formerly called aminohydroxypropylidenediphosphonate disodium (APD)

Cautions cardiac disease; previous thyroid surgery (risk of hypocalcaemia); monitor serum electrolytes, calcium, and phosphate—possibility of convulsions due to electrolyte changes; ensure adequate hydration; avoid concurrent use with other bisphosphonates; consider dental check-up before initiating bisphosphonate (risk of osteonecrosis of the jaw, see MHRA/CHM advice, p. 475); **interactions:** Appendix 1 (bisphosphonates)

Skilled tasks Patients should be warned against driving, cycling, or performing skilled tasks immediately after treatment (somnolence or dizziness can occur)

Hepatic impairment use with caution in severe impairment—no information available

Renal impairment monitor renal function in renal disease or predisposition to renal impairment (e.g. in tumour-induced hypercalcaemia)

Pregnancy avoid—toxicity in *animal* studies

Breast-feeding avoid

Side-effects hypophosphataemia, transient rise in body temperature, fever and influenza-like symptoms (sometimes accompanied by malaise, rigors, fatigue, and flushes); arthralgia, myalgia, bone pain, nausea, vomiting, headache, lymphocytopenia, hypomagnesaemia; *rarely* muscle cramps, anorexia, abdominal pain, diarrhoea, constipation, dyspepsia, agitation, confusion,

dizziness, insomnia, somnolence, lethargy, anaemia, leucopenia, hypotension or hypertension, rash, pruritus, symptomatic hypocalcaemia (paraesthesia, tetany), hyperkalaemia or hypokalaemia, hypernatraemia; osteonecrosis of the jaw (see MHRA/CHM advice, p. 475); isolated cases of seizures, hallucinations, thrombocytopenia, haematuria, acute renal failure, deterioration of renal disease, conjunctivitis and other ocular symptoms; atrial fibrillation, and reactivation of herpes simplex and zoster also reported; also local reactions at injection site

Licensed use not licensed for use in children

Indication and dose

See notes above, specialist use only

Disodium pamidronate (Non-proprietary) (PoM)
Concentrate for intravenous infusion, disodium pamidronate 3 mg/mL, net price 5-mL vial = £27.50, 10-mL vial = £55.00; 6 mg/mL, 10-mL vial = £95.00; 9 mg/mL, 10-mL vial = £165.00; 15 mg/mL, 1-mL vial = £29.83, 2-mL vial = £59.66, 4-mL vial = £119.32, 6-mL vial £170.46

Aredia Dry Powder® (Novartis) (PoM)
Injection, powder for reconstitution, disodium pamidronate, for use as an infusion. Net price 15-mg vial = £29.83; 30-mg vial = £59.66; 90-mg vial = £170.45 (all with diluent)

▌ RISEDRONATE SODIUM

Cautions oesophageal abnormalities and other factors which delay transit or emptying (e.g. stricture or achalasia—see also under Side-effects); correct hypocalcaemia before starting, correct other disturbances of bone and mineral

metabolism (e.g. Vitamin-D deficiency) at onset of treatment; consider dental check-up before initiating bisphosphonate (risk of osteonecrosis of the jaw, see MHRA/CHM advice, p. 475); **interactions:** Appendix 1 (bisphosphonates)

◁ **RISEDRONATE SODIUM** (*continued*)

Contra-indications hypocalcaemia (see Cautions above)

Renal impairment avoid if estimated glomerular filtration rate is less than 30 mL/minute/1.73 m²

Pregnancy avoid

Breast-feeding avoid

Side-effects gastro-intestinal effects (including abdominal pain, dyspepsia, nausea, diarrhoea, constipation); dizziness, headache; influenza-like symptoms, musculoskeletal pain; *rarely* oesophageal stricture, oesophagitis, oesophageal ulcer, dysphagia, gastritis, duodenitis, glossitis, peripheral oedema, weight loss, myasthenia, arthralgia, apnoea, bronchitis, sinusitis, rash, nocturia, amblyopia, corneal lesion, dry eye, tinnitus, iritis; *very rarely* hypersensitivity reactions including angioedema, osteonecrosis of the jaw (see MHRA/CHM advice, p. 475)

Licensed use not licensed for use in children

Indication and dose

See notes above, specialist use only

Counselling Swallow tablets whole with full glass of water; on rising, take on an empty stomach at least 30 minutes before first food or drink of the day **or**, if taking at any other time of the day, avoid food and drink for at least 2 hours before or after risedronate (particularly avoid calcium containing products e.g. milk; also avoid iron and mineral supplements and antacids); stand or sit upright for at least 30 minutes; do not take tablets at bedtime or before rising

Actonel® (Procter & Gamble Pharm.) [PoM]
Tablets, f/c, risedronate sodium 5 mg (yellow), net price 28-tab pack = £18.36; 30 mg (white), 28-tab pack = £146.85. Counselling, administration, food, and calcium (see above)

Actonel Once a Week® (Procter & Gamble Pharm.) [PoM]
Tablets, f/c, risedronate sodium 35 mg (orange), net price 4-tab pack = £19.51. Counselling, administration, food and calcium (see above)

▌SODIUM CLODRONATE

Cautions monitor renal and hepatic function and white cell count; also monitor serum calcium and phosphate periodically; renal dysfunction reported in patients receiving concomitant NSAIDs; maintain adequate fluid intake during treatment; consider dental check-up before initiating bisphosphonate (risk of osteonecrosis of the jaw, see MHRA/CHM advice, p. 475); **interactions**: Appendix 1 (bisphosphonates)

Contra-indications acute gastro-intestinal inflammatory conditions

Renal impairment use half normal dose if estimated glomerular filtration rate 10–30 mL/minute/1.73 m²; avoid if estimated glomerular filtration rate less than 10 mL/minute/1.73 m²

Pregnancy avoid

Breast-feeding no information available

Side-effects nausea, diarrhoea; skin reactions; bronchospasm; *very rarely* osteonecrosis of the jaw (see MHRA/CHM advice, p. 475)

Licensed use not licensed for use in children

Indication and dose

See notes above, specialist use only

Counselling Avoid food for 1 hour before and after oral treatment, particularly calcium-containing products e.g. milk; also avoid iron and mineral supplements and antacids; maintain adequate fluid intake

Bonefos® (Bayer Schering) [PoM]
Capsules, yellow, sodium clodronate 400 mg. Net price 120-cap pack = £142.53. Counselling, food and calcium

Tablets, f/c, scored, sodium clodronate 800 mg. Net price 60-tab pack = £149.27. Counselling, food and calcium

Clasteon® (Beacon) [PoM]
Capsules, blue/white, sodium clodronate 400 mg, net price 30-cap pack = £40.49, 120-cap pack = £161.97. Counselling, food and calcium

Loron® (Roche) [PoM]
Loron 520® tablets, f/c, scored, sodium clodronate 520 mg. Net price 60-tab pack = £155.67. Label: 10, patient information leaflet., Counselling, food and calcium

6 Endocrine system

6.7 Other endocrine drugs

6.7.1 Bromocriptine and other dopaminergic drugs

Classification not used in *BNF for Children*.

6.7.2 Drugs affecting gonadotrophins

Classification not used in *BNF for Children*. See section 6.4.2 for use in precocious puberty.

6.7.3 Metyrapone

Metyrapone is a competitive inhibitor of 11β-hydroxylation in the adrenal cortex; the resulting inhibition of cortisol (and to a lesser extent aldosterone) production leads to an increase in ACTH production which, in turn, leads to increased synthesis and release of cortisol precursors. It is used as a test of anterior pituitary function.

Most types of *Cushing's syndrome* are treated surgically. Metyrapone may be useful to control the symptoms of the disease or to prepare the child for surgery. The dosages used are either low, and tailored to cortisol production, or high, in which case corticosteroid replacement therapy is also needed.

Ketoconazole (section 5.2) is also used by specialists for the management of *Cushing's syndrome* [unlicensed indication].

METYRAPONE

Cautions gross hypopituitarism (risk of precipitating acute adrenal failure); hypertension on long-term administration; hypothyroidism (delayed response); many drugs interfere with diagnostic estimation of steroids; avoid in acute porphyria (section 9.8.2)

Skilled tasks Drowsiness may affect the performance of skilled tasks (e.g. driving)

Contra-indications adrenocortical insufficiency (see Cautions)

Hepatic impairment use with caution (delayed response)

Pregnancy avoid (may impair biosynthesis of fetal-placental steroids)

Breast-feeding avoid—no information available

Side-effects occasional nausea, vomiting, dizziness, headache, hypotension, sedation; rarely abdominal pain, allergic skin reactions, hypoadrenalism, hirsutism

Licensed use licensed for use in children

Indication and dose

Differential diagnosis of ACTH-dependent Cushing's syndrome
- By mouth

  Child 1 month–18 years 15 mg/kg (or 300 mg/m^2) every 4 hours for 6 doses; minimum dose 250 mg every 4 hours, max. 750 mg every 4 hours

Management of Cushing's syndrome
- By mouth

  Range 250 mg–6 g daily, adjusted according to cortisol production; see notes above

Metopirone® (Alliance) PoM

Capsules, ivory, metyrapone 250 mg, net price 100-tab pack = £38.88. Label: 21, counselling, driving

6.7.4 Somatomedins

Somatomedins are a group of polypeptide hormones structurally related to insulin and commonly known as insulin-like growth factors (IGFs). **Mecasermin**, a human insulin-like growth factor-I (rhIGF-I), is the principal mediator of the somatotropic effects of human growth hormone and is used to treat growth failure in children with severe primary insulin-like growth factor-I deficiency.

MECASERMIN

(Recombinant human insulin-like growth factor-I; rhIGF-I)

Cautions correct hypothyroidism before initiating treatment; diabetes mellitus (adjustment of antidiabetic therapy may be necessary), monitor ECG before and on termination of treatment (and during treatment if ECG abnormal), papilloedema (see under Side-effects), monitor for disorders of the epiphysis of the hip (monitor for limping), monitor for signs of tonsillar hypertrophy (snoring, sleep apnoea, and chronic middle ear effusions)

Contra-indications evidence of tumour activity (discontinue treatment)

Pregnancy avoid unless essential; contraception advised in women of child-bearing potential

Breast-feeding avoid

Side-effects headache, funduscopy for papilloedema recommended if severe or recurrent headache, visual problems, nausea and vomiting occur—if papilloedema confirmed consider benign intracranial hypertension (rare cases reported); cardiomegaly, ventricular hypertrophy, tachycardia; convulsions, sleep apnoea, night terrors, dizziness, nervousness; tonsillar hypertrophy (see Cautions above); hypoglycaemia (especially in first month, and in younger children), hyperglycaemia, gynaecomastia; arthralgia, myalgia; visual disturbance, impaired

◁ **MECASERMIN (continued)**

hearing; antibody formation; injection-site reactions (rotate site)

Indication and dose

Growth failure in children with severe primary insulin-like growth factor-I deficiency

• **By subcutaneous injection**

Child 2–18 years initially 40 micrograms/kg twice daily for 1 week, if tolerated increase dose in steps of 40 micrograms/kg to max.

120 micrograms/kg twice daily; discontinue if no response within 1 year

Counselling Dose should be administered just before or after food; do not increase dose if a dose is missed
Note Reduce dose if hypoglycaemia occurs despite adequate food intake; withhold injection if patient unable to eat

Increlex® (Ipsen) ▼ PoM
Injection, mecasermin 10 mg/mL, net price 4-mL vial = £605.00. Counselling, administration
Excipients include benzyl alcohol (avoid in neonates, see Excipients, p. 3)

6
Endocrine system

7 Obstetrics, gynaecology, and urinary-tract disorders

7.1 Drugs used in obstetrics

This section is not included in *BNF for Children*. See BNF for management of obstetrics.

For the management of ductus arteriosus, see section 2.14.

7.2 Treatment of vaginal and vulval conditions

7.2.1 Preparations for vaginal and vulval changes
7.2.2 Vaginal and vulval infections

Pre-pubertal girls may be particularly susceptible to vulvovaginitis. Barrier preparations (section 13.2.2) applied after cleansing can be useful when the symptoms are due to non-specific irritation, but systemic drugs are required in the treatment of bacterial infection (section 5.1) or threadworm infestation (section 5.5.1). Intravaginal preparations, particularly those that require the use of an applicator, are not generally suitable for young girls; topical preparations may be useful in some adolescent girls.

In older girls symptoms are often restricted to the vulva, but infections almost invariably involve the vagina, which should also be treated; treatment should be as for adults, see BNF section 7.2.2.

7.2.1 Preparations for vaginal and vulval changes

Topical oestrogen creams containing **estriol** 0.01% (*Gynest*®) are used in the treatment of labial adhesions (for details of preparation, see BNF section 7.2.1); treatment is usually restricted to symptomatic cases. Estriol cream should be applied to the adhesions once or twice daily for 2–6 weeks; adhesions may recur following treatment.

7.2.2 Vaginal and vulval infections

Effective specific treatments are available for the common vaginal infections.

Fungal infections

Vaginal fungal infections are not normally a problem in younger girls but can occur in adolescents. *Candidal vulvitis* can be treated locally with cream, but is almost invariably associated with vaginal infection which should also be treated. *Vaginal candidiasis*, rare in girls before puberty, can be treated with antifungal pessaries or cream inserted high into the vagina (including during menstruation); however, these are not recommended for pre-pubertal girls and treatment with an external cream may be more appropriate. Single-dose intravaginal preparations offer an advantage when compliance is a problem. Local irritation can occur on application of vaginal antifungal products.

Imidazole drugs (clotrimazole, econazole, and miconazole) are effective against candida in short courses of 1 to 3 days according to the preparation used; treatment can be repeated if initial course fails to control symptoms or if symptoms recur. Vaginal applications may be supplemented with antifungal cream for vulvitis and to treat other superficial sites of infection.

Oral treatment of vaginal infection with fluconazole (section 5.2) may be considered for girls post-puberty.

Vulvovaginal candidiasis in pregnancy Vulvovaginal candidiasis is common during pregnancy and can be treated with vaginal application of an imidazole (such as clotrimazole), and a topical imidazole cream for vulvitis. Pregnant women need a longer duration of treatment, usually about 7 days, to clear the infection. There is limited absorption of imidazoles from the skin and vagina. Oral antifungal treatment should be avoided during pregnancy.

Recurrent vulvovaginal candidiasis Recurrent vulvovaginal candidiasis is very rare in children, but can occur if there are predisposing factors such as antibacterial therapy, pregnancy, diabetes mellitus, and possibly oral contraceptive use. Reservoirs of infection can also lead to recontamination and should be treated; these include other skin sites such as the digits, nail beds, and umbilicus, as well as the gastro-intestinal tract and the bladder. The sexual partner may also be the source of re-infection and, if symptomatic, should be treated with cream at the same time.

Treatment against candida may need to be extended for 6 months in recurrent vulvovaginal candidiasis. Some recommended regimens suitable for older children [all unlicensed] include:

- fluconazole (section 5.2) by mouth 100 mg (as a single dose) once every week for 6 months;
- clotrimazole vaginally 500-mg pessary (as a single dose) once every week for 6 months.

PREPARATIONS FOR VAGINAL AND VULVAL CANDIDIASIS

Cautions avoid intravaginal preparations (particularly those that require use of an applicator) in young girls unless there is no alternative

Pregnancy see notes above

Side-effects occasional local irritation

Licensed use consult product literature for individual preparations

Indication and dose

See notes above and under preparations below

Clotrimazole (Non-proprietary)
Cream (topical), clotrimazole 1%, net price 20 g = £1.77, 50 g = £4.79
Condoms effect on latex condoms and diaphragms not yet known

Dose

Apply to anogenital area 2–3 times daily

Pessary, clotrimazole 500 mg, net price 1 pessary with applicator = £3.04

Dose

Insert 1 pessary at night as a single dose; can be repeated once if necessary

Canesten® (Bayer Consumer Care)
Cream (topical), clotrimazole 1%, net price 20 g = £2.14; 50 g = £3.50
Excipients include benzyl alcohol, cetostearyl alcohol, polysorbates
Condoms damages latex condoms and diaphragms

Dose

Apply to anogenital area 2–3 times daily

Thrush Cream (topical), clotrimazole 2%, net price 20 g = £3.99
Excipients include benzyl alcohol, cetostearyl alcohol, polysorbates
Condoms damages latex condoms and diaphragms

Dose

Apply to anogenital area 2–3 times daily

Vaginal cream (*10% VC®*) (PoM), clotrimazole 10%, net price 5-g applicator pack = £4.90
Excipients include benzyl alcohol, cetostearyl alcohol, polysorbates
Condoms damages latex condoms and diaphragms

Dose

Insert 5 g at night as a single dose; may be repeated once if necessary

Note Brands for sale to the public include *Canesten® Internal Cream*

7

Obstetrics, gynaecology, and urinary-tract disorders

◻ **PREPARATIONS FOR VAGINAL AND VULVAL CANDIDIASIS (continued)**

Cream Combi, clotrimazole 10% vaginal cream and 2% topical cream, net price 5-g vaginal cream (with applicator) and 10-g topical cream = £6.81
Excipients include benzyl alcohol, cetostearyl alcohol, polysorbates
Condoms damages latex condoms and diaphragms

Dose
> See under individual components

Pessaries, clotrimazole 200 mg, 3 pessaries with applicator = £3.63
Condoms damages latex condoms and diaphragms

Dose
> Insert 200 mg for 3 nights; course may be repeated once if necessary

Pessary, clotrimazole 500 mg, net price 1 pessary with applicator = £3.18
Excipients none as listed in section 13.1.3
Condoms damages latex condoms and diaphragms

Dose
> Insert 1 pessary at night as a single dose; may be repeated once if necessary

Combi, clotrimazole 500-mg pessary and cream (topical) 2%, net price 1 pessary and 10-g cream = £5.51
Condoms damages latex condoms and diaphragms

Dose
> See under individual components

Gyno-Daktarin® (Janssen-Cilag) [PoM]
Ovule (= vaginal capsule) (*Gyno-Daktarin 1®*),

miconazole nitrate 1.2 g in a fatty basis, net price 1 ovule = £3.00
Excipients include hydroxybenzoates (parabens)
Condoms damages latex condoms and diaphragms

Dose
> Insert 1 ovule at night as a single dose; can be repeated once if necessary

Gyno-Pevaryl® (Janssen-Cilag) [PoM]
Pessaries, econazole nitrate 150 mg, net price 3 pessaries = £2.83
Excipients none as listed in section 13.1.3
Condoms damages latex condoms and diaphragms

Dose
> Insert 1 pessary for 3 nights; course can be repeated once if necessary

Pessary (*Gyno-Pevaryl 1®*), econazole nitrate 150 mg, formulated for single-dose therapy, net price 1 pessary with applicator = £3.01
Excipients none as listed in section 13.1.3
Condoms damages latex condoms and diaphragms

Dose
> Insert 1 pessary at night as a single dose; can be repeated once if necessary

Nizoral® (Janssen-Cilag) [PoM]
Cream (topical), ketoconazole 2%, net price 30 g = £3.40
Excipients include polysorbates, propylene glycol, stearyl alcohol
Condoms effect on latex condoms and diaphragms not yet known

Dose
> Apply to anogenital area once or twice daily

Other infections

Trichomonal infections commonly involve the lower urinary tract as well as the genital system and need systemic treatment with metronidazole (section 5.1.11) or tinidazole (section 5.4.2).

Bacterial infections with Gram-negative organisms are particularly common in association with gynaecological operations and trauma. Metronidazole is effective against certain Gram-negative organisms, especially *Bacteroides* spp. and can be used prophylactically in gynaecological surgery.

Clindamycin cream and metronidazole gel are indicated for bacterial vaginosis.

The antiviral drugs aciclovir, famciclovir, and valaciclovir can be used in the treatment of genital infection due to *herpes simplex virus*, the HSV type 2 being a major cause of genital ulceration. They have a beneficial effect on virus shedding and healing, generally giving relief from pain and other symptoms. See section 5.3 for systemic preparations, and section 13.10.3 for topical preparations.

PREPARATIONS FOR OTHER VAGINAL INFECTIONS

Dalacin® (Pharmacia) [PoM]
Cream, clindamycin 2% (as phosphate), net price 40-g pack with 7 applicators = £10.86
Excipients include benzyl alcohol, cetostearyl alcohol, polysorbates, propylene glycol
Condoms damages latex condoms and diaphragms
Side-effects irritation, cervicitis and vaginitis; poorly absorbed into the blood—low risk of systemic effects, see section 5.1.6
Licensed use not licensed for use in pre-pubertal children

Dose
> **Bacterial vaginosis**
> Insert 5-g applicatorful at night for 3–7 nights

Zidoval® (Meda) [PoM]
Vaginal gel, metronidazole 0.75%, net price 40-g pack with 5 applicators = £4.31
Excipients include disodium edetate, hydroxybenzoates (parabens), propylene glycol
Cautions not recommended during menstruation; some absorption may occur, see section 5.1.11 for systemic effects
Side-effects local effects including irritation, candidiasis, abnormal discharge, pelvic discomfort
Licensed use not licensed for use in pre-pubertal children

Dose
> **Bacterial vaginosis**
> Insert 5-g applicatorful at night for 5 nights

7.3 Contraceptives

The Fraser Guidelines[1] should be followed when prescribing contraception for women under 16 years. The UK Medical Eligibility Criteria for Contraceptive Use (available at www.ffprhc.org.uk) is published by the Faculty of Sexual and Reproductive Healthcare; it categorises the risks of using contraceptive methods with pre-existing medical conditions.

Hormonal contraception is the most effective method of fertility control, but has major and minor side-effects, especially for certain groups of women. Hormonal contraception should only be used by adolescents after menarche.

Intra-uterine devices are a highly effective method of contraception but may produce undesirable local side-effects. They may be used in women of all ages irrespective of parity but are less appropriate for those with an increased risk of pelvic inflammatory disease.

Barrier methods alone (condoms, diaphragms, and caps) are less effective but can be very reliable for well-motivated couples if used in conjunction with a **spermicide**. Occasionally sensitivity reactions occur. A female condom (*Femidom®*) is also available; it is prelubricated but does not contain a spermicide.

7.3.1 Combined hormonal contraceptives

Oral contraceptives containing an oestrogen and a progestogen ('combined oral contraceptives') are effective preparations for general use. Advantages of combined oral contraceptives include:

- reliable and reversible;
- reduced dysmenorrhoea and menorrhagia;
- reduced incidence of premenstrual tension;
- reduced risk of symptomatic fibroids and functional ovarian cysts;
- less benign breast disease;
- reduced risk of ovarian and endometrial cancer;
- reduced risk of pelvic inflammatory disease.

Combined oral contraceptives containing a fixed amount of an oestrogen and a progestogen in each active tablet are termed 'monophasic'; those with varying amounts of the two hormones according to the stage of the cycle are termed 'phasic'. A transdermal patch and a vaginal ring, both containing an oestrogen with a progestogen, are also available.

Choice   The majority of combined oral contraceptives contain ethinylestradiol as the oestrogen component; mestranol and estradiol valerate are also used. The ethinylestradiol content of combined oral contraceptives ranges from 20 to 40 micrograms. Generally a preparation with the lowest oestrogen and progestogen content which gives good cycle control and minimal side-effects in the individual woman is chosen.

- *Low strength preparations* (containing ethinylestradiol 20 micrograms) are particularly appropriate for women with risk factors for circulatory disease, provided a combined oral contraceptive is otherwise suitable.

- *Standard strength preparations* (containing ethinylestradiol 30 or 35 micrograms or in 30–40 microgram *phased* preparations) are appropriate for standard use—but see Risk of Venous Thromboembolism below. Phased preparations are generally reserved for women who *either* do not have withdrawal bleeding *or* who have breakthrough bleeding with monophasic products.

The progestogens desogestrel, drospirenone, and gestodene (in combination with ethinylestradiol) may be considered for women who have side-effects (such as

---

1. See Department of Health Guidance (July 2004): Best practice guidance for doctors and other health professionals on the provision of advice and treatment to young people under 16 on contraception, sexual and reproductive health. Available at www.dh.gov.uk

acne, headache, depression, weight gain, breast symptoms, and breakthrough bleeding) with other progestogens. However, women should be advised that desogestrel and gestodene have also been associated with an increased risk of *venous thromboembolism*. Drospirenone, a derivative of spironolactone, has anti-androgenic and anti-mineralocorticoid activity; it should be used with care if an increased plasma-potassium concentration might be hazardous.

The progestogen norelgestromin is combined with ethinylestradiol in a transdermal patch (*Evra*®).

The vaginal contraceptive ring contains the progestogen etonogestrel combined with ethinylestradiol (*NuvaRing*®).

Risk of venous thromboembolism   There is an increased risk of venous thromboembolic disease (particularly during the first year) in users of oral contraceptives, but this risk is considerably smaller than that associated with pregnancy (about 60 cases of venous thromboembolic disease per 100 000 pregnancies). In all cases the risk of venous thromboembolism increases with age and in the presence of other risk factors for venous thromboembolism, such as obesity.

The incidence of venous thromboembolism in healthy, non-pregnant women who are not taking an oral contraceptive is about 5–10 cases per 100 000 women per year. For those using combined oral contraceptives containing second-generation progestogens, such as levonorgestrel, this incidence is about 15 per 100 000 women per year of use. The risk of venous thromboembolism with transdermal patches may be slightly increased compared with combined oral contraceptives that contain levonorgestrel. Some studies have reported a greater risk of venous thromboembolism in women using combined oral contraceptives containing the third-generation progestogens desogestrel and gestodene; the incidence in these women is about 25 per 100 000 women per year of use. The absolute risk of venous thromboembolism in women using combined oral contraceptives containing these third-generation progestogens is very small and well below the risk associated with pregnancy. The risk of venous thromboembolism in women using a combined oral contraceptive containing drospirenone may be between that associated with combined oral contraceptives containing second-generation progestogens and combined oral contraceptives containing third-generation progestogens. The risk of venous thromboembolism with vaginal ring use compared to the risk with other combined hormonal contraceptives is unknown.

Provided that women are informed of the relative risks of venous thromboembolism and accept them, the choice of oral contraceptive is for the woman together with the prescriber jointly to make in light of her individual medical history and any contra-indications.

Travel   Women taking oral contraceptives or using the patch or vaginal ring are at an increased risk of deep-vein thrombosis during travel involving long periods of immobility (over 5 hours). The risk may be reduced by appropriate exercise during the journey and possibly by wearing graduated compression hosiery.

Missed pill   The critical time for loss of contraceptive protection is when a pill is omitted at the *beginning* or *end* of a cycle (which lengthens the pill-free interval).

If a woman forgets to take a pill, it should be taken as soon as she remembers, and the next one taken at the normal time (even if this means taking 2 pills together). A missed pill is one that is 24 or more hours late; for women taking *Qlaira*®, see below. If a woman misses only one pill, she should take an active pill as soon as she remembers and then resume normal pill-taking. No additional precautions are necessary.

If a woman misses 2 or more pills (especially from the first 7 in a packet), she may not be protected. She should take an active pill as soon as she remembers and then resume normal pill-taking. In addition, she must either abstain from sex or use an additional method of contraception such as a condom for the next 7 days. If these 7 days run beyond the end of the packet, the next packet should be started at once, omitting the pill-free interval (or, in the case of *everyday* (ED) pills, omitting the 7 inactive tablets).

A missed pill for a woman taking *Qlaira*® is one that is 12 hours or more late; for information on how to manage missed pills in women taking *Qlaira*®, refer to product literature.

Emergency contraception (section 7.3.5) is recommended if 2 or more combined oral contraceptive tablets are missed from the first 7 tablets in a packet and unprotected intercourse has occurred since finishing the last packet.

Note The Faculty of Sexual and Reproductive Healthcare offers 2 different types of missed pill advice depending on the ethinylestradiol content of the contraceptive pill. The missed pill information above offers the same advice regardless of the ethinylestradiol content of the contraceptive pill; it is a simplified, more cautious version of advice issued by the Faculty of Sexual and Reproductive Healthcare.

Delayed application or detached patch   If a patch is partly detached for less than 24 hours, reapply to the same site or replace with a new patch immediately; no additional contraception is needed and the next patch should be applied on the usual 'change day'. If a patch remains detached for more than 24 hours or if the user is not aware when the patch became detached then stop the current contraceptive cycle and start a new cycle by applying a new patch, giving a new 'Day 1'; an additional non-hormonal contraceptive must be used concurrently for the first 7 days of the new cycle.

If application of a new patch at the start of a new cycle is delayed, contraceptive protection is lost. A new patch should be applied as soon as remembered giving a new 'Day 1'; additional non-hormonal methods of contraception should be used for the first 7 days of the new cycle. If intercourse has occurred during this extended patch-free interval, a possibility of fertilisation should be considered. If application of a patch in the middle of the cycle is delayed (i.e. the patch is not changed on day 8 or day 15):

- for up to 48 hours, apply a new patch immediately; next patch change day remains the same and no additional contraception is required;

- for more than 48 hours, contraceptive protection may have been lost. Stop the current cycle and start a new 4-week cycle immediately by applying a new patch giving a new 'Day 1'; additional non-hormonal contraception should be used for the first 7 days of the new cycle.

If the patch is not removed at the end of the cycle (day 22), remove it as soon as possible and start the next cycle on the usual 'change day', the day after day 28; no additional contraception is required.

Expulsion, delayed insertion or removal, or broken vaginal ring   If the vaginal ring is expelled for *less than 3 hours*, rinse the ring with cool water and reinsert immediately; no additional contraception is needed.

If the ring remains outside the vagina for *more than 3 hours* or if the user does not know when the ring was expelled, contraceptive protection may be reduced:

- if ring expelled during week 1 or 2 of cycle, rinse ring with cool water and reinsert; use additional precautions (barrier methods) for next 7 days;

- if ring expelled during week 3 of cycle, either insert a new ring to start a new cycle *or* allow a withdrawal bleed and insert a new ring no later than 7 days after ring was expelled; latter option only available if ring was used continuously for at least 7 days prior to expulsion.

If insertion of a new ring at the start of a new cycle is delayed, contraceptive protection is lost. A new ring should be inserted as soon as possible; additional precautions (barrier methods) should be used for the first 7 days of the new cycle. If intercourse occurred during the extended ring-free interval, pregnancy should be considered.

No additional contraception is required if the removal of the ring is delayed by up to 1 week (4 weeks of continuous use). The 7-day ring-free interval should be observed and subsequently a new ring should be inserted. Contraceptive protection may be reduced with continuous use of the ring for more than 4 weeks—pregnancy should be ruled out before inserting a new ring.

If the ring breaks during use, remove it and insert a new ring immediately; additional precautions (barrier methods) should be used for the first 7 days of the new cycle.

Diarrhoea and vomiting   Vomiting and persistent, severe diarrhoea can interfere with the absorption of combined oral contraceptives. If vomiting occurs within 2 hours of taking a combined oral contraceptive another pill should be taken as soon as possible. In cases of persistent vomiting or severe diarrhoea lasting more than 24 hours, additional precautions should be used during and for 7 days (9 days for *Qlaira*®) after recovery (see also under Missed pill, above). If the vomiting and diarrhoea occurs during the last 7 tablets, the next pill-free interval should be omitted (in the case of ED tablets the inactive ones should be omitted).

Interactions   The effectiveness of *combined* oral contraceptives, *progestogen-only* oral contraceptives (section 7.3.2.1), contraceptive patches, and vaginal rings can be considerably reduced by interaction with drugs that induce hepatic enzyme activity (e.g. **carbamazepine, griseofulvin, modafinil, nelfinavir, nevirapine, oxcarbazepine, phenytoin, phenobarbital, primidone, ritonavir, St John's Wort, topiramate**, and, above all, **rifabutin** and **rifampicin**). A condom together with a long-acting method, such as an injectable contraceptive, may be more suitable for patients with HIV infection or at risk of HIV infection; advice on the possibility of interaction with antiretroviral drugs should be sought from HIV specialists.

For a *short course of an enzyme-inducing drug*, the dose of combined oral contraceptives should be adjusted to provide ethinylestradiol 50 micrograms or more daily [unlicensed use]; furthermore, additional contraceptive precautions should be taken whilst taking the enzyme-inducing drug and for 4 weeks after stopping it. Additional contraceptive precautions are also required for women using contraceptive patches and vaginal rings whilst taking the enzyme-inducing drug and for 4 weeks after stopping. If concomitant administration runs beyond the 3 weeks of patch or vaginal ring use, a new treatment cycle should be started immediately without a patch-free or ring-free break.

Women requiring a *long-term course of an enzyme-inducing drug* should be encouraged to consider a contraceptive method that is unaffected by the interacting drug. In women unable to use an alternative method of contraception (for rifampicin and rifabutin see also below), a regimen of combined oral contraceptives should be taken which provides a daily intake of ethinylestradiol 50 micrograms or more [unlicensed use]; 'tricycling' (i.e. taking 3 or 4 packets of monophasic tablets without a break followed by a short tablet-free interval of 4 days) may be recommended. **Rifampicin** and **rifabutin** are such potent enzyme-inducing drugs that an alternative method of contraception (such as an IUD) is **always** recommended. Since enzyme activity does not return to normal for several weeks after stopping an enzyme-inducing drug, appropriate contraceptive measures are required for 4 to 8 weeks after stopping. Contraceptive patches and vaginal rings are not recommended for women taking enzyme-inducing drugs over a long period.

Some antibacterials that do not induce liver enzymes (e.g. ampicillin, doxycycline) may reduce the efficacy of *combined* oral contraceptives by impairing the bacterial flora responsible for recycling ethinylestradiol from the large bowel. Additional contraceptive precautions should be taken whilst taking a short course of an antibacterial drug that is not enzyme-inducing and for 7 days after stopping. If these 7 days run beyond the end of a packet the next packet should be started immediately without a break (in the case of ED tablets the inactive ones should be omitted). If the antibacterial course *exceeds 3 weeks*, the bacterial flora develop antibacterial resistance and additional precautions become unnecessary unless a new antibacterial is prescribed; additional precautions are also unnecessary if a woman starting a *combined* oral contraceptive has been on a course of antibacterial therapy for 3 weeks or more.

It is possible that some antibacterials reduce the efficacy of contraceptive patches and vaginal rings. Additional contraceptive precautions are recommended during concomitant use and for 7 days after discontinuation of an antibacterial that is not enzyme-inducing (except tetracycline with contraceptive patch use, and amoxicillin or doxycycline with vaginal ring use). If concomitant administration runs beyond the 3 weeks of patch or vaginal ring use, a new treatment cycle should be started immediately without a patch-free or ring-free break. If the antibacterial course exceeds 3 weeks, additional precautions become unnecessary unless a new antibacterial is prescribed; additional precautions are also unnecessary if a woman starting a contraceptive patch or vaginal ring has been on a course of antibacterial therapy for 3 weeks or more.

Surgery   Oestrogen-containing contraceptives should preferably be discontinued (and adequate alternative contraceptive arrangements made) 4 weeks before major elective surgery and all surgery to the legs or surgery which involves prolonged immobilisation of a lower limb; they should normally be recommenced at the first menses occurring at least 2 weeks after full mobilisation. A depot injection of a progestogen-only contraceptive may be offered and the oestrogen-containing contraceptive restarted later—if preferred before the next injection would be due. When discontinuation of an oestrogen-containing contraceptive is not possible, e.g. after trauma or if a patient admitted for an elective procedure is still on an oestrogen-containing contraceptive, thromboprophylaxis (with unfractionated or low molecular weight heparin and graduated compression hosiery) is advised. These recommendations do not apply to minor surgery with short duration of anaesthesia, e.g. laparoscopic sterilisation or tooth extraction, or to women using oestrogen-free hormonal contraceptives (whether by mouth or by injection).

Reason to stop immediately Combined hormonal contraceptives should be stopped (pending investigation and treatment), if any of the following occur:

- sudden severe chest pain (even if not radiating to left arm);
- sudden breathlessness (or cough with blood-stained sputum);
- unexplained swelling or severe pain in calf of one leg;
- severe stomach pain;
- serious neurological effects including unusual severe, prolonged headache especially if first time or getting progressively worse *or* sudden partial or complete loss of vision *or* sudden disturbance of hearing or other perceptual disorders *or* dysphasia *or* bad fainting attack or collapse *or* first unexplained epileptic seizure *or* weakness, motor disturbances, very marked numbness suddenly affecting one side or one part of body;
- hepatitis, jaundice, liver enlargement;
- very high blood pressure;
- prolonged immobilisation after surgery or leg injury;
- detection of a risk factor which contra-indicates treatment (see Cautions and Contra-indications under Combined Hormonal Contraceptives below).

COMBINED HORMONAL CONTRACEPTIVES

Cautions see notes above; also risk factors for venous thromboembolism (see below and also notes above), arterial disease and migraine, see below; personal or family history of hypertriglyceridaemia (increased risk of pancreatitis); hyperprolactinaemia (seek specialist advice); history of severe depression especially if induced by hormonal contraceptive; undiagnosed breast mass; gene mutations associated with breast cancer (e.g. BRCA 1); sickle-cell disease; inflammatory bowel disease including Crohn's disease; reduced efficacy of contraceptive patch in women with body-weight $\geq$ 90 kg; **interactions:** see above and Appendix 1 (oestrogens, progestogens)

Risk factors for venous thromboembolism See also notes above. Use with **caution** if any of following factors present but **avoid** if two or more factors present:

- *family history of venous thromboembolism* in first-degree relative aged under 45 years (avoid contraceptive containing desogestrel or gestodene, *or* avoid if known prothrombotic coagulation abnormality e.g. factor V Leiden or antiphospholipid antibodies (including lupus anticoagulant));
- *obesity*—caution if overweight according to BMI (adjusted for age and gender), avoid if obese;
- *long-term immobilisation* e.g. in a wheelchair (avoid if confined to bed or leg in plaster cast);
- *history of superficial thrombophlebitis*;
- *smoking*.

Risk factors for arterial disease Use with **caution** if any one of following factors present but **avoid** if two or more factors present:

- *family history of arterial disease* in first degree relative aged under 45 years (avoid if atherogenic lipid profile);
- *diabetes mellitus* (avoid if diabetes complications present);
- *hypertension* (avoid if blood pressure very high);
- *smoking* (avoid if smoking 40 or more cigarettes daily);

- *obesity*—caution if overweight according to BMI (adjusted for age and gender), avoid if obese;
- *migraine without aura* (avoid if *migraine with aura* (focal symptoms), *or* severe migraine frequently lasting over 72 hours despite treatment, *or* migraine treated with ergot derivatives).

Migraine Women should report any increase in headache frequency or onset of focal symptoms (discontinue immediately and refer urgently to neurology expert if focal neurological symptoms not typical of aura persist for more than 1 hour—see also Reason to stop immediately in notes above)

Contra-indications see notes above; also personal history of venous or arterial thrombosis, severe or multiple risk factors for arterial disease or for venous thromboembolism (see above), heart disease associated with pulmonary hypertension or risk of embolus; sclerosing treatment for varicose veins; migraine (but see above); transient cerebral ischaemic attacks without headaches; systemic lupus erythematosus; acute porphyria (section 9.8.2); gallstones; active trophoblastic disease (until return to normal of urine- and plasma-gonadotrophin concentration); history of haemolytic uraemic syndrome or history during pregnancy of pruritus, cholestatic jaundice, chorea, pemphigoid gestationis; history of breast cancer but can be used after 5 years if no evidence of disease and non-hormonal methods unacceptable; undiagnosed vaginal bleeding

Hepatic impairment avoid in active liver disease including disorders of hepatic excretion (e.g. Dubin-Johnson or Rotor syndromes), infective hepatitis (until liver function returns to normal), and liver tumours

Pregnancy not known to be harmful

Breast-feeding avoid until weaning or for 6 months after birth (adverse effects on lactation)

Side-effects see notes above; also nausea, vomiting, abdominal cramps, changes in body-weight,

◻ **COMBINED HORMONAL CONTRACEPTIVES (*continued*)**

liver impairment, hepatic tumours; fluid retention, thrombosis (more common when factor V Leiden present or in blood groups A, B, and AB; see also notes above), hypertension, changes in lipid metabolism; headache, depression, chorea, nervousness, irritability; changes in libido, breast tenderness, enlargement, and secretion; reduced menstrual loss, 'spotting' in early cycles, absence of withdrawal bleeding, amenorrhoea after discontinuation, changes in vaginal discharge, cervical erosion; contact lenses may irritate, visual disturbances; leg cramps; skin reactions, chloasma, photosensitivity; rarely gallstones and systemic lupus erythematosus

Breast cancer There is a small increase in the risk of having breast cancer diagnosed in women taking the combined oral contraceptive pill; this relative risk may be due to an earlier diagnosis. In users of combined oral contraceptive pills the cancers are more likely to be localised to the breast. The most important factor for diagnosing breast cancer appears to be the age at which the contraceptive is stopped rather than the duration of use; any increase in the rate of diagnosis diminishes gradually during the 10 years after stopping and disappears by 10 years

Cervical cancer Use of combined oral contraceptives for 5 years or longer is associated with a small increased risk of cervical cancer; the risk diminishes after stopping and disappears by about 10 years. The risk of cervical cancer with transdermal patches and vaginal rings is not yet known

Note The possible small increase in the risk of breast cancer and cervical cancer should be weighed against the protective effect against cancers of the ovary and endometrium

Licensed use consult product literature for the licensing status of individual preparations

Indication and dose

Contraception, menstrual symptoms (section 6.4.1.2)

- **By mouth**

Each tablet should be taken at approximately same time each day; if delayed by longer than 24 hours (12 hours for *Qlaira*®) contraceptive protection may be lost

21-Day combined (monophasic) preparations, 1 tablet daily for 21 days; subsequent courses repeated after a 7-day interval (during which withdrawal bleeding occurs); first course usually started on day 1 of cycle—if starting on day 4 of cycle or later, additional precautions (barrier methods) necessary during first 7 days

Every day (ED) combined (monophasic) preparations, 1 *active* tablet starting on day 1 of cycle (see also under preparations below)—if starting on day 4 of cycle or later, additional precautions (barrier methods) necessary during first 7 days; withdrawal bleeding occurs when *inactive* tablets being taken; subsequent courses repeated without interval

Phasic preparations, see under individual preparations below

Changing to combined preparation containing different progestogen *21-day combined preparations:* continue current pack until last tablet and start first tablet of new brand the next day. If a 7-day break is taken before starting new brand, additional precautions (barrier methods) should be used during first 7 days (9 days for *Qlaira*®) of taking the new brand

Every Day (ED) combined preparations: start the new brand (first tablet of a *21-day preparation* or the first

active tablet of an *ED preparation*) the day after taking the last *active* tablet of previous brand (omitting the *inactive* tablets)

Changing from progestogen-only tablet Start on day 1 of menstruation or any day if amenorrhoea present and pregnancy has been excluded

Secondary amenorrhoea (exclude pregnancy) Start any day, additional precautions (barrier methods) necessary during first 7 days (9 days for *Qlaira*®)

After childbirth (not breast-feeding) Start 3 weeks after birth (increased risk of thrombosis if started earlier); later than 3 weeks postpartum additional precautions (barrier methods) necessary for first 7 days (9 days for *Qlaira*®)

After abortion or miscarriage Start same day

- **By transdermal application**

Apply first patch on day 1 of cycle, change patch on days 8 and 15; remove third patch on day 22 and apply new patch after 7-day patch-free interval to start subsequent contraceptive cycle

Note If first patch applied later than day 1, additional precautions (abstinence or barrier methods) should be used for the next 7 days

Changing from combined oral contraception Apply patch on the first day of withdrawal bleeding; if no withdrawal bleeding within 5 days of taking last *active* tablet, rule out pregnancy before applying first patch. Unless patch is applied on first day of withdrawal bleeding, additional precautions (barrier methods) should be used concurrently for first 7 days

Changing from progestogen-only method From an implant, apply first patch on the day implant removed; from an injection, apply first patch when next injection due; from oral progestogen, first patch may be started on any day after stopping pill. For all methods additional precautions (barrier methods) should be used concurrently for first 7 days

After childbirth (not breast-feeding) Start 4 weeks after birth; if started later than 4 weeks after birth additional precautions (barrier methods) should be used for first 7 days

After abortion or miscarriage Before 20 weeks' gestation start immediately; no additional contraception required if started immediately. After 20 weeks' gestation start on day 21 after abortion or on the first day of first spontaneous menstruation; additional precautions (barrier methods) should be used for first 7 days after applying the patch

- **By vagina**

Insert ring into vagina on day 1 of cycle and leave in for 3 weeks; remove ring on day 22; subsequent courses repeated after 7-day ring-free interval (during which withdrawal bleeding occurs)

Note If first ring inserted later than day 1, additional precaution (abstinence or barrier methods) should be used for the next 7 days

Changing from combined hormonal contraception Insert ring at the latest on the day after the usual tablet-free, patch-free, or placebo-tablet interval. If previous contraceptive used correctly and pregnancy unlikely, can switch to ring on any day of cycle

Changing from progestogen-only method From an implant or intra-uterine progestogen-only device, insert ring on the day implant or intra-uterine progestogen-only device removed; from an injection, insert ring when injection next due; from oral preparation, first ring may be inserted on any day after stopping pill. For all methods additional precautions (barrier methods) should be used concurrently for first 7 days

After first trimester abortion Start immediately

After childbirth (not breast-feeding) or second trimester abortion Start 4 weeks after birth or abortion; if started later than 4 weeks after birth or abortion additional precautions (barrier methods) should be used for first 7 days

◻ **COMBINED HORMONAL CONTRACEPTIVES** (*continued*)

Low strength (oral)
◢**Ethinylestradiol with Norethisterone**
Loestrin 20® (Galen) ℗ℴ𝕄
Tablets, blue, ethinylestradiol 20 micrograms, nor-ethisterone acetate 1 mg, net price 3 × 21-tab pack = £2.75
Dose
> 1 tablet daily for 21 days; subsequent courses repeated after 7-day tablet-free interval (during which with-drawal bleeding occurs); for starting routines see under Dose above

◢**Ethinylestradiol with Desogestrel**
See Risk of Venous Thromboembolism in notes above before prescribing

Mercilon® (Organon) ℗ℴ𝕄
Tablets, ethinylestradiol 20 micrograms, desogestrel 150 micrograms, net price 3 × 21-tab pack = £7.97
Dose
> 1 tablet daily for 21 days; subsequent courses repeated after 7-day tablet-free interval (during which with-drawal bleeding occurs); for starting routines see under Dose above

◢**Ethinylestradiol with Gestodene**
See Risk of Venous Thromboembolism in notes above before prescribing

Femodette® (Bayer Schering) ℗ℴ𝕄
Tablets, s/c, ethinylestradiol 20 micrograms, gestodene 75 micrograms, net price 3 × 21-tab pack = £9.08
Dose
> 1 tablet daily for 21 days; subsequent courses repeated after 7-day tablet-free interval (during which with-drawal bleeding occurs); for starting routines see under Dose above

Sunya 20/75® (Stragen) ℗ℴ𝕄
Tablets, s/c, ethinylestradiol 20 micrograms, gestodene 75 micrograms, net price 3 × 21-tab pack = £6.62
Dose
> 1 tablet daily for 21 days; subsequent courses repeated after 7-day tablet-free interval (during which with-drawal bleeding occurs); for starting routines see under Dose above

Low strength (vaginal)
◢**Ethinylestradiol with Etonogestrel**
NuvaRing® (Organon) ▼ ℗ℴ𝕄
Vaginal ring, releasing ethinylestradiol approx. 15 micrograms/24 hours and etonogestrel approx. 120 micrograms/24 hours, net price 3-ring pack = £27.00. Counselling, administration
Dose
> 1 ring to be inserted into the vagina for 3 weeks, removed on day 22; subsequent courses repeated after 7-day ring-free interval (during which withdrawal bleeding occurs); for starting routines see under Dose above

Counselling The presence of the ring should be checked regularly. In case of expulsion see Expulsion, Delayed Insertion or Removal, or Broken Vaginal Ring, p. 485

Standard strength (oral)
◢**Ethinylestradiol with Levonorgestrel**
Levest (Morningside) ℗ℴ𝕄
Tablets, ethinylestradiol 30 micrograms, levonor-gestrel 150 micrograms, net price 3 × 21-tab pack = £2.64
Dose
> 1 tablet daily for 21 days; subsequent courses repeated after 7-day tablet-free interval (during which with-drawal bleeding occurs); for starting routines see under Dose above

Logynon® (Bayer Schering) ℗ℴ𝕄
6 light brown tablets, ethinylestradiol 30 micr-ograms, levonorgestrel 50 micrograms;
5 white tablets, ethinylestradiol 40 micrograms, levonorgestrel 75 micrograms;
10 ochre tablets, ethinylestradiol 30 micrograms, levonorgestrel 125 micrograms.
Net price 3 × 21-tab pack = £3.96
Dose
> 1 tablet daily for 21 days, starting with light brown tablet marked 1 on day 1 of cycle; repeat after 7-day tablet-free interval; for starting routines see under Dose above

Logynon ED® (Bayer Schering) ℗ℴ𝕄
6 light brown tablets, ethinylestradiol 30 micr-ograms, levonorgestrel 50 micrograms;
5 white tablets, ethinylestradiol 40 micrograms, levonorgestrel 75 micrograms;
10 ochre tablets, ethinylestradiol 30 micrograms, levonorgestrel 125 micrograms;
7 white, inactive tablets.
Net price 3 × 28-tab pack = £3.96
Dose
> 1 tablet daily for 28 days, starting on day 1 of cycle with active tablet (withdrawal bleeding occurs when inactive tablets being taken); subsequent courses repeated without interval; for starting routines see under Dose above

Microgynon 30® (Bayer Schering) ℗ℴ𝕄
Tablets, s/c, ethinylestradiol 30 micrograms, levo-norgestrel 150 micrograms, net price 3 × 21-tab pack = £2.87
Dose
> 1 tablet daily for 21 days; subsequent courses repeated after 7-day tablet-free interval (during which with-drawal bleeding occurs); for starting routines see under Dose above

Microgynon 30 ED® (Bayer Schering) ℗ℴ𝕄
Tablets, beige, ethinylestradiol 30 micrograms, levonorgestrel 150 micrograms, white inactive tablets, net price 3 × 28-tab (7 are inactive) pack = £2.59
Dose
> 1 tablet daily for 28 days starting on day 1 of cycle with active tablet (withdrawal bleeding occurs when inac-tive tablets being taken); subsequent courses repeated without interval; for starting routines see also under Dose above

7 Obstetrics, gynaecology, and urinary-tract disorders

◻ **COMBINED HORMONAL CONTRACEPTIVES (*continued*)**

Ovranette® (Wyeth) [PoM]
Tablets, ethinylestradiol 30 micrograms, levonorgestrel 150 micrograms, net price 3 × 21-tab pack = £2.20

Dose

> 1 tablet daily for 21 days; subsequent courses repeated after 7-day tablet-free interval (during which withdrawal bleeding occurs); for starting routines see under Dose above

▲**Ethinylestradiol with Norethisterone**
BiNovum® (Janssen-Cilag) [PoM]
7 white tablets, ethinylestradiol 35 micrograms, norethisterone 500 micrograms;

14 peach tablets, ethinylestradiol 35 micrograms, norethisterone 1 mg.
Net price 3 × 21-tab pack = £2.00

Dose

> 1 tablet daily for 21 days, starting with white tablet on day 1 of cycle; repeat after 7-day tablet-free interval; for starting routines see under Dose above

Brevinor® (Pharmacia) [PoM]
Tablets, blue, ethinylestradiol 35 micrograms, norethisterone 500 micrograms, net price 3 × 21-tab pack = £1.99

Dose

> 1 tablet daily for 21 days; subsequent courses repeated after 7-day tablet-free interval (during which withdrawal bleeding occurs); for starting routines see under Dose above

Loestrin 30® (Galen) [PoM]
Tablets, pale green, ethinylestradiol 30 micrograms, norethisterone acetate 1.5 mg, net price 3 × 21-tab pack = £3.95

Dose

> 1 tablet daily for 21 days; subsequent courses repeated after 7-day tablet-free interval (during which withdrawal bleeding occurs); for starting routines see under Dose above

Norimin® (Pharmacia) [PoM]
Tablets, ethinylestradiol 35 micrograms, norethisterone 1 mg, net price 3 × 21-tab pack = £2.28

Dose

> 1 tablet daily for 21 days; subsequent courses repeated after 7-day tablet-free interval (during which withdrawal bleeding occurs); for starting routines see under Dose above

Ovysmen® (Janssen-Cilag) [PoM]
Tablets, ethinylestradiol 35 micrograms, norethisterone 500 micrograms, net price 3 × 21-tab pack = £1.52

Dose

> 1 tablet daily for 21 days; subsequent courses repeated after 7-day tablet-free interval (during which withdrawal bleeding occurs); for starting routines see under Dose above

Synphase® (Pharmacia) [PoM]
7 blue tablets, ethinylestradiol 35 micrograms, norethisterone 500 micrograms;

9 white tablets, ethinylestradiol 35 micrograms, norethisterone 1 mg;

5 blue tablets, ethinylestradiol 35 micrograms, norethisterone 500 micrograms.
Net price 21-tab pack = £1.20

Dose

> 1 tablet daily for 21 days, starting with blue tablet marked 1 on day 1 of cycle; repeat after 7-day tablet-free interval; for starting routines see under Dose above

TriNovum® (Janssen-Cilag) [PoM]
7 white tablets, ethinylestradiol 35 micrograms, norethisterone 500 micrograms;

7 light peach tablets, ethinylestradiol 35 micrograms, norethisterone 750 micrograms;

7 peach tablets, ethinylestradiol 35 micrograms, norethisterone 1 mg.
Net price 3 × 21-tab pack = £2.78

Dose

> 1 tablet daily for 21 days, starting with white tablet on day 1 of cycle; repeat after 7-day tablet-free interval; for starting routines see under Dose above

▲**Ethinylestradiol with Norgestimate**
Cilest® (Janssen-Cilag) [PoM]
Tablets, blue, ethinylestradiol 35 micrograms, norgestimate 250 micrograms, net price 3 × 21-tab pack = £2.99, 6 × 21-tab pack = £5.97

Dose

> 1 tablet daily for 21 days; subsequent courses repeated after 7-day tablet-free interval (during which withdrawal bleeding occurs); for starting routines see under Dose above

▲**Ethinylestradiol with Desogestrel**
See Risk of Venous Thromboembolism in notes above before prescribing

Marvelon® (Organon) [PoM]
Tablets, ethinylestradiol 30 micrograms, desogestrel 150 micrograms, net price 3 × 21-tab pack = £6.57

Dose

> 1 tablet daily for 21 days; subsequent courses repeated after 7-day tablet-free interval (during which withdrawal bleeding occurs); for starting routines see under Dose above

▲**Ethinylestradiol with Drospirenone**
See Risk of Venous Thromboembolism in notes above before prescribing

Yasmin® (Bayer Schering) [PoM]
Tablets, f/c, yellow, ethinylestradiol 30 micrograms, drospirenone 3 mg, net price 3 × 21-tab pack = £14.70

Cautions use with care if increased concentration of plasma-potassium might be hazardous

Renal impairment avoid if estimated glomerular filtration rate less than 30 mL/minute/1.73m²

Dose

> 1 tablet daily for 21 days; subsequent courses repeated after 7-day tablet-free interval (during which withdrawal bleeding occurs); for starting routines see under Dose above

◻ **COMBINED HORMONAL CONTRACEPTIVES** (*continued*)

◢**Ethinylestradiol with Gestodene**
See Risk of Venous Thromboembolism in notes
above before prescribing

Femodene® (Bayer Schering) PoM
Tablets, s/c, ethinylestradiol 30 micrograms,
gestodene 75 micrograms, net price 3 × 21-tab
pack = £6.90

Dose
1 tablet daily for 21 days; subsequent courses repeated
after 7-day tablet-free interval (during which withdrawal bleeding occurs); for starting routines see
under Dose above

Femodene® ED (Bayer Schering) PoM
Tablets, s/c, ethinylestradiol 30 micrograms,
gestodene 75 micrograms, net price 3 × 28-tab (7
are inactive) pack = £6.90

Dose
1 tablet daily for 28 days, starting on day 1 of cycle
with active tablet (withdrawal bleeding occurs when
inactive tablets being taken); subsequent courses
repeated without interval; for starting routines see
under Dose above

Katya 30/75® (Stragen) PoM
Tablets, s/c, ethinylestradiol 30 micrograms,
gestodene 75 micrograms, net price 3 × 21-tab
pack = £5.03

Dose
1 tablet daily for 21 days; subsequent courses repeated
after 7-day tablet-free interval (during which withdrawal bleeding occurs); for starting routines see
under Dose above

Triadene® (Bayer Schering) PoM
6 beige tablets, ethinylestradiol 30 micrograms,
gestodene 50 micrograms;

5 dark brown tablets, ethinylestradiol 40 micrograms, gestodene 70 micrograms;

10 white tablets, ethinylestradiol 30 micrograms,
gestodene 100 micrograms.
Net price 3 × 21-tab pack = £9.17

Dose
1 tablet daily for 21 days, starting with beige tablet
marked 'start' on day 1 of cycle; repeat after 7-day
tablet-free interval; for starting routines see under
Dose above

◢**Mestranol with Norethisterone**
Norinyl-1® (Pharmacia) PoM
Tablets, mestranol 50 micrograms, norethisterone
1 mg, net price 3 × 21-tab pack = £2.19

Dose
1 tablet daily for 21 days; subsequent courses repeated
after 7-day tablet-free interval (during which withdrawal bleeding occurs); for starting routines see
under Dose above

◢**Ethinylestradiol with cyproterone acetate**
See Co-cyprindiol (section 13.6.2)

◢**Estradiol valerate with Dienogest**
Qlaira® (Bayer Schering) ▼ PoM
2 dark yellow tablets, estradiol valerate 3 mg;

5 red tablets, estradiol valerate 2 mg, dienogest
2 mg;

17 light yellow tablets, estradiol valerate 2 mg,
dienogest 3 mg;

2 dark red tablets, estradiol valerate 1 mg;

2 white, inactive tablets.
Net price 3 × 28-tab pack = £25.18

Dose
1 tablet daily for 28 days starting on day 1 of cycle with
active tablet (withdrawal bleeding occurs when inactive tablets being taken); subsequent courses repeated
without interval; for starting routines see under Dose
above

Standard strength (transdermal)
◢**Ethinylestradiol with Norelgestromin**
Evra® (Janssen-Cilag) PoM
Patches, self-adhesive (releasing ethinylestradiol
approx. 33.9 micrograms/24 hours and norelgestromin approx. 203 micrograms/24 hours); net
price 9-patch pack = £15.63. Counselling, administration

Dose
1 patch to be applied once weekly for three weeks,
followed by a 7-day patch-free interval; subsequent
courses repeated after 7-day patch-free interval (during which withdrawal bleeding occurs); for starting
routines see under Dose above

Note Adhesives or bandages should not be used to hold
patch in place. If patch no longer sticky do not reapply but
use a new patch.
The *Scottish Medicines Consortium* has advised (September
2003) that *Evra®* patches should be restricted for use in
women who are likely to comply poorly with combined
oral contraceptives

7.3.2 **Progestogen-only contraceptives**

7.3.2.1 Oral progestogen-only contraceptives

7.3.2.2 Parenteral progestogen-only contraceptives

7.3.2.3 Intra-uterine progestogen-only device

7.3.2.1 **Oral progestogen-only contraceptives**
Oral progestogen-only preparations may offer a suitable alternative when oestrogens are contra-indicated (including those patients with venous thrombosis or a
past history or predisposition to venous thrombosis), but have a higher failure rate
than combined preparations. They are suitable for heavy smokers, and for those
with hypertension, valvular heart disease, diabetes mellitus, and migraine. Men-

7

Obstetrics, gynaecology, and urinary-tract disorders

strual irregularities (oligomenorrhoea, menorrhagia) are more common but tend to resolve on long-term treatment.

Interactions   Effectiveness of oral progestogen-only preparations is not affected by antibacterials that do not induce liver enzymes. The efficacy of oral progestogen-only preparations is, however, reduced by enzyme-inducing drugs and an additional or alternative contraceptive method is recommended during treatment with an enzyme-inducing drug and for at least 4 weeks afterwards—see p. 486 and Appendix 1 (progestogens).

Surgery   All progestogen-only contraceptives (including those given by injection) are suitable for use as an alternative to combined oral contraceptives before major elective surgery, before all surgery to the legs, or before surgery which involves prolonged immobilisation of a lower limb.

Starting routine   One tablet daily, on a continuous basis, starting on day 1 of cycle and taken at the same time each day (if delayed by longer than 3 hours (12 hours for *Cerazette*®) contraceptive protection may be lost). Additional contraceptive precautions are not necessary when initiating treatment.

Changing from a combined oral contraceptive   Start on the day following completion of the combined oral contraceptive course without a break (or in the case of ED tablets omitting the inactive ones).

After childbirth   Start any time after 3 weeks postpartum (increased risk of breakthrough bleeding if started earlier).

Missed pill   The following advice is now recommended by family planning organisations:

'If you forget a pill, take it as soon as you remember and carry on with the next pill at the right time. If the pill was more than 3 hours (12 hours for *Cerazette*®) overdue you are not protected. Continue normal pill-taking but you must also use another method, such as the condom, for the next 2 days.'

The Faculty of Sexual and Reproductive Healthcare recommends emergency contraception (see p. 498) if one or more progestogen-only contraceptive tablets are missed or taken more than 3 hours (12 hours for *Cerazette*®) late and unprotected intercourse has occurred before 2 further tablets have been correctly taken.

Diarrhoea and vomiting   Vomiting and persistent, severe diarrhoea can interfere with the absorption of oral progestogen-only contraceptives. If vomiting occurs within 2 hours of taking an oral progestogen-only contraceptive, another pill should be taken as soon as possible. If a replacement pill is not taken within 3 hours (12 hours for *Cerazette*®) of the normal time for taking the progestogen-only pill, or in cases of persistent vomiting or very severe diarrhoea, additional precautions should be used during illness and for 2 days after recovery (see also under Missed pill above).

ORAL PROGESTOGEN-ONLY CONTRACEPTIVES

(Progestogen-only pill, 'POP')

Cautions   arterial disease; sex-steroid dependent cancer; past ectopic pregnancy; malabsorption syndromes; active trophoblastic disease (until return to normal of urine- and plasma-gonadotrophin concentration); functional ovarian cysts; history of jaundice in pregnancy; **interactions:** see notes above and Appendix 1 (progestogens)

Other conditions The product literature advises caution in patients with history of thromboembolism, hypertension, diabetes mellitus and migraine; evidence for caution in these conditions is unsatisfactory

Contra-indications   undiagnosed vaginal bleeding; severe arterial disease; acute porphyria (section 9.8.2); history of breast cancer but can be used after 5 years if no evidence of disease and non-hormonal contraceptive methods unacceptable

Hepatic impairment   caution in active liver disease; and recurrent cholestatic jaundice, avoid in liver tumour

Pregnancy   not known to be harmful

Breast-feeding   progestogen-only contraceptives do not affect lactation; see also After Childbirth above

Side-effects   menstrual irregularities (see also notes above); nausea, vomiting, headache, dizziness, breast discomfort, depression, skin disorders, disturbance of appetite, weight changes, changes in libido

Breast cancer There is a small increase in the risk of having breast cancer diagnosed in women using, or who have recently used, a progestogen-only contraceptive pill; this relative risk may be due to an earlier diagnosis. The most important risk factor appears to be the age at which the contraceptive is stopped rather than the duration of use; the risk disappears gradually during the 10 years after stopping and there is no excess risk by 10 years. A possible small increase in the risk of breast cancer should be weighed against the benefits

Licensed use   consult product literature for the licensing status of individual preparations

◻ **ORAL PROGESTOGEN-ONLY CONTRACEPTIVES (*continued*)**

Indication and dose

Contraception

• **By mouth**

1 tablet daily at same time each day, starting on day 1 of cycle then continuously; if administration delayed for 3 hours (12 hours for *Cerazette®*) or more it should be regarded as a 'missed pill', see notes above

Cerazette® (Organon) [PoM]
Tablets, f/c, desogestrel 75 micrograms, net price 3 × 28-tab pack = £8.68
The *Scottish Medicines Consortium* has advised (September 2003) that *Cerazette®* should be restricted for use in women who cannot tolerate oestrogen-containing contraceptives or in whom such preparations are contra-indicated

Femulen® (Pharmacia) [PoM]
Tablets, etynodiol diacetate 500 micrograms, net price 3 × 28-tab pack = £3.31

Micronor® (Janssen-Cilag) [PoM]
Tablets, norethisterone 350 micrograms, net price 3 × 28-tab pack = £1.69

Norgeston® (Bayer Schering) [PoM]
Tablets, s/c, levonorgestrel 30 micrograms, net price 35-tab pack = 94p

Noriday® (Pharmacia) [PoM]
Tablets, norethisterone 350 micrograms, net price 3 × 28-tab pack = £2.10

7.3.2.2 Parenteral progestogen-only contraceptives

Medroxyprogesterone acetate (*Depo-Provera®*) is a long-acting progestogen given by intramuscular injection; it is as effective as the combined oral preparations but because of its prolonged action it should never be given without *full counselling backed by the patient information leaflet*. It may be used as a short-term or long-term contraceptive for women who have been counselled about the likelihood of menstrual disturbance and the potential for a delay in return to full fertility. Delayed return of fertility and irregular cycles may occur after discontinuation of treatment but there is no evidence of permanent infertility. Heavy bleeding has been reported in patients given medroxyprogesterone acetate in the immediate puerperium; delaying the first injection until 6 weeks after the birth may minimise bleeding problems. If the woman is not breast-feeding, the first injection may be given within 5 days postpartum (she should be warned that the risk of heavy or prolonged bleeding may be increased). The manufacturer advises that in women who are breast-feeding, the first dose should be delayed until 6 weeks after the birth; however, evidence suggests no harmful effect to infant if given earlier. The benefits of using medroxyprogesterone acetate in breast-feeding women outweigh any risks.

Reduction in bone mineral density and, rarely, osteoporosis and osteoporotic fractures have also been reported with medroxyprogesterone acetate. The reduction in bone mineral density occurs in the first 2–3 years of use and then stabilises. See also below.

- In adolescents, medroxyprogesterone acetate (*Depo-Provera®*) should be used only when other methods of contraception are inappropriate;
- in all women, the benefits of using medroxyprogesterone acetate beyond 2 years should be evaluated against the risks;
- in women with risk factors for osteoporosis, a method of contraception other than medroxyprogesterone acetate should be considered.

Norethisterone enantate (*Noristerat®*) is a long-acting progestogen given as an oily injection which provides contraception for 8 weeks; it is used as short-term interim contraception e.g. before vasectomy becomes effective.

An **etonogestrel-releasing implant** (*Implanon®*) is also available. It consists of a single flexible rod that is inserted subdermally into the lower surface of the upper arm and provides effective contraception for up to 3 years. The manufacturer advises that in heavier women, blood etonogestrel concentrations are lower and therefore the implant may not provide effective contraception during the third year; they advise that earlier replacement may be considered in such patients, however, evidence to support this recommendation is lacking. Local reactions such as bruising and itching can occur at the insertion site. The contraceptive effect of *Implanon®* is rapidly reversed on removal of the implant. *The doctor or nurse administering (or removing) the system should be fully trained in the technique and should provide full counselling reinforced by the patient information leaflet.*

The cautions, contra-indications, and side-effects of oral progestogen-only contraceptives apply to parenteral progestogen-only contraceptives, except that

7 Obstetrics, gynaecology, and urinary-tract disorders

parenteral preparations reliably inhibit ovulation and therefore protect against ectopic pregnancy and functional ovarian cysts.

Interactions Effectiveness of parenteral progestogen-only contraceptives is not affected by antibacterials that do not induce liver enzymes. However, effectiveness of norethisterone and etonogestrel (but not medroxyprogesterone acetate) may be reduced by enzyme-inducing drugs; additional contraceptive precautions should be taken whilst taking the enzyme-inducing drug and for 4 weeks after stopping it *or* an alternative contraceptive method should be considered if *long-term* use of the enzyme-inducing drug is contemplated.

PARENTERAL PROGESTOGEN-ONLY CONTRACEPTIVES

Cautions see notes above and under preparations; possible risk of breast cancer, see oral progestogen-only contraceptives (section 7.3.2.1); history during pregnancy of pruritus or of deterioration of otosclerosis, disturbances of lipid metabolism; **interactions:** see notes above and Appendix 1 (progestogens)

Counselling Full counselling backed by *patient information leaflet* required before administration

Contra-indications see notes above; history of breast cancer but can be used after 5 years if no evidence of disease and non-hormonal contraceptive methods unacceptable

Hepatic impairment see Oral Progestogen-only Contraceptives, section 7.3.2.1

Pregnancy not known to be harmful; for *Implanon*® if pregnancy occurs remove implant

Breast-feeding progestogen-only contraceptives do not affect lactation; see also notes above

Side-effects see notes above; injection-site reactions

Cervical cancer Use of injectable progestogen-only contraceptives is associated with a small increased risk of cervical cancer; this increased risk may be similar to that seen with combined oral contraceptives, see p. 487. The risk of cervical cancer with other progestogen-only contraceptives is not yet known.

Licensed use consult product literature for the licensing status of individual preparations

Indication and dose

Contraception see also notes above and under preparations (roles vary according to preparation)

For dose see under preparations

◀Injectable preparations

Depo-Provera® (Pfizer) PoM

Injection (aqueous suspension), medroxyprogesterone acetate 150 mg/mL, net price 1-mL prefilled syringe = £6.01, 1-mL vial = £6.01. Counselling, see patient information leaflet

Dose

• By deep intramuscular injection

150 mg within first 5 days of cycle or within first 5 days after parturition (delay until 6 weeks after parturition if breast-feeding); for long-term contraception, repeated every 12 weeks (if interval greater than 12 weeks and 5 days, rule out pregnancy before next injection and advise patient to use additional contraceptive measures (e.g. barrier) for 14 days after the injection)

Noristerat® (Bayer Schering) PoM

Injection (oily), norethisterone enantate 200 mg/mL, net price 1-mL amp = £3.45. Counselling, see patient information leaflet

Dose

• By deep intramuscular injection

Given very slowly *into gluteal muscle*, short-term contraception, 200 mg within first 5 days of cycle or immediately after parturition (duration 8 weeks); may be repeated once after 8 weeks (withhold breast-feeding for neonates with severe or persistent jaundice requiring medical treatment)

◀Implants

Implanon® (Organon) PoM

Implant, containing etonogestrel 68 mg in each flexible rod, net price = £79.46. Counselling, see patient information leaflet

Dose

• By subdermal implantation

No previous hormonal contraceptive, 1 implant inserted during first 5 days of cycle; parturition or abortion in second trimester, 1 implant inserted between days 21–28 after delivery or abortion (if inserted after 28 days additional precautions necessary for next 7 days); abortion in first trimester, 1 implant inserted immediately; changing from another method of contraception, consult product literature; remove within 3 years of insertion

7.3.2.3 Intra-uterine progestogen-only device

The progestogen-only intra-uterine system, *Mirena*®, releases **levonorgestrel** directly into the uterine cavity. It is used as a contraceptive, for the treatment of primary menorrhagia and for the prevention of endometrial hyperplasia during oestrogen replacement therapy. This may therefore be a contraceptive method of choice for women who have excessively heavy menses.

The effects of the progestogen-only intra-uterine system are mainly local and hormonal including prevention of endometrial proliferation, thickening of cervical mucus, and suppression of ovulation in some women (in some cycles). In addition to the progestogenic activity, the intra-uterine system itself may contribute slightly to the contraceptive effect. Return of fertility after removal is rapid and appears to be complete.

Advantages of the progestogen-only intra-uterine system over copper intra-uterine devices are that there may be an improvement in any dysmenorrhoea and a reduction in blood loss; there is also evidence that the frequency of pelvic inflammatory disease may be reduced (particularly in the youngest age groups who are most at risk).

In primary menorrhagia, menstrual bleeding is reduced significantly within 3–6 months of inserting the progestogen-only intra-uterine system, probably because it prevents endometrial proliferation. Another treatment should be considered if menorrhagia does not improve within this time (section 6.4.1.2).

Cautions and contra-indications   Generally the cautions and contra-indications for the progestogen-only intra-uterine system are as for standard intra-uterine devices (section 7.3.4), but the risk of ectopic pregnancy is considerably smaller. Although the progestogen-only intra-uterine system produces little systemic progestogenic activity, it is usually avoided for 5 years after any evidence of breast cancer. However, the system can be considered for a woman in long-term remission from breast cancer who has menorrhagia and requires effective contraception. Since levonorgestrel is released close to the site of the main contraceptive action (on cervical mucus and endometrium) progestogenic side-effects and interactions are less likely; in particular, enzyme-inducing drugs are unlikely to significantly reduce the contraceptive effect of the progestogen-only intra-uterine system and additional contraceptive precautions are not required.

Side-effects   Initially, changes in the pattern and duration of menstrual bleeding (spotting or prolonged bleeding) are common; endometrial disorders should be ruled out before insertion and the patient should be fully counselled (and provided with a patient information leaflet). Improvement in progestogenic side-effects, such as mastalgia and mood changes, and in the bleeding pattern usually occurs a few months after insertion and bleeding may often become very light or absent. Functional ovarian cysts (usually asymptomatic) can occur and usually resolve spontaneously (ultrasound monitoring recommended).

INTRA-UTERINE PROGESTOGEN-ONLY SYSTEM

Cautions see notes above; advanced uterine atrophy; not suitable for emergency contraception; **interactions:** see notes above and Appendix 1 (progestogens)

Contra-indications see notes above

Hepatic impairment see Oral Progestogen-only Contraceptives, section 7.3.2.1

Pregnancy avoid; if pregnancy occurs remove system

Breast-feeding progestogen-only contraceptives do not affect lactation

Side-effects see notes above; also abdominal pain; peripheral oedema; nervousness; salpingitis and pelvic inflammatory disease; pelvic pain, back pain; *rarely* hirsutism, hair loss, pruritus, migraine, rash

Licensed use not licensed for use in women under 18 years

Indication and dose

See under preparation

Mirena® (Bayer Schering) [PoM]
Intra-uterine system, T-shaped plastic frame (impregnated with barium sulphate and with threads attached to base) with polydimethylsiloxane reservoir releasing levonorgestrel 20 micrograms/24 hours, net price = £87.32. Counselling, see patient information leaflet

Dose

Contraception and menorrhagia
Insert into uterine cavity within 7 days of onset of menstruation, or anytime if replacement, or anytime if reasonably certain the women is not pregnant and there is no risk of conception (additional precautions (e.g barrier methods) necessary for next 7 days), or immediately after first-trimester termination by curettage; postpartum insertions should be delayed until at least 4 weeks after delivery; effective for 5 years

Prevention of endometrial hyperplasia during oestrogen replacement therapy
Insert during last days of menstruation or withdrawal bleeding or anytime if amenorrhoeic; effective for 4 years

---

7.3.3 Spermicidal contraceptives

Spermicidal contraceptives are useful additional safeguards but do **not** give adequate protection if used alone unless fertility is already significantly diminished. They have two components: a spermicide and a vehicle which itself may have some inhibiting effect on sperm activity. They are suitable for use with barrier methods, such as diaphragms or caps; however spermicidal contraceptives are not generally recommended for use with condoms, as there is no evidence of any additional protection compared with non-spermicidal lubricants.

Spermicidal contraceptives are not suitable for use in those with or at high risk of sexually transmitted diseases (including HIV); high frequency use of the spermi-

7 Obstetrics, gynaecology, and urinary-tract disorders

cide nonoxinol '9' has been associated with genital lesions, which may increase the risk of acquiring these infections.

> Products such as petroleum jelly (*Vaseline*®), baby oil and oil-based vaginal and rectal preparations are likely to damage condoms and contraceptive diaphragms made from latex rubber, and may render them less effective as a barrier method of contraception and as a protection from sexually transmitted diseases (including HIV).

Gygel® (Marlborough)
Gel, nonoxinol '9' 2%, net price 30 g = £4.25
Excipients include hydroxybenzoates (parabens), propylene glycol, sorbic acid

Condoms No evidence of harm to latex condoms and diaphragms
Breast-feeding present in milk in *animal* studies

7.3.4 Contraceptive devices

Intra-uterine devices

The intra-uterine device (IUD) is a suitable contraceptive for women of all ages irrespective of parity; however, it is less appropriate for those with an increased risk of pelvic inflammatory disease e.g. women under 25 years (see below). The most effective intra-uterine devices have at least 380 mm^2 of copper and have banded copper on the arms.

Smaller devices have been introduced to minimise side-effects; these consist of a plastic carrier wound with copper wire or fitted with copper bands; some also have a central core of silver to prevent fragmentation of the copper.

A frameless, copper-bearing intra-uterine device (*GyneFix*®) is also available. It consists of a knotted, polypropylene thread with 6 copper sleeves; the device is anchored in the uterus by inserting the knot into the uterine fundus. The intra-uterine devices *Multiload*® *Cu250* and *Multiload*® *Cu250 Short* (Organon) have been discontinued, but some women may have the devices in place until 2011.

The timing and technique of fitting an intra-uterine device are critical for its subsequent performance. *The healthcare professional inserting (or removing) the device should be fully trained in the technique and should provide full counselling, backed, where available, by the patient information leaflet.* Devices should not be fitted during the heavy days of the period; they are best fitted after the end of menstruation and before the calculated time of implantation. The main excess risk of infection occurs in the first 20 days after insertion and is believed to be related to existing carriage of a sexually transmitted disease. Women under 25 years are at a higher risk of sexually transmitted diseases, and pre-insertion screening (for chlamydia, and depending on sexual history and local prevalence of disease, *Neisseria gonorrhoeae*) should be performed. If results are unavailable at the time of fitting an intra-uterine device for emergency contraception, appropriate prophylactic antibacterial cover should be given. The woman should be advised to attend *as an emergency* if she experiences sustained pain during the next 20 days.

An intra-uterine device should not be removed in mid-cycle unless an additional contraceptive was used for the previous 7 days. If removal is essential post-coital contraception should be considered.

If an intra-uterine device fails and the woman wishes to continue to full-term the device should be removed in the first trimester if possible.

INTRA-UTERINE CONTRACEPTIVE DEVICES

Cautions see notes above; also anaemia, menorrhagia (progestogen intra-uterine system might be preferable, section 7.3.2.3), endometriosis, severe primary dysmenorrhoea, history of pelvic inflammatory disease, diabetes, fertility problems, nulliparity and young age, severely scarred uterus (including after endometrial resection) or severe cervical stenosis; drug- or disease-induced immunosuppression (risk of infection—avoid if marked immunosuppression); epilepsy (risk of seizure at time of insertion);

increased risk of expulsion if inserted before uterine involution; gynaecological examination before insertion, 6–8 weeks after then annually but counsel women to see doctor promptly in case of significant symptoms, especially pain; anticoagulant therapy (avoid if possible)

Contra-indications severe anaemia, recent sexually transmitted infection (if not fully investigated and treated), unexplained uterine bleeding, distorted or small uterine cavity, genital malignancy, active trophoblastic disease (until return to nor-

◻ **INTRA-UTERINE CONTRACEPTIVE DEVICES** (*continued*)

mal of urine- and plasma-gonadotrophin concentration), pelvic inflammatory disease, established or marked immunosuppression; *copper devices:* copper allergy, Wilson's disease, medical diathermy

Pregnancy remove device; if pregnancy occurs, increased likelihood that it may be ectopic

Breast-feeding not known to be harmful

Side-effects uterine or cervical perforation, displacement, expulsion; pelvic infection may be exacerbated, menorrhagia, dysmenorrhoea, allergy; *on insertion:* pain (alleviated by NSAID such as ibuprofen 30 minutes before insertion) and bleeding, occasionally epileptic seizure and vasovagal attack

Indication and dose

See notes above

Cu-Safe® T300 (Williams) ⃞
Intra-uterine device, copper wire, wound on vertical stem of T-shaped plastic carrier, surface area approx. 300 mm², impregnated with barium sulphate for radio-opacity, monofilament thread attached to base of vertical stem; preloaded in inserter, net price = £9.11

For uterine length over 5 cm; replacement every 5 years (see notes above)

Flexi-T 300® (Durbin)
Intra-uterine device, copper wire, wound on vertical stem of T-shaped plastic carrier, surface area approx. 300 mm², impregnated with barium sulphate for radio-opacity, monofilament thread attached to base of vertical stem; preloaded in inserter, net price = £9.47

For uterine length over 5 cm; replacement every 5 years (see also notes above)

Flexi-T® + 380 (Durbin)
Intra-uterine device, copper wire, wound on vertical stem of T-shaped plastic carrier with copper sleeve on each arm, total surface area approx. 380 mm², impregnated with barium sulphate for radio-opacity, monofilament thread attached to base of vertical stem; preloaded in inserter, net price = £10.06

For uterine length over 6 cm; replacement every 5 years (see also notes above)

GyneFix® (Williams)
Intra-uterine device, 6 copper sleeves with surface area of 330 mm² on polypropylene thread, net price = £26.64
Suitable for all uterine sizes; replacement every 5 years

Load® 375 (Durbin)
Intra-uterine device, copper wire, wound on vertical stem of U-shaped plastic carrier, surface area approx. 375 mm², impregnated with barium sulphate for radio-opacity, monofilament thread attached to base of vertical stem; preloaded in inserter, net price = £8.52

For uterine length over 7 cm; replacement every 5 years (see also notes above)

Mini TT 380® Slimline (Durbin)
Intra-uterine device, copper wire, wound on vertical stem of T-shaped plastic carrier with copper sleeves fitted flush on to distal portion of each horizontal arm, total surface area approx. 380 mm², impregnated with barium sulphate for radio-opacity, thread attached to base of vertical stem; easy-loading system, no capsule, net price = £12.46

For minimum uterine length 5 cm; replacement every 5 years (see also notes above)

Multiload® Cu375 (Organon)
Intra-uterine device, as *Load® 375*, with copper surface area approx. 375 mm² and vertical stem length 3.5 cm, net price = £9.24

For uterine length 6–9 cm; replacement every 5 years (see also notes above)

Multi-Safe® 375 (Williams)
Intra-uterine device, copper wire, wound on vertical stem of U-shaped plastic carrier, surface area approx. 375 mm², impregnated with barium sulphate for radio-opacity, monofilament thread attached to base of vertical stem; preloaded in inserter, net price = £8.80

For uterine length 6–9 cm; replacement every 5 years (see also notes above)

MultiSafe® 375 Short Stem (Williams) ⃞
Intra-uterine device, copper wire, wound on vertical stem of U-shaped plastic carrier, surface area approx. 375 mm², impregnated with barium sulphate for radio-opacity, monofilament thread attached to base of vertical stem; preloaded in inserter, net price = £8.80

For uterine length 5–7 cm; replacement every 5 years (see also notes above)

Neo-Safe® T380 (Williams)
Intra-uterine device, copper wire, wound on vertical stem of T-shaped plastic carrier, surface area approx. 380 mm², impregnated with barium sulphate for radio-opacity, threads attached to base of vertical stem, net price = £13.08

For uterine length 6.5–9 cm; replacement every 5 years (see also notes above)

Nova-T® 380 (Bayer Schering)
Intra-uterine device, copper wire with silver core, wound on vertical stem of T-shaped plastic carrier, surface area approx. 380 mm², impregnated with barium sulphate for radio-opacity, threads attached to base of vertical stem, net price = £12.97

For uterine length 6.5–9 cm; replacement every 5 years (see also notes above)

T-Safe® 380A Quickload (Williams)
Intra-uterine device, copper wire, wound on vertical stem of T-shaped plastic carrier with copper collar on the distal portion of each arm, total surface area approx. 380 mm², impregnated with barium sulphate for radio-opacity, threads attached to base of vertical stem, net price = £10.29; available with a capsule loading device (*T-Safe® CU 380A* ⃞), net price £10.29

For uterine length 6.5–9 cm; replacement every 10 years (see also notes above)

TT 380® Slimline (Durbin)
Intra-uterine device, copper wire, wound on vertical stem of T-shaped plastic carrier, with copper sleeves fitted flush on to distal portion of each horizontal arm, total surface area approx. 380 mm², impregnated with barium sulphate for radio-opacity, thread attached to base of vertical stem; easy-loading system, no capsule, net price = £12.46

For uterine length 6.5–9 cm; replacement every 10 years (see also notes above)

UT 380 Short® (Durbin)
Intra-uterine device, copper wire, wound on vertical stem of T-shaped plastic carrier, surface area approx. 380 mm², impregnated with barium sulphate for radio-opacity, thread attached to base of vertical stem; net price = £11.22

For uterine length 5–7 cm; replacement every 5 years (see also notes above)

UT 380 Standard® (Durbin)
Intra-uterine device, copper wire, wound on vertical stem of T-shaped plastic carrier, surface area approx. 380 mm², impregnated with barium sulphate for radio-opacity, thread attached to base of vertical stem; net price = £11.22

For uterine length 6.5–9 cm; replacement every 5 years (see also notes above)

7

Obstetrics, gynaecology, and urinary-tract disorders

Obstetrics, gynaecology, and urinary-tract disorders

7

Other contraceptive devices

▲Rubber contraceptive caps
Type A Contraceptive Pessary
Opaque rubber, sizes 1 (50 mm), 2 (55 mm), 3 (60 mm), 4 (65 mm), 5 (75 mm), net price = £6.85

Type B Contraceptive Pessary
Opaque rubber, sizes 22 to 31 mm (rising in steps of 3 mm), net price = £8.46

Type C Contraceptive Pessary
Opaque rubber, sizes 1 to 3 (42, 48, and 54 mm), net price = £7.26

▲Silicone contraceptive caps
Silicone Contraceptive Pessary
Silicone, sizes 22, 26, and 30 mm, net price = £15.00
Brands include *FemCap*®

▲Rubber contraceptive diaphragms
Type A Diaphragm with Flat Metal Spring
Transparent rubber with flat metal spring, sizes 55–95 mm (rising in steps of 5 mm), net price = £5.78
Brands include *Reflexions*®

Type B Diaphragm with Coiled Metal Spring
Opaque rubber with coiled metal spring, sizes 60–100 mm (rising in steps of 5 mm), net price = £6.79

Type C Arcing Spring Diaphragm
Opaque rubber with arcing spring, sizes 60–95 mm (rising in steps of 5 mm), net price = £7.72

▲Silicone contraceptive diaphragms
Type B Diaphragm with Coiled Metal Spring
Silicone with coiled metal spring, sizes 60–90 mm (rising in steps of 5 mm), net price = £8.35
Brands include *Milex Omniflex*®

Type C Arching Spring diaphragm
Silicone with arcing spring, sizes 60–90 mm (rising in steps of 5 mm), net price = £8.35
Brands include *Milex Arcing Style*®, *Ortho All-Flex*®

7.3.5 Emergency contraception

Hormonal methods

Hormonal emergency contraceptives include **levonorgestrel** and **ulipristal**; either drug should be taken as soon as possible after unprotected intercourse to increase efficacy.

Levonorgestrel is effective if taken within 72 hours (3 days) of unprotected intercourse and may also be used between 72 and 120 hours after unprotected intercourse [unlicensed use], but efficacy decreases with time. Ulipristal, a progesterone receptor modulator, is effective if taken within 120 hours (5 days) of unprotected intercourse.

Levonorgestrel is less effective than insertion of an intra-uterine device (see below). Ulipristal is as effective as levonorgestrel but it's efficacy compared to an intra-uterine device is not yet known.

If vomiting occurs within 2 hours of taking levonorgestrel or within 3 hours of taking ulipristal, a replacement dose should be given. If an anti-emetic is required domperidone is preferred.

When prescribing hormonal emergency contraception the doctor should explain:

*   that the next period may be early or late;
*   that a barrier method of contraception needs to be used until the next period;
*   the need to return promptly if any lower abdominal pain occurs because this could signify an ectopic pregnancy (and also in 3 to 4 weeks if the subsequent menstrual bleed is abnormally light, heavy or brief, or is absent, or if she is otherwise concerned).

Interactions The effectiveness of levonorgestrel, and possibly ulipristal is reduced in women taking enzyme-inducing drugs (and possibly for 4 weeks after stopping); a copper intra-uterine device can be offered instead or the dose of levonorgestrel should be increased to a total of 3 mg taken as a single dose [unlicensed dose—advise women accordingly]. There is no need to increase the dose for emergency contraception if the patient is taking antibacterials that are not enzyme inducers.

LEVONORGESTREL

Cautions see notes above; past ectopic pregnancy; severe malabsorption syndromes; active trophoblastic disease (until return to normal of urine- and plasma-gonadotrophin concentration); **interactions:** see notes above and Appendix 1 (progestogens)

Contra-indications acute porphyria (section 9.8.2)

Pregnancy not known to be harmful

Breast-feeding progestogen-only contraceptives do not affect lactation

◻ **LEVONORGESTREL (continued)**

Side-effects menstrual irregularities (see also notes above), nausea, low abdominal pain, fatigue, headache, dizziness, breast tenderness, vomiting

Licensed use consult product literature

Indication and dose

> **Emergency contraception**
> - **By mouth**
>   1.5 mg as a single dose as soon as possible after coitus (preferably within 12 hours but no later than after 72 hours)

[1] **Levonelle® One Step** (Bayer Schering)
Tablets, levonorgestrel 1.5 mg, net price 1-tab pack = £13.83

1. Can be sold to women over 16 years; when supplying emergency contraception to the public, pharmacists should refer to guidance issued by the Royal Pharmaceutical Society of Great Britain

Levonelle® 1500 (Bayer Schering) [PoM]
Tablets, levonorgestrel 1.5 mg, net price 1-tab pack = £5.37

▮ **ULIPRISTAL ACETATE**

Cautions see notes above; uncontrolled severe asthma; effectiveness of combined hormonal and progestogen-only contraceptives may be reduced—additional precautions (barrier methods) required; repeated use within a menstrual cycle; **interactions:** see notes above and Appendix 1 (ulipristal)

Hepatic impairment manufacturer advises avoid in severe impairment—no information available

Pregnancy limited information available

Breast-feeding manufacturer advises avoid for at least 36 hours—no information available

Side-effects gastro-intestinal disturbances (including nausea, vomiting, diarrhoea, and abdominal pain); dizziness, fatigue, headache; menstrual irregularities (see notes above); back pain, muscle spasms; *less commonly* tremor, hot flushes, uterine spasm, breast tenderness, dry mouth, blurred vision, pruritus, and rash

Licensed use not licensed in women under 18 years

Indication and dose

> **Emergency contraception**
> - **By mouth**
>   30 mg as a single dose as soon as possible after coitus, but no later than after 120 hours

EllaOne® (HRA Pharma) ▼ [PoM]
Tablets, ulipristal acetate 30 mg, net price 1-tab pack = £16.95

▮ **Intra-uterine device**

Insertion of an intra-uterine device is more effective than oral levonorgestrel for emergency contraception, see also notes above. A copper intra-uterine contraceptive device (section 7.3.4) can be inserted up to 120 hours (5 days) after unprotected intercourse; sexually transmitted diseases should be tested for and insertion of the device should usually be covered by antibacterial prophylaxis (e.g. azithromycin 1 g as a single dose). If intercourse has occurred more than 5 days previously, the device can still be inserted up to 5 days after the earliest likely calculated ovulation (i.e. within the minimum period before implantation), regardless of the number of episodes of unprotected intercourse earlier in the cycle.

7.4 Drugs for genito-urinary disorders

- **7.4.1** Drugs for urinary retention
- **7.4.2** Drugs for urinary frequency, enuresis, and incontinence
- **7.4.3** Drugs used in urological pain
- **7.4.4** Bladder instillations and urological surgery
- **7.4.5** Drugs for erectile dysfunction

For drugs used in the treatment of urinary-tract infections see section 5.1.13.

7.4.1 Drugs for urinary retention

Acute retention is painful and is treated by catheterisation.

Chronic retention is painless and often long-standing. Clean intermittent catheterisation may be considered. After the cause has been established and treated, drugs may be required to increase detrusor muscle tone.

Alpha-blockers such as doxazosin and tamsulosin can be used in some cases of dysfunctional voiding.

▮ **Alpha-blockers**

The selective alpha-blockers **doxazosin** and **tamsulosin** can be used to improve bladder emptying in children with dysfunctional voiding where the post-void residual urine volume is significant; treatment should be under specialist advice only. Alpha-blockers can reduce blood pressure rapidly after the first dose and should be introduced with caution.

DOXAZOSIN

Cautions see under Doxazosin (section 2.5.4)

Contra-indications see under Doxazosin (section 2.5.4)

Hepatic impairment see under Doxazosin (section 2.5.4)

Pregnancy see under Doxazosin (section 2.5.4)

Breast-feeding see under Doxazosin (section 2.5.4)

Side-effects see under Doxazosin (section 2.5.4)

Licensed use not licensed for use in children

Indication and dose

Dysfunctional voiding (see notes above)

• By mouth

Child 4–12 years initially 0.5 mg daily increased at monthly intervals according to response; maximum 2 mg daily

Child 12–18 years initially 1 mg daily, dose may be doubled at intervals of 1 month according to response; usual maintenance 2–4 mg daily; max. 8 mg daily

Hypertension section 2.5.4

◢Preparations
Section 2.5.4

TAMSULOSIN HYDROCHLORIDE

Cautions care with initial dose (postural hypotension); cataract surgery (risk of intra-operative floppy iris syndrome); **interactions:** Appendix 1 (alpha-blockers)

Driving May affect performance of skilled tasks e.g. driving

Contra-indications history of postural hypotension

Hepatic impairment avoid in severe impairment

Renal impairment use with caution if estimated glomerular filtration rate less than 10 mL/minute/1.73 m^2

Side-effects dizziness, headache, asthenia; abnormal ejaculation; *less commonly* nausea, vomiting, constipation, diarrhoea, palpitation, postural hypotension, syncope, rhinitis, rash, pruritus, and urticaria; *very rarely* angioedema and priapism; also drowsiness, blurred vision, dry mouth, and oedema; *also reported* intra-operative floppy iris syndrome

Licensed use not licensed for use in children

Indication and dose

Dysfunctional voiding (see notes above)

• By mouth

Child 12–18 years 400 micrograms once daily

Tamsulosin hydrochloride (Non-proprietary) ℗ₒ𝗠
Capsules, m/r, tamsulosin hydrochloride 400 micrograms, net price 30-cap pack = £4.55. Label: 25, counselling, driving
Brands include *Bazetham® MR, Contiflo® XL, Diffundox® XL, Stronazon® MR, Tabphyn® MR*

Flomaxtra® XL (Astellas) ℗ₒ𝗠
Tablets, m/r, tamsulosin hydrochloride 400 micrograms, net price 30-tab pack = £11.00. Label: 25, counselling, driving

7.4.2 Drugs for urinary frequency, enuresis, and incontinence

Urinary incontinence

Involuntary detrusor contractions cause urgency and urge incontinence, usually with frequency and nocturia. Antimuscarinic drugs reduce these contractions and increase bladder capacity; **oxybutynin** also has a direct relaxant effect on urinary smooth muscle. Oxybutynin can be considered first for children under 12 years. Side-effects limit the use of oxybutynin, but they may be reduced by starting at a lower dose and then slowly titrating upwards; alternatively oxybutynin can be given by intravesicular instillation. **Tolterodine** is also effective for urinary incontinence; it can be considered for children over 12 years, or for younger children who have failed to respond to oxybutynin. Modified-release preparations of oxybutynin and tolterodine are available; they may have fewer side-effects. Antimuscarinic treatment should be reviewed soon after it is commenced, and then at regular intervals; a response generally occurs within 6 months but occasionally may take longer. Children with nocturnal enuresis may require specific additional measures if night-time symptoms also need to be controlled (see p. 502).

Cautions   Antimuscarinic drugs should be used with caution in autonomic neuropathy. Antimuscarinics can worsen hyperthyroidism, congestive heart failure, arrhythmias, and tachycardia. For **interactions**, see Appendix 1 (antimuscarinics).

Contra-indications   Antimuscarinic drugs should be avoided in myasthenia gravis, significant bladder outflow obstruction or urinary retention, severe ulcerative colitis, toxic megacolon, and in gastro-intestinal obstruction or intestinal atony.

Side-effects   Side-effects of antimuscarinic drugs include dry mouth, gastro-intestinal disturbances including constipation, blurred vision, dry eyes, drowsiness, difficulty in micturition (less commonly urinary retention), palpitation, and skin reactions (including dry skin, rash, and photosensitivity); also headache, diarrhoea, angioedema, arrhythmias, and tachycardia. Central nervous system stimulation, such as restlessness, disorientation, hallucination, and convulsions may occur. Antimuscarinic drugs may reduce sweating leading to heat sensations and fainting in hot environments or in patients with fever.

OXYBUTYNIN HYDROCHLORIDE

Cautions   see notes above; acute porphyria (section 9.8.2)

Contra-indications   see notes above

Hepatic impairment   manufacturer advises caution

Renal impairment   manufacturer advises caution

Pregnancy   manufacturer advises avoid unless essential—toxicity in *animal* studies

Breast-feeding   manufacturer advises avoid—present in milk in *animal* studies

Side-effects   see notes above; also dizziness; *less commonly* anorexia, facial flushing; *rarely* night terrors

Licensed use   not licensed for use in children under 5 years; intravesical instillation not licensed for use in children

Indication and dose

> Urinary frequency, urgency and incontinence, neurogenic bladder instability
> - By mouth
>
>   **Child 2–5 years** 1.25–2.5 mg 2–3 times daily;
>
>   **Child 5–12 years** 2.5–3 mg twice daily, increased to 5 mg 2–3 times daily
>
>   **Child 12–18 years** 5 mg 2–3 times daily, increased if necessary to max. 5 mg 4 times daily
>
> - By intravesical instillation
>
>   **Child 2–18 years** 5 mg 2–3 times daily

> Nocturnal enuresis associated with overactive bladder
> - By mouth
>
>   **Child 7–18 years** 2.5–3 mg twice daily increased to 5 mg 2–3 times daily (last dose before bedtime)

Oxybutynin Hydrochloride (Non-proprietary) ᴘᴏᴍ
Tablets, oxybutynin hydrochloride 2.5 mg, net price 56-tab pack = £7.36; 3 mg, 56-tab pack = £9.15; 5 mg, 56-tab pack = £5.89, 84-tab pack = £12.82. Label: 3

Intravesical instillation, oxybutynin (as hydrochloride) 5 mg/30 mL.
Available from 'special-order' manufacturers or specialist importing companies, see p. 957

Cystrin® (Sanofi-Aventis) ᴘᴏᴍ
Tablets, oxybutynin hydrochloride 3 mg, net price 56-tab pack = £9.15; 5 mg (scored), 84-tab pack = £21.99. Label: 3

Ditropan® (Sanofi-Aventis) ᴘᴏᴍ
Tablets, both blue, scored, oxybutynin hydrochloride 2.5 mg, net price 84-tab pack = £6.59; 5 mg, 84-tab pack = £12.82. Label: 3

Elixir, oxybutynin hydrochloride 2.5 mg/5 mL, net price 150-mL pack = £6.88. Label: 3

◢ Modified release

Lyrinel® XL (Janssen-Cilag) ᴘᴏᴍ
Tablets, m/r, oxybutynin hydrochloride 5 mg (yellow), net price 30-tab pack = £11.03; 10 mg (pink), 30-tab pack = £22.05. Label: 3, 25

Dose
> Neurogenic bladder instability
> - By mouth
>
>   **Child 6–18 years** initially 5 mg once daily adjusted according to response in steps of 5 mg at weekly intervals; max. 15 mg once daily

Note Children taking immediate-release oxybutynin may be transferred to the nearest equivalent daily dose of *Lyrinel® XL*

TOLTERODINE TARTRATE

Cautions   see notes above; history of QT-interval prolongation; concomitant use with other drugs known to prolong QT interval

Contra-indications   see notes above

Hepatic impairment   reduce dose; avoid *Detrusitol® XL*

Renal impairment   reduce dose if estimated glomerular filtration rate less than 30 mL/minute/1.73 m²; avoid *Detrusitol® XL* if estimated glomerular filtration rate less than 30 mL/minute/1.73 m²

Pregnancy   manufacturer advises avoid—toxicity in *animal* studies

7

Obstetrics, gynaecology, and urinary-tract disorders

◻ **TOLTERODINE TARTRATE** (*continued*)

Breast-feeding manufacturer advises avoid—no information available

Side-effects see notes above; also chest pain, peripheral oedema; sinusitis; bronchitis; paraesthesia, fatigue, vertigo, weight gain; flushing also reported

Licensed use not licensed for use in children

Indication and dose

Urinary frequency, urgency, incontinence
• By mouth
Child 2–18 years 1 mg once daily, increased according to response; max. 2 mg twice daily

Nocturnal enuresis associated with overactive bladder
• By mouth
Child 7–18 years 1 mg once daily at bedtime, increased according to response; max. 2 mg twice daily

Detrusitol® (Pharmacia) (PoM)
Tablets, f/c, tolterodine tartrate 1 mg, net price 56-tab pack = £29.03; 2 mg, 56-tab pack = £30.56

◀ **Modified release**
Detrusitol® XL (Pharmacia) (PoM)
Capsules, blue, m/r, tolterodine tartrate 4 mg, net price 28-cap pack = £25.78. Label: 25
Note Children stabilised on immediate-release tolteridone 2 mg twice daily may be transferred to *Detrusitol® XL* 4 mg once daily

Nocturnal enuresis

Nocturnal enuresis is common in young children, but persists in as many as 5% by 10 years of age. Treatment is not appropriate in children under 5 years and it is usually not needed in those aged under 7 years and in cases where the child and parents are not anxious about the bedwetting; however, children over 10 years usually require prompt treatment. An **enuresis alarm** should be first-line treatment for well-motivated, well supported children aged over 7 years because alarms have a lower relapse rate than drug treatment when discontinued. Use of an alarm can be combined with drug therapy if either method alone is unsuccessful.

Drug therapy is not usually appropriate for children under 7 years of age; it can be used when alternative measures have failed, preferably on a short-term basis, for example to cover periods away from home, or if the child and family are anxious about the condition.

Desmopressin (section 6.5.2), an analogue of vasopressin, is used for nocturnal enuresis; it is given by oral or by sublingual administration. Particular care is needed to avoid fluid overload and treatment should not be continued for longer than 3 months without interrupting treatment for one week for full reassessment. When stopping treatment with desmopressin gradual withdrawal may be considered. Desmopressin should not be given intranasally for nocturnal enuresis due to an increased incidence of side-effects.

Tricyclic antidepressants (section 4.3.1) such as **imipramine**, and rarely **amitriptyline** and **nortriptyline**, are used but behavioural disturbances can occur and relapse is common after withdrawal. Treatment should not normally exceed 3 months unless a full physical examination is made and the child is fully reassessed; toxicity following overdosage with tricyclics is of particular concern.

Nocturnal enuresis associated with daytime symptoms (overactive bladder) can be managed by antimuscarinic drugs (see Urinary incontinence, p. 500), with the addition of desmopressin if necessary.

7.4.3 Drugs used in urological pain

Lidocaine (lignocaine) gel is a useful topical application in *urethral pain* or to relieve the discomfort of catheterisation (section 15.2).

Alkalinisation of urine

Alkalinisation of urine can be undertaken with **potassium citrate**. The alkalinising action may relieve the discomfort of *cystitis* caused by lower urinary tract infections.

POTASSIUM CITRATE

Cautions cardiac disease; **interactions**: Appendix 1 (potassium salts)

Renal impairment close monitoring required—high risk of hyperkalaemia; avoid in severe impairment

▱ **POTASSIUM CITRATE** (*continued*)

Side-effects hyperkalaemia on prolonged high dosage, mild diuresis

Indication and dose

> Relief of discomfort in mild urinary-tract infections, alkalinisation of urine for dose see preparations below

Potassium Citrate Mixture BP
(Potassium Citrate Oral Solution)
Oral solution, potassium citrate 30%, citric acid monohydrate 5% in a suitable vehicle with a lemon flavour. Extemporaneous preparations should be recently prepared according to the following for-

mula: potassium citrate 3 g, citric acid monohydrate 500 mg, syrup 2.5 mL, quillaia tincture 0.1 mL, lemon spirit 0.05 mL, double-strength chloroform water 3 mL, water to 10 mL. Contains about 28 mmol K^+/10 mL. Label: 27

Dose

> • By mouth
>
> **Child 1–6 years** 5 mL 3 times daily well diluted with water
>
> **Child 6–18 years** 10 mL 3 times daily well diluted with water

Note Proprietary brands of potassium citrate are on sale to the public for the relief of discomfort in mild urinary-tract infections

7.4.4 Bladder instillations and urological surgery

Bladder infection   Various solutions are available as irrigations or washouts.

Aqueous **chlorhexidine** (section 13.11.2) can be used in the management of common infections of the bladder but it is ineffective against most *Pseudomonas* spp. Solutions containing chlorhexidine 1 in 5000 (0.02%) are used, but they may irritate the mucosa and cause burning and haematuria (in which case they should be discontinued); sterile **sodium chloride solution 0.9%** (physiological saline) is usually adequate and is preferred as a mechanical irrigant.

Dissolution of blood clots   Clot retention is usually treated by irrigation with sterile **sodium chloride solution 0.9%** but sterile **sodium citrate solution for bladder irrigation 3%** may also be helpful.

Maintenance of indwelling urinary catheters

The deposition which occurs in catheterised patients is usually chiefly composed of phosphate and to minimise this the catheter (if latex) should be changed at least as often as every 6 weeks. If the catheter is to be left for longer periods a silicone catheter should be used together with the appropriate use of catheter maintenance solutions. Repeated blockage usually indicates that the catheter needs to be changed.

CATHETER PATENCY SOLUTIONS

Chlorhexidine 0.02%
Brands include *Uro-Tainer Chlorhexidine*®, 100-mL sachet = £2.60

Sodium chloride 0.9%
Brands include *OptiFlo S*®, 50- and 100-mL sachets = £3.20; *Uriflex S*®, 100-mL sachet = £2.40; *Uriflex SP*®, with integral drug additive port, 100-mL sachet = £2.40; *Uro-Tainer Sodium Chloride*®, 50- and 100-mL sachets = £3.25; *Uro-Tainer M*®, with integral drug additive port, 50- and 100-mL sachets = £2.90

Solution G
Citric acid 3.23%, magnesium oxide 0.38%, sodium bicarbonate 0.7%, disodium edetate 0.01%. Brands include *OptiFlo G*®, 50- and 100-mL sachets = £3.40; *Uriflex G*®, 100-mL sachet = £2.40; *Uro-Tainer*® Twin Suby G, 2 × 30-mL = £4.46

Solution R
Citric acid 6%, gluconolactone 0.6%, magnesium carbonate 2.8%, disodium edetate 0.01%. Brands include *OptiFlo R*®, 50- and 100-mL sachets = £3.40; *Uriflex R*®, 100-mL sachet = £2.40; *Uro-Tainer*® Twin Solutio R, 2 × 30-mL = £4.46

7.4.5 Drugs for erectile dysfunction

This section is not included in *BNF for Children*. Adolescents presenting with erectile dysfunction should be referred to a specialist.

7 Obstetrics, gynaecology, and urinary-tract disorders

8 Malignant disease and immunosuppression

8.1 Cytotoxic drugs

8.1.1 Alkylating drugs
8.1.2 Cytotoxic antibiotics
8.1.3 Antimetabolites
8.1.4 Vinca alkaloids and etoposide
8.1.5 Other antineoplastic drugs

The management of childhood cancer is complex and is generally confined to specialist regional centres, and some associated shared-care units, affiliated to the Children's Cancer and Leukaemia Group (CCLG). The Group, together with other national and international organisations, develops and co-ordinates treatment protocols.

Cytotoxic drugs have both anti-cancer activity and the potential for damage to normal tissue. In children, chemotherapy is almost always started with curative intent, but may be continued as palliation if the disease is refractory.

Chemotherapy with a combination of two or more cytotoxic drugs aims to reduce the development of resistance and to improve cytotoxic effect. Treatment protocols generally incorporate a series of treatment courses at defined intervals with clear criteria for starting each course, such as adequate bone-marrow recovery and renal or cardiac function. The principal component of treatment for leukaemias in children is cytotoxic therapy, whereas solid tumours may be managed with surgery or radiotherapy in addition to chemotherapy.

> **Guidelines for handling cytotoxic drugs**
> - Trained personnel should reconstitute cytotoxics;
> - Reconstitution should be carried out in designated pharmacy areas;
> - Protective clothing (including gloves, gowns, and masks) should be worn;
> - The eyes should be protected and means of first aid should be specified;
> - Pregnant staff should avoid exposure to cytotoxic drugs (all females of child-bearing age should be informed of the reproductive hazard);
> - Use local procedures for dealing with spillages and safe disposal of waste material, including syringes, containers, and absorbent material;
> - Staff exposure to cytotoxic drugs should be monitored.

Only medical or nursing staff who have received appropriate training should administer parenteral cytotoxics. In most instances central venous access will be required for the intravenous administration of cytotoxics to children; care is required to avoid the risk of extravasation (see Side-effects of Cytotoxic Drugs and their Management).

> **Intrathecal chemotherapy**
> A Health Service Circular (HSC 2008/001) provides guidance on the introduction of safe practice in NHS Trusts where intrathecal chemotherapy is administered; written local guidance covering all aspects of national guidance should be available. Support for training programmes is also available.
> Copies, and further information may be obtained from:
> Department of Health
> PO Box 777
> London SE1 6XH
> Fax: 01623 724524
> www.dh.gov.uk

Safe system requirements for cytotoxic medicines:

- Cytotoxic drugs for the treatment of cancer should be given as part of a wider pathway of care that is co-ordinated by a multi-disciplinary team;
- Cytotoxic drugs should be prescribed, dispensed and administered only in the context of a written protocol or treatment plan;
- Injectable cytotoxic drugs should only be dispensed if they are prepared for administration;
- Oral cytotoxic medicines should be dispensed with clear directions for use.

> **Risks of incorrect dosing of oral anti-cancer medicines**
> The National Patient Safety Agency has advised (January 2008) that the prescribing and use of oral cytotoxic medicines should be carried out to the same standard as parenteral cytotoxic therapy. Standards to be followed to achieve this include:
> - non-specialists who prescribe or administer oral cytotoxic medication should have access to written protocols and treatment plans, including guidance on the monitoring and treatment of toxicity
> - staff dispensing oral cytotoxic medicines should confirm that the prescribed dose is appropriate for the patient. Patients and their carers should have written information that includes details of the intended oral anti-cancer regimen, the treatment plan, and arrangements for monitoring, taken from the original protocol from the initiating hospital. Staff dispensing oral cytotoxic medicines should also have access to this information, and to advice from an experienced cancer pharmacist in the initiating hospital

> **Doses**
> Doses of cytotoxic drugs are determined using a variety of different methods including age, body-surface area, or body-weight. Alternatively, doses may be fixed. Doses may be further adjusted following consideration of a patient's neutrophil count, renal and hepatic function, and history of previous adverse effects to the cytotoxic drug. Doses may also differ depending on whether a drug is used alone or in combination.
> Because of the complexity of dosage regimens in the treatment of malignant disease, dose statements have been omitted from many of the drug entries in this chapter.

Side-effects of cytotoxic drugs and their management

Side-effects common to most cytotoxic drugs are discussed below whilst side-effects characteristic of a particular drug or class of drugs (e.g. neurotoxicity with vinca alkaloids) are mentioned in the appropriate sections. Manufacturers' product literature, hospital-trust protocols, and treatment protocols should be consulted for full details of side-effects of individual drugs.

Side-effects of cytotoxic drugs often do not occur at the time of administration, but days or weeks later. It is therefore important that children, their carers, and healthcare professionals can identify symptoms that cause concern and can contact an expert for advice. Toxicities should be accurately recorded using a recognised scoring system such as the Common Toxicity Criteria for Adverse Events (CTCAE) developed by the National Cancer institute.

Extravasation of intravenous drugs A number of cytotoxic drugs will cause severe local tissue irritation and necrosis if leakage into the extravascular compartment occurs. For information on the prevention and management of extravasation injury, see section 10.3.

Gastro-intestinal effects Management of gastro-intestinal effects of cytotoxic drugs includes the use of antacids, H₂-receptor antagonists, and proton pump inhibitors to protect the gastric mucosa, laxatives to treat constipation, and enteral and parenteral nutritional support.

Oral mucositis Good oral hygiene keeps the mouth clean and moist and helps to prevent mucositis; prevention is more effective than treatment of the complication. Good oral hygiene measures for children over 6 months include brushing teeth with a soft small brush with fluoride toothpaste 2–3 times daily, and rinsing the mouth frequently. Daily fluoride supplements (section 9.5.3) can be used on the advice of the child's dental team. For children under 6 months or when it is not possible to brush teeth, carers should be instructed how to clean the mouth using an oral sponge moistened with water or with an antimicrobial solution such as diluted chlorhexidine. Mucositis related to chemotherapy can be extremely painful and may, in some circumstances, require opioid analgesia (section 4.7.2). Secondary infection with candida is frequent; treatment with a systemically absorbed antifungal, such as fluconazole (section 5.2), is effective.

Nausea and vomiting Nausea and vomiting cause considerable distress to many children who receive chemotherapy, and to a lesser extent abdominal radiotherapy, and may lead to refusal of further treatment; prophylaxis of nausea and vomiting is therefore extremely important. Symptoms may be acute (occurring within 24 hours of treatment), delayed (first occurring more than 24 hours after treatment), or anticipatory (occurring prior to subsequent doses). Delayed and anticipatory symptoms are more difficult to control than acute symptoms and require different management.

Susceptibility to nausea and vomiting may increase with repeated exposure to the cytotoxic drug.

Drugs may be divided according to their emetogenic potential and some examples are given below, but the symptoms vary according to the dose, to other drugs administered, and to the individual's susceptibility to emetogenic stimuli.

Mildly emetogenic treatment—fluorouracil, etoposide, low doses of methotrexate, the vinca alkaloids, and abdominal radiotherapy.

Moderately emetogenic treatment—carboplatin, doxorubicin, intermediate and low doses of cyclophosphamide, mitoxantrone (mitozantrone), and high doses of methotrexate.

Highly emetogenic treatment—cisplatin, dacarbazine, and high doses of alkylating drugs.

Anti-emetic drugs, when given regularly, help prevent or ameliorate emesis associated with chemotherapy in children.

Prevention of acute symptoms For patients at *low risk of emesis*, pretreatment with metoclopramide (or less commonly domperidone) continued for up to 24 hours after chemotherapy, is often effective (section 4.6); a 5HT₃ antagonist (section 4.6) may also be of benefit.

For patients at *high risk of emesis* or when other treatment is inadequate, a 5HT₃ antagonist (section 4.6) is often highly effective. The addition of dexamethasone and other anti-emetics may also be required.

Prevention of delayed symptoms Dexamethasone, given by mouth, is the drug of choice for preventing delayed symptoms; it is used alone or with metoclopramide. The 5HT₃ antagonists may have a role in preventing uncontrolled symptoms.

Prevention of anticipatory symptoms Good symptom control is the best way to prevent anticipatory symptoms. Lorazepam can be helpful for its amnesiac, sedative, and anxiolytic effects.

Bone-marrow suppression All cytotoxic drugs except vincristine and bleomycin cause bone-marrow depression. This commonly occurs 7 to 10 days after administration, but is delayed for certain drugs, such as melphalan. Peripheral blood counts must be checked before each treatment. The duration and severity of neutropenia can be reduced by the use of granulocyte-colony stimulating factors (section 9.1.6); their use should be reserved for children who have previously experienced severe neutropenia.

Infection in a child with neutropenia requires immediate broad-spectrum antibacterial treatment that covers all likely pathogens (Table 1, section 5.1). Appropriate bacteriological investigations should be conducted as soon as possible. All children should be investigated and treated under the supervision of an appropriate oncology or haematology specialist. Antifungal treatment (section 5.2) may be required in a child with prolonged neutropenia or fever lasting longer than 4–5 days. Chickenpox and measles can be particularly hazardous in immunocompromised children. Varicella–zoster immunoglobulin (section 14.5.2) is indicated if the child does not have immunity against varicella and has had close contact with infectious chickenpox or herpes zoster. Antiviral prophylaxis (section 5.3.2.1) can be considered in addition to varicella–zoster immunoglobulin or as an alternative if varicella–zoster immunoglobulin is inappropriate. If an immunocompromised child has come into close contact with an infectious individual with measles, normal immunoglobulin (section 14.5.1) should be given.

Alopecia Reversible hair loss is a common complication, although it varies in degree between drugs and individual patients.

Pregnancy and reproductive function Before using cytotoxic drugs during pregnancy consideration should be given to both the prognosis of the patient and the fetal risk. The rapidly dividing cells of the fetus are potentially susceptible to the effects of cytotoxic drugs. Although antimetabolites are thought to be the strongest teratogens, specific risk assessment of individual cytotoxics is not possible with the available data. All of the long-term effects of cytotoxic exposure are not fully known.

The use of cytotoxic drugs during the first trimester is associated with the greatest risk of harm to the fetus; spontaneous abortion and teratogenicity are possible. If at all possible cytotoxic drugs should be avoided before week 10 of pregnancy.

In the second and third trimesters the risk of teratogenicity is negligible, but growth and developmental effects are possible. In the third trimester early induction of delivery may be considered. If cytotoxic drugs are unavoidable in older girls with reproductive potential, contraceptive advice should be offered where appropriate. Regimens containing an alkylating drug carry the risk of causing permanent male sterility (but may not affect sexual potency).

Long-term and delayed toxicity Cytotoxic drugs may produce specific organ-related toxicity in children (e.g. cardiotoxicity with doxorubicin or nephrotoxicity with cisplatin and ifosfamide). Manifestations of such toxicity may not appear for several months or even years after cancer treatment. Careful follow-up of survivors of childhood cancer is therefore vital; national and local guidelines have been developed to facilitate this.

Thromboembolism Venous thromboembolism can be a complication of cancer itself, but chemotherapy increases the risk.

Tumour lysis syndrome Tumour lysis syndrome occurs secondary to spontaneous or treatment related rapid destruction of malignant cells. Patients at risk of tumour lysis syndrome include those with non-Hodgkin's lymphoma (especially if high grade and bulky disease), Burkitt's lymphoma, acute lymphoblastic leukaemia and acute myeloid leukaemia (particularly if high white blood cell counts or bulky disease), and occasionally those with solid tumours. Pre-existing hyperuricaemia, dehydration and renal impairment are also predisposing factors. Features, include hyperkalaemia, hyperuricaemia, and hyperphosphataemia with hypocalcaemia; renal damage and arrhythmias can follow. Early recognition of patients at risk, and initiation of prophylaxis or therapy for tumour lysis syndrome, is essential.

8 Malignant disease and immunosuppression

Drugs for cytotoxic-induced side-effects

Anthracycline-induced cardiotoxicity

The anthracycline cytotoxic drugs are associated with dose-related, cumulative, and potentially life-threatening cardiotoxic side-effects.

Dexrazoxane, an iron chelator, is licensed in adults for the prevention of chronic cumulative cardiotoxicity caused by doxorubicin or epirubicin treatment in advanced or metastatic cancer patients who have previously received anthracycline therapy. In practice, dexrazoxane is used for any patient receiving anthracycline therapy with evidence of subclinical cardiotoxicity thought to be secondary to anthracycline therapy, or for those children at risk of anthracycline-induced cardiotoxicity. Children receiving dexrazoxane should continue to be monitored for cardiac toxicity. The myelosuppresive effects of dexrazoxane may be additive to those of chemotherapy.

DEXRAZOXANE

Cautions see notes above; monitor full blood count

Hepatic impairment monitor liver function

Renal impairment use with caution—risk of accumulation; manufacturer of *Cardioxane®* advises reduce dose by 50% if creatinine clearance less than 40 mL/minute/1.73 m^2

Pregnancy avoid unless essential (toxicity in *animal* studies); ensure effective contraception during and for 3 months after treatment in men and women

Breast-feeding discontinue breast-feeding

Side-effects nausea, vomiting, dyspepsia, abdominal pain, diarrhoea, stomatitis, dry mouth, anorexia; dyspnoea; dizziness, syncope, asthenia, paraesthesia, tremor, fatigue, drowsiness; pyrexia; vaginal haemorrhage; myalgia; blood disorders (including anaemia, leucopenia, neutropenia, and thrombocytopenia); alopecia, pruritus; peripheral oedema, injection-site reactions including phlebitis

Licensed use not licensed for use in children

Indication and dose

> Prevention of anthracycline-induced cardiotoxicity (see notes above)
>
> • By intravenous infusion, 30 minutes prior to anthracycline administration
> 10–20 times the doxorubicin-equivalent dose (depending on treatment protocol) *or* 10 times the epirubicin-equivalent dose

Administration for *intravenous infusion* of *Cardioxane®* reconstitute each vial with 25 mL Water for Injections then dilute contents of each vial with 25–100 mL Compound sodium lactate; give over 15 minutes. For *intravenous infusion* of *Savene®*, reconstitute each vial with 25 mL of Water for Injections then dilute in 500 mL *Savene®* diluent provided; give over 1–2 hours

Cardioxane® (Novartis) ▼ PoM
Intravenous infusion, powder for reconstitution, dexrazoxane (as hydrochloride), net price 500-mg vial = £156.57

Savene® (SpePharm) ▼ PoM
Intravenous infusion, powder for reconstitution, dexrazoxane (as hydrochloride), net price 500-mg vial = £675.00

Hyperuricaemia

Hyperuricaemia, which may be present in high-grade lymphoma and leukaemia, can be markedly worsened by chemotherapy and is associated with acute renal failure.

Allopurinol is used routinely in children at low to moderate risk of hyperuricaemia. It should be started 24 hours before treatment; patients should be adequately hydrated (consideration should be given to omitting phosphate and potassium from hydration fluids). The dose of mercaptopurine or azathioprine should be reduced if allopurinol is given concomitantly (see Appendix 1).

Rasburicase is a recombinant urate oxidase used in children who are at high-risk of developing hyperuricaemia. It rapidly reduces plasma uric acid and may be of particular value in preventing complications following treatment of leukaemias or bulky lymphomas.

ALLOPURINOL

Cautions ensure adequate fluid intake; for hyperuricaemia associated with cancer therapy, allopurinol treatment should be started before cancer therapy; **interactions:** Appendix 1 (allopurinol)

Hepatic impairment reduce dose, monitor hepatic function

Renal impairment manufacturer advises reduce dose or increase dose interval in severe impairment; adjust dose to maintain plasma-oxipurinol concentration below 100 micromol/litre

Pregnancy toxicity not reported; manufacturer advises use only if no safer alternative and disease carries risk for mother or child

△ **ALLOPURINOL (continued)**

Breast-feeding present in milk—not known to be harmful

Side-effects rashes (**withdraw** therapy; if rash mild re-introduce cautiously but **discontinue** immediately if recurrence—hypersensitivity reactions occur rarely and include exfoliation, fever, lymphadenopathy, arthralgia, and eosinophilia resembling Stevens-Johnson or Lyell's syndrome, vasculitis, hepatitis, renal impairment, and very rarely seizures); gastro-intestinal disorders; rarely malaise, headache, vertigo, drowsiness, visual and taste disturbances, hypertension, alopecia, hepatotoxicity, paraesthesia and neuropathy, blood disorders (including leucopenia, thrombocytopenia, haemolytic anaemia and aplastic anaemia)

Indication and dose

Prophylaxis of hyperuricaemia associated with cancer chemotherapy, prophylaxis of hyperuricaemic nephropathy, enzyme disorders causing increased serum urate e.g. Lesch-Nyhan syndrome

- By mouth

  Child 1 month–15 years 10–20 mg/kg daily (max. 400 mg daily), preferably after food

  Child 15–18 years initially 100 mg daily, increased according to response; max. 900 mg daily (doses over 300 mg daily given in divided doses); preferably after food

Allopurinol (Non-proprietary) ℗ₒₘ
Tablets, allopurinol 100 mg, net price 28-tab pack = £1.08; 300 mg, 28-tab pack = £1.33. Label: 8, 21, 27
Brands include *Caplenal®*, *Cosuric®*, *Rimapurinol®*

Zyloric® (GSK) ℗ₒₘ
Tablets, allopurinol 100 mg, net price 100-tab pack = £10.19; 300 mg, 28-tab pack = £7.31. Label: 8, 21, 27

◢Extemporaneous formulations available see Extemporaneous Preparations, p. 8

RASBURICASE

Cautions monitor closely for hypersensitivity; atopic allergies; may interfere with test for uric acid—consult product literature

Contra-indications G6PD deficiency (section 9.1.5)

Pregnancy manufacturer advises avoid—no information available

Breast-feeding manufacturer advises avoid—no information available

Side-effects fever; nausea, vomiting; less frequently diarrhoea, headache, hypersensitivity reactions (including rash, bronchospasm and anaphylaxis); haemolytic anaemia, methaemoglobinaemia

Licensed use not licensed for use in children

Indication and dose

Prophylaxis and treatment of acute hyperuricaemia with initial chemotherapy for haematological malignancy

- By intravenous infusion
  Consult local treatment protocol for details

Fasturtec® (Sanofi-Aventis) ℗ₒₘ
Intravenous infusion, powder for reconstitution, rasburicase, net price 1.5-mg vial (with solvent) = £57.88; 7.5-mg vial (with solvent) = £241.20

Methotrexate-induced mucositis and myelosuppression

Folinic acid (given as calcium folinate) is used to counteract the folate-antagonist action of methotrexate and thus speed recovery from methotrexate-induced mucositis or myelosuppression ('folinic acid rescue').

The calcium salt of **levofolinic acid**, a single isomer of folinic acid, is also used following methotrexate administration. The dose of calcium levofolinate is generally half that of calcium folinate.

The disodium salts of folinic acid and levofolinic acid are also used for rescue therapy following methotrexate administration.

The efficacy of high dose methotrexate is enhanced by delaying initiation of folinic acid for at least 24 hours, local protocols define the correct time. Folinic acid is normally continued until the plasma-methotrexate concentration falls to 100–200 nanomol/litre (45–90 micrograms/mL).

In the treatment of methotrexate overdose, folinate should be administered immediately; other measures to enhance the elimination of methotrexate are also necessary.

FOLINIC ACID

Cautions avoid simultaneous administration of methotrexate; **not** indicated for pernicious anaemia or other megaloblastic anaemias due to vit-

amin B_{12} deficiency; **interactions:** Appendix 1 (folates)

Safe Practice Intrathecal injection **contra-indicated**

◁ **FOLINIC ACID** *(continued)*

Pregnancy not known to be harmful; benefit outweighs risk

Breast-feeding presence in milk unknown but benefit outweighs risk

Side-effects *rarely* pyrexia after parenteral use; gastro-intestinal disturbances, insomnia, agitation, and depression after high doses

Licensed use consult product literature for licensing status of individual preparations

Indication and dose

See under preparation

▲Calcium folinate
(Calcium leucovorin)

Calcium Folinate (Non-proprietary) ᴾᵒᴹ
Tablets, scored, folinic acid (as calcium salt) 15 mg, net price 10-tab pack = £39.20, 30-tab pack = £85.74
Brands include *Refolinon*®
Note Not all strengths and pack sizes are available from all manufacturers

Injection, folinic acid (as calcium salt) 3 mg/mL, net price 1-mL amp = £4.00, 10-mL amp = £4.62; 7.5 mg/mL, net price 2-mL amp = £7.80; 10 mg/mL, net price 5-mL vial = £19.41, 10-mL vial = £35.09, 30-mL vial = £94.69, 35-mL vial = £90.98
Brands include *Refolinon*®
Note Not all strengths and pack sizes are available from all manufacturers

Injection, powder for reconstitution, folinic acid (as calcium salt), net price 15-mg vial = £4.46; 30-mg vial = £8.36

Dose

Reduction of methotrexate-induced toxicity
• By mouth, by intravenous injection or by intravenous infusion
See notes above. Consult local treatment protocol for details

Methotrexate overdose
• By intravenous injection or by intravenous infusion
See notes above. Consult local treatment protocol for details

Megaloblastic anaemia due to folate deficiency
• By mouth
Child up to 12 years 250 microgram/kg once daily
Child 12–18 years 15 mg once daily

Metabolic disorders leading to folate deficiency
• By mouth or by intravenous infusion
Child up to 18 years 15 mg once daily; larger doses may be required in older children

Prevention of megaloblastic anaemia associated with pyrimethamine and sulfadiazine treatment of congenital toxoplasmosis
• By mouth
Neonate 5 mg 3 times a week (increased up to 20 mg 3 times a week if neutropenic)
Child 1 month–1 year 10 mg 3 times a week

▲Disodium folinate
Sodiofolin® (Medac) ᴾᵒᴹ
Injection, folinic acid (as disodium salt) 50 mg/mL, net price 2-mL vial = £35.09, 8-mL vial = £126.25, 18-mL vial = £284.07
Dose
Antidote to methotrexate
• By intravenous injection or by intravenous infusion
Consult local treatment protocols for details

LEVOFOLINIC ACID

Note Levofolinic acid is an isomer of folinic acid
Cautions see Folinic acid

Safe Practice Intrathecal injection **contra-indicated**

Pregnancy see Folinic acid
Breast-feeding see Folinic acid
Side-effects see Folinic acid

Indication and dose

Reduction of methotrexate-induced toxicity
• By intramuscular injection or by intravenous injection or by intravenous infusion
See notes above. Consult local treatment protocol for details

Methotrexate overdose
• By intramuscular injection or by intravenous injection or by intravenous infusion
See notes above. Consult local treatment protocol for details

▲Calcium levofolinate
(Calcium levoleucovorin)

Calcium Levofolinate (Non-proprietary)
Injection, levofolinic acid (as calcium salt) 10 mg/mL, net price 17.5-mL vial = £84.63

Isovorin® (Wyeth) ᴾᵒᴹ
Injection, levofolinic acid (as calcium salt) 10 mg/mL, net price 2.5-mL vial = £11.62, 5-mL vial = £26.00, 17.5-mL vial = £81.33

▲Disodium levofolinate
Levofolinic Acid (Non-proprietary) ᴾᵒᴹ
Injection, levofolinic acid (as disodium salt) 50 mg/mL, net price 1-mL vial = £24.70, 4-mL vial = £80.40

Urothelial toxicity

Haemorrhagic cystitis is a common manifestation of urothelial toxicity which occurs with the oxazaphosphorines, cyclophosphamide and ifosfamide; it is caused by the metabolite acrolein. Adequate hydration is essential to reduce the risk of urothelial toxicity. **Mesna** reacts specifically with acrolein in the urinary tract, preventing toxicity. Mesna is given for the same duration as cyclophosphamide or ifosfamide. It is generally given intravenously; the dose of mesna is equal to or greater than that of the oxazaphosphorine. For the role of nebulised mesna as a mucolytic in cystic fibrosis, see section 3.7.

MESNA

Contra-indications hypersensitivity to thiol-containing compounds

Pregnancy not known to be harmful

Side-effects nausea, vomiting, colic, diarrhoea, fatigue, headache, limb and joint pains, depression, irritability, rash, hypotension and tachycardia; rarely hypersensitivity reactions (more common in patients with auto-immune disorders)

Licensed use not licensed for use in children

Indication and dose

Urothelial toxicity following oxazaphosphorine therapy

- **By intravenous injection or by continuous intravenous infusion**
  See notes above. Consult local treatment protocol for details

Mucolytic in cystic fibrosis section 3.7

Mesna (Non-proprietary) PoM
Tablets, f/c, mesna 400 mg, net price 10-tab pack = £42.90; 600 mg, 10-tab pack = £61.10

Injection, mesna 100 mg/mL, net price 4-mL amp = £3.95; 10-mL amp = £9.77

Note For oral administration contents of ampoule are taken in a flavoured drink such as orange juice or cola which may be stored in a refrigerator for up to 24 hours in a sealed container

8.1.1 Alkylating drugs

Extensive experience is available with these drugs, which are among the most widely used in cancer chemotherapy. They act by damaging DNA, thus interfering with cell replication. In addition to the side-effects common to many cytotoxic drugs (section 8.1), problems associated specifically with alkylating drugs include:

- an adverse effect on gametogenesis which may be reversible, particularly in females; amenorrhoea may also occur, which also may be reversible;

- a marked increase in the incidence of secondary tumours and leukaemia, particularly when alkylating drugs are combined with extensive irradiation;

- fluid retention with oedema and dilutional hyponatraemia in younger children; the risk of this complication is higher in the first 2 days and also when given with concomitant vinca alkaloids;

- urothelial toxicity with intravenous use; adequate hydration may reduce this risk; mesna (section 8.1) provides further protection against urotoxic effects of cyclophosphamide and ifosfamide.

BUSULFAN
(Busulphan)

Cautions see section 8.1 and notes above; monitor full blood count regularly throughout treatment; monitor liver function; previous mediastinal or pulmonary radiation therapy; avoid in acute porphyria (but see section 9.8.2); **interactions:** Appendix 1 (busulfan)

Hepatic impairment manufacturer advises monitor hepatic function—no information available

Pregnancy avoid (teratogenic in *animals*); manufacturers advise effective contraception during and for 6 months after treatment in men or women; see also Pregnancy and Reproductive Function, p. 507

Breast-feeding discontinue breast-feeding

Side-effects see section 8.1 and notes above; also hepatotoxicity (including hepatic veno-occlusive disease, hyperbilirubinaemia, jaundice, and fibrosis); cardiac tamponade in thalassaemia; pneumonia, skin hyperpigmentation; *rarely* progressive pulmonary fibrosis, seizures, aplastic anaemia, visual disturbances, hypersensitivity reactions (including urticaria, erythema); *very rarely* myasthenia gravis, gynaecomastia

Indication and dose

Conditioning treatment before haematopoietic stem-cell transplantation

- **By mouth or by intravenous infusion**
  Consult local treatment protocol for details

Busilvex® (Fabre) ▼ PoM
Concentrate for intravenous infusion, busulfan 6 mg/mL, net price 10-mL vial = £201.25

◁ **BUSULFAN** *(continued)*

Myleran® (GSK) ⓅⓄⓂ
Tablets, f/c, busulfan 2 mg, net price 25-tab pack = £5.20

Busulfan
Capsules, busulfan 25 mg
Available from 'special-order' manufacturers or specialist importing companies, p. 957

◢Extemporaneous formulations available see Extemporaneous Preparations, p. 8

CHLORAMBUCIL

Cautions see section 8.1 and notes above; monitor full blood count regularly throughout treatment; increased seizure risk in children with nephrotic syndrome or history of epilepsy; avoid in acute porphyria (but see section 9.8.2)

Hepatic impairment manufacturer advises consider dose reduction in severe impairment—limited information available

Pregnancy avoid; manufacturer advises effective contraception during treatment in men or women; see also Pregnancy and Reproductive Function, p. 507

Breast-feeding discontinue breast-feeding

Side-effects see section 8.1 and notes above; also *less commonly* skin rash (possible progression to Stevens-Johnson syndrome and toxic epidermal necrolysis); *rarely* seizures, hepatotoxicity and jaundice; *very rarely* irreversible bone-marrow suppression, pulmonary fibrosis, tremor, peripheral neuropathy, sterile cystitis, sterility in pre-pubertal and pubertal males

Licensed use not licensed for use in nephrotic syndrome

Indication and dose

Hodgkin's disease
• By mouth
Consult local treatment protocol for details

Non-Hodgkin's lymphoma
• By mouth
Consult local treatment protocol for details

Relapsing steroid-sensitive nephrotic syndrome; initiated in specialist centres (see also section 6.3.2, p. 452)
• By mouth
Child 3 months–18 years 200 micrograms/kg once daily for 8 weeks

Leukeran® (GSK) ⓅⓄⓂ
Tablets, f/c, brown, chlorambucil 2 mg, net price 25-tab pack = £8.36

◢Extemporaneous formulations available see Extemporaneous Preparations, p. 8

CYCLOPHOSPHAMIDE

Cautions see section 8.1 and notes above; previous or concurrent mediastinal irradiation—risk of cardiotoxicity; diabetes mellitus; avoid in acute porphyria (but see section 9.8.2); **interactions:** Appendix 1 (cyclophosphamide)

Contra-indications haemorrhagic cystitis

Hepatic impairment reduce dose—consult local treatment protocol for details

Renal impairment reduce dose—consult local treatment protocol for details

Pregnancy avoid; manufacturer advises effective contraception during and for at least 3 months after treatment in men or women; see also Pregnancy and Reproductive Function, p. 507

Breast-feeding discontinue breast-feeding during and for 36 hours after stopping treatment

Side-effects see section 8.1 and notes above; *also* anorexia; pancreatitis; cardiotoxicity at high doses; interstitial pulmonary fibrosis; inappropriate secretion of anti-diuretic hormone, disturbances of carbohydrate metabolism; urothelial toxicity; pigmentation of palms, nails and soles; *rarely* hepatotoxicity and renal dysfunction

Licensed use not licensed for use in children

Indication and dose

Acute lymphoblastic leukaemia, non-Hodgkin's lymphoma, retinoblastoma, neuroblastoma, rhabdomyosarcoma, soft-tissue sarcomas, Ewing tumour, neuroectodermal tumours (including medulloblastoma), infant brain tumours, ependymona, high-dose conditioning for bone marrow transplantation, lupus nephritis
• By mouth or by intravenous infusion
Consult local treatment protocol for details

Steroid-sensitive nephrotic syndrome see also section 6.3.2, p. 452
• By mouth
Child 3 months–18 years 2–3 mg/kg once daily for eight weeks
• By intravenous infusion
Child 3 months–18 years 500 mg/m² once a month for six months

Administration Consult local treatment protocol for details

Cyclophosphamide (Non-proprietary) ⓅⓄⓂ
Tablets, s/c, cyclophosphamide (anhydrous) 50 mg, net price 100 = £10.58. Label: 25, 27

Injection, powder for reconstitution, cyclophosphamide, net price 500-mg vial = £2.88; 1-g vial = £5.04

◢Extemporaneous formulations available see Extemporaneous Preparations, p. 8

IFOSFAMIDE

Cautions see section 8.1 and notes above; ensure satisfactory electrolyte balance, and renal function before each course (risk of tubular dysfunction, Fanconi's syndrome, or diabetes insipidus if renal toxicity not treated promptly); avoid in acute porphyria (but see section 9.8.2); **interactions:** Appendix 1 (ifosfamide)

Contra-indications urinary tract obstruction; acute infection (including urinary-tract infection); urothelial damage

Hepatic impairment avoid

Renal impairment avoid

Pregnancy avoid (teratogenic and carcinogenic in *animals*); manufacturer advises adequate contraception during and for at least 6 months after treatment in men or women; see also Pregnancy and Reproductive Function, p. 507

Breast-feeding discontinue breast-feeding

Side-effects see section 8.1 and notes above; *also* drowsiness, confusion, disorientation, restlessness, psychosis; urothelial toxicity causing haemorrhagic cystitis and dysuria, renal toxicity (see Cautions above); *less commonly* severe encephalopathy; *rarely* diarrhoea, constipation, convulsions, anorexia; *very rarely* jaundice, thrombophlebitis, syndrome of inappropriate antidiuretic hormone secretion

Indication and dose

Rhabdomyosarcoma, soft-tissue sarcomas, Ewing tumour, germ cell tumour, osteogenic sarcoma

• By intravenous infusion
  Consult local treatment protocol for details

Ifosfamide (Non-proprietary) ▣PoM▢
Injection, powder for reconstitution, ifosfamide, net price 1-g vial = £43.53; 2-g vial = £88.62 (hosp. only)

MELPHALAN

Cautions see section 8.1 and notes above; monitor full blood count before and throughout treatment; for high-dose intravenous administration establish adequate hydration (see notes above), consider use of prophylactic anti-infective agents; haematopoietic stem cell transplantation essential for high dose treatment (consult local treatment protocol for details); avoid in acute porphyria (but see section 9.8.2); **interactions:** Appendix 1 (melphalan)

Renal impairment reduce dose initially—consult product literature

Pregnancy avoid; manufacturer advises adequate contraception during treatment in men or women; see also Pregnancy and Reproductive Function, p. 507

Breast-feeding discontinue breast-feeding

Side-effects see section 8.1 and notes above

Licensed use childhood neuroblastoma

Indication and dose

High intravenous dose with haematopoietic stem cell transplantation in the treatment of childhood neuroblastoma and some other advanced embryonal tumours

• Intravenous infusion
  Consult local treatment protocol for details

Alkeran® (GSK) ▣PoM▢
Injection, powder for reconstitution, melphalan 50 mg (as hydrochloride). Net price 50-mg vial (with solvent-diluent) = £33.13

8.1.2 Cytotoxic antibiotics

Cytotoxic antibiotics are widely used. Many act as radiomimetics and simultaneous use of radiotherapy should be **avoided** as it may enhance toxicity markedly.

Daunorubicin, **doxorubicin**, and **epirubicin** are anthracycline antibiotics. **Mitoxantrone** (mitozantrone) is an anthracycline derivative.

All anthracycline antibiotics have been associated with varying degrees of cardiac toxicity—this may be idiosyncratic and reversible, but is commonly related to total cumulative dose and is irreversible. Cardiac function should be monitored before and at regular intervals throughout treatment and afterwards. Anthracycline antibiotics should not normally be used in children with left ventricular dysfunction. Epirubicin and mitoxantrone are considered less toxic, and may be suitable for children who have received high cumulative doses of other anthracyclines. **Dexrazoxane** can be used to prevent chronic cumulative cardiotoxicity, see section 8.1.

BLEOMYCIN

Cautions see section 8.1; ensure monitoring of pulmonary function—investigate any shortness of breath before initiation; caution in handling—irritant to tissues

Contra-indications acute pulmonary infection or significantly reduced lung function

Renal impairment reduce dose—consult local treatment protocol for details

Pregnancy avoid (teratogenic and carcinogenic in *animal* studies); see also Pregnancy and Reproductive Function, p. 507

Breast-feeding discontinue breast-feeding

8

Malignant disease and immunosuppression

◁ **BLEOMYCIN (continued)**

Side-effects see section 8.1, less bone marrow suppression; anorexia; pulmonary toxicity e.g. pulmonary fibrosis (usually dose-related and delayed); fever (directly following administration), fatigue; dermatological and mucous membrane toxicity, localised skin hyperpigmentation; rarely cardiorespiratory collapse and hyperpyrexia

Licensed use not licensed for use in children

Indication and dose

> Some germ cell tumours, Hodgkin's lymphoma
> * By intravenous infusion
>   Consult local treatment protocol for details

Bleomycin (Non-proprietary) [PoM]
Injection, powder for reconstitution, bleomycin (as sulphate), net price 15 000-unit vial = £15.56

Note To conform to the European Pharmacopoeia vials previously labelled as containing '15 units' of bleomycin are now labelled as containing 15 000 units. The amount of bleomycin in the vial has not changed.
Brands include *Bleo-Kyowa*®

DACTINOMYCIN

(Actinomycin D)

Cautions see section 8.1 and notes above; caution in handling—irritant to tissues

Hepatic impairment consider dose reduction if raised serum bilirubin or biliary obstruction—consult local treatment protocol for details

Pregnancy avoid (teratogenic in *animal* studies); see also Pregnancy and Reproductive Function, p. 507

Breast-feeding discontinue breast-feeding

Side-effects see section 8.1 and notes above; *less commonly* cheilitis, dysphagia; fever, malaise, lethargy; anaemia, hypoglycaemia; myalgia; acne; *rarely* hepatotoxicity (possibly dose-related)

Licensed use not licensed for use in children under 12 years

Indication and dose

> Wilms' tumour, childhood rhabdomyosarcoma and other soft tissue sarcomas, Ewing's sarcoma
> * By intravenous injection
>   Consult local treatment protocol for details

Cosmegen Lyovac® (Ovation) [PoM]
Injection, powder for reconstitution, dactinomycin, net price 500-microgram vial = £6.75

DAUNORUBICIN

Cautions see section 8.1 and notes above; caution in handling—irritant to tissues

Hepatic impairment reduce dose according to serum bilirubin concentration—consult local treatment protocol for details

Renal impairment reduce dose—consult local treatment protocol for details

Pregnancy avoid (teratogenic and carcinogenic in *animal* studies), see also Pregnancy and Reproductive Function, p. 507

Breast-feeding discontinue breast-feeding

Side-effects see section 8.1 and notes above, leucopenia, less commonly mucositis; cardiac toxicity (usually 1–6 months after initiation of therapy); fever; red urine discolouration

Licensed use *DaunoXome*® not licensed for use in children

Indication and dose

> Acute myelogenous leukaemia, acute lymphocytic leukaemia
> * By intravenous infusion
>   Consult local treatment protocol for details

Daunorubicin (Non-proprietary) [PoM]
Injection, powder for reconstitution, daunorubicin (as hydrochloride), net price 20-mg vial = £44.76

▲**Lipid formulation**
DaunoXome® (Diatos) [PoM]
Concentrate for intravenous infusion, daunorubicin encapsulated in liposomes. For dilution before use, net price 50-mg vial = £137.67

DOXORUBICIN HYDROCHLORIDE

Cautions see section 8.1 and notes above; caution in handling—irritant to tissues; **interactions:** Appendix 1 (doxorubicin)

Hepatic impairment reduce dose according to bilirubin concentration—consult local treatment protocol for details

Pregnancy avoid (teratogenic and toxic in *animal* studies); manufacturer of liposomal product advises effective contraception during and for at least 6 months after treatment in men or women; see also Pregnancy and Reproductive Function, p. 507

Breast-feeding discontinue breast-feeding

Side-effects see section 8.1 and notes above; red urine discoloration; thrombophlebitis over injection site; less commonly bronchospasm, fever, amenorrhoea, and skin rash

Licensed use not licensed for use in children

△ **DOXORUBICIN HYDROCHLORIDE** (*continued*)

Indication and dose

Paediatric malignancies including Ewing's sarcoma, osteogenic sarcoma, Wilms' tumour, neuroblastoma, retinoblastoma, some liver tumours, acute lymphoblastic leukaemia, Hodgkin's lymphoma, non-Hodgkin's lymphoma
• By intravenous infusion
  Consult local treatment protocol for details

Doxorubicin (Non-proprietary) ⓅⓄⓂ
Injection, powder for reconstitution, doxorubicin hydrochloride, net price 10-mg vial = £18.72; 50-mg vial = £96.86

Note The brand name *Adriamycin*® was formerly used

Injection, doxorubicin hydrochloride 2 mg/mL, net price 5-mL vial = £20.50, 25-mL vial = £102.00, 100-mL vial = £275.00

EPIRUBICIN HYDROCHLORIDE

Cautions see section 8.1 and notes above; caution in handling—irritant to tissues

Hepatic impairment reduce dose according to bilirubin concentration—consult local treatment protocol for details

Pregnancy avoid (carcinogenic in *animal* studies); see also Pregnancy and Reproductive Function, p. 507

Breast-feeding discontinue breast-feeding

Side-effects see section 8.1 and notes above; red urine discolouration; anaphylaxis

Licensed use not licensed for use in children

Indication and dose

Recurrent acute lymphoblastic leukaemia, rhabdomyosarcoma, other soft tissue tumours of childhood
• Intravenous infusion
  Consult local treatment protocol for details

Epirubicin hydrochloride (Non-proprietary) ⓅⓄⓂ
Injection, epirubicin hydrochloride 2 mg/mL, net price 5-mL vial = £16.99, 25-mL vial = £84.95, 50-mL vial = £169.92, 100-mL vial = £308.93

Pharmorubicin® Rapid Dissolution (Pharmacia) ⓅⓄⓂ
Injection, powder for reconstitution, epirubicin hydrochloride, net price 50-mg vial = £96.54

Pharmorubicin® Solution for Injection (Pharmacia) ⓅⓄⓂ
Injection, epirubicin hydrochloride 2 mg/mL, net price 5-mL vial = £19.31, 25-mL vial = £96.54, 100-mL vial = £386.16

MITOXANTRONE
(Mitozantrone)

Cautions see section 8.1 and notes above

Hepatic impairment manufacturer advises caution in severe impairment—consult local treatment protocol for details

Renal impairment manufacturer advises caution in severe impairment

Pregnancy avoid; manufacturer advises effective contraception during and for at least 6 months after treatment in men or women; see also Pregnancy and Reproductive Function, p. 507

Breast-feeding discontinue breast-feeding

Side-effects see section 8.1 and notes above; transient blue-green discoloration of urine; less commonly gastro-intestinal bleeding, anorexia, allergic reactions, dyspnoea, fatigue, fever, amenorrhoea, and transient blue discoloration of skin and nails

Licensed use not licensed for use in children

Indication and dose

Acute myeloid leukaemia, recurrent acute lymphoblastic leukaemia
• By intravenous infusion
  Consult local treatment protocol for details

Mitoxantrone (Non-proprietary) ⓅⓄⓂ
Concentrate for intravenous infusion, mitoxantrone (as hydrochloride) 2 mg/mL, net price 10-mL vial = £100.00

Onkotrone® (Baxter) ⓅⓄⓂ
Concentrate for intravenous infusion, mitoxantrone (as hydrochloride) 2 mg/mL, net price 10-mL vial = £121.85, 12.5-mL vial = £152.33, 15-mL vial = £203.04

8.1.3 Antimetabolites

Antimetabolites are incorporated into new nuclear material or they combine irreversibly with cellular enzymes and prevent normal cellular division. **Cytarabine**, **fludarabine**, **mercaptopurine**, **methotrexate**, and **tioguanine** are commonly used in paediatric chemotherapy.

Methotrexate inhibits the enzyme dihydrofolate reductase, essential for the synthesis of purines and pyrimidines. It is given by mouth, intravenously, intramuscularly, or intrathecally. Methotrexate causes myelosuppression, mucositis, and rarely pneumonitis. It is **contra-indicated** in significant renal impairment because it is excreted primarily by the kidney. It is also contra-indicated in

8 Malignant disease and immunosuppression

patients with severe hepatic impairment. It should also be **avoided** in the presence of significant pleural effusion or ascites because it can accumulate in these fluids, and its subsequent return to the circulation may cause myelosuppression. Systemic toxicity may follow intrathecal administration and blood counts should be carefully monitored. Folinic acid (section 8.1) following methotrexate administration helps to prevent methotrexate-induced mucositis and myelosuppression.

Cytarabine acts by interfering with pyrimidine synthesis. It is given subcutaneously, intravenously, or intrathecally. It is a potent myelosuppressant and requires careful haematological monitoring. A liposomal formulation of cytarabine for intrathecal use is available for lymphomatous meningitis.

Fludarabine is generally well tolerated but does cause myelosuppression, which may be cumulative.

> **Fludarabine** has a potent and prolonged immunosuppressive effect. Children treated with fludarabine are more prone to serious bacterial, opportunistic fungal, and viral infections, and prophylactic therapy is recommended in children at risk. To prevent potentially fatal transfusion-related graft-versus-host reaction, only irradiated blood products should be administered. Prescribers should consult specialist literature when using highly immunosuppressive drugs.

Clofarabine is licensed for the treatment of acute lymphoblastic leukaemia in children who have relapsed or are refractory after receiving at least two previous regimens. It is given by intravenous infusion.

Nelarabine is licensed for the treatment of T-cell acute lymphoblastic leukaemia and T-cell lymphoblastic lymphoma in children who have relapsed or who are refractory after receiving at least two previous regimens. It is given by intravenous infusion. Neurotoxicity is common with nelarabine, and close monitoring for neurological events is strongly recommended—discontinue treatment if neurotoxicity occurs.

Mercaptopurine is used as maintenance therapy for acute lymphoblastic leukaemia and in the management of ulcerative colitis and Crohn's disease (section 1.5). Azathioprine, which is metabolised to mercaptopurine, is generally used as an immunosuppressant (section 8.2.1 and section 10.1.3). The dose of both drugs should be reduced if the child is receiving allopurinol since it interferes with their metabolism. For the role of thiopurine methyltransferase (TPMT) in the metabolism of azathioprine see section 8.2.1.

Tioguanine (thioguanine) is given by mouth for the treatment of acute lymphoblastic leukaemia; it is given at various stages of treatment in short-term cycles. Tioguanine has a lower incidence of gastro-intestinal side-effects than mercaptopurine. Long-term therapy with tioguanine is no longer recommended because of the high risk of liver toxicity.

◣ CLOFARABINE

Cautions see section 8.1; cardiac disease

Hepatic impairment manufacturer advises caution in mild to moderate impairment; avoid in severe impairment

Renal impairment manufacturer advises caution in mild to moderate impairment; avoid in severe impairment

Pregnancy manufacturer advises avoid (teratogenic in *animal* studies; see also Pregnancy and Reproductive Function, p. 507

Breast-feeding discontinue breast-feeding

Side-effects see section 8.1; also diarrhoea, abdominal pain, jaundice; tachycardia, flushing, hypotension, pericardial effusion, oedema, haematoma; dyspnoea, cough; anxiety, agitation, dizziness, drowsiness, headache, paraesthesia, peripheral neuropathy, restlessness; haematuria; arthralgia, myalgia; rash, pruritus, hand-foot (desquamative) syndrome, increased sweating; pancreatitis also reported

Licensed use not licensed for use in children under 1 year

Indication and dose

> **Relapsed or refractory acute lymphoblastic leukaemia**
> • By intravenous infusion
>   Consult local treatment protocol for details

Evoltra® (Genzyme) ▼ (PoM)
Concentrate for intravenous infusion, clofarabine 1 mg/mL, net price 20-mL vial = £1200.00
Electrolytes Na⁺ 3.08 mmol/vial

▲ CYTARABINE

Cautions see section 8.1 and notes above; **inter-actions**: Appendix 1 (cytarabine)

Hepatic impairment reduce dose

Renal impairment reduce dose for high dose regimens or avoid—consult local treatment protocol for details

Pregnancy avoid (teratogenic in *animal* studies); see also Pregnancy and Reproductive Function, p. 507

Breast-feeding discontinue breast-feeding

Side-effects see section 8.1 and notes above; 'cytarabine syndrome'—6–12 hours after intravenous administration—characterised by fever and malaise, myalgia, bone pain, maculopapular rash, and occasionally chest pain; *less commonly* conjunctivitis (consider prophylactic corticosteroid eye drops), neurotoxicity, renal and hepatic dysfunction, jaundice; *rarely* severe spinal cord toxicity following intrathecal administration

Licensed use *Depocyte®* intrathecal injection not licensed for use in children

Indication and dose

> **Acute lymphoblastic leukaemia, acute myeloid leukaemia, non-Hodgkin's lymphoma**
> • By intravenous injection, by intravenous infusion, or by subcutaneous injection
>   Consult local treatment protocol for details

> **Meningeal leukaemia, meningeal neoplasms**
> • By intrathecal injection
>   Consult local treatment protocol for details

Note Based on weight or body-surface area, children may tolerate higher doses of cytarabine than adults

---

Cytarabine (Non-proprietary) ℗ℴ𝕄
Injection (for intravenous, subcutaneous or intrathecal use), cytarabine 20 mg/mL, net price 5-mL vial = £4.00

Injection (for intravenous or subcutaneous use), cytarabine 20 mg/mL, net price 5-mL vial = £3.90, 25-mL vial = £19.50

Injection (for intravenous or subcutaneous use), cytarabine 100 mg/mL, net price 1-mL vial = £4.00; 5-mL vial = £20.00; 10-mL vial = £39.00; 20-mL vial = £77.50

◢ **Lipid formulation for intrathecal use**
DepoCyte® (Napp) ℗ℴ𝕄
Intrathecal injection, cytarabine encapsulated in liposomes, net price 50-mg vial = £1223.75

▲ FLUDARABINE PHOSPHATE

Cautions see section 8.1 and notes above; monitor for signs of haemolysis; monitor for neurological toxicity; worsening of existing and increased susceptibility to skin cancer; **interactions**: Appendix 1 (fludarabine)

Contra-indications haemolytic anaemia

Renal impairment reduce dose by up to 50% if creatinine clearance 30–70 mL/minute/1.73 m²; avoid if creatinine clearance less than 30 mL/minute/1.73 m²

Pregnancy avoid (embryotoxic and teratogenic in *animal* studies); manufacturer advises effective contraception during and for at least 6 months after treatment in men or women; see also Pregnancy and Reproductive Function, p. 507

Breast-feeding discontinue breast-feeding

Side-effects see section 8.1 and notes above; also diarrhoea, anorexia; oedema; pneumonia, cough; peripheral neuropathy, visual disturbances; chills, fever, malaise, weakness; rash; *less commonly* gastro-intestinal haemorrhage, pulmonary toxicity (including pulmonary infiltrates, pneumonitis, and fibrosis), and confusion; *rarely* heart failure, arrhythmia, coma, seizures, agitation,

myelodysplastic syndrome, acute myeloid leukaemia, optic neuropathy, blindness, Stevens-Johnson syndrome, toxic epidermal necrolysis, skin cancer, and haemorrhagic cystitis

Licensed use not licensed for use in children

Indication and dose

> **Poor prognosis or relapsed acute myeloid leukaemia, relapsed acute lymphoblastic leukaemia, conditioning before bone marrow transplantation**
> • By mouth, by intravenous injection, or by intravenous infusion
>   Consult local treatment protocol for details

Fludarabine phosphate (Non-proprietary) ℗ℴ𝕄
Injection, powder for reconstitution, fludarabine phosphate, net price 50-mg vial = £140.40

Fludara® (Genzyme) ℗ℴ𝕄
Tablets, f/c, pink, fludarabine phosphate 10 mg, net price 15-tab pack = £268.12, 20-tab pack = £357.49
Injection, powder for reconstitution, fludarabine phosphate, net price 50-mg vial = £149.92

▲ MERCAPTOPURINE

Cautions see section 8.1 and notes above; monitor liver function—discontinue if jaundice develops; **interactions**: Appendix 1 (mercaptopurine)

Hepatic impairment may need dose reduction

Renal impairment manufacturer advises consider reducing dose

Pregnancy avoid (teratogenic); see also Pregnancy and Reproductive Function, p. 507

Breast-feeding discontinue breast-feeding

Side-effects see section 8.1 and notes above; gastro-intestinal effects less common; hepatotoxicity (more frequent at higher doses); rarely intestinal ulceration, pancreatitis, fever, crystal-

8

Malignant disease and immunosuppression

◁ **MERCAPTOPURINE** (*continued*)

luria with haematuria, rash, and hyperpigmentation

Licensed use not licensed for use in children for acute lymphoblastic lymphoma or T-cell non-Hodgkins lymphoma

Indication and dose

> **Acute lymphoblastic leukaemia, lymphoblastic lymphomas**
> • By mouth
> Consult local treatment protocol for details

> **Severe ulcerative colitis and Crohn's disease** section 1.5.3

Puri-Nethol® (GSK) PoM
Tablets, yellow, scored, mercaptopurine 50 mg, net price 25-tab pack = £22.54

Mercaptopurine
Capsules, mercaptopurine 10 mg
Available from 'special-order' manufacturers or specialist importing companies, p. 957

◢ Extemporaneous formulations available see Extemporaneous Preparations, p. 8

▌ **METHOTREXATE**

Cautions see section 8.1 and section 10.1.3; monitor renal and hepatic function; peptic ulceration, ulcerative colitis, diarrhoea, and ulcerative stomatitis; porphyria (section 9.8.2); **interactions:** Appendix 1 (methotrexate)

Hepatic impairment avoid in severe impairment—consult local treatment protocol for details

Renal impairment reduce dose—risk of nephrotoxicity at high doses; avoid in severe impairment

Pregnancy avoid (teratogenic; fertility may be reduced during therapy but this may be reversible); manufacturer advises effective contraception during and for at least 3 months after treatment in men or women; see also Pregnancy and Reproductive Function, p. 507

Breast-feeding discontinue breast-feeding—present in milk

Side-effects see section 8.1; also anorexia, abdominal discomfort, dyspepsia, gastro-intestinal ulceration and bleeding, diarrhoea, toxic megacolon, hepatotoxicity (see Cautions above); hypotension, pericarditis, pericardial tamponade, thrombosis; pulmonary oedema, pleuritic pain, pulmonary fibrosis, interstitial pneumonitis (see also Pulmonary Toxicity, p. 620); anaphylactic reactions, urticaria; dizziness, fatigue, chills, fever, drowsiness, malaise, headache, mood changes, abnormal cranial sensations, neurotoxicity, confusion, psychosis, paraesthesia, cerebral oedema; precipitation of diabetes; menstrual disturbances, vaginitis, cystitis, reduced libido, impotence; haematuria, dysuria, renal failure; osteoporosis, arthralgia, myalgia, vasculitis; conjunctivitis, blepharitis, visual disturbances; rash, pruritus, Stevens-Johnson syndrome, toxic epidermal necrolysis, photosensitivity, changes in nail and skin pigmentation, telangiectasia, acne, furunculosis, ecchymosis; injection-site reactions

Indication and dose

> **Maintenance and remission of acute lymphoblastic leukaemia, lymphoblastic lymphoma**
> • By mouth
> Consult local treatment protocol for details

Safe Practice To avoid error with low-dose methotrexate, it is recommended that:
- the child or their carer is carefully advised of the **dose** and **frequency** and the reason for taking methotrexate and any other prescribed medicine (e.g. folic acid);
- only one strength of methotrexate tablet (usually 2.5 mg) is prescribed and dispensed;
- the prescription and the dispensing label clearly show the dose and frequency of methotrexate administration;
- the child or their carer is warned to report immediately the onset of any feature of blood disorders (e.g. sore throat, bruising, and mouth ulcers), liver toxicity (e.g. nausea, vomiting, abdominal discomfort, and dark urine), and respiratory effects (e.g. shortness of breath).

> **Treatment of early stage Burkitt's lymphoma, non-Hodgkin's lymphoma, osteogenic sarcoma, some CNS tumours including infant brain tumours, acute lymphoblastic leukaemia**
> • By intravenous injection or infusion
> Consult local treatment protocol for details

> **Meningeal leukaemia, treatment and prevention of CNS involvement of leukaemia**
> • By intrathecal injection
> Consult local treatment protocol for details

> **Severe Crohn's disease** section 1.5.3

> **Rheumatic disease** section 10.1.3

> **Psoriasis** section 13.5.3

Methotrexate (Non-proprietary) PoM
Injection, methotrexate (as sodium salt) 2.5 mg/mL, net price 2-mL vial = £1.68

Injection, methotrexate (as sodium salt) 25 mg/mL, net price 2-mL vial = £3.00, 20-mL vial = £30.00

Injection, methotrexate 100 mg/mL (not for intrathecal use), net price 10-mL vial = £78.33, 50-mL vial = £380.07

◢ **Oral preparations**
Section 10.1.3

◢ NELARABINE

Cautions see section 8.1 and notes above; previous or concurrent intrathecal chemotherapy or craniospinal irradiation (increased risk of neurotoxicity)

Skilled tasks Drowsiness may affect performance of skilled tasks (e.g. cycling or driving)

Pregnancy avoid (teratogenic in *animal* studies); manufacturer advises effective contraception during and for at least 3 months after treatment in men and women; see also Pregnancy and Reproductive Function, p. 507

Breast-feeding discontinue breast-feeding

Side-effects see section 8.1 and notes above; also constipation, diarrhoea; confusion, seizures, drowsiness, peripheral neurological disorders, demyelination, hypoesthesia, paraesthesia, ataxia, tremor, headache, asthenia, fatigue; pyrexia; hypoglycaemia, electrolyte disturbances; arthralgia; benign and malignant tumours also reported

Indication and dose

T-cell acute lymphoblastic leukaemia, T-cell lymphoblastic lymphoma
- **By intravenous infusion**
  Consult local treatment protocol for details

Atriance® (GSK) ▼ PoM
Intravenous infusion, nelarabine 5 mg/mL, net price 50-mL vial = £222.00
Electrolytes Na$^+$ 3.75 mmol/vial

◢ TIOGUANINE
(Thioguanine)

Cautions see section 8.1 and notes above; monitor liver function weekly—discontinue if liver toxicity develops; **interactions**: Appendix 1 (tioguanine)

Hepatic impairment reduce dose

Renal impairment reduce dose

Pregnancy avoid (teratogenicity reported when men receiving tioguanine have fathered children); ensure effective contraception during treatment in men or women; see also Pregnancy and Reproductive Function, p. 507

Breast-feeding discontinue breast-feeding

Side-effects see section 8.1; also stomatitis and hepatotoxicity; *rarely* intestinal necrosis and perforation

Indication and dose

Infant acute lymphoblastic leukaemia
- **By mouth**
  Consult local treatment protocol for details

Lanvis® (GSK) PoM
Tablets, yellow, scored, tioguanine 40 mg. Net price 25-tab pack = £54.49

◢Extemporaneous formulations available see Extemporaneous Preparations, p. 8

■ 8.1.4   Vinca alkaloids and etoposide

The vinca alkaloids, **vinblastine** and **vincristine** are used to treat a variety of cancers including leukaemias, lymphomas, and some solid tumours.

Neurotoxicity, usually as peripheral or autonomic neuropathy, occurs with all vinca alkaloids and is a limiting side-effect of vincristine; it occurs less often with vinblastine. Children with neurotoxicity commonly have peripheral paraesthesia, loss of deep tendon reflexes, abdominal pain, and constipation; ototoxicity has been reported. If symptoms of neurotoxicity are severe, doses should be reduced, but children generally tolerate vincristine better than adults. Motor weakness can also occur and dose reduction or discontinuation of therapy may be appropriate if motor weakness increases. Recovery from neurotoxic effects is usually slow but complete.

Myelosuppression is the dose-limiting side-effect of vinblastine; vincristine causes negligible myelosuppression. The vinca alkaloids may cause reversible alopecia. They cause severe local irritation and care must be taken to avoid extravasation. Constipation is common with vinblastine and vincristine; prophylactic use of laxatives may be considered.

> **Safe Practice**
> Vinblastine and vincristine are for **intravenous administration only**. Inadvertent intrathecal administration can cause severe neurotoxicity, which is usually fatal.
> The National Patient Safety Agency has advised (August 2008) that teenage patients treated in an adolescent unit should receive their vinca alkaloid dose in a 50 mL minibag. Teenagers and children treated in a child unit may receive their vinca alkaloid dose in a syringe.

Etoposide, usually given by slow intravenous infusion, is used to treat acute leukaemias, lymphomas, and some solid tumours. Etoposide may also be given by mouth but it is unpredictably absorbed.

ETOPOSIDE

Cautions see section 8.1 and notes above; **interactions**: Appendix 1 (etoposide)

Hepatic impairment avoid in severe impairment

Renal impairment consider dose reduction—consult local treatment protocol for details

Pregnancy avoid (teratogenic in *animal* studies); see also Pregnancy and Reproductive Function, p. 507

Breast-feeding discontinue breast-feeding

Side-effects see section 8.1, dose limiting myelosuppression, mucositis more common if given with doxorubicin; anaphylaxis associated with concentrated infusions; hypotension associated with rapid infusion; irritant to tissues if extravasated

Licensed use not licensed for use in children

Indication and dose

Stage 4 neuroblastoma, germ-cell tumours, intracranial germ-cell tumours, rhabdomyosarcoma, soft-tissue sarcomas, neuroectodermal tumours (including medulloblastoma), relapsed Hodgkin's disease, non-Hodgkin's lymphoma, Ewing tumour, acute lymphoblastic leukaemia, acute myeloid leukaemia

* By mouth or by intravenous infusion
  Consult local treatment protocol for details

Etoposide (Non-proprietary) ⓅⓄⓂ
Concentrate for intravenous infusion, etoposide 20 mg/mL, net price 5-mL vial = £12.15, 10-mL vial = £29.00, 25-mL vial = £60.75
Brands include *Eposin®*

Etopophos® (Bristol-Myers Squibb) ⓅⓄⓂ
Injection, powder for reconstitution, etoposide (as phosphate), net price 100-mg vial = £26.70 (hosp. only)

Vepesid® (Bristol-Myers Squibb) ⓅⓄⓂ
Capsules, both pink, etoposide 50 mg, net price 20 = £101.84; 100 mg, 10-cap pack = £88.99 (hosp. only). Label: 23

VINBLASTINE SULPHATE

Cautions see section 8.1 and notes above; caution in handling; **interactions**: Appendix 1 (vinblastine)

Contra-indications see notes above

> Safe Practice Intrathecal injection **contra-indicated**

Hepatic impairment dose reduction may be necessary—consult local treatment protocol for details

Pregnancy avoid (limited experience suggests fetal harm; teratogenic in *animal* studies); see also Pregnancy and Reproductive Function, p. 507

Breast-feeding discontinue breast-feeding

Side-effects see section 8.1 and notes above; abdominal pain, constipation, leucopenia, muscle pain; less commonly peripheral neuropathy; rarely paralytic ileus; irritant to tissues if extravasated

Licensed use licensed for use in children (age range not specified by manufacturer)

Indication and dose

Hodgkin's disease and other lymphomas
* By intravenous injection
  Consult local treatment protocol for details

Vinblastine (Non-proprietary) ⓅⓄⓂ
Injection, vinblastine sulphate 1 mg/mL, net price 10-mL vial = £13.09

Velbe® (Genus) ⓅⓄⓂ
Injection, powder for reconstitution, vinblastine sulphate, net price 10-mg amp = £14.15

VINCRISTINE SULPHATE

Cautions see section 8.1 and notes above; neuromuscular disease; ileus; caution in handling; **interactions**: Appendix 1 (vincristine)

Contra-indications see notes above

> Safe Practice Intrathecal injection **contra-indicated**

Hepatic impairment dose reduction may be necessary—consult local treatment protocol for details

Pregnancy avoid (teratogenicity and fetal loss in *animal* studies); see also Pregnancy and Reproductive Function, p. 507

Breast-feeding discontinue breast-feeding

Side-effects see section 8.1 and notes above; constipation (see notes above), diarrhoea, intestinal necrosis, paralytic ileus may occur in young children; dose-limiting neuromuscular effects (see notes above); urinary retention, rarely convulsions followed by coma; inappropriate secretion of antidiuretic hormone; irritant to tissues if extravasated

Licensed use licensed for use in children (age range not specified by manufacturer)

Indication and dose

Acute leukaemias, lymphomas, paediatric solid tumours
* By intravenous injection
  Consult local treatment protocol for details

Vincristine (Non-proprietary) ⓅⓄⓂ
Injection, vincristine sulphate 1 mg/mL, net price 1-mL vial = £13.47; 2-mL vial = £26.66; 5-mL vial = £44.16

◁ **VINCRISTINE SULPHATE (***continued***)**

Oncovin® (Genus) [PoM]
  Injection, vincristine sulphate 1 mg/mL, net price
  1-mL vial = £14.18; 2-mL vial = £28.05

8.1.5 Other antineoplastic drugs

Amsacrine

Amsacrine has an action and toxic effects similar to those of doxorubicin (section 8.1.2) and is given *intravenously*. It is occasionally used in acute myeloid leukaemia.

AMSACRINE

Cautions see section 8.1 and notes above; consider monitoring cardiac function; monitor electrolytes (fatal arrhythmias possible if hypokalaemia); previous treatment with anthracyclines; also caution in handling—irritant to skin and tissues

Hepatic impairment manufacturer advises reduce initial dose by 20–30%

Renal impairment manufacturer advises reduce initial dose by 20–30%

Pregnancy avoid (teratogenic and toxic in *animal* studies); may reduce fertility; see also Pregnancy and Reproductive Function, p. 507

Breast-feeding discontinue breast-feeding

Side-effects see section 8.1; mucositis, phlebitis; *less commonly* diarrhoea, cardiotoxicity, haematuria, renal impairment, hepatotoxicity, skin rash; *rarely* acute renal failure, grand mal seizures

Licensed use not licensed for use in children

Indication and dose

Acute myeloid leukaemia
• By intravenous infusion
  Consult local treatment protocol for details

Amsidine® (Goldshield) [PoM]
Concentrate for intravenous infusion, amsacrine 5 mg (as lactate)/mL, when reconstituted by mixing two solutions. Net price 1.5-mL (75-mg) amp with 13.5-mL diluent vial = £54.08 (hosp. only)

Asparaginase

Asparaginase is used almost exclusively in the treatment of acute lymphoblastic leukaemia. Hypersensitivity reactions may occur and facilities for the management of anaphylaxis should be available. A number of different preparations of asparaginase exist and only the product specified in the treatment protocol should be used.

Crisantaspase is the enzyme asparaginase produced by *Erwinia chrysanthemi*. Preparations of asparaginase derived from *Escherichia coli* are also available. Children who are hypersensitive to asparaginase derived from one organism may tolerate asparaginase derived from another organism but cross-sensitivity occurs in about 20–30% of individuals.

CRISANTASPASE

Cautions see section 8.1 and notes above

Contra-indications history of pancreatitis related to asparaginase therapy

Pregnancy avoid; see also Pregnancy and Reproductive Function, p. 507

Breast-feeding discontinue breast-feeding

Side-effects see section 8.1, also liver dysfunction, pancreatitis; diarrhoea; coagulation disorders; lethargy, drowsiness, confusion, dizziness, neurotoxicity, convulsions, headache; *less commonly* changes in blood lipids, anaphylaxis, hyperglycaemia; *rarely* CNS depression; *very rarely* myalgia; abdominal pain and hypertension also reported

Indication and dose

Acute lymphoblastic leukaemia, acute myeloid leukaemia, non-Hodgkin's lymphoma
• By intravenous, intramuscular or subcutaneous injection
  Consult local treatment protocol for details

Erwinase® (EUSA Pharma) [PoM]
Injection, powder for reconstitution, crisantaspase, net price 10 000-unit vial = £232.88

◢**Preparations**
Preparations of asparaginase derived from *Escherichia coli* are available but they are not licensed, they include: *Medac®* asparaginase, *Elspar®* asparaginase, and *Oncaspar®* pegaspargase.

Dacarbazine and temozolomide

Dacarbazine is a component of a commonly used combination for Hodgkin's disease (ABVD—doxorubicin [previously *Adriamycin®*], bleomycin, vinblastine, and dacarbazine). It is given *intravenously*.

8 Malignant disease and immunosuppression

Temozolomide is structurally related to dacarbazine and is used in children for second-line treatment of malignant glioma.

DACARBAZINE

Cautions see section 8.1; caution in handling

Hepatic impairment dose reduction may be required in combined hepatic and renal impairment; avoid in severe impairment

Renal impairment dose reduction may be required in combined renal and hepatic impairment; avoid in severe impairment

Pregnancy avoid (carcinogenic and teratogenic in *animal* studies); ensure effective contraception during and for at least 6 months after treatment in men or women; see also Pregnancy and Reproductive Function, p. 507

Breast-feeding discontinue breast-feeding

Side-effects see section 8.1; *also* anorexia; *less commonly* facial flushing, confusion, headache, seizures, facial paraesthesia, influenza-like symptoms, blurred vision, renal impairment,

rash; *rarely* diarrhoea, hepatotoxicity including liver necrosis and hepatic vein thrombosis, photosensitivity, irritant to skin and tissues, injection-site reactions

Indication and dose

Hodgkin's disease, paediatric solid tumours
• By intravenous injection or by intravenous infusion
  Consult local treatment protocol for details

Dacarbazine (Non-proprietary) ⒫
Injection, powder for reconstitution, dacarbazine (as citrate), net price 100-mg vial = £5.05; 200-mg vial = £7.16; 500-mg vial = £16.50; 600-mg vial = £22.50; 1-g vial = £31.80

TEMOZOLOMIDE

Cautions see section 8.1; **interactions:** Appendix 1 (temozolomide)

Hepatic impairment use with caution in severe impairment—no information available

Renal impairment manufacturer advises caution—no information available

Pregnancy avoid (teratogenic and embryotoxic in *animal* studies); manufacturer advises adequate contraception during treatment; see also Pregnancy and Reproductive Function, p. 507; also men should avoid fathering a child during and for at least 6 months after treatment

Breast-feeding discontinue breast-feeding

Side-effects see section 8.1

Licensed use not licensed for treatment of malignant gliomas in children under 3 years

Indication and dose

Treatment of malignant gliomas
• By mouth
  Consult local treatment protocol for details

Temodal® (Schering-Plough) ⒫
Capsules, temozolomide 5 mg (green/white), net price 5-cap pack = £16.97; 20 mg (yellow/white), 5-cap pack = £67.88; 100 mg (pink/white), 5-cap pack = £339.40; 140 mg (blue/white), 5-cap pack = £475.16; 180 mg (orange/white), 5-cap pack = £610.92; 250 mg (white), 5-cap pack = £848.50. Label: 23, 25

Imatinib

Imatinib, a tyrosine kinase inhibitor, has recently been licensed in children for the treatment of newly diagnosed Philadelphia-chromosome-positive chronic myeloid leukaemia when bone marrow transplantation is not considered first line treatment, and for Philadelphia-chromosome-positive chronic myeloid leukaemia in chronic phase after failure of interferon alfa, or in accelerated phase, or in blast crisis.

IMATINIB

Cautions see section 8.1; cardiac disease; monitor for fluid retention; monitor liver function (see also Hepatic Impairment, below); **interactions:** Appendix 1 (imatinib)

Hepatic impairment start with minimum recommended dose; reduce dose further if not tolerated; consult local treatment protocol

Renal impairment start with minimum recommended dose; reduce dose further if not tolerated; consult local treatment protocol

Pregnancy manufacturer advises avoid unless potential benefit outweighs risk; effective contraception required during treatment; see also Pregnancy and Reproductive Function, p. 507

Breast-feeding discontinue breast-feeding

Side-effects see section 8.1; also abdominal pain, appetite changes, constipation, diarrhoea, flatulence, gastro-oesophageal reflux, taste disturbance, weight changes, dry mouth; oedema (including pulmonary oedema, pleural effusion, and ascites), flushing, haemorrhage; cough, dyspnoea; dizziness, headache, insomnia, hypoaesthesia, paraesthesia, fatigue; influenza-like symptoms; cramps, arthralgia; visual disturbances, lacrimation, conjunctivitis, dry eyes; epistaxis; dry skin, sweating, rash, pruritus, photosensitivity; *less commonly* gastric ulceration, pancreatitis, hepatic dysfunction (rarely hepatic failure, hepatic necrosis), dysphagia, heart failure,

◁ **IMATINIB** (*continued*)

tachycardia, palpitation, syncope, hypertension, hypotension, cold extremities, cough, acute respiratory failure, depression, drowsiness, anxiety, peripheral neuropathy, tremor, migraine, impaired memory, vertigo, gynaecomastia, menorrhagia, irregular menstruation, sexual dysfunction, electrolyte disturbances, renal failure, urinary frequency, gout, tinnitus, hearing loss; skin hyperpigmentation; *rarely* intestinal obstruction, gastro-intestinal perforation, inflammatory bowel disease, arrhythmia, atrial fibrillation, myocardial infarction, angina, pulmonary fibrosis, pulmonary hypertension, increased intracranial pressure, convulsions, confusion, haemolytic anaemia, rhabdomyolysis, myopathy, aseptic necrosis of bone, cataract, glaucoma, angioedema, exfoliative dermatitis, and Stevens-Johnson syndrome

Indication and dose

Chronic phase and advanced phase chronic myeloid leukaemia
* By mouth
  Consult local treatment protocol for details

Glivec® (Novartis) ▼ PoM
Tablets, f/c, imatinib (as mesilate) 100 mg (yellow-brown, scored), net price 60-tab pack = £802.04; 400 mg (yellow), 30-tab pack = £1604.08. Label: 21, 27

Counselling Tablets may be dispersed in water or apple juice

Mitotane

Mitotane is used in children for the symptomatic treatment of advanced or inoperable adrenocortical carcinoma. It selectively inhibits the activity of the adrenal cortex, necessitating corticosteroid replacement therapy (section 6.3.1); the dose of glucocorticoid should be increased in case of shock, trauma, or infection. Neuro-psychological impairment can occur, possibly secondary to hypothyroidism, and growth retardation has also been reported in children treated with mitotane.

MITOTANE

Cautions see notes above; risk of accumulation in overweight patients; monitor plasma-mitotane concentration—consult product literature; **interactions**: Appendix 1 (mitotane)

Skilled tasks Central nervous system toxicity may affect performance of skilled tasks

Counselling Children and their carers should be warned to contact doctor immediately if injury, infection, or illness occurs (because of the risk of acute adrenal insufficiency)

Hepatic impairment manufacturer advises caution in mild to moderate impairment—monitoring of plasma-mitotane concentration recommended; avoid in severe impairment

Renal impairment manufacturer advises caution in mild to moderate renal impairment—monitoring of plasma-mitotane concentration recommended; avoid in severe impairment

Pregnancy manufacturer advises avoid—women of child-bearing age should use effective contraception during and after treatment; see also Pregnancy and Reproductive Function, p. 507

Breast-feeding discontinue breast-feeding

Side-effects see section 8.1 and notes above; also gastro-intestinal disturbances (including nausea, vomiting, diarrhoea, epigastric discomfort), anorexia, liver disorders; hypercholesterolaemia, hypertriglyceridaemia; ataxia, confusion, asthenia, myasthenia, paraesthesia, drowsiness, neuropathy, cognitive impairment, movement disorder, dizziness, headache; gynaecomastia; prolonged bleeding time, leucopenia, thrombocytopenia, anaemia; rash; *rarely* hypersalivation, hypertension, postural hypotension, flushing, pyrexia, haematuria, proteinuria, haemorrhagic cystitis, hypouricaemia, visual disturbances and ocular disorders

Licensed use not licensed for use in children

Indication and dose

Symptomatic treatment of advanced or inoperable adrenocortical carcinoma
* By mouth
  Consult local treatment protocol for details

Lysodren® (HRA Pharma) PoM
Tablets, scored, mitotane 500 mg, net price 100-tab pack = £460.40. Label: 2, 10, 21, counselling, skilled tasks, adrenal suppression

---

Platinum compounds

Carboplatin is used in the treatment of a variety of paediatric malignancies; it is given by intravenous infusion. Carboplatin can be given in an outpatient setting and is better tolerated than cisplatin; nausea and vomiting are less severe and nephrotoxicity, neurotoxicity, and ototoxicity are much less of a problem. Carboplatin is, however, more myelosuppressive than cisplatin.

Cisplatin is of value in children with a variety of malignancies; it is given by intravenous infusion. Cisplatin requires intensive intravenous hydration; routine use of intravenous fluids containing potassium or magnesium may also be required to help control hypokalaemia and hypomagnesaemia. Treatment may be complicated by severe nausea and vomiting; delayed vomiting may occur and is difficult to control. Cisplatin has dose-related and potentially cumulative side-effects including nephrotoxicity, neurotoxicity, and ototoxicity. Baseline testing of renal function and hearing is required; for children with pre-existing renal or hearing impairment or marked bone-marrow suppression, consideration should be given to withholding treatment or using another drug.

CARBOPLATIN

Cautions see section 8.1 and notes above; consider therapeutic drug monitoring; **interactions**: Appendix 1 (platinum compounds)

Renal impairment reduce dose and monitor haematological parameters and renal function; avoid if creatinine clearance less than 20 mL/minute/1.73 m²

Pregnancy avoid (teratogenic and embryotoxic in *animal* studies); see also Pregnancy and Reproductive Function, p. 507

Breast-feeding discontinue breast-feeding

Side-effects see section 8.1 and notes above

Licensed use not licensed for use in children

Indication and dose

Stage 4 neuroblastoma, germ cell tumours, low-grade gliomas (including astrocytomas), neuroectodermal tumours (including medulloblastoma), rhabdomyosarcoma (metastatic and non-metastatic disease), soft-tissue sarcomas, retinoblastoma, high risk Wilms' tumour, some liver tumours

• By intravenous infusion
Consult local treatment protocol for details

Carboplatin (Non-proprietary) ▣
Injection, carboplatin 10 mg/mL, net price 5-mL vial = £22.04, 15-mL vial = £56.29, 45-mL vial = £168.85, 60-mL vial = £260.00

CISPLATIN

Cautions see section 8.1 and notes above; monitor full blood count, renal function, audiology, and plasma electrolytes; **interactions**: Appendix 1 (platinum compounds)

Renal impairment avoid if possible—nephrotoxic

Pregnancy avoid (teratogenic and toxic in *animal* studies); manufacturer advises effective contraception during and for at least 3 months after treatment in men or women; see also Pregnancy and Reproductive Function, p. 507

Breast-feeding discontinue breast-feeding

Side-effects see section 8.1 and notes above; also peripheral neuropathy; hypophosphataemia, hypocalcaemia, hyperuricaemia also reported

Licensed use not licensed for use in children

Indication and dose

Osteogenic sarcoma, stage 4 neuroblastoma, some liver tumours, infant brain tumours, intracranial germ-cell tumours

• By intravenous infusion
Consult local treatment protocol for details

Cisplatin (Non-proprietary) ▣
Injection, cisplatin 1 mg/mL, net price 10-mL vial = £5.85, 50-mL vial = £24.50, 100-mL vial = £50.22

Injection, powder for reconstitution, cisplatin, net price 50-mg vial = £17.00

Procarbazine

Procarbazine is most often used in Hodgkin's disease. It is given *by mouth*. It is a weak monoamine-oxidase inhibitor and dietary restriction is rarely considered necessary. Alcohol ingestion may cause a disulfiram-like reaction.

PROCARBAZINE

Cautions see section 8.1 and notes above; **interactions**: Appendix 1 (procarbazine)

Hepatic impairment caution in mild to moderate impairment; avoid in severe impairment

Renal impairment caution in mild to moderate impairment; avoid in severe impairment

Pregnancy avoid (teratogenic in *animal* studies and isolated reports in humans); see also Pregnancy and Reproductive Function, p. 507

Breast-feeding discontinue breast-feeding

Side-effects see section 8.1 and notes above; hypersensitivity rash (discontinue treatment)

Indication and dose

Hodgkin's lymphoma, gliomas
• By mouth
Consult local treatment protocol for details

Procarbazine (Non-proprietary) ▣
Capsules, ivory, procarbazine (as hydrochloride) 50 mg, net price 50-cap pack = £190.09. Label: 4

◢Extemporaneous formulations available see Extemporaneous Preparations, p. 8

Tretinoin

Tretinoin is licensed for the induction of remission in acute promyelocytic leukaemia. It is used in previously untreated children as well as in those who have relapsed after standard chemotherapy or who are refractory to it.

▲ TRETINOIN

Note Tretinoin is the acid form of vitamin A

Cautions exclude pregnancy before starting treatment, see also Pregnancy below; monitor full blood count and coagulation profile, liver function, serum calcium and plasma lipids before and during treatment; increased risk of thromboembolism during first month of treatment; **interactions:** Appendix 1 (retinoids)

Hepatic impairment reduce dose—consult local treatment protocol for details

Renal impairment reduce dose—consult local treatment protocol for details

Pregnancy teratogenic; effective contraception must be used for at least 1 month before oral treatment, during treatment and for at least 1 month after stopping (oral progestogen-only contraceptives **not** considered effective); see also Pregnancy and Reproductive Function, p. 507

Breast-feeding discontinue breast-feeding

Side-effects retinoic acid syndrome (fever, dyspnoea, acute respiratory distress, pulmonary infiltrates, pleural effusion, hyperleukocytosis, hypotension, oedema, weight gain, hepatic, renal and multi-organ failure) requires immediate treatment—consult product literature; gastrointestinal disturbances, pancreatitis; arrhythmias, flushing, oedema; headache, benign intracranial hypertension (children particularly susceptible—consider dose reduction if intractable headache), shivering, dizziness, confusion, anxiety, depression, insomnia, paraesthesia, visual and hearing disturbances (children particularly susceptible to nervous system effects); raised liver enzymes, serum creatinine and lipids; bone and chest pain, alopecia, erythema, rash, pruritus, sweating, dry skin and mucous membranes, cheilitis; thromboembolism, hypercalcaemia, and genital ulceration reported

Indication and dose

Acute promyelocytic leukaemia
- By mouth
  Consult treatment protocol for details

Vesanoid® (Roche) [PoM]
Capsules, yellow/brown, tretinoin 10 mg, net price 100-cap pack = £163.87. Label: 21, 25

8.2 Drugs affecting the immune response

- 8.2.1 Antiproliferative immunosuppressants
- 8.2.2 Corticosteroids and other immunosuppressants
- 8.2.3 Rituximab and alemtuzumab
- 8.2.4 Other immunomodulating drugs

Immunosuppressant therapy

Immunosuppressants are used to suppress rejection in organ transplant recipients and to treat a variety of chronic inflammatory and autoimmune diseases. Solid organ transplant patients are usually maintained on a calcineurin inhibitor (ciclosporin or tacrolimus), combined with an antiproliferative drug (azathioprine or mycophenolate mofetil) and a corticosteroid. Specialist management is required and other immunomodulators may be used to initiate treatment or to treat rejection.

> **Bioavailability**
> Different formulations of the same immunosuppressant may vary in bioavailability and to avoid reduced effect or excessive side-effects, it is important not to change formulation except on the advice of a transplant specialist.

Impaired immune responsiveness   Infections in the immunocompromised child can be severe and show atypical features. Specific local protocols should be followed for the management of infection. Corticosteroids may suppress clinical signs of infection and allow diseases such as septicaemia or tuberculosis to reach an advanced stage before being recognised. Children should be up-to-date with their childhood vaccinations before initiation of immunosuppressant therapy (e.g. before transplantation); vaccination with varicella-zoster vaccine (section 14.4) is also necessary during this period—**important:** for advice on measles exposure, see section 14.5.1, and chickenpox (varicella) exposure, see section 14.5.2. For advice on the use of live vaccines in individuals with impaired immune response, see section 14.1. For general comments and warnings relating to corticosteroids and immunosuppressants, see section 6.3.2.

Pregnancy   Transplant patients immunosuppressed with azathioprine should not discontinue it on becoming pregnant. However, there have been reports of premature birth and low birth-weight following exposure to azathioprine, particularly in combination with corticosteroids. Spontaneous abortion has been reported following maternal or paternal exposure. Azathioprine is teratogenic in *animal* studies.

There is less experience of ciclosporin in pregnancy but it does not appear to be any more harmful than azathioprine. The use of these drugs during pregnancy needs to be supervised in specialist units.

8.2.1 Antiproliferative immunosuppressants

Azathioprine is widely used for transplant recipients and it is also used to treat a number of auto-immune conditions (see section 10.1.3), usually when cortico-steroid therapy alone provides inadequate control. It is metabolised to mercapto-purine, and doses should be reduced to one quarter of the original dose when allopurinol is given concurrently.

Blood tests and monitoring for signs of myelosuppression are essential in long-term treatment with azathioprine. The enzyme thiopurine methyltransferase (TPMT) metabolises azathioprine; the risk of myelosuppression is increased in those with reduced activity of the enzyme, particularly in the few individuals who are deficient for TPMT activity. Consider measuring TPMT activity before starting azathioprine therapy. Patients with deficient TPMT activity should not receive azathioprine; those with reduced TPMT activity may be treated under specialist supervision.

Mycophenolate mofetil is metabolised to mycophenolic acid which has a more selective mode of action than azathioprine. It is used in combination with a corticosteroid and either ciclosporin or tacrolimus for the prophylaxis of acute rejection in transplant recipients. Compared with similar regimens incorporating azathioprine, mycophenolate mofetil may reduce the risk of acute rejection episodes; the risk of opportunistic infections (particularly due to tissue-invasive cytomegalovirus) and the occurrence of blood disorders such as leucopenia may be higher. Children may suffer a high incidence of side-effects, particularly gastro-intestinal effects, calling for temporary reduction in dose or interruption of treatment. Cases of pure red cell aplasia have been reported with mycophenolate mofetil; dose reduction or discontinuation of mycophenolate mofetil should be considered under specialist supervision.

> **NICE guidance (immunosuppressive therapy for renal transplantation in children and adolescents)**
> See p. 528

Cyclophosphamide (section 8.1.1) is less commonly prescribed as an immuno-suppressant.

AZATHIOPRINE

Cautions monitor for toxicity throughout treatment; monitor full blood count weekly (more frequently with higher doses or if hepatic or renal impairment) for first 4 weeks (manufacturer advises weekly monitoring for 8 weeks but evidence of practical value unsatisfactory), thereafter reduce frequency of monitoring to at least every 3 months; **interactions**: Appendix 1 (azathioprine)

Bone marrow suppression Children and their carers should be warned to report immediately any signs or symptoms of bone marrow suppression e.g. inexplicable bruising or bleeding, infection

Contra-indications hypersensitivity to azathioprine or mercaptopurine

Hepatic impairment may need dose reduction

Renal impairment reduce dose and monitor full blood count

Pregnancy see section 8.2; treatment should not normally be initiated during pregnancy

Breast-feeding teratogenic metabolite present in milk in low concentration but no evidence of harm in small studies—consider if potential benefit outweighs risk

Side-effects hypersensitivity reactions (including malaise, dizziness, vomiting, diarrhoea, fever, rigors, myalgia, arthralgia, rash, hypotension and interstitial nephritis—calling for immediate withdrawal); dose-related bone marrow suppression (see also Cautions); liver impairment, cholestatic jaundice, hair loss and increased susceptibility to infections and colitis in patients also receiving corticosteroids; nausea; rarely pancreatitis, pneumonitis, hepatic veno-occlusive disease

Indication and dose

Suppression of transplant rejection
- By mouth, or (if oral route not possible) by intravenous infusion (see also note below)
  Consult local treatment protocol for details
  Child 1 month–18 years maintenance, 1–3 mg/kg once daily, adjusted according to response; total daily dose may alternatively be given in 2 divided doses

Severe ulcerative colitis and Crohn's disease section 1.5.3

◻ **AZATHIOPRINE** (*continued*)

> **Systemic lupus erythematosus, vasculitis, auto-immune conditions when corticosteroid therapy alone has proved inadequate** section 10.1.3

Administration Consult local treatment protocol for details

For *intravenous injection*, give over at least 1 minute

For *intravenous infusion*, dilute to a concentration of 0.25–2.5 mg/mL in Glucose 5% *or* Sodium Chloride 0.9% *or* Sodium Chloride and Glucose; give over 30–60 minutes

Note Intravenous injection is alkaline and very irritant. Intravenous route should therefore be used **only** if oral route not feasible and discontinued as soon as oral route

can be tolerated. To reduce irritation flush line with sodium chloride 0.9% *or* glucose 4%/sodium chloride 0.18%.

Azathioprine (Non-proprietary) ▣PoM
Tablets, azathioprine 25 mg, net price 28-tab pack = £9.88; 50 mg, 56-tab pack = £8.22. Label: 21
Brands include *Azamune*®

Imuran® (Aspen) ▣PoM
Tablets, both f/c, azathioprine 25 mg (orange), net price 100-tab pack = £10.99; 50 mg (yellow), 100-tab pack = £7.99. Label: 21

Injection, powder for reconstitution, azathioprine (as sodium salt), net price 50-mg vial = £15.38

◢ Extemporaneous formulations available see Extemporaneous Preparations, p. 8

◢ **MYCOPHENOLATE MOFETIL**

Cautions full blood counts every week for 4 weeks then twice a month for 2 months then every month in the first year (consider interrupting treatment if neutropenia develops); active gastro-intestinal disease (risk of haemorrhage, ulceration and perforation); delayed graft function; increased susceptibility to skin cancer (avoid exposure to strong sunlight); possible decreased effectiveness of vaccination—avoid live vaccines; **interactions:** Appendix 1 (mycophenolate mofetil)

Bone marrow suppression Children and their carers should be warned to report immediately any signs or symptoms of bone marrow suppression e.g. infection or inexplicable bruising or bleeding

Renal impairment manufacturer advises consider dose reduction if estimated glomerular filtration rate less than 25 mL/minute/1.73 m²

Pregnancy manufacturer advises avoid—congenital malformations reported; effective contraception required before treatment, during treatment, and for 6 weeks after discontinuation of treatment

Breast-feeding manufacturer advises avoid—present in milk in *animal* studies

Side-effects gastro-intestinal disturbances (including diarrhoea, vomiting, and abdominal pain), gastro-intestinal ulceration and bleeding, oesophagitis, abnormal liver function tests, hepatitis, jaundice, pancreatitis; oedema, tachycardia, hypertension, hypotension, vasodilation; cough, dyspnoea; insomnia, agitation, tremor, dizziness, headache; influenza-like syndrome, infections (viral, bacterial and fungal); hyperglycaemia; renal impairment; increased risk of malignancies particularly of the skin; blood disorders (including leucopenia, anaemia, thrombocytopenia, pancytopenia, and red cell aplasia—see notes above), disturbances of electrolytes and blood lipids; arthralgia; alopecia, acne, and rash; progressive multifocal leucoencephalopathy, interstitial lung disease, and pulmonary fibrosis reported

Licensed use by mouth, in combination with a corticosteroid and ciclosporin, for children 2 years and older for the prophylaxis of acute transplant rejection in renal transplantation

Indication and dose

> **Prophylaxis of acute rejection in renal transplantation in combination with a corticosteroid and ciclosporin**
> • By mouth or by intravenous infusion
> Consult local treatment protocol for details
> **Child 1 month–18 years** 600 mg/m² twice daily (max. 2 g daily)

> **Prophylaxis of acute rejection in renal transplantation in combination with a corticosteroid and tacrolimus**
> • By mouth or by intravenous infusion
> Consult local treatment protocol for details
> **Child 1 month–18 years** 300 mg/m² twice daily (max. 2 g daily)

> **Prophylaxis of acute rejection in hepatic transplantation in combination with a corticosteroid and ciclosporin or tacrolimus**
> • By mouth or by intravenous infusion
> Consult local treatment protocol for details
> **Child 1 month–18 years** 10 mg/kg twice daily, increased to 20 mg/kg twice daily (max. 2 g daily)

Note Tablets and capsules not appropriate for dose titration in children with body surface area less than 1.25 m²

Administration For *intravenous infusion*, dilute reconstituted solution to a concentration of 6 mg/mL in Glucose 5%; infuse over 2 hours

CellCept® (Roche) ▣PoM
Capsules, blue/brown, mycophenolate mofetil 250 mg, net price 100-cap pack = £83.92

Tablets, lavender, mycophenolate mofetil 500 mg, net price 50-tab pack = £83.92

Oral suspension, mycophenolate mofetil 1 g/5 mL when reconstituted with water, net price 175 mL = £117.48
Excipients include aspartame (section 9.4.1)

Intravenous infusion, powder for reconstitution, mycophenolate mofetil (as hydrochloride), net price 500-mg vial = £9.31

8

Malignant disease and immunosuppression

8.2.2 Corticosteroids and other immunosuppressants

The corticosteroids prednisolone and dexamethasone are widely used in paediatric oncology; they have a marked antitumour effect. Dexamethasone is preferred for acute lymphoblastic leukaemia whilst prednisolone may be used for Hodgkin's disease, non-Hodgkin's lymphoma, and B-cell lymphoma and leukaemia.

Dexamethasone is the corticosteroid of choice in paediatric supportive and palliative care. For children who are not receiving a corticosteroid as a component of their chemotherapy, dexamethasone may be used to reduce raised intracranial pressure (see p. 28), or to help control emesis when combined with an appropriate anti-emetic (see p. 27). For more information on glucocorticoid therapy, including the disadvantages of treatment, see section 6.3.2.

The corticosteroids are also powerful immunosuppressants. They are used to prevent organ transplant rejection, and in high dose to treat rejection episodes.

Ciclosporin (cyclosporin), a calcineurin inhibitor, is a potent immunosuppressant which is virtually non-myelotoxic but markedly nephrotoxic. It may be used in organ and tissue transplantation, for prevention of graft rejection following bone marrow, kidney, liver, pancreas, heart, lung, and heart-lung transplantation, and for prophylaxis and treatment of graft-versus-host disease. Ciclosporin also has a role in steroid-sensitive and steroid-resistant nephrotic syndrome; in corticosteroid-sensitive nephrotic syndrome it may be given with prednisolone (section 6.3).

Tacrolimus is also a calcineurin inhibitor. Although not chemically related to ciclosporin it has a similar mode of action and side-effects.

Sirolimus is a potent non-calcineurin inhibiting immunosuppressant.

Basiliximab is a monoclonal antibody that prevents T-lymphocyte proliferation; it is used for prophylaxis of acute rejection in allogeneic renal transplantation. It is given with ciclosporin and corticosteroid immunosuppression regimens; its use should be confined to specialist centres.

Antithymocyte immunoglobulin (rabbit) is used for the prophylaxis of organ rejection in renal and heart allograft recipients and for the treatment of corticosteroid-resistant allograft rejection in renal transplantation. Tolerability is increased by pretreatment with an intravenous corticosteroid and antihistamine; an antipyretic drug such as paracetamol may also be beneficial.

> **NICE guidance**
>
> **Immunosuppressive therapy for renal transplantation in children and adolescents (April 2006)**
>
> NICE has recommended that for induction therapy in the prophylaxis of organ rejection, either basiliximab or daclizumab [discontinued] are options for combining with a calcineurin inhibitor. For each individual, ciclosporin or tacrolimus is chosen as the calcineurin inhibitor on the basis of side-effects. Mycophenolate mofetil is recommended as part of an immunosuppressive regimen **only if**:
>
> - the calcineurin inhibitor is not tolerated, particularly if nephrotoxicity endangers the transplanted kidney; *or*
> - there is very high risk of nephrotoxicity from the calcineurin inhibitor, requiring a reduction in the dose of the calcineurin inhibitor or its avoidance.
>
> Mycophenolic acid is not recommended as part of an immunosuppressive regimen for renal transplantation in children or adolescents.
>
> Sirolimus [not licensed for use in children] is recommended as a component of immunosuppressive regimen **only if** intolerance necessitates the withdrawal of a calcineurin inhibitor.
>
> These recommendations may not be consistent with the marketing authorisation of some of the products.

ANTITHYMOCYTE IMMUNOGLOBULIN (RABBIT)

Cautions see notes above; monitor blood count

Contra-indications infection

Pregnancy manufacturer advises use only if potential benefit outweighs risk—no information available

◁ **ANTITHYMOCYTE IMMUNOGLOBULIN (RABBIT)** *(continued)*

Breast-feeding manufacturer advises avoid—no information available

Side-effects nausea, vomiting, dysphagia, diarrhoea; hypotension; infusion-related reactions (including cytokine release syndrome and anaphylaxis, see notes above), serum sickness; fever, shivering, increased susceptibility to infection; increased susceptibility to malignancy; lymphopenia, neutropenia, thrombocytopenia; myalgia; pruritus, rash

Indication and dose

Heart transplantation
- **By intravenous infusion over at least 6 hours**
  Child 1 month–18 years 1–2.5 mg/kg daily for 3–5 days starting the day of transplantation
  Note To avoid excessive dosage in obese patients, calculate dose on the basis of ideal body weight

Renal transplantation
- **By intravenous infusion over at least 6 hours**
  Child 1–18 years 1–1.5 mg/kg daily for 3–9 days starting the day of transplantation
  Note To avoid excessive dosage in obese patients, calculate dose on the basis of ideal body weight

Corticosteroid-resistant renal graft rejection
- **By intravenous infusion over at least 6 hours**
  Child 1–18 years 1.5 mg/kg daily for 7–14 days
  Note To avoid excessive dosage in obese patients, calculate dose on the basis of ideal body weight

Administration For *continuous intravenous infusion* reconstitute each vial with 5 mL water for injection to produce a solution of 5 mg/mL; gently rotate to dissolve. Dilute requisite dose with Glucose 5% *or* Sodium Chloride 0.9% to an approx. concentration of 0.5 mg/mL; begin infusion immediately after dilution; give through an in-line filter (pore size 0.22 micron); incompatible with unfractionated heparin and hydrocortisone in glucose infusion—precipitation reported

Thymoglobuline® (Genzyme) ▼ PoM
Intravenous infusion, powder for reconstitution, rabbit anti-human thymocyte immunoglobulin, net price 25-mg vial = £168.18

■ **BASILIXIMAB**

Pregnancy manufacturer advises avoid—no information available; adequate contraception must be used during treatment and for 16 weeks after last dose

Breast-feeding manufacturer advises avoid—no information available

Side-effects severe hypersensitivity reactions and cytokine release syndrome reported

Indication and dose

Prophylaxis of acute rejection in allogeneic renal transplantation used in combination with ciclosporin and corticosteroid-containing immunosuppression regimens
- **By intravenous injection or by intravenous infusion**
  Consult local treatment protocol for details
  Child over 1 year, body-weight under 35 kg 10 mg within 2 hours before transplant surgery and 10 mg 4 days after surgery

Child body-weight over 35 kg 20 mg within 2 hours before transplant surgery and 20 mg 4 days after surgery

Note withhold second dose if severe hypersensitivity or graft loss occurs

Administration For *intravenous infusion*, dilute reconstituted solution to a concentration not exceeding 400 micrograms/mL, with Glucose 5% *or* Sodium Chloride 0.9%; give over 20–30 minutes

Simulect® (Novartis) PoM
Injection, powder for reconstitution, basiliximab, net price 10-mg vial = £758.69, 20-mg vial = £842.38 (both with water for injections). For intravenous infusion

■ **CICLOSPORIN**

(Cyclosporin)

Cautions monitor kidney function—dose dependent increase in serum creatinine and urea during first few weeks may necessitate discontinuation (exclude rejection of kidney transplant); monitor liver function (see also Hepatic Impairment below); monitor blood pressure—discontinue if hypertension develops that cannot be controlled by antihypertensives; hyperuricaemia; monitor serum potassium especially in renal dysfunction (risk of hyperkalaemia); monitor serum magnesium; measure blood lipids before treatment and thereafter as appropriate; monitor whole blood ciclosporin concentration (trough level depen-

dent on indication—consult local treatment protocol for details); use with tacrolimus specifically contra-indicated; for patients other than transplant recipients, preferably avoid other immunosuppressants (increased risk of infection and malignancies, including lymphoma and skin cancer); avoid excessive exposure to UV light, including sunlight; **interactions:** Appendix 1 (ciclosporin)

Additional cautions in nephrotic syndrome *Contra-indicated* in uncontrolled hypertension, uncontrolled infections, and malignancy; in long-term management, perform renal biopsies every 1–2 years

Additional cautions Atopic Dermatitis and Psoriasis, section 13.5.3; Rheumatoid Arthritis, section 10.1.3

8 *Malignant disease and immunosuppression*

◁ **CICLOSPORIN** (*continued*)

Hepatic impairment dosage adjustment based on bilirubin and liver enzymes may be needed

Renal impairment dose as in normal renal function but see Cautions above; in *nephrotic syndrome* reduce dose by 25–50% if serum creatinine more than 30% above baseline on more than one measurement

Pregnancy crosses placenta; see Immunosuppressant Therapy, p. 525

Breast-feeding present in milk—manufacturer advises avoid

Side-effects gastro-intestinal disturbances, gingival hyperplasia, hepatic dysfunction, anorexia; hypertension; tremor, headache, paraesthesia, fatigue; renal dysfunction (renal structural changes on long-term administration; see also under Cautions), hyperuricaemia, hyperkalaemia, hypomagnesaemia, hyperlipidaemia, hypercholesterolaemia; muscle cramps, myalgia; hypertrichosis; *less commonly* oedema, weight gain, encephalopathy, anaemia, thrombocytopenia, rash; *rarely* pancreatitis, motor polyneuropathy, menstrual disturbances, gynaecomastia, micro-angiopathic haemolytic anaemia, haemolytic uraemic syndrome, hyperglycaemia, muscle weakness, myopathy; visual disturbances secondary to benign intracranial hypertension (discontinue), also anaphylaxis reported with infusion

Licensed use not licensed for use in children under 3 months

Indication and dose

Prevention of graft rejection following bone-marrow, kidney, liver, pancreas, heart, lung, and heart-lung transplantation, prophylaxis and treatment of graft-versus-host disease
• By mouth or by intravenous infusion
   Consult local treatment protocols for details

Nephrotic syndrome see also section 6.3.2, p. 452
• By mouth
   Child 1 month–18 years 3 mg/kg twice daily, increase if necessary in corticosteroid-resistant disease; for maintenance reduce to lowest effective dose according to whole blood-ciclosporin concentrations, proteinuria, and renal function

Refractory ulcerative colitis section 1.5.3

Severe psoriasis, severe eczema section 13.5.3

Important Patients should be stabilised on a particular brand and formulation of oral ciclosporin because switching between formulations without close monitoring may lead to clinically important changes in blood-ciclosporin concentration. Prescribing and dispensing of ciclosporin should be by brand name to avoid inadvertent switching. If it is necessary to switch a patient to a different brand or formulation of ciclosporin, the patient should be monitored closely for changes in blood-ciclosporin concentration, serum-creatinine, blood pressure, and transplant function.

Deximune® (Dexcel) [PoM]
Capsules, grey, ciclosporin 25 mg, net price 30-cap pack = £15.76; 50 mg 30-cap pack = £30.86; 100 mg 30-cap pack = £58.57. Counselling, administration
Note Contains ethyl lactate which is metabolised to ethanol
Counselling Total daily dose should be taken in 2 divided doses. Avoid grapefruit or grapefruit juice 1 hour before dose

Neoral® (Novartis) [PoM]
Capsules, ciclosporin 10 mg (yellow/white), net price 60-cap pack = £20.88; 25 mg (blue/grey), 30-cap pack = £21.01; 50 mg (yellow/white), 30-cap pack = £41.14; 100 mg (blue/grey), 30-cap pack = £78.09. Counselling, administration
Excipients include propylene glycol (see Excipients, p. 3)
Note Contains ethanol

Oral solution, yellow, sugar-free, ciclosporin 100 mg/mL, net price 50 mL = £117.00. Counselling, administration
Excipients include propylene glycol (see Excipients, p. 3)
Note Contains ethanol
Counselling Total daily dose should be taken in 2 divided doses. Avoid grapefruit or grapefruit juice for 1 hour before dose
Mix solution with orange juice (or squash) or apple juice (to improve taste) or with water immediately before taking (and rinse with more to ensure total dose). Do not mix with grapefruit juice. Keep medicine measure away from other liquids (including water)

Sandimmun® (Novartis) [PoM]
Concentrate for intravenous infusion (oily), ciclosporin 50 mg/mL. To be diluted before use, net price 1-mL amp = £1.94; 5-mL amp = £9.17
Excipients include polyoxyl castor oil (risk of anaphylaxis, see Excipients, p. 3)
Note Contains ethanol
Administration For *intravenous infusion*, dilute to a concentration of 0.5–2.5 mg/mL with Glucose 5% *or* Sodium Chloride 0.9%; give over 2–6 hours; not to be used with PVC equipment; observe patient for signs of anaphylaxis for at least 30 minutes after starting infusion and at frequent intervals thereafter
Note Capsules and oral solution available direct from Novartis for children who cannot be transferred to a different oral preparation

▌ **SIROLIMUS**

Cautions monitor renal function when given with ciclosporin; Afro-Caribbean patients may require higher doses; **interactions:** Appendix 1 (sirolimus)

Hepatic impairment dose reduction may be necessary, consult local treatment protocol for details; monitor blood-sirolimus trough concentration

Pregnancy avoid unless essential—toxicity in *animal* studies; effective contraception must be used during treatment and for 12 weeks after stopping

Breast-feeding discontinue breast-feeding

Side-effects abdominal pain, diarrhoea, stomatitis, abnormal liver-function tests (elevated transaminases); oedema, tachycardia, hypercholesterolaemia, hypertriglyceridaemia, venous

◻ **SIROLIMUS (continued)**

thromboembolism; pneumonitis; pyrexia, increased susceptibility to infection (especially urinary-tract infection); proteinuria, haemolytic uraemic syndrome; anaemia, thrombocytopenia, thrombotic thrombocytopenic purpura, leucopenia, neutropenia, hypokalaemia, hypophosphataemia, hyperglycaemia, lymphocele; arthralgia, osteonecrosis; epistaxis; acne, rash, impaired healing; *less commonly* pancreatitis, pulmonary embolism, pulmonary haemorrhage, pericardial effusion, nephrotic syndrome, increased susceptibility to lymphoma and other malignancies particularly of the skin, and pancytopenia; *rarely* interstitial lung disease, hepatic necrosis, lymphoedema, and hypersensitivity reactions including anaphylactic reactions, angiodema, exfoliative dermatitis, and hypersensitivity vasculitis

Licensed use not licensed for use in children

Indication and dose

See NICE guidance, p. 528

● **By mouth**
Consult local treatment protocols for details

Rapamune® (Wyeth) PoM
Tablets, coated, sirolimus 1 mg (white), net price 30-tab pack = £86.49; 2 mg (yellow), 30-tab pack = £172.98. Counselling, administration

Oral solution, sirolimus 1 mg/mL, net price 60 mL = £162.41. Counselling, administration

Administration food may affect absorption (give at the same time with respect to food). Mix solution with at least 60 mL water or orange juice in a glass or plastic container immediately before taking; refill container with at least 120 mL of water or orange juice and drink immediately (to ensure total dose). Do not mix with any other liquids

---

▮ TACROLIMUS

Cautions monitor blood pressure, ECG (**important**: see cardiomyopathy below), fasting blood-glucose concentration, haematological and neurological, including visual, parameters, electrolytes, hepatic and renal function; monitor whole blood-tacrolimus trough concentration (especially during episodes of diarrhoea)—consult local treatment protocol for details; QT-interval prolongation; neurotoxicity; increased risk of infections, malignancies, and lymphoproliferative disorders; avoid excessive exposure to UV light (including sunlight); pregnancy (exclude before starting—if contraception needed non-hormonal methods should be used); **interactions**: Appendix 1 (tacrolimus)

Skilled tasks May affect performance of skilled tasks (e.g. driving)

Contra-indications hypersensitivity to macrolides; avoid concurrent administration with ciclosporin (care if patient has previously received ciclosporin)

Hepatic impairment dose reduction may be necessary in severe impairment

Pregnancy avoid unless potential benefit outweighs risk—risk of premature delivery, intra-uterine growth restriction, and hyperkalaemia; toxicity in *animal* studies

Breast-feeding avoid—present in milk

Side-effects gastro-intestinal disturbances (including nausea, vomiting, diarrhoea, constipation, dyspepsia, inflammatory and ulcerative disorders), hepatic dysfunction, jaundice, bile-duct and gall-bladder abnormalities; tachycardia, hypertension, thromboembolic and ischaemic events; dyspnoea, pleural effusion, and parenchymal lung disorders; insomnia, tremor, headache, mood changes, depression, confusion, seizures, paraesthesia, dizziness, nightmares; hyperglycaemia; renal impairment; electrolyte disturbances (including hyperkalaemia and hyperuricaemia); anaemia, leucopenia, thrombocytopenia, coagulation disorders; arthralgia, muscle cramps; visual disturbances; tinnitus; alopecia, acne; *less commonly* hypoglycaemia, pancreatitis, respiratory failure, heart failure, arrhythmias, cerebrovascular accidents, encephalopathy, psychosis, photosensitivity, dermatitis; *rarely* cardiomyopathy (**important**: see cardiomyopathy below), pericardial effusion, toxic epidermal necrolysis, hirsutism; *very rarely* myasthenia

Cardiomyopathy Cardiomyopathy has been reported in children given tacrolimus after transplantation. Children should be monitored carefully by echocardiography for hypertrophic changes; dose reduction or discontinuation should be considered if these occur

Licensed use *Advagraf®* not licensed for use in children

Indication and dose

See under preparations and consult local treatment protocols

Atopic eczema (topical use) section 13.5.3

> **Important** *Prograf®*, *Modigraf®*, and *Advagraf®* (tacrolimus): serious medication errors.
> It is important to note the correct use of these medicines:
> ● *Prograf®* is an immediate-release formulation that is taken twice daily, once in the morning and once in the evening;
> ● *Modigraf®* granules are used to prepare an immediate-release suspension which is taken twice daily, once in the morning and once in the evening;
> ● *Advagraf®* is a prolonged-release formulation that is taken once daily in the morning.
> Switching between *Prograf®*, *Modigraf®*, and *Advagraf®* requires careful therapeutic monitoring. Substitution should be made only under the close supervision of a transplant specialist.

Administration For *continuous intravenous infusion* over 24 hours, dilute to a concentration of 4–100 micrograms/mL with Glucose 5% *or* Sodium Chloride 0.9%, to a total volume between 20–500 mL; incompatible with PVC

Modigraf® (Astellas) ▼ PoM
Granules, tacrolimus (as monohydrate), 200 micrograms, net price 50-sachet pack = £71.30; 1 mg,

◻ **TACROLIMUS** (*continued*)

50-sachet pack = £356.65. Label: 13, 23, counselling, skilled tasks

Note Tacrolimus is incompatible with PVC

Dose

> Prophylaxis of graft rejection following liver transplantation, starting 12 hours after transplantation
> • By mouth
> > **Child 1 month–18 years** 150 micrograms/kg twice daily, adjusted according to whole blood concentration

> Prophylaxis of graft rejection following kidney transplantation, starting within 24 hours of transplantation
> • By mouth
> > **Child 1 month–18 years** 150 micrograms/kg twice daily, adjusted according to whole blood concentration

> Prophylaxis of graft rejection following heart transplantation *without antibody induction* starting within 5 days of transplantation
> • By mouth
> > **Child 1 month–18 years** 150 micrograms/kg twice daily as soon as clinically possible (8–12 hours after discontinuing intravenous infusion), adjusted according to whole blood concentration

> Prophylaxis of graft rejection following heart transplantation *following antibody induction* starting within 5 days of transplantation
> • By mouth
> > **Child 1 month–18 years** 50–150 micrograms/kg twice daily, adjusted according to whole blood concentration

> Allograft rejection resistant to conventional immunosuppressive therapy Consult local treatment protocol

Prograf® (Astellas) [PoM]

Capsules, tacrolimus (as monohydrate) 500 micrograms (yellow), net price 50-cap pack = £63.13; 1 mg (white), 50-cap pack = £81.90, 100-cap pack = £163.78; 5 mg (greyish-red), 50-cap pack = £302.56. Label: 23, counselling, driving

Concentrate for intravenous infusion, tacrolimus 5 mg/mL. To be diluted before use. Net price 1-mL amp = £59.63
Excipients include polyoxyl castor oil (risk of anaphylaxis, see Excipients, p. 3)

Dose

> Prophylaxis of graft rejection following liver transplantation, starting 12 hours after transplantation
> • By mouth
> > **Child 1 month–18 years** initially 150 micrograms/kg twice daily, adjusted according to whole blood concentration

> • By continuous intravenous infusion (only if oral route inappropriate)
> > **Child 1 month–18 years** 50 micrograms/kg over 24 hours for up to 7 days (then transfer to oral therapy), adjusted according to whole blood concentration

> Prophylaxis of graft rejection following kidney transplantation, starting within 24 hours of transplantation
> • By mouth
> > **Child 1 month–18 years** initially 150 micrograms/kg twice daily adjusted according to whole blood concentration
> > Note A lower dose of 100 micrograms/kg twice daily has been used in adolescents to prevent very high 'trough' concentrations

> • By continuous intravenous infusion (only if oral route inappropriate)
> > **Child 1 month–18 years** 75–100 micrograms/kg over 24 hours for up to 7 days (then transfer to oral therapy), adjusted according to whole blood concentration

> Prophylaxis of graft rejection following heart transplantation *without antibody induction*, starting within 5 days of transplantation
> • By mouth
> > **Child 1 month–18 years** 150 micrograms/kg twice daily as soon as clinically possible (8–12 hours after discontinuation of intravenous infusion), adjusted according to whole blood concentration

> • By continuous intravenous infusion
> > **Child 1 month–18 years** initially 30–50 micrograms/kg daily over 24 hours for up to 7 days (then transfer to oral therapy), adjusted according to whole blood concentration

> Prophylaxis of graft rejection following heart transplantation *following antibody induction*, starting within 5 days of transplantation
> • By mouth
> > **Child 1 month–18 years** 50–150 micrograms/kg twice daily, adjusted according to whole blood concentration

> Allograft rejection resistant to conventional immunosuppressive therapy Consult local treatment protocol

◢**Modified release**
Advagraf® is not licensed for use in children

Advagraf® (Astellas) [PoM]

Capsules, m/r, tacrolimus (as monohydrate) 500 micrograms (yellow/orange), net price 50-cap pack = £35.79; 1 mg (white/orange), 50-cap pack = £71.59, 100-cap pack = £143.17; 3 mg (red/orange), 50-cap pack = £214.76; 5 mg (red/orange), 50-cap pack = £266.92. Label: 23, 25, counselling, driving

◢Extemporaneous formulations available see Extemporaneous Preparations, p. 8

Rituximab, a monoclonal antibody which causes lysis of B lymphocytes, has been used as a component of the treatment of post-transplantation lymphoproliferative disease, non-Hodgkin's lymphoma, Hodgkin's lymphoma, and severe cases of resistant immune modulated disease including idiopathic thrombocytopenia purpura, haemolytic anaemia, and systemic lupus erythematosus. Full resuscitation facilities should be at hand and as with other cytotoxics, treatment should be undertaken under the close supervision of a specialist.

Rituximab should be used with caution in children receiving cardiotoxic chemotherapy or with a history of cardiovascular disease; in adults exacerbation of angina, arrhythmia, and heart failure have been reported. Transient hypotension occurs frequently during infusion and antihypertensives may need to be withheld for 12 hours before infusion. Progressive multifocal leucoencephalopathy (which is usually fatal or causes severe disability) has been reported in association with rituximab; children treated with rituximab should be monitored for cognitive, neurological, or psychiatric signs and symptoms. If progressive multifocal leucoencephalopathy is suspected, suspend treatment until it has been excluded.

Infusion-related side-effects (including cytokine release syndrome) are reported commonly with rituximab and occur predominantly during the first infusion; they include fever and chills, nausea and vomiting, allergic reactions (such as rash, pruritus, angioedema, bronchospasm and dyspnoea), flushing and tumour pain. Children should be given an analgesic and an antihistamine before each dose of rituximab to reduce these effects. Premedication with a corticosteroid should also be considered. The infusion may have to be stopped temporarily and the infusion-related effects treated—consult product literature or local treatment protocol for appropriate management. Evidence of pulmonary infiltration and features of tumour lysis syndrome should be sought if infusion-related effects occur.

Fatalities following **severe** cytokine release syndrome (characterised by severe dyspnoea) and associated with features of tumour lysis syndrome have occurred 1–2 hours after infusion of rituximab. Children with a high tumour burden as well as those with pulmonary insufficiency or infiltration are at increased risk and should be monitored **very closely** (and a slower rate of infusion considered).

Alemtuzumab, another monoclonal antibody that causes lysis of B lymphocytes, has been used in children for conditioning therapy before allogeneic bone marrow transplantation. In common with rituximab, it causes infusion-related side-effects including cytokine release syndrome (see above) and premedication with an analgesic, an antihistamine, and a corticosteroid is recommended.

▚ ALEMTUZUMAB

Cautions see notes above—for full details (including monitoring) consult product literature or local treatment protocol

Contra-indications for full details consult product literature or local treatment protocol

Pregnancy avoid; manufacturer advises effective contraception during and for 6 months after treatment in men or women

Breast-feeding manufacturer advises avoid breast-feeding during treatment and for at least 4 weeks after treatment

Side-effects see notes above—for full details (including monitoring and management of side-effects) consult product literature

Licensed use not licensed for use in children under 17 years

Indication and dose

See notes above
● By intravenous infusion
Consult local treatment protocol for details

MabCampath® (Genzyme) PoM
Concentrate for intravenous infusion, alemtuzumab 30 mg/mL, net price 1-mL amp = £264.11

▚ RITUXIMAB

Cautions see notes above—but for full details (including monitoring) consult product literature or local treatment protocol

Pregnancy avoid unless potential benefit to mother outweighs risk of B-lymphocyte depletion in fetus—effective contraception (in both sexes) required during and for 12 months after treatment

Breast-feeding avoid breast-feeding during and for 12 months after treatment

Side-effects see notes above—but for full details (including monitoring and management of side-effects) consult product literature

Licensed use not licensed for use in children

Indication and dose

See notes above
● By intravenous infusion
Consult local treatment protocol for details

MabThera® (Roche) PoM
Concentrate for intravenous infusion, rituximab 10 mg/mL, net price 10-mL vial = £174.63, 50-mL vial = £873.15

Malignant disease and immunosuppression

8

8.2.4 Other immunomodulating drugs

Interferon alfa

Interferon alfa has shown some antitumour effect and may have a role in inducing early regression of life-threatening corticosteroid-resistant haemangiomas of infancy. Interferon alfa preparations are also used in the treatment of chronic hepatitis B, and chronic hepatitis C ideally in combination with ribavirin (section 5.3.3). Interferon alfa should always be used under the close supervision of a specialist. Side-effects are dose-related, but commonly include anorexia, nausea, influenza-like symptoms, and lethargy. Ocular side-effects and depression (including suicidal behaviour) have also been reported. Myelosuppression may occur, particularly affecting granulocyte counts. Cardiovascular problems (hypotension, hypertension, and arrhythmias), nephrotoxicity and hepatotoxicity have been reported and monitoring of hepatic function is recommended. Hypertriglyceridaemia, sometimes severe, has been observed; monitoring of lipid concentration is recommended. Other side-effects include hypersensitivity reactions, thyroid abnormalities, hyperglycaemia, alopecia, psoriasiform rash, confusion, coma and seizures, and reversible motor problems in young children. Rarely pulmonary infiltrates, pneumonitis, and pneumonia have occurred; respiratory symptoms should be investigated and if pulmonary infiltrates are suspected or lung function is impaired the discontinuation of interferon alfa should be considered.

INTERFERON ALFA

Cautions consult product literature and local treatment protocol for details; **interactions:** Appendix 1 (interferons)

Contra-indications consult product literature and local treatment protocol for details; avoid injections containing benzyl alcohol in neonates (see under preparations below)

Hepatic impairment close monitoring in mild to moderate impairment; manufacturers advise avoid if severe

Renal impairment close monitoring required in mild to moderate impairment; manufacturers advise avoid in severe impairment

Pregnancy manufacturers advise avoid unless potential benefit outweighs risk (toxicity in *animal* studies); effective contraception required during treatment—consult product literature

Breast-feeding manufacturers advise avoid

Side-effects see notes above, consult product literature and local treatment protocols for details

Licensed use not licensed for use in children for chronic active hepatitis B; *Roferon-A*® not licensed for use in children

Indication and dose

Induction of early regression of life-threatening corticosteroid resistant haemangiomata of infancy

• By subcutaneous injection
  Consult local treatment protocol for details

Chronic active hepatitis B infection see under preparations below

Chronic active hepatitis C infection see under preparations below

IntronA® (Schering-Plough) ℗ₒ𝗠
Injection, interferon alfa-2b (rbe) 10 million units/mL, net price 1-mL vial = £42.35, 2.5-mL vial =

£105.95. For subcutaneous injection or intravenous infusion

Injection pen, interferon alfa-2b (rbe), net price 15 million units/mL, 1.5-mL cartridge = £76.28; 25 million units/mL, 1.5-mL cartridge = £127.14; 50 million units/mL, 1.5-mL cartridge = £254.28. For subcutaneous injection

Note Each 1.5-mL multidose cartridge delivers 6 doses of 0.2 mL i.e. a total of 1.2 mL

Dose

> **Chronic active hepatitis B**
> • By subcutaneous injection
>   **Child 2–18 years** 5–10 million units/m² 3 times weekly

> **Chronic active hepatitis C** (in combination with oral ribavirin, see p. 399)
> • By subcutaneous injection
>   **Child 3–18 years** 3 million units/m² 3 times weekly

Roferon-A® (Roche) ℗ₒ𝗠
Injection, interferon alfa-2a (rbe). Net price 6 million units/mL, 0.5-mL (3 million-unit) prefilled syringe = £14.48; 9 million units/mL, 0.5-mL (4.5 million-unit) prefilled syringe = £21.72; 12 million units/mL, 0.5-mL (6 million-unit) prefilled syringe = £28.95; 18 million units/mL, 0.5-mL (9 million-unit) prefilled syringe = £43.43; 36 million units/mL, 0.5-mL (18 million-unit) prefilled syringe = £86.86; 30 million units/mL, 0.6-mL (18 million-unit) cartridge = £86.86, for use with *Roferon* pen device. For subcutaneous injection (cartridges, vials, and prefilled syringes) and intramuscular injection (cartridges and vials)
Excipients include benzyl alcohol (avoid in neonates, see Excipients, p. 3)

Dose

> **Chronic active hepatitis B**
> • By subcutaneous injection
>   **Child 2–18 years** 2.5–5 million units/m² 3 times weekly; up to 10 million units/m² has been used 3 times weekly

Interferon gamma

Interferon gamma-1b is used to reduce the frequency of serious infection in chronic granulomatous disease and in severe malignant osteopetrosis.

INTERFERON GAMMA-1b

(Immune interferon)

Cautions seizure disorders (including seizures associated with fever); cardiac disease (including ischaemia, congestive heart failure, and arrhythmias; monitor before and during treatment: haematological tests (including full blood count, differential white cell count, and platelet count), blood chemistry tests (including renal and liver function tests) and urinalysis; avoid simultaneous administration of foreign proteins including immunological products (risk of exaggerated immune response); **interactions:** Appendix 1 (interferons)

Driving May impair ability to perform skilled tasks; effects may be enhanced by alcohol

Hepatic impairment manufacturer advises caution in severe impairment—risk of accumulation

Renal impairment manufacturer advises caution in severe impairment—risk of accumulation

Pregnancy manufacturers advise avoid unless potential benefit outweighs risk (toxicity in *animal* studies); effective contraception required during treatment—consult product literature

Breast-feeding manufacturer advises avoid—no information available

Side-effects nausea, vomiting; headache, fatigue, fever; myalgia, arthralgia; rash, injection-site reactions; *rarely* confusion and systemic lupus erythematosus; also reported, neutropenia, thrombocytopenia, and raised liver enzymes

Indication and dose

See notes above and under Preparations below

Immukin® (Boehringer Ingelheim) [PoM]
Injection, recombinant human interferon gamma-1b 200 micrograms/mL, net price 0.5-mL vial = £66.67

Dose
- **By subcutaneous injection**
 Body surface area 0.5 m² or less 1.5 micrograms/kg 3 times a week

 Body surface area greater than 0.5 m² 50 micrograms/m² 3 times a week

 Not recommended for infant under 6 months with chronic granulomatous disease

Canakinumab

Canakinumab is a recombinant human monoclonal antibody that selectively inhibits interleukin-1beta receptor binding. It is licensed for the treatment of cryopyrin-associated periodic syndromes, including severe forms of familial cold auto-inflammatory syndrome (or familial cold urticaria), Muckle-Wells syndrome, and neonatal-onset multisystem inflammatory disease (also known as chronic infantile neurological, cutaneous, articular syndrome), which are rare inherited auto-inflammatory disorders.

CANAKINUMAB

Cautions history of recurrent infection or predisposition to infection; monitor neutrophil count before starting treatment, 1–2 months after starting treatment, and periodically thereafter; children should receive all recommended vaccinations (including pneumococcal and inactivated influenza vaccine) before starting treatment; avoid live vaccines unless potential benefit outweighs risk—consult product literature for further information and section 14.1, p. 733

Tuberculosis Children should be evaluated for latent and active tuberculosis before starting treatment and monitored for signs and symptoms of tuberculosis during and after treatment

Contra-indications severe active infection (see also Cautions); neutropenia; concomitant use with tumour necrosis factor inhibitors (possible increased risk of infections)

Hepatic impairment no information available

Renal impairment limited information available but manufacturer advises no dose adjustment required

Pregnancy manufacturer advises avoid unless potential benefit outweighs risk; effective contraception required during treatment and for up to 3 months after last dose

Breast-feeding consider if benefit outweighs risk—not known if present in human milk

Side-effects vertigo, increased susceptibility to infection, injection-site reactions

Indication and dose

Cryopyrin-associated periodic syndromes
- **By subcutaneous injection**
 Child 4–18 years

 Body-weight 15–40 kg 2 mg/kg every 8 weeks. If clinical response not achieved 7 days after starting treatment, a repeat dose of 2 mg/kg can be considered; if a full response is then achieved, subsequent dosing should be 4 mg/kg every 8 weeks

 Body-weight over 40 kg 150 mg every 8 weeks. If clinical response not achieved 7 days after starting treatment, a repeat dose of 150 mg can be considered; if a full response is then achieved, subsequent dosing should be 300 mg every 8 weeks

8

Malignant disease and immunosuppression

◻ **CANAKINUMAB** (*continued*)

Ilaris® (Novartis) ▼ PoM
  Injection, powder for reconstitution, canakinumab,
  net price 150-mg vial = £9927.80

Mifamurtide

Mifamurtide is licensed in children and adolescents for the treatment of high-grade, resectable, non-metastatic osteosarcoma after complete surgical resection. It is used in combination with chemotherapy.

MIFAMURTIDE

Cautions asthma and chronic obstructive pulmonary disease—consider prophylactic bronchodilator therapy; history of autoimmune, inflammatory, or collagen disease; monitor renal function, hepatic function and clotting parameters; monitor patients with history of venous thrombosis, vasculitis, or unstable cardiovascular disorders for persistent or worsening symptoms during administration—consult product literature **interactions:** Appendix 1 (mifamurtide)

Hepatic impairment use with caution—no information available

Renal impairment use with caution—no information available

Pregnancy avoid; effective contraception required

Breast-feeding avoid—no information available

Side-effects gastro-intestinal disturbances (including anorexia, nausea, vomiting, diarrhoea, constipation, abdominal pain, dyspepsia); tachycardia, hypertension, palpitations, hypotension, phlebitis; oedema, respiratory disorders (including dyspnoea, epistaxis, cough, tachypnoea, haemoptysis, pleural effusion); confusion, depression, insomnia, headache, dizziness, paraesthesia, hypoaesthesia, tremor, drowsiness, anxiety; hypokalaemia, anaemia, leucopenia, thrombocytopenia, granulocytopenia; haematuria, dysuria, pollakiuria; musculoskeletal pain; blurred vision; vertigo, tinnitus, hearing loss; sweating, alopecia, rash, dry skin, flushing

Indication and dose

  See notes above
  • **By intravenous infusion** (over 1 hour)
  Consult local treatment protocols for details

Mepact® (Takeda) ▼ PoM
  Intravenous infusion, powder for reconstitution, mifamurtide, net price 4-mg vial = £2375.00

8.3 Sex hormones and hormone antagonists in malignant disease

Classification not used in *BNF for Children*.

9 Nutrition and blood

9 Nutrition and blood

9.1 Anaemias and some other blood disorders

9.1.1 Iron-deficiency anaemias
9.1.2 Drugs used in megaloblastic anaemias
9.1.3 Drugs used in hypoplastic, haemolytic, and renal anaemias
9.1.4 Drugs used in platelet disorders
9.1.5 G6PD deficiency
9.1.6 Drugs used in neutropenia

Before initiating treatment for anaemia it is essential to determine which type is present. Iron salts may be harmful and result in iron overload if given alone to patients with anaemias other than those due to iron deficiency.

9.1.1 Iron-deficiency anaemias

9.1.1.1 Oral iron
9.1.1.2 Parenteral iron

Treatment with an iron preparation is justified only in the presence of a demonstrable iron-deficiency state. Before starting treatment, it is important to exclude any serious underlying cause of the anaemia (e.g. gastro-intestinal bleeding). The possibility of thalassaemia should be considered in children of Mediterranean or Indian subcontinent descent.

Prophylaxis with an iron preparation may be appropriate in those with a poor diet, malabsorption, menorrhagia, pregnancy, in haemodialysis patients, and in the management of low birth-weight infants such as preterm neonates.

9.1.1.1 Oral iron

Iron salts should be given by mouth unless there are good reasons for using another route.

Ferrous salts show only marginal differences between one another in efficiency of absorption of iron. Haemoglobin regeneration rate is little affected by the type of salt used provided sufficient iron is given, and in most patients the speed of response is not critical. Choice of preparation is thus usually decided by formulation, palatability, incidence of side-effects, and cost.

Treatment of iron-deficiency anaemia   The oral dose of **elemental iron** to treat deficiency is 3–6 mg/kg (max. 200 mg) daily given in 2–3 divided doses. Iron supplementation may also be required to produce an optimum response to erythropoietins in iron-deficient children with chronic renal failure or in preterm neonates. (See also Prophylaxis of iron deficiency, below.)

Prescribing Express the dose in terms of elemental iron and iron salt and select the most appropriate preparation; specify both the iron salt and formulation on the prescription. The iron content of artificial formula feeds should also be considered.

Iron content of different iron salts		
Iron salt	Amount	Content of ferrous iron
Ferrous fumarate	200 mg	65 mg
Ferrous gluconate	300 mg	35 mg
Ferrous sulphate	300 mg	60 mg
Ferrous sulphate, dried	200 mg	65 mg
Sodium feredetate	190 mg	27.5 mg

Therapeutic response   The haemoglobin concentration should rise by about 100–200 mg/100 mL (1–2 g/litre) per day *or* 2 g/100 mL (20 g/litre) over 3–4 weeks. When the haemoglobin is in the normal range, treatment should be continued for a further 3 months to replenish the iron stores. Epithelial tissue changes such as atrophic glossitis and koilonychia are usually improved, but the response is often slow. The most common reason for lack of response in children is poor compliance; poor absorption is rare in children.

Prophylaxis of iron deficiency   In neonates, haemoglobin and haematocrit concentrations change rapidly. These changes are not due to iron deficiency and cannot be corrected by iron supplementation. Similarly, neonatal anaemia resulting from repeated blood sampling does not respond to iron therapy.

All babies, including preterm neonates, are born with substantial iron stores but these stores can become depleted unless dietary intake is adequate. All babies require an iron intake of 400–700 nanograms daily to maintain body stores. Iron in breast milk is well absorbed but that in artificial feeds or in cow's milk is less so. Most artificial formula feeds are sufficiently fortified with iron to prevent deficiency and their iron content should be taken into account when considering further iron supplementation.

Dose   Prophylactic iron supplementation (elemental iron 5 mg daily) may be required in babies of low birth-weight who are solely breast-fed; supplementation is started 4–6 weeks after birth and continued until mixed feeding is established.

Infants with a poor diet may become anaemic in the second year of life, particularly if cow's milk, rather than fortified formula feed, is a major part of the diet.

Compound preparations   Some oral preparations contain **ascorbic acid** to aid absorption of the iron, but the therapeutic advantage of such preparations is minimal and cost may be increased.

There is no justification for the inclusion of other ingredients, such as the **B group of vitamins**, except **folic acid** for pregnant women, see p. 543.

Side-effects   Gastro-intestinal irritation can occur with iron salts. Nausea and epigastric pain are dose-related, but the relationship between dose and altered bowel habit (constipation or diarrhoea) is less clear. Oral iron can exacerbate diarrhoea in patients with inflammatory bowel disease.

Iron preparations taken orally can be constipating and occasionally lead to faecal impaction.

If side-effects occur, the dose may be reduced; alternatively, another iron salt may be used, but an improvement in tolerance may simply be a result of a lower content of elemental iron. The incidence of side-effects due to ferrous sulphate is no greater than with other iron salts when compared on the basis of equivalent amounts of elemental iron.

Iron preparations are an important cause of accidental overdose in children and as little as 20 mg/kg of elemental iron can lead to symptoms of toxicity. For the treatment of **iron overdose**, see Emergency Treatment of Poisoning, p. 42.

Counselling   Although iron preparations are best absorbed on an empty stomach, they can be taken after food to reduce gastro-intestinal side-effects; they may discolour stools.

FERROUS SULPHATE

Cautions interactions: Appendix 1 (iron)
Side-effects see notes above

Indication and dose

Iron-deficiency anaemia, prophylaxis of iron deficiency see notes above and preparations

Ferrous Sulphate (Non-proprietary)
Tablets, coated, dried ferrous sulphate 200 mg (65 mg iron), net price 28-tab pack = £1.20

Dose
Child 6–18 years prophylactic, 1 tablet daily; therapeutic, 1 tablet 2–3 times daily, see notes above

Ironorm® Drops (Wallace Mfg)
Oral drops, ferrous sulphate 125 mg (25 mg iron)/ mL, net price 15 mL = £4.95

Dose
Child 1 month–6 years prophylactic 0.3 mL daily, but see notes above

Child 6–18 years prophylactic 0.6 mL daily

FERROUS FUMARATE

Cautions interactions: Appendix 1 (iron)
Side-effects see notes above

Indication and dose

Iron-deficiency anaemia, prophylaxis of iron deficiency see notes above and preparations

Fersaday® (Goldshield)
Tablets, brown, f/c, ferrous fumarate 322 mg (100 mg iron). Net price 28-tab pack = 79p

Dose
Child 12–18 years prophylactic, 1 tablet daily; therapeutic, 1 tablet twice daily

Fersamal® (Goldshield)
Tablets, brown, ferrous fumarate 210 mg (68 mg iron), net price 100 = £1.44

Dose
Child 12–18 years 1–2 tablets 3 times daily, but see notes above

Syrup, brown, ferrous fumarate approx. 140 mg (45 mg iron)/5 mL. Net price 200 mL = £3.11

Dose
Preterm neonate see notes above

Neonate see notes above

Child 1 month–6 years 2.5–5 mL twice daily, but see notes above

Child 6–18 years 10 mL twice daily, but see notes above

9

Nutrition and blood

◁ **FERROUS FUMARATE (continued)**

Galfer® (Thornton & Ross)
Capsules, red/green, ferrous fumarate 305 mg
(100 mg iron), net price 100 = £1.80

Dose

> **Child 12–18 years** prophylactic, 1 capsule daily;
> therapeutic, 1 capsule twice daily

Syrup, brown, sugar-free ferrous fumarate 140 mg
(45 mg iron)/5 mL. Net price 300 mL = £4.86

Dose

> **Preterm neonate and body-weight up to 3 kg** prophy-
> lactic, 0.5 mL daily, see notes above

> **Neonate** prophylactic and therapeutic, 0.25 mL/kg
> twice daily (total daily dose may alternatively be
> given in 3 divided doses), see notes above

> **Child 1 month–12 years** prophylactic and therapeutic,
> 0.25 mL/kg twice daily (total daily dose may alterna-
> tively be given in 3 divided doses); max 20 mL daily,
> see notes above

> **Child 12–18 years** prophylactic, 10 mL once daily;
> therapeutic, 10 mL 1–2 times daily

FERROUS GLUCONATE

Cautions interactions: Appendix 1 (iron)
Side-effects see notes above

Indication and dose

> Iron-deficiency anaemia see notes above and
> preparation

Ferrous Gluconate (Non-proprietary)
Tablets, red, coated, ferrous gluconate 300 mg
(35 mg iron), net price 28 = £2.65

Dose

> **Child 6–12 years** prophylactic and therapeutic, 1–3
> tablets daily

> **Child 12–18 years** prophylactic, 2 tablets daily; ther-
> apeutic, 4–6 tablets daily in divided doses

POLYSACCHARIDE-IRON COMPLEX

Cautions interactions: Appendix 1 (iron)
Side-effects see notes above

Indication and dose

> Iron-deficiency anaemia, prophylaxis of iron
> deficiency see notes above and preparation

Niferex® (Tillomed)
Elixir, brown, sugar-free, polysaccharide-iron complex equivalent to 100 mg of iron/5 mL. Net price
240-mL pack = £6.06; (NHS)[1] 30-mL dropper bottle
for paediatric use = £2.16. Counselling, use of
dropper

Dose

> **Neonate** (from dropper bottle) 1 drop (approx.
> 500 micrograms iron) per 450 g body-weight 3 times
> daily, see notes above

> **Child 1 month–2 years** (from dropper bottle) 1 drop
> (approx. 500 micrograms iron) per 450 g body-weight
> 3 times daily, see notes above

> **Child 2–6 years** therapeutic, 2.5 mL daily

> **Child 6–12 years** therapeutic, 5 mL daily

> **Child 12–18 years** prophylactic, 2.5 mL daily; thera-
> peutic, 5 mL 1–2 times daily (5 mL once daily if
> required during second and third trimester of
> pregnancy)

1. except 30 mL paediatric dropper bottle for prophylaxis
and treatment of iron deficiency in infants born prematurely; endorse prescription 'SLS'

SODIUM FEREDETATE
(Sodium ironedetate)

Cautions interactions: Appendix 1 (iron)
Side-effects see notes above
Licensed use not licensed for prophylaxis of iron
deficiency

Indication and dose

> Iron-deficiency anaemia, prophylaxis of iron
> deficiency see notes above and preparation

Sytron® (Archimedes)
Elixir, sugar-free, sodium feredetate 190 mg
equivalent to 27.5 mg of iron/5 mL. Net price
100 mL = £1.07

Dose

> **Neonate** prophylactic, 1 mL daily, see notes above;
> therapeutic, up to 2.5 mL twice daily (smaller doses
> should be used initially), see notes above

> **Child 1 month–1 year** prophylactic, 1 mL daily, see
> notes above; therapeutic, up to 2.5 mL twice daily
> (smaller doses should be used initially), see notes
> above

> **Child 1–5 years** therapeutic, 2.5 mL 3 times daily

> **Child 5–12 years** therapeutic, 5 mL 3 times daily

> **Child 12–18 years** therapeutic, 5 mL increasing gra-
> dually to 10 mL 3 times daily

9.1.1.2 Parenteral iron

Iron can be administered parenterally as **iron dextran**, **iron sucrose**, or **ferric carboxymaltose**. Parenteral iron is generally reserved for use when oral therapy is unsuccessful because the child cannot tolerate oral iron, or does not take it reliably, or if there is continuing blood loss, or in malabsorption.

Many children with chronic renal failure who are receiving haemodialysis (and some who are receiving peritoneal dialysis) also require iron by the intravenous route on a regular basis (see also Erythropoietins, section 9.1.3).

With the exception of children with severe renal failure receiving haemodialysis, parenteral iron does not produce a faster haemoglobin response than oral iron provided that the oral iron preparation is taken reliably and is absorbed adequately.

Anaphylactic reactions can occur with parenteral iron complexes; facilities for cardiopulmonary resuscitation must be available. Depending on the preparation, a small test dose may be required. If children complain of acute symptoms particularly nausea, back pain, breathlessness, or develop hypotension, the infusion should be stopped.

FERRIC CARBOXYMALTOSE

A ferric carboxymaltose complex containing 5% (50 mg/mL) of iron

Cautions hypersensitivity can occur with parenteral iron and facilities for cardiopulmonary resuscitation must be available; oral iron should not be given concomitantly; allergic disorders including asthma and eczema; infection (discontinue if ongoing bacteraemia); **interactions**: Appendix 1 (iron)

Hepatic impairment use with caution; avoid in conditions where iron overload increases risk of impairment

Pregnancy avoid in first trimester; crosses the placenta in *animal* studies; may influence skeletal development

Side-effects gastro-intestinal disturbances; headache, dizziness; rash; injection-site reactions; *less commonly* hypotension, flushing, chest pain, peripheral oedema, hypersensitivity reactions (including anaphylaxis), fatigue, paraesthesia, malaise, pyrexia, rigors, myalgia, arthralgia, back pain, pruritus, and urticaria; *rarely* dyspnoea

Licensed use not licensed for use in children under 14 years

Indication and dose

Iron-deficiency anaemia see notes above

- **By slow intravenous injection or by intravenous infusion**
  Calculated according to body-weight and iron deficit, consult product literature

Ferinject® (Syner-Med) ▼ PoM
Injection, iron (as ferric carboxymaltose) 50 mg/mL, net price 2-mL vial = £21.75, 10-mL vial = £108.75
Electrolytes Na+ 0.24 mmol/mL

IRON DEXTRAN

A complex of ferric hydroxide with sucrose containing 5% (50 mg/mL) of iron

Cautions oral iron not to be given until 5 days after last injection; **interactions**: Appendix 1 (iron)

Anaphylaxis Anaphylactic reactions can occur with parenteral iron and a test dose is recommended before *each* dose; the patient should be carefully observed for 60 minutes after the first test dose and for 15 minutes after subsequent test doses. Facilities for cardiopulmonary resuscitation must be available; risk of allergic reactions increased in immune or inflammatory conditions

Contra-indications history of allergic disorders including asthma, and eczema; infection; active rheumatoid arthritis

Hepatic impairment avoid in severe impairment

Renal impairment avoid in acute renal failure

Pregnancy avoid in first trimester

Side-effects *less commonly* nausea, vomiting, abdominal pain, flushing, dyspnoea, anaphylactic reactions (see Anaphylaxis above), numbness, cramps, blurred vision, pruritus, and rash; *rarely* diarrhoea, chest pain, hypotension, angioedema, arrhythmias, tachycardia, dizziness, restlessness, fatigue, seizures, tremor, impaired consciousness, myalgia, arthralgia, sweating, and injection-site reactions; *very rarely* hypertension, palpitation, headache, paraesthesia, haemolysis, and transient deafness

Licensed use not licensed for use in children under 14 years

Indication and dose

Iron-deficiency anaemia see notes above

- **By slow intravenous injection or by intravenous infusion**
  Calculated according to body-weight and iron deficit, consult product literature

CosmoFer® (Vitaline) PoM
Injection, iron (as iron dextran) 50 mg/mL, net price 2-mL amp = £7.97; 10-mL amp = £39.85

9

Nutrition and blood

IRON SUCROSE

A complex of ferric hydroxide with sucrose containing 2% (20 mg/mL) of iron

Cautions oral iron therapy should not be given until 5 days after last injection; infection (discontinue if ongoing bacteraemia); **interactions**: Appendix 1 (iron)

Anaphylaxis Anaphylactic reactions can occur with parenteral iron and a test dose is recommended before the first dose; the patient should be carefully observed for 15 minutes. Facilities for cardiopulmonary resuscitation must be available

Contra-indications history of allergic disorders including asthma, eczema, and anaphylaxis

Hepatic impairment use with caution; avoid in conditions where iron overload increases risk of impairment

Pregnancy avoid in first trimester

Side-effects taste disturbances; *less commonly* nausea, vomiting, abdominal pain, diarrhoea, hypotension, tachycardia, flushing, palpitation, chest pain, bronchospasm, dyspnoea, headache, dizziness, fever, myalgia, pruritus, rash, and injection-site reactions; *rarely* peripheral oedema, anaphylactic reactions (see Anaphylaxis above), fatigue, asthenia, and paraesthesia; confusion, arthralgia, and increased sweating also reported

Licensed use not licensed for use in children

Indication and dose

Iron-deficiency anaemia see notes above

● **By slow intravenous injection or by intravenous infusion**

Calculated according to body-weight and iron deficit, consult product literature

Venofer® (Syner-Med) (PoM)
Injection, iron (as iron sucrose) 20 mg/mL, net price 5-mL amp = £8.50

9.1.2 Drugs used in megaloblastic anaemias

Megaloblastic anaemias are rare in children; they may result from a lack of either vitamin B_{12} or folate, and it is essential to establish in every case which deficiency is present and the underlying cause. In emergencies, when delay might be dangerous, it is sometimes necessary to administer both substances after the bone marrow test while plasma assay results are awaited. Normally, however, appropriate treatment should not be instituted until the results of tests are available.

Vitamin B_{12} is used in the treatment of megaloblastosis caused by *prolonged nitrous oxide anaesthesia*, which inactivates the vitamin, and in the rare disorders of *congenital transcobalamin II deficiency, methylmalonic acidaemia* and *homocystinuria* (see section 9.8.1).

Vitamin B_{12} should be given prophylactically after *total ileal resection*.

Apart from dietary deficiency, all other causes of vitamin B_{12} deficiency are attributable to malabsorption. There is little place for the use of low-dose vitamin B_{12} orally and none for vitamin B_{12} intrinsic factor complexes given by mouth. Vitamin B_{12} in large oral doses [unlicensed] may be effective.

Hydroxocobalamin has completely replaced cyanocobalamin as the form of vitamin B_{12} of choice for therapy; it is retained in the body longer than cyanocobalamin and thus for maintenance therapy can be given at intervals of up to 3 months. Treatment is generally initiated with frequent administration of intramuscular injections to replenish the depleted body stores. Thereafter, maintenance treatment, which is usually for life, can be instituted. There is no evidence that doses larger than those recommended provide any additional benefit in vitamin B_{12} neuropathy.

Folic acid has few indications for long-term therapy since most causes of folate deficiency are self-limiting or will yield to a short course of treatment. It should not be used in undiagnosed megaloblastic anaemia unless vitamin B_{12} is administered concurrently otherwise neuropathy may be precipitated (see above).

In *folate-deficient megaloblastic anaemia* (e.g. because of poor nutrition, pregnancy, or treatment with antiepileptics), daily folic acid supplementation for 4 months brings about haematological remission and replenishes body stores; higher doses may be necessary in malabsorption states. In pregnancy, folic acid 5 mg daily is continued to term.

For prophylaxis in *chronic haemolytic states, malabsorption* or *in renal dialysis*, folic acid is given daily or sometimes weekly, depending on the diet and the rate of haemolysis.

For *prophylaxis in pregnancy*, see Prevention of Neural Tube Defects below.

Folic acid is actively excreted in breast milk and is well absorbed by the infant. It is also present in cow's milk and artificial formula feeds but is heat labile. Serum and red cell folate concentrations fall after delivery and urinary losses are high, particularly in low birth-weight neonates. Although symptomatic deficiency is rare in the absence of malabsorption or prolonged diarrhoea, it is common for neonatal units to give supplements of folic acid to all preterm neonates from 2 weeks of age until full-term corrected age is reached, particularly if heated breast milk is used without an artificial formula fortifier.

Folinic acid is also effective in the treatment of folate-deficient megaloblastic anaemia but it is normally only used in association with cytotoxic drugs (see section 8.1); it is given as calcium folinate.

Prevention of neural tube defects   Folic acid supplements taken before and during pregnancy can reduce the occurrence of neural tube defects. The risk of a neural tube defect occurring in a child should be assessed and folic acid given as follows:

> Women at a low risk of conceiving a child with a neural tube defect should be advised to take folic acid as a medicinal or food supplement at a dose of 400 micrograms daily before conception and until week 12 of pregnancy. Women who have not been taking folic acid and who suspect they are pregnant should start at once and continue until week 12 of pregnancy.

> Couples are at a high risk of conceiving a child with a neural tube defect if either partner has a neural tube defect (or either partner has a family history of neural tube defects), if they have had a previous pregnancy affected by a neural tube defect, or if the woman has coeliac disease (or other malabsorption state), diabetes mellitus, sickle-cell anaemia, or is taking antiepileptic medicines (see also section 4.8.1).

> Women in the high-risk group who wish to become pregnant (or who are at risk of becoming pregnant) should be advised to take folic acid 5 mg daily and continue until week 12 of pregnancy (women with sickle-cell disease should continue taking their normal dose of folic acid 5 mg daily throughout pregnancy).

> There is **no** justification for prescribing multiple-ingredient vitamin preparations containing vitamin B_{12} or folic acid.

HYDROXOCOBALAMIN

Cautions   should not be given before diagnosis fully established but see also notes above; **interactions** Appendix 1 (hydroxocobalamin)

Breast-feeding   present in milk but not known to be harmful

Side-effects   nausea, headache, dizziness; fever, hypersensitivity reactions (including rash and pruritus); injection-site reactions; hypokalaemia and thrombocytosis during initial treatment; chromaturia

Licensed use   licensed for use in children (age not specified by manufacturers); not licensed for use in inborn errors of metabolism

Indication and dose

Macrocytic anaemia without neurological involvement
- **By intramuscular injection**

  Child 1 month–18 years initially 250 micrograms–1 mg 3 times a week for 2 weeks then 250 micrograms once weekly until blood count normal, then 1 mg every 3 months

Macrocytic anaemia with neurological involvement
- **By intramuscular injection**

  Child 1 month–18 years initially 1 mg on alternate days until no further improvement, then 1 mg every 2 months

Prophylaxis of macrocytic anaemias associated with vitamin B_{12} deficiency
- **By intramuscular injection**

  Child 1 month–18 years 1 mg every 2–3 months

Leber's optic atrophy
- **By intramuscular injection**

  Initially 1 mg daily for 2 weeks, then 1 mg twice weekly until no further improvement, thereafter 1 mg every 1–3 months

Congenital transcobalamin II deficiency
- **By intramuscular injection**

  Neonate 1 mg 3 times a week, reduce after 1 year to 1 mg once weekly or as appropriate

  Child 1 month–18 years 1 mg 3 times a week, reduce after 1 year to 1 mg once weekly or as appropriate

9

Nutrition and blood

⌷ **HYDROXOCOBALAMIN** (*continued*)

Methylmalonic acidaemia and homocystinuria
- **By intramuscular injection**

  Child 1 month–18 years initially 1 mg daily for 5–7 days, reduce according to response to maintenance dose of up to 1 mg once or twice weekly

Methylmalonic acidaemia, maintenance once intramuscular response established
- **By mouth**

  Child 1 month–18 years 5–10 mg once or twice weekly

Note Some children do not respond to the oral route

Hydroxocobalamin (Non-proprietary) PoM
Injection, hydroxocobalamin 1 mg/mL. Net price 1-mL amp = 92p
Brands include *Cobalin-H*® JHS, *Neo-Cytamen*® JHS

Injection, hydroxocobalamin 2.5 mg/mL, 2 mL
Available from 'special-order' manufacturers or specialist importing companies, see p. 957
Administration For administration *by mouth*, injection solution may be given orally; it will not have prolonged effect via this route
Note The BP directs that when Vitamin B$_{12}$ injection is prescribed or demanded hydroxocobalamin injection shall be dispensed or supplied
Powder available from specialist importing companies

▌FOLIC ACID

Cautions should never be given alone for vitamin B$_{12}$ deficiency states (may precipitate subacute combined degeneration of the spinal cord); **interactions**: Appendix 1 (folates)
Side-effects rarely gastro-intestinal disturbances
Licensed use unlicensed for limiting methotrexate toxicity

Indication and dose

Folate supplementation in neonates (see notes above)
- **By mouth**

  Neonate 50 micrograms once daily *or* 500 micrograms once weekly

Megaloblastic anaemia due to folate deficiency (see notes above)
- **By mouth**

  Neonate initially 500 micrograms/kg once daily for up to 4 months

  Child 1 month–1 year initially 500 micrograms/kg once daily (max. 5 mg) for up to 4 months; up to 10 mg daily may be required in malabsorption states

  Child 1–18 years 5 mg daily for 4 months (until term in pregnant women); up to 15 mg daily may be required in malabsorption states

Haemolytic anaemia; metabolic disorders
- **By mouth**

  Child 1 month–12 years 2.5–5 mg once daily

  Child 12–18 years 5–10 mg once daily

Prophylaxis of folate deficiency in dialysis
- **By mouth**

  Child 1 month–12 years 250 microgram/kg (max. 10 mg) once daily

  Child 12–18 years 5–10 mg once daily

Prevention of methotrexate side-effects in juvenile idiopathic arthritis
- **By mouth**

  Child 2–18 years 1 mg daily *or* 5 mg once weekly, adjusted according to local guidelines

Prevention of methotrexate side-effects in severe Crohn's disease or severe psoriasis
- **By mouth**

  See section 1.5.3 and section 13.5.3

Prevention of neural tube defects
- **By mouth**

  See notes above

[1]**Folic Acid** (Non-proprietary) PoM
Tablets, folic acid 400 micrograms, net price 90-tab pack = £2.37; 5 mg, 28-tab pack = 99p

Syrup, folic acid 2.5 mg/5 mL, net price 150 mL = £9.16; 400 micrograms/5 mL, 150 mL = £1.40
Brands include *Folicare*®, *Lexpec*® (sugar-free)
1. Can be sold to the public provided daily doses do not exceed 500 micrograms

---

▌9.1.3 Drugs used in hypoplastic, haemolytic, and renal anaemias

Anabolic steroids (see BNF, section 6.4.3), pyridoxine, antilymphocyte immunoglobulin, and various corticosteroids are used in hypoplastic and haemolytic anaemias.

Antilymphocyte immunoglobulin given intravenously through a central line over 12–18 hours each day for 5 days produces a response in about 50% of cases of acquired *aplastic anaemia*; the response rate may be increased when ciclosporin is given as well. Severe reactions are common in the first 2 days and profound immunosuppression can occur; antilymphocyte immunoglobulin should be given under specialist supervision with appropriate resuscitation facilities. Alternatively, oxymetholone tablets (available from 'special-order' manufacturers or specialist importing companies, see p. 957) may be used in aplastic anaemia at a dose of 1–5 mg/kg daily for 3 to 6 months.

It is unlikely that dietary deficit of **pyridoxine** (section 9.6.2) produces clinically relevant haematological effects. However, certain forms of *sideroblastic anaemia* respond to pharmacological doses, possibly reflecting its role as a co-enzyme during haemoglobin synthesis. Pyridoxine is indicated in both *idiopathic acquired* and *hereditary sideroblastic anaemias*. Although complete cures have not been reported, some increase in haemoglobin can occur with high doses. *Reversible sideroblastic anaemias* respond to treatment of the underlying cause but pyridoxine is indicated in pregnancy, haemolytic anaemias, or during isoniazid treatment.

Corticosteroids (section 6.3) have an important place in the management of haematological disorders including *autoimmune haemolytic anaemia*, *idiopathic thrombocytopenias* (section 9.1.4) and *neutropenias*, and *major transfusion reactions*. They are also used in chemotherapy schedules for many types of *lymphoma*, *lymphoid leukaemias*, and *paraproteinaemias*, including *multiple myeloma*.

Erythropoietins

Epoetins (recombinant human erythropoietins) are used to treat the anaemia associated with erythropoietin deficiency in chronic renal failure, see below.

Epoetin beta is also used for the prevention of anaemia in preterm neonates of low birth-weight; a therapeutic response may take several weeks. Only unpreserved formulations should be used as other preparations may contain benzyl alcohol (see Excipients, p. 3).

There is insufficient information to support the use of erythropoietins in children with leukaemia or in those receiving cancer chemotherapy.

Darbepoetin is a glycosylated derivative of epoetin; it persists longer in the body and can be administered less frequently than epoetin.

Other factors, such as iron or folate deficiency, that contribute to the anaemia of chronic renal failure should be corrected before treatment and monitored during therapy. Supplemental iron may improve the response in resistant patients and in preterm neonates (see section 9.1.1.1). Aluminium toxicity, concurrent infection, or other inflammatory disease can impair the response to erythropoietin.

> **Erythropoietins—haemoglobin concentration**
> In chronic kidney disease, the use of erythropoietins can be considered in a child with anaemia. The aim of treatment is to relieve symptoms of anaemia and to avoid the need for blood transfusion. The optimum haemoglobin concentration is dependent on the child's age and factors such as symptoms, co-morbidities, and patient preferences. The haemoglobin concentration should not be increased beyond that which provides adequate control of symptoms of anaemia. In *adults*, overcorrection of haemoglobin concentration with erythropoietins in those with chronic kidney disease may increase the risk of serious cardiovascular events and death; haemoglobin concentrations higher than 12 g/100 mL should be avoided in children.
> For MHRA/CHM advice relating to adults, see BNF section 9.1.3.

> **CSM advice (pure red cell aplasia)**
> There have been very rare reports of pure red cell aplasia in patients treated with epoetin alfa. The CSM has advised that in patients developing lack of efficacy with epoetin alfa, with a diagnosis of pure red cell aplasia, treatment with epoetin alfa must be discontinued and testing for erythropoietin antibodies considered. Patients who develop pure red cell aplasia should **not** be switched to another form of erythropoietin.

9 Nutrition and blood

◢ DARBEPOETIN ALFA

Cautions see Epoetin

Contra-indications see Epoetin

Hepatic impairment manufacturer advises caution

Pregnancy no evidence of harm in *animal* studies—manufacturer advises caution

Breast-feeding manufacturer advises avoid—no information available

Side-effects see Epoetin; also, oedema, injection-site pain; isolated reports of pure red cell aplasia particularly following subcutaneous administration in patients with chronic renal failure (discontinue therapy)—see also CSM advice above

◿ **DARBEPOETIN ALFA (continued)**

Indication and dose

Symptomatic anaemia associated with chronic renal failure in children on dialysis (see also notes above)

• By intravenous or subcutaneous injection

  Child 11–18 years initially 450 nanograms/kg once weekly adjusted according to response by approx. 25% at intervals of at least 4 weeks; maintenance dose, given once weekly or once every 2 weeks

Symptomatic anaemia associated with chronic renal failure in children not on dialysis (see also notes above)

• By intravenous or subcutaneous injection

  Child 11–18 years by subcutaneous or intravenous injection, initially 450 nanograms/kg once weekly or by subcutaneous injection, initially 750 nanograms/kg once every 2 weeks; adjusted according to response by approx. 25% at intervals of at least 4 weeks; maintenance dose, given subcutaneously or intravenously once weekly or subcutaneously once every 2 weeks or subcutaneously once every month

Note Subcutaneous route preferred in patients not on haemodialysis. Reduce dose by approximately 25% if rise in haemoglobin concentration exceeds 2 g/100 mL over 4 weeks or if haemoglobin concentration exceeds 12 g/100 mL; if haemoglobin concentration continues to rise, despite dose reduction, suspend treatment until haemoglobin concentration decreases and then restart at a dose approximately 25% lower than the previous dose. When changing route give same dose then adjust according to weekly or fortnightly haemoglobin measurements. Adjust doses not more frequently than every 2 weeks during maintenance treatment.

Aranesp® (Amgen) ᴾᴼᴹ
Injection, prefilled syringe, darbepoetin alfa, 25 micrograms/mL, net price 0.4 mL (10 micrograms) = £14.98; 40 micrograms/mL, 0.375 mL (15 micrograms) = £22.47, 0.5 mL (20 micrograms) = £29.96; 100 micrograms/mL, 0.3 mL (30 micrograms) = £44.93, 0.4 mL (40 micrograms) = £59.91, 0.5 mL (50 micrograms) = £74.89; 200 micrograms/mL, 0.3 mL (60 micrograms) = £89.86, 0.4 mL (80 micrograms) = £119.82, 0.5 mL (100 micrograms) = £149.77, 0.65 mL (130 micrograms) = £194.70; 500 micrograms/mL, 0.3 mL (150 micrograms) = £224.66, 0.6 mL (300 micrograms) = £449.32, 1 mL (500 micrograms) = £748.86

Injection (Aranesp® SureClick), prefilled disposable injection device, darbepoetin alfa, 40 micrograms/mL, net price 0.5 mL (20 micrograms) = £29.95; 100 micrograms/mL, net price 0.4 mL (40 micrograms) = £59.91; 200 micrograms/mL, net price 0.3 mL (60 micrograms) = £89.86, 0.4 mL (80 micrograms) = £119.82, 0.5 mL (100 micrograms) = £149.77; 500 micrograms/mL, net price 0.3 mL (150 micrograms) = £224.66, 0.6 mL (300 micrograms) = £449.32, 1 mL (500 micrograms) = £748.86

◤ **EPOETIN ALFA, BETA, and ZETA**
(Recombinant human erythropoietins)
Note The prescriber must specify which epoetin is required, see also Biosimilar medicines, p. 2

Cautions see notes above; also inadequately treated or poorly controlled blood pressure (monitor closely blood pressure, reticulocyte counts, haemoglobin, and electrolytes; interrupt treatment if blood pressure uncontrolled; sudden stabbing migraine-like pain is warning of hypertensive crisis; sickle-cell disease (lower target haemoglobin concentration may be appropriate); ischaemic vascular disease; thrombocytosis (monitor platelet count for first 8 weeks); epilepsy; malignant disease; increase in unfractionated or low molecular weight heparin dose may be needed during dialysis

Contra-indications pure red cell aplasia following erythropoietin therapy (see also CSM advice above); uncontrolled hypertension; avoid injections containing benzyl alcohol in neonates (see under preparations, below)

Hepatic impairment manufacturers advise caution in chronic hepatic failure

Pregnancy no evidence of harm; benefits probably outweigh risks of anaemia and blood transfusion

Breast-feeding unlikely to be present in milk; effect on infant minimal

Side-effects diarrhoea, nausea, vomiting; dose-dependent increase in blood pressure or aggravation of hypertension; in isolated patients with normal or low blood pressure, hypertensive crisis with encephalopathy-like symptoms and generalised tonic-clonic seizures requiring immediate medical attention; dose-dependent increase in platelet count (but thrombocytosis rare) regressing during treatment; influenza-like symptoms (may be reduced if intravenous injection given over 5 minutes); cardiovascular events; shunt thrombosis especially if tendency to hypotension or arteriovenous shunt complications; very rarely sudden loss of efficacy because of pure red cell aplasia, particularly following subcutaneous administration in patients with chronic renal failure (discontinue erythropoietin therapy)—see also CSM advice above, hyperkalaemia, hypersensitivity reactions (including anaphylaxis and angioedema), skin reactions, and peripheral oedema also reported

Licensed use Eprex® 20 000-unit, 30 000-unit, and 40 000-unit prefilled syringes not licensed for use in children

Indication and dose
See under preparations, below

◂**Epoetin alfa**
Binocrit® (Sandoz) ▼ ᴾᴼᴹ
Injection, prefilled syringe, epoetin alfa, net price 1000 units = £5.09; 2000 units = £10.18; 3000 units = £15.27; 4000 units = £20.36; 5000 units =

◻ **EPOETIN ALFA, BETA, and ZETA (continued)**

£25.46; 6000 units = £30.55; 8000 units = £40.73; 10 000 units = £50.91

Note Biosimilar Medicine, p. 2

Dose

> **Symptomatic anaemia associated with chronic renal failure in children on haemodialysis (see also notes above)**
> • By intravenous injection over 1–5 minutes
>> **Child 1 month–18 years** initially 50 units/kg 3 times weekly adjusted according to response in steps of 25 units/kg 3 times weekly at intervals of at least 4 weeks; maintenance dose, body-weight under 10 kg usually 75–150 units/kg 3 times weekly, body-weight 10–30 kg usually 60–150 units/kg 3 times weekly, body-weight over 30 kg usually 30–100 units/kg 3 times weekly

Note Reduce dose by approximately 25 % if rise in haemoglobin concentration exceeds 2 g/100 mL over 4 weeks or if haemoglobin concentration exceeds 12 g/100 mL; if haemoglobin concentration continues to rise, despite dose reduction, suspend treatment until haemoglobin concentration decreases and then restart at a dose approximately 25 % lower than the previous dose

Eprex® (Janssen-Cilag) ℗ℴ𝕄
Injection, prefilled syringe, epoetin alfa, net price 1000 units = £5.72; 2000 units = £11.44; 3000 units = £17.16; 4000 units = £22.88; 5000 units = £28.60; 6000 units = £34.32; 8000 units = £45.76; 10 000 units = £57.19; 20 000 units = £114.39; 30 000 units = £205.90; 40 000 units = £274.53. An auto-injector device is available for use with pre-filled syringes

Dose

> **Symptomatic anaemia associated with chronic renal failure in children on haemodialysis (see also notes above)**
> • By intravenous injection over 1–5 minutes
>> **Child 1 month–18 years** initially 50 units/kg 3 times weekly adjusted according to response in steps of 25 units/kg 3 times weekly at intervals of at least 4 weeks; maintenance dose, body-weight under 10 kg usually 75–150 units/kg 3 times weekly, body-weight 10–30 kg usually 60–150 units/kg 3 times weekly, body-weight 30–60 kg usually 30–100 units/kg 3 times weekly, body-weight over 60 kg usually 75–300 units/kg weekly (as a single dose or in divided doses)

Note Reduce dose by approximately 25% if rise in haemoglobin concentration exceeds 2 g/100 mL over 4 weeks or if haemoglobin concentration exceeds 12 g/100 mL; if haemoglobin concentration continues to rise, despite dose reduction, suspend treatment until haemoglobin concentration decreases and then restart at a dose approximately 25% lower than the previous dose

◢**Epoetin beta**

NeoRecormon® (Roche) ℗ℴ𝕄
Injection, prefilled syringe, epoetin beta, net price 500 units = £3.75; 2000 units = £14.98; 3000 units = £22.47; 4000 units = £29.96; 5000 units = £37.47; 6000 units = £44.94; 10 000 units = £74.90; 20 000 units = £149.79; 30 000 units = £224.69
Excipients include phenylalanine up to 300 micrograms/syringe (section 9.4.1)

Dose

> **Symptomatic anaemia associated with chronic renal failure (see also notes above)**
> • By subcutaneous injection
>> **Neonate** initially 20 units/kg 3 times weekly for 4 weeks, increased according to response at intervals of 4 weeks in steps of 20 units/kg 3 times weekly; total weekly dose may be divided into daily doses; maintenance dose, initially reduce dose by half then adjust according to response at intervals of 1–2 weeks; total

weekly maintenance dose may be given as a single dose or in 3 or 7 divided doses; max. 720 units/kg weekly

>> **Child 1 month–18 years** initially 20 units/kg 3 times weekly for 4 weeks, increased according to response at intervals of 4 weeks in steps of 20 units/kg 3 times weekly; total weekly dose may be divided into daily doses; maintenance dose, initially reduce dose by half then adjust according to response at intervals of 1–2 weeks; total weekly maintenance dose may be given as a single dose or in 3 or 7 divided doses; max. 720 units/kg weekly

> • By intravenous injection over 2 minutes
>> **Neonate** initially 40 units/kg 3 times weekly for 4 weeks, increased according to response to 80 units/kg 3 times weekly after 4 weeks, with further increases if needed at intervals of 4 weeks in steps of 20 units/kg 3 times weekly; maintenance dose, initially reduce dose by half then adjust according to response at intervals of 1–2 weeks; max. 720 units/kg weekly

>> **Child 1 month–18 years** initially 40 units/kg 3 times weekly for 4 weeks, increased according to response to 80 units/kg 3 times weekly after 4 weeks, with further increases if needed at intervals of 4 weeks in steps of 20 units/kg 3 times weekly; maintenance dose, initially reduce dose by half then adjust according to response at intervals of 1–2 weeks; max. 720 units/kg weekly

Note Subcutaneous route preferred in patients not on haemodialysis. Reduce dose by approximately 25% if rise in haemoglobin concentration exceeds 2 g/100 mL over 4 weeks or if haemoglobin concentration approaches or exceeds 12 g/100 mL; if haemoglobin concentration continues to rise, despite dose reduction, suspend treatment until haemoglobin concentration decreases and then restart at a dose approximately 25% lower than the previous dose.

> **Prevention of anaemias of prematurity in neonates with birth-weight of 0.75–1.5 kg and gestational age under 34 weeks**
> • By subcutaneous injection (of single-dose, unpreserved injection)
>> **Neonate** 250 units/kg 3 times weekly preferably starting within 3 days of birth and continued for 6 weeks

Multidose injection, powder for reconstitution, epoetin beta, net price 50 000-unit vial = £374.48 (with solvent)
Excipients include phenylalanine up to 5 mg/vial (section 9.4.1), benzyl alcohol (avoid in neonates, see Excipients p. 3)

Note Avoid contact of reconstituted injection with glass; use only plastic materials

Dose

> **Symptomatic anaemia associated with chronic renal failure (see also notes above)**
> • By subcutaneous injection
>> **Child 3–18 years** initially 20 units/kg 3 times weekly for 4 weeks, increased according to response at intervals of 4 weeks in steps of 20 units/kg 3 times weekly; total weekly dose may be divided into daily doses; maintenance dose, initially reduce dose by half then adjust according to response at intervals of 1–2 weeks; total weekly maintenance dose may be given as a single dose or in 3 or 7 divided doses; max. 720 units/kg weekly

> • By intravenous injection over 2 minutes
>> **Child 3–18 years** initially 40 units/kg 3 times weekly for 4 weeks, increased according to response to 80 units/kg 3 times weekly after 4 weeks, with further increases if needed at intervals of 4 weeks in steps of 20 units/kg 3 times weekly; maintenance dose, initially reduce dose by half then adjust according to response at intervals of 1–2 weeks; max. 720 units/kg weekly

Note Subcutaneous route preferred in patients not on haemodialysis. Reduce dose by approximately 25% if rise

9

Nutrition and blood

◻ **EPOETIN ALFA, BETA, and ZETA (continued)**

in haemoglobin concentration exceeds 2 g/100 mL over 4 weeks or if haemoglobin concentration approaches or exceeds 12 g/100 mL; if haemoglobin concentration continues to rise, despite dose reduction, suspend treatment until haemoglobin concentration decreases and then restart at a dose approximately 25% lower than the previous dose.

◢**Epoetin zeta**

Retacrit® (Hospira) ▼ PoM

Injection, prefilled syringe, epoetin zeta, net price 1000 units = £5.66; 2000 units = £11.31; 3000 units = £16.97; 4000 units = £22.63; 5000 units = £28.28; 6000 units = £33.94; 8000 units = £45.25; 10 000 units = £56.57; 20 000 units = £113.13; 30 000 units = £169.70; 40 000 units = £226.26

Excipients include phenylalanine up to 500 micrograms/syringe (section 9.4.1)

Note Biosimilar Medicine, p. 2

Dose

> Symptomatic anaemia associated with chronic renal failure in children on haemodialysis (see also notes above)
>
> • By intravenous injection over 1–5 minutes
>
> **Child 1 month–18 years** initially 50 units/kg 3 times weekly adjusted according to response in steps of 25 units/kg 3 times weekly at intervals of at least 4 weeks; maintenance dose, body-weight under 10 kg usually 75–150 units/kg 3 times weekly, body-weight 10–30 kg usually 60–150 units/kg 3 times weekly, body-weight over 30 kg usually 30–100 units/kg 3 times weekly

Note Avoid increasing haemoglobin concentration at a rate exceeding 2 g/100 mL over 4 weeks

Sickle-cell disease

Sickle-cell disease is caused by a structural abnormality of haemoglobin resulting in deformed, less flexible red blood cells. Acute complications in the more severe forms include *sickle-cell crisis*, where infarction of the microvasculature and blood supply to organs results in severe pain. Sickle-cell crisis requires hospitalisation, intravenous fluids, analgesia (section 4.7), and treatment of any concurrent infection. Chronic complications include skin ulceration, renal failure, and increased susceptibility to infection. Pneumococcal vaccine (section 14.4), haemophilus influenzae type b vaccine (section 14.4), an annual influenza vaccine (section 14.4), and prophylactic penicillin (Table 2, section 5.1) reduce the risk of infection. Hepatitis B vaccine (section 14.4) should be considered if the child is not immune.

In most forms of sickle-cell disease, varying degrees of haemolytic anaemia are present accompanied by increased erythropoiesis; this may increase folate requirements and folate supplementation may be necessary (section 9.1.2).

Hydroxycarbamide (hydroxyurea) can reduce the frequency of crises and the need for blood transfusions. Hydroxycarbamide should be considered, in consultation with a specialist centre, for children who have recurrent episodes of acute pain (more than 3 admissions in the previous 12 months, or who are very symptomatic in the community) or who have had 2 or more episodes of acute sickle chest syndrome in the last 2 years (or 1 episode requiring ventilatory support). Beneficial effects of hydroxycarbamide may not become evident for several months. Myelosuppression, and skin reactions are the most common side-effects.

HYDROXYCARBAMIDE

(Hydroxyurea)

Cautions see section 8.1 and notes above; also monitor renal and hepatic function before and during treatment; monitor full blood count before treatment, then every 2 weeks for the first 2 months and then every 2 months thereafter (or every 2 weeks if on max. dose); leg ulcers (review treatment if cutaneous vasculitic ulcerations develop); **interactions:** Appendix 1 (hydroxycarbamide)

Hepatic impairment manufacturer advises caution in mild to moderate impairment; avoid in severe impairment

Renal impairment reduce initial dose by 50% if estimated glomerular filtration rate less than 60 mL/minute/1.73 m^2; avoid if estimated glomerular filtration rate less than 30 mL/minute/1.73 m^2

Pregnancy avoid (teratogenic in *animal* studies); manufacturer advises effective contraception before and during treatment; see also section 8.1

Breast-feeding discontinue breast-feeding

Side-effects see section 8.1 and notes above; also headache; *less commonly* dizziness, and rash; *rarely* reduced sperm count and activity; fever, amenorrhoea, bleeding, and hypomagnesaemia also reported

Indication and dose

> Sickle-cell disease (see notes above)
>
> • By mouth
>
> **Child 2–18 years** initially 10–15 mg/kg once daily, increased every 12 weeks in steps of 5 mg/kg daily according to response; usual dose 15–30 mg/kg daily (max. 35 mg/kg daily)

9 Nutrition and blood

◻ **HYDROXYCARBAMIDE (continued)**

Siklos® (Nordic) ▼ PoM
Tablets, scored, f/c, hydroxycarbamide 1 g, net price 30-tab pack = £500.00

▲Extemporaneous formulations available see Extemporaneous Preparations, p. 8

Iron overload

Severe tissue iron overload can occur in aplastic and other refractory anaemias, mainly as the result of repeated blood transfusions. It is a particular problem in refractory anaemias with hyperplastic bone marrow, especially *thalassaemia major*, where excessive iron absorption from the gut and inappropriate iron therapy can add to the tissue siderosis.

Iron overload associated with haemochromatosis can be treated with repeated venesection. Venesection may also be used for patients who have received multiple transfusions and whose bone marrow has recovered. Where venesection is contra-indicated, and in thalassaemia, the long-term administration of the iron chelating compound **desferrioxamine mesilate** is useful. Subcutaneous infusions of desferrioxamine are given over 8–12 hours, 3–7 times a week; the dose should reflect the degree of iron overload. The initial dose should not exceed 30 mg/kg. For established overload the dose is usually between 20 and 50 mg/kg daily. Desferrioxamine (up to 2 g per unit of blood) may also be given at the time of blood transfusion, provided that the desferrioxamine is **not** added to the blood and is **not** given through the same line as the blood (but the two may be given through the same cannula).

Iron excretion induced by desferrioxamine is enhanced by ascorbic acid (vitamin C, section 9.6.3) 100–200 mg daily by mouth; it should be given separately from food since it also enhances iron absorption. Ascorbic acid should not be given to children with cardiac dysfunction; in children with normal cardiac function ascorbic acid should be introduced 1 month after starting desferrioxamine.

Desferrioxamine infusion can be used to treat *aluminium overload* in dialysis patients; theoretically 100 mg of desferrioxamine binds with 4.1 mg of aluminium.

Deferasirox, an oral iron chelator, is licensed for the treatment of chronic iron overload in children over 6 years with thalassaemia major who receive frequent blood transfusions (more than 7 mL/kg/month of packed blood cells). It is also licensed for chronic iron overload when desferrioxamine is contra-indicated or inadequate in children with thalassaemia major who receive infrequent blood transfusions (less than 7 mL/kg/month of packed red blood cells), in children with other anaemias, and in children aged 2 to 5 years.

The *Scottish Medicines Consortium* (p. 4) has advised (January 2007) that deferasirox is accepted for restricted use within NHS Scotland for the treatment of chronic iron overload associated with the treatment of rare acquired or inherited anaemias requiring recurrent blood transfusions. It is not recommended for patients with myelodysplastic syndromes.

Deferiprone, an oral iron chelator, is licensed for the treatment of iron overload in children over 6 years of age with thalassaemia major in whom desferrioxamine is contra-indicated or is inadequate. Blood dyscrasias, particularly agranulocytosis, have been reported with deferiprone.

◣ DEFERASIROX

Cautions eye and ear examinations required before treatment and annually during treatment; monitor body-weight, height and sexual development annually; monitor serum-ferritin concentration monthly; risk of gastro-intestinal ulceration and haemorrhage; platelet count less than 50×10^9/litre; consider treatment interruption if unexplained cytopenia occurs; not recommended in conditions which may reduce life expectancy (e.g. high-risk myelodysplastic syndromes); history of liver cirrhosis; test liver function before treatment, then every 2 weeks during the first month, and then monthly; measure baseline serum-creatinine and monitor renal function weekly during the first month of treatment and monthly thereafter; test for proteinuria monthly; **interactions:** Appendix 1 (deferasirox)

Hepatic impairment manufacturer advises caution—no information available; avoid in severe impairment

Renal impairment reduce dose by 10 mg/kg if serum-creatinine increased above age-appropriate limits *or* estimated glomerular filtration rate less than 90 mL/minute/1.73 m² on 2 consecutive occasions—interrupt treatment if deterioration in renal function persists after dose reduction; avoid if estimated glomerular filtration rate less than 60 mL/minute/1.73 m²

9

Nutrition and blood

⌐ **DEFERASIROX** *(continued)*

Pregnancy manufacturer advises avoid unless essential—toxicity in *animal* studies

Breast-feeding manufacturer advises avoid—present in milk in *animal* studies

Side-effects gastro-intestinal disturbances (including ulceration and fatal haemorrhage); headache; proteinuria; pruritus; rash; *less commonly* oedema, hepatitis, cholelithiasis, fatigue, anxiety, sleep disorder, dizziness, pyrexia, pharyngitis, glucosuria, renal tubulopathy, disturbances of hearing and vision (including lens opacity and maculopathy), and skin pigmentation; hepatic failure, acute renal failure, blood disorders (including agranulocytosis, neutropenia, pancytopenia, and thrombocytopenia), hypersensitivity reactions (including anaphylaxis and angioedema), and alopecia also reported

Licensed use see notes above

Indication and dose

Chronic iron overload
- **By mouth**

    Child 2–18 years initially 10–30 mg/kg once daily according to serum-ferritin concentration and amount of transfused blood (consult product literature); maintenance, adjust dose every 3–6 months in steps of 5–10 mg/kg according to serum-ferritin concentration; usual max. 30 mg/kg daily, but may be increased to max. 40 mg/kg daily and reduced in steps of 5–10 mg/kg once control achieved

    Note Dose should be rounded to nearest whole tablet size

Exjade® (Novartis) ▼ PoM

Dispersible tablets, deferasirox 125 mg, net price 28-tab pack = £117.60; 250 mg, 28-tab pack = £235.20; 500 mg, 28-tab pack = £470.40. Label: 13, 22, counselling, administration

Counselling Tablets should be dispersed in water, orange juice, or apple juice; if necessary, resuspend residue and swallow

DEFERIPRONE

Cautions monitor neutrophil count weekly and discontinue treatment if neutropenia develops

Blood disorders Patients or their carers should be told how to recognise signs of neutropenia and advised to seek immediate medical attention if symptoms such as fever or sore throat develop

Contra-indications history of agranulocytosis or recurrent neutropenia

Hepatic impairment manufacturer advises monitor liver function—interrupt treatment if persistent elevation in serum alanine aminotransferase

Renal impairment manufacturer advises caution—no information available

Pregnancy manufacturer advises avoid before intended conception and during pregnancy—teratogenic and embryotoxic in *animal* studies; contraception advised in girls of child-bearing potential

Breast-feeding manufacturer advises avoid—no information available

Side-effects gastro-intestinal disturbances (reducing dose and increasing gradually may improve tolerance), increased appetite; headache; red-brown urine discoloration; neutropenia, agranulocytosis; zinc deficiency; arthropathy

Licensed use see notes above

Indication and dose

Iron overload in thalassaemia major
- **By mouth**

    Child 6–18 years 25 mg/kg 3 times daily (max. 100 mg/kg daily)

Ferriprox® (Swedish Orphan) PoM

Tablets, f/c, scored, deferiprone 500 mg, net price 100-tab pack = £152.39. Label: 14, counselling, blood disorders

Oral solution, red, deferiprone 100 mg/mL, net price 500 mL = £152.39. Label: 14, counselling, blood disorders

DESFERRIOXAMINE MESILATE
(Deferoxamine Mesilate)

Cautions eye and ear examinations before treatment and at 3-month intervals during treatment; monitor body-weight and height in children at 3-month intervals—risk of growth restriction with excessive doses; aluminium-related encephalopathy (may exacerbate neurological dysfunction); **interactions:** Appendix 1 (desferrioxamine)

Renal impairment use with caution

Pregnancy teratogenic in *animal* studies, manufacturer advises use only if potential benefit outweighs risk

Breast-feeding manufacturer advises use only if potential benefit outweighs risk—no information available

Side-effects hypotension (especially when given too rapidly by intravenous injection), disturbances of hearing and vision (including lens opacity and retinopathy); injection site reactions, gastro-intestinal disturbances, asthma, fever, headache, arthralgia and myalgia; very rarely anaphylaxis, acute respiratory distress syndrome, neurological disturbances (including dizziness, neuropathy and paraesthesia), Yersinia and mucormycosis infections, rash, renal impairment, and blood dyscrasias

Indication and dose

Chronic iron overload see notes above

Aluminium overload in dialysis patients
- **By intravenous infusion**

    Child 1 month–18 years 5 mg/kg once weekly

▱ **DESFERRIOXAMINE MESILATE** (*continued*)

Iron poisoning

See Emergency Treatment of Poisoning, p. 42

Administration For *intravenous* or *subcutaneous infusion*, reconstitute powder with Water for Injection to a concentration of 100 mg/mL; dilute with Glucose 5% *or* Sodium Chloride 0.9%. In *haemodialysis* or *haemofiltration* administer over the last hour of dialysis (may be given via the dialysis fistula). *Intraperitoneal*: may be added to dialysis fluid. In CAPD give prior to the last exchange of the day.

Note For full details and warnings relating to administration, consult product literature

Desferrioxamine mesilate (Non-proprietary) [PoM]
Injection, powder for reconstitution, desferrioxamine mesilate, net price 500-mg vial = £4.26; 2-g vial = £17.05

Desferal® (Novartis) [PoM]
Injection, powder for reconstitution, desferrioxamine mesilate, net price 500-mg vial = £4.44, 2-g vial = £17.77

9.1.4 Drugs used in platelet disorders

Idiopathic thrombocytopenic purpura   Acute idiopathic thrombocytopenic purpura is usually self-limiting in children. A **corticosteroid**, such as prednisolone (p. 460), is sometimes used if idiopathic thrombocytopenic purpura does not resolve spontaneously or if it is associated with severe cutaneous symptoms or mucous membrane bleeding; corticosteroid treatment should not be continued longer than 14 days regardless of the response.

Immunoglobulin preparations (section 14.5) may be used in idiopathic thrombocytopenic purpura or where a temporary rapid rise in platelets is needed, as in pregnancy or pre-operatively; they are often used in preference to a corticosteroid. Anti-D immunoglobulin is licensed for the management of idiopathic thrombocytopenic purpura.

Other therapy that has been tried under specialist supervision in refractory idiopathic thrombocytopenic purpura includes azathioprine (section 8.2.1), cyclophosphamide (section 8.1.1), vincristine (section 8.1.4), and ciclosporin (section 8.2.2). Rituximab is also used in specialist centres but experience of its use in children is limited. For patients with chronic severe thrombocytopenia refractory to other therapy, tranexamic acid (section 2.11) may be given to reduce the severity of haemorrhage.

Splenectomy is considered in chronic thrombocytopenic purpura if a satisfactory platelet count is not achieved with regular immunoglobulin infusions, if there is a relapse on withdrawing or reducing the dose of corticosteroid, and if other therapies are considered inappropriate.

Essential thrombocythaemia   **Anagrelide** reduces platelets in essential thrombocythaemia in patients at risk of thrombo-haemorrhagic events who have not responded adequately to other drugs or who cannot tolerate other drugs.

◢ ANAGRELIDE

Cautions cardiovascular disease—assess cardiac function before and during treatment; concomitant aspirin in patients at risk of haemorrhage; monitor full blood count (monitor platelet count every 2 days for 1 week, then weekly until maintenance dose established), liver function, serum creatinine, and urea; **interactions:** Appendix 1 (anagrelide)

Skilled tasks Dizziness may affect performance of skilled tasks (e.g. driving)

Hepatic impairment manufacturer advises caution in mild impairment; avoid in moderate to severe impairment

Renal impairment manufacturer advises avoid if estimated glomerular filtration rate less than 50 mL/minute/1.73 m^2

Pregnancy manufacturer advises avoid (toxicity in *animal* studies)

Breast-feeding manufacturer advises avoid—no information available

Side-effects gastro-intestinal disturbances; palpitation, tachycardia, fluid retention; headache, dizziness, fatigue; anaemia; rash; *less commonly* pancreatitis, gastro-intestinal haemorrhage, congestive heart failure, hypertension, arrhythmias, syncope, chest pain, dyspnoea, sleep disturbances, paraesthesia, hypoaesthesia, depression, nervousness, confusion, amnesia, fever, weight changes, impotence, blood disorders, myalgia, arthralgia, epistaxis, dry mouth, alopecia, skin discoloration, and pruritus; *rarely* gastritis, colitis, postural hypotension, angina, myocardial infarction, vasodilatation, pulmonary infiltrates, migraine, drowsiness, impaired co-ordination, dysarthria, asthenia, tinnitus, renal failure, noc-

9

Nutrition and blood

◌ **ANAGRELIDE (continued)**

turia, visual disturbances, and gingival bleeding; allergic alveolitis also reported

Licensed use not licensed for use in children

Indication and dose

> Essential thrombocythaemia in at-risk children who have not responded adequately to other therapy or who are intolerant of it (initiated under specialist supervision)
>
> • By mouth
>
> **Child 7–18 years** initially 500 micrograms daily adjusted according to response in steps of

500 micrograms daily at weekly intervals to max. 10 mg daily (max. single dose 2.5 mg); usual dose range 1–3 mg daily in divided doses

Xagrid® (Shire) ▼ PoM
Capsules, anagrelide (as hydrochloride), 500 micrograms, net price 100–cap pack= £337.14. Counselling, skilled tasks, see above

---

9.1.5 G6PD deficiency

Glucose 6-phosphate dehydrogenase (G6PD) deficiency is highly prevalent in individuals originating from most parts of Africa, from most parts of Asia, from Oceania, and from Southern Europe; it can also occur, rarely, in any other individuals. G6PD deficiency is more common in males than it is in females.

Individuals with G6PD deficiency are susceptible to developing acute haemolytic anaemia when they take a number of common drugs. They are also susceptible to developing acute haemolytic anaemia when they eat fava beans (broad beans, *Vicia faba*); this is termed *favism* and can be more severe in children or when the fresh fava beans are eaten raw.

When prescribing drugs for children with G6PD deficiency, the following three points should be kept in mind:

• G6PD deficiency is genetically heterogeneous; susceptibility to the haemolytic risk from drugs varies; thus, a drug found to be safe in some G6PD-deficient individuals may not be equally safe in others;

• manufacturers do not routinely test drugs for their effects in G6PD-deficient individuals;

• the risk and severity of haemolysis is almost always dose-related.

The lists below should be read with these points in mind. Ideally, information about G6PD deficiency should be available before prescribing a drug listed below. However, in the absence of this information, the possibility of haemolysis should be considered, especially if the child belongs to a group in which G6PD deficiency is common.

A very few G6PD-deficient individuals with chronic non-spherocytic haemolytic anaemia have haemolysis even in the absence of an exogenous trigger. These children must be regarded as being at high risk of severe exacerbation of haemolysis following administration of any of the drugs listed below.

> **Drugs with *definite* risk of haemolysis in most G6PD-deficient individuals**
> **Dapsone** and other sulphones (higher doses for dermatitis herpetiformis more likely to cause problems)
> **Methylthioninium chloride** (methylene blue)
> **Niridazole** [not on UK market]
> **Nitrofurantoin**
> **Pamaquin** [not on UK market]
> **Primaquine** (30 mg weekly for 8 weeks has been found to be without undue harmful effects in African and Asian people, see section 5.4.1)
> **Quinolones** (including ciprofloxacin, moxifloxacin, nalidixic acid, norfloxacin, and ofloxacin)
> **Sulphonamides** (including co-trimoxazole; some sulphonamides, e.g. sulfadiazine, have been tested and found not to be haemolytic in many G6PD-deficient individuals)

> **Drugs with *possible* risk of haemolysis in some G6PD-deficient individuals**
> **Aspirin** (acceptable up to a dose of at least 1 g daily in most G6PD-deficient individuals)
> **Chloroquine** (acceptable in acute malaria and malaria chemoprophylaxis)
> **Menadione**, water-soluble derivatives (e.g. menadiol sodium phosphate)
> **Probenecid** [not on UK market]
> **Quinidine** (acceptable in acute malaria) [not on UK market]
> **Quinine** (acceptable in acute malaria)
> **Rasburicase**

Note Naphthalene in mothballs also causes haemolysis in individuals with G6PD-deficiency.

9.1.6 Drugs used in neutropenia

Recombinant human granulocyte-colony stimulating factor (rhG-CSF) stimulates the production of neutrophils and may reduce the duration of chemotherapy-induced neutropenia and thereby reduce the incidence of associated sepsis; there is as yet no evidence that it improves overall survival. **Filgrastim** (unglycosylated rhG-CSF) and **lenograstim** (glycosylated rhG-CSF) have similar effects; both have been used in a variety of clinical settings, including cytotoxic-induced neutropenia, and neutropenia following bone marrow transplantation, but they do not have any clear-cut routine indications. In congenital neutropenia filgrastim usually increases the neutrophil count with an appropriate clinical response. Prolonged use may be associated with an increased risk of myeloid malignancy.

Treatment with granulocyte-colony stimulating factors should only be prescribed by those experienced in their use.

Neonatal neutropenia   Filgrastim has been used to treat sepsis-induced neutropenia in preterm neonates. There is no clear evidence that granulocyte-colony stimulating factors improve survival or long-term outcomes.

Cautions   Granulocyte-colony stimulating factors should be used with caution in patients with pre-malignant or malignant myeloid conditions. Full blood counts (including differential white cell count and platelet count) should be monitored. Treatment should be withdrawn in patients who develop signs of pulmonary infiltration. There have been reports of pulmonary infiltrates leading to acute respiratory distress syndrome—patients with a history of pulmonary infiltrates or pneumonia may be at higher risk. Granulocyte-colony stimulating factors should be used with caution in children with sickle-cell disease. Spleen size should be monitored during treatment as there is a risk of splenomegaly and rupture.

Pregnancy and breast-feeding   There have been reports of toxicity in *animal* studies and manufacturers advise to not use granulocyte-colony stimulating factors during pregnancy unless the potential benefit outweighs the risk. There is no evidence for the use of granulocyte-colony stimulating factors during breast-feeding and manufacturers advise avoiding use.

Side-effects   Side-effects of granulocyte-colony stimulating factors include gastro-intestinal disturbances, anorexia, headache, asthenia, fever, musculoskeletal pain, bone pain, rash, alopecia, injection-site reactions, thrombocytopenia, and leucocytosis. *Less commonly* chest pain can occur. Pulmonary side-effects, particularly interstitial pneumonia (see Cautions above), cutaneous vasculitis, and acute febrile neutrophilic dermatosis have *rarely* been reported.

9

Nutrition and blood

FILGRASTIM

(Recombinant human granulocyte-colony stimulating factor, G-CSF)

Cautions see notes above; also regular morphological and cytogenetic bone-marrow examinations recommended in severe congenital neutropenia (possible risk of myelodysplastic syndromes or leukaemia); secondary acute myeloid leukaemia; osteoporotic bone disease (monitor bone density if given for more than 6 months); **interactions:** Appendix 1 (filgrastim)

Contra-indications severe congenital neutropenia (Kostman's syndrome) with abnormal cytogenetics

Pregnancy see notes above

Breast-feeding see notes above

Side-effects see notes above; also mucositis, splenic enlargement, hepatomegaly, transient hypotension, epistaxis, urinary abnormalities (including dysuria, proteinuria, and haematuria), osteoporosis, exacerbation of rheumatoid arth-

◁ FILGRASTIM (*continued*)

ritis, anaemia, transient decrease in blood glucose, pseudogout, and raised uric acid; *very rarely* splenic rupture

Licensed use not licensed for treatment of glycogen storage disease or neonatal neutropenia

Indication and dose

Cytotoxic-induced neutropenia

- Preferably by subcutaneous injection or by intravenous infusion (over 30 minutes)

  Child 1 month–18 years 5 micrograms/kg daily started not less than 24 hours after cytotoxic chemotherapy, continued until neutrophil count in normal range, usually for up to 14 days (up to 38 days in acute myeloid leukaemia)

Myeloablative therapy followed by bone-marrow transplantation

- By intravenous infusion over 30 minutes or over 24 hours or by subcutaneous infusion over 24 hours

  Child 1 month–18 years 10 micrograms/kg daily, started not less than 24 hours following cytotoxic chemotherapy (and within 24 hours of bone-marrow infusion), then adjusted according to absolute neutrophil count (consult product literature and local protocol)

Mobilisation of peripheral blood progenitor cells for autologous infusion, used alone

- By subcutaneous injection or by subcutaneous infusion over 24 hours

  Child 1 month–18 years 10 micrograms/kg daily for 5–7 days

Mobilisation of peripheral blood progenitor cells for autologous infusion following adjunctive myelosuppressive chemotherapy (to improve yield)

- By subcutaneous injection

  Child 1 month–18 years 5 micrograms/kg daily, started the day after completion of chemotherapy and continued until neutrophil count in normal range; for timing of leucopheresis consult product literature

Mobilisation of peripheral blood progenitor cells in normal donors for allogeneic infusion

- By subcutaneous injection

  Child over 16 years 10 micrograms/kg daily for 4–5 days; for timing of leucopheresis consult product literature

Severe chronic neutropenia

- By subcutaneous injection

  Child 1 month–18 years in severe congenital neutropenia, initially 12 micrograms/kg daily in single or divided doses (initially 5 micrograms/kg daily in idiopathic or cyclic neutropenia), adjusted according to response (consult product literature and local protocol)

Persistent neutropenia in HIV infection

- By subcutaneous injection

  Child 1 month–18 years initially 1 microgram/kg daily, increased as necessary until absolute neutrophil count in normal range (usual max. 4 micrograms/kg daily), then adjusted to maintain absolute neutrophil count in normal range (consult product literature)

Neonatal neutropenia

- By subcutaneous injection

  Neonate 10 micrograms/kg daily, discontinue if white cell count exceeds 50×10^9/litre

Glycogen storage disease type 1b

- By subcutaneous injection

  5 micrograms/kg daily, adjusted as necessary

Administration For *subcutaneous* or *intravenous infusion*, dilute with Glucose 5% to a concentration of not less than 15 micrograms/mL (concentration of 100 micrograms/mL adequate for *subcutaneous injection* in neonates); to dilute to a concentration of 2–15 micrograms/mL, add albumin solution (human albumin solution) to produce a final albumin solution of 2 mg/mL; not compatible with Sodium Chloride solutions

Neupogen® (Amgen) ℗ℴℳ
Injection, filgrastim 30 million units (300 micrograms)/mL; net price 1-mL vial = £65.74

Injection (Singleject®), filgrastim 60 million units (600 micrograms)/mL, net price 0.5-mL prefilled syringe = £65.74; 96 million units (960 micrograms)/mL, 0.5-mL prefilled syringe = £104.85

Ratiograstim® (Ratiopharm UK) ▼ ℗ℴℳ
Injection, prefilled syringe, filgrastim, net price 30 million units (300 micrograms)/0.5 ml = £62.25; 48 million units (480 micrograms)/0.8 ml = £99.29
Note Biosimilar medicine , p. 2

Zarzio® (Sandoz) ▼ ℗ℴℳ
Injection, prefilled syringe, filgrastim, net price 30 million-units (300 micrograms)/0.5 mL = £59.00; 48 million-units (480 micrograms)/0.5 mL = £94.00
Note Biosimilar medicine , p. 2

LENOGRASTIM

(Recombinant human granulocyte-colony stimulating factor, rHuG-CSF)

Cautions see notes above

Pregnancy see notes above

Breast-feeding see notes above

Side-effects see notes above; also splenic rupture and toxic epidermal necrolysis

Licensed use not licensed for use in children for cytotoxic-induced neutropenia, mobilisation of peripheral blood progenitor cells (monotherapy or adjunctive therapy), or following peripheral stem cells transplantation

◁ **LENOGRASTIM (continued)**

Indication and dose

Following peripheral stem cells or bone-marrow transplantation

- By intravenous infusion over 30 minutes or by subcutaneous injection

  Child 2–18 years 150 micrograms/m² daily started the day after transplantation, continued until neutrophil count stable in acceptable range (max. 28 days)

Cytotoxic-induced neutropenia

- By subcutaneous injection

  Child 2–18 years 150 micrograms/m² daily started the day after completion of chemotherapy, continued until neutrophil count stable in acceptable range (max. 28 days)

Mobilisation of peripheral blood progenitor cells, used alone

- By subcutaneous injection

  Child 2–18 years 10 micrograms/kg daily for 4–6 days (5–6 days in healthy donors)

Mobilisation of peripheral blood progenitor cells following adjunctive myelosuppressive chemotherapy (to improve yield)

- By subcutaneous injection

  Child 2–18 years 150 micrograms/m² daily, started 1–5 days after completion of chemotherapy and continued until neutrophil count in acceptable range; for timing of leucopheresis consult product literature

Administration for *intravenous infusion*, dilute reconstituted solution to a concentration of not less than 2 micrograms/mL (*Granocyte-13*) or 2.5 micrograms/mL (*Granocyte-34*) with Sodium Chloride 0.9%

Granocyte® (Chugai) PoM

Injection, powder for reconstitution, lenograstim, net price 13.4 million-unit (105-microgram) vial = £40.11; 33.6 million-unit (263-microgram) vial = £64.47 (both with 1-mL prefilled syringe water for injections)
Excipients include phenylalanine (section 9.4.1)

9.2 Fluids and electrolytes

9.2.1 Oral preparations for fluid and electrolyte imbalance
9.2.2 Parenteral preparations for fluid and electrolyte imbalance

The following tables give a selection of useful electrolyte values:

Electrolyte concentrations—intravenous fluids

Intravenous infusion	Millimoles per litre				
	Na^+	K^+	HCO_3^-	Cl^-	Ca^{2+}
Normal plasma values	142	4.5	26	103	2.5
Sodium Chloride 0.9%	150	—	—	150	—
Compound Sodium Lactate (Hartmann's)	131	5	29	111	2
Sodium Chloride 0.45% and Glucose 5%	75	—	—	75	—
Potassium Chloride 0.15% and Glucose 5%	—	20	—	20	—
Potassium Chloride 0.15% and Sodium Chloride 0.9%	150	20	—	170	—
Potassium Chloride 0.3% and Glucose 5%	—	40	—	40	—
Potassium Chloride 0.3% and Sodium Chloride 0.9%	150	40	—	190	—
To correct metabolic acidosis					
Sodium Bicarbonate 1.26%	150	—	150	—	—
Sodium Bicarbonate 8.4% for cardiac arrest	1000	—	1000	—	—
Sodium Lactate (m/6)	167	—	167	—	—

Electrolyte content—gastro-intestinal secretions

Type of fluid	Millimoles per litre				
	H^+	Na^+	K^+	HCO_3^-	Cl^-
Gastric	40–60	20–80	5–20	—	100–150
Biliary	—	120–140	5–15	30–50	80–120
Pancreatic	—	120–140	5–15	70–110	40–80
Small bowel	—	120–140	5–15	20–40	90–130

Faeces, vomit, or aspiration should be saved and analysed where possible if abnormal losses are suspected; where this is impracticable the approximations above may be helpful in planning replacement therapy

9

Nutrition and blood

9.2.1 Oral preparations for fluid and electrolyte imbalance

9.2.1.1 Oral potassium
9.2.1.2 Oral sodium and water
9.2.1.3 Oral bicarbonate

Sodium and potassium salts, which may be given by mouth to prevent deficiencies or to treat established deficiencies of mild or moderate degree, are discussed in this section. Oral preparations for removing excess potassium and preparations for oral rehydration therapy are also included here. Oral bicarbonate, for metabolic acidosis, is also described in this section.

For reference to calcium, magnesium, and phosphate, see section 9.5.

9.2.1.1 Oral potassium

Compensation for potassium loss is especially necessary:

- in children in whom secondary hyperaldosteronism occurs, e.g. renal artery stenosis, renal tubule disorder, the nephrotic syndrome, and severe heart failure;
- in children with excessive losses of potassium in the faeces, e.g. chronic diarrhoea associated with intestinal malabsorption or laxative abuse;
- in those taking digoxin or anti-arrhythmic drugs, where potassium depletion may induce arrhythmias.

Measures to compensate for potassium loss may be required during long-term administration of drugs known to induce potassium loss (e.g. corticosteroids). Potassium supplements are **seldom required** with the small doses of diuretics given to treat hypertension; **potassium-sparing diuretics** (rather than potassium supplements) are recommended for prevention of hypokalaemia due to diuretics such as furosemide (frusemide) or the thiazides when these are given to eliminate oedema.

Dosage If potassium salts are used for the *prevention of hypokalaemia*, then doses of potassium chloride 1–2 mmol/kg (usual max. 50 mmol potassium) daily by mouth are suitable in patients taking a normal diet. *Smaller doses* must be used if there is *renal insufficiency* to reduce the **risk** of **hyperkalaemia**. Potassium salts cause nausea and vomiting and poor compliance is a major limitation to their effectiveness (small divided doses may minimise gastric irritation); when appropriate, potassium-sparing diuretics are preferable (see also above). Regular monitoring of plasma-potassium concentration is essential in those taking potassium supplements. When there is *established potassium depletion* larger doses may be necessary, the quantity depending on the severity of any continuing potassium loss (monitoring of plasma-potassium concentration and specialist advice would be required). Potassium depletion is frequently associated with chloride depletion and with metabolic alkalosis, and these disorders require correction.

Administration Potassium salts are preferably given as a liquid (or effervescent) preparation, rather than modified-release tablets; they should be given as the chloride (the use of effervescent potassium tablets BPC 1968 should be restricted to *hyperchloraemic states*, section 9.2.1.3). Potassium chloride solutions suitable for use by mouth in neonates are available from 'special-order' manufacturers or specialist importing companies, see p. 957; they should be used with care because they are hypertonic and can damage the gastric mucosa.

Salt substitutes A number of salt substitutes which contain significant amounts of potassium chloride are readily available as health food products (e.g. *LoSalt®* and *Ruthmol®*). These should not be used by patients with renal failure as potassium intoxication may result.

POTASSIUM CHLORIDE

Cautions see notes above; cardiac disease; intestinal stricture, history of peptic ulcer, hiatus hernia (*with modified-release preparations*); **interactions:** Appendix 1 (potassium salts)

Contra-indications plasma-potassium concentration above 5 mmol/litre

Renal impairment close monitoring required—risk of hyperkalaemia; avoid in severe impairment

Side-effects nausea, vomiting, abdominal pain, diarrhoea, flatulence; *with modified-release pre-parations*, gastro-intestinal obstruction, ulceration, and bleeding also reported

Indication and dose

Potassium depletion
- By mouth

    Neonate 0.5–1 mmol/kg K^+ twice daily (total daily dose may alternatively be given in 3 divided doses), adjusted according to plasma-potassium concentration

9 Nutrition and blood

◻ **POTASSIUM CHLORIDE** (*continued*)

Child 1 month–18 years 0.5–1 mmol/kg K$^+$ twice daily (total daily dose may alternatively be given in 3 divided doses), adjusted according to plasma-potassium concentration

Note Do not confuse Effervescent Potassium Tablets BPC 1968 (section 9.2.1.3) with effervescent potassium chloride tablets. Effervescent Potassium Tablets BPC 1968 do not contain chloride ions and their use should be restricted to hyperchloraemic states (section 9.2.1.3).

Kay-Cee-L® (Geistlich)
Syrup, sugar-free, red, potassium chloride 7.5% (1 mmol/mL each of K$^+$ and Cl$^-$), net price 500 mL = £3.74. Label: 21

Sando-K® (HK Pharma)
Tablets, effervescent, potassium bicarbonate and chloride equivalent to potassium 470 mg (12 mmol of K$^+$) and chloride 285 mg (8 mmol of Cl$^-$), net price 20 = £1.53. Label: 13, 21

◢**Modified-release preparations**
Avoid unless effervescent tablets or liquid preparations inappropriate

Slow-K® (Alliance) ◢
Tablets, m/r, orange, s/c, potassium chloride 600 mg (8 mmol each of K$^+$ and Cl$^-$), net price 100 = £2.14. Label: 25, 27, counselling, swallow whole with fluid during meals while sitting or standing

Management of hyperkalaemia

Acute severe hyperkalaemia calls for urgent treatment with intravenous infusion of **soluble insulin** (0.3–0.6 units/kg/hour in neonates and 0.05–0.2 units/kg/hour in children over 1 month) with **glucose** 0.5–1 g/kg/hour (5–10 mL/kg of glucose 10%; 2.5–5 mL/kg of glucose 20% via a central venous catheter may also be considered). If insulin cannot be used, **salbutamol** (section 3.1.1.1) can be given by intravenous injection, but it has a slower onset of action and may be less effective for reducing plasma-potassium concentration.

Calcium gluconate (section 9.5.1.1) is given by slow intravenous injection to manage cardiac excitability caused by hyperkalaemia.

The correction of causal or compounding acidosis with sodium bicarbonate infusion (section 9.2.2.1) should be considered (**important**: preparations of sodium bicarbonate and calcium salts should not be administered in the same line—risk of precipitation). Intravenous furosemide can also be given but is less effective in children with renal impairment. Drugs exacerbating hyperkalaemia should be reviewed and stopped as appropriate; dialysis may occasionally be required.

Ion-exchange resins may be used to remove excess potassium in *mild hyperkalaemia* or in *moderate hyperkalaemia* when there are no ECG changes. Calcium polystyrene sulphonate is preferred unless plasma-calcium concentrations are high.

POLYSTYRENE SULPHONATE RESINS

Cautions impaction of resin with excessive dosage or inadequate dilution; monitor for electrolyte disturbances (stop if plasma-potassium concentration below 5 mmol/litre); sodium-containing resin in congestive heart failure, hypertension, and oedema; **interactions**: Appendix 1 (polystyrene sulphonate resins)

Contra-indications obstructive bowel disease; neonates with reduced gut motility; calcium-containing resin in hyperparathyroidism, multiple myeloma, sarcoidosis, or metastatic carcinoma

Renal impairment use sodium-containing resin with caution

Pregnancy manufacturers advise use only if potential benefit outweighs risk—no information available

Breast-feeding manufacturers advise use only if potential benefit outweighs risk—no information available

Side-effects rectal ulceration following rectal administration; colonic necrosis reported following enemas containing sorbitol; sodium retention, hypercalcaemia, gastric irritation, anorexia, nausea, vomiting, constipation (discontinue treatment—avoid magnesium-containing laxa-

tives), diarrhoea; calcium-containing resin can cause hypercalcaemia (in dialysed patients and occasionally in those with renal impairment), hypomagnesaemia

Indication and dose

Hyperkalaemia associated with anuria or severe oliguria, and in dialysis patients
- By mouth
  Child 1 month–18 years 125–250 mg/kg (max. 15 g) 3–4 times daily
- By rectum
  Neonate 125–250 mg/kg repeated as necessary every 6–8 hours. Irrigate colon to remove resin after 6–12 hours

  Child 1 month–18 years 125–250 mg/kg repeated as necessary every 6–8 hours. Irrigate colon to remove resin after 6–12 hours

Administration By mouth: administer in water or as a paste—do not give with fruit squash, which has a high potassium content.
By rectum: mix 1 g of resin with 5–10 mL of a methylcellulose solution. Water may be used but retention is more difficult.

9

Nutrition and blood

◿ **POLYSTYRENE SULPHONATE RESINS (continued)**

Calcium Resonium® (Sanofi-Aventis)
Powder, buff, calcium polystyrene sulphonate, net price 300 g = £68.47. Label: 13

Resonium A® (Sanofi-Aventis)
Powder, buff, sodium polystyrene sulphonate, net price 454 g = £67.50. Label: 13

9.2.1.2 Oral sodium and water

Sodium chloride is indicated in states of sodium depletion. In preterm neonates in the first few weeks of life and in chronic conditions associated with mild or moderate degrees of sodium depletion, e.g. in salt-losing bowel or renal disease, oral supplements of sodium chloride (section 9.2.1.3) may be sufficient. Sodium chloride solutions suitable for use by mouth in neonates are available from 'special-order' manufacturers or specialist importing companies, see p. 957; they should be used with care because they are hypertonic. Supplementation with sodium chloride may be required to replace losses in children with cystic fibrosis particularly in warm weather.

▍SODIUM CHLORIDE

Indication and dose

See also section 9.2.2

Sodium supplementation in neonates
• By mouth

Preterm neonate 2 mmol/100 mL of formula feed or 3–4 mmol/100 mL of breast milk, consult dietician

Sodium replacement
• By mouth

Child 1 month–18 years according to requirements, generally 1–2 mmol/kg daily in divided doses, higher doses may be needed in severe depletion

Chronic renal loss
• By mouth

Child 1 month–18 years 1–2 mmol/kg daily in divided doses, adjusted according to requirements

Slow Sodium® (HK Pharma)
Tablets, m/r, sodium chloride 600 mg (approx. 10 mmol each of Na^+ and Cl^-). Net price 100-tab pack = £6.05. Label: 25

Capsules available from 'special-order' manufacturers or specialist importing companies, see p. 957

◢ Extemporaneous formulations available see Extemporaneous Preparations, p. 8

Oral rehydration therapy (ORT)

Diarrhoea in children is usually self-limiting, however, in children under 6 months of age, and more particularly in those under 3 months, symptoms of dehydration may be less obvious and there is a risk of rapid and severe deterioration. Intestinal absorption of sodium and water is enhanced by glucose (and other carbohydrates). Replacement of fluid and electrolytes lost through diarrhoea can therefore be achieved by giving solutions containing sodium, potassium, and glucose or another carbohydrate such as rice starch.

Oral rehydration solutions should:

• enhance the absorption of water and electrolytes;

• replace the electrolyte deficit adequately and safely;

• contain an alkalinising agent to counter acidosis;

• be slightly hypo-osmolar (about 250 mmol/litre) to prevent the possible induction of osmotic diarrhoea;

• be simple to use in hospital and at home;

• be palatable and acceptable, especially to children;

• be readily available.

It is the policy of the World Health Organization (WHO) to promote a single oral rehydration solution but to use it flexibly (e.g. by giving extra water between drinks of oral rehydration solution to moderately dehydrated infants).

9 Nutrition and blood

Oral rehydration solutions used in the UK are lower in sodium (50–60 mmol/litre) than the WHO formulation since, in general, patients suffer less severe sodium loss.

Rehydration should be rapid over 3 to 4 hours (except in hypernatraemic dehydration in which case rehydration should occur more slowly over 12 hours). The patient should be reassessed after initial rehydration and if still dehydrated rapid fluid replacement should continue.

Once rehydration is complete further dehydration is prevented by encouraging the patient to drink normal volumes of an appropriate fluid and by replacing continuing losses with an oral rehydration solution; in infants, breast-feeding or formula feeds should be offered between oral rehydration drinks.

For intravenous rehydration see section 9.2.2.

◢ ORAL REHYDRATION SALTS (ORS)

Licensed use *Dioralyte® Relief* not licensed for use in children under 3 months

Indication and dose

Fluid and electrolyte loss in diarrhoea see notes above

• By mouth

Child 1 month–1 year 1–1½ times usual feed volume

Child 1–12 years 200 mL after every loose motion

Child 12–18 years 200–400 mL after every loose motion

◢ UK formulations

Note After reconstitution any unused solution should be discarded no later than 1 hour after preparation unless stored in a refrigerator when it may be kept for up to 24 hours.

Dioralyte® (Sanofi-Aventis)

Oral powder, sodium chloride 470 mg, potassium chloride 300 mg, disodium hydrogen citrate 530 mg, glucose 3.56 g/sachet, net price 6-sachet pack = £2.25, 20-sachet pack (black currant- or citrus-flavoured or natural) = £6.72

Note Reconstitute 1 sachet with 200 mL of water (freshly boiled and cooled for infants); 5 sachets reconstituted with 1 litre of water provide Na^+ 60 mmol, K^+ 20 mmol, Cl^- 60 mmol, citrate 10 mmol, and glucose 90 mmol

Dioralyte® Relief (Sanofi-Aventis)

Oral powder, sodium chloride 350 mg, potassium chloride 300 mg, sodium citrate 580 mg, cooked

rice powder 6 g/sachet, net price 6-sachet pack (apricot-, black currant- or raspberry-flavoured) = £2.50, 20-sachet pack (apricot-flavoured) = £7.13

Note Reconstitute 1 sachet with 200 mL of water (freshly boiled and cooled for infants); 5 sachets when reconstituted with 1 litre of water provide Na^+ 60 mmol, K^+ 20 mmol, Cl^- 50 mmol and citrate 10 mmol; contains aspartame (section 9.4.1)

Electrolade® (Actavis)

Oral powder, sodium chloride 236 mg, potassium chloride 300 mg, sodium bicarbonate 500 mg, anhydrous glucose 4 g/sachet (banana-, black currant-, lemon and lime-, or orange-flavoured). Net price 6-sachet (plain or multiflavoured) pack = £1.33, 20-sachet (single- or multiflavoured) pack = £4.99

Note Reconstitute 1 sachet with 200 mL of water (freshly boiled and cooled for infants); 5 sachets when reconstituted with 1 litre of water provide Na^+ 50 mmol, K^+ 20 mmol, Cl^- 40 mmol, HCO_3^- 30 mmol, and glucose 111 mmol

◢ WHO formulation

Oral Rehydration Salts (Non-proprietary)

Oral powder, sodium chloride 2.6 g, potassium chloride 1.5 g, sodium citrate 2.9 g, anhydrous glucose 13.5 g. To be dissolved in sufficient water to produce 1 litre (providing Na^+ 75 mmol, K^+ 20 mmol, Cl^- 65 mmol, citrate 10 mmol, glucose 75 mmol/litre)

Note Recommended by the WHO and the United Nations Children's Fund but not commonly used in the UK

9.2.1.3 Oral bicarbonate

Sodium bicarbonate is given by mouth for *chronic acidotic states* such as uraemic acidosis or renal tubular acidosis. The dose for correction of metabolic acidosis is not predictable and the response must be assessed. For severe *metabolic acidosis*, sodium bicarbonate can be given intravenously (section 9.2.2).

Sodium supplements may increase blood pressure or cause fluid retention and pulmonary oedema in those at risk; hypokalaemia may be exacerbated.

Sodium bicarbonate may affect the stability or absorption of other drugs if administered at the same time. If possible, allow 1–2 hours before administering other drugs orally.

Where *hyperchloraemic acidosis* is associated with potassium deficiency, as in some renal tubular and gastro-intestinal disorders it may be appropriate to give oral **potassium bicarbonate**, although acute or severe deficiency should be managed by intravenous therapy.

9

Nutrition and blood

▌SODIUM BICARBONATE

Cautions see notes above; avoid in respiratory acidosis; **interactions:** Appendix 1 (antacids)

Indication and dose

Renal acidosis (see also notes above)
* By mouth

    Neonate initially 1–2 mmol/kg daily in divided doses, adjusted according to response

    Child 1 month–18 years initially 1–2 mmol/kg daily in divided doses, adjusted according to response

Metabolic acidosis section 9.2.2.1

Renal hyperkalaemia section 9.2.2.1

Sodium Bicarbonate (Non-proprietary)
Capsules, sodium bicarbonate 500 mg (approx. 6 mmol each of Na^+ and HCO_3^-), net price 56-cap pack = £7.79

Tablets, sodium bicarbonate 600 mg, net price 100-tab pack = £2.48

Important Oral solutions of sodium bicarbonate are required occasionally; these need to be obtained from 'special-order' manufacturers or specialist importing companies, see p. 957, and the strength of sodium bicarbonate should be stated on the prescription

▌POTASSIUM BICARBONATE

Cautions cardiac disease, **interactions:** Appendix 1 (potassium salts)

Contra-indications hypochloraemia; plasma-potassium concentration above 5 mmol/litre

Renal impairment close monitoring required—high risk of hyperkalaemia; avoid in severe impairment

Side-effects nausea, vomiting, abdominal pain, diarrhoea, and flatulence

Potassium Tablets, Effervescent (Non-proprietary)
Effervescent tablets, potassium bicarbonate 500 mg, potassium acid tartrate 300 mg, each tablet providing 6.5 mmol of K^+. To be dissolved in water before administration. Net price 56 = £29.93. Label: 13, 21

Note These tablets do not contain chloride; for effervescent tablets containing potassium and chloride, see under Potassium Chloride, section 9.2.1.1

9.2.2 Parenteral preparations for fluid and electrolyte imbalance

9.2.2.1   Electrolytes and water
9.2.2.2   Plasma and plasma substitutes

9.2.2.1 Electrolytes and water

Solutions of electrolytes are given intravenously, to meet normal fluid and electrolyte requirements or to replenish substantial deficits or continuing losses when it is not possible or desirable to use the oral route. When intravenous administration is not possible, fluid (as sodium chloride 0.9% or glucose 5%) can also be given subcutaneously by hypodermoclysis.

In an individual patient the nature and severity of the electrolyte imbalance must be assessed from the history and clinical and biochemical examination. Sodium, potassium, chloride, magnesium, phosphate, and water depletion can occur singly and in combination with or without disturbances of acid-base balance; for reference to the use of magnesium and phosphates, see section 9.5.

Isotonic solutions may be infused safely into a peripheral vein. Solutions more concentrated than plasma, for example 15% glucose, are best given through an indwelling catheter positioned in a large vein.

Maintenance fluid requirements in children are usually derived from the relationship that exists between body-weight and metabolic rate; the figures in the table below may be used as a guide outside the neonatal period. The glucose requirement is that needed to minimise gluconeogenesis from amino acids obtained as substrate from muscle breakdown. Maintenance fluids are intended only to provide hydration for a short period until enteral or parenteral nutrition can be established.

It is usual to meet these requirements by using a standard solution of sodium chloride and glucose. Solutions containing 20 mmol/litre of potassium chloride meet usual potassium requirements when given in the suggested volumes; adjustments may be needed if there is an inability to excrete fluids or electrolytes, excessive renal loss or continuing extra-renal losses. The exact requirements depend upon the nature of the clinical situation and types of losses incurred; see Caution on dilutional hyponatraemia below.

Fluid requirements for children over 1 month:	
Body-weight	**24-hour fluid requirement**
Under 10 kg	100 mL/kg
10–20 kg	100 mL/kg for the first 10 kg + 50 mL/kg for each 1 kg body-weight over 10 kg
Over 20 kg	100 mL/kg for the first 10 kg + 50 mL/kg for each 1 kg body-weight between 10–20 kg + 20 mL/kg for each 1 kg body-weight over 20 kg (max. 2 litres in females, 2.5 litres in males)

Important The baseline fluid requirements shown in the table above should be adjusted to take account of factors that reduce water loss (e.g. increased antidiuretic hormone, renal failure, hypothermia, and high ambient humidity) or increase water loss (e.g. pyrexia or burns).

Caution During parenteral hydration, fluids and electrolytes should be monitored closely and any disturbance corrected by slow infusion of an appropriate solution. The volume of fluid infused should take into account the possibility of reduced fluid loss owing to increased antidiuretic hormone and factors such as renal failure, hypothermia, and high humidity.

Dilutional hyponatraemia is a rare but potentially fatal risk of parenteral hydration. It may be caused by inappropriate use of hypotonic fluids such as sodium chloride 0.18% and glucose 4% intravenous infusion, especially in the postoperative period when antidiuretic hormone secretion is increased. Dilutional hyponatraemia is characterized by a rapid fall in plasma-sodium concentration leading to cerebral oedema and seizures; any child with severe hyponatraemia or rapidly changing plasma-sodium concentration should be referred urgently to a paediatric high dependency facility.

> **Safe practice**
> Sodium chloride 0.18% and glucose 4% intravenous infusion fluid should not generally be used for fluid replacement in children because of the risk of hyponatraemia; availability of this infusion should be restricted to critical care and specialist wards, such as renal, liver, and cardiac units. Local guidelines on intravenous fluids should be consulted.

Replacement therapy: initial intravenous replacement fluid is generally required if the child is over 10% dehydrated, or if 5–10% dehydrated and oral or enteral rehydration is not tolerated or possible. Oral rehydration is adequate, if tolerated, in the majority of those less than 10% dehydrated. Subsequent fluid and electrolyte requirements are determined by clinical assessment of fluid balance.

Neonates Neonates lose water through the skin and nose, particularly if preterm or if the skin is damaged. The basic fluid requirement for a term baby in average ambient humidity is 40–60 mL/kg/day plus urinary losses. Preterm babies have very high transepidermal losses particularly in the first few days of life; they may need more fluid replacement than full term babies and up to 180 mL/kg/day may be required. Local guidelines for fluid management in the neonatal period should be consulted.

Intravenous sodium

Intravenous sodium chloride in isotonic (0.9%) solution provides the most important extracellular ions in near physiological concentrations and is indicated in *sodium depletion*. It may be given for initial treatment of acute fluid loss and to replace ongoing gastro-intestinal losses from the upper gastro-intestinal tract. Intravenous sodium chloride is commonly given as a component of maintenance and replacement therapy, usually in combination with other electrolytes and glucose, see notes above. Sodium chloride solutions should be used cautiously in renal insufficiency, cardiac failure, cardio-respiratory diseases, hepatic cirrhosis and in children receiving glucocorticoids. Hyponatraemia with serious consequences may occur if maintenance and replacement fluids do not meet sodium requirements (see Caution, dilutional hyponatraemia, above).

9

Nutrition and blood

Chronic hyponatraemia should ideally be corrected by fluid restriction. However, if sodium chloride is required, the deficit should be corrected slowly to avoid the risk of osmotic demyelination syndrome; the rise in plasma-sodium concentration should be no more than 10 mmol/litre in 24 hours.

Sodium chloride and glucose solutions are indicated when there is combined *water and sodium depletion*. A 1:1 mixture of isotonic sodium chloride and 5% glucose allows some of the water (free of sodium) to enter body cells which suffer most from dehydration while the sodium salt with a volume of water determined by the normal plasma Na$^+$ remains extracellular. Maintenance fluid should accurately reflect daily requirements and close monitoring is required to avoid fluid and electrolyte imbalance. Illness or injury increase the secretion of anti-diuretic hormone and therefore the ability to excrete excess water may be impaired. Injudicious use of hypotonic solutions such as sodium chloride 0.18% and glucose 4% may also cause dilutional hyponatraemia especially in children (see Caution on dilutional hyponatraemia, above); if necessary, guidance should be sought from a clinician experienced in the management of fluid and electrolytes.

Combined sodium, potassium, chloride, and water depletion may occur, for example, with severe diarrhoea or persistent vomiting; replacement is carried out with sodium chloride intravenous infusion 0.9% and glucose intravenous infusion 5% with potassium as appropriate.

Compound sodium lactate (Hartmann's solution) can be used instead of isotonic sodium chloride solution during or after surgery, or in the initial management of the injured or wounded.

Neonates   The sodium requirement for most healthy neonates is 3 mmol/kg daily. Preterm neonates, particularly below 30 weeks gestation, may require up to 6 mmol/kg daily. *Hyponatraemia* may be caused by excessive renal loss of sodium; it may also be dilutional and restriction of fluid intake may be appropriate. Sodium supplementation is likely to be required if the serum sodium concentration is significantly reduced.

Hypernatraemia may also occur, most often due to dehydration (e.g. breast milk insufficiency). Severe hypernatraemia and hyponatraemia can cause fits and rarely brain damage. Sodium in drug preparations, delivered via continuous infusions, or in infusions to maintain the patency of intravascular or umbilical lines, can result in significant amounts of sodium being delivered, (e.g. 1 mL/hour of 0.9% sodium chloride infused over 24 hours is equivalent to 3.6 mmol/day of sodium).

SODIUM CHLORIDE

Cautions   restrict intake in impaired renal function, cardiac failure, hypertension, peripheral and pulmonary oedema, toxaemia of pregnancy; see also notes above

Side-effects   administration of large doses may give rise to sodium accumulation and oedema

Indication and dose

Electrolyte imbalance see notes above, also section 9.2.1.2

Sodium Chloride (Non-proprietary) [PoM]
Intravenous infusion, usual strength sodium chloride 0.9% (9 g, 150 mmol each of Na$^+$ and Cl$^-$/litre), this strength being supplied when normal saline for injection is requested. Net price 2-mL amp = 28p; 5-mL amp = 34p; 10-mL amp = 46p; 20-mL amp = £1.04; 50-mL amp = £2.01
In hospitals, 500- and 1000-mL packs, and sometimes other sizes, are available

Note The term 'normal saline' should **not** be used to describe sodium chloride intravenous infusion 0.9%; the term 'physiological saline' is acceptable but it is preferable to give the composition (i.e. sodium chloride intravenous infusion 0.9%).

◢With other ingredients
Note See above for warning on hyponatraemia

Sodium Chloride and Glucose (Non-proprietary) [PoM]
Intravenous infusion, sodium chloride 0.18% (Na$^+$ and Cl$^-$ each 30 mmol/litre), glucose 4%
In hospitals, usually 500-mL packs and sometimes other sizes are available

Intravenous infusion, sodium chloride 0.45% (Na$^+$ and Cl$^-$ each 75 mmol/litre), glucose 5%
In hospitals, usually 500-mL packs and sometimes other sizes are available

Intravenous infusion, sodium chloride 0.9% (Na$^+$ and Cl$^-$ each 150 mmol/litre), glucose 5%
In hospitals, usually 500-mL packs and sometimes other sizes are available

Ringer's Solution (Non-proprietary) [PoM]
Calcium chloride (dihydrate) 322 micrograms, potassium chloride 300 micrograms, sodium chloride 8.6 mg/mL, providing the following ions (in mmol/litre), Ca^{2+} 2.2, K$^+$ 4, Na$^+$ 147, Cl$^-$ 156
In hospitals, 500- and 1000-mL packs, and sometimes other sizes, are available

⌐ **SODIUM CHLORIDE** *(continued)*

Sodium Lactate, Compound (Non-proprietary) ▣
(Hartmann's Solution; Ringer-Lactate Solution)
Intravenous infusion, sodium chloride 0.6%, sodium lactate 0.32%, potassium chloride 0.04%, calcium chloride 0.027% (containing Na$^+$ 131 mmol,

K$^+$ 5 mmol, Ca^{2+} 2 mmol, HCO$_3^-$ (as lactate) 29 mmol, Cl$^-$ 111 mmol/litre)
In hospitals, 500- and 1000-mL packs, and sometimes other sizes, are available

Intravenous glucose

Glucose solutions are used mainly to replace water deficit and should not be given alone except when there is no significant loss of electrolytes; prolonged administration of glucose solutions without electrolytes can lead to hyponatraemia and other electrolyte disturbances. Water depletion (dehydration) tends to occur when losses are not matched by a comparable intake, as may occur in coma or dysphagia.

Water loss rarely exceeds electrolyte losses but this can occur in fevers, hyperthyroidism, and in uncommon water-losing renal states such as diabetes insipidus or hypercalcaemia. The volume of glucose solution needed to replace deficits varies with the severity of the disorder; the rate of infusion should be adjusted to return the plasma-sodium concentration to normal over 48 hours.

Glucose solutions are also used to correct and prevent hypoglycaemia and to provide a source of energy in those too ill to be fed adequately by mouth; glucose solutions are a key component of parenteral nutrition (section 9.3).

Glucose solutions are given with insulin for the emergency management of *hyperkalaemia* (see p. 557). They are also given, after correction of hyperglycaemia, during treatment of diabetic ketoacidosis, when they must be accompanied by continuous insulin infusion (section 6.1.3).

Injections containing more than 10% glucose can be irritant and should be given into a central venous line; however, solutions containing up to 12.5% can be administered for a short period into a peripheral line.

GLUCOSE

(Dextrose Monohydrate)
Note Glucose BP is the monohydrate but Glucose Intravenous Infusion BP is a sterile solution of anhydrous glucose or glucose monohydrate, potency being expressed in terms of anhydrous glucose

Side-effects glucose injections especially if hypertonic may have a low pH and may cause venous irritation and thrombophlebitis

Indication and dose

Fluid replacement see notes above

Provision of energy section 9.3

Hypoglycaemia section 6.1.4

Glucose (Non-proprietary) ▣
Intravenous infusion, glucose or anhydrous glucose (potency expressed in terms of anhydrous glucose), usual strengths 5% (50 mg/mL) and 10% (100 mg/mL); 25% solution, net price 25-mL amp = £2.21; 50% solution[1], 20-mL amp = 95 p, 50-mL amp = £2.61
In hospitals, 500- and 1000-mL packs, and sometimes other sizes and strengths, are available; also available *Minijet® Glucose*, 50% in 50-mL disposable syringe[1]
1. ▣ restriction does not apply where administration is for saving life in emergency

Intravenous potassium

Potassium chloride and sodium chloride intravenous infusion is the initial treatment for the correction of *severe hypokalaemia* and when sufficient potassium cannot be taken by mouth. Ready-mixed infusion solutions should be used when possible (see under Safe Practice below); for peripheral intravenous infusion, the concentration of potassium should not usually exceed 40 mmol/litre. Potassium infusions should be given slowly over at least 2–3 hours and at a rate not exceeding 0.2 mmol/kg/hour with specialist advice and ECG monitoring in difficult cases. Higher concentrations of potassium chloride or faster infusion rates may be given in very severe depletion, but require specialist advice.

Repeated measurements of plasma-potassium concentration are necessary to determine whether further infusions are required and to avoid the development of hyperkalaemia, which is especially likely in renal impairment.

Initial potassium replacement therapy should **not** involve glucose infusions, because glucose may cause a further decrease in the plasma-potassium concentration.

> **Safe Practice**
> Potassium overdose can be fatal. Ready-mixed infusion solutions containing potassium should be used. Exceptionally, if potassium chloride concentrate is used for preparing an infusion, the infusion solution should be **thoroughly mixed**. Local policies on avoiding inadvertent use of potassium chloride concentrate should be followed.

POTASSIUM CHLORIDE

Cautions for peripheral intravenous infusion the concentration of solution should not usually exceed 3 g (40 mmol)/litre; specialist advice and ECG monitoring (see notes above); **interactions:** Appendix 1 (potassium salts)

Contra-indications plasma-potassium concentration above 5 mmol/litre

Renal impairment close monitoring required—high risk of hyperkalaemia; avoid in severe impairment

Side-effects rapid infusion toxic to heart

Indication and dose

Electrolyte imbalance see also oral potassium supplements, section 9.2.1.1
- **By slow intravenous infusion**
  depending on the deficit or the daily maintenance requirements, see also notes above

  Neonate 1–2 mmol/kg daily

  Child 1 month–18 years 1–2 mmol/kg daily

Administration see notes above

Potassium Chloride and Glucose (Non-proprietary) PoM
Intravenous infusion, usual strengths potassium chloride 0.3% (3 g, 40 mmol each of K^+ and Cl^-/litre) or 0.15% (1.5 g, 20 mmol each of K^+ and Cl^-/litre) with 5% of anhydrous glucose
In hospitals, 500- and 1000-mL packs, and sometimes other sizes, are available

Potassium Chloride and Sodium Chloride (Non-proprietary) PoM
Intravenous infusion, usual strength potassium chloride 0.15% (1.5 g/litre) with sodium chloride 0.9% (9 g/litre), containing K^+ 20 mmol, Na^+ 150 mmol, and Cl^- 170 mmol/litre
In hospitals, 500- and 1000-mL packs, and sometimes other sizes, are available

Potassium Chloride, Sodium Chloride, and Glucose (Non-proprietary) PoM
Intravenous infusion, sodium chloride 0.45% (4.5 g, Na^+ 75 mmol/litre) with 5% of anhydrous glucose and usually sufficient potassium chloride to provide K^+ 10–40 mmol/litre (to be specified by the prescriber)
In hospitals, 500- and 1000-mL packs, and sometimes other sizes are available

Potassium Chloride (Non-proprietary) PoM
Sterile concentrate, potassium chloride 15% (150 mg, approximately 2 mmol each of K^+ and Cl^-/mL). Net price 10-mL amp = 48p
Solutions containing 10 and 20% of potassium chloride are also available in both 5- and 10-mL ampoules
Important Must be diluted with **not less** than 50 times its volume of Sodium Chloride 0.9% or other suitable diluent and **mixed well**; see Safe Practice, above

Bicarbonate and trometamol

Sodium bicarbonate is used to control severe *metabolic acidosis* (pH < 7.1) particularly that caused by loss of bicarbonate (as in renal tubular acidosis or from excessive gastro-intestinal losses). Mild metabolic acidosis associated with volume depletion should first be managed by appropriate fluid replacement because acidosis usually resolves as tissue and renal perfusion are restored. In more severe metabolic acidosis or when the acidosis remains unresponsive to correction of anoxia or hypovolaemia, sodium bicarbonate (1.26%) can be infused over 3–4 hours with plasma-pH and electrolyte monitoring. In severe shock (section 2.7.1), for example in cardiac arrest, metabolic acidosis can develop without sodium depletion; in these circumstances sodium bicarbonate is best given intravenously as a small volume of hypertonic solution, such as 8.4%; plasma pH and electrolytes should be monitored. For *chronic acidotic states*, sodium bicarbonate can be given by mouth (section 9.2.1.3).

Trometamol (tris(hydroxymethyl)aminomethane, THAM), an organic buffer, corrects metabolic acidosis by causing an increase in urinary pH and an osmotic diuresis. It is indicated when sodium bicarbonate is unsuitable as in carbon dioxide retention, hypernatraemia, or renal impairment. Respiratory support may be required because trometamol induces respiratory depression. It is also used during cardiac bypass surgery and, very rarely, in cardiac arrest.

◢ SODIUM BICARBONATE

Indication and dose

> **Metabolic acidosis** see also notes above
> * By slow intravenous injection of a strong solution (up to 8.4%), or by continuous intravenous infusion of a weaker solution (usually 1.26%)
>
>   An amount appropriate to the body base deficit

> **Renal hyperkalaemia**
> * By slow intravenous injection
>
>   **Neonate** 1 mmol/kg daily
>
>   **Child 1 month–18 years** 1 mmol/kg daily

> **Renal acidosis** section 9.2.1.3

Sodium Bicarbonate [PoM]

Intravenous infusion, usual strength sodium bicarbonate 1.26% (12.6 g, 150 mmol each of Na^+ and HCO_3^-/litre); various other strengths available In hospitals, 500- and 1000-mL packs, and sometimes other sizes, are available

Administration For *peripheral infusion* dilute 8.4% solution at least 1 in 10; for *central line infusion* dilute 1 in 5 with Glucose 5% or 10% *or* Sodium Chloride 0.9%. Extravasation can cause severe tissue damage

Minijet® Sodium Bicarbonate (UCB Pharma) [PoM]

Intravenous injection, sodium bicarbonate in disposable syringe, net price 4.2%, 10 mL = £8.92; 8.4%, 10 mL = £9.95, 50 mL = £11.45

◢ TROMETAMOL

(Tris(hydroxymethyl)aminomethane, THAM)

Cautions see notes above; extravasation can cause severe tissue damage

Contra-indications anuria; chronic respiratory acidosis

Renal impairment use with caution, may cause hyperkalaemia

Pregnancy limited information available, hypoglycaemia may harm fetus

Breast-feeding no information available

Side-effects respiratory depression; hypoglycaemia; hyperkalaemia in renal impairment; liver necrosis reported following administration via umbilical vein in neonates

Licensed use unlicensed preparation

Indication and dose

> **Metabolic acidosis**
> * By intravenous infusion
>
>   An amount appropriate to the body base deficit

◢ **Preparations**

Available from 'special-order' manufacturers or specialist importing companies, see p. 957

◢ Water

Water for Injections [PoM]

Net price 1-mL amp = 18p; 2-mL amp = 18p; 5-mL amp = 32p; 10-mL amp = 33p; 20-mL amp = 92p; 50-mL amp = £1.91; 100-mL vial= £2.07

9.2.2.2 Plasma and plasma substitutes

Albumin solutions, prepared from whole blood, contain soluble proteins and electrolytes but no clotting factors, blood group antibodies, or plasma cholinesterases; they may be given without regard to the recipient's blood group.

Albumin is usually used after the acute phase of illness to correct a plasma-volume deficit; hypoalbuminaemia itself is not an appropriate indication. The use of albumin solutions in acute plasma or blood loss may be wasteful; plasma substitutes are more appropriate. Concentrated albumin solutions may also be used to obtain a diuresis in hypoalbuminaemic patients (e.g. in nephrotic syndrome).

Recent evidence does not support the previous view that the use of albumin increases mortality.

> Plasma and plasma substitutes are often used in very ill children whose condition is unstable. Therefore, close monitoring is required and fluid and electrolyte therapy should be adjusted according to the child's condition at all times.

◢ ALBUMIN SOLUTION

(Human Albumin Solution)

A solution containing protein derived from plasma, serum, or normal placentas; at least 95% of the protein is albumin. The solution may be isotonic (containing 3.5–5% protein) or concentrated (containing 15–25% protein).

9

Nutrition and blood

◻ **ALBUMIN SOLUTION (*continued*)**

Cautions history of cardiac or circulatory disease (administer slowly to avoid rapid rise in blood pressure and cardiac failure, and monitor cardiovascular and respiratory function); increased capillary permeability; correct dehydration when administering concentrated solution

Contra-indications cardiac failure; severe anaemia

Side-effects hypersensitivity reactions (including anaphylaxis) with nausea, vomiting, increased salivation, fever, tachycardia, hypotension and chills reported

Indication and dose

See notes above and under preparations, below

◢**Isotonic solutions**
Indications: acute or sub-acute loss of plasma volume e.g. in burns, pancreatitis, trauma, and complications of surgery; plasma exchange

Available as: Human Albumin Solution 4.5% (50-, 100-, 250- and 400-mL bottles—Baxter); *Human Albumin Solution 5%* (250- and 500-mL bottles—Baxter); *Albunorm®* 5% (100-, 250-, and 500-mL bottles—Octapharma); *Octalbin®* 5% (100- and 250-mL bottles—Octapharma); *Zenalb®* 4.5% (50-, 100-, 250-, and 500-mL bottles—BPL)

◢**Concentrated solutions (20%)**
Indications: severe hypoalbuminaemia associated with low plasma volume and generalised oedema where salt and water restriction with plasma volume expansion are required; adjunct in the treatment of hyperbilirubinaemia by exchange transfusion in the newborn; paracentesis of large volume ascites associated with portal hypertension
Available as: Human Albumin Solution 20% (50- and 100-mL vials—Baxter); *Albunorm®* 20% (50- and 100-mL bottles—Octapharma); *Flexbumin®* 20% (50- and 100-mL bags—Baxter); *Octalbin®* 20% (50- and 100-mL bottles—Octapharma); *Zenalb®* 20% (50- and 100-mL bottles—BPL)

Plasma substitutes

Gelatin and the **etherified starches** (**pentastarch** and **tetrastarch**) are macromolecular substances which are metabolised slowly; they may be used at the outset to expand and maintain blood volume in shock arising from conditions such as burns or septicaemia. Plasma substitutes may be used as an immediate short-term measure to treat haemorrhage until blood is available. They are rarely needed when shock is due to sodium and water depletion because, in these circumstances, the shock responds to water and electrolyte repletion; see also section 2.7.1 for the management of shock.

Plasma substitutes should **not** be used to maintain plasma volume in conditions such as burns or peritonitis where there is loss of plasma protein, water, and electrolytes over periods of several days or weeks. In these situations, plasma or plasma protein fractions containing large amounts of albumin should be given.

Large volumes of *some* plasma substitutes can increase the risk of bleeding through depletion of coagulation factors.

> Plasma and plasma substitutes are often used in very ill children whose condition is unstable. Therefore, close monitoring is required and fluid and electrolyte therapy should be adjusted according to the child's condition at all times.
> The use of plasma substitutes in children requires specialist supervision due to the risk of fluid overload; use is best restricted to an intensive care setting.

Cautions Plasma substitutes should be used with caution in cardiac disease, liver disease, or renal impairment; urine output should be monitored. Care should be taken to avoid haematocrit concentration from falling below 25–30% and the child should be monitored for hypersensitivity reactions.

Side-effects Hypersensitivity reactions may occur including, rarely, severe anaphylactic reactions. Transient increase in bleeding time may occur.

◢ **GELATIN**

Note The gelatin is partially degraded
Cautions see notes above
Pregnancy manufacturer of *Geloplasma®* advises avoid at the end of pregnancy
Side-effects see notes above

Indication and dose

Low blood volume in hypovolaemic shock, burns and cardiopulmonary bypass
• By intravenous infusion
  Initially 10–20 mL/kg of a 3.5–4% solution (see notes above)

Nutrition and blood **9**

◁ **GELATIN** *(continued)*

Gelofusine® (Braun) [PoM]
Intravenous infusion, succinylated gelatin (modified fluid gelatin, average molecular weight 30 000) 40 g (4%), Na^+ 154 mmol, Cl^- 124 mmol/litre, net price 500-mL *Ecobag®* = £5.15; 1-litre *Ecobag®* = £9.67
Contains traces of calcium

Geloplasma® (Fresenius Kabi) [PoM]
Intravenous infusion, partially hydrolysed and succinylated gelatin (modified liquid gelatin) (as anhydrous gelatin) 30 g (3%), Na^+ 150 mmol, K^+ 5 mmol, Mg^{2+} 1.5 mmol, Cl^- 100 mmol, lactate 30 mmol/litre, net price 500-mL bag = £5.05

Isoplex® (IS Pharmaceuticals) [PoM]
Intravenous infusion, succinylated gelatin (modified fluid gelatin, average molecular weight 30 000) 40 g (4%), Na^+ 145 mmol, K^+ 4 mmol, Mg^{2+} 0.9 mmol, Cl^- 105 mmol, lactate 25 mmol/litre, net price 500-mL bag = £7.53; 1-litre bag = £14.54

Volplex® (IS Pharmaceuticals) [PoM]
Intravenous infusion, succinylated gelatin (modified fluid gelatin, average molecular weight 30 000) 40 g (4%), Na^+ 154 mmol, Cl^- 125 mmol/litre, net price 500-mL bag = £4.70; 1-litre bag = £9.09

ETHERIFIED STARCH

A starch composed of more than 90% of amylopectin that has been etherified with hydroxyethyl groups; the terms tetrastarch and pentastarch reflect the degree of etherification

Cautions see notes above

Side-effects see notes above; also pruritus, raised serum amylase

Indication and dose

Low blood volume
• **By intravenous infusion**
According to the child's condition (see notes above)

◢**Pentastarch**

HAES-steril® (Fresenius Kabi) [PoM]
Intravenous infusion, pentastarch (weight average molecular weight 200 000) 10% in sodium chloride intravenous infusion 0.9%, net price, 500 mL = £16.50

Hemohes® (Braun) [PoM]
Intravenous infusion, pentastarch (weight average molecular weight 200 000), net price (both in sodium chloride intravenous infusion 0.9%) 6%, 500 mL = £12.50; 10%, 500 mL = £16.50

◢**Tetrastarch**

Tetraspan® (Braun) [PoM]
Intravenous infusion, hydroxyethyl starch (weight average molecular weight 130 000) 6% in sodium chloride 0.625%, containing Na^+ 140 mmol, K^+ 4 mmol, Mg^{2+} 1 mmol, Cl^- 118 mmol, Ca^{2+} 2.5 mmol, acetate 24 mmol, malate 5 mmol/litre, net price 500-mL bag = £13.50

Volulyte® (Fresenius Kabi) [PoM]
Intravenous infusion, hydroxyethyl starch (weight average molecular weight 130 000) 6% in sodium chloride intravenous infusion 0.6%, containing Na^+ 137 mmol, K^+ 4 mmol, Mg^{2+} 1.5 mmol, Cl^- 110 mmol, acetate 34 mmol/litre, net price 500-mL bag = £13.50

Voluven® (Fresenius Kabi) [PoM]
Intravenous infusion, hydroxyethyl starch (weight average molecular weight 130 000) 6% in sodium chloride intravenous infusion 0.9%, net price 500-mL bag = £12.50

◢**Hypertonic solution**

HyperHAES® (Fresenius Kabi) [PoM]
Intravenous infusion, hydroxyethyl starch (weight average molecular weight 200 000) 6% in sodium chloride intravenous infusion 7.2%, net price 250-mL bag = £28.00
Cautions see notes above; also diabetes

9

Nutrition and blood

9.3 Intravenous nutrition

When adequate feeding through the alimentary tract is not possible, nutrients may be given by intravenous infusion. This may be in addition to oral or enteral tube feeding—**supplemental parenteral nutrition**, or may be the sole source of nutrition—**total parenteral nutrition** (TPN). Complete enteral starvation is undesirable and total parenteral nutrition is a last resort.

Indications for parenteral nutrition include prematurity; severe or prolonged disorders of the gastro-intestinal tract; preparation of undernourished patients for surgery, chemotherapy, or radiation therapy; major surgery, trauma, or burns; prolonged coma or inability to eat; and some patients with renal or hepatic failure. The composition of proprietary preparations used in children is given in the table Proprietary Infusion Fluids for Parenteral Feeding, p. 568.

Parenteral nutrition requires the use of a solution containing amino acids, glucose, lipids, electrolytes, trace elements, and vitamins. This is now commonly provided by the pharmacy in the form of an amino-acid, glucose, electrolyte bag, and a separate lipid infusion or, in older children a single 'all-in-one' bag. If the patient is able to take small amounts by mouth, vitamins may be given orally.

Proprietary Infusion Fluids for Parenteral Feeding

Preparation	Nitrogen g/litre	1,2 Energy kJ/litre	Electrolytes mmol/litre					Other components/litre
			K⁺	Mg²⁺	Na⁺	Acet⁻	Cl⁻	
ClinOleic 20% (Baxter) Net price 100 mL = £6.28; 250 mL = £10.08; 500 mL = £13.88		8360						purified olive and soya oil 200 g, glycerol 22.5 g, egg phosphatides 12 g
Glamin (Fresenius Kabi) Net price 250 mL = £14.16; 500 mL = £26.38	22.4				62			
Intralipid 10% (Fresenius Kabi) Net price 100 mL = £4.70; 500 mL = £10.30		4600						soya oil 100 g, glycerol 22 g, purified egg phospholipids 12 g, phosphate 15 mmol
Intralipid 20% (Fresenius Kabi) Net price 100 mL = £7.05; 250 mL = £11.60; 500 mL = £15.45		8400						soya oil 200 g, glycerol 22 g, purified egg phospholipids 12 g, phosphate 15 mmol
Intralipid 30% (Fresenius Kabi) Net price 333 mL = £17.30		12600						soya oil 300 g, glycerol 16.7 g, purified egg phospholipids 12 g, phosphate 15 mmol
Lipofundin MCT/LCT 10% (Braun) Net price 100 mL = £7.70; 500 mL = £12.90		4430						soya oil 50 g, medium chain triglycerides 50 g
Lipofundin MCT/LCT 20% (Braun) Net price 100 mL = £12.51; 250 mL = £11.30; 500 mL = £19.18		8000						soya oil 100 g, medium chain triglycerides 100 g
³Primene 10% (Baxter) Net price 100 mL = £5.78, 250 mL = £7.92	15						19	
Synthamin 9 (Baxter) Net price 500 mL = £6.66; 1000 mL = £12.34	9.1		60	5	70	100	70	acid phosphate 30 mmol
Synthamin 9 EF (electrolyte-free) (Baxter) Net price 500 mL = £6.66; 1000 mL = £12.34	9.1					44	22	
Vamin 9 Glucose (Fresenius Kabi) Net price 100 mL = £3.80; 500 mL = £7.70; 1000 mL = £13.40	9.4	1700	20	1.5	50		50	Ca²⁺ 2.5 mmol, anhydrous glucose 100 g
Vaminolact (Fresenius Kabi) Net price 100 mL = £4.20; 500 mL = £9.70	9.3							

1. *Note.* 1000 kcal = 4200 kJ; 1000 kJ= 238.8 kcal. All entries are [PoM]
2. Excludes protein- or amino acid-derived energy
3. For use in neonates and children only

The nutrition solution is infused through a central venous catheter inserted under full surgical precautions. Alternatively, infusion through a peripheral vein may be used for supplementary as well as total parenteral nutrition, depending on the availability of peripheral veins; factors prolonging cannula life and preventing thrombophlebitis include the use of soft polyurethane paediatric cannulas and use of nutritional solutions of low osmolality and neutral pH. Nutritional fluids should be given by a dedicated intravenous line; if not possible, compatibility with any drugs or fluids should be checked as precipitation of components may occur. Extravasation of parenteral nutrition solution can cause severe tissue damage and injury; the infusion site should be regularly monitored.

Before starting intravenous nutrition the patient should be clinically stable and renal function and acid-base status should be assessed. Appropriate biochemical tests should have been carried out beforehand and serious deficits corrected. Nutritional and electrolyte status must be monitored throughout treatment. The nutritional components of parenteral nutrition regimens are usually increased gradually over a number of days to prevent metabolic complications and to allow metabolic adaptation to the infused nutrients. The solutions are usually infused over 24 hours but this may be gradually reduced if long-term nutrition is required. Home parenteral nutrition is usually infused over 12 hours overnight.

Complications of long-term parenteral nutrition include gall bladder sludging, gall stones, cholestasis and abnormal liver function tests. For details of the prevention and management of parenteral nutrition complications, specialist literature should be consulted.

Protein (nitrogen) is given as mixtures of essential and non-essential synthetic L-amino acids. Ideally, all essential amino acids should be included with a wide variety of non-essential ones to provide sufficient nitrogen together with electrolytes (see also section 9.2.2). Solutions vary in their composition of amino acids; they often contain an energy source (usually glucose) and electrolytes. Solutions for use in neonates and children under 1 year of age are based on the amino acid profile of umbilical cord blood (*Primene®*) or breast milk (*Vaminolact®*) and contain amino acids that are essential in this age group; these amino acids may not be present in sufficient quantities in preparations designed for older children and adults.

Energy requirements must be met if amino acids are to be utilised for tissue maintenance. An appropriate energy to protein ratio is essential and requirements will vary depending on the child's age and condition. A mixture of carbohydrate and fat energy sources (usually 30–50% as fat) gives better utilisation of amino acids than glucose alone.

Glucose is the preferred source of carbohydrate, but frequent monitoring of blood glucose is required particularly during initiation and build-up of the regimen; insulin may be necessary. Glucose above a concentration of 12.5% must be infused through a central venous catheter to avoid thrombosis; the maximum concentration of glucose that should normally be infused in fluid restricted children is 20–25%.

In parenteral nutrition regimens, it is necessary to provide adequate **phosphate** in order to allow phosphorylation of glucose and to prevent hypophosphataemia. Neonates, particularly preterm neonates, and young children also require phosphorus and calcium to ensure adequate bone mineralisation. The compatibility and solubility of calcium and phosphorus salts is complex and unpredictable; precipitation is a risk and specialist pharmacy advice should be sought.

Fat (lipid) emulsions have the advantages of a high energy to fluid volume ratio, neutral pH, and iso-osmolarity with plasma, and provide essential fatty acids. Several days of adaptation may be required to attain maximal utilisation. Reactions include occasional febrile episodes (usually only with 20% emulsions) and rare anaphylactic responses. Interference with biochemical measurements such as those for blood gases and calcium may occur if samples are taken before fat has been cleared. Regular monitoring of plasma cholesterol and triglyceride is necessary to ensure clearance from the plasma, particularly in conditions where fat metabolism may be disturbed e.g. infection. Emulsions containing 20% or 30% fat should be used in neonates as they are cleared more efficiently. **Additives should not be mixed with fat emulsions unless compatibility is known.**

Electrolytes are usually provided as the chloride salts of potassium and sodium. Acetate salts can be used to reduce the amount of chloride infused; hyperchloraemic acidosis or hypochloraemic alkalosis can occur in preterm neonates or children with renal impairment.

9

Nutrition and blood

Administration. Because of the complex requirements relating to parenteral nutrition full details relating to administration have been omitted. In all cases *specialist pharmacy advice, product literature and other specialist literature should be consulted.*

9 Nutrition and blood

Supplementary preparations

> Compatibility with the infusion solution must be ascertained before adding supplementary preparations.

Addiphos® (Fresenius Kabi) PoM
Solution, sterile, phosphate 40 mmol, K^+ 30 mmol, Na^+ 30 mmol/20 mL. For addition to *Vamin®* solutions and glucose intravenous infusions. Net price 20-mL vial = £1.53

Additrace® (Fresenius Kabi) PoM
Solution, trace elements for addition to *Vamin®* solutions and glucose intravenous infusions, traces of Fe^{3+}, Zn^{2+}, Mn^{2+}, Cu^{2+}, Cr^{3+}, Se^{4+}, Mo^{6+}, F^-, I^-. For children over 40 kg. Net price 10-mL amp = £2.31

Cernevit® (Baxter) PoM
Solution, *dl*-alpha tocopherol 11.2 units, ascorbic acid 125 mg, biotin 69 micrograms, colecalciferol 220 units, cyanocobalamin 6 micrograms, folic acid 414 micrograms, glycine 250 mg, nicotinamide 46 mg, pantothenic acid (as dexpanthenol) 17.25 mg, pyridoxine hydrochloride 5.5 mg, retinol (as palmitate) 3500 units, riboflavin (as dihydrated sodium phosphate) 4.14 mg, thiamine (as cocarboxylase tetrahydrate) 3.51 mg. Dissolve in 5 mL water for injections. Net price per vial = £3.32

Decan® (Baxter) PoM
Solution, trace elements for addition to infusion solutions, Fe^{2+}, Zn^{2+}, Cu^{2+}, Mn^{2+}, F^-, Co^{2+} I^-, Se^{4+}, Mo^{6+}, Cr^{3+}. For children over 40 kg. Net price 40-mL vial = £2.00

Dipeptiven® (Fresenius Kabi) PoM
Solution, *N*(2)-L-alanyl-L-glutamine 200 mg/mL (providing L-alanine 82 mg, L-glutamine 134.6 mg). For addition to infusion solutions containing amino acids. Net price 50 mL = £16.40, 100 mL = £30.50

Dose
Amino acid supplement for hypercatabolic or hypermetabolic states
300–400 mg/kg daily; max. 400 mg/kg daily, dose not to exceed 20% of total amino acid intake

Glycophos® Sterile Concentrate (Fresenius Kabi) PoM
Solution, sterile, phosphate 20 mmol, Na^+ 40 mmol/20 mL. For addition to *Vamin®* and

Vaminolact® solutions, and glucose intravenous infusions. Net price 20-mL vial = £4.60

Peditrace® (Fresenius Kabi) PoM
Solution, trace elements for addition to *Vaminolact®*, *Vamin® 14 Electrolyte-Free* solutions and glucose intravenous infusions, traces of Zn^{2+}, Cu^{2+}, Mn^{2+}, Se^{4+}, F^-, I^-. For use in neonates (when kidney function established, usually second day of life), infants, and children. Net price 10-mL vial = £4.18

Cautions reduced biliary excretion especially in cholestatic liver disease or in markedly reduced urinary excretion (careful biochemical monitoring required); total parenteral nutrition exceeding 1 month (measure serum manganese concentration and check liver function before commencing treatment and regularly during treatment)—discontinue if manganese concentration raised or if cholestasis develops

Solivito N® (Fresenius Kabi) PoM
Solution, powder for reconstitution, biotin 60 micrograms, cyanocobalamin 5 micrograms, folic acid 400 micrograms, glycine 300 mg, nicotinamide 40 mg, pyridoxine hydrochloride 4.9 mg, riboflavin sodium phosphate 4.9 mg, sodium ascorbate 113 mg, sodium pantothenate 16.5 mg, thiamine mononitrate 3.1 mg. Dissolve in water for injections or glucose intravenous infusion for adding to glucose intravenous infusion or *Intralipid®*; dissolve in *Vitlipid N®* or *Intralipid®* for adding to *Intralipid®* only. Net price per vial = £2.32

Vitlipid N® (Fresenius Kabi) PoM
Emulsion, adult, vitamin A 330 units, ergocalciferol 20 units, *dl*-alpha tocopherol 1 unit, phytomenadione 15 micrograms/mL. For addition to *Intralipid®*. For adults and children over 11 years. Net price 10-mL amp = £2.32

Emulsion, infant, vitamin A 230 units, ergocalciferol 40 units, *dl*-alpha tocopherol 0.7 unit, phytomenadione 20 micrograms/mL. For addition to *Intralipid®*. Net price 10-mL amp = £2.32

9.4 Oral nutrition

9.4.1 Foods for special diets
9.4.2 Enteral nutrition

9.4.1 Foods for special diets

These are preparations that have been modified to eliminate a particular constituent from a food or that are nutrient mixtures formulated as food substitutes for children who either cannot tolerate or cannot metabolise certain common constituents of food.

Coeliac disease   Intolerance to gluten in coeliac disease is managed by completely eliminating gluten from the diet. A range of gluten-free products is available for prescription—see Appendix 2 (p. 926).

Phenylketonuria   Phenylketonuria (hyperphenylalaninaemia, PKU), which results from the inability to metabolise phenylalanine, is managed by restricting dietary intake of phenylalanine to a small amount sufficient for tissue building and repair.

Aspartame (used as a sweetener in some foods and medicines) contributes to the phenylalanine intake and may affect control of phenylketonuria. If alternatives are unavailable, children with phenylketonuria should not be denied access to appropriate medication; the amount of aspartame consumed can be taken in to account in the management of the condition. Where the presence of aspartame in a preparation is specified in the product literature, aspartame is listed as an excipient in the relevant product entry in *BNF for Children*; the child or carer should be informed of this.

For further information on special dietary products used in the management of metabolic diseases, see Appendix 2.

Some rare forms of phenylketonuria are caused by a deficiency of tetrahydrobiopterin. Treatment involves oral supplementation of **tetrahydrobiopterin**; in some severe cases, the addition of the neurotransmitter precursors, levodopa (section 4.9.1) and 5-hydroxytryptophan, is also necessary.

Sapropterin, a synthetic form of tetrahydrobiopterin, is licensed as an adjunct to dietary restriction of phenylalanine in the management of patients with phenylketonuria and tetrahydrobiopterin deficiency.

TETRAHYDROBIOPTERIN

Renal impairment   use with caution—accumulation of metabolites

Pregnancy   crosses the placenta; use only if benefit outweighs risk

Breast-feeding   present in milk, effects unknown

Side-effects   diarrhoea, urinary frequency, disturbed sleep

Licensed use   not licensed

Indication and dose

Monotherapy in tetrahydrobiopterin-sensitive phenylketonuria (specialist use only)
- By mouth

   Child 1 month–18 years 10 mg/kg twice daily (total daily dose may alternatively be given in 3 divided doses), adjusted according to response

In combination with neurotransmitter precursors for tetrahydrobiopterin-sensitive phenylketonuria (specialist use only)
- By mouth

   Child 1 month–2 years initially 250–750 micrograms/kg 4 times daily (total daily dose may alternatively be given in 3 divided doses), adjusted according to response; max. 7 mg/kg daily

   Child 2–18 years initially 250–750 micrograms/kg 4 times daily (total daily dose may alternatively be given in 3 divided doses), adjusted according to response; usual max. 10 mg/kg daily

Tetrahydrobiopterin (Non-proprietary)
Tablets, tetrahydrobiopterin 10 mg and 50 mg
Available from 'special-order' manufacturers or specialist importing companies, see p. 957

SAPROPTERIN DIHYDROCHLORIDE

Note Sapropterin is a synthetic form of tetrahydrobiopterin

Cautions   monitor blood-phenylalanine concentration before and after first week of treatment—if unsatisfactory response increase dose at weekly intervals to max. dose and monitor blood-phenylalanine concentration weekly; discontinue treatment if unsatisfactory response after 1 month; monitor blood-phenylalanine and tyrosine concentrations 1–2 weeks after dose adjustment and during treatment; history of convulsions

Hepatic impairment   manufacturer advises caution—no information available

Renal impairment   manufacturer advises caution—no information available

Pregnancy   manufacturer advises caution—consider only if strict dietary management inadequate

Breast-feeding   manufacturer advises avoid—no information available

Side-effects   diarrhoea, vomiting, abdominal pain; nasal congestion, cough, pharyngolaryngeal pain; headache

Indication and dose

Phenylketonuria (specialist use only)
- By mouth

   Child 4–18 years initially 10 mg/kg once daily, preferably in the morning, adjusted according to response; usual dose 5–20 mg/kg daily

◻ **SAPROPTERIN DIHYDROCHLORIDE (continued)**

Tetrahydrobiopterin deficiency (specialist use only)
• By mouth

Neonate initially 2–5 mg/kg once daily, preferably in the morning, adjusted according to response; max. 20 mg/kg daily; total daily dose may alternatively be given in 2–3 divided doses

Child 1 month–18 years initially 2–5 mg/kg once daily, preferably in the morning, adjusted according to response; max. 20 mg/kg daily;

total daily dose may alternatively be given in 2–3 divided doses

Kuvan® (Merck Serono) ▼ PoM
Dispersible tablets, sapropterin dihydrochloride 100 mg, net price 30-tab pack = £597.22, 120-tab pack = £2388.88. Label: 13, 21, counselling, tablets should be dissolved in water and taken within 20 minutes

9.4.2 Enteral nutrition

Children have higher nutrient requirements per kg body-weight, different metabolic rates, and physiological responses compared to adults. They have low nutritional stores and are particularly vulnerable to growth and nutritional problems during critical periods of development. Major illness, operations, or trauma impose increased metabolic demands and can rapidly exhaust nutritional reserves.

Every effort should be made to optimise oral food intake before beginning enteral tube feeding; this may include change of posture, special seating, feeding equipment, oral desensitisation, food texture changes, thickening of liquids, increasing energy density of food, treatment of reflux or oesophagitis, as well as using age-specific nutritional supplements.

Enteral tube feeding has a role in both short-term rehabilitation and long-term nutritional management in paediatrics. It can be used as supportive therapy, in which the enteral feed supplies a proportion of the required nutrients, or as primary therapy, in which the enteral feed delivers all the necessary nutrients. Most children receiving tube feeds should also be encouraged to take oral food and drink. Tube feeding should be considered in the following situations:

• unsafe swallowing and risk of aspiration;
• inability to consume at least 60% of energy needs by mouth;
• total feeding time of more than 4 hours per day;
• weight loss or no weight gain for a period of 3 months (less for younger children and infants);
• weight for height (or length) less than 2nd percentile for age and sex.

Most feeds for enteral use (Appendix 2) contain protein derived from cows' milk or soya. Elemental feeds containing protein hydrolysates or free amino acids can be used for children who have diminished ability to break down protein, for example in inflammatory bowel disease or pancreatic insufficiency.

Even when nutritionally complete feeds are given, water and electrolyte balance should be monitored. Haematological and biochemical parameters should also be monitored, particularly in the clinically unstable child. Extra minerals (e.g. magnesium and zinc) may be needed in patients where gastro-intestinal secretions are being lost. Additional vitamins may also be needed. Feeds containing vitamin K may affect the INR in children receiving warfarin—see **interactions**: Appendix 1 (vitamins).

Choosing the best formula for children depends on several factors including: nutritional requirements, gastro-intestinal function, underlying disease, nutrient restrictions, age, and feed characteristics (nutritional composition, viscosity, osmolality, availability and cost). Children have specific dietary requirements and in many situations liquid feeds prepared for adults are totally unsuitable and should not be given. Expert advice from a dietician should be sought before prescribing enteral feeds for a child.

Infant formula feeds   Child 0–12 months. Term infants with normal gastro-intestinal function are given either breast milk or normal infant formula during the first year of life. The average intake is between 150 mL and 200 mL/kg/day. Infant milk formulas are based on whey- or casein-dominant protein, lactose with or without maltodextrin, amylose, vegetable oil and milk fat. The composition of all normal and soya infant formulas have to meet The Infant Formula and Follow-on

Formula Regulations (England and Wales) 2007, which enact the European Community Regulations 2006/141/EC; the composition of other enteral and specialist feeds has to meet the Commission Directive (1999/21/EC) on Dietary Foods for Special Medical Purposes.

A high-energy feed (Appendix 2, p. 901), which contains 9–11% of energy derived from protein can be used for infants who fail to grow adequately. Alternatively, energy supplements (Appendix 2, p. 919) may be added to normal infant formula to achieve a higher energy content (but this will reduce the protein to energy ratio) or the normal infant formula concentration may be increased slightly. Care should be taken not to present an osmotic load of more than 500 milliosmols/kg water to the normal functioning gut, otherwise osmotic diarrhoea will result. Concentrating or supplementing feeds should not be attempted without the advice of a paediatric dietician.

Enteral feeds   **Child 1–6 years (body-weight 8–20 kg).** Ready-to-use feeds (Appendix 2, p. 901) based on caseinates, maltodextrin and vegetable oils (with or without added medium chain triglyceride (MCT) oil or fibre) are well tolerated and effective in improving nutritional status in this age group. Although originally designed for children 1–6 years (body-weight 8–20 kg), some products have ACBS approval for use in children weighing up to 30 kg (approx. 10 years of age). Enteral feeds formulated for children 1–6 years are low in sodium and potassium; electrolyte intake and biochemical status should be monitored. Older children in this age range taking small feed volumes may need to be given additional micronutrients. Fibre-enriched feeds may be helpful for children with chronic constipation or diarrhoea.

Child 7–12 years (body-weight 21–45 kg). Depending on age, weight, clinical condition and nutritional requirements, ready-to-use feeds (Appendix 2, p. 901) formulated for 7–12 year olds may be given at appropriate rates.

Child over 12 years (body-weight over 45 kg). As there are no standard enteral feeds formulated for this age group, adult formulations are used. The intake of protein, electrolytes, vitamins, and trace minerals should be carefully assessed and monitored.

Note Adult feeds containing more than 6 g/100 mL protein or 2 g/100 mL fibre should be used with caution and expert advice.

Specialised formula   It is essential that any infant who is intolerant of breast milk or normal infant formula, or whose condition requires nutrient-specific adaptation, is prescribed an adequate volume of a nutritionally complete replacement formula (see Appendix 2, p. 911). In the first 4 months of life, a volume of 150–200 mL/kg/day is recommended. After 6 months, should the formula still be required, a volume of 600 mL/day should be maintained, in addition to solid food.

Products for cow's milk protein intolerance or lactose intolerance. There are a number of infant formulas formulated for cow's milk protein intolerance or lactose intolerance; these feeds may contain a residual amount of lactose (less than 1 g/100 mL formula)—sometimes described as clinically lactose-free or 'lactose-free' by manufacturers. If the total daily intake of these formulas is low, it may be necessary to supplement with calcium, and a vitamin and mineral supplement.

Soya-based infant formulas have a high phytoestrogen content and this may be a long-term reproductive health risk. The Chief Medical Officer has advised that soya-based infant formulas should not be used as the first choice for the management of infants with proven cow's milk sensitivity, lactose intolerance, galacto-kinase deficiency and galactosaemia. Most UK paediatricians with expertise in inherited metabolic disease still advocate soya-based formulations for infants with galactosaemia as there are concerns about the residual lactose content of low lactose formulas and protein hydrolysates based on cow's milk protein.

Low lactose infant formulations, based on whole cow's milk protein, are unsuitable for children with cow's milk protein intolerance. Liquid soya milks purchased from supermarkets and health food stores are not nutritionally complete and should never be used for infants under 1 year of age.

Protein hydrolysate formulas. Non-milk, peptide-based feeds containing hydrolysates of casein, whey, meat and soya protein, are suitable for infants with disaccharide or whole protein intolerance. The total daily intake of electrolytes, vitamins and minerals should be carefully assessed and modified to meet the

9

Nutrition and blood

child's nutritional requirements; these feeds have a high osmolality when given at recommended dilution and need gradual and careful introduction.

Elemental (amino acid based formula). Specially formulated elemental feeds containing essential and non-essential amino acids are available for use in infants and children under 6 years with proven whole protein intolerance. Adult elemental formula may be used for children over 6 years; the intake of electrolytes, vitamins and minerals should be carefully assessed and modified to meet nutritional requirements. These feeds have a high osmolality when given at the recommended concentration and therefore need gradual and careful introduction.

Modular feeds. Modular feeds (see Specialised Formulas for Specific Clinical Conditions, p. 916) are based on individual protein, fat, carbohydrate, vitamin and mineral components or modules which can be combined to meet the specific needs of a child. Modular feeds are used when nutritionally complete specialised formula are not tolerated, or if the fluid and nutrient requirements change e.g. in gastro-intestinal, renal or liver disease. The main advantage of modular feeds is their flexibility; disadvantages include their complexity and preparation difficulties. Modular feeds should not be used without the supervision of a paediatric dietician.

Specialised formula. Highly specialised formulas are designed to meet the specific requirements in various clinical conditions such as renal and liver diseases. When using these formulas, both the biochemical status of the child and their growth parameters need to be monitored.

Feed thickeners   Carob based thickeners (Appendix 2, p. 925) may be used to thicken feeds for infants under 1 year with significant gastro-oesophageal reflux. Breast-fed infants can be given the thickener mixed to a paste with water or breast-milk prior to feeds.

Pre-thickened formula Milk-protein- or casein-dominant infant formula, which contains small quantities of pre-gelatinized starch, is recommended primarily for infants with mild gastro-oesophageal reflux. Pre-thickened formula is prepared in the same way as normal infant formula and flows through a standard teat. The feeds do not thicken on standing but thicken in the stomach when exposed to acid pH.

Starched based thickeners can be used to thicken liquids and feeds for children over 1 year of age with dysphagia.

Dietary supplements for oral use   (Appendix 2, p. 906) Three types of prescribable fortified dietary supplements are available: fortified milk and non-milk tasting (juice-style) drinks, and fortified milk-based semi-solid preparations. The recommended daily quantity is age-dependent. The following is a useful guide: 1–2 years, 200 kcal (840 kJ); 3–5 years, 400 kcal (1680 kJ); 6–11 years, 600 kcal (2520 kJ); and over 12 years, 800 kcal (3360 kJ). Supplements containing 1.5 kcal/mL are high in protein and should not be used for children under 3 years of age. Many supplements are high in sugar or maltodextrin; care should be taken to prevent prolonged contact with teeth. Ideally supplements should be administered after meals or at bedtime so as not to affect appetite.

Products for metabolic diseases   There is a large range of disease-specific infant formulas and amino acid-based supplements available for use in children with metabolic diseases (see under specific metabolic diseases, Appendix 2, p. 930). Some of these formulas are nutritionally incomplete and supplementation with vitamins and other nutrients may be necessary. Many of the product names are similar; to prevent metabolic complications in children who cannot tolerate specific amino acids it is important to ensure the correct supplement is supplied.

Preparations (Borderline substances)   See Appendix 2.

9.5 Minerals

9.5.1 **Calcium and magnesium**

9.5.2 **Phosphorus**

9.5.3 **Fluoride**

9.5.4 **Zinc**

See section 9.1.1 for iron salts.

9.5.1 Calcium and magnesium

9.5.1.1 Calcium supplements
9.5.1.2 Hypercalcaemia and hypercalciuria
9.5.1.3 Magnesium

9.5.1.1 Calcium supplements

Calcium supplements are usually only required where dietary calcium intake is deficient. This dietary requirement varies with age and is relatively greater in childhood, pregnancy, and lactation, due to an increased demand. Hypocalcaemia may be caused by vitamin D deficiency (section 9.6.4), impaired metabolism, a failure of secretion (hypoparathyroidism), or resistance to parathyroid hormone (pseudohypoparathyroidism).

Mild asymptomatic hypocalcaemia may be managed with oral calcium supplements. *Severe symptomatic hypocalcaemia* requires an intravenous infusion of calcium gluconate 10% over 5 to 10 minutes, repeating the dose if symptoms persist; in exceptional cases it may be necessary to maintain a continuous calcium infusion over a day or more. Calcium chloride injection is also available, but is more irritant; care should be taken to prevent extravasation.

For the role of calcium gluconate in temporarily reducing the toxic effects of *hyperkalaemia*, see p. 557.

Persistent hypocalcaemia requires oral calcium supplements and either a vitamin D analogue (alfacalcidol or calcitriol) for hypoparathyroidism and pseudohypoparathyroidism or natural vitamin D (calciferol) if due to vitamin D deficiency (section 9.6.4). It is important to monitor plasma and urinary calcium during long-term maintenance therapy.

Neonates   Hypocalcaemia is common in the first few days of life, particularly following birth asphyxia or respiratory distress. Late onset at 4–10 days after birth may be secondary to vitamin D deficiency, hypoparathyroidism or hypomagnesaemia and may be associated with seizures.

◢ CALCIUM SALTS

Cautions   see notes above; sarcoidosis; history of nephrolithiasis; avoid calcium chloride in respiratory acidosis or respiratory failure; **interactions**: Appendix 1 (antacids, calcium salts)

Contra-indications   conditions associated with hypercalcaemia and hypercalciuria (e.g. some forms of malignant disease)

Renal impairment   use with caution; risk of hypercalcaemia and renal calculi

Side-effects   gastro-intestinal disturbances, constipation; bradycardia, arrhythmias; with injection, peripheral vasodilatation, fall in blood pressure, injection-site reactions, severe tissue damage with extravasation

Indication and dose

See notes above; calcium deficiency
• By mouth

> **Neonate** 0.25 mmol/kg 4 times a day, adjusted to response

> **Child 1 month–4 years** 0.25 mmol/kg 4 times a day, adjusted to response

> **Child 5–12 years** 0.2 mmol/kg 4 times a day, adjusted to response

> **Child 12–18 years** 10 mmol 4 times a day, adjusted to response

Acute hypocalcaemia, urgent correction; hyperkalaemia (prevention of arrhythmias)
• By slow intravenous injection over 5–10 minutes

> **Neonate** 0.11 mmol/kg (0.5 mL/kg of calcium gluconate 10%) as a single dose. [Some units use a dose of 0.46 mmol/kg (2 mL/kg calcium gluconate 10%) for hypocalcaemia in line with US practice]

> **Child 1 month–18 years** 0.11 mmol/kg (0.5 mL/kg calcium gluconate 10%), max 4.5 mmol (20 mL calcium gluconate 10%)

Acute hypocalcaemia, maintenance
• By continuous intravenous infusion

> **Neonate** 0.5 mmol/kg daily over 24 hours, adjusted to response, use oral route as soon as possible due to risk of extravasation

> **Child 1 month–2 years** 1 mmol/kg daily (usual max 8.8 mmol) over 24 hours, use oral route as soon as possible due to risk of extravasation

> **Child 2–18 years** 8.8 mmol over 24 hours, use oral route as soon as possible due to risk of extravasation

9

Nutrition and blood

◻ **CALCIUM SALTS** *(continued)*

◢**Oral preparations**

Calcium Gluconate (Non-proprietary)

Effervescent tablets, calcium gluconate 1 g (calcium 89 mg or Ca^{2+} 2.23 mmol), net price 28-tab pack = £14.31. Label: 13

Note Each tablet usually contains 4.46 mmol Na^+

Calcium Lactate (Non-proprietary)

Tablets, calcium lactate 300 mg (calcium 39 mg or Ca^{2+} 1 mmol), net price 84 = £2.63

Adcal® (ProStrakan)

Chewable tablets, fruit flavour, calcium carbonate 1.5 g (calcium 600 mg or Ca^{2+} 15 mmol), net price 100-tab pack = £7.25. Label: 24

Cacit® (Procter & Gamble Pharm.)

Tablets, effervescent, pink, calcium carbonate 1.25 g, providing calcium citrate when dispersed in water (calcium 500 mg or Ca^{2+} 12.5 mmol), net price 76-tab pack = £12.05. Label: 13

Calcichew® (Shire)

Tablets (chewable), orange flavour, calcium carbonate 1.25 g (calcium 500 mg or Ca^{2+} 12.5 mmol), net price 100-tab pack = £9.33. Label: 24

Forte tablets (chewable), orange flavour, scored, calcium carbonate 2.5 g (calcium 1 g or Ca^{2+} 25 mmol), net price 60-tab pack = £13.16. Label: 24
Excipients include aspartame (section 9.4.1)

Calcium-500 (Martindale)

Tablets, pink, f/c, calcium carbonate 1.25 g (calcium 500 mg or Ca^{2+} 12.5 mmol), net price 100-tab pack = £9.46. Label: 25

Calcium-Sandoz® (Alliance)

Syrup, orange flavour, calcium glubionate 1.09 g, calcium lactobionate 727 mg (calcium 108.3 mg or Ca^{2+} 2.7 mmol)/5 mL, net price 300 mL = £3.14

Sandocal® (Novartis Consumer Health)

Sandocal 400 tablets, effervescent, orange flavour, calcium lactate gluconate 930 mg, calcium carbonate 700 mg, providing calcium 400 mg (Ca^{2+} 10 mmol), net price 5 × 20-tab pack = £6.87. Label: 13
Excipients include aspartame (section 9.4.1)

Sandocal 1000 tablets, effervescent, orange flavour, calcium lactate gluconate 2.263 g, calcium carbonate 1.75 g, providing 1 g calcium (Ca^{2+} 25 mmol), net price 3 × 10-tab pack = £6.17. Label: 13
Excipients include aspartame (section 9.4.1)

◢**Parenteral preparations**

Calcium Gluconate (Non-proprietary) ⃞PoM

Injection, calcium gluconate 10% (calcium 8.4 mg or Ca^{2+} 226 micromol)/mL. Net price 10-mL amp = 60p

Administration For *intravenous infusion* dilute to at least 45 micromol/mL with Glucose 5% *or* Sodium Chloride 0.9%. Maximum administration rate 45 micromol/kg/hour (or in neonates max. 22 micromol/kg/hour). May be given more concentrated via a central venous catheter. May be used undiluted (10% calcium gluconate) in emergencies. Avoid extravasation; should not be given by intramuscular injection. Incompatible with sodium bicarbonate and phosphate solutions.

Calcium Chloride (Non-proprietary) ⃞PoM

Injection, calcium chloride dihydrate 10% (calcium 27.3 mg or Ca^{2+} 680 micromol/mL), net price 10-mL disposable syringe = £5.10
Brands include *Minijet® Calcium Chloride 10%*

Injection, calcium chloride dihydrate 13.4% (calcium 36 mg or Ca^{2+} 910 micromol/mL), net price 10–mL amp = £14.94

◢**With vitamin D**

Section 9.6.4

9.5.1.2 **Hypercalcaemia and hypercalciuria**

Severe hypercalcaemia Severe hypercalcaemia calls for urgent treatment before detailed investigation of the cause. Dehydration should be corrected first with intravenous infusion of **sodium chloride 0.9%**. Drugs (such as thiazides and vitamin D compounds) which promote hypercalcaemia, should be discontinued and dietary calcium should be restricted.

If *severe hypercalcaemia persists* drugs which inhibit mobilisation of calcium from the skeleton may be required. The **bisphosphonates** are useful and disodium pamidronate (section 6.6.2) is probably the most effective.

Corticosteroids (section 6.3) are widely given, but may only be useful where hypercalcaemia is due to sarcoidosis or vitamin D intoxication; they often take several days to achieve the desired effect.

Calcitonin (section 6.6.1) is relatively non-toxic, but its effect can wear off after a few days despite continued use; it is rarely effective where bisphosphonates have failed to reduce serum calcium adequately.

After treatment of severe hypercalcaemia the underlying cause must be established. *Further treatment* is governed by the same principles as for initial therapy. Salt and water depletion and drugs promoting hypercalcaemia should be avoided; oral administration of a bisphosphonate may be useful. Parathyroidectomy may be indicated for hyperparathyroidism.

Hypercalciuria Hypercalciuria should be investigated for an underlying cause, which should be treated. Reducing dietary calcium intake may be beneficial but severe restriction of calcium intake has not proved beneficial and may even be harmful.

9.5.1.3 Magnesium

Magnesium is an essential constituent of many enzyme systems, particularly those involved in energy generation; the largest stores are in the skeleton.

Magnesium salts are not well absorbed from the gastro-intestinal tract, which explains the use of magnesium sulphate (section 1.6.4) as an osmotic laxative.

Magnesium is excreted mainly by the kidneys and is therefore retained in renal failure, but significant *hypermagnesaemia* (causing muscle weakness and arrhythmias) is rare.

Hypomagnesaemia Since magnesium is secreted in large amounts in the gastro-intestinal fluid, excessive losses in diarrhoea, stoma or fistula are the most common causes of *hypomagnesaemia*; deficiency may also occur as a result of treatment with certain drugs. Hypomagnesaemia often causes secondary hypocalcaemia (with which it may be confused), particularly in neonates, and also hypokalaemia and hyponatraemia.

Symptomatic *hypomagnesaemia* is associated with a deficit of 0.5–1 mmol/kg. Magnesium is given initially by intravenous infusion or by intramuscular injection of **magnesium sulphate**; the intramuscular injection is painful. Plasma magnesium concentration should be measured to determine the rate and duration of infusion and the dose should be reduced in renal impairment. To prevent *recurrence of the deficit*, magnesium may be given by mouth in divided doses. For maintenance (e.g. in intravenous nutrition), parenteral doses of magnesium are of the order of 0.2–0.4 mmol/kg (usual max. 20 mmol) Mg^{2+} daily.

Arrhythmias Magnesium sulphate has also been recommended for the emergency treatment of *serious arrhythmias*, especially in the presence of hypokalaemia (when hypomagnesaemia may also be present) and when salvos of rapid ventricular tachycardia show the characteristic twisting wave front known as *torsade de pointes* (see also section 2.3.1).

MAGNESIUM SULPHATE

Cautions see notes above; in severe hypomagnesaemia administer initially via controlled infusion device (preferably syringe pump); monitor blood pressure, respiratory rate, urinary output and for signs of overdosage (loss of patellar reflexes, weakness, nausea, sensation of warmth, flushing, drowsiness, double vision, and slurred speech); **interactions**: Appendix 1 (magnesium, parenteral)

Hepatic impairment avoid in hepatic coma if risk of renal failure

Renal impairment avoid or reduce dose; increased risk of toxicity

Pregnancy sufficient may cross the placenta in mothers treated with high doses e.g. in pre-eclampsia, causing hypotonia and respiratory depression in newborns

Breast-feeding present in breast milk; may cause diarrhoea in breast-fed babies

Side-effects generally associated with hypermagnesaemia, nausea, vomiting, thirst, flushing of skin, hypotension, arrhythmias, coma, respiratory depression, drowsiness, confusion, loss of tendon reflexes, muscle weakness

Licensed use 20% injection licensed for use in children. Other strengths unlicensed

Indication and dose

Neonatal hypocalcaemia
- **By deep intramuscular injection or intravenous infusion**

Neonate 0.4 mmol/kg Mg^{2+} (100 mg/kg magnesium sulphate) 12 hourly for 2–3 doses

Hypomagnesaemia
- **By intravenous injection over at least 10 minutes**

Neonate 0.4 mmol/kg Mg^{2+} (100 mg/kg magnesium sulphate) 6–12 hourly as necessary

Child 1 month–12 years 0.2 mmol/kg Mg^{2+} (50 mg/kg magnesium sulphate) 12 hourly as necessary

Child 12–18 years 4 mmol Mg^{2+} (1 g magnesium sulphate) 12 hourly as necessary

Torsade de pointes (consult local guidelines)
- **By intravenous injection over 10–15 minutes**
  Child 1 month–18 years 0.1–0.2 mmol/kg (25–50 mg/kg magnesium sulphate); max. 8 mmol (2 g magnesium sulphate); dose repeated once if necessary

Persistent pulmonary hypertension section 2.5.1

Severe acute asthma section 3.1

Administration Dilute to 10% (100 mg in 1 mL) with Glucose 5 *or* 10%, Sodium Chloride 0.45 *or* 0.9% *or* Glucose and Sodium Chloride combinations. Up to 20% solution may be given in fluid restriction. Rate of administration should not exceed 10 mg/kg/minute of magnesium sulphate

Note Magnesium sulphate 1 g equivalent to Mg^{2+} approx. 4 mmol

9

Nutrition and blood

◁ **MAGNESIUM SULPHATE** (*continued*)

Magnesium Sulphate (Non-proprietary) [PoM]
Injection, magnesium sulphate 20% (Mg^{2+} approx. 0.8 mmol/mL), net price 20-mL (4-g) amp = £2.75; 50% (Mg^{2+} approx. 2 mmol/mL), 2-mL (1-g) amp = £2.80, 4-mL (2-g) prefilled syringe = £7.39; 5-mL (2.5-g) amp = £3.00, 10-mL (5-g) amp = 96p; 10-mL (5-g) prefilled syringe = £4.95
Brands include *Minijet® Magnesium Sulphate 50%*

MAGNESIUM-L-ASPARTATE

Cautions see under Magnesium Sulphate

Renal impairment avoid or reduce dose; increased risk of toxicity

Side-effects see under Magnesium Sulphate; also diarrhoea

Licensed use classified as a Food for Special Medical Purposes for use in children over 2 years

Indication and dose

Hypomagnesaemia
• By mouth

Child 1 month–2 years initially 0.2 mmol/kg of Mg^{2+} 3 times daily dissolved in water, dose adjusted as required

Child 2–10 years half a sachet (5 mmol Mg^{2+}) daily dissolved in 100 mL of water, dose adjusted as required

Child 10–18 years one sachet (10 mmol Mg^{2+}) daily dissolved in 200 mL of water, dose adjusted as required

Magnaspartate® (KoRa)
Oral powder, magnesium-L-aspartate 6.5 g (10 mmol Mg^{2+})/sachet, net price 10-sachet pack = £7.95
Excipients include sucrose

MAGNESIUM GLYCEROPHOSPHATE

Cautions see under Magnesium Sulphate

Renal impairment avoid or reduce dose; increased risk of toxicity

Side-effects see under Magnesium Sulphate; also diarrhoea

Licensed use not licensed

Indication and dose

Hypomagnesaemia
• By mouth

Child 1 month–12 years initially 0.2 mmol/kg Mg^{2+} 3 times daily, dose adjusted as required

Child 12–18 years initially 4–8 mmol Mg^{2+} 3 times daily, dose adjusted as required

Administration tablets may be dispersed in water

Magnesium Glycerophosphate (Non-proprietary)
Tablets, magnesium glycerophosphate 1 g (approximately magnesium 97 mg or Mg^{2+} 4 mmol)
Available from 'special-order' manufacturers or specialist importing companies, see p. 957

Liquid, magnesium glycerophosphate 250 mg/mL (approximately magnesium 24.25 mg or Mg^{2+} 1 mmol/mL)
Available from 'special-order' manufacturers or specialist importing companies, see p. 957

◀ Extemporaneous formulations available see Extemporaneous Preparations, p. 8

9.5.2 Phosphorus

9.5.2.1 Phosphate supplements
9.5.2.2 Phosphate-binding agents

9.5.2.1 Phosphate supplements

Oral phosphate supplements may be required in addition to vitamin D in children with hypophosphataemic vitamin D-resistant rickets (section 9.6.4). Diarrhoea is a common side-effect and should prompt a reduction in dosage.

Phosphate infusion is occasionally needed in phosphate deficiency arising from use of parenteral nutrition deficient in phosphate supplements; phosphate depletion also occurs in severe diabetic ketoacidosis. It is difficult to provide detailed guidelines for the treatment of *severe hypophosphatemia* because the extent of total body deficits and response to therapy are difficult to predict. High doses of phosphate may result in a transient serum elevation followed by redistribution into intracellular compartments or bone tissue; excessive doses may cause hypocalcaemia and metastatic calcification. It is essential to monitor plasma concentrations of calcium, phosphate, potassium and other electrolytes. It is recommended that severe hypophosphataemia be treated intravenously as large doses of oral phosphate may cause diarrhoea; intestinal absorption may be unreliable and dose adjustment may be necessary.

9 Nutrition and blood

Phosphate is not the first choice for the treatment of hypercalcaemia because of the risk of precipitation of calcium phosphate in the kidney and other tissues. If used, the child should be well hydrated and electrolytes monitored.

Neonates   Phosphate deficiency may occur in very low-birthweight infants and may compromise bone growth if not corrected. Parenterally fed infants may be at risk of phosphate deficiency due to the limited solubility of phosphate. Some units routinely supplement expressed breast milk with phosphate, although the effect on the osmolality of the milk should be considered.

◢ PHOSPHATE

Cautions   see notes above, also cardiac disease, diabetes mellitus, dehydration; avoid extravasation with parenteral forms, severe tissue necrosis; sodium and potassium concentrations of preparations

Renal impairment   reduce dose; monitor closely

Side-effects   nausea, diarrhoea; hypotension, oedema; hypocalcaemia; acute renal failure; phlebitis; tissue necrosis on extravasation

Indication and dose

Hypophosphataemia, including hypophosphataemic rickets and osteomalacia (see notes above)

• By mouth

Neonate 1 mmol/kg daily in 1–2 divided doses, or as a supplement in breast milk

Child 1 month–5 years 2–3 mmol/kg (max. 48 mmol) phosphate daily in 2–4 divided doses, adjusted as necessary

Child 5–18 years 2–3 mmol/kg (max. 97 mmol) phosphate daily in 2–4 divided doses, adjusted as necessary

Administration Caution, solubility in breast milk is limited to 1.2 mmol in 100 mL if calcium also added, contact pharmacy department for details

• By intravenous infusion (see administration below)

Neonate 1 mmol/kg phosphate daily, adjusted as necessary

Child 1 month–2 years 0.7 mmol/kg phosphate daily, adjusted as necessary

Child 2–18 years 0.4 mmol/kg phosphate daily, adjusted as necessary

Administration (see also Important, below) Dilute injection with Sodium Chloride 0.9% or 0.45% or Glucose 5% or 10%. Administration rate of phosphate should not exceed 0.05 mmol/kg/hour. In emergencies in intensive care faster rates may be used—seek specialist advice

> **Important**   Some phosphate injection preparations also contain potassium. For peripheral intravenous administration the *concentration* of potassium should not usually exceed 40 mmol/litre. The infusion solution should be **thoroughly mixed.** Local policies on avoiding inadvertent use of potassium concentrate should be followed. The potassium content of some phosphate preparations may also limit the *rate* at which they may be administered, see section 9.2.2.1.

◢ Oral

Phosphate-Sandoz® (HK Pharma)

Tablets, effervescent, anhydrous sodium acid phosphate 1.936 g, sodium bicarbonate 350 mg, potassium bicarbonate 315 mg, equivalent to phosphorus 500 mg (phosphate 16.1 mmol), sodium 468.8 mg (Na$^+$ 20.4 mmol), potassium 123 mg (K$^+$ 3.1 mmol). Net price 20 = £3.29. Label: 13

◢ Extemporaneous formulations available see Extemporaneous Preparations, p. 8

Various strengths and salts available, caution electrolyte load

◢ Injection

Phosphates (Fresenius Kabi) [PoM]

Intravenous infusion, phosphates (providing phosphate 100 mmol/litre, potassium 19 mmol/litre, sodium 162 mmol/litre), net price 500 mL (*Polyfusor®*) = £3.75.

Potassium acid phosphate (Non-proprietary) [PoM]

Injection, 13.6% (1 mmol/mL phosphate, 1 mmol/mL potassium) 10 mL ampoule

Note See also Important, above

Dipotassium hydrogen phosphate (Non-proprietary) [PoM]

Injection, 17.42% (1 mmol/mL phosphate and 2 mmol/mL potassium) 10 mL ampoule

Note See also Important, above

Disodium hydrogen phosphate (Non-proprietary) [PoM]

Injection, 17.42% (0.6 mmol/mL phosphate and 1.2 mmol/mL sodium) 10 mL ampoule

9

Nutrition and blood

9.5.2.2   Phosphate-binding agents

Calcium-containing preparations are used as phosphate-binding agents in the management of hyperphosphataemia complicating renal failure. Aluminium-containing preparations are rarely used as phosphate-binding agents and can cause aluminium accumulation.

Sevelamer is licensed for the treatment of hyperphosphataemia in adults on haemodialysis or peritoneal dialysis. Although experience is limited in children sevelamer may be useful when hypercalcaemia prevents the use of calcium carbonate.

ALUMINIUM HYDROXIDE

Cautions see notes above; **interactions:** Appendix 1 (antacids)

Side-effects constipation; hyperaluminaemia

Alu-Cap® (3M)
Capsules, green/red, dried aluminium hydroxide 475 mg (low Na^+), net price 120-cap pack = £3.75

Dose
> **Hyperphosphataemia**
> • By mouth
> **Child 5–12 years** 1–2 capsules 3–4 times daily, adjusted as necessary
> **Child 12–18 years** 1–5 capsules 3–4 times daily, adjusted as necessary

CALCIUM SALTS

Cautions **interactions:** Appendix 1 (antacids, calcium salts)

Contra-indications hypercalcaemia, hypercalciuria

Side-effects hypercalcaemia

Indication and dose
> **Phosphate binding in renal failure and hyperphosphataemia**
> • By mouth
> **Child 1 month–1 year** 120 mg calcium carbonate 3–4 times daily with feeds, adjusted as necessary
> **Child 1–6 years** 300 mg calcium carbonate 3–4 times daily prior to or with meals, adjusted as necessary
> **Child 6–12 years** 600 mg calcium carbonate 3–4 times daily prior to or with meals, adjusted as necessary
> **Child 12–18 years** 1.25 g calcium carbonate 3–4 times daily prior to or with meals, adjusted as necessary

Adcal®
Section 9.5.1.1

Calcichew®
Section 9.5.1.1

Calcium-500
Section 9.5.1.1

Phosex® (Vitaline)
Tablets, yellow, calcium acetate 1 g (calcium 250 mg or Ca^{2+} 6.2 mmol), net price 180-tab pack = £19.79. Label: 25, counselling, with meals

Dose
> Phosphate-binding agent (with meals) in renal failure, according to the requirements of the patient

◢ Extemporaneous formulations available see Extemporaneous Preparations, p. 8

SEVELAMER

Cautions gastro-intestinal disorders; **interactions:** Appendix 1 (sevelamer)

Contra-indications bowel obstruction

Pregnancy manufacturer advises use only if potential benefit outweighs risk

Breast-feeding manufacturer advises use only if potential benefit outweighs risk

Side-effects gastro-intestinal disturbances; *very rarely* intestinal obstruction; *also reported* intestinal perforation, pruritus, and rash

Licensed use not licensed for use in children under 18 years

Indication and dose
> **Hyperphosphataemia in patients on haemodialysis or peritoneal dialysis**
> • By mouth
> **Child 12–18 years** initially 0.8–1.6 g 3 times daily with meals, then adjusted according to plasma-phosphate concentration

Renagel® (Genzyme) PoM
Tablets, f/c, sevelamer 800 mg, net price 180-tab pack = £117.97. Label: 25, counselling, with meals

9.5.3 Fluoride

Availability of adequate fluoride confers significant resistance to dental caries. It is now considered that the topical action of fluoride on enamel and plaque is more important than the systemic effect.

When the fluoride content of drinking water is less than 700 micrograms per litre (0.7 parts per million), daily administration of fluoride tablets or drops provide suitable supplementation. Systemic fluoride supplements should not be prescribed without reference to the fluoride content of the local water supply. Infants need not receive fluoride supplements until the age of 6 months.

Dentifrices which incorporate sodium fluoride or monofluorophosphate are also a convenient source of fluoride.

Individuals who are either particularly caries prone or medically compromised may be given additional protection by use of fluoride rinses or by application of fluoride gels. Rinses may be used daily or weekly; daily use of a less concentrated rinse is more effective than weekly use of a more concentrated one. High-strength gels must be applied regularly under professional supervision; extreme caution is necessary to prevent the child from swallowing any excess. Less concentrated gels are available for home use. Varnishes are also available and are particularly valuable for young or disabled children since they adhere to the teeth and set in the presence of moisture.

Fluoride mouthwash, oral drops, tablets, and toothpaste are prescribable on form FP10D (GP14 in Scotland, WP10D in Wales; for details see preparations below).

There are also arrangements for health authorities to supply fluoride tablets in the course of pre-school dental schemes, and they may also be supplied in school dental schemes.

Fluoride gels are not prescribable on form FP10D (GP14 in Scotland, WP10D in Wales).

■ FLUORIDES

Note Sodium fluoride 2.2 mg provides approx. 1 mg fluoride ion

Contra-indications not for areas where drinking water is fluoridated

Side-effects occasional white flecks on teeth with recommended doses; *rarely* yellowish-brown discoloration if recommended doses are exceeded

Indication and dose

Prophylaxis of dental caries—see notes above

Note Dose expressed as fluoride ion (F^-):
Water content less than F^- 300 micrograms/litre (0.3 parts per million)

• By mouth

Child 6 months–3 years F^- 250 micrograms daily

Child 3–6 years F^- 500 micrograms daily

Child 6 years and over F^- 1 mg daily

Water content between F^- 300 and 700 micrograms/litre (0.3–0.7 parts per million)

Child 3–6 years F^- 250 micrograms daily

Child 6 years and over F^- 500 micrograms daily

Water content above F^- 700 micrograms/litre (0.7 parts per million), supplements not advised

Note These doses reflect the recommendations of the British Dental Association, the British Society of Paediatric Dentistry and the British Association for the Study of Community Dentistry (*Br Dent J* 1997; **182**: 6–7)

■Tablets

Counselling Tablets should be sucked or dissolved in the mouth and taken preferably in the evening
There are arrangements for health authorities to supply fluoride tablets in the course of pre-school dental schemes, and they may also be supplied in school dental schemes.

En-De-Kay® (Manx)
Fluotabs 3–6 years, orange-flavoured, scored, sodium fluoride 1.1 mg (F^- 500 micrograms), net price 200-tab pack = £2.38

Dental prescribing on NHS May be prescribed as Sodium Fluoride Tablets

Fluotabs 6+ years, orange-flavoured, scored, sodium fluoride 2.2 mg (F^- 1 mg), net price 200-tab pack = £2.38

Dental prescribing on NHS May be prescribed as Sodium Fluoride Tablets

Fluor-a-day® (Dental Health)
Tablets, buff, sodium fluoride 1.1 mg (F^- 500 micrograms), net price 200-tab pack = £2.54; 2.2 mg (F^- 1 mg), 200-tab pack = £2.54

Dental prescribing on NHS May be prescribed as Sodium Fluoride Tablets

FluoriGard® (Colgate-Palmolive)
Tablets 0.5, purple, grape-flavoured, scored, sodium fluoride 1.1 mg (F^- 500 micrograms), net price 200-tab pack = £1.91

Dental prescribing on NHS May be prescribed as Sodium Fluoride Tablets

Tablets 1.0, orange, orange-flavoured, scored, sodium fluoride 2.2 mg (F^- 1 mg), net price 200-tab pack = £1.91

Dental prescribing on NHS May be prescribed as Sodium Fluoride Tablets

■Oral drops

Note Fluoride supplements not considered necessary below 6 months of age (see notes above)

En-De-Kay® (Manx)
Fluodrops® (= paediatric drops), sugar-free, sodium fluoride 550 micrograms (F^- 250 micrograms)/0.15 mL. Net price 60 mL = £2.38

Dental prescribing on NHS Corresponds to Sodium Fluoride Oral Drops DPF 0.37% equivalent to sodium fluoride 80 micrograms (F^- 36 micrograms)/drop

■Mouthwashes

Rinse mouth for 1 minute and spit out
Counselling Avoid eating, drinking, or rinsing mouth for 15 minutes after use

Duraphat® (Colgate-Palmolive)
Weekly dental rinse (= mouthwash), blue, sodium fluoride 0.2%. Net price 150 mL = £2.37. Counselling, see above

Dose

Child 6 years and over for *weekly* use, rinse with 10 mL

Dental prescribing on NHS May be prescribed as Sodium Fluoride Mouthwash 0.2%

9
Nutrition and blood

◁ **FLUORIDES** (*continued*)

En-De-Kay® (Manx)
Daily fluoride mouthrinse (= mouthwash), blue, sodium fluoride 0.05%. Net price 250 mL = £1.51

Dose

> **Child 6 years and over** for *daily* use, rinse with 10 mL

Dental prescribing on NHS May be prescribed as Sodium Fluoride Mouthwash 0.05%

Fluorinse PoM (= mouthwash), red, sodium fluoride 2%. Net price 100 mL = £4.97. Counselling, see above

Dose

> **Child 8 years and over** for *daily* use, dilute 5 drops to 10 mL of water; for *weekly* use, dilute 20 drops to 10 mL

Dental prescribing on NHS May be prescribed as Sodium Fluoride Mouthwash 2%

FluoriGard® (Colgate-Palmolive)
Daily dental rinse (= mouthwash), blue, sodium fluoride 0.05%. Net price 500 mL = £3.46. Counselling, see above

Dose

> **Child 6 years and over** for *daily* use, rinse with 10 mL

Dental prescribing on NHS May be prescribed as Sodium Fluoride Mouthwash 0.05%

◀ **Gels**

FluoriGard® (Colgate-Palmolive)
Gel-Kam (= gel), stannous fluoride 0.4% in glycerol basis. Net price 100 mL = £2.97. Counselling, see below

Dose

> **Child over 3 years** for *daily* use, using a toothbrush, apply on to all tooth surfaces
>
> **Counselling** Swish between teeth for 1 minute before spitting out. Avoid eating, drinking, or rinsing mouth for at least 30 minutes after use

◀ **Toothpastes**

Duraphat® (Colgate-Palmolive) PoM
Duraphat® '2800 ppm' toothpaste, sodium fluoride 0.619%. Net price 75 mL = £3.26. Counselling, see below

Dose

> **Child over 10 years** apply 1 cm twice daily using a toothbrush
>
> **Counselling** Brush teeth for 1 minute before spitting out. Avoid drinking or rinsing mouth for 30 minutes after use

Dental prescribing on NHS May be prescribed as Sodium Fluoride Toothpaste 0.619%

Duraphat® '5000 ppm' toothpaste, sodium fluoride 1.1%. Net price 51 g = £4.45. Counselling, see below

Dose

> **Child over 16 years** apply 2 cm 3 times daily after meals using a toothbrush
>
> **Counselling** Brush teeth for 3 minutes before spitting out

Dental prescribing on NHS May be prescribed as Sodium Fluoride Toothpaste 1.1%

9.5.4 Zinc

Zinc supplements should not be given unless there is good evidence of deficiency (hypoproteinaemia spuriously lowers plasma-zinc concentration) or in zinc-losing conditions. Zinc deficiency can occur as a result of inadequate diet or malabsorption; excessive loss of zinc can occur in trauma, burns, and protein-losing conditions. A zinc supplement is given until clinical improvement occurs, but it may need to be continued in severe malabsorption, metabolic disease, or in zinc-losing states. Zinc is used in the treatment of Wilson's disease (section 9.8.1) and acrodermatitis enteropathica, a rare inherited abnormality of zinc absorption.

Parenteral nutrition regimens usually include trace amounts of zinc (section 9.3). If necessary, further zinc can be added to some intravenous feeding regimens.

◢ **ZINC SULPHATE**

Cautions interactions: Appendix 1 (zinc)

Renal impairment accumulation may occur in acute renal failure

Pregnancy crosses placenta; risk theoretically minimal, but no information available

Breast-feeding present in milk; risk theoretically minimal, but no information available

Side-effects abdominal pain, dyspepsia, nausea, vomiting, diarrhoea, gastric irritation, gastritis; irritability, headache, lethargy

Licensed use *Solvazinc®* not licensed for use in acrodermatitis enteropathica

Solvazinc® (Galen)
Effervescent tablets, zinc sulphate monohydrate 125 mg (45 mg zinc), net price 30 = £4.32. Label: 13, 21

Dose

> **Zinc deficiency** (see notes above)
> • By mouth
>
> **Neonate** 1 mg/kg elemental zinc daily
>
> **Child under 10 kg** half a tablet daily in water after food, adjusted as necessary
>
> **Child 10–30 kg** half a tablet 1–3 times daily in water after food, adjusted as necessary
>
> **Child over 30 kg** 1 tablet 1–3 times daily in water after food, adjusted as necessary

9 Nutrition and blood

◻ **ZINC SULPHATE (*continued*)**

Acrodermatitis enteropathica
● By mouth

> **Neonate** 0.5–1 mg/kg elemental zinc twice daily (total daily dose may alternatively be given in 3 divided doses), adjusted as necessary

> **Child 1 month–18 years** 0.5–1 mg/kg elemental zinc twice daily (total daily dose may alternatively be given in 3 divided doses), adjusted as necessary

9.6 Vitamins

9.6.1 Vitamin A
9.6.2 Vitamin B group
9.6.3 Vitamin C
9.6.4 Vitamin D
9.6.5 Vitamin E
9.6.6 Vitamin K
9.6.7 **Multivitamin preparations**

Vitamins are used for the prevention and treatment of specific deficiency states or where the diet is known to be inadequate; they may be prescribed in the NHS to prevent or treat deficiency but not as dietary supplements. Except for iron-deficiency anaemia, a primary vitamin or mineral deficiency due to simple dietary inadequacy is rare in the developed world. Some children may be at risk of developing deficiencies because of an inadequate intake, impaired vitamin synthesis or malabsorption in disease states such as cystic fibrosis and Crohn's disease.

The use of vitamins as general 'pick-me-ups' is of unproven value and the 'fad' for mega-vitamin therapy with water-soluble vitamins, such as ascorbic acid and pyridoxine, is unscientific and can be harmful. Many vitamin supplements are described as 'multivitamin' but few contain the whole range of essential vitamins and many contain relatively high amounts of vitamins A and D. Care should be taken to ensure the correct dose is not exceeded.

Dietary reference values for vitamins are available in the Department of Health publication:

> Dietary Reference Values for Food Energy and Nutrients for the United Kingdom: Report of the Panel on Dietary Reference Values of the Committee on Medical Aspects of Food Policy. *Report on Health and Social Subjects 41.* London: HMSO, 1991

Dental patients It is unjustifiable to treat stomatitis or glossitis with mixtures of vitamin preparations; this delays diagnosis and correct treatment.

Most patients who develop a nutritional deficiency despite an adequate intake of vitamins have malabsorption and if this is suspected the patient should be referred to a medical practitioner.

9.6.1 Vitamin A

Deficiency of vitamin A (retinol) is associated with ocular defects (particularly xerophthalmia) and an increased susceptibility to infections, but deficiency is rare in the UK (even in disorders of fat absorption).

Vitamin A supplementation may be required in children with liver disease, particularly cholestatic liver disease, due to the malabsorption of fat soluble vitamins. In those with complete biliary obstruction an intramuscular dose once a month may be appropriate.

Treatment is sometimes initiated with very high doses of vitamin A and the child should be monitored closely; very high doses are associated with acute toxicity.

Preterm neonates have low plasma concentrations of vitamin A and are usually given vitamin A supplements, often as part of an oral multivitamin preparation (section 9.6.7) once enteral feeding has been established.

Massive overdose can cause rough skin, dry hair, an enlarged liver, and a raised erythrocyte sedimentation rate and raised serum calcium and serum alkaline phosphatase concentrations.

Pregnancy In view of evidence suggesting that high levels of vitamin A may cause birth defects, women who are (or may become) pregnant are advised not to

9

Nutrition and blood

take vitamin A supplements (including tablets and fish-liver oil drops), except on the advice of a doctor or an antenatal clinic; nor should they eat liver or products such as liver paté or liver sausage.

▍VITAMIN A
(Retinol)

Cautions see notes above; **interactions:** Appendix 1 (vitamins)

Pregnancy teratogenic; see notes above

Breast-feeding toxicity likely if mother taking high doses

Side-effects see notes above

Licensed use preparations containing only vitamin A are not licensed

Indication and dose

See also notes above

Vitamin A deficiency
• By mouth

Neonate 5000 units daily

Child 1 month–1 year 5000 units daily with or after food

Child 1–18 years 10 000 units daily with or after food

Note Higher doses may be used initially for treatment of severe deficiency

---

Prevention of deficiency in complete biliary obstruction
• By intramuscular injection

Neonate 50 000 units once a month

Child 1 month–1 year 50 000 units once a month

Arovit® (Non-proprietary)
Oral solution, vitamin A 150 000 units/mL
Available from 'special-order' manufacturers or specialist importing companies, see p. 957

Aquasol-A® (Non-proprietary)
Injection, vitamin A (as palmitate) 50 000 units/mL, 2-mL amp
Available from 'special-order' manufacturers or specialist importing companies, see p. 957

▍VITAMINS A and D

Cautions see notes above and section 9.6.4; prolonged excessive ingestion of vitamins A and D can lead to hypervitaminosis; **interactions:** Appendix 1 (vitamins)

Pregnancy see notes above

Side-effects see notes above and section 9.6.4

Licensed use not licensed in children under 6 months of age

Indication and dose

See notes above and section 9.6.4

Prevention of vitamin A and D deficiency see individual preparations for dose information

---

◢Vitamins A and D
Vitamins A and D (Non-proprietary)
Capsules, vitamin A 4000 units, vitamin D 400 units. Net price 84 = £3.10

Note May be difficult to obtain

Dose

Child 1–18 years 1 capsule daily

◢Vitamins A, C and D
Healthy Start Children's Vitamin Drops (Non-proprietary)
Oral drops, vitamin A 5000 units, vitamin D 2000 units, ascorbic acid 150 mg/mL
Available free of charge to children under 4 years through the Healthy Start Scheme; otherwise available direct to the public from maternity and child health clinics; community pharmacists may have difficulty obtaining supplies

Dose

Prevention of vitamin deficiency
• By mouth

Child 1 month–5 years 5 drops daily (5 drops contain vitamin A approx. 700 units, vitamin D approx. 300 units, ascorbic acid approx. 20 mg)

Note *Healthy Start Vitamins for women* (containing ascorbic acid, vitamin D, and folic acid) are also available to women during pregnancy and until their baby is one year old, through the Healthy Start Scheme

9.6.2 Vitamin B group

Deficiency of the B vitamins, other than vitamin B_{12} (section 9.1.2), is rare in the UK and is usually treated by preparations containing thiamine (B_1), and riboflavin (B_2). Other members (or substances traditionally classified as members) of the vitamin B complex such as aminobenzoic acid, biotin, choline, inositol, and pantothenic acid or panthenol may be included in vitamin B preparations, but there is no evidence of their value as supplements; however, they can be used in the management of certain metabolic disorders (section 9.8.1). Anaphylaxis has been reported with parenteral B vitamins (see MHRA/CHM advice, below).

As with other vitamins of the B group, pyridoxine (B$_6$) deficiency is rare, but it may occur during isoniazid therapy (section 5.1.9) or penicillamine treatment in Wilson's disease (section 9.8.1) and is characterised by peripheral neuritis. High doses of **pyridoxine** are given in some metabolic disorders, such as hyperoxaluria, cystathioninuria and homocystinuria; folic acid supplementation may also be beneficial in these disorders (section 9.1.2). Pyridoxine is also used in sideroblastic anaemia (section 9.1.3). Rarely, seizures in the neonatal period or during infancy respond to pyridoxine treatment; pyridoxine should be tried in all cases of early-onset intractable seizures and status epilepticus. Pyridoxine has been tried for a wide variety of other disorders, but there is little sound evidence to support the claims of efficacy, and overdosage induces toxic effects.

A number of mitochondrial disorders may respond to treatment with certain B vitamins but these disorders require specialist management. **Thiamine** is used in the treatment of maple syrup urine disease, mitochondrial respiratory chain defects and, together with riboflavin, in the treatment of congenital lactic acidosis; riboflavin is also used in glutaric acidaemias and cytochrome oxidase deficiencies; biotin (section 9.8.1) is used in carboxylase defects.

Folic acid and vitamin B$_{12}$ are used in the treatment of megaloblastic anaemia (section 9.1.2). Folinic acid (available as calcium folinate) is used in association with cytotoxic therapy (section 8.1).

RIBOFLAVIN
(Riboflavine, vitamin B$_2$)

Cautions see notes above

Pregnancy crosses the placenta but no adverse effects reported, information at high doses limited

Breast-feeding present in breast milk but no adverse effects reported, information at high doses limited

Side-effects bright yellow urine

Licensed use not licensed in children

Indication and dose

See also notes above

Metabolic diseases
• By mouth

Neonate 50 mg 1–2 times daily, adjusted according to response

Child 1 month–18 years 50–100 mg 1–2 times daily, adjusted according to response, up to 400 mg daily has been used

Riboflavin (Non-proprietary)
Tablets, 10 mg, 50 mg and 100 mg
Available from 'special-order' manufacturers or specialist importing companies, see p. 957

◀ Oral vitamin B complex preparations
See below

◀ Extemporaneous formulations available see Extemporaneous Preparations, p. 8

THIAMINE
(Vitamin B$_1$)

MHRA/CHM advice (September 2007) Although potentially serious allergic adverse reactions may rarely occur during, or shortly after, parenteral administration, the CHM has recommended that:

1. This should not preclude the use of parenteral thiamine in patients where this route of administration is required, particularly in patients at risk of Wernicke-Korsakoff syndrome where treatment with thiamine is essential;

2. Intravenous administration should be by infusion over 30 minutes;

3. Facilities for treating anaphylaxis (including resuscitation facilities) should be available when parenteral thiamine is administered.

Cautions anaphylactic shock may occasionally follow injection (see MHRA/CHM advice above)

Breast-feeding severely thiamine-deficient mothers should avoid breast-feeding as toxic methyl-glyoxal present in milk

Side-effects hypersensitivity reactions to injection

Licensed use not licensed in children

Indication and dose

See also notes above

Maple syrup urine disease
• By mouth

Neonate 5 mg/kg daily, adjusted as necessary

Child 1 month–18 years 5 mg/kg daily, adjusted as necessary

Metabolic disorders including congenital lactic acidosis
• By mouth or by intravenous infusion over 30 minutes

Neonate 50–200 mg once daily (total dose may alternatively be given in 2–3 divided doses), adjusted as necessary

Child 1 month–18 years 100–300 mg once daily (total dose may alternatively be given in 2–3 divided doses), adjusted as necessary; up to 2 g daily may be necessary

◁ **THIAMINE (continued)**

Thiamine (Non-proprietary)
Tablets, thiamine hydrochloride 50 mg, net price
100 = £3.98; 100 mg, 100 = £6.16
Brands include *Benerva®* ᴶᴴˢ

Injection, 50 mg/mL, 2-mL vial; 100 mg/mL, 2-mL
vial

Injection (intramuscular), 100 mg/mL, 5-mL vial
Available from 'special-order' manufacturers or specialist
importing companies, see p. 957
Note Some preparations may contain phenol as a preservative

◢ **Oral vitamin B complex preparations**
See below

PYRIDOXINE HYDROCHLORIDE
(Vitamin B₆)

Cautions see notes above; risk of cardiovascular
collapse with intravenous injection—resuscitation facilities must be available, monitor closely; **interactions:** Appendix 1 (vitamins)

Side-effects sensory neuropathy reported with
high doses given for extended periods

Licensed use not licensed for use in children

Indication and dose

See also notes above

**Metabolic diseases including cystathioninuria
and homocystinuria**
• By mouth
Neonate 50–100 mg 1–2 times daily

Child 1 month–18 years 50–250 mg 1–2 times
daily

Treatment of isoniazid-induced neuropathy
• By mouth
Neonate 5–10 mg daily

Child 1 month–12 years 10–20 mg 2–3 times
daily

Child 12–18 years 30–50 mg 2–3 times daily

Prevention of isoniazid-induced neuropathy
• By mouth
Neonate 5 mg daily

Child 1 month–12 years 5–10 mg daily

Child 12–18 years 10 mg daily

Prevention of penicillamine-induced neuropathy in Wilson's disease (see notes above)
• By mouth
Child 1–12 years 5–10 mg daily

Child 12–18 years 10 mg daily

Pyridoxine-dependent seizures
• By intravenous injection or by mouth
Neonate initial test dose 50–100 mg by intravenous injection, may be repeated; if responsive
followed by an oral maintenance dose of 50–
100 mg once daily, adjusted as necessary

Child 1 month–12 years initial test dose 50–
100 mg daily; if responsive followed by an oral
dose of 20–50 mg 1–2 times daily, adjusted as
necessary; doses up to 30 mg/kg or 1 g daily
have been used

Pyridoxine (Non-proprietary)
Tablets, pyridoxine hydrochloride 10 mg, net price
500 = £8.53; 20 mg, 500 = £8.53; 50 mg, 28 = £1.08

Injection, 25 mg/mL, 2 mL vial
Available from 'special-order' manufacturers or specialist
importing companies, see p. 957

◢ Extemporaneous formulations available see
Extemporaneous Preparations, p. 8

Oral vitamin B complex preparations
Note Other multivitamin preparations are in section 9.6.7.

Vitamin B Tablets, Compound ◢
Tablets, nicotinamide 15 mg, riboflavin 1 mg, thiamine hydrochloride 1 mg, net price 28 = £1.00

Vitamin B Tablets, Compound, Strong ◢
Tablets, brown, f/c or s/c, nicotinamide 20 mg,
pyridoxine hydrochloride 2 mg, riboflavin 2 mg,
thiamine hydrochloride 5 mg. Net price 28-tab pack
= £2.22

Vigranon B® (Wallace Mfg) ᴶᴴˢ ◢
Syrup, thiamine hydrochloride 5 mg, riboflavin
2 mg, nicotinamide 20 mg, pyridoxine hydrochloride 2 mg, panthenol 3 mg/5 mL. Net price
150 mL = £2.41
Dose

Treatment of deficiency
• By mouth
Child 1 month–1 year 5 mL 3 times daily
Child 1–12 years 10 mL 3 times daily
Child 12–18 years 10–15 mL 3 times daily

Prophylaxis of deficiency
• By mouth
Child 1 month–1 year 5 mL once daily
Child 1–12 years 5 mL twice daily
Child 12–18 years 5 mL 3 times daily

9.6.3 Vitamin C
(Ascorbic acid)

Vitamin C therapy is essential in scurvy, but less florid manifestations of vitamin C deficiency have been reported. Vitamin C is used to enhance the excretion of iron one month after starting desferrioxamine therapy (section 9.1.3); it is given separately from food as it also enhances iron absorption. Vitamin C is also used in the treatment of some inherited metabolic disorders, particularly mitochondrial disorders; specialist management of these conditions is required.

Severe scurvy causes gingival swelling and bleeding margins as well as petechiae on the skin. This is, however, exceedingly rare and a child with these signs is more likely to have leukaemia. Investigation should not be delayed by a trial period of vitamin treatment.

Claims that vitamin C ameliorates colds or promotes wound healing have not been proved.

ASCORBIC ACID
(Vitamin C)

Cautions interactions: Appendix 1 (vitamins)

Contra-indications hyperoxaluria

Side-effects nausea, diarrhoea; headache, fatigue; hyperoxaluria

Licensed use not licensed for metabolic disorders

Indication and dose

Treatment of scurvy
* By mouth

    Child 1 month–4 years 125–250 mg daily in 1–2 divided doses

    Child 4–12 years 250–500 mg daily in 1–2 divided doses

    Child 12–18 years 500 mg–1 g daily in 1–2 divided doses

Adjunct to desferrioxamine (see notes above)
* By mouth

    Child 1 month–18 years 100–200 mg daily 1 hour before food

Metabolic disorders (tyrosinaemia type III; transient tyrosinaemia of the newborn; glutathione synthase deficiency; Hawkinsinuria)
* By mouth

    Neonate 50–200 mg daily, adjusted as necessary

    Child 1 month–18 years 200–400 mg daily in 1–2 divided doses, adjusted as necessary; up to 1 g daily may be required

Ascorbic Acid (Non-proprietary)
Tablets, ascorbic acid 50 mg, net price 28 = £1.21; 100 mg, 28 = £1.26; 200 mg, 28 = £1.27; 500 mg (label: 24), 28 = £2.76
Excipients may include aspartame
Brands include *Redoxon*® [NHS]

Injection, ascorbic acid 100 mg/mL, net price 5-mL amp = £3.25
Excipients include metabisulphite

9.6.4 Vitamin D

Note The term Vitamin D is used for a range of compounds including ergocalciferol (calciferol, vitamin D_2), colecalciferol (vitamin D_3), dihydrotachysterol, alfacalcidol (1α-hydroxycholecalciferol), and calcitriol (1,25-dihydroxycholecalciferol).

Symptomatic deficiency of vitamin D is uncommon in the United Kingdom, but may occur in certain ethnic groups, and rarely in association with malabsorption. The amount of vitamin D required in infancy is related to the stores built up *in-utero* and subsequent exposure to sunlight. The amount of vitamin D in breast milk varies and some breast-fed babies, particularly if preterm or born to vitamin D deficient mothers, may become deficient. Most formula milk and supplement feeds contain adequate vitamin D to prevent deficiency.

Simple, nutritional vitamin D deficiency can be prevented by oral supplementation of 400 units of **ergocalciferol** (calciferol, vitamin D_2) or **colecalciferol** (vitamin D_3) daily, using multi-vitamin drops (section 9.6.7), manufactured 'special' solutions, or as calcium and ergocalciferol tablets (although the calcium is unnecessary); excessive supplementation may cause hypercalcaemia.

Inadequate bone mineralisation can be caused by a deficiency, or a lack of action of vitamin D or its active metabolite. In childhood this causes bowing and distortion of bones (rickets); initial high doses of vitamin D should be reduced after a few weeks, as there is a significant risk of hypercalcaemia (see caution below).

9 Nutrition and blood

Poor bone mineralisation in neonates and young children may also be due to inadequate intake of phosphate or calcium particularly during long-term parenteral nutrition—supplementation with phosphate (section 9.5.2.1) or calcium (section 9.5.1.1) may be required.

Hypophosphataemic rickets occurs due to abnormal phosphate excretion; treatment with high doses of oral phosphate (section 9.5.2.1), and hydroxylated (activated) forms of vitamin D allow bone mineralisation and optimise growth.

Nutritional deficiency of vitamin D is best treated with colecalciferol or ergocalciferol. Preparations containing calcium and colecalciferol are also occasionally used in children where there is evidence of combined calcium and vitamin D deficiency. Vitamin D deficiency caused by *intestinal malabsorption* or *chronic liver disease* usually requires vitamin D in pharmacological doses, such as **ergocalciferol** in doses of up to 40 000 units daily; the hypocalcaemia of *hypoparathyroidism* often requires higher doses in order to achieve normocalcaemia and alfacalcidol is generally preferred.

Vitamin D supplementation is often given in combination with calcium supplements for persistent hypocalcaemia in neonates, and in chronic renal disease.

Vitamin D requires hydroxylation, by the kidney and liver, to its active form therefore the hydroxylated derivatives **alfacalcidol** or **calcitriol** should be prescribed if patients with *severe liver or renal impairment* require vitamin D therapy. Alfacalcidol is generally preferred in children as there is more experience of its use and appropriate formulations are available. Calcitriol is unlicensed for use in children and is generally reserved for those with severe liver disease.

Important. All patients receiving pharmacological doses of vitamin D or its analogues should have their plasma-calcium concentration checked at intervals (initially once or twice weekly) and whenever nausea or vomiting occur. Breast milk from women taking pharmacological doses of vitamin D can cause hypercalcaemia if given to an infant.

■ ERGOCALCIFEROL
(Calciferol, Vitamin D₂)

Cautions see notes above; monitor plasma-calcium concentration in patients receiving high doses and in renal impairment; **interactions**: Appendix 1 (vitamins)

Contra-indications hypercalcaemia; metastatic calcification

Pregnancy avoid excessive supplementation; high doses teratogenic in *animals* but therapeutic doses unlikely to be harmful

Breast-feeding avoid excessive supplementation; may cause hypercalcaemia in infant—monitor serum-calcium concentration

Side-effects symptoms of overdosage include anorexia, lassitude, nausea and vomiting, diarrhoea, constipation, weight loss, polyuria, sweating, headache, thirst, vertigo, and raised concentrations of calcium and phosphate in plasma and urine

Licensed use Calcium and Ergocalciferol tablets not licensed for use in children under 6 years

Indication and dose
See also notes above

Nutritional vitamin-D deficiency rickets
• By mouth
Child 1–6 months 3000 units daily, adjusted as necessary
Child 6 months–12 years 6000 units daily, adjusted as necessary
Child 12–18 years 10 000 units daily, adjusted as necessary

Nutritional or physiological supplement; prevention of rickets
• By mouth
Neonate 400 units daily
Child 1 month–18 years 400–600 units daily

Vitamin D deficiency in intestinal malabsorption or in chronic liver disease
• By mouth or by intramuscular injection
Child 1–12 years 10 000–25 000 units daily, adjusted as necessary
Child 12–18 years 10 000–40 000 units daily, adjusted as necessary

◢ **Pharmacological strengths**
(see notes above)
The BP directs that when calciferol is prescribed or demanded, colecalciferol or ergocalciferol should be dispensed or supplied

Ergocalciferol (Non-proprietary)
Tablets, ergocalciferol 250 micrograms (10 000 units), net price 100 = £21.99; 1.25 mg (50 000 units), 100 = £30.34
Note May be difficult to obtain
Important When the strength of the tablets ordered or prescribed is not clear, the intention of the prescriber or purchaser with respect to the strength (expressed in micrograms or milligrams per tablet) should be ascertained.

Solution ergocalciferol 3000 units/mL
Excipients may include peanut oil
Available from 'special-order' manufacturers or specialist importing companies, see p. 957

Nutrition and blood

9

◁ **ERGOCALCIFEROL** (*continued*)

Injection, colecalciferol or ergocalciferol, 7.5 mg (300 000 units)/mL in oil. Net price 1-mL amp = £8.50, 2-mL amp = £9.18

◢**Daily supplements**

Note There is no plain vitamin D tablet available for treating simple deficiency (see notes above). Alternatives include vitamins capsules (section 9.6.7), preparations of vitamins A and D (section 9.6.1), and calcium and ergocalciferol tablets (see below).

For prescribing information on calcium, see section 9.5.1

Calcium and Ergocalciferol (Non-proprietary) **(Calcium and Vitamin D)**

Tablets, calcium lactate 300 mg, calcium phosphate 150 mg (calcium 97 mg or Ca²⁺ 2.4 mmol), ergocalciferol 10 micrograms (400 units). Net price 28-tab pack = £3.28. Counselling, crush before administration or may be chewed

---

◢ **ALFACALCIDOL**

(1α-Hydroxycholecalciferol)

Cautions see under Ergocalciferol; also nephrolithiasis

Contra-indications see under Ergocalciferol

Pregnancy see under Ergocalciferol

Breast-feeding see under Ergocalciferol

Side-effects see under Ergocalciferol; also *rarely* nephrocalcinosis, pruritus, rash, and urticaria

Indication and dose

See also notes above

Hypophosphataemic rickets; persistent hypocalcaemia due to hypoparathyroidism or pseudohypoparathyroidism

• **By mouth or by intravenous injection**

Child 1 month–12 years 25–50 nanograms/kg (max. 1 microgram) once daily, adjusted as necessary

Child 12–18 years 1 microgram once daily, adjusted as necessary

---

Persistent neonatal hypocalcaemia

• **By mouth or by intravenous injection**

Neonate 50–100 nanograms/kg once daily, adjusted as necessary (up to 2 micrograms/kg daily may be needed in resistant cases)

Prevention of vitamin D deficiency in renal or cholestatic liver disease

• **By mouth or by intravenous injection**

Neonate 20 nanograms/kg once daily, adjusted as necessary

Child 1 month–12 years, body-weight under 20 kg 15–30 nanograms/kg (max. 500 nanograms) once daily; **body-weight over 20 kg** 250–500 nanograms once daily, adjusted as necessary

Child 12–18 years 250–500 nanograms once daily, adjusted as necessary

Alfacalcidol (Non-proprietary) PoM

Capsules, alfacalcidol 250 nanograms, net price 30-cap pack = £5.32; 500 nanograms 30-cap pack = £10.43; 1 microgram 30-cap pack = £14.26

One-Alpha® (LEO) PoM

Capsules, alfacalcidol 250 nanograms (white), net price 30-cap pack = £3.37; 500 nanograms (red), 30-cap pack = £6.27; 1 microgram (brown), 30-cap pack = £8.75

Excipients include sesame oil

Oral drops, sugar-free, alfacalcidol 2 micrograms/mL (1 drop contains approx. 100 nanograms), net price 10 mL = £22.49

Excipients include alcohol

Note The concentration of alfacalcidol in *One-Alpha®* *drops* is **10 times greater** than that of the former preparation *One-Alpha®* *solution*.

Injection, alfacalcidol 2 micrograms/mL, net price 0.5-mL amp = £2.16, 1-mL amp = £4.11

Excipients include alcohol, propylene glycol (caution in neonates, see, p. 3)

Note Shake ampoule for at least 5 seconds before use

◢ **CALCITRIOL**

(1,25-Dihydroxycholecalciferol)

Cautions see under Ergocalciferol; monitor plasma calcium, phosphate, and creatinine during dosage titration

Contra-indications see under Ergocalciferol

Pregnancy see under Ergocalciferol

Breast-feeding see under Ergocalciferol

Side-effects see under Ergocalciferol

Licensed use not licensed for use in children

Indication and dose

See also notes above

Vitamin D dependent rickets; hypophosphataemic rickets; persistent hypocalcaemia due to hypoparathyroidism or pseudo-hypoparathyroidism (limited experience)

• **By mouth**

Child 1 month–12 years initially 15 nanograms/kg (max. 250 nanograms) once daily, increased if necessary in steps of 5 nanograms/kg daily (max. 250 nanograms) every 2–4 weeks

Child 12–18 years initially 250 nanograms once daily increased if necessary in steps of 5 nanograms/kg daily (max. 250 nanograms step) every 2–4 weeks; usual dose 0.5–1 microgram daily

9

Nutrition and blood

◁ **CALCITRIOL (continued)**

Hypocalcaemia in dialysis patients (limited experience)
- **By intravenous injection**

    Child 12–18 years initially 250–500 nanograms (approx. 10 nanograms/kg) 3 times a week, increased if necessary in steps of 2–5 nanograms/kg every 2–4 weeks; usual dose 0.5–3 micrograms 3 times a week

Administration For administration *by mouth*, injection solution may be given orally or contents of capsule administered by oral syringe; capsules contain approx. 0.168 mL of fluid

For administration *by intravenous injection*, injection may be given via catheter after dialysis

Calcitriol (Non-proprietary) ℞
Capsules, calcitriol 250 nanograms, net price 30-cap pack = £5.87, 100-cap pack = £19.15; 500 nanograms, 30-cap pack =£10.50, 100-cap pack = £25.76

Rocaltrol® (Roche) ℞
Capsules, calcitriol 250 nanograms (red/white), net price 100 = £18.40; 500 nanograms (red), 100 = £32.90

Calcijex® (Abbott) ℞
Injection, calcitriol 1 microgram/mL, net price 1-mL amp = £5.14; 2 micrograms/mL, 1-mL amp = £10.28

◾ COLECALCIFEROL

(Cholecalciferol, vitamin D₃)

Cautions see under Ergocalciferol

Contra-indications see under Ergocalciferol

Pregnancy see under Ergocalciferol

Breast-feeding see under Ergocalciferol

Side-effects see under Ergocalciferol

Licensed use *Sandocal® + D 600* not licensed for use in children under 2 years; *Adcal-D3®*, *Calceos®*, *Calcichew®D3*, and *Sandocal® + D 1200* not licensed for use in children under 12 years; *Cacit®D3* not licensed for use in children (age range not specified by manufacturers); *Calcichew®D3 Forte*, *Calfovit D3®*, and *Natecal D3®* not licensed for use in children under 18 years

Indication and dose

See under Ergocalciferol and notes above—alternative to Ergocalciferol, see also Pharmacological Strengths

◢Extemporaneous formulations available see Extemporaneous Preparations, p. 8

◢With calcium
For prescribing information on calcium, see section 9.5.1

Adcal-D₃® (ProStrakan)
Tablets (chewable), lemon or tutti-frutti flavour, calcium carbonate 1.5 g (calcium 600 mg or Ca²⁺ 15 mmol), colecalciferol 10 micrograms (400 units), net price 56-tab pack = £3.89, 112-tab pack = £7.78. Label: 24

Dissolve (effervescent tablets), lemon flavour, calcium carbonate 1.5 g (calcium 600 mg or Ca²⁺ 15 mmol), colecalciferol 10 micrograms (400 units), net price 56-tab pack = £4.99. Label: 13

Cacit® D3 (Procter & Gamble Pharm.)
Granules, effervescent, lemon flavour, calcium carbonate 1.25 g (calcium 500 mg or Ca²⁺ 12.5 mmol), colecalciferol 11 micrograms (440 units)/sachet, net price 30-sachet pack = £4.14. Label: 13

Calceos® (Galen)
Tablets (chewable), lemon flavour, calcium carbonate 1.25 g (calcium 500 mg or Ca²⁺ 12.5 mmol), colecalciferol 10 micrograms (400 units), net price 60-tab pack = £3.69. Label: 24

Calcichew® D3 (Shire)
Tablets (chewable), orange flavour, calcium carbonate 1.25 g (calcium 500 mg or Ca²⁺ 12.5 mmol), colecalciferol 5 micrograms (200 units), net price 100-tab pack = £14.43. Label: 24
Excipients include aspartame (section 9.4.1)

Calcichew® D3 Forte (Shire)
Tablets (chewable), lemon flavour, calcium carbonate 1.25 g (calcium 500 mg or Ca²⁺ 12.5 mmol), colecalciferol 10 micrograms (400 units), net price 100-tab pack = £7.21. Label: 24
Excipients include aspartame (section 9.4.1)

Calfovit D3® (Menarini)
Powder, lemon flavour, calcium phosphate 3.1 g (calcium 1.2 g or Ca²⁺ 30 mmol), colecalciferol 20 micrograms (800 units), net price 30-sachet pack = £4.32. Label: 13, 21

Natecal D3® (Chiesi)
Tablets (chewable), (aniseed, peppermint, and molasses flavour), calcium carbonate 1.5 g (calcium 600 mg or Ca²⁺ 15 mmol), colecalciferol 10 micrograms (400 units), net price 60-tab pack = £3.70. Label: 24
Excipients include aspartame (section 9.4.1)

Sandocal®+D (Novartis Consumer Health)
Sandocal® +D 600 tablets, effervescent, orange flavour, calcium lactate gluconate 1.36 g, calcium carbonate 1.05 g, providing calcium 600 mg (Ca²⁺ 15 mmol), colecalciferol concentrate 4 mg, providing colecalciferol 10 micrograms (400 units), net price 60-tab pack = £5.35, 100-tab pack = £8.75. Label: 13
Excipients include aspartame (section 9.4.1)

Sandocal® +D 1200 tablets, effervescent, orange flavour, calcium lactate gluconate 2.72 g, calcium carbonate 2.1 g, providing calcium 1200 mg (Ca²⁺ 30 mmol), colecalciferol concentrate 8 mg, providing colecalciferol 20 micrograms (800 units), net price 30-tab pack = £4.32. Label: 13
Excipients include aspartame (section 9.4.1)

9 Nutrition and blood

9.6.5 Vitamin E
(Tocopherols)

The daily requirement of vitamin E has not been well defined. Vitamin E supplements are given to children with fat malabsorption such as in cystic fibrosis and cholestatic liver disease. In children with abetalipoproteinaemia abnormally low vitamin E concentrations may occur in association with neuromuscular problems; this usually responds to high doses of vitamin E. Some neonatal units still administer a single intramuscular dose of vitamin E at birth to preterm neonates to reduce the risk of complications; no trials of long-term outcome have been carried out. The intramuscular route should also be considered in children with severe liver disease when response to oral therapy is inadequate.

Vitamin E has been tried for various other conditions but there is little scientific evidence of its value.

ALPHA TOCOPHERYL ACETATE

Cautions predisposition to thrombosis; increased risk of necrotising enterocolitis in preterm neonates (see administration); **interactions:** Appendix 1 (vitamins)

Pregnancy no evidence of safety of high doses

Breast-feeding excreted in breast milk, minimal risk although caution with large doses

Side-effects diarrhoea and abdominal pain, particularly with high doses

Indication and dose

Vitamin E deficiency
• By mouth
  Neonate 10 mg/kg once daily

  Child 1 month–18 years 2–10 mg/kg daily, up to 20 mg/kg has been used

Malabsorption in cystic fibrosis
• By mouth (with food and pancreatic enzymes)
  Child 1 month–1 year 50 mg once daily, adjusted as necessary

  Child 1–12 years 100 mg once daily, adjusted as necessary

  Child 12–18 years 100–200 mg once daily, adjusted as necessary

Vitamin E deficiency in cholestasis and severe liver disease
• By mouth
  Neonate 10 mg/kg daily

  Child 1 month–12 years initially 100 mg daily, adjusted according to response; up to 200 mg/kg daily may be required

  Child 12–18 years initially 200 mg daily, adjusted according to response; up to 200 mg/kg daily may be required

• By intramuscular injection
  Neonate 10 mg/kg once a month

  Child 1 month–18 years 10 mg/kg (max. 100 mg) once a month

Malabsorption in abetalipoproteinaemia
• By mouth
  Neonate 100 mg/kg once daily

  Child 1 month–18 years 50–100 mg/kg once daily

Vitamin E Suspension (Non-proprietary)
Suspension, alpha tocopheryl acetate 100 mg/mL. Net price 100 mL = £27.59
Excipients include sucrose

Administration consider dilution in neonates due to high osmolality (see Cautions)

Note Tablets containing tocopheryl acetate are available from 'special-order' manufacturers or specialist importing companies, see p. 957

Vitamin E Injection (Roche)
Injection tocopheryl acetate 50 mg/mL, 2-mL ampoule
Available from 'special-order' manufacturers or specialist importing companies, see p. 957

ALPHA TOCOPHEROL

Cautions predisposition to thrombosis; **interactions:** Appendix 1 (vitamins)

Contra-indications preterm neonates

Hepatic impairment manufacturer advises caution and monitor closely—no information available

Renal impairment manufacturer advises caution and monitor closely; risk of renal toxicity due to polyethylene glycol content

Pregnancy manufacturer advises caution; no evidence of harm in *animal* studies

Breast-feeding manufacturer advises use only if potential benefit outweighs risk—no information available

Side-effects diarrhoea; *less commonly* asthenia, headache, pruritus, disturbances in serum-potassium and serum-sodium concentrations, alopecia, and rash

9

Nutrition and blood

◻ **ALPHA TOCOPHEROL (continued)**

Vedrop® (Orphan Europe) PoM

Oral solution, yellow, D-alpha tocopherol (as tocofersolan) 50 mg/mL, net price 20 mL = £54.55, 60 mL = £163.65 (all with oral syringe)

Note Tocofersolan is a water-soluble form of D-alpha tocopherol

Dose

Vitamin E deficiency because of malabsorption in congenital or hereditary chronic cholestasis
• By mouth
Neonate 17 mg/kg daily, adjusted as necessary
Child 1 month–18 years 17 mg/kg daily, adjusted as necessary

9.6.6 Vitamin K

Vitamin K is necessary for the production of blood clotting factors and proteins necessary for the normal calcification of bone.

Because vitamin K is fat soluble, children with fat malabsorption, especially in biliary obstruction or hepatic disease, may become deficient. For oral administration to prevent vitamin K deficiency in malabsorption syndromes, a water-soluble preparation, **menadiol sodium phosphate** (see Contra-indications below) must be used.

Oral coumarin anticoagulants act by interfering with vitamin K metabolism in the hepatic cells and their effects can be antagonised by giving vitamin K; for advice on the use of vitamin K in haemorrhage, see section 2.8.2.

Vitamin K deficiency bleeding Neonates are relatively deficient in vitamin K and those who do not receive supplements are at risk of serious bleeds (haemorrhagic disease), including intracranial bleeding. The Chief Medical Officer and the Chief Nursing Officer have recommended that all newborn babies should receive vitamin K to prevent vitamin K deficiency bleeding (haemorrhagic disease of the newborn). Local protocols may vary and an appropriate regimen should be selected after discussion with parents in the antenatal period.

Vitamin K (as phytomenadione) 1 mg may be given by a single intramuscular injection at birth; this prevents vitamin K deficiency bleeding in virtually all babies; preterm neonates may be given 400 micrograms/kg (max. 1 mg). The intravenous route is preferred by some in preterm neonates of very low birth-weight but it does not provide the prolonged protection of the intramuscular injection, and any babies receiving intravenous vitamin K should be given subsequent oral doses, as described below.

Babies considered at particular risk of vitamin K deficiency bleeding should receive intramuscular vitamin K at birth; this includes those experiencing birth asphyxia or bleeding problems, those born to mothers with liver disease or taking enzyme inducing anticonvulsant drugs (carbamazepine, phenobarbital, phenytoin), rifampicin or warfarin. In infants with cholestatic disease, vitamin K must be given either intramuscularly or intravenously because oral absorption is likely to be impaired.

Alternatively, in healthy babies who are not at particular risk of bleeding disorders, vitamin K may be given by mouth, and arrangements must be in place to ensure the appropriate regimen is followed. Two doses of a colloidal (mixed micelle) preparation of phytomenadione 2 mg should be given in the first week, the first dose being given at birth. For exclusively breast-fed babies, a third dose of phytomenadione 2 mg is given at 1 month of age; the third dose is omitted in formula-fed babies because formula feeds contain vitamin K.

◼ MENADIOL SODIUM PHOSPHATE

Cautions G6PD deficiency (section 9.1.5) and vitamin E deficiency (risk of haemolysis); **interactions:** Appendix 1 (vitamins)

Contra-indications neonates and infants

Pregnancy avoid in late pregnancy and labour; risk of neonatal haemolytic anaemia, hyperbilirubinaemia, and kernicterus in neonate

Indication and dose

See notes above

Supplementation in vitamin K malabsorption
• By mouth
Child 1–12 years 5–10 mg daily, adjusted as necessary
Child 12–18 years 10–20 mg daily, adjusted as necessary

9 Nutrition and blood

◁ **MENADIOL SODIUM PHOSPHATE** (*continued*)

Menadiol Phosphate (Non-proprietary)
Tablets, menadiol sodium phosphate equivalent to
10 mg of menadiol phosphate, net price 100-tab
pack = £53.08

◢Extemporaneous formulations available see
Extemporaneous Preparations, p. 8

◢ PHYTOMENADIONE

(Vitamin K₁)

Cautions intravenous injections should be given
very slowly—risk of vascular collapse (see also
below); **interactions:** Appendix 1 (vitamins)

Pregnancy manufacturer advises use only if
potential benefit outweighs risk

Breast-feeding present in milk, but see notes
above

Indication and dose

> Neonatal prophylaxis of vitamin-K deficiency
> bleeding see notes above

> Neonatal hypoprothrombinaemia or vitamin-K
> deficiency bleeding
> • **By intravenous injection**
>
> > **Neonate** 1 mg repeated 8 hourly if necessary

> Neonatal biliary atresia and liver disease
> • **By mouth**
>
> > **Neonate** 1 mg daily

> Reversal of coumarin anticoagulation when
> continued anticoagulation required or if no
> significant bleeding (see also section 2.8.2)—
> seek specialist advice
> • **By intravenous injection**
>
> > **Child 1 month–18 years** 15–30 micrograms/kg
> > (max. 1 mg) as a single dose, repeated as
> > necessary

> Reversal of coumarin anticoagulation when
> anticoagulation not required or if significant
> bleeding; treatment of haemorrhage asso-
> ciated with vitamin-K deficiency (see also sec-
> tion 2.8.2)—seek specialist advice
> • **By intravenous injection**
>
> > **Child 1 month–18 years** 250–300 micrograms/
> > kg (max. 10 mg) as a single dose

◢Colloidal formulation

Konakion® MM (Roche) [PoM]
Injection, phytomenadione 10 mg/mL in a mixed
micelles vehicle. Net price 1-mL amp = 39p
Excipients include glycocholic acid 54.6 mg/amp, lecithin
Cautions reduce dose in liver impairment (glycocholic
acid may displace bilirubin); reports of anaphylactoid
reactions
Administration *Konakion® MM* may be administered by
slow intravenous injection or by intravenous infusion in
glucose 5%; **not** for intramuscular injection

Konakion® MM Paediatric (Roche) ▼ [PoM]
Injection, phytomenadione 10 mg/mL in a mixed
micelles vehicle, net price 0.2-mL amp = 96p
Excipients include glycocholic acid 10.9 mg/amp, lecithin
Cautions parenteral administration in premature infants
body-weight less than 2.5 kg (increased risk of kernicterus)
Administration *Konakion® MM Paediatric* may be administered *by mouth* or *by intramuscular injection* or *by
intravenous injection*. For *intravenous injection*, may be
diluted with Glucose 5% if necessary

9.6.7 Multivitamin preparations

Multivitamin supplements are used in children with vitamin deficiencies and also
in malabsorption conditions such as cystic fibrosis or liver disease. To avoid
potential toxicity, the content of all vitamin preparations, particularly vitamin A,
should be considered when used together with other supplements. Supplementation is not required if nutrient enriched feeds are used; consult a dietician for
further advice.

◢ MULTIVITAMIN PREPARATIONS

Cautions see individual vitamins; vitamin A concentration of preparations varies

Contra-indications see individual vitamins

Side-effects see individual vitamins

Licensed use *Dalivit®* not licensed for use in
children under 6 weeks

Indication and dose

> See under preparations below

Vitamins
Capsules, ascorbic acid 15 mg, nicotinamide
7.5 mg, riboflavin 500 micrograms, thiamine

hydrochloride 1 mg, vitamin A 2500 units, vitamin
D 300 units, net price 28-cap pack = £1.50
Dose
> Prevention of deficiency
> • **By mouth**
>
> > **Child 1–12 years** 1 capsule daily
> >
> > **Child 12–18 years** 2 capsules daily

> Cystic fibrosis: prevention of deficiency
> • **By mouth**
>
> > **Child 1–18 years** 2–3 capsules daily

◁ **MULTIVITAMIN PREPARATIONS (continued)**

Abidec® (Chefaro UK)

Drops, vitamins A, B group, C, and D. Net price 25 mL (with dropper) = £2.20

Note Contains 1333 units of vitamin A (as palmitate) per 0.6 mL dose

Excipients include arachis (peanut) oil and sucrose

Dose

> Prevention of deficiency
> • By mouth
>
> Preterm neonate 0.6 mL daily
>
> Neonate 0.3 mL daily
>
> Child 1 month–1 year 0.3 mL daily
>
> Child 1–18 years 0.6 mL daily

> Cystic fibrosis: prevention of deficiency
> • By mouth
> Child 1 month–1 year 0.6 mL daily
>
> Child 1–18 years 1.2 mL daily

Dalivit® (LPC)

Oral drops, vitamins A, B group, C, and D, net price 25 mL = £2.98, 50 mL = £4.85

Note Contains 5000 units of vitamin A (as palmitate) per 0.6 mL dose

Excipients include sucrose

Dose

> Prevention of deficiency
> • By mouth
>
> Neonate (including preterm) 0.3 mL daily
>
> Child 1 month–1 year 0.3 mL daily
>
> Child 1–18 years 0.6 mL daily

> Cystic fibrosis: prevention of deficiency
> • By mouth
> Child 1 month–1 year 0.6 mL daily
>
> Child 1–18 years 1 mL daily

Vitamin and mineral supplements and adjuncts to synthetic diets

Forceval® (Alliance)

Capsules, brown/red, vitamins (ascorbic acid 60 mg, biotin 100 micrograms, cyanocobalamin 3 micrograms, folic acid 400 micrograms, nicotinamide 18 mg, pantothenic acid 4 mg, pyridoxine 2 mg, riboflavin 1.6 mg, thiamine 1.2 mg, vitamin A 2500 units, vitamin D_2 400 units, vitamin E 10 mg, minerals and trace elements (calcium 100 mg, chromium 200 micrograms, copper 2 mg, iodine 140 micrograms, iron 12 mg, magnesium 30 mg, manganese 3 mg, molybdenum 250 micrograms, phosphorus 77 mg, potassium 4 mg, selenium 50 micrograms, zinc 15 mg), net price 15-cap pack = £2.83, 30-cap pack = £5.19, 90-cap pack = £12.53. Label: 25

Dose

> Vitamin and mineral deficiency and as adjunct in synthetic diets
> Child 12–18 years 1 capsule daily one hour after a meal

Junior capsules, brown, vitamins (ascorbic acid 25 mg, biotin 50 micrograms, cyanocobalamin 2 micrograms, folic acid 100 micrograms, nicotinamide 7.5 mg, pantothenic acid 2 mg, pyridoxine 1 mg, riboflavin 1 mg, thiamine 1.5 mg, vitamin A 1250 units, vitamin D_2 200 units, vitamin E 5 mg, vitamin K_1 25 micrograms), minerals and trace elements (chromium 50 micrograms, copper 1 mg, iodine 75 micrograms, iron 5 mg, magnesium 1 mg, manganese 1.25 mg, molybdenum 50 micrograms, selenium 25 micrograms, zinc 5 mg), net price 30-cap pack = £3.52, 60-cap pack = £6.69

Dose

> Vitamin and mineral deficiency and as adjunct in synthetic diets
> Child 5–12 years 2 junior capsules daily

Ketovite® (Paines & Byrne)

Tablets [PoM], yellow, ascorbic acid 16.6 mg, riboflavin 1 mg, thiamine hydrochloride 1 mg, pyridoxine hydrochloride 330 micrograms, nicotinamide 3.3 mg, calcium pantothenate 1.16 mg, alpha tocopheryl acetate 5 mg, inositol 50 mg, biotin 170 micrograms, folic acid 250 micrograms, acetomenaphthone 500 micrograms, net price 100-tab pack = £4.17

Dose

> Prevention of vitamin deficiency in disorders of carbohydrate or amino-acid metabolism and adjunct in restricted, specialised, or synthetic diets
> Child 1 month–18 years 1 tablet 3 times daily; dose adjusted according to condition, diet, or age; use with *Ketovite®* Liquid for complete vitamin supplementation

Administration may be crushed immediately before use

Liquid, pink, sugar-free, vitamin A 2500 units, ergocalciferol 400 units, choline chloride 150 mg, cyanocobalamin 12.5 micrograms/5 mL, net price 150-mL pack = £2.70

Dose

> Prevention of vitamin deficiency in disorders of carbohydrate or amino-acid metabolism and adjunct in restricted, specialised, or synthetic diets
> Child 1 month–18 years 5 mL daily; dose adjusted according to condition, diet, or age; use with *Ketovite®* Tablets for complete vitamin supplementation

Administration may be mixed with milk, cereal, or fruit juice

9.7 Bitters and tonics

Classification not included in *BNF for Children*.

9.8 Metabolic disorders

9.8.1 Drugs used in metabolic disorders
9.8.2 Acute porphyrias

This section covers drugs used in metabolic disorders and not readily classified elsewhere.

9.8.1 Drugs used in metabolic disorders

Metabolic disorders should be managed under the guidance of a specialist. As many preparations are unlicensed and may be difficult to obtain, arrangements for continued prescribing and supply should be made in primary care.

General advice on the use of medicines in metabolic disorders can be obtained from:
Alder Hey Children's Hospital
Medicines Information Centre
Tel: (0151) 252 5381

and

Great Ormond Street Hospital for Children
Pharmacy
Tel: (020) 7405 9200

Wilson's disease

Penicillamine is used in Wilson's disease (hepatolenticular degeneration) to aid the elimination of copper ions; it is also used for cystinuria. Children who are hypersensitive to penicillin may react rarely to penicillamine.

Trientine is used for the treatment of Wilson's disease only, in patients intolerant of penicillamine; it is **not** an alternative to penicillamine in other diseases such as cystinuria. Penicillamine-induced systemic lupus erythematosus may not resolve on transfer to trientine.

Zinc prevents the absorption of copper in Wilson's disease. Symptomatic patients should be treated initially with a chelating agent because zinc has a slow onset of action. When transferring from chelating treatment to zinc maintenance therapy, chelating treatment should be co-administered for 2–3 weeks until zinc produces its maximal effect.

PENICILLAMINE

Cautions concomitant nephrotoxic drugs (increased risk of toxicity); monitor urine for proteinuria; monitor blood and platelet count regularly (see below); neurological involvement in Wilson's disease; **interactions:** Appendix 1 (penicillamine)

Blood counts and urine tests Consider withdrawal if platelet count falls below 120 000/mm³ or white blood cells below 2500/mm³ or if 3 successive falls within reference range (can restart at reduced dose when counts return to within reference range but permanent withdrawal necessary if recurrence of leucopenia or thrombocytopenia)

Counselling Warn child and carer to tell doctor immediately if sore throat, fever, infection, non-specific illness, unexplained bleeding and bruising, purpura, mouth ulcers, or rashes develop

Contra-indications lupus erythematosus

Renal impairment reduce dose and monitor renal function or avoid—consult product literature

Pregnancy fetal abnormalities reported rarely; avoid if possible

Breast-feeding manufacturer advises avoid unless potential benefit outweighs risk—no information available

Side-effects initially nausea, anorexia, fever, and skin reactions; taste loss (mineral supplements not recommended); blood disorders including thrombocytopenia, leucopenia, agranulocytosis and aplastic anaemia; proteinuria, rarely haematuria (withdraw immediately and seek specialist advice); haemolytic anaemia, pancreatitis, cholestatic jaundice, nephrotic syndrome, lupus erythematosus-like syndrome, myasthenia gravis-like syndrome, neuropathy (especially if neurological involvement in Wilson's disease—prophylactic pyridoxine recommended, see section 9.6.2, polymyositis (rarely with cardiac involvement), dermatomyositis, mouth ulcers, stomatitis, alopecia, bronchiolitis and pneumoni-

◁ **PENICILLAMINE** (*continued*)

tis, pemphigus, Goodpasture's syndrome, and Stevens-Johnson syndrome also reported; male and female breast enlargement reported; in non-rheumatoid conditions rheumatoid arthritis-like syndrome also reported; late rashes (consider withdrawing treatment)

Indication and dose

> **Wilson's disease**
> * By mouth
>
> **Child 1 month–12 years** 2.5 mg/kg twice daily before food, increased at 1–2 week intervals to 10 mg/kg twice daily
>
> **Child 12–18 years** 0.75–1 g twice daily before food, max. 2 g daily for 1 year; usual maintenance dose 0.75–1 g daily

> **Cystinuria**
> * By mouth
>
> **Child 1 month–12 years** 5–10 mg/kg twice daily before food, adjusted to maintain urinary cystine below 200 mg/litre; maintain adequate fluid intake
>
> **Child 12–18 years** 0.5–1.5 g twice daily before food, adjusted to maintain urinary cystine below 200 mg/litre; maintain adequate fluid intake

Penicillamine (Non-proprietary) PoM
Tablets, penicillamine 125 mg, net price 56-tab pack = £13.63; 250 mg, 56-tab pack = £21.04. Label: 6, 22, counselling, blood disorder symptoms (see above)

Distamine® (Alliance) PoM
Tablets, all f/c, penicillamine 125 mg, net price 100 = £10.34; 250 mg, 100 = £17.78. Label: 6, 22, counselling, blood disorder symptoms (see above)

◤ **TRIENTINE DIHYDROCHLORIDE**

Cautions see notes above; **interactions:** Appendix 1 (trientine)

Pregnancy teratogenic in *animal* studies—use only if benefit outweighs risk; monitor maternal and neonatal serum-copper concentrations

Side-effects nausea, rash; *very rarely* anaemia; duodenitis and colitis also reported

Indication and dose

> **Wilson's disease in patients intolerant of penicillamine**
> * By mouth
>
> **Child 2–12 years** 0.6–1.5 g daily in 2–4 divided doses before food, adjusted according to response; reduce dose and increase frequency if nausea is a problem
>
> **Child 12–18 years** 1.2–2.4 g daily in 2–4 divided doses before food, adjusted according to response; reduce dose and increase frequency if nausea is a problem

Trientine Dihydrochloride (Univar) PoM
Capsules, trientine dihydrochloride 300 mg. Label: 6, 22

◤ **ZINC ACETATE**

Cautions portal hypertension (risk of hepatic decompensation when switching from chelating agent); monitor full blood count and serum cholesterol; **interactions:** Appendix 1 (zinc)

Pregnancy usual dose 25 mg 3 times daily adjusted according to plasma-copper concentration and urinary copper excretion

Breast-feeding manufacturer advises avoid; present in milk—may cause zinc-induced copper deficiency in infant

Side-effects gastric irritation (usually transient; may be reduced if first dose taken mid-morning or with a little protein); *less commonly* sideroblastic anaemia and leucopenia

Indication and dose

> **Wilson's disease**
>
> Note dose expressed as elemental zinc
>
> * By mouth
>
> **Child 1–6 years** 25 mg twice daily
>
> **Child 6–16 years** body-weight under 57 kg, 25 mg 3 times daily; body-weight 57 kg or over, 50 mg 3 times daily
>
> **Child 16–18 years** 50 mg 3 times daily

Wilzin® (Orphan Europe) ▼ PoM
Capsules, zinc (as acetate) 25 mg (blue), net price 250-cap pack = £132.00; 50 mg (orange), 250-cap pack = £242.00. Label: 23
Administration capsules may be opened and the contents mixed with water

---

◤ **Carnitine deficiency**

Carnitine is available for the management of primary carnitine deficiency due to inborn errors of metabolism, or of secondary deficiency in haemodialysis patients.

Carnitine is also used in the treatment of some organic acidaemias; however, use in fatty acid oxidation is controversial.

CARNITINE

Cautions diabetes mellitus; monitoring of free and acyl carnitine in blood and urine recommended

Renal impairment accumulation of metabolites may occur with chronic oral administration in severe impairment

Pregnancy appropriate to use; no evidence of teratogenicity in *animal* studies

Side-effects nausea, vomiting, abdominal pain, diarrhoea, fishy body odour; side-effects may be dose-related—monitor tolerance during first week and after any dose increase

Licensed use not licensed for use by intravenous infusion; tablets, chewable tablets, and oral liquid (10%) not licensed in children under 12 years; paediatric oral solution (30%) not licensed in children over 12 years; not licensed for use in organic acidaemias

Indication and dose

Primary deficiency and organic acidaemias
- **By mouth**

  Neonate 50 mg/kg twice daily, higher doses up to 200 mg/kg daily occasionally required

  Child 1 month–18 years 50 mg/kg twice daily, higher doses up to 200 mg/kg daily occasionally required; usual max. 3 g daily

- **By intravenous infusion**

  Neonate initially 100 mg/kg over 30 minutes followed by a continuous infusion of 4 mg/kg/hour

  Child 1 month–18 years initially 100 mg/kg over 30 minutes followed by a continuous infusion of 4 mg/kg/hour

- **By slow intravenous injection over 2–3 minutes**

  Neonate up to 100 mg/kg/daily in 2–4 divided doses

  Child 1 month–18 years up to 100 mg/kg/daily in 2–4 divided doses

Secondary deficiency in dialysis patients
- **By slow intravenous injection over 2–3 minutes**

  Child 1 month–18 years 20 mg/kg after each dialysis session, adjusted according to plasma-carnitine concentration

- **By mouth**
  (maintenance therapy if benefit gained from first intravenous course)

  Child 1 month–18 years 1 g daily

Administration for *intravenous infusion*, dilute injection with Sodium Chloride 0.9% *or* Glucose 5% or 10%.

Carnitor® (Sigma-Tau) PoM
Tablets, L-carnitine 330 mg, net price 90-tab pack = £103.95

Chewable tablets, L-carnitine 1 g, net price 10-tab pack = £35.00

Oral liquid, L-carnitine 100 mg/mL (10%), net price 10 × 10-mL (1-g) single-dose bottle = £35.00

Paediatric oral solution, L-carnitine 300 mg/mL (30%), net price 20 mL = £21.00

Injection, L-carnitine 200 mg/mL, net price 5-mL amp = £11.90

Fabry's disease

Agalsidase alfa and **agalsidase beta**, enzymes produced by recombinant DNA technology, are licensed for long-term enzyme replacement therapy in Fabry's disease (a lysosomal storage disorder caused by deficiency of alpha-galactosidase A).

AGALSIDASE ALFA and BETA

Cautions interactions: Appendix 1 (agalsidase alfa and beta)

Infusion-related reactions Infusion-related reactions very common; manage by slowing the infusion rate or interrupting the infusion, or minimise by pre-treatment with an antihistamine, antipyretic, or corticosteroid—consult product literature

Pregnancy use with caution

Breast-feeding use with caution—no information available

Side-effects gastro-intestinal disturbances, taste disturbances; tachycardia, bradycardia, palpitation, hypertension, hypotension, chest pain, oedema, flushing; dyspnoea, cough, wheezing, hoarseness, rhinorrhoea; headache, fatigue, dizziness, asthenia, paraesthesia, syncope, neuropathic pain, tremor, sleep disturbances; influenza-like symptoms, nasopharyngitis; pain in extremities, muscle spasms, myalgia, arthralgia; eye irritation; tinnitus, vertigo; hypersensitivity reactions, angioedema, pruritus, urticaria, rash, acne; *less commonly* bronchospasm, cold extremities, parosmia, ear pain and swelling, skin discoloration, and injection-site reactions

Indication and dose

Fabry's disease (specialist use only)
see under preparations

Fabrazyme® (Genzyme) PoM
Intravenous infusion, powder for reconstitution, agalsidase beta, net price 5-mg vial = £325.50; 35-mg vial = £2269.20

Dose

Fabry's disease (specialist use only)
- **By intravenous infusion**
  Child 8–18 years 1 mg/kg every 2 weeks

Administration for *intravenous infusion*, reconstitute initially with Water for Injections (5 mg in 1.1 mL, 35 mg in 7.2 mL) to produce a solution containing 5 mg/mL; dilute with Sodium Chloride 0.9% (for doses less than 35 mg dilute with at least 50 mL; doses 35–70 mg dilute with at least 100 mL; doses 70–100 mg dilute with at least

9

Nutrition and blood

◁ **AGALSIDASE ALFA and BETA (continued)**

250 mL; doses greater than 100 mg dilute with 500 mL)
and give through an in-line low protein-binding 0.2 micron
filter at an initial rate of no more than 15 mg/hour; for
subsequent infusions, infusion rate may be increased
gradually once tolerance has been established

Replagal® (Shire) ℞
Concentrate for intravenous infusion, agalsidase
alfa 1 mg/mL, net price 1-mL vial = £356.85; 3.5-
mL vial = £1068.64

Dose
> **Fabry's disease** (specialist use only)
> • By intravenous infusion
>   **Child 7–18 years** 200 micrograms/kg every 2 weeks

Administration for *intravenous infusion*, dilute requisite
dose with 100 mL Sodium Chloride 0.9% and give over 40
minutes using an in-line filter; use within 3 hours of
dilution

Gaucher's disease

Imiglucerase, an enzyme produced by recombinant DNA technology, is administered as enzyme replacement therapy in Gaucher's disease, a familial disorder
affecting principally the liver, spleen, bone marrow, and lymph nodes.

Miglustat, an inhibitor of glucosylceramide synthase, is licensed in adults for the
treatment of mild to moderate type I Gaucher's disease in patients for whom
imiglucerase is unsuitable; it is given by mouth.

IMIGLUCERASE

Cautions monitor for imiglucerase antibodies;
when stabilised, monitor all parameters and
response to treatment at intervals of 6–12 months
Pregnancy manufacturer advises use with caution—limited information available
Breast-feeding no information available
Side-effects hypersensitivity reactions (including
urticaria, angioedema, hypotension, flushing,
tachycardia, backache); *less commonly* nausea,
vomiting, diarrhoea, abdominal cramps, fatigue,
headache, dizziness, paraesthesia, fever, arthralgia, injection-site reactions

Indication and dose

Gaucher's disease type I (specialist use only)
• By intravenous infusion

> **Neonate** initially 60 units/kg once every 2
> weeks, adjusted according to response; doses as
> low as 30 units/kg once every 2 weeks may be
> appropriate

> **Child 1 month–18 years** initially 60 units/kg
> once every 2 weeks, adjusted according to
> response; doses as low as 30 units/kg once
> every 2 weeks may be appropriate

Gaucher's disease type III (specialist use only)
• By intravenous infusion

> **Neonate** 60–120 units/kg once every 2 weeks,
> adjusted according to response

> **Child 1 month–18 years** 60–120 units/kg once
> every 2 weeks, adjusted according to response

Administration For *intravenous infusion*, initially
reconstitute with Water for Injections (200 units
in 5.1 mL, 400 units in 10.2 mL) to a concentration of 40 units/mL; dilute requisite dose with
Sodium Chloride 0.9% to a final volume of 100–
200 mL; give initial dose at a rate not exceeding
0.5 units/kg/minute, subsequent doses to be
given at a rate not exceeding 1 unit/kg/minute;
administer within 3 hours of reconstitution

Cerezyme® (Genzyme) ℞
Intravenous infusion, powder for reconstitution,
imiglucerase, net price 200-unit vial = £553.35;
400-unit vial = £1106.70
Electrolytes Na⁺ 0.62 mmol/200-unit vial, 1.24 mmol/400-
unit vial

Mucopolysaccharidosis

Laronidase, an enzyme produced by recombinant DNA technology, is licensed
for long-term replacement therapy in the treatment of non-neurological manifestations of mucopolysaccharidosis I, a lysosomal storage disorder caused by
deficiency of alpha-L-iduronidase.

Idursulfase, an enzyme produced by recombinant DNA technology, is licensed
for long-term replacement therapy in mucopolysaccharidosis II (Hunter
syndrome), a lysosomal storage disorder caused by deficiency of iduronate-2-
sulfatase.

Galsulfase, a recombinant form of human N-acetylgalactosamine-4-sulfatase, is
licensed for long-term replacement therapy in mucopolysaccharidosis VI (Mar-
oteaux-Lamy syndrome).

Infusion-related reactions Infusion-related reactions often occur with administration of laronidase, idursulfase, and galsulfase; they can be managed by slowing

the infusion rate or interrupting the infusion, and can be minimised by pre-treatment with an antihistamine and an antipyretic. Recurrent infusion-related reactions may require pre-treatment with a corticosteroid—consult product literature for details.

GALSULFASE

Cautions respiratory disease; acute febrile or respiratory illness (consider delaying treatment)
Infusion-related reactions See notes above

Pregnancy manufacturer advises avoid unless essential

Breast-feeding manufacturer advises avoid—no information available

Side-effects abdominal pain, umbilical hernia, gastroenteritis; chest pain, hypertension; dyspnoea, apnoea, nasal congestion; rigors, malaise, areflexia; pharyngitis; conjunctivitis, corneal opacity; ear pain; facial oedema

Indication and dose

Mucopolysaccharidosis VI (specialist use only)
• By intravenous infusion
Child 5–18 years 1 mg/kg once weekly

Administration for *intravenous infusion*, dilute requisite dose with Sodium Chloride 0.9% to a final volume of 250 mL and mix gently; infuse through a 0.2 micron in-line filter; give approx. 2.5% of the total volume over 1 hour, then infuse remaining volume over next 3 hours; if body-weight under 20 kg and at risk of fluid overload, dilute requisite dose in 100 mL Sodium Chloride 0.9% and give over at least 4 hours

Naglazyme® (BioMarin) ▼ PoM
Concentrate for intravenous infusion, galsulfase 1 mg/mL, net price 5-mL vial = £982.00

IDURSULFASE

Cautions severe respiratory disease; acute febrile respiratory illness (consider delaying treatment)
Infusion-related reactions See notes above

Contra-indications women of child-bearing potential

Pregnancy manufacturer advises avoid—no information available

Breast-feeding no information available

Side-effects gastro-intestinal disturbances, swollen tongue; arrhythmia, chest pain, cyanosis; peripheral oedema, hypertension, hypotension, flushing, pulmonary embolism; bronchospasm, cough, wheezing, tachypnoea, dyspnoea; headache, dizziness, tremor; pyrexia; arthralgia; increased lacrimation; facial oedema, urticaria, pruritus, rash, infusion-site swelling, erythema, and eczema; anaphylaxis also reported

Indication and dose

Mucopolysaccharidosis II (specialist use only)
• By intravenous infusion
Child 5–18 years 500 micrograms/kg once weekly

Administration for *intravenous infusion*, dilute requisite dose in 100 mL Sodium Chloride 0.9% and mix gently (do not shake); give over 3 hours (gradually reduced to 1 hour if no infusion-related reactions)

Elaprase® (Shire) ▼ PoM
Concentrate for intravenous infusion, idursulfase 2 mg/mL, net price 3-mL vial = £1985.00

LARONIDASE

Cautions monitor immunoglobulin G (IgG) antibody concentration; **interactions:** Appendix 1 (laronidase)
Infusion-related reactions See notes above

Pregnancy manufacturer advises avoid unless essential—no information available

Breast-feeding manufacturer advises avoid—no information available

Side-effects nausea, vomiting, diarrhoea, abdominal pain; cold extremities, pallor, flushing, tachycardia, blood pressure changes; dyspnoea, cough, angioedema, anaphylaxis; headache, paraesthesia, dizziness, fatigue, restlessness; influenza-like symptoms; musculoskeletal pain, pain in extremities; rash, pruritus, urticaria, alopecia, infusion-site reactions; bronchospasm and respiratory arrest also reported

Indication and dose

Non-neurological manifestations of mucopolysaccharidosis I (specialist use only)
• By intravenous infusion
Child 1 month–18 years 100 units/kg once weekly

Administration for *intravenous infusion*, dilute with Sodium Chloride 0.9%; body-weight under 20 kg, dilute to 100 mL, body-weight over 20 kg dilute to 250 mL; give through in-line filter (0.22 micron) initially at a rate of 2 units/kg/hour then increase gradually every 15 minutes to max. 43 units/kg/hour

Aldurazyme (Genzyme) PoM
Concentrate for intravenous infusion, laronidase 100 units/mL, net price 5-mL vial = £460.35
Electrolytes Na⁺ 1.29 mmol /5-mL vial

9

Nutrition and blood

Nephropathic cystinosis

Mercaptamine (cysteamine) is available for the treatment of nephropathic cystinosis. The oral dose is increased over several weeks to avoid intolerance.

Mercaptamine eye drops are used in the management of ocular symptoms arising from the deposition of cystine crystals in the eye.

Phosphocysteamine is a pro-drug of mercaptamine; it is available from specialist centres only, as a powder or specially manufactured capsule. Mercaptamine does not contain phosphate, therefore, if transferring from phosphocysteamine to mercaptamine phosphate supplements may need to be initiated or adjusted. Mercaptamine 1 mg is approximately equivalent to 3 mg of phosphocysteamine.

Both mercaptamine and phosphocysteamine have a very unpleasant taste and smell, which can affect compliance.

All patients receiving mercaptamine and phosphocysteamine should be registered (contact local specialist centre for details).

> **Safe Practice**
> Mercaptamine has been confused with mercaptopurine; care must be taken to ensure the correct drug is prescribed and dispensed.

MERCAPTAMINE
(Cysteamine)

Cautions leucocyte-cystine concentration and haematological monitoring required—consult product literature; dose of phosphate supplement may need to be adjusted

Contra-indications hypersensitivity to mercaptamine or penicillamine

Pregnancy avoid—teratogenic and toxic in *animal* studies

Breast-feeding avoid

Side-effects breath and body odour, nausea, vomiting, diarrhoea, anorexia, lethargy, fever, rash; also reported dehydration, hypertension, abdominal discomfort, gastroenteritis, drowsiness, encephalopathy, headache, nervousness, depression; anaemia, leucopenia, *rarely* gastrointestinal ulceration and bleeding, seizures, hallucinations, urticaria, interstitial nephritis

Licensed use eye drops not licensed

Indication and dose

Nephropathic cystinosis (specialist use only)
- **By mouth**

  Neonate initially 2–3 mg/kg 4 times daily, increased over 4–6 weeks to 12.5 mg/kg 4 times daily

  Child 1 month–12 years or under 50 kg initially 2–3 mg/kg 4 times daily, increased over 4–6 weeks to 12.5 mg/kg 4 times daily

  Child 12–18 years or over 50 kg initially 100 mg 4 times daily, increased over 4–6 weeks to 500 mg 4 times daily

Cystagon® (Orphan Europe) ℗ℴℳ
Capsules, mercaptamine (as bitartrate) 50 mg, net price 100-cap pack = £59.00; 150 mg, 100-cap pack = £162.00

Note For child under 6 years at risk of aspiration, capsules can be opened and contents sprinkled on food (at a temperature suitable for eating); avoid adding to acidic drinks (e.g. orange juice)

◀ Eye drops
Mercaptamine (Non-proprietary)
Eye drops, mercaptamine 0.11%, 10 mL
Available from 'special-order' manufacturers or specialist importing companies, see p. 957

Pompe disease

Alglucosidase alfa, an enzyme produced by recombinant DNA technology, is licensed for long-term replacement therapy in Pompe disease, a lysosomal storage disorder caused by deficiency of acid alpha-glucosidase.

ALGLUCOSIDASE ALFA

Cautions cardiac and respiratory dysfunction—monitor closely; monitor immunoglobulin G (IgG) antibody concentration

Infusion-related reactions Infusion-related reactions very common, calling for use of antihistamine, antipyretic, or corticosteroid; consult product literature for details

Pregnancy toxicity in *animal* studies, but treatment should not be withheld

Breast-feeding manufacturer advises avoid—no information available

Side-effects nausea, vomiting, diarrhoea; flushing, tachycardia, blood pressure changes, cold extremities, cyanosis, facial oedema, chest discomfort; cough, tachypnoea, bronchospasm; headache, agitation, tremor, irritability, restless-

Nutrition and blood — 9

◁ **ALGLUCOSIDASE ALFA** (*continued*)

ness, paraesthesia, dizziness, fatigue; pyrexia; antibody formation; myalgia, muscle spasms; sweating, rash, pruritus, urticaria, injection-site reactions; hypersensitivity reactions (including anaphylaxis)

Indication and dose

Pompe disease (specialist use only)
• By intravenous infusion

> **Neonate** 20 mg/kg every 2 weeks

> **Child 1 month –18 years** 20 mg/kg every 2 weeks

Administration For *intravenous infusion*, reconstitute 50 mg with 10.3 mL Water for Injections to produce 5 mg/mL solution; gently rotate vial without shaking; dilute requisite dose with Sodium Chloride 0.9% to give a final concentration of 0.5–4 mg/mL; give through a low protein-binding in-line filter (0.2 micron) at an initial rate of 1 mg/kg/hour increased by 2 mg/kg/hour every 30 minutes to max. 7 mg/kg/hour

Myozyme® (Genzyme) ▼ PoM
Intravenous infusion, powder for reconstitution, alglucosidase alfa, net price 50-mg vial = £368.59

Urea cycle disorders

Sodium benzoate and **sodium phenylbutyrate** are used in the management of urea cycle disorders. Both, either singly or in combination, are indicated as adjunctive therapy in all patients with neonatal-onset disease and in those with late-onset disease who have a history of hyperammonaemic encephalopathy. Sodium benzoate is also used in non-ketotic hyperglycinaemia.

Gastro-intestinal side-effects of sodium benzoate or sodium phenylbutyrate may be reduced by giving smaller doses more frequently. The preparations contain significant amounts of sodium; therefore, they should be used with caution in children with congestive heart failure, renal insufficiency and clinical conditions involving sodium retention with oedema.

The long-term management of urea cycle disorders includes oral maintenance treatment with sodium benzoate and sodium phenylbutyrate combined with a low protein diet and other drugs such as **arginine** or **citrulline**, depending on the specific disorder.

Carglumic acid is licensed for the treatment of hyperammonaemia due to *N*-acetylglutamate synthase deficiency.

ARGININE

Cautions monitor plasma pH and chloride

Contra-indications not to be used in the treatment of arginase deficiency

Pregnancy no information available

Breast-feeding no information available

Side-effects intravenous injection only: nausea, vomiting; flushing, hypotension; headache, numbness; hyperchloraemic metabolic acidosis; irritation at injection-site

Licensed use injection and tablets not licensed in children; powder licensed for urea cycle disorders in children

Indication and dose

Acute hyperammonaemia in carbamylphosphate synthetase deficiency, ornithine carbamyl transferase deficiency (specialist use only)
• By intravenous infusion

> **Neonate** initially 200 mg/kg over 90 minutes followed by 8 mg/kg/hour

> **Child 1 month–18 years** initially 200 mg/kg over 90 minutes followed by 8 mg/kg/hour

Maintenance treatment of hyperammonaemia in carbamylphosphate synthetase deficiency, ornithine carbamyl transferase deficiency (specialist use only)
• By mouth

> **Neonate** 100 mg/kg daily in 3–4 divided doses

> **Child 1 month–18 years** 100 mg/kg daily in 3–4 divided doses

Acute hyperammonaemia in citrullinaemia, arginosuccinic aciduria (specialist use only)
• By intravenous infusion

> **Neonate** initially 600 mg/kg over 90 minutes followed by 25 mg/kg/hour

> **Child 1 month–18 years** initially 600 mg/kg over 90 minutes followed by 25 mg/kg/hour

Maintenance treatment of hyperammonaemia in citrullinaemia, arginosuccinic aciduria (specialist use only)
• By mouth

> **Neonate** 100–175 mg/kg 3–4 times daily, with food, adjusted according to response

> **Child 1 month–18 years** 100–175 mg/kg 3–4 times daily, with food, adjusted according to response

9

Nutrition and blood

◻ ARGININE (*continued*)

L-Arginine (Non-proprietary)
Tablets, L-arginine (as hydrochloride) 500 mg,

Oral solution, L-arginine 100 mg/mL
Available from 'special-order' manufacturers or specialist importing companies, see p. 957

Powder, L-arginine (as hydrochloride), net price 100 g = £11.70
Prescribe as a borderline substance (ACBS). For use as a supplement in urea cycle disorders other than arginase deficiency, such as hyperammonaemia types I and II, citrullinaemia, arginosuccinic aciduria, and deficiency of N-acetyl glutamate synthetase

Injection, L-arginine (as hydrochloride) 500 mg/mL, 10-mL ampoules; 100 mg/mL, 200-mL amp
Available from 'special-order' manufacturers or specialist importing companies, see p. 957

Note Other strengths may be available from 'special-order' manufacturers or specialist importing companies, see p. 957

Administration dilute to a concentration of 20 mg/mL with Sodium Chloride 0.9% or 0.45%, *or* Glucose 5% or 10%; max. concentration 100 mg/mL; may be given orally

CARGLUMIC ACID

Pregnancy manufacturer advises avoid unless essential—no information available

Breast-feeding manufacturer advises avoid—present in milk in *animal* studies

Side-effects sweating

Indication and dose

Hyperammonaemia due to *N*-acetyl glutamate synthase deficiency (initiated under specialist supervision)
• By mouth

Neonate initially 50–125 mg/kg twice daily immediately before feeds, adjusted according to plasma-ammonia concentration; maintenance

5–50 mg/kg twice daily; total daily dose may alternatively be given in 3–4 divided doses

Child 1 month–18 years initially 50–125 mg/kg twice daily immediately before food, adjusted according to plasma-ammonia concentration; maintenance 5–50 mg/kg twice daily; total daily dose may alternatively be given in 3–4 divided doses

Carbaglu® (Orphan Europe) PoM
Dispersible tablets, carglumic acid 200 mg, net price 5-tab pack = £243.00, 60-tab pack = £2914.00. Label: 13

CITRULLINE

Pregnancy no information available

Breast-feeding no information available

Indication and dose

Carbamyl phosphate synthase deficiency, ornithine carbamyl transferase deficiency
• By mouth

Neonate 150 mg/kg daily in 3–4 divided doses, adjusted according to response

Child 1 month–18 years 150 mg/kg daily in 3–4 divided doses, adjusted according to response

Citrulline Powder (Non-proprietary)
Powder, L-citrulline 100 g
Available from 'special-order' manufacturers or specialist importing companies, see p. 957

Administration May be mixed with drinks or taken as a paste

SODIUM BENZOATE

Cautions see notes above; neonates (risk of kernicterus and increased side-effects); **interactions**: Appendix 1 (sodium benzoate)

Renal impairment see notes above

Pregnancy no information available

Breast-feeding no information available

Side-effects nausea, vomiting, anorexia; irritability, lethargy, coma

Licensed use not licensed for use in children

Indication and dose

Acute hyperammonaemia due to urea cycle disorders (specialist use only)
• By intravenous infusion

Neonate initially 250 mg/kg over 90 minutes followed by 20 mg/kg/hour, adjusted according to response

Child 1 month–18 years initially 250 mg/kg over 90 minutes followed by 20 mg/kg/hour, adjusted according to response

Maintenance treatment of hyperammonaemia due to urea cycle disorders; non-ketotic hyperglycinaemia (specialist use only)
• By mouth

Neonate 50–150 mg/kg 3–4 times daily, with food, adjusted according to response

Child 1 month–18 years 50–150 mg/kg 3–4 times daily, with food, adjusted according to response

Administration for administration *by mouth*, oral solution or powder may be administered in fruit drinks; less soluble in acidic drinks

Sodium Benzoate (Non-proprietary) PoM
Tablets, sodium benzoate 500 mg
Available from 'special-order' manufacturers or specialist importing companies, see p. 957

Capsules, sodium benzoate 50 mg; 250 mg; 400 mg; 500 mg
Available from 'special-order' manufacturers or specialist importing companies, see p. 957

◻ **SODIUM BENZOATE** (*continued*)

Oral solution, sodium benzoate 100 mg/mL; 200 mg/mL; 300 mg/mL
Available from 'special-order' manufacturers or specialist importing companies, see p. 957

Powder
Available from 'special-order' manufacturers or specialist importing companies, see p. 957

Injection, sodium benzoate 200 mg/mL, 5-mL amp
Note Contains Na^+ 1.4 mmol /mL
Available from 'special-order' manufacturers or specialist importing companies, see p. 957
Administration for *intravenous infusion*, dilute to a concentration of 20 mg/mL with Sodium Chloride 0.9% or 0.45%, *or* Glucose 5% or 10%; max. concentration 50 mg/mL

�})SODIUM PHENYLBUTYRATE

Cautions see notes above; congestive heart failure; **interactions**: Appendix 1 (sodium phenylbutyrate)

Hepatic impairment manufacturer advises use with caution

Renal impairment manufacturer advises use with caution; see also notes above

Pregnancy avoid—toxicity in *animal* studies; manufacturer advises adequate contraception in women of child-bearing potential

Breast-feeding manufacturer advises avoid—no information available

Side-effects amenorrhoea and irregular menstrual cycles, decreased appetite, body odour, taste disturbances; less commonly nausea, vomiting, abdominal pain, peptic ulcer, pancreatitis, rectal bleeding, arrhythmia, oedema, syncope, depression, headache, rash, weight gain, renal tubular acidosis, aplastic anaemia, ecchymoses

Licensed use injection not licensed for use in children

Indication and dose

> Acute hyperammonaemia due to urea cycle disorders (specialist use only)
> • By continuous intravenous infusion
>
> **Neonate** initially 250 mg/kg over 90 minutes followed by 20 mg/kg/hour adjusted according to response

> **Child 1 month–18 years** initially 250 mg/kg over 90 minutes followed by 20 mg/kg/hour adjusted according to response

> Maintenance treatment of hyperammonaemia due to urea cycle disorders (specialist use only)
> • By mouth
>
> **Neonate** 75–150 mg/kg 3–4 times daily, with food

> **Child 1 month–18 years** 75–150 mg/kg 3–4 times daily, with food (max. 20 g daily)
> **Administration** Oral dose may be mixed with fruit drinks, milk, or feeds

Sodium Phenylbutyrate (Non-proprietary) PoM
Injection, sodium phenylbutyrate 200 mg/mL, 5-mL amp
Note Contains Na^+ 1.1 mmol /mL
Available from 'special-order' manufacturers or specialist importing companies, see p. 957
Administration for *intravenous infusion*, dilute to a concentration of 20 mg/mL (max. 50 mg/mL) with Glucose 5% or 10%

Ammonaps® (Swedish Orphan) PoM
Tablets, sodium phenylbutyrate 500 mg. Contains Na^+ 2.7 mmol/tablet. Net price 250-tab pack = £493.00

Granules, sodium phenylbutyrate 940 mg/g. Contains Na^+ 5.4 mmol/g. Net price 266-g pack = £860.00

Note Granules should be mixed with food before taking

▎Other metabolic disorders

Other metabolic disorders and the drugs used in their management include:

Amino acid disorders: maple syrup urine disease (thiamine section 9.6.2); tyrosinaemia type III, hawkinsinuria (Vitamin C, section 9.6.3); tyrosinaemia type I (nitisinone).

Mitochondrial disorders: isolated carboxylase defects, defects of biotin metabolism (biotin, see below); mitochondrial myopathies (ubidecarenone); congenital lactic acidosis (riboflavine and thiamine, section 9.6.2); respiratory chain defects (thiamine, section 9.6.2); pyruvate dehydrogenase defects (sodium dichloroacetate)

Neimann-Pick type C disease: miglustat is available for the treatment of progressive neurological manifestations of Neimann-Pick type C disease, a neurodegenerative disorder characterised by impaired intracellular lipid trafficking.

Homocystinuria and defects in cobalamin metabolism: betaine, pyridoxine (section 9.6.2), hydroxocobalamin (section 9.1.2)

Tetrahydrofolate reductase deficiency: betaine, folic acid (section 9.1.2)

The *Scottish Medicines Consortium* (p. 4) has advised (February 2009) that betaine anhydrous powder (*Cystadane®*) is **not** recommended for use as adjunctive treatment of homocystinuria.

9

Nutrition and blood

◢ BETAINE

Cautions monitor plasma-methionine concentration before and during treatment—interrupt treatment if symptoms of cerebral oedema occur

Pregnancy manufacturer advises avoid unless essential—limited information available

Breast-feeding manufacturer advises caution—no information available

Side-effects *less commonly* gastro-intestinal disorders, anorexia, reversible cerebral oedema (see Cautions), agitation, depression, personality disorder, sleep disturbances, urinary incontinence, alopecia, and urticaria

Indication and dose

> Adjunctive treatment of homocystinuria (specialist use only)
> - By mouth
>
> > **Neonate** 50 mg/kg twice daily, dose and frequency adjusted according to response; max. 75 mg/kg twice daily
>
> > **Child 1 month–10 years** 50 mg/kg twice daily, dose and frequency adjusted according to response; max. 75 mg/kg twice daily
>
> > **Child 10–18 years** 3 g twice daily, adjusted according to response; max. 10 g twice daily

Administration Powder should be mixed with water, juice, milk, formula, or food until completely dissolved and taken immediately; measuring spoons are provided to measure 1 g, 150 mg, and 100 mg of *Cystadane*® powder

Betaine (Non-proprietary) ⒫ⓞⓜ
Powder (for oral solution), betaine anhydrous 500 mg/mL when reconstituted.
Available from 'special-order' manufacturers or specialist importing companies, see p. 957

Tablets, betaine anhydrous 500 mg
Available from 'special-order' manufacturers or specialist importing companies, see p. 957

Cystadane® (Orphan Europe) ⒫ⓞⓜ
Powder, betaine (anhydrous), net price 180 g = £314.00

◢ BIOTIN
(Vitamin H)

Pregnancy no information available

Breast-feeding no information available

Indication and dose

> Isolated carboxylase defects
> - By mouth or by slow intravenous injection
>
> > **Neonate** 5 mg once daily, adjusted according to response; usual maintenance 10–50 mg daily, higher doses may be required
>
> > **Child 1 month–18 years** 10 mg once daily, adjusted according to response; usual maintenance 10–50 mg daily but up to 100 mg daily may be required

> Defects of biotin metabolism
> - By mouth or by slow intravenous injection
>
> > **Neonate** 10 mg once daily adjusted according to response; usual maintenance 5–20 mg daily but higher doses may be required
>
> > **Child 1 month–18 years** 10 mg once daily adjusted according to response; usual maintenance 5–20 mg daily but higher doses may be required

Biotin (Non-proprietary) ⒫ⓞⓜ
Tablets, biotin 5 mg, 20-tab pack

Injection, biotin 5 mg/mL
Available from 'special order' manufacturers or specialist importing companies, see p. 957

Administration For administration *by mouth*, tablets may be crushed and mixed with food or drink

◢ MIGLUSTAT

Cautions monitor cognitive and neurological function, growth, and platelet count

Hepatic impairment manufacturer advises caution—no information available

Renal impairment child 12–18 years, initially 200 mg twice daily if estimated glomerular filtration rate 50–70 mL/minute/1.73 m^2; child 12–18 years, initially 100 mg twice daily if estimated glomerular filtration rate 30–50 mL/minute/1.73 m^2; avoid if estimated glomerular filtration rate less than 30 mL/minute/1.73 m^2; child under 12 years—consult product literature

Pregnancy manufacturer advises avoid (toxicity in *animal* studies)—effective contraception must be used during treatment; also men should avoid fathering a child during and for 3 months after treatment

Breast-feeding manufacturer advises avoid—no information available

Side-effects diarrhoea, flatulence, abdominal pain, dyspepsia, constipation, nausea, vomiting, anorexia, weight changes; tremor, dizziness, headache, peripheral neuropathy, ataxia, hypoaesthesia, paraesthesia, insomnia, fatigue, asthenia; decreased libido; thrombocytopenia; muscle spasm

Indication and dose

> Neimann-Pick type C disease (specialist supervision only)
> - By mouth
>
> > **Child 4–12 years**
> >
> > **Body surface area less than 0.47 m^2** 100 mg once daily
> >
> > **Body surface area 0.47–0.73 m^2** 100 mg twice daily
> >
> > **Body surface area 0.73–0.88 m^2** 100 mg three times daily

9 Nutrition and blood

◁ **MIGLUSTAT (***continued***)**

Body surface area 0.88–1.25 m² 200 mg twice daily

Body surface area greater than 1.25 m² 200 mg three times daily

Child 12–18 years 200 mg three times daily

Zavesca® (Actelion) [PoM]
Capsules, miglustat 100 mg, net price 84-cap pack = £3890.13 (hospital only)

NITISINONE
(NTBC)

Cautions slit-lamp examination of eyes recommended before treatment; monitor liver function regularly; monitor platelet and white blood cell count every 6 months

Pregnancy manufacturer advises avoid unless potential benefit outweighs risk—toxicity in *animal* studies

Breast-feeding manufacturer advises avoid— adverse effect in *animal* studies

Side-effects thrombocytopenia, leucopenia, granulocytopenia; conjunctivitis, photophobia, corneal opacity, keratitis, eye pain; *less commonly* leucocytosis, blepharitis, pruritus, exfoliative dermatitis, and erythematous rash

Indication and dose

Hereditary tyrosinaemia type I (in combination with dietary restriction of tyrosine and phenylalanine)
● By mouth

Neonate initially 500 micrograms/kg twice daily, adjusted according to response; max. 2 mg/kg daily

Child 1 month–18 years initially 500 micrograms/kg twice daily, adjusted according to response; max. 2 mg/kg daily

Administration capsules can be opened and the contents suspended in a small amount of water or formula diet and taken immediately

Orfadin® (Swedish Orphan) [PoM]
Capsules, nitisinone 2 mg, net price 60-cap pack = £564.00; 5 mg, 60-cap pack = £1127.00; 10 mg, 60-cap pack = £2062.00

SODIUM DICHLOROACETATE

Pregnancy no information available

Breast-feeding no information available

Side-effects polyneuropathy on prolonged use; abnormal oxalate metabolism; metabolic acidosis

Indication and dose

Pyruvate dehydrogenase defects
● By mouth

Neonate initially 12.5 mg/kg 4 times daily, adjusted according to response; up to 200 mg/ kg daily may be required

Child 1 month–18 years initially 12.5 mg/kg 4 times daily, adjusted according to response; up to 200 mg/kg daily may be required

Sodium dichloroacetate (Non-proprietary) [PoM]
Powder (for oral solution), sodium dichloroacetate 50 mg/mL when reconstituted with water
Available from 'special-order' manufacturers or specialist importing companies, see p. 957

UBIDECARENONE
(Ubiquinone, Co-enzyme Q10)

Cautions may reduce insulin requirement in diabetes mellitus; **interactions**: Appendix 1 (ubidecarenone)

Hepatic impairment reduce dose in moderate and severe impairment

Side-effects nausea, diarrhoea, heartburn; *rarely* headache, irritability, agitation, dizziness

Licensed use not licensed

Indication and dose

Mitochondrial disorders
● By mouth

Neonate initially 5 mg once or twice daily with food, adjusted according to response, up to 200 mg daily may be required

Child 1 month–18 years initially 5 mg once or twice daily with food, adjusted according to response, up to 300 mg daily may be required

Ubidecarenone (Non-proprietary) [PoM]
Oral solution, ubidecarenone 50 mg/10 mL

Tablets, ubidecarenone 10 mg

Capsules, ubidecarenone 10 mg, 30 mg
Available from 'special-order' manufacturers or specialist importing companies, see p. 957

9

Nutrition and blood

9.8.2 Acute porphyrias

The acute porphyrias (acute intermittent porphyria, variegate porphyria, hereditary coproporphyria, and 5-aminolaevulinic acid dehydratase deficiency porphyria) are hereditary disorders of haem biosynthesis; they have a prevalence of about 1 in 10 000 of the population.

Great care must be taken when prescribing for patients with acute porphyria, since certain drugs can induce acute porphyric crises. Since acute porphyrias are hereditary, relatives of affected individuals should be screened and advised about the potential danger of certain drugs. Acute attacks of porphyria are exceptionally rare before puberty. When acute porphyria is suspected in a child, support from an expert porphyria service should be sought.

Treatment of serious or life-threatening conditions should not be withheld from patients with acute porphyria. When there is no safe alternative, treatment should be started and urinary porphobilinogen excretion should be measured regularly; if it increases or symptoms occur, the drug can be withdrawn and the acute attack treated. If an acute attack of porphyria occurs during pregnancy, contact an expert porphyria service for further advice.

Haem arginate is administered by short intravenous infusion as haem replacement in moderate, severe, or unremitting acute porphyria crises.

Supplies of haem arginate may be obtained outside office hours from the on-call pharmacist at:

St Thomas' Hospital, London
Tel: (020) 7188 7188

HAEM ARGINATE
(Human hemin)

Pregnancy manufacturer advises avoid unless essential

Breast-feeding manufacturer advises avoid unless essential—no information available

Side-effects *rarely* hypersensitivity reactions and fever; pain and thrombophlebitis at injection site

Indication and dose

Acute porphyrias (acute intermittent porphyria, porphyria variegata, hereditary coproporphyria)
• By intravenous infusion
    Child 1 month–18 years 3 mg/kg once daily (max. 250 mg daily) for 4 days; if response inadequate, repeat 4-day course with close biochemical monitoring

Normosang® (Orphan Europe) ▼ PoM
Concentrate for intravenous infusion, haem arginate 25 mg/mL, net price 10-mL amp = £338.50
Administration administer over at least 30 minutes; dilute requisite dose in 100 mL Sodium Chloride 0.9% in glass bottle; administer within 1 hour after dilution; max. concentration 2.5 mg/mL

Drugs unsafe for use in acute porphyrias

The following list contains drugs on the UK market that have been classified as 'unsafe' in porphyria because they have been shown to be porphyrinogenic in animals or *in vitro*, or have been associated with acute attacks in patients. Absence of a drug from the following lists does not necessarily imply that the drug is safe. For many drugs no information about porphyria is available.

An up-to-date list of drugs considered **safe** in acute porphyrias is available at www.wmic.wales.nhs.uk/porphyria_info.php.

Further information may be obtained from www.porphyria-europe.org and also from:

Welsh Medicines Information Centre
University Hospital of Wales
Cardiff, CF14 4XW.
Tel: (029) 2074 2979/3877

Note Quite modest changes in chemical structure can lead to changes in porphyrinogenicity but where possible general statements have been made about groups of drugs; these should be checked first.

Unsafe drug groups (check first)

Alkylating drugs[1]	Ergot derivatives[7]	Statins[9]
Amphetamines	Gold salts	Sulphonamides[10]
Anabolic steroids	Hormone replacement therapy[6]	Sulphonylureas[11]
Antidepressants[2]	Imidazole antifungals[8]	Taxanes[1]
Antihistamines[3]	Non-nucleoside reverse tran-	Tetracyclines
Barbiturates[4]	scriptase inhibitors[1]	Thiazolidinediones[1]
Calcium channel blockers[5]	Progestogens[6]	Triazole antifungals[8]
Contraceptives, hormonal[6]	Protease inhibitors[1]	

Unsafe drugs (check groups above first)

Aceclofenac	Griseofulvin	Phenoxybenzamine
Alcohol	Halothane	Phenytoin
Amiodarone	Hydralazine	Pivmecillinam
Azapropazone	Indapamide	Porfimer
Bosentan	Isometheptene mucate	Potassium canrenoate[18]
Bromocriptine	Isoniazid	Probenecid
Buspirone	Ketamine	Pyrazinamide
Cabergoline	Ketorolac	Rifabutin [19]
Carbamazepine	Lidocaine (lignocaine)[15]	Rifampicin [19]
Chloral hydrate [12]	Mebeverine	Risperidone
Chloramphenicol	Mefenamic acid[16]	Spironolactone
Chloroform[13]	Meprobamate	Sulfinpyrazone
Clindamycin	Methyldopa	Sulpiride
Clonidine	Metoclopramide[16]	Tamoxifen
Cocaine	Metolazone	Telithromycin
Colistin	Metronidazole[16]	Temoporfin
Cycloserine	Metyrapone	Theophylline[20]
Danazol	Mifepristone	Tiagabine
Dapsone	Minoxidil [16]	Tinidazole
Dexfenfluramine	Nalidixic acid	Topiramate
Diazepam[14]	Nitrazepam	Toremifene
Diclofenac	Nitrofurantoin	Triclofos[12]
Erythromycin	Orphenadrine	Trimethoprim
Etamsylate	Oxcarbazepine	Valproate[14]
Ethosuximide	Oxybutynin	Xipamide
Etomidate	Oxycodone[17]	Zidovudine[1]
Fenfluramine	Pentazocine[17]	Zuclopenthixol
Flupentixol	Pentoxifylline (oxpentifylline)	

1. Contact Welsh Medicines Information Centre for further advice.
2. Includes tricyclic (and related) and MAOIs; fluoxetine, mianserin and venlafaxine thought to be safe.
3. Alimemazine (trimeprazine), chlorphenamine, desloratadine, fexofenadine, ketotifen, loratadine, and promethazine thought to be safe.
4. Includes primidone and thiopental.
5. Amlodipine, felodipine, and nifedipine may be used with caution.
6. Progestogens are more porphyrinogenic than oestrogens; oestrogens may be safe at least in replacement doses. Progestogens should be avoided whenever possible by all young women susceptible to acute porphyria; however, when non-hormonal contraception is inappropriate, progestogens may be used with extreme caution if the potential benefit outweighs risk. The risk of an acute attack is greatest in young women who have had a previous attack. Long-acting progestogen preparations should never be used in those at risk of acute porphyria.
7. Includes ergometrine (oxytocin probably safe) and pergolide.
8. Applies to oral and intravenous use; topical antifungals are thought to be safe due to low systemic exposure.
9. Rosuvastatin thought to be safe.
10. Includes co-trimoxazole and sulfasalazine.
11. Glipizide is thought to be safe.
12. Although evidence of hazard is uncertain, manufacturer advises avoid.
13. Small amounts in medicines probably safe.
14. Status epilepticus has been treated successfully with intravenous diazepam.
15. When used for local anaesthesia, articaine, bupivacaine, lidocaine (lignocaine), prilocaine, and tetracaine are thought to be safe.
16. May be used with caution if safer alternative not available.
17. Buprenorphine, codeine, diamorphine, dihydrocodeine, fentanyl, methadone, morphine, pethidine, and tramadol are thought to be safe.
18. Evidence of hazard uncertain—contact Welsh Medicines Information Centre for further advice.
19. Rifamycins have been used in a few patients without evidence of harm—use with caution if safer alternative not available.
20. Includes aminophylline.

10 Musculoskeletal and joint diseases

This chapter also includes advice on the drug management of the following:
dental and orofacial pain, p. 609
extravasation, p. 628
myasthenia gravis, p. 624
soft-tissue and other musculoskeletal disorders, below
juvenile idiopathic arthritis and other inflammatory disorders, below

For treatment of septic arthritis see Table 1, section 5.1.

10.1 Drugs used in rheumatic diseases

10.1.1 Non-steroidal anti-inflammatory drugs
10.1.2 Corticosteroids
10.1.3 Drugs that suppress the rheumatic disease process
10.1.4 Gout and cytotoxic-induced hyperuricaemia
10.1.5 Other drugs for rheumatic diseases

Juvenile idiopathic arthritis and other inflammatory disorders

Rheumatic diseases require symptomatic treatment to relieve pain, swelling, and stiffness, together with treatment to control and suppress disease activity. Treatment of juvenile idiopathic arthritis may involve non-steroidal anti-inflammatory drugs (NSAIDs) (section 10.1.1), a disease modifying antirheumatic drug (DMARD) (section 10.1.3) such as methotrexate or a cytokine modulator, and intra-articular, intravenous, or oral corticosteroids (section 10.1.2).

Soft-tissue and musculoskeletal disorders

The management of children with soft-tissue injuries and strains, and musculoskeletal disorders, may include temporary rest together with the local application of heat or cold, local massage and physiotherapy. For pain relief, **paracetamol** (section 4.7.1) is often adequate and should be used first. Alternatively, the lowest effective dose of a **NSAID** (e.g. ibuprofen) can be used. If pain relief with either drug is inadequate, both paracetamol (in a full dose appropriate for the child) and a low dose of a NSAID may be required.

10.1.1 Non-steroidal anti-inflammatory drugs

In *single doses* non-steroidal anti-inflammatory drugs (NSAIDs) have analgesic activity comparable to that of paracetamol (section 4.7.1), but paracetamol is preferred.

In regular *full dosage* NSAIDs have both a lasting analgesic and an anti-inflammatory effect which makes them particularly useful for the treatment of continuous or regular pain associated with inflammation.

Choice   Generally, differences in anti-inflammatory activity between NSAIDs are small, but there is considerable variation in individual response and tolerance to these drugs. A large proportion of children will respond to any NSAID; of the others, those who do not respond to one may well respond to another. Pain relief starts soon after taking the first dose and a full analgesic effect should normally be obtained within a week, whereas an anti-inflammatory effect may not be achieved (or may not be clinically assessable) for up to 3 weeks. However, in juvenile idiopathic arthritis NSAIDs may take 4–12 weeks to be effective. If appropriate responses are not obtained within these times, another NSAID should be tried. The availability of appropriate formulations needs to be considered when prescribing NSAIDs for children.

NSAIDs reduce the production of prostaglandins by inhibiting the enzyme cyclo-oxygenase. They vary in their selectivity for inhibiting different types of cyclo-oxygenase; selective inhibition of cyclo-oxygenase-2 is associated with less gastro-intestinal intolerance. However, in children gastro-intestinal symptoms are rare in those taking NSAIDs for short periods. The role of selective inhibitors of cyclo-oxygenase-2 is undetermined in children.

Ibuprofen and **naproxen** are propionic acid derivatives used in children:

Ibuprofen combines anti-inflammatory, analgesic, and antipyretic properties. It has fewer side-effects than other NSAIDs but its anti-inflammatory properties are weaker.

Naproxen combines good efficacy with a low incidence of side-effects.

Diclofenac, **indometacin**, **mefenamic acid**, and **piroxicam** have properties similar to those of propionic acid derivatives:

Diclofenac has actions and side-effects similar to those of naproxen.

Indometacin (indomethacin) has an action equal to or superior to that of naproxen, but with a high incidence of side-effects including headache, dizziness, and gastro-intestinal disturbances. It is rarely used in children and should be reserved for when other NSAIDs have been unsuccessful.

Mefenamic acid has minor anti-inflammatory properties. It has occasionally been associated with diarrhoea and haemolytic anaemia which require discontinuation of treatment.

Piroxicam is as effective as naproxen and has a long duration of action which permits once-daily administration. However, it has more gastro-intestinal side-effects than most other NSAIDs, and is associated with more frequent serious skin reactions (**important**: see CHMP advice, p. 615).

Meloxicam is a selective inhibitor of cyclo-oxygenase-2. Its use may be considered in adolescents intolerant to other NSAIDs.

Ketorolac can be used for the short-term management of postoperative pain (section 15.1.4.2).

Etoricoxib, a selective inhibitor of cyclo-oxygenase-2, is licensed for the relief of pain in osteoarthritis, rheumatoid arthritis, ankylosing spondylitis, and acute gout in children aged 16 years and over. For concerns about the cardiovascular safety of cyclo-oxygenase-2 selective inhibitors (see below).

For the role of **aspirin** in children, see section 2.9.

Dental and orofacial pain   Most mild to moderate dental pain and inflammation is effectively relieved by **ibuprofen** or **diclofenac**. In an appraisal of the relative safety in adults of 7 non-selective NSAIDs, the CSM assessed ibuprofen to have the lowest risk of serious gastro-intestinal side-effects (see below).

For further information on the management of dental and orofacial pain, see p. 253.

10

Musculoskeletal and joint diseases

Cautions and contra-indications NSAIDs should be used with caution in children with a history of hypersensitivity to any NSAID—which includes those in whom attacks of asthma, angioedema, urticaria or rhinitis have been precipitated by any NSAID. NSAIDs should also be used with caution in coagulation defects. Caution may also be required in children with allergic disorders, and also in children with connective-tissue disorders, see Side-effects below.

In children with cardiac impairment, caution is required since NSAIDs may impair renal function (see also Side-effects below). All NSAIDs are contra-indicated in severe heart failure. The selective inhibitor of cyclo-oxygenase-2, etoricoxib, is contra-indicated in ischaemic heart disease, cerebrovascular disease, peripheral arterial disease, and moderate or severe heart failure. Etoricoxib should be used with caution in children with a history of cardiac failure, left ventricular dysfunction, hypertension, in children with oedema for any other reason, and in children with risk factors for heart disease.

> **NSAIDs and cardiovascular events**
> The role of cyclo-oxygenase-2 selective inhibitors is undetermined in children. Cyclo-oxygenase-2 selective inhibitors are associated with an increased risk of thrombotic events (e.g. myocardial infarction and stroke) in adults, and they should not be used in preference to non-selective NSAIDs, except when specifically indicated (i.e. for children at a particularly high risk of developing gastroduodenal ulcers or bleeding) *and* after assessing their cardiovascular risk.
>
> In adults, non-selective NSAIDs are also associated with a small increased risk of thrombotic events even when used short-term in those with no cardiovascular risk factors. In adults, **diclofenac** (150 mg daily) and **ibuprofen** (2.4 g daily) are associated with an increased risk of thrombotic events. The increased risk for diclofenac is similar to that of **etoricoxib**. **Naproxen** (in adults, 1 g daily) is associated with a lower thrombotic risk, and lower doses of ibuprofen (in adults, 1.2 g daily or less) have not been associated with an increased risk of myocardial infarction. A small increased thrombotic risk cannot be excluded in children.
>
> The lowest effective dose of NSAID or cyclo-oxygenase-2 selective inhibitor should be prescribed for the shortest period of time to control symptoms, and the need for long-term treatment should be reviewed periodically.

NSAIDs are generally contra-indicated if there is active or previous gastro-intestinal ulceration or bleeding; however, some children may require NSAIDs for effective relief of pain and stiffness. For advice on the prophylaxis and treatment of NSAID-associated gastro-intestinal ulcers, see section 1.3.

For **interactions** of NSAIDs, see Appendix 1 (NSAIDs).

Hepatic impairment NSAIDs should be used with caution in children with hepatic impairment; there is an increased risk of gastro-intestinal bleeding and fluid retention. NSAIDs should be avoided in severe liver disease; see also individual drugs.

Renal impairment NSAIDs should be avoided if possible or used with caution in children with renal impairment; the **lowest effective dose** should be used for the **shortest possible duration**, and renal function should be **monitored**. Sodium and water retention may occur and renal function may deteriorate, possibly leading to renal failure; deterioration in renal function has also been reported after topical use; see also individual drugs.

Pregnancy Most manufacturers advise avoiding NSAIDs during pregnancy or avoiding them unless the potential benefit outweighs risk. NSAIDs should be avoided during the third trimester because use is associated with a risk of closure of fetal ductus arteriosus *in utero* and possibly persistent pulmonary hypertension of the newborn; also, the onset of labour may be delayed and the duration may be increased.

Breast-feeding NSAIDs should be used with caution during breast-feeding; see also individual drugs.

Side-effects The side-effects of NSAIDs vary in severity and frequency. Gastro-intestinal disturbances including discomfort, nausea, diarrhoea, and occasionally bleeding and ulceration may occur (see also notes below and Cautions above).

> **Gastro-intestinal side-effects**
>
> All NSAIDs are associated with gastro-intestinal toxicity. In adults, evidence on the relative safety of NSAIDs indicates differences in the risks of serious upper gastro-intestinal side-effects. **Ibuprofen** is associated with the *lowest risk*; **piroxicam**, **indometacin**, **naproxen**, and **diclofenac** are associated with *intermediate risks* (possibly higher in the case of piroxicam, see also CHMP advice, p. 615). **Selective inhibitors of cyclo-oxygenase-2** are associated with a *lower risk* of serious upper gastro-intestinal side-effects than non-selective NSAIDs.
>
> Children appear to tolerate NSAIDs better than adults and gastro-intestinal side-effects are less common; use of gastro-protective drugs may not be necessary (see also section 1.3).

Other side-effects include hypersensitivity reactions (particularly rashes, angio-edema, and bronchospasm), headache, dizziness, nervousness, depression, drowsiness, insomnia, vertigo, hearing disturbances such as tinnitus, photosensitivity, and haematuria. Blood disorders have also occurred. Fluid retention may occur (rarely precipitating congestive heart failure); blood pressure may be raised.

> **Asthma**
>
> All NSAIDs have the potential to worsen asthma, either acutely or as a gradual worsening of symptoms; consider both prescribed NSAIDs and those that are purchased over the counter.

Renal failure may be provoked by NSAIDs, especially in patients with pre-existing renal impairment (**important**, see Renal impairment above). Rarely, papillary necrosis or interstitial fibrosis associated with NSAIDs can lead to renal failure. Hepatic damage, alveolitis, pulmonary eosinophilia, pancreatitis, visual disturbances, Stevens-Johnson syndrome, and toxic epidermal necrolysis are other rare side-effects. Induction of or exacerbation of colitis or Crohn's disease has been reported. Aseptic meningitis has been reported rarely with NSAIDs—children with connective tissue disorders such as systemic lupus erythematosus may be especially susceptible.

Overdosage: see Emergency Treatment of Poisoning, p. 36.

◢ DICLOFENAC SODIUM

Cautions see notes above; avoid in acute porphyria (section 9.8.2)

Contra-indications see notes above; avoid injections containing benzyl alcohol in neonates (see preparations below)

Intravenous use Additional contra-indications include concomitant NSAID or anticoagulant use (including low-dose heparins), history of haemorrhagic diathesis, history of confirmed or suspected cerebrovascular bleeding, operations with high risk of haemorrhage, history of asthma, moderate or severe renal impairment, hypovolaemia, dehydration

Hepatic impairment see notes above

Renal impairment avoid in severe impairment; see also Intravenous Use and notes above

Pregnancy see notes above

Breast-feeding amount too small to be harmful; see also notes above

Side-effects see notes above; suppositories may cause rectal irritation; injection site reactions

Licensed use not licensed for use in children under 1 year; *suppositories* not licensed for use in children under 6 years except for use in children over 1 year for juvenile idiopathic arthritis; solid dose forms containing more than 25 mg not licensed for use in children; *diclofenac potassium tablets* not licensed for use in children under 14 years; *injection* not licensed for use in children

Indication and dose

Inflammation and mild to moderate pain
- By mouth or by rectum

    Child 6 months–18 years 0.3–1 mg/kg (max. 50 mg) 3 times daily

Postoperative pain
- By rectum

    Child 6–18 years 0.5–1 mg/kg (max. 75 mg) twice daily for max. 4 days; total daily dose may alternatively be given in 3 divided doses

- By intravenous infusion or deep intramuscular injection into gluteal muscle

    Child 2–18 years 0.3–1 mg/kg once or twice daily for max. 2 days (max. 150 mg daily)

Pain and inflammation in rheumatic disease including juvenile idiopathic arthritis
- By mouth

    Child 6 months–18 years 1.5–2.5 mg/kg (max. 75 mg) twice daily; total daily dose may alternatively be given in 3 divided doses

Administration for *intravenous infusion*, dilute 75 mg with 100–500 mL Glucose 5% *or* Sodium Chloride 0.9% (previously buffered with 0.5 mL Sodium Bicarbonate 8.4% solution *or* with 1 mL Sodium Bicarbonate 4.2% solution); give over 30–120 minutes

10 Musculoskeletal and joint diseases

◻ **DICLOFENAC SODIUM** (*continued*)

Diclofenac Sodium (Non-proprietary) [PoM]
Tablets, both e/c, diclofenac sodium 25 mg, net price 84-tab pack = £1.27; 50 mg, 84-tab pack = £1.43. Label: 5, 25
Brands include *Defenac®*, *Dicloflex®*, *Diclozip®*, *Fenactol®*, *Flamrase®*

Dispersible tablets, sugar-free, diclofenac sodium 10 mg
Available from 'special-order' manufacturers or specialist importing companies, see p. 957

Suppositories, diclofenac sodium 100 mg, net price 10 = £3.06
Brands include *Econac®*

Voltarol® (Novartis) [PoM]
Tablets, e/c, diclofenac sodium 25 mg (yellow), net price 84-tab pack = £2.94; 50 mg (brown), 84-tab pack = £4.57. Label: 5, 25

Dispersible tablets, sugar-free, pink, diclofenac, equivalent to diclofenac sodium 50 mg, net price 21-tab pack = £6.19. Label: 13, 21

Injection, diclofenac sodium 25 mg/mL, net price 3-mL amp = 83p
Excipients include benzyl alcohol (avoid in neonates unless there is no safer alternative, see Excipients, p. 3), propylene glycol

Suppositories, diclofenac sodium 12.5 mg, net price 10 = 58p; 25 mg, 10 = £1.03; 50 mg, 10 = £1.70; 100 mg, 10 = £3.03

◢**Diclofenac potassium**
¹**Voltarol® Rapid** (Novartis) [PoM]
Tablets, s/c, diclofenac potassium 25 mg (red), net price 30-tab pack = £4.33; 50 mg (brown), 30-tab pack = £8.28

Dose

> **Rheumatic disease, musculoskeletal disorders, postoperative pain**
> • By mouth
> **Child 14–18 years** 75–100 mg daily in 2–3 divided doses

1. 12.5 mg tablets can be sold to the public for the treatment of headache, dental pain, period pain, rheumatic and muscular pain, backache and the symptoms of cold and flu (including fever), in patients aged over 14 years subject to max. single dose of 25 mg, max. daily dose of 75 mg for max. 3 days, and max. pack size of 18 × 12.5 mg

◢**Modified release**
Diclomax SR® (Galen) [PoM]
Capsules, m/r, yellow, diclofenac sodium 75 mg, net price 56-cap pack = £11.63. Label: 21, 25

Diclomax Retard® (Galen) [PoM]
Capsules, m/r, diclofenac sodium 100 mg, net price 28-cap pack = £8.36. Label: 21, 25

Motifene® 75 mg (Daiichi Sankyo) [PoM]
Capsules, e/c, m/r, diclofenac sodium 75 mg (enclosing e/c pellets containing diclofenac sodium 25 mg and m/r pellets containing diclofenac sodium 50 mg), net price 56-cap pack = £8.00. Label: 25

Voltarol® 75 mg SR (Novartis) [PoM]
Tablets, m/r, pink, diclofenac sodium 75 mg, net price 28-tab pack = £6.46; 56-tab pack = £12.92. Label: 21, 25

Note Other brands of modified-release tablets containing diclofenac sodium 75 mg include *Defenac®* SR, *Dexomon® 75 SR*, *Dicloflex® 75 SR*, *Fenactol® 75 mg SR*, *Flamatak® 75 MR*, *Flamrase® SR*, *Flexotard® MR 75*, *Rheumatac® Retard 75*, *Rhumalgan® CR*, *Slofenac® SR*, *Volsaid® Retard 75*

Voltarol® Retard (Novartis) [PoM]
Tablets, m/r, red, diclofenac sodium 100 mg, net price 28-tab pack = £9.47. Label: 21, 25

Note Other brands of modified-release tablets containing diclofenac sodium 100 mg include *Defenac® Retard*, *Dexomon® Retard 100*, *Dicloflex® Retard*, *Fenactol® Retard 100 mg*, *Flamatak® 100 MR*, , *Rhumalgan® CR*, *Slofenac® SR*, *Volsaid® Retard 100*

━━━━━━━━

◤ **ETORICOXIB**

Cautions see notes above; also dehydration; monitor blood pressure before treatment, 2 weeks after initiation and periodically during treatment

Contra-indications see notes above; inflammatory bowel disease; uncontrolled hypertension (persistently above 140/90 mmHg)

Hepatic impairment max. 60 mg daily in mild impairment; max. 60 mg on alternate days or 30 mg once daily in moderate impairment; see also notes above

Renal impairment avoid if estimated glomerular filtration rate less than 30 mL/minute/1.73 m²; see also notes above

Pregnancy manufacturer advises avoid (teratogenic in *animal* studies); see also notes above

Breast-feeding manufacturer advises avoid—present in milk in *animal* studies; see also notes above

Side-effects see notes above; also palpitation, fatigue, influenza-like symptoms, ecchymosis; *less commonly* dry mouth, taste disturbance, mouth ulcer, appetite and weight change, atrial fibrillation, transient ischaemic attack, chest pain, flushing, cough, dyspnoea, epistaxis, anxiety, mental acuity impaired, paraesthesia, electrolyte disturbance, myalgia and arthralgia; *very rarely* confusion and hallucinations

Musculoskeletal and joint diseases

10

◻ ETORICOXIB (continued)

Indication and dose

Osteoarthritis
- By mouth

  Child 16–18 years 30 mg once daily, increased if necessary to 60 mg once daily

Rheumatoid arthritis and ankylosing spondylitis
- By mouth

  Child 16–18 years 90 mg once daily

Acute gout
- By mouth

  Child 16–18 years 120 mg once daily for max. 8 days

Arcoxia® (MSD) ▼ [PoM]

Tablets, f/c, etoricoxib 30 mg (blue-green), net price 28-tab pack = £13.99; 60 mg (dark green), 28-tab pack = £20.11; 90 mg (white), 28-tab pack = £22.96; 120 mg (pale green), 7-tab pack = £5.74

▌ IBUPROFEN

Cautions see notes above

Contra-indications see notes above

Hepatic impairment see notes above

Renal impairment avoid in severe impairment; see also notes above

Pregnancy see notes above

Breast-feeding amount too small to be harmful, but some manufacturers advise avoid; see also notes above

Side-effects see notes above

Licensed use not licensed for use in children under 3 months or body-weight under 5 kg

Indication and dose

Mild to moderate pain, pain and inflammation of soft-tissue injuries, pyrexia with discomfort
- By mouth

  Child 1–3 months 5 mg/kg 3–4 times daily

  Child 3–6 months 50 mg 3 times daily; max. 30 mg/kg daily in 3–4 divided doses

  Child 6 months–1 year 50 mg 3–4 times daily; max. 30 mg/kg daily in 3–4 divided doses

  Child 1–4 years 100 mg 3 times daily; max. 30 mg/kg daily in 3–4 divided doses

  Child 4–7 years 150 mg 3 times daily; max. 30 mg/kg daily in 3–4 divided doses

  Child 7–10 years 200 mg 3 times daily; max. 30 mg/kg (max. 2.4 g) daily in 3–4 divided doses

  Child 10–12 years 300 mg 3 times daily; max. 30 mg/kg (max. 2.4 g) daily in 3–4 divided doses

  Child 12–18 years initially 300–400 mg 3–4 times daily; increased if necessary to max. 600 mg 4 times daily; maintenance dose of 200–400 mg 3 times daily may be adequate

Pain and inflammation in rheumatic disease including juvenile idiopathic arthritis
- By mouth

  Child 3 months–18 years 30–40 mg/kg (max. 2.4 g) daily in 3–4 divided doses; in systemic juvenile idiopathic arthritis up to 60 mg/kg (max. 2.4 g) daily [unlicensed] in 4–6 divided doses

Post-immunisation pyrexia in infants (see also p. 734)
- By mouth

  Child 2–3 months 50 mg as a single dose repeated once after 6 hours if necessary

Closure of patent ductus arteriosus in neonates
see section 2.14

¹Ibuprofen (Non-proprietary) [PoM]

Tablets, coated, ibuprofen 200 mg, net price 84-tab pack = £2.13; 400 mg, 84-tab pack = £1.87; 600 mg, 84-tab pack = £3.63. Label: 21
Brands include *Arthrofen®*, *Ebufac®*, *Rimafen®*
Dental prescribing on NHS Ibuprofen Tablets may be prescribed

Oral suspension, ibuprofen 100 mg/5 mL, net price 100 mL = £1.47, 150 mL = £2.71, 500 mL = £8.88. Label: 21

Note Sugar-free versions are available and can be ordered by specifying 'sugar-free' on the prescription
Brands include *Calprofen®*, *Feverfen®*, *Nurofen® for Children*, *Orbifen® for Children*

Dental prescribing on NHS Ibuprofen Oral Suspension Sugar-free may be prescribed

1. Can be sold to the public under certain circumstances; for exemptions see *Medicines, Ethics and Practice*, No. 33, London, Pharmaceutical Press, 2009 (and subsequent editions as available)

Brufen® (Abbott) [PoM]

Tablets, f/c, ibuprofen 200 mg, net price 100-tab pack = £3.92; 400 mg, 100-tab pack = £8.16; 600 mg, 100-tab pack = £12.24. Label: 21

Syrup, orange, ibuprofen 100 mg/5 mL, net price 500 mL (orange-flavoured) = £8.88. Label: 21

Granules, effervescent, ibuprofen 600 mg/sachet, net price 20–sachet pack = £6.53. Label: 13, 21
Contains sodium approx. 9 mmol/sachet

◢Modified release

Brufen Retard® (Abbott) [PoM]

Tablets, m/r, ibuprofen 800 mg, net price 56-tab pack = £6.48. Label: 25, 27

Dose

Pain and inflammation
- By mouth

  Child 12–18 years 2 tablets daily as a single dose, preferably in the early evening, increased in severe cases to 3 tablets daily in 2 divided doses

Fenbid® (Goldshield) [PoM]

Spansule® (= capsule m/r), maroon/pink, enclosing off-white pellets, ibuprofen 300 mg, net price 120-cap pack = £9.64. Label: 25

Dose

Pain and inflammation
- By mouth

  Child 12–18 years initially 2 capsules twice daily, increased in severe cases to 3 capsules twice daily; then 1–2 capsules twice daily

10

Musculoskeletal and joint diseases

INDOMETACIN
(Indomethacin)

Cautions see notes above; also epilepsy, psychiatric disturbances; during prolonged therapy ophthalmic and blood examinations particularly advisable; avoid rectal administration in proctitis and haemorrhoids

Skilled tasks Dizziness may affect performance of skilled tasks (e.g. driving)

Contra-indications see notes above

Hepatic impairment see notes above

Renal impairment avoid in severe impairment; see also notes above

Pregnancy see notes above

Breast-feeding amount probably too small to be harmful—manufacturer advises avoid; see also notes above

Side-effects see notes above; *rarely* confusion, convulsions, psychiatric disturbances, syncope, blood disorders (particularly thrombocytopenia), hyperglycaemia, peripheral neuropathy, and intestinal strictures; suppositories may cause rectal irritation and occasional bleeding

Licensed use not licensed for use in children

Indication and dose

> **Relief of pain and inflammation in rheumatic diseases including juvenile idiopathic arthritis**
> - By mouth
>   **Child 1 month–18 years** 0.5–1 mg/kg twice daily; higher doses may be used under specialist supervision

> **Closure of patent ductus arteriosus in premature babies** section 2.14

Indometacin (Non-proprietary) ᴾᵒᴹ
Capsules, indometacin 25 mg, net price 28-cap pack = £1.60; 50 mg, 28-cap pack = £1.78. Label: 21, counselling, driving, see above
Brands include *Rimacid*®

Suppositories, indometacin 100 mg, net price 10 = £15.52. Counselling, driving, see above

Suspension, indometacin 5 mg/mL
Available from 'special-order' manufacturers or specialist importing companies, see p. 957

◢ **Modified release**
Indometacin m/r preparations ᴾᵒᴹ
Capsules, m/r, indometacin 75 mg. Label: 21, 25, counselling, driving, see above
Brands include *Indolar SR*®, *Pardelprin*®

MEFENAMIC ACID

Cautions see notes above; epilepsy; acute porphyria (section 9.8.2)

Contra-indications see notes above; inflammatory bowel disease

Hepatic impairment see notes above

Renal impairment avoid in severe impairment; see also notes above

Pregnancy see notes above

Breast-feeding amount too small to be harmful but manufacturer advises avoid; see also notes above

Side-effects see notes above; also diarrhoea or rashes (withdraw treatment), stomatitis; *less commonly* paraesthesia and fatigue; *rarely* hypotension, palpitation, glucose intolerance, thrombocytopenia, haemolytic anaemia (positive Coombs' test), and aplastic anaemia

Indication and dose

> **Acute pain including dysmenorrhoea, menorrhagia**
> - By mouth
>   **Child 12–18 years** 500 mg 3 times daily

Mefenamic Acid (Non-proprietary) ᴾᵒᴹ
Capsules, mefenamic acid 250 mg, net price 100 = £3.65. Label: 21

Tablets, mefenamic acid 500 mg, net price 28-tab pack = £2.18. Label: 21

Suspension, mefenamic acid 50 mg/5 mL, net price 125 mL = £79.99. Label: 21
Excipients include ethanol

Ponstan® (Chemidex) ᴾᵒᴹ
Capsules, blue/ivory, mefenamic acid 250 mg, net price 100-cap pack = £8.17. Label: 21

Forte tablets, yellow, mefenamic acid 500 mg, net price 100-tab pack = £15.72. Label: 21

MELOXICAM

Cautions see notes above

Contra-indications see notes above

Hepatic impairment see notes above

Renal impairment avoid if estimated glomerular filtration rate less than 25 mL/minute/1.73 m²; see also notes above

Pregnancy see notes above

Breast-feeding present in milk in *animal* studies—manufacturer advises avoid; see also notes above

Side-effects see notes above

Licensed use not licensed for use in children under 16 years

Indication and dose

> **Relief of pain and inflammation in juvenile idiopathic arthritis and other musculoskeletal disorders in children intolerant to other NSAIDs**
> - By mouth
>   **Child 12–18 years and body-weight under 50 kg** 7.5 mg once daily

Musculoskeletal and joint diseases

10

◿ **MELOXICAM** (*continued*)

Child 12–18 years and body-weight over 50 kg
15 mg once daily

Administration *Mobic®* tablets may be dispersed in water

Meloxicam (Non-proprietary) ℞
Tablets, meloxicam 7.5 mg, net price 30-tab pack = £2.64; 15 mg, 30-tab pack = £3.13

Mobic® (Boehringer Ingelheim) ℞
Tablets, yellow, scored, meloxicam 7.5 mg, net price 30-tab pack = £9.30; 15 mg, 30-tab pack = £12.93. Label: 21

▮ **NAPROXEN**

Cautions see notes above; **interactions:** Appendix 1 (NSAIDs)

Contra-indications see notes above

Hepatic impairment see notes above

Renal impairment avoid if estimated glomerular filtration rate less than 30 mL/minute/1.73 m²; see also notes above

Pregnancy see notes above

Breast-feeding amount too small to be harmful but manufacturer advises avoid; see also notes above

Side-effects see notes above

Licensed use not licensed for use in children under 5 years for juvenile idiopathic arthritis; not licensed for use in children under 16 years for musculoskeletal disorders or dysmenorrhoea

Indication and dose

Pain and inflammation in musculoskeletal disorders, dysmenorrhoea
• By mouth
Child 1 month–18 years 5 mg/kg twice daily (max. 1 g daily)

Juvenile idiopathic arthritis
• By mouth
Child 2–18 years 5–7.5 mg/kg twice daily (max. 1 g daily)

¹Naproxen (Non-proprietary) ℞
Tablets, naproxen 250 mg, net price 28-tab pack = £1.42; 500 mg, 28-tab pack = £1.90. Label: 21
Brands include *Arthroxen®*

Tablets, e/c, naproxen 250 mg, net price 56-tab pack = £5.72; 375 mg, 56-tab pack = £26.82; 500 mg, 56-tab pack = £8.47. Label: 5, 25

Suspension, naproxen 25 mg/mL
Available from 'special-order' manufacturers or specialist importing companies, see p. 957

1. Can be sold to the public for the treatment of primary dysmenorrhoea in women aged 15–50 years subject to max. single dose of 500 mg, max. daily dose of 750 mg for max. 3 days, and a max. pack size of 9 × 250 mg tablets; for exemptions see *Medicines, Ethics and Practice*, No. 33, London, Pharmaceutical Press, 2009 (and subsequent editions as available)

Naprosyn® (Roche) ℞
Tablets, yellow, scored, naproxen 250 mg, net price 56-tab pack = £4.37; 500 mg, 56-tab pack = £8.74. Label: 21

Tablets, e/c, (*Naprosyn EC®*), naproxen 250 mg, net price 56-tab pack = £4.37; 375 mg, 56-tab pack = £6.55; 500 mg, 56-tab pack = £8.74. Label: 5, 25

Synflex® (Roche) ℞
Tablets, blue, naproxen sodium 275 mg, net price 60-tab pack = £7.25. Label: 21

Note 275 mg naproxen sodium ≡ 250 mg naproxen

▮ **PIROXICAM** ◿

Cautions see notes above and CHMP advice below

Contra-indications inflammatory gastro-intestinal disease; see also notes above

Hepatic impairment see notes above

Renal impairment see notes above

Pregnancy see notes above

Breast-feeding amount too small to be harmful; see also notes above

Side-effects see notes above

Licensed use not licensed for use in children

Indication and dose

Relief of pain and inflammation in juvenile idiopathic arthritis
• By mouth
Child 6–18 years and body-weight under 15 kg
5 mg daily

Child 6–18 years and body-weight 16–25 kg
10 mg daily

Child 6–18 years and body-weight 26–45 kg
15 mg daily

Child 6–18 years and body-weight over 46 kg
20 mg daily

CHMP advice

Piroxicam (June 2007) The CHMP has recommended restrictions on the use of piroxicam because of the increased risk of gastro-intestinal side effects and serious skin reactions. The CHMP has advised that:

• piroxicam should be initiated only by physicians experienced in treating inflammatory or degenerative rheumatic diseases

• piroxicam should not be used as first-line treatment

• in adults, use of piroxicam should be limited to the symptomatic relief of osteoarthritis, rheumatoid arthritis, and ankylosing spondylitis

• piroxicam dose should not exceed 20 mg daily

• piroxicam should no longer be used for the treatment of acute painful and inflammatory conditions

• treatment should be reviewed 2 weeks after initiating piroxicam, and periodically thereafter

• concomitant administration of a gastro-protective agent (section 1.3) should be considered

Note Topical preparations containing piroxicam are not affected by these restrictions

10 Musculoskeletal and joint diseases

◁ **PIROXICAM (continued)**

Piroxicam (Non-proprietary) PoM ◢

Capsules, piroxicam 10 mg, net price 56-cap pack = £1.99; 20 mg, 28-cap pack = £1.99. Label: 21

Dispersible tablets, piroxicam 10 mg, net price 56-tab pack = £9.96; 20 mg, 28-tab pack = £32.41. Label: 13, 21

Brexidol® (Chiesi) PoM ◢

Tablets, yellow, scored, piroxicam (as betadex) 20 mg, net price 30-tab pack = £14.09. Label: 21

Feldene® (Pfizer) PoM ◢

Capsules, piroxicam 10 mg (maroon/blue), net price 56-cap pack = £7.20; 20 mg (maroon), 28-cap pack = £7.20. Label: 21

Tablets, (*Feldene Melt®*), piroxicam 20 mg, net price 30-tab pack = £9.83. Label: 10, patient information leaflet, 21

Excipients include aspartame equivalent to phenylalanine 140 micrograms/tablet (section 9.4.1)

Note Tablets may be halved [unlicensed] to give 10-mg dose; tablet placed on tongue and allowed to dissolve or may be swallowed

10.1.2 Corticosteroids

10.1.2.1 Systemic corticosteroids

The general actions, uses, and cautions of corticosteroids are described in section 6.3. In children with rheumatic diseases corticosteroids should be reserved for specific indications (e.g. when other anti-inflammatory drugs are unsuccessful) and should be used only under the supervision of a specialist.

Systemic corticosteroids may be considered for the management of juvenile idiopathic arthritis in systemic disease or when several joints are affected. Systemic corticosteroids may also be considered in severe, possibly life-threatening conditions such as systemic lupus erythematosus, systemic vasculitis, juvenile dermatomyositis, Behçet's disease, and polyarticular joint disease.

In severe conditions, short courses ('pulses') of high-dose intravenous methylprednisolone or a pulsed oral corticosteroid may be particularly effective for providing rapid relief, and has fewer long-term adverse effects than continuous treatment.

Corticosteroid doses should be reduced with care because of the possibility of relapse if the reduction is too rapid. If complete discontinuation of corticosteroids is not possible, consideration should be given to alternate-day (or alternate high-dose, low-dose) administration; on days when no corticosteroid is given, or a lower dose is given, an additional dose of a NSAID may be helpful. In some conditions, alternative treatment using an antimalarial or concomitant use of an immunosuppressant drug, such as azathioprine, methotrexate or cyclophosphamide may prove useful; in less severe conditions treatment with a NSAID alone may be adequate.

Administration of corticosteroids may result in suppression of growth and may affect the development of puberty. The risk of corticosteroid-induced osteoporosis should be considered for those on long-term corticosteroid treatment (section 6.6); corticosteroids may also increase the risk of osteopenia in those unable to exercise. For the disadvantages of corticosteroid treatment see section 6.3.2.

10.1.2.2 Local corticosteroid injections

Corticosteroids are injected locally for an anti-inflammatory effect. In inflammatory conditions of the joints, including juvenile idiopathic arthritis, they are given by *intra-articular injection* as an adjunct to long-term therapy to reduce swelling and deformity in one or a few joints. Aseptic precautions (e.g. a no-touch technique) are essential, as is a clinician skilled in the technique; infected areas should be avoided and general anaesthesia, or local anaesthesia, or conscious sedation should be used. Occasionally an acute inflammatory reaction develops after an intra-articular or soft-tissue injection of a corticosteroid. This may be a reaction to the microcrystalline suspension of the corticosteroid used, but must be distinguished from sepsis introduced into the injection site.

Triamcinolone hexacetonide [unlicensed] is preferred for intra-articular injection because it is almost insoluble and has a long-acting (depot) effect. Triamcinolone acetonide and methylprednisolone may also be considered for intra-articular injection into larger joints, whilst hydrocortisone acetate should be reserved for smaller joints or for soft-tissue injections. Intra-articular corticosteroid injections can cause flushing and may affect the hyaline cartilage. Each joint should usually be treated no more than 3–4 times in one year.

A smaller amount of corticosteroid may also be injected directly into soft tissues for the relief of inflammation in conditions such as *tennis* or *golfer's elbow* or *compression neuropathies*, which occur rarely in children. In *tendinitis*, injections should be made into the tendon sheath and not directly into the tendon (due to the absence of a true tendon sheath and a high risk of rupture, the Achilles tendon should not be injected).

Corticosteroid injections are also injected into soft tissues for the treatment of skin lesions (see section 13.4).

◀ LOCAL CORTICOSTEROID INJECTIONS

Cautions see notes above and consult product literature; see also section 6.3.2

Contra-indications see notes above and consult product literature; avoid injections containing benzyl alcohol in neonates (see preparation below)

Side-effects see notes above and consult product literature

Licensed use triamcinolone acetonide not licensed for use in children under 6 years

Indication and dose

See under preparations

◀Hydrocortisone acetate
Hydrocortistab® (Sovereign) PoM
Injection (aqueous suspension), hydrocortisone acetate 25 mg/mL, net price 1-mL amp = £5.72

Dose

• By intra-articular injection
(For details consult product literature)

Child 1 month–12 years 5–30 mg according to size of child and joint

Child 12–18 years 5–50 mg according to size of child and joint

Note Where appropriate may be repeated at intervals of 21 days; not more than 3 joints should be treated on any one day

◀Methylprednisolone acetate
Depo-Medrone® (Pharmacia) PoM
Injection (aqueous suspension), methylprednisolone acetate 40 mg/mL, net price 1-mL vial = £2.87; 2-mL vial = £5.15; 3-mL vial = £7.47

Depo-Medrone® with Lidocaine (Pharmacia) PoM
Injection (aqueous suspension), methylprednisolone acetate 40 mg, lidocaine hydrochloride

10 mg/mL, net price 1-mL vial = £3.28; 2-mL vial = £5.88

◀Triamcinolone hexacetonide
Triamcinolone hexacetonide (Non-proprietary) PoM
Injection, various strengths available from 'special order' manufacturers or specialist importing companies, see, p. 957

Dose

• By intra-articular injection
(For details consult product literature)

Child 1–18 years for larger joints 1 mg/kg (usual max. 20 mg, but higher doses have been used); if appropriate repeat treatment for relapse

◀Triamcinolone acetonide
Adcortyl® Intra-articular/Intradermal (Squibb) PoM
Injection (aqueous suspension), triamcinolone acetonide 10 mg/mL, net price 1-mL amp = 91p; 5-mL vial = £3.70
Excipients include benzyl alcohol (avoid in neonates, see Excipients, p. 3)

Dose

• By intra-articular injection
(For details consult product literature)

Child 1–18 years for larger joints 2 mg/kg (max. 15 mg); for doses above 15 mg use *Kenalog® Intra-articular/Intramuscular*, if appropriate repeat treatment for relapse

Kenalog® Intra-articular/Intramuscular (Squibb) PoM
Injection (aqueous suspension), triamcinolone acetonide 40 mg/mL, net price 1-mL vial = £1.52

Dose

• By intra-articular injection
(For details consult product literature)

Child 1–18 years for larger joints 2 mg/kg (usual max. 40 mg, but higher doses have been used); if appropriate repeat treatment for relapse

10.1.3 Drugs that suppress the rheumatic disease process

Certain drugs, such as methotrexate, cytokine modulators, and sulfasalazine, are used to suppress the disease process in *juvenile idiopathic arthritis* (juvenile chronic arthritis); these drugs are known as disease-modifying antirheumatic drugs (DMARDs). In children, disease-modifying antirheumatic drugs should generally be used under specialist supervision.

Some children with juvenile idiopathic arthritis do not require disease-modifying antirheumatic drugs. Methotrexate is effective in juvenile idiopathic arthritis; sulfasalazine is an alternative but should be avoided in *systemic-onset juvenile idiopathic arthritis*. Gold and penicillamine are no longer used. For the role of cytokine modulators in *polyarticular juvenile idiopathic arthritis*, see p. 620.

Unlike NSAIDs, disease-modifying antirheumatic drugs can affect the progression of disease but they may require 3–6 months of treatment for a full therapeutic response. Response to a disease-modifying antirheumatic drug may allow the dose of the NSAID to be reduced.

Disease-modifying antirheumatic drugs can improve not only the symptoms of inflammatory joint disease but also extra-articular manifestations such as vasculitis. They reduce the erythrocyte sedimentation rate and C-reactive protein.

Antimalarials

The antimalarial **hydroxychloroquine** is rarely used to treat juvenile idiopathic arthritis. Hydroxychloroquine can also be useful for systemic or discoid lupus erythematosus, particularly involving the skin and joints, and in sarcoidosis.

Retinopathy (see below) rarely occurs provided that the recommended doses are not exceeded.

Mepacrine is used on rare occasions to treat discoid lupus erythematosus [unlicensed].

Cautions   Hydroxychloroquine should be used with caution in moderate to severe hepatic impairment and in renal impairment (see Hydroxychloroquine Sulphate, below). Hydroxychloroquine should be used with caution in neurological disorders (especially in those with a history of epilepsy), in severe gastro-intestinal disorders, in G6PD deficiency (section 9.1.5), and in acute porphyria. Hydroxychloroquine may exacerbate psoriasis and aggravate myasthenia gravis. Concurrent use of hepatotoxic drugs should be avoided; other **interactions**: Appendix 1 (chloroquine and hydroxychloroquine).

Pregnancy   It is not necessary to withdraw an antimalarial drug during pregnancy if the rheumatic disease is well controlled; however, the manufacturer of hydroxychloroquine advises avoiding use.

Breast-feeding   Hydroxychloroquine is present in breast milk and breast-feeding should be avoided when it is used to treat rheumatic disease.

> Screening for ocular toxicity
> Hydroxychloroquine is rarely associated with ocular toxicity. The British Society for Paediatric and Adolescent Rheumatology recommends that children should have their vision tested before long-term treatment with hydroxychloroquine and have an annual review of visual acuity. Children should be referred to an ophthalmologist if there is visual impairment, changes in visual acuity, or blurred vision. The Royal College of Ophthalmologists has recommended that a locally agreed protocol between the prescribing doctor and ophthalmologist be established to monitor the vision of these children.

> Important
> To avoid excessive dosage in obese children, the dose of hydroxychloroquine should be calculated on the basis of ideal body-weight; ocular toxicity is unlikely with doses under 5–6.5 mg/kg or max. 400 mg daily.

Side-effects   The side-effects of hydroxychloroquine include gastro-intestinal disturbances, headache, and skin reactions (rashes, pruritus); those occurring less frequently include ECG changes, convulsions, visual changes, retinal damage (see above), keratopathy, ototoxicity, hair depigmentation, hair loss, and discoloration of skin, nails, and mucous membranes. Side-effects that occur rarely include blood disorders (including thrombocytopenia, agranulocytosis, and aplastic anaemia), mental changes (including emotional disturbances and psychosis), myopathy (including cardiomyopathy and neuromyopathy), acute generalised exanthematous pustulosis, exfoliative dermatitis, Stevens-Johnson syndrome, photosensitivity, and hepatic damage; angioedema and bronchospasm have also been reported. **Important**: very toxic in overdosage—immediate advice from poisons centres essential (see also p. 41).

HYDROXYCHLOROQUINE SULPHATE

Cautions see notes above

Hepatic impairment use with caution in moderate to severe impairment

Renal impairment manufacturer advises caution and monitoring of plasma-hydroxychloroquine concentration in severe impairment

Pregnancy see notes above

Breast-feeding avoid—risk of toxicity in infant

Side-effects see notes above

Indication and dose

Juvenile idiopathic arthritis, systemic and discoid lupus erythematosus, dermatological conditions caused or aggravated by sunlight
* By mouth
  Child 1 month–18 years based on ideal body-weight, 5–6.5 mg/kg (max. 400 mg) once daily

Plaquenil® (Sanofi-Aventis) [PoM]
Tablets, f/c, hydroxychloroquine sulphate 200 mg, net price 60-tab pack = £5.25. Label: 5, 21

▲Extemporaneous formulations available see Extemporaneous Preparations, p. 8

Drugs affecting the immune response

Methotrexate, given as a once weekly dose, is the disease-modifying antirheumatic drug of choice in the treatment of juvenile idiopathic arthritis and also has a role in juvenile dermatomyositis, vasculitis, uveitis, systemic lupus erythematosus, localised scleroderma, and sarcoidosis. For these indications it is given by the intramuscular, subcutaneous, or oral routes. Absorption from intramuscular or subcutaneous routes may be more predictable than from the oral route; if the oral route is ineffective subcutaneous administration is generally preferred. Regular full blood counts (including differential white cell count and platelet count), renal and liver function tests are required. Folic acid may reduce mucosal or gastro-intestinal side-effects of methotrexate. The dosage regimen for folic acid has not been established—in children over 2 years a dose of 5 mg weekly may be given, usually at least 24 hours after the dose of methotrexate.

Azathioprine may be used in children for vasculitis which has failed to respond to other treatments, for the management of severe cases of *systemic lupus erythematosus* and other connective tissue disorders, in conjunction with corticosteroids for patients with severe or progressive renal disease, and in cases of *polymyositis* which are resistant to corticosteroids. Azathioprine has a corticosteroid-sparing effect in patients whose corticosteroid requirements are excessive.

Ciclosporin (cyclosporin) is rarely used in juvenile idiopathic arthritis, connective tissue diseases, vasculitis, and uveitis; it may be considered if the condition has failed to respond to other treatments.

AZATHIOPRINE

Cautions section 8.2.1

Contra-indications section 8.2.1

Hepatic impairment section 8.2.1

Renal impairment section 8.2.1

Pregnancy section 8.2.1

Breast-feeding section 8.2.1

Side-effects section 8.2.1

Indication and dose

Systemic lupus erythematosus, vasculitis, auto-immune conditions usually when corticosteroid therapy alone has proved inadequate
see also notes above
* By mouth
  Child 1 month–18 years initially 1 mg/kg daily, adjusted according to response to max. 3 mg/kg daily (consider withdrawal if no improvement within 3 months)

Inflammatory bowel disease section 1.5.3

Transplantation rejection section 8.2.1

▲Preparations
Section 8.2.1

METHOTREXATE

Cautions section 8.1.3; see advice below (blood count, gastro-intestinal, liver, and pulmonary toxicity); extreme caution in blood disorders (avoid if severe); risk of accumulation in pleural effusion or ascites—drain before treatment; full blood count and liver function tests before starting treatment repeated fortnightly for at least the first 4 weeks and at this frequency after any

◁ **METHOTREXATE** *(continued)*

change in dose until therapy stabilised, thereafter monthly; renal function tests before starting treatment and then regularly during treatment; children or their carers should report all symptoms and signs suggestive of infection, especially sore throat; treatment with folinic acid (as calcium folinate, section 8.1) may be required in acute toxicity; check immunity to varicella-zoster and consider vaccination (section 14.4) before initiating therapy; acute porphyria (section 9.8.2); **interactions:** see below and Appendix 1 (methotrexate)

Blood count Bone marrow suppression can occur abruptly; factors likely to increase toxicity include renal impairment and concomitant use with another anti-folate drug. A clinically significant drop in white cell count or platelet count calls for immediate withdrawal of methotrexate and introduction of supportive therapy

Gastro-intestinal toxicity Withdraw treatment if stomatitis develops—may be first sign of gastro-intestinal toxicity

Liver toxicity Persistent 2–fold rise in liver transaminases may necessitate dose reduction or rarely discontinuation; abrupt withdrawal should be avoided as this can lead to disease flare

Pulmonary toxicity Acute pulmonary toxicity is rare in children treated for juvenile idiopathic arthritis, but children and carers should seek medical attention if dyspnoea, cough or fever develops; discontinue if pneumonitis suspected.

NSAIDs Children and carers should be advised to avoid self-medication with over-the-counter ibuprofen

Contra-indications see section 8.1.3 and cautions above

Hepatic impairment avoid—dose-related toxicity; see also Cautions above

Renal impairment section 8.1.3

Pregnancy section 8.1.3

Breast-feeding section 8.1.3

Side-effects section 8.1.3; chronic pulmonary fibrosis; blood dyscrasias (including fatalities); liver cirrhosis

Licensed use not licensed for use in children for non-malignant conditions

Indication and dose

> Juvenile idiopathic arthritis, juvenile dermatomyositis, vasculitis, uveitis, systemic lupus erythematosus, localised scleroderma, sarcoidosis
> • By mouth, subcutaneous injection, or intramuscular injection
> **Child 1 month–18 years** 10–15 mg/m^2 once weekly initially, increased if necessary to max. 25 mg/m^2 once weekly

---

Safe Practice Note that the above dose is a **weekly** dose. To avoid error with low-dose methotrexate, it is recommended that:

- the child or their carer is carefully advised of the **dose** and **frequency** and the reason for taking methotrexate and any other prescribed medicine (e.g. folic acid);
- only one strength of methotrexate tablet (usually 2.5 mg) is prescribed and dispensed;
- the prescription and the dispensing label clearly show the dose and frequency of methotrexate administration;
- the child or their carer is warned to report immediately the onset of any feature of blood disorders (e.g. sore throat, bruising, and mouth ulcers), liver toxicity (e.g. nausea, vomiting, abdominal discomfort, and dark urine), and respiratory effects (e.g. shortness of breath).

Severe Crohn's disease section 1.5.3

Malignant disease section 8.1.3

Psoriasis section 13.5.3

Methotrexate (Non-proprietary) ▣PoM▣
Tablets, yellow, methotrexate 2.5 mg, net price 28-tab pack = £3.27. Counselling, dose, NSAIDs
Brands include *Maxtrex*®

Tablets, yellow, methotrexate 10 mg, net price 100-tab pack = £55.19. Counselling, dose, NSAIDs

Suspension, various strengths available from 'special-order' manufacturers or specialist importing companies, see p. 957

◂**Parenteral preparations**
See also section 8.1.3

Metoject® (Medac) ▣PoM▣
Injection, prefilled syringe, methotrexate (as disodium salt) 50 mg/mL, net price 0.15 mL (7.5 mg) = £14.85, 0.2 mL (10 mg) = £15.29, 0.3 mL (15 mg) = £16.57, 0.4 mL (20 mg) = £17.84, 0.5 mL (25 mg) = £18.48
Note Strength and volume of prefilled syringe has changed

Cytokine modulators

Cytokine modulators should be used under specialist supervision.

Adalimumab, **etanercept**, and **infliximab** inhibit the activity of tumour necrosis factor alpha (TNF-α). Adalimumab and etanercept can be used for the management of active polyarticular juvenile idiopathic arthritis. Infliximab has been used in refractory polyarticular juvenile idiopathic arthritis [unlicensed indication] when other treatments, such as etanercept, have failed.

> ### NICE guidance
>
> **Etanercept for the treatment of juvenile idiopathic arthritis (March 2002)**
> Etanercept is recommended in children aged 4–17 years with active poly-articular-course juvenile idiopathic arthritis who have not responded adequately to methotrexate or who are intolerant of it. Etanercept should be used under specialist supervision according to the guidelines of the British Society for Paediatric and Adolescent Rheumatology [previously the British Paediatric Rheumatology Group].
>
> Etanercept should be withdrawn if severe side-effects develop or if there is no response after 6 months or if the initial response is not maintained. A decision to continue therapy beyond 2 years should be based on disease activity and clinical effectiveness in individual cases.
>
> Prescribers of etanercept should register consenting patients with the Biologics Registry of the British Society for Paediatric and Adolescent Rheumatology.

Side-effects Adalimumab, etanercept, and infliximab have been associated with infections, sometimes severe, including tuberculosis, septicaemia, and hepatitis B reactivation. Other side-effects include nausea, abdominal pain, worsening heart failure, hypersensitivity reactions (including angioedema, bronchospasm, urticaria, and anaphylaxis), fever, headache, depression, antibody formation (including lupus erythematosus-like syndrome), pruritus, injection-site reactions, and blood disorders (including anaemia, leucopenia, thrombocytopenia, pancytopenia, aplastic anaemia).

Abatacept prevents the full activation of T-lymphocytes; it can be used for the management of active polyarticular juvenile idiopathic arthritis. Abatacept is not recommended for use in combination with TNF inhibitors.

◢ ABATACEPT

Cautions predisposition to infection (screen for latent tuberculosis and viral hepatitis); do not initiate until active infections are controlled; children should be brought up to date with current immunisation schedule (section 14.1) before initiating therapy; progressive multifocal leucoencephalopathy—discontinue treatment if neurological symptoms present; **interactions:** Appendix 1 (abatacept)

Contra-indications severe infection (see also Cautions)

Pregnancy manufacturer advises avoid unless essential—effective contraception required during treatment and for 14 weeks after last dose

Breast-feeding present in milk in *animal* studies—manufacturer advises avoid breast-feeding during treatment and for 14 weeks after last dose

Side-effects abdominal pain, diarrhoea, dyspepsia, nausea; flushing, hypertension; cough; dizziness, fatigue, headache; infection, rhinitis; rash; *less commonly* gastritis, stomatitis, tachycardia, bradycardia, palpitation, hypotension, dyspnoea, paraesthesia, weight gain, depression, anxiety, amenorrhoea, basal cell carcinoma, thrombocytopenia, leucopenia, arthralgia, pain in extremities, conjunctivitis, visual disturbance, vertigo, bruising, alopecia, and dry skin

Indication and dose

> Moderate to severe active polyarticular juvenile idiopathic arthritis (in combination with methotrexate) in children who have not responded adequately to other disease-modifying antirheumatic drugs (including at least one tumour necrosis factor (TNF) inhibitor)
>
> • By intravenous infusion
>
> **Child 6–17 years**
>
> **Body-weight less than 75 kg** 10 mg/kg, repeated 2 weeks and 4 weeks after initial infusion, then every 4 weeks
>
> **Body-weight 75–100 kg** 750 mg, repeated 2 weeks and 4 weeks after initial infusion, then every 4 weeks
>
> **Body-weight over 100 kg** 1 g, repeated 2 weeks and 4 weeks after initial infusion, then every 4 weeks
>
> Note Review treatment if no response within 6 months

Administration for *intravenous infusion*, reconstitute each vial with 10 mL water for injections using the silicone-free syringe provided; dilute requisite dose in Sodium Chloride 0.9% to 100 mL (using the same silicone-free syringe); give over 30 minutes through a low protein-binding filter (pore size 0.2–1.2 micron)

Orencia® (Bristol-Myers Squibb) ▼ [PoM]
Intravenous infusion, powder for reconstitution, abatacept, net price 250-mg vial = £242.17
Electrolytes Na⁺<0.5 mmol/vial

10 Musculoskeletal and joint diseases

ADALIMUMAB

Cautions predisposition to infection; monitor for infections before, during, and for 5 months after treatment (see also Tuberculosis below); do not initiate until active infections are controlled; discontinue if new serious infection develops; hepatitis B virus—monitor for active infection; children should be brought up to date with current immunisation schedule (section 14.1) before initiating therapy; mild heart failure (discontinue if symptoms develop or worsen—avoid in moderate or severe heart failure); demyelinating CNS disorders (risk of exacerbation); history of malignancy; monitor for non-melanoma skin cancer before and during treatment, especially in children with history of PUVA treatment for psoriasis or extensive immunosuppressant therapy; **interactions**: Appendix 1 (adalimumab)

Tuberculosis Children should be evaluated for tuberculosis before treatment. Active tuberculosis should be treated with standard treatment (section 5.1.9) for at least 2 months before starting adalimumab. Children who have previously received adequate treatment for tuberculosis can start adalimumab but should be monitored every 3 months for possible recurrence. In those without active tuberculosis but who were previously not treated adequately, chemoprophylaxis should ideally be completed before starting adalimumab. In children at high risk of tuberculosis who cannot be assessed by tuberculin skin test, chemoprophylaxis can be given concurrently with adalimumab. Children and their carers should be advised to seek medical attention if symptoms suggestive of tuberculosis (e.g. persistent cough, weight loss, and fever) develop

Contra-indications severe infection (see also Cautions)

Pregnancy avoid; manufacturer advises effective contraception required during treatment and for at least 5 months after last dose

Breast-feeding avoid; manufacturer advises avoid for at least 5 months after last dose

Side-effects see under Cytokine Modulators, p. 621 and Cautions above; also vomiting, dyspepsia, gastro-intestinal haemorrhage; dizziness, hyperlipidaemia, hypertension, oedema, flushing, chest pain, tachycardia; cough, dyspnoea; mood changes, sleep disturbances, anxiety, paraesthesia; haematuria, renal impairment; benign tumours, non-melanoma skin cancers; electrolyte disturbances, hyperuricaemia; musculoskeletal pain; eye disorders; rash, dermatitis, onycholysis, impaired healing; *less commonly* dysphagia, pancreatitis, cholelithiasis, hepatic steatosis, cholecystitis, arrhythmias, interstitial lung disease, pneumonitis, tremor, erectile dysfunction, nocturia, malignancy, rhabdomyolysis, hearing loss, tinnitus; *rarely* vascular occlusion, myocardial infarction, demyelinating disorders; Stevens-Johnson syndrome, cutaneous vasculitis, new onset or worsening psoriasis, and hepatosplenic T-cell lymphoma also reported

Indication and dose

Active polyarticular juvenile idiopathic arthritis (in combination with methotrexate or alone if methotrexate inappropriate) in children who have not responded adequately to one or more disease-modifying antirheumatic drug

• By subcutaneous injection

   Child 13–17 years 40 mg on alternate weeks; review treatment if no response within 12 weeks

Humira® (Abbott) ▼ PoM
Injection, adalimumab, net price 40-mg prefilled pen or prefilled syringe = £357.50. Counselling, tuberculosis

ETANERCEPT

Cautions predisposition to infection (avoid if predisposition to septicaemia); significant exposure to herpes zoster virus—interrupt treatment and consider varicella–zoster immunoglobulin; hepatitis B virus—monitor for active infection; monitor for worsening hepatitis C infection; children should be brought up to date with current immunisation schedule (section 14.1) before initiating therapy; heart failure (risk of exacerbation); demyelinating CNS disorders (risk of exacerbation); history of malignancy; monitor for non-melanoma skin cancer in those at risk, including children with psoriasis or a history of PUVA treatment; history of blood disorders; **interactions**: Appendix 1 (etanercept)

Tuberculosis Children should be evaluated for tuberculosis before treatment. Active tuberculosis should be treated with standard treatment (section 5.1.9) for at least 2 months before starting etanercept. Children who have previously received adequate treatment for tuberculosis can start etanercept but should be monitored every 3 months for possible recurrence. In those without active tuberculosis but who were previously not treated adequately, chemoprophylaxis should ideally be completed before starting etanercept. In children at high risk of tuberculosis who cannot be assessed by tuberculin skin test, chemoprophylaxis can be given concurrently with etanercept. Children and their carers should be advised to seek medical attention if symptoms suggestive of tuber-

culosis (e.g. persistent cough, weight loss, and fever) develop

Blood disorders Children and their carers should be advised to seek medical attention if symptoms suggestive of blood disorders (such as fever, sore throat, bruising, or bleeding) develop

Contra-indications active infection; avoid injections containing benzyl alcohol in neonates (see preparations below)

Hepatic impairment use with caution in moderate to severe alcoholic hepatitis

Pregnancy manufacturer advises avoid—no information available

Breast-feeding manufacturer advises avoid—present in milk in *animal* studies

Side-effects see under Cytokine Modulators, p. 621; also *less commonly* interstitial lung disease, non-melanoma skin cancer, rash; *rarely* demyelinating disorders, seizures, Stevens-Johnson syndrome, and cutaneous vasculitis; *very rarely* toxic epidermal necrolysis; *also reported* appendicitis, cholecystitis, gastritis, gastro-intestinal haemorrhage, intestinal obstruction, liver damage, oesophagitis, pancreatitis, ulcerative colitis, vomiting, cerebral ischaemia, hypertension, hypotension, myocardial infarction, thrombophlebitis, thromboembolism, asthma,

ETANERCEPT (continued)

dyspnoea, aseptic meningitis, confusion, paresis, paraesthesia, vertigo, lymphadenopathy, diabetes mellitus, haematuria, malignancy, renal calculi, renal impairment, bone fracture, bursitis, polymyositis, scleritis, and cutaneous ulcer

Indication and dose

Active polyarticular juvenile idiopathic arthritis in children who have had an inadequate response to methotrexate or who cannot tolerate it

- **By subcutaneous injection**

  Child 4–17 years 400 micrograms/kg (max. 25 mg) twice weekly, with an interval of 3–4 days between doses

Severe plaque psoriasis section 13.5.3

Enbrel® (Wyeth) ▼ PoM

Injection, powder for reconstitution, etanercept, net price 25-mg vial (with solvent) = £89.38. Label: 10, alert card, counselling, tuberculosis and blood disorders

Paediatric injection, powder for reconstitution, etanercept, net price 25-mg vial (with solvent) = £89.38. Label: 10, alert card, counselling, tuberculosis and blood disorders
Excipients include benzyl alcohol (avoid in neonates, see Excipients, p. 3)

Injection, etanercept, net price 25-mg prefilled syringe = £89.38; 50-mg prefilled pen or prefilled syringe = £178.75. Label: 10, alert card, counselling, tuberculosis and blood disorders

---

Sulfasalazine

Sulfasalazine (sulphasalazine) has a beneficial effect in suppressing the inflammatory activity associated with some forms of juvenile idiopathic arthritis; it is generally not used in systemic-onset disease. Sulfasalazine may cause haematological abnormalities including leucopenia, neutropenia, and thrombocytopenia and close monitoring of full blood counts (including differential white cell count and platelet count) is necessary initially, and at monthly intervals during the first 3 months (liver-function tests also being performed at monthly intervals for the first 3 months). Although the manufacturer recommends renal function tests, evidence of practical value is unsatisfactory. For use of sulfasalazine also see section 1.5.1, aminosalicylates.

SULFASALAZINE

(Sulphasalazine)

Cautions see section 1.5.1 and notes above
Contra-indications see section 1.5.1
Hepatic impairment section 1.5.1
Renal impairment section 1.5.1
Pregnancy section 1.5.1
Breast-feeding section 1.5.1
Side-effects see section 1.5.1 and notes above
Licensed use not licensed for use in children for juvenile idiopathic arthritis

Indication and dose

Juvenile idiopathic arthritis (see also notes above)

- **By mouth**

  Child 2–18 years initially 5 mg/kg twice daily for 1 week, then 10 mg/kg twice daily for 1 week, then 20 mg/kg twice daily for 1 week, maintenance dose 20–25 mg/kg twice daily; Child 2–12 years max. 2 g daily, Child 12–18 years max. 3 g daily

Preparations
Section 1.5.1

10.1.4 Gout and cytotoxic-induced hyperuricaemia

This section is not included in *BNF for Children*. For the role of allopurinol and rasburicase in the prophylaxis of hyperuricaemia associated with cancer chemotherapy and in enzyme disorders causing increased serum urate, see section 8.1. The management of gout in adolescents requires specialist supervision.

10.1.5 Other drugs for rheumatic diseases

Classification not used in *BNF for Children*.

10 Musculoskeletal and joint diseases

10.2 Drugs used in neuromuscular disorders

10.2.1 Drugs that enhance neuromuscular transmission
10.2.2 Skeletal muscle relaxants

10.2.1 Drugs that enhance neuromuscular transmission

Anticholinesterases are used as first-line treatment in *ocular myasthenia gravis* and as an adjunct to immunosuppressant therapy for *generalised myasthenia gravis*.

Corticosteroids are used when anticholinesterases do not control symptoms completely. A second-line immunosuppressant such as azathioprine is frequently used to reduce the dose of corticosteroid.

Plasmapheresis or infusion of intravenous immunoglobulin [unlicensed indication] may induce temporary remission in severe relapses, particularly where bulbar or respiratory function is compromised or before thymectomy.

Anticholinesterases

Anticholinesterase drugs enhance neuromuscular transmission in voluntary and involuntary muscle in myasthenia gravis. They prolong the action of acetylcholine by inhibiting the action of the enzyme acetylcholinesterase. Excessive dosage of these drugs can impair neuromuscular transmission and precipitate cholinergic crises by causing a depolarising block. This may be difficult to distinguish from a worsening myasthenic state.

Muscarinic side-effects of anticholinesterases include increased sweating, increased salivary and gastric secretions, increased gastro-intestinal and uterine motility, and bradycardia. These parasympathomimetic effects are antagonised by atropine.

Edrophonium has a very brief action and it is therefore used mainly for the diagnosis of myasthenia gravis. However, such testing should be performed only by those experienced in its use; other means of establishing the diagnosis are available. A single test-dose usually causes substantial improvement in muscle power (lasting about 5 minutes) in patients with the disease (if respiration already impaired, *only* in conjunction with someone skilled at intubation).

Edrophonium can also be used to determine whether a patient with myasthenia is receiving inadequate or excessive treatment with cholinergic drugs. If treatment is excessive an injection of edrophonium will either have no effect or will intensify symptoms (if respiration already impaired, give *only* in conjunction with someone skilled at intubation). Conversely, transient improvement may be seen if the patient is being inadequately treated. The test is best performed just before the next dose of anticholinesterase.

Neostigmine produces a therapeutic effect for up to 4 hours. Its pronounced muscarinic action is a disadvantage, and simultaneous administration of an antimuscarinic drug such as atropine or propantheline may be required to prevent colic, excessive salivation, or diarrhoea. In severe disease neostigmine can be given every 2 hours. In infants, neostigmine by either subcutaneous or intramuscular injection is preferred for the short-term management of myasthenia.

Pyridostigmine is less powerful and slower in action than neostigmine but it has a longer duration of action. It is preferable to neostigmine because of its smoother action and the need for less frequent dosage. It is particularly preferred in patients whose muscles are weak on waking. It has a comparatively mild gastro-intestinal effect but an antimuscarinic drug may still be required. It is inadvisable to use excessive doses because acetylcholine receptor down regulation may occur. Immunosuppressant therapy may be considered if high doses of pyridostigmine are needed. Neostigmine and pyridostigmine should be given to neonates 30 minutes before feeds to improve suckling.

Neostigmine and edrophonium are also used to reverse the actions of the non-depolarising neuromuscular blocking drugs (section 15.1.6).

NEOSTIGMINE

Cautions asthma (*extreme* caution), bradycardia, arrhythmias, recent myocardial infarction, epilepsy, hypotension, parkinsonism, vagotonia, peptic ulceration, hyperthyroidism; atropine or

▱ **NEOSTIGMINE (continued)**

other antidote to muscarinic effects may be necessary (particularly when neostigmine is given by injection), but not given routinely because it may mask signs of overdosage; **interactions:** Appendix 1 (parasympathomimetics)

Contra-indications intestinal or urinary obstruction

Renal impairment may need dose reduction

Pregnancy manufacturer advises use only if potential benefit outweighs risk

Breast-feeding amount probably too small to be harmful

Side-effects nausea, vomiting, increased salivation, diarrhoea, abdominal cramps (more marked with higher doses); signs of overdosage include bronchoconstriction, increased bronchial secretions, lacrimation, excessive sweating, involuntary defaecation and micturition, miosis, nystagmus, bradycardia, heart block, arrhythmias, hypotension, agitation, excessive dreaming, and weakness eventually leading to fasciculation and paralysis

Indication and dose

Treatment of myasthenia gravis
• By mouth (as neostigmine bromide)

Neonate initially 1–2 mg, then 1–5 mg every 4 hours, give 30 minutes before feeds

Child up to 6 years initially 7.5 mg repeated at suitable intervals throughout the day, total daily dose 15–90 mg

Child 6–12 years initially 15 mg repeated at suitable intervals throughout the day, total daily dose 15–90 mg

Child 12–18 years initially 15–30 mg repeated at suitable intervals throughout the day, total daily dose 75–300 mg (but max. most can tolerate is 180 mg daily)

• By subcutaneous or intramuscular injection (as neostigmine metilsulfate)

Neonate 150 micrograms/kg every 6–8 hours, 30 minutes before feeds, increased to max. 300 micrograms/kg every 4 hours, if necessary [unlicensed]

Child 1 month–12 years 200–500 micrograms repeated at suitable intervals throughout the day

Child 12–18 years 1–2.5 mg repeated at suitable intervals throughout the day

Neostigmine (Non-proprietary) [PoM]
Tablets, scored, neostigmine bromide 15 mg, net price 140 = £56.10

◢ Injection
Section 15.1.6

◢ **EDROPHONIUM CHLORIDE**

Cautions see under Neostigmine; have resuscitation facilities; *extreme* caution in respiratory distress (see notes above) and in asthma
Note Severe cholinergic reactions can be counteracted by injection of atropine sulphate (which should always be available)

Contra-indications see under Neostigmine
Pregnancy see under Neostigmine
Breast-feeding see under Neostigmine
Side-effects see under Neostigmine

Indication and dose

Diagnostic test for myasthenia gravis
• By intravenous injection

Child 1 month–12 years 20 micrograms/kg followed after 30 seconds (if no adverse reaction has occurred) by 80 micrograms/kg

Child 12–18 years 2 mg followed after 30 seconds (if no adverse reaction has occurred) by 8 mg

Detection of overdosage or underdosage of cholinergic drugs
• By intravenous injection

Child 1 month–12 years 20 micrograms/kg (preferably just before next dose of anticholinesterase, see notes above)

Child 12–18 years 2 mg (preferably just before next dose of anticholinesterase, see notes above)

Edrophonium (Non-proprietary) [PoM]
Injection, edrophonium chloride 10 mg/mL, net price 1-mL amp = £8.65

◢ **PYRIDOSTIGMINE BROMIDE**

Cautions see under Neostigmine; weaker muscarinic action
Contra-indications see under Neostigmine
Renal impairment reduce dose; excreted by kidney
Pregnancy see under Neostigmine
Breast-feeding see under Neostigmine
Side-effects see under Neostigmine

Indication and dose

Treatment of myasthenia gravis
• By mouth

Neonate initially 1–1.5 mg/kg, increased gradually to max. 10 mg, repeated throughout the day, give 30–60 minutes before feeds

Child 1 month–12 years initially 1–1.5 mg/kg/day, increased gradually to 7 mg/kg/day in 6 divided doses; usual total daily dose 30–360 mg

Child 12–18 years 30–120 mg, repeated throughout the day; usual total daily dose 300–600 mg (but consider immunosuppressant ther-

10

Musculoskeletal and joint diseases

○ **PYRIDOSTIGMINE BROMIDE** (*continued*)

apy if total daily dose exceeds 360 mg, down-regulation of acetylcholine receptors possible if total daily dose exceeds 450 mg; see notes above)

Mestinon® (Meda) PoM
Tablets, scored, pyridostigmine bromide 60 mg, net price 200 = £48.12

◢ Extemporaneous formulations available see Extemporaneous Preparations, p. 8

Immunosuppressant therapy

A course of **corticosteroids** (section 6.3) is an established treatment in severe cases of myasthenia gravis and may be particularly useful when antibodies to the acetylcholine receptor are present in high titre. Short courses of high-dose ('pulsed') methylprednisolone followed by maintenance therapy with oral corticosteroids may also be useful.

Corticosteroid treatment is usually initiated under specialist supervision. For disadvantages of corticosteroid treatment, see section 6.3.2. Transient but very serious worsening of symptoms can occur in the first 2–3 weeks, especially if the corticosteroid is started at a high dose. Once remission has occurred (usually after 2–6 months), the dose of prednisolone should be reduced slowly to the minimum effective dose.

10.2.2 Skeletal muscle relaxants

The drugs described below are used for the relief of chronic muscle spasm or spasticity associated with neurological damage; they are not indicated for spasm associated with minor injuries. They act principally on the central nervous system with the exception of dantrolene, which has a peripheral site of action. They differ in action from the muscle relaxants used in anaesthesia (section 15.1.5), which block transmission at the neuromuscular junction.

The underlying cause of spasticity should be treated and any aggravating factors (e.g. pressure sores, infection) remedied. Skeletal muscle relaxants are effective in most forms of spasticity except the rare alpha variety. The major disadvantage of treatment with these drugs is that reduction in muscle tone can cause a loss of splinting action of the spastic leg and trunk muscles and sometimes lead to an increase in disability.

Dantrolene acts directly on skeletal muscle and produces fewer central adverse effects. It is generally used in resistant cases. The dose should be increased slowly.

Baclofen inhibits transmission at spinal level and also depresses the central nervous system. The dose should be increased slowly to avoid the major side-effects of sedation and muscular hypotonia (other adverse events are uncommon).

Diazepam has undoubted efficacy in some children. Sedation and occasionally extensor hypotonus are disadvantages. Other benzodiazepines also have muscle-relaxant properties.

▌ BACLOFEN

Cautions psychiatric illness; respiratory impairment; epilepsy; history of peptic ulcer (avoid oral route in active peptic ulceration); diabetes; hypertonic bladder sphincter; avoid abrupt withdrawal (risk of hyperactive state, may exacerbate spasticity, and precipitate autonomic dysfunction including hyperthermia, psychiatric reactions and convulsions, see also under Withdrawal below); **interactions**: Appendix 1 (muscle relaxants)

Withdrawal CSM has advised that serious side-effects can occur on abrupt withdrawal; to minimise risk, discontinue by gradual dose reduction over at least 1–2 weeks (longer if symptoms occur)

Skilled tasks Drowsiness may affect performance of skilled tasks (e.g. driving); effects of alcohol enhanced

Hepatic impairment manufacturer advises use by mouth with caution

Renal impairment risk of toxicity—use smaller oral doses and if necessary increase dosage interval; if estimated glomerular filtration rate less than 15 mL/minute/1.73m² use by mouth only if potential benefit outweighs risk; excreted by kidney

Pregnancy manufacturer advises use only if potential benefit outweighs risk (toxicity in *animal* studies)

Breast-feeding present in milk—amount probably too small to be harmful

Side-effects gastro-intestinal disturbances, dry mouth; hypotension, respiratory or cardiovascular depression; sedation, drowsiness, confusion, dizziness, ataxia, hallucinations, nightmares, headache, euphoria, insomnia, depression,

◻ BACLOFEN (*continued*)

anxiety, agitation, tremor; seizure; urinary disturbances; myalgia; visual disorders; rash, hyperhidrosis; *rarely* taste disturbances, abdominal pain, changes in hepatic function, paraesthesia, erectile dysfunction, dysarthria; *very rarely* hypothermia

Indication and dose

Chronic severe spasticity of voluntary muscle
• By mouth

Child 1–2 years initially 300 micrograms/kg daily in 4 divided doses, increased gradually to usual maintenance dose of 0.75–2 mg/kg daily in divided doses (*or* 10–20 mg daily in divided doses); review treatment if no benefit within 6 weeks

Child 2–6 years initially 300 micrograms/kg daily in 4 divided doses, increased gradually to usual maintenance dose of 0.75–2 mg/kg daily in divided doses (*or* 20–30 mg daily in divided doses); review treatment if no benefit within 6 weeks

Child 6–8 years initially 300 micrograms/kg daily in 4 divided doses, increased gradually to usual maintenance dose of 0.75–2 mg/kg daily in divided doses (*or* 30–40 mg daily in divided doses); review treatment if no benefit within 6 weeks

Child 8–10 years initially 300 micrograms/kg daily in 4 divided doses, increased gradually to usual maintenance dose of 0.75–2 mg/kg daily in divided doses (*or* up to 60 mg daily in divided doses); review treatment if no benefit within 6 weeks

Child 10–18 years initially 5 mg 3 times daily increased gradually; usual maintenance dose up to 60 mg daily in divided doses (max. 100 mg daily); review treatment if no benefit within 6 weeks

Severe chronic spasticity of cerebral origin unresponsive to oral antispastic drugs (or oral therapy not tolerated), as alternative to ablative neurosurgical procedures—specialist use only
• By intrathecal injection

Child 4–18 years initial *test dose* 25 micrograms over at least 1 minute via catheter or lumbar puncture, increased in 25-microgram steps (not more often than every 24 hours) to max. 100 micrograms to determine appropriate dose *then dose-titration phase*, most often using infusion pump (implanted into chest wall or abdominal wall tissues) to establish *maintenance dose* (ranging from 24 micrograms to 1.2 mg daily in children under 12 years or 1.4 mg daily for those over 12 years) retaining some spasticity to avoid sensation of paralysis

Safe Practice Consult product literature for details on dose testing and titration—important to monitor patients closely in appropriately equipped and staffed environment during screening and immediately after pump implantation. Resuscitation equipment must be available for immediate use

Baclofen (Non-proprietary) PoM
Tablets, baclofen 10 mg, net price 84-tab pack = £1.59. Label: 2, 8, 21

Oral solution, baclofen 5 mg/5 mL, net price 300 mL = £10.00. Label: 2, 8, 21
Brands include *Lyflex®* (sugar-free)

Lioresal® (Novartis) PoM
Tablets, scored, baclofen 10 mg, net price 84-tab pack = £10.84. Label: 2, 8, 21
Excipients include gluten

Liquid, sugar-free, raspberry–flavoured, baclofen 5 mg/5 mL, net price 300 mL = £8.95. Label: 2, 8, 21

◀By intrathecal injection
Lioresal® (Novartis) PoM
Intrathecal injection, baclofen, 50 micrograms/mL, net price 1-mL amp (for test dose) = £2.74; 500 micrograms/mL, 20-mL amp (for use with implantable pump) = £60.77; 2 mg/mL, 5-mL amp (for use with implantable pump) = £60.77

◢ DANTROLENE SODIUM

Cautions impaired cardiac and pulmonary function; therapeutic effect may take a few weeks to develop—discontinue if no response within 45 days; **interactions:** Appendix 1 (muscle relaxants)

Hepatotoxicity Potentially life-threatening hepatotoxicity reported, usually if doses greater than 400 mg daily used, in females, if history of liver disorders, or concomitant use of hepatotoxic drugs; test liver function before and at intervals during therapy—discontinue if abnormal liver function tests or symptoms of liver disorder (counselling, see below); re-introduce only if complete reversal of hepatotoxicity

Counselling Children and their carers should be told how to recognise signs of liver disorder and advised to seek prompt medical attention if symptoms such as anorexia,

nausea, vomiting, fatigue, abdominal pain, dark urine, or pruritus develop

Skilled tasks Drowsiness may affect performance of skilled tasks (eg. driving); effects of alcohol enhanced

Contra-indications acute muscle spasm; avoid when spasticity is useful, for example, locomotion

Hepatic impairment avoid—may cause severe liver damage; injection may be used in an emergency for malignant hyperthermia

Pregnancy avoid use in chronic spasticity—embryotoxic in *animal* studies

Breast-feeding present in milk—manufacturer advises avoid use in chronic spasticity

Side-effects diarrhoea (withdraw if severe, discontinue treatment if recurs on re-introduction),

10

Musculoskeletal and joint diseases

◁ **DANTROLENE SODIUM** *(continued)*

nausea, vomiting, anorexia, hepatotoxicity (see above), abdominal pain; pericarditis; pleural effusion, respiratory depression; headache, drowsiness, dizziness, asthenia, fatigue, seizures, fever, chills; speech and visual disturbances; rash; *less commonly* dysphagia, constipation, exacerbation of cardiac insufficiency, tachycardia, erratic blood pressure, dyspnoea, depression, confusion, nervousness, insomnia, increased urinary frequency, urinary incontinence or retention, haematuria, crystalluria, and increased sweating

Licensed use not licensed for use in children

Indication and dose

Chronic severe spasticity of voluntary muscle
• By mouth
  Child 5–12 years initially 500 micrograms/kg once daily; after 7 days increase to 500 micr-

ograms/kg/dose 3 times daily; every 7 days increase by further 500 micrograms/kg/dose until satisfactory response; max. 2 mg/kg 3–4 times daily (max. total daily dose 400 mg)

  Child 12–18 years initially 25 mg once daily; increase to 3 times daily after 7 days; every 7 days increase by further 500 micrograms/kg/dose until satisfactory response; max. 2 mg/kg 3–4 times daily (max. total daily dose 400 mg)

Malignant hyperthermia section 15.1.8

Dantrium® (SpePharm) [PoM]
Capsules, orange/brown, dantrolene sodium 25 mg, net price 100 = £16.87; 100 mg, 100 = £43.07. Label: 2, counselling, driving, hepatotoxicity

---

DIAZEPAM

Cautions section 4.8.2
Contra-indications section 4.8.2
Hepatic impairment section 4.8.2
Renal impairment section 4.8.2
Pregnancy section 4.8.2
Breast-feeding section 4.8.2
Side-effects section 4.8.2; also hypotonia

Indication and dose

Muscle spasm in cerebral spasticity or in postoperative skeletal muscle spasm
• By mouth
  Child 1–12 months initially 250 microgram/kg twice daily
  Child 1–5 years initially 2.5 mg twice daily
  Child 5–12 years initially 5 mg twice daily
  Child 12–18 years initially 10 mg twice daily; max. total daily dose 40 mg

Tetanus
• By intravenous injection
  Child 1 month–18 years 100–300 micrograms/kg repeated every 1–4 hours

• By intravenous infusion (or by nasoduodenal tube)
  Child 1 month–18 years 3–10 mg/kg over 24 hours, adjusted according to response

Status epilepticus section 4.8.2

Febrile convulsions section 4.8.3

Peri-operative use section 15.1.4.1

Administration for *continuous intravenous infusion* of diazepam emulsion, dilute to a concentration of max. 400 micrograms/mL with Glucose 5% or 10%; max. 6 hours between addition and completion of infusion; diazepam adsorbed by plastics of infusion bags and giving sets
For *continuous intravenous infusion* of diazepam solution, dilute to a concentration of max. 50 micrograms/mL with Glucose 5% or Sodium Chloride 0.9%; diazepam adsorbed by plastics of infusion bags and giving sets

◢ Oral preparations
Section 15.1.4.1

◢ Parenteral preparations
Section 4.8.2

10.3 Drugs for the relief of soft-tissue inflammation

10.3.1 Enzymes
10.3.2 Rubefacients and other topical antirheumatics

Extravasation

Local guidelines for the management of extravasation should be followed where they exist or specialist advice sought.

Extravasation injury follows leakage of drugs or intravenous fluids from the veins or inadvertent administration into the subcutaneous or subdermal tissue. It must be dealt with **promptly** to prevent tissue necrosis.

10 Musculoskeletal and joint diseases

Acidic or alkaline preparations and those with an osmolarity greater than that of plasma can cause extravasation injury; excipients including alcohol and poly-ethylene glycol have also been implicated. Cytotoxic drugs commonly cause extravasation injury. Very young children are at increased risk. Those receiving anticoagulants are more likely to lose blood into surrounding tissues if extravasa-tion occurs, while those receiving sedatives or analgesics may not notice the early signs or symptoms of extravasation.

Prevention of extravasation   Precautions should be taken to avoid extravasa-tion; ideally, drugs likely to cause extravasation injury should be given through a central line and children receiving repeated doses of hazardous drugs peripherally should have the cannula resited at regular intervals. Attention should be paid to the manufacturers' recommendations for administration. Placing a glyceryl tri-nitrate patch or using glyceryl trinitrate ointment distal to the cannula may improve the patency of the vessel in children with small veins or in those whose veins are prone to collapse.

Children or their carers should be asked to report any pain or burning at the site of injection immediately.

Management of extravasation   If extravasation is suspected the infusion should be stopped immediately but the cannula should not be removed until after an attempt has been made to aspirate the area (through the cannula) in order to remove as much of the drug as possible. Aspiration is sometimes possible if the extravasation presents with a raised bleb or blister at the injection site and is surrounded by hardened tissue, but it is often unsuccessful if the tissue is soft or soggy. **Corticosteroids** are usually given to treat inflammation, although there is little evidence to support their use in extravasation. Hydrocortisone or dexa-methasone (section 6.3.2) can be given either locally by subcutaneous injection or intravenously at a site distant from the injury. **Antihistamines** (section 3.4.1) and **analgesics** (section 4.7) may be required for symptom relief.

The management of extravasation beyond these measures is not well standar-dised and calls for specialist advice. Treatment depends on the nature of the offending substance; one approach is to localise and neutralise the substance whereas another is to spread and dilute it. The first method may be appropriate following extravasation of vesicant drugs and involves administration of an antidote (if available) and the application of cold compresses 3–4 times a day (consult specialist literature for details of specific antidotes). Spreading and diluting the offending substance involves infiltrating the area with physiological saline, applying warm compresses, elevating the affected limb, and administering hyaluronidase (section 10.3.1). A saline flush-out technique (involving flushing the subcutaneous tissue with physiological saline) may be effective but requires specialist advice. Hyaluronidase should **not** be administered following extravasa-tion of vesicant drugs (unless it is either specifically indicated or used in the saline flush-out technique).

10.3.1 Enzymes

Hyaluronidase is used for the management of extravasation For preparations, see *BNF section 10.3.1.*

10.3.2 Rubefacients and other topical antirheumatics

Classification not used in *BNF for Children.*

10 Musculoskeletal and joint diseases

11 Eye

11.1 Administration of drugs to the eye

Drugs are most commonly administered to the eye by topical application as eye drops or eye ointments. When a higher drug concentration is required within the eye, a local injection may be necessary.

Eye-drop dispenser devices are available to aid the instillation of eye drops from plastic bottles; they are particularly useful for children in whom normal application is difficult, for the visually impaired, or otherwise physically limited patients.

Eye drops and eye ointments Eye drops are generally instilled into the pocket formed by gently pulling down the lower eyelid and keeping the eye closed for as long as possible after application; in neonates and infants it may be more appropriate to administer the drop in the inner angle of the open eye. One drop is all that is needed; instillation of more than one drop at a time should be discouraged because it may increase systemic side-effects. A small amount of eye ointment is applied similarly; the ointment melts rapidly and blinking helps to spread it.

When two different eye-drop preparations are used at the same time of day, dilution and overflow may occur when one immediately follows the other. The carer or child should therefore leave an interval of at least 5 minutes between the two. Eye ointment should be applied after drops. Both drops and ointment may cause transient blurred vision.

Systemic effects may arise from absorption of drugs into the general circulation from conjunctival vessels or from the nasal mucosa after the excess preparation has drained down through the tear ducts. The extent of systemic absorption following ocular administration is highly variable; nasal drainage of drugs is associated with eye drops much more often than with eye ointments. Pressure on the lacrimal punctum for at least a minute after applying eye drops reduces nasolacrimal drainage and therefore decreases systemic absorption from the nasal mucosa.

For warnings relating to eye drops and contact lenses, see section 11.9.

Eye lotions These are solutions for the irrigation of the conjunctival sac. They act mechanically to flush out irritants or foreign bodies as a first-aid treatment.

Sterile sodium chloride 0.9% solution (section 11.8.1) is usually used. Clean water will suffice in an emergency.

Other preparations   Subconjunctival injection may be used to administer anti-infective drugs, mydriatics, or corticosteroids for conditions not responding to topical therapy. The drug diffuses through the cornea and sclera to the anterior and posterior chambers and vitreous humour. However, because the dose-volume is limited, this route is suitable only for drugs which are readily soluble.

Drugs such as antimicrobials and corticosteroids may be administered systemically to treat an eye condition.

Preservatives and sensitisers   Information on preservatives and on substances identified as skin sensitisers (section 13.1.3) is provided under preparation entries.

11.2 Control of microbial contamination

Preparations for the eye should be sterile when issued. Eye drops in multiple-application containers include a preservative but care should nevertheless be taken to avoid contamination of the contents during use.

Eye drops in multiple-application containers for *home use* should not be used for more than 4 weeks after first opening (unless otherwise stated).

Eye drops for use in *hospital wards* are normally discarded 1 week after first opening (24 hours if preservative-free). Individual containers should be provided for each child, and for each eye if there are special concerns about contamination. Containers used before an operation should be discarded at the time of the operation and fresh containers supplied. A fresh supply should also be provided upon discharge from hospital; in specialist ophthalmology units it may be acceptable to issue eye-drop bottles that have been dispensed to the patient on the day of discharge.

In *out-patient departments* single-application packs should preferably be used; if multiple-application packs are used, they should be discarded at the end of each day. In clinics for eye diseases and in accident and emergency departments, where the dangers of infection are high, single-application packs should be used; if a multiple-application pack is used, it should be discarded after single use.

Diagnostic dyes (section 11.8.2) should be used only from single-application packs.

In *eye surgery*   single-application containers should be used if possible; if a multiple-application pack is used, it should be discarded after single use. Preparations used during intra-ocular procedures and others that may penetrate into the anterior chamber must be isotonic and without preservatives and buffered if necessary to a neutral pH. Specially formulated fluids should be used for intra-ocular surgery; large volume intravenous infusion preparations are not suitable for this purpose. For all surgical procedures, a previously unopened container is used for each patient.

11.3 Anti-infective eye preparations

11.3.1 Antibacterials
11.3.2 Antifungals
11.3.3 Antivirals

Eye infections   Most acute superficial eye infections can be treated topically. Blepharitis and conjunctivitis are often caused by staphylococci; keratitis and endophthalmitis may be bacterial, viral, or fungal.

Bacterial *blepharitis* is treated by lid hygiene and application of antibacterial eye drops to the conjunctival sac or to the lid margins. Systemic treatment may be required and may be necessary for 3 months or longer.

Most cases of acute bacterial conjunctivitis are self-limiting; where treatment is appropriate, antibacterial eye drops or an eye ointment are used. A poor response might indicate viral or allergic conjunctivitis or antibiotic resistance.

Corneal ulcer and *keratitis* require specialist treatment, usually under inpatient care, and may call for intensive topical, subconjunctival, or systemic administration of antimicrobials.

Endophthalmitis is a medical emergency which also calls for specialist management and often requires parenteral, subconjunctival, or intra-ocular administration of antimicrobials.

For reference to the treatment of *crab lice of the eyelashes*, see section 13.10.4

11.3.1 Antibacterials

Bacterial infections are generally treated topically with eye drops and eye ointments; systemic treatment is sometimes appropriate in blepharitis.

Chloramphenicol has a broad spectrum of activity and is the drug of choice for *superficial eye infections*. Chloramphenicol eye drops are well tolerated and the recommendation that chloramphenicol eye drops should be avoided because of an increased risk of aplastic anaemia is not well founded.

Other antibacterials with a broad spectrum of activity include the quinolones, **ciprofloxacin**, **levofloxacin**, and **ofloxacin**; the aminoglycosides, **gentamicin** and **neomycin** are also active against a wide variety of bacteria. Gentamicin, quinolones, and **polymyxin B** are effective for infections caused by *Pseudomonas aeruginosa*.

Ciprofloxacin eye drops are licensed for *corneal ulcers*; intensive application (especially in the first 2 days) is required throughout the day and night.

Trachoma, which results from chronic infection with *Chlamydia trachomatis*, can be treated with **azithromycin** by mouth [unlicensed indication].

Fusidic acid is useful for staphylococcal infections.

Propamidine isetionate is of little value in bacterial infections but is specific for the rare but potentially devastating condition of *acanthamoeba keratitis* (see also section 11.9).

Other antibacterial eye drops may be prepared aseptically in a specialist manufacturing unit from material supplied for injection, see section 11.8.

Neonates   Antibacterial eye drops are used to treat acute bacterial conjunctivitis in neonates (ophthalmia neonatorum); where possible the causative micro-organism should be identified. **Chloramphenicol** or **neomycin** eye drops are used to treat mild conjunctivitis; more serious infections also require a systemic antibacterial. Failure to respond to initial treatment requires further investigation; chlamydial infection is one of the most frequent causes of neonatal conjunctivitis and should be considered.

Gonococcal eye infections are treated with a single-dose of parenteral **cefotaxime** *or* **ceftriaxone**. *Chlamydial eye infections* should be managed with oral **erythromycin**. **Gentamicin** eye drops together with appropriate systemic antibacterials are used in the treatment of *pseudomonal eye infections*; high-strength gentamicin eye drops (1.5%) [unlicensed] are available for severe infections.

With corticosteroids   Many antibacterial preparations also incorporate a corticosteroid but such mixtures should **not** be used unless a patient is under close specialist supervision. In particular they should not be prescribed for undiagnosed 'red eye' which is sometimes caused by the herpes simplex virus and may be difficult to diagnose (section 11.4).

Administration   Frequency of application depends on the severity of the infection and the potential for irreversible ocular damage; antibacterial eye preparations are usually administered as follows.

Eye drops. Apply 1 drop at least every 2 hours in severe infection then reduce frequency as infection is controlled and continue for 48 hours after healing. For less severe infection 3–4 times daily is generally sufficient.

Eye ointment. Apply *either* at night (if eye drops used during the day) *or* 3–4 times daily (if eye ointment used alone).

11 Eye

CHLORAMPHENICOL

Side-effects transient stinging; see also notes above

Indication and dose

See notes above

Chloramphenicol (Non-proprietary) PoM
Eye drops, chloramphenicol 0.5%. Net price 10 mL = £2.02

Eye ointment, chloramphenicol 1%. Net price 4 g = £2.18

Note Chloramphenicol 0.5% eye drops (max. pack size 10 mL) and 1% eye ointment (max. pack size 4 g) can be sold to the public for treatment of acute bacterial conjunctivitis in children over 2 years; max. duration of treatment 5 days

Chloromycetin® (Goldshield) PoM
Redidrops (= eye drops), chloramphenicol 0.5%. Net price 5 mL = £1.65; 10 mL = 90p
Excipients include phenylmercuric acetate

Ophthalmic ointment (= eye ointment), chloramphenicol 1%. Net price 4 g = £1.08

◀ Single use
Minims® Chloramphenicol (Bausch & Lomb) PoM
Eye drops, chloramphenicol 0.5%. Net price 20 × 0.5 mL = £8.61

CIPROFLOXACIN

Cautions not recommended for children under 1 year
Pregnancy manufacturer advises use only if potential benefit outweighs risk
Breast-feeding manufacturer advises caution
Side-effects local burning and itching; lid margin crusting; hyperaemia; taste disturbances; corneal staining, keratitis, lid oedema, lacrimation, photophobia, corneal infiltrates; nausea and visual disturbances reported
Licensed use not licensed for use in children under 1 year

Indication and dose

Superficial bacterial infections

See notes above

Corneal ulcer

Apply eye drops throughout day and night, day 1 apply every 15 minutes for 6 hours then every 30 minutes, day 2 apply every hour, days 3–14 apply every 4 hours (max. duration of treatment 21 days)

Apply eye ointment throughout day and night; apply 1.25 cm ointment every 1–2 hours for 2 days then every 4 hours for next 12 days

Ciloxan® (Alcon) PoM
Ophthalmic solution (= eye drops), ciprofloxacin (as hydrochloride) 0.3%. Net price 5 mL = £4.79
Excipients include benzalkonium chloride

Eye ointment, ciprofloxacin (as hydrochloride) 0.3%. Net price 3.5 g = £5.32

FUSIDIC ACID

Indication and dose

See notes above and under preparation below

Fucithalmic® (LEO) PoM
Eye drops, m/r, fusidic acid 1% in gel basis (liquifies on contact with eye). Net price 5 g = £2.00
Excipients include benzalkonium chloride, disodium edetate
Dose
Apply twice daily

GENTAMICIN

Indication and dose

See notes above

Genticin® (Roche) PoM
Drops (for ear or eye), gentamicin 0.3% (as sulphate). Net price 10 mL = £2.13
Excipients include benzalkonium chloride

Gentamicin (Non-proprietary) PoM
Eye drops, gentamicin 1.5%, 10 mL, available as a manufactured special from Moorfields Eye Hospital, see also 'special-order' manufacturers or specialist importing companies, p. 957

LEVOFLOXACIN

Pregnancy manufacturer advises avoid—systemic quinolones have caused arthropathy in *animal* studies
Breast-feeding manufacturer advises avoid
Side-effects transient ocular irritation, visual disturbances, lid margin crusting, lid or conjunctival oedema, hyperaemia, conjunctival follicles, photophobia, headache, rhinitis

Licensed use not licensed for use in children under 1 year

Indication and dose

See notes above

Oftaquix® (Kestrel Ophthalmics) ▼ PoM
Eye drops, levofloxacin 0.5%, net price 5 mL = £6.95

11
Eye

NEOMYCIN SULPHATE

Licensed use *Neosporin®* not licensed for use in children under 2 years

Indication and dose

See notes above and under preparations below

Neomycin (Non-proprietary) PoM
Eye drops, neomycin sulphate 0.5% (3500 units/mL). Net price 10 mL = £3.11
Available from 'special-order' manufacturers or specialist importing companies, see p. 957

Eye ointment, neomycin sulphate 0.5% (3500 units/g). Net price 3 g = £2.44
Available from 'special-order' manufacturers or specialist importing companies, see p. 957

◢With other antibacterials
Neosporin® (TEVA UK) PoM
Eye drops, gramicidin 25 units, neomycin sulphate 1700 units, polymyxin B sulphate 5000 units/mL. Net price 5 mL = £4.86
Excipients include thiomersal

Dose

Apply 2–4 times daily or more frequently if required

OFLOXACIN

Cautions not to be used for more than 10 days

Pregnancy manufacturer advises use only if benefit outweighs risk; systemic quinolones have caused arthropathy in *animal* studies

Breast-feeding manufacturer advises avoid

Side-effects local irritation including photophobia; dizziness, numbness, nausea and headache reported

Licensed use not licensed for use in neonates

Indication and dose

Local treatment of infections (but see notes above)

Apply every two to four hours for the first two days then reduce frequency to four times daily (max. 10 days treatment)

Exocin® (Allergan) PoM
Ophthalmic solution (= eye drops), ofloxacin 0.3%. Net price 5 mL = £2.17
Excipients include benzalkonium chloride

POLYMYXIN B SULPHATE

Indication and dose

See notes above

◢With other antibacterials
Polyfax® (TEVA UK) PoM
Eye ointment, polymyxin B sulphate 10 000 units, bacitracin zinc 500 units/g. Net price 4 g = £3.26

PROPAMIDINE ISETIONATE

Indication and dose

See under preparations below

Brolene® (Sanofi-Aventis)
Eye drops, propamidine isetionate 0.1%. Net price 10 mL = £2.80
Excipients include benzalkonium chloride

Dose

Local treatment of infections (but see notes above)

Apply 4 times daily

Note Eye drops containing propamidine isetionate 0.1% also available from Typharm (*Golden Eye Drops*)

Eye ointment, dibrompropamidine isetionate 0.15%. Net price 5 g = £2.92

Dose

Local treatment of infections (but see notes above)

Apply 1–2 times daily

Note Eye ointment containing dibrompropamidine isetionate 0.15% also available from Typharm (*Golden Eye Ointment*)

11.3.2 Antifungals

Fungal infections of the cornea are rare. Orbital mycosis is rarer, and when it occurs it is usually because of direct spread of infection from the paranasal sinuses. Debility or immunosuppression can encourage fungal proliferation. The spread of infection through blood occasionally produces metastatic endophthalmitis.

Many different fungi are capable of producing ocular infection; they can be identified by appropriate laboratory procedures.

Antifungal preparations for the eye are not generally available. Treatment is normally carried out at specialist centres, but requests for information about supplies of preparations not available commercially should be addressed to the Strategic Health Authority (or equivalent in Scotland or Northern Ireland), or to the nearest hospital ophthalmology unit, or to Moorfields Eye Hospital, 162 City Road, London EC1V 2PD (tel. (020) 7253 3411) or www.moorfields.nhs.uk

11.3.3 Antivirals

Herpes simplex infections producing, for example, dendritic corneal ulcers can be treated with **aciclovir**.

For systemic treatment of CMV retinitis, see section 5.3.2.2.

ACICLOVIR

(Acyclovir)

Side-effects local irritation and inflammation, superficial punctate keratopathy; *rarely* blepharitis; *very rarely* hypersensitivity reactions including angioedema

Indication and dose

Local treatment of herpes simplex infections

Apply 5 times daily (continue for at least 3 days after complete healing)

Herpes simplex skin infections section 13.10.3

Herpes simplex and varicella–zoster infections section 5.3.2.1

Zovirax® (GSK) PoM
Eye ointment, aciclovir 3%. Net price 4.5 g = £9.53

11.4 Corticosteroids and other anti-inflammatory preparations

11.4.1 Corticosteroids
11.4.2 Other anti-inflammatory preparations

11.4.1 Corticosteroids

Corticosteroids administered locally to the eye or given by mouth are effective for treating anterior segment inflammation in uveitis (section 11.5) and following surgery.

Topical corticosteroids should normally only be used under expert supervision; three main dangers are associated with their use:

- a 'red eye', when the diagnosis is unconfirmed, may be due to herpes simplex virus, and a corticosteroid may aggravate the condition, leading to corneal ulceration, with possible damage to vision and even loss of the eye. Bacterial, fungal, and amoebic infections pose a similar hazard;
- 'steroid glaucoma' may follow the use of corticosteroid eye preparations in susceptible individuals;
- a 'steroid cataract' may follow prolonged use.

Other side-effects of ocular corticosteroids include thinning of the cornea and sclera. Prolonged use in neonates and infants can cause adrenal suppression.

Products combining a corticosteroid with an antimicrobial are used after ocular surgery to reduce inflammation and prevent infection: use of combination products is otherwise rarely justified.

Systemic corticosteroids (section 6.3.2) may be useful for ocular conditions. The risk of producing a 'steroid cataract' increases with the dose and duration of corticosteroid use.

11
Eye

BETAMETHASONE

Cautions see notes above
Side-effects see notes above

Indication and dose

Local treatment of inflammation (short-term)

Apply eye drops every 1–2 hours until controlled then reduce frequency; eye ointment 2–4 times daily or at night when used with eye drops

Betnesol® (UCB Pharma) PoM
Drops (for ear, eye, or nose), betamethasone sodium phosphate 0.1%. Net price 10 mL = £2.23
Excipients include benzalkonium chloride, disodium edetate

Eye ointment, betamethasone sodium phosphate 0.1%. Net price 3 g = £1.36

Vistamethasone® (Martindale) PoM
Drops (for ear, eye, or nose), betamethasone sodium phosphate 0.1%. Net price 5 mL = £1.02; 10 mL = £1.16
Excipients include benzalkonium chloride

◀With neomycin

Betnesol-N® (UCB Pharma) PoM
Drops (for ear, eye, or nose), see section 12.1.1

Eye ointment, betamethasone sodium phosphate 0.1%, neomycin sulphate 0.5%. Net price 3 g = £1.28
Note May be difficult to obtain

DEXAMETHASONE

Cautions see notes above
Side-effects see notes above

Indication and dose

Local treatment of inflammation (short-term)

Apply eye drops 4–6 times daily; severe conditions every 30–60 minutes until controlled then reduce frequency

Maxidex® (Alcon) PoM
Eye drops, dexamethasone 0.1%, hypromellose 0.5%. Net price 5 mL = £1.44; 10 mL = £2.86
Excipients include benzalkonium chloride, disodium edetate, polysorbate 80

◢ Single use
Minims® Dexamethasone (Bausch & Lomb) PoM
Eye drops, dexamethasone sodium phosphate 0.1%. Net price 20 × 0.5 mL = £9.04
Excipients include disodium edetate

◢ With antibacterials
Maxitrol® (Alcon) PoM ◢
Eye drops, dexamethasone 0.1%, hypromellose 0.5%, neomycin 0.35% (as sulphate), polymyxin B sulphate 6000 units/mL. Net price 5 mL = £1.72
Excipients include benzalkonium chloride, polysorbate 20

Eye ointment, dexamethasone 0.1%, neomycin 0.35% (as sulphate), polymyxin B sulphate 6000 units/g. Net price 3.5 g = £1.47
Excipients include hydroxybenzoates (parabens), wool fat

Sofradex® (Sanofi-Aventis) PoM ◢
Drops (for ear or eye), see section 12.1.1

FLUOROMETHOLONE

Cautions see notes above
Side-effects see notes above
Licensed use not licensed for use in children under 2 years

Indication and dose

Local treatment of inflammation (short-term)

Apply 2–4 times daily (initially every hour for 24–48 hours then reduce frequency)

FML® (Allergan) PoM
Ophthalmic suspension (= eye drops), fluorometholone 0.1%, polyvinyl alcohol (*Liquifilm®*) 1.4%. Net price 5 mL = £1.71; 10 mL = £2.95
Excipients include benzalkonium chloride, disodium edetate, polysorbate 80

HYDROCORTISONE ACETATE

Cautions see notes above
Side-effects see notes above

Indication and dose

Local treatment of inflammation (short-term)

Apply eye drops 4 times daily; apply eye ointment twice daily or at night

Hydrocortisone (Non-proprietary) PoM
Eye drops, hydrocortisone acetate 1%. Net price 10 mL = £3.21

Eye ointment, hydrocortisone acetate 0.5%, net price 3 g = £2.88; 1%, 3 g = £6.71; 2.5%, 3 g = £7.86

PREDNISOLONE

Cautions see notes above
Side-effects see notes above

Indication and dose

Local treatment of inflammation (short-term)

Apply every 1–2 hours until controlled then reduce frequency

Pred Forte® (Allergan) PoM
Eye drops, prednisolone acetate 1%. Net price 5 mL = £1.52; 10 mL = £3.05
Excipients include benzalkonium chloride, disodium edetate, polysorbate 80

Predsol® (UCB Pharma) PoM
Drops (for ear or eye), prednisolone sodium phosphate 0.5%. Net price 10 mL = £1.92
Excipients include benzalkonium chloride, disodium edetate

◢ Single use
Minims® Prednisolone Sodium Phosphate (Bausch & Lomb) PoM
Eye drops, prednisolone sodium phosphate 0.5%. Net price 20 × 0.5 mL = £9.78
Excipients include disodium edetate

◢ With neomycin
Predsol-N® (UCB Pharma) PoM ◢
Drops (for ear or eye), see section 12.1.1

11.4.2 Other anti-inflammatory preparations

Eye drops containing **antihistamines**, such as **antazoline** (with xylometazoline as *Otrivine-Antistin®*), **azelastine**, **epinastine**, **ketotifen**, and **olopatadine**, can be used for allergic conjunctivitis.

Sodium cromoglicate and **nedocromil sodium** eye drops may be useful for vernal keratoconjunctivitis and other allergic forms of conjunctivitis.

Lodoxamide eye drops are used for allergic conjunctival conditions including seasonal allergic conjunctivitis.

Emedastine eye drops are licensed for seasonal allergic conjunctivitis.

ANTAZOLINE SULPHATE

Indication and dose

Allergic conjunctivitis

See preparation below

Otrivine-Antistin® (Novartis Consumer Health)
Eye drops, antazoline sulphate 0.5%, xylometazoline hydrochloride 0.05%. Net price 10 mL = £2.35
Excipients include benzalkonium chloride, disodium edetate

Dose

Child 12–18 years apply 2–3 times daily (max. duration 7 days)

Note Xylometazoline is a sympathomimetic; it should be used with caution in patients susceptible to angle-closure glaucoma; absorption of antazoline and xylometazoline may result in systemic side-effects and the possibility of interaction with other drugs, see Appendix 1 (antihistamines and sympathomimetics)

AZELASTINE HYDROCHLORIDE

Side-effects mild transient irritation; bitter taste reported

Indication and dose

Allergic conjunctivitis, seasonal allergic conjunctivitis

Child 4–18 years apply twice daily, increased if necessary to 4 times daily

Perennial conjunctivitis

Child 12–18 years apply twice daily, increased if necessary to 4 times daily; max. duration of treatment 6 weeks

Optilast® (Meda) (PoM)
Eye drops, azelastine hydrochloride 0.05%. Net price 8 mL = £6.40
Excipients include benzalkonium chloride, disodium edetate

EMEDASTINE

Side-effects transient burning or stinging; blurred vision, local oedema, keratitis, irritation, dry eye, lacrimation, corneal infiltrates (discontinue) and staining; photophobia; headache, and rhinitis occasionally reported

Indication and dose

Seasonal allergic conjunctivitis

Child 3–18 years apply twice daily

Emadine® (Alcon) (PoM)
Eye drops, emedastine 0.05% (as difumarate), net price 5 mL = £7.45
Excipients include benzalkonium chloride

EPINASTINE HYDROCHLORIDE

Side-effects burning; *less commonly* dry mouth, taste disturbance; nasal irritation, rhinitis; headache, blepharoptosis, conjunctival oedema and hyperaemia, dry eye, local irritation, photophobia, visual disturbance; pruritus

Indication and dose

Seasonal allergic conjunctivitis

Child 12–18 years apply twice daily; max. duration of treatment 8 weeks

Relestat® (Allergan) (PoM)
Eye drops, epinastine hydrochloride 500 micrograms/mL, net price 5 mL = £9.90
Excipients include benzalkonium chloride, disodium edetate

KETOTIFEN

Side-effects transient burning or stinging, punctate corneal epithelial erosion; *less commonly* dry eye, subconjunctival haemmorhage, photophobia; headache, drowsiness, skin reactions, and dry mouth also reported

Indication and dose

Seasonal allergic conjunctivitis

Child 3–18 years apply twice daily

11 Eye

△ **KETOTIFEN** (*continued*)

Zaditen® (Novartis) PoM
Eye drops, ketotifen (as fumarate) 250 micrograms/
mL, net price 5 mL = £9.75
Excipients include benzalkonium chloride

LODOXAMIDE

Side-effects burning, stinging, itching, blurred
vision, tear production disturbance, and ocular
discomfort; *less commonly*, flushing, nasal dryness, dizziness, drowsiness, headache, blepharitis,
and keratitis

Indication and dose

Allergic conjunctivitis

Child 4–18 years apply 4 times daily

Note Improvement of symptoms may sometimes require
treatment for up to 4 weeks

Alomide® (Alcon) PoM
Ophthalmic solution (= eye drops), lodoxamide
0.1% (as trometamol). Net price 10 mL = £5.31
Excipients include benzalkonium chloride, disodium edetate
Note Lodoxamide 0.1% eye drops can be sold to the
public for treatment of allergic conjunctivitis in children
over 4 years

NEDOCROMIL SODIUM

Side-effects transient burning and stinging; distinctive taste reported

Indication and dose

Seasonal and perennial allergic conjunctivitis

Child 6–18 years apply twice daily increased if
necessary to 4 times daily; max. 12 weeks
treatment for seasonal allergic conjunctivitis

Vernal keratoconjunctivitis

Child 6–18 years apply 4 times daily

Rapitil® (Sanofi-Aventis) PoM
Eye drops, nedocromil sodium 2%. Net price 5 mL
= £4.92
Excipients include benzalkonium chloride, disodium edetate

OLOPATADINE

Side-effects local irritation; less commonly
keratitis, dry eye, local oedema, photophobia;
headache, asthenia, dizziness; dry nose also
reported

Indication and dose

Seasonal allergic conjunctivitis

Child 3–18 years apply twice daily; max. duration of treatment 4 months

Opatanol® (Alcon) PoM
Eye drops, olopatadine (as hydrochloride) 1 mg/
mL, net price 5 mL = £3.98
Excipients include benzalkonium chloride

SODIUM CROMOGLICATE
(Sodium cromoglycate)

Side-effects transient burning and stinging

Indication and dose

Allergic conjunctivitis, vernal keratoconjunctivitis

Apply eye drops 4 times daily

Sodium Cromoglicate (Non-proprietary) PoM
Eye drops, sodium cromoglicate 2%. Net price
13.5 mL = £1.94
Brands include *Hay-Crom® Aqueous, Opticrom® Aqueous,
Vividrin®*
Note Sodium cromoglicate 2% eye drops can be sold to
the public (in max. pack size of 10 mL) for treatment of
acute seasonal and perennial allergic conjunctivitis

11.5 Mydriatics and cycloplegics

Antimuscarinics dilate the pupil and paralyse the ciliary muscle; they vary in
potency and duration of action.

Short-acting, relatively weak mydriatics, such as **tropicamide** 0.5% (action lasts
for 4–6 hours), facilitate the examination of the fundus of the eye. **Cyclopentolate**
1% (action up to 24 hours) or **atropine** (action up to 7 days) are preferable for
producing cycloplegia for refraction in young children; tropicamide may be
preferred in neonates. Atropine ointment 1% is sometimes preferred for children
under 5 years because systemic absorption from the ointment is reduced. **Phenylephrine** 2.5% is used for mydriasis in diagnostic or therapeutic procedures;

mydriasis occurs within 60–90 minutes and lasts up to 5–7 hours. Phenylephrine 10% drops are contra-indicated in children owing to the risk of systemic effects.

Mydriatics and cycloplegics are used in the treatment of anterior uveitis, usually as an adjunct to corticosteriods (section 11.4.1). Atropine is used in anterior uveitis mainly to prevent posterior synechiae and to relieve ciliary spasm, often in combination with phenylphrine eye drops; cyclopentolate or **homatropine** (action up to 3 days) can also be used and may be preferred because they have a shorter duration of action.

Cautions and contra-indications   Darkly pigmented irides are more resistant to pupillary dilatation and caution should be exercised to avoid overdosage. Mydriasis can precipitate acute angle-closure glaucoma in the very few children who are predisposed to the condition because of a shallow anterior chamber. Atropine, cyclopentolate, and homatropine should be used with caution in children under 3 months owing to the possible association between cycloplegia and the development of amblyopia; also, neonates are at increased risk of systemic toxicity.
Skilled tasks Children may not be able to undertake skilled tasks for 1–2 hours after mydriasis.

Side-effects   Ocular side-effects of mydriatics and cycloplegics include transient stinging and raised intra-ocular pressure; on prolonged administration, local irritation, hyperaemia, oedema, and conjunctivitis can occur. Contact dermatitis can occur with the antimuscarinic mydriatic drugs, especially atropine.

Toxic systemic reactions to atropine and cyclopentolate can occur in neonates and children; see section 1.2 for systemic side-effects of antimuscarinic drugs.

Antimuscarinics

ATROPINE SULPHATE

Cautions   risk of systemic effects with eye drops in infants under 3 months—eye ointment preferred; see also notes above

Side-effects   see notes above

Licensed use   not licensed for use in children for uveitis

Indication and dose

Cycloplegia

  Child 3 months–18 years apply drops or ointment twice daily for 3 days before procedure

Anterior uveitis

  Child 2–18 years 1 drop up to 4 times daily

Atropine (Non-proprietary) PoM
Eye drops, atropine sulphate 0.5%, net price 10 mL = £2.78; 1%, 10 mL = £1.11

Eye ointment, atropine sulphate 1%. Net price 3 g = £2.97

◢Single use
Minims® Atropine Sulphate (Bausch & Lomb) PoM
Eye drops, atropine sulphate 1%. Net price 20 × 0.5 mL = £9.59

CYCLOPENTOLATE HYDROCHLORIDE

Cautions   see notes above
Side-effects   see notes above

Indication and dose

See notes above

Cycloplegia

  Child 3 months–12 years 1 drop of 1% eye drops 30–60 minutes before examination

  Child 12–18 years 1 drop of 0.5% eye drops 30–60 minutes before examination

Uveitis

  Child 3 months–18 years 1 drop of 0.5% eye drops (1% for deeply pigmented eyes) 2–4 times daily

Mydrilate® (Intrapharm) PoM
Eye drops, cyclopentolate hydrochloride 0.5%, net price 5 mL = £6.73; 1%, 5 mL = £6.73
Excipients include benzalkonium chloride

◢Single use
Minims® Cyclopentolate Hydrochloride (Bausch & Lomb) PoM
Eye drops, cyclopentolate hydrochloride 0.5% and 1%. Net price 20 × 0.5 mL (both) = £9.35

HOMATROPINE HYDROBROMIDE

Cautions   see notes above
Side-effects   see notes above

Licensed use   not licensed for use in children under 3 months

11
Eye

◻ **HOMATROPINE HYDROBROMIDE** (*continued*)

Indication and dose

See notes above

> **Child 3 months–2 years** (0.5% only) 1 drop daily or on alternate days adjusted according to response
>
> **Child 2–18 years** 1 drop twice daily adjusted according to response

Homatropine (Non-proprietary) ℞
Eye drops, homatropine hydrobromide 1%, net price 10 mL = £2.55; 2%, 10 mL = £2.69
Available without preservatives as manufactured specials from Moorfields Eye Hospital

Eye drops, homatropine 0.125% and 0.5%, 10 mL, available as a manufactured special from Moorfields Eye Hospital, see also 'special-order' manufacturers or specialist importing companies, p. 957
Excipients include chlorhexidine

TROPICAMIDE

Cautions see notes above
Side-effects see notes above

Indication and dose

See notes above

> **Funduscopy**
>
> **Neonate and child** apply 0.5% eye drops 20 minutes before examination

Mydriacyl® (Alcon) ℞
Eye drops, tropicamide 0.5%, net price 5 mL = £1.32; 1%, 5 mL = £1.63
Excipients include benzalkonium chloride, disodium edetate

◢ **Single use**
Minims® Tropicamide (Bausch & Lomb) ℞
Eye drops, tropicamide 0.5% and 1%. Net price 20 × 0.5 mL (both) = £8.63

Sympathomimetics

PHENYLEPHRINE HYDROCHLORIDE

Cautions cardiovascular disease (avoid or use 2.5% strength only); tachycardia; hyperthyroidism; diabetes; susceptibility to angle-closure glaucoma; see also notes above
Contra-indications 10% drops in neonates and children
Side-effects eye pain and stinging; blurred vision, photophobia; systemic effects include palpitations, arrhythmias, hypertension, coronary artery spasm; *very rarely* angle-closure glaucoma

Indication and dose

> **Mydriasis**
>
> See notes above

◢ **Single use**
Minims® Phenylephrine Hydrochloride (Bausch & Lomb)
Eye drops, phenylephrine hydrochloride 2.5%, net price 20 × 0.5 mL = £9.20
Excipients include disodium edetate, sodium metabisulphite

11.6 Treatment of glaucoma

Glaucoma describes a group of disorders characterised by a loss of visual field associated with cupping of the optic disc and optic nerve damage and is generally associated with raised intra-ocular pressure.

Glaucoma is rare in children and should always be managed by a specialist. *Primary congenital glaucoma* is the most common form of glaucoma in children, followed by *secondary glaucomas*, such as following hereditary anterior segment malformations; *juvenile open-angle glaucoma* is less common and usually occurs in older children. *Primary angle closure glaucoma* (acute closed-angle glaucoma, narrow angle glaucoma) is very rare in children; it results from blockage of aqueous humour flow into the anterior chamber and is a medical emergency that requires urgent reduction of intra-ocular pressure, see below.

Treatment of glaucoma is determined by the pathophysiology and usually involves controlling raised intra-ocular pressure with surgery and drug therapy. Drugs that reduce intra-ocular pressure by different mechanisms are available for managing glaucoma. A topical beta-blocker or a prostaglandin analogue can be used. It may be necessary to combine these drugs or add others, such as miotics, sympathomimetics, or carbonic anhydrase inhibitors, to control intra-ocular pressure.

For urgent reduction of intra-ocular pressure and before surgery, **mannitol** 20% (up to 500 mL) is given by slow intravenous infusion until the intra-ocular pressure has been satisfactorily reduced (see section 2.2.5). **Acetazolamide** by intravenous injection can also be used for the emergency management of raised intra-ocular pressure.

Standard antiglaucoma therapy is used if supplementary treatment is required after iridotomy, iridectomy, or a drainage operation in either primary open-angle or acute closed-angle glaucoma.

Beta-blockers

Topical application of a beta-blocker to the eye reduces intra-ocular pressure effectively in *primary open-angle glaucoma*, probably by reducing the rate of production of aqueous humour. Administration by mouth also reduces intra-ocular pressure but this route is not used since side-effects may be troublesome.

Cautions, contra-indications, and side-effects Systemic absorption can follow topical application to the eye; therefore, eye drops containing a beta-blocker are contra-indicated in bradycardia, heart block, or uncontrolled heart failure. **Important**: for a warning to avoid in asthma, see below. Consider also other cautions, contra-indications, and side-effects of beta-blockers (p. 114). Local side-effects of eye drops include ocular stinging, burning, pain, itching, erythema, dry eyes and allergic reactions including anaphylaxis and blepharoconjunctivitis; occasionally corneal disorders have been reported.

Important Beta-blockers, even those with apparent cardioselectivity, should not be used in patients with asthma or a history of obstructive airways disease, unless no alternative treatment is available. In such cases the risk of inducing bronchospasm should be appreciated and appropriate precautions taken.

Interactions Since systemic absorption may follow topical application the possibility of interactions, in particular with drugs such as verapamil, should be borne in mind. See also Appendix 1 (beta-blockers).

◢ BETAXOLOL HYDROCHLORIDE

Cautions see notes above
Contra-indications see notes above
Side-effects see notes above
Licensed use not licensed for use in children

Indication and dose
See notes above
   Apply twice daily

Betoptic® (Alcon) (PoM)
Ophthalmic solution (= eye drops), betaxolol (as hydrochloride) 0.5%, net price 5 mL = £1.94
Excipients include benzalkonium chloride, disodium edetate

Ophthalmic suspension (= eye drops), betaxolol (as hydrochloride) 0.25%, net price 5 mL = £2.71
Excipients include benzalkonium chloride, disodium edetate

Unit dose eye drop suspension, betaxolol (as hydrochloride) 0.25%, net price 50 × 0.25 mL = £14.04

◢ CARTEOLOL HYDROCHLORIDE

Cautions see notes above
Contra-indications see notes above
Side-effects see notes above
Licensed use not licensed for use in children

Indication and dose
See notes above
   Apply twice daily

Teoptic® (Spectrum) (PoM)
Eye drops, carteolol hydrochloride 1%, net price 5 mL = £4.60; 2%, 5 mL = £5.40
Excipients include benzalkonium chloride

◢ LEVOBUNOLOL HYDROCHLORIDE

Cautions see notes above
Contra-indications see notes above
Side-effects see notes above; anterior uveitis occasionally reported
Licensed use not licensed for use in children

Indication and dose
See notes above
   Apply once or twice daily

Levobunolol (Non-proprietary) (PoM)
Eye drops, levobunolol hydrochloride 0.5%. Net price 5 mL = £2.72

Betagan® (Allergan) (PoM)
Eye drops, levobunolol hydrochloride 0.5%, polyvinyl alcohol (*Liquifilm®*) 1.4%. Net price 5-mL = £1.85
Excipients include benzalkonium chloride, disodium edetate, sodium metabisulphite

11
Eye

◁ **LEVOBUNOLOL HYDROCHLORIDE** (*continued*)

Unit dose eye drops, levobunolol hydrochloride
0.5%, polyvinyl alcohol (*Liquifilm®*) 1.4%. Net price
30 × 0.4 mL = £9.98
Excipients include disodium edetate

TIMOLOL MALEATE

Cautions see notes above
Contra-indications see notes above
Side-effects see notes above
Licensed use not licensed for use in children

Indication and dose

See notes above
Apply twice daily; long-acting preparations, see
under preparations below

Timolol (Non-proprietary) PoM
Eye drops, timolol (as maleate) 0.25%, net price
5 mL = £1.52; 0.5%, 5 mL = £1.67

Timoptol® (MSD) PoM
Eye drops, in *Ocumeter®* metered-dose unit, timolol
(as maleate) 0.25%, net price 5 mL = £3.12; 0.5%,
5 mL = £3.12
Excipients include benzalkonium chloride

Unit dose eye drops, timolol (as maleate) 0.25%,
net price 30 × 0.2 mL = £8.45; 0.5%, 30 × 0.2 mL =
£9.65

◢ **Once-daily preparations**
Nyogel® (Novartis) PoM
Eye gel (= eye drops), timolol (as maleate) 0.1%, net
price 5 g = £2.85
Excipients include benzalkonium chloride

Dose

Child 12–18 years apply once daily

Timoptol®-LA (MSD) PoM
Ophthalmic gel-forming solution (= eye drops),
timolol (as maleate) 0.25%, net price 2.5 mL =
£3.12; 0.5%, 2.5 mL = £3.12
Excipients include benzododecinium bromide

Dose

Apply eye drops once daily

◢ **With dorzolamide**
See under Dorzolamide

Prostaglandin analogues

The prostaglandin analogues **latanoprost**, and **travoprost**, and the synthetic
prostamide, **bimatoprost**, increase uveoscleral outflow and subsequently reduce
intra-ocular pressure. They are used to reduce intra-ocular pressure. They are not
licensed for use in children. Children receiving prostaglandin analogues should be
managed by a specialist and monitored for any changes to eye coloration since an
increase in the brown pigment in the iris can occur; particular care is required in
those with mixed coloured irides and those receiving treatment to one eye only.

Sympathomimetics

Apraclonidine (section 11.8.2) is an alpha₂-adrenoceptor agonist. Eye drops
containing apraclonidine 0.5% are used for a short period to delay laser treatment
or surgery for glaucoma in patients not adequately controlled by another drug;
eye drops containing 1% are used for control of intra-ocular pressure after
anterior segment laser surgery.

Brimonidine is an alpha₂-adrenoceptor agonist that reduces intra-ocular pressure; it should be used with caution in children because it has been associated
with severe systemic side-effects.

Carbonic anhydrase inhibitors and systemic drugs

The **carbonic anhydrase inhibitors**, acetazolamide, brinzolamide, and dorzolamide, reduce intra-ocular pressure by reducing aqueous humour production.
Systemic use of acetazolamide also produces weak diuresis.

Acetazolamide is given by mouth or, rarely in children, by intravenous injection
(intramuscular injections are painful because of the alkaline pH of the solution). It
is used as an adjunct to other treatment for reducing intra-ocular pressure.
Acetazolamide is a sulphonamide; blood disorders, rashes, and other sulphonamide-related side-effects occur occasionally. It is not generally recommended for
long-term use; electrolyte disturbances and metabolic acidosis that occur can be
corrected by administering potassium bicarbonate (as effervescent potassium
tablets, section 9.2.1.3).

Dorzolamide and **brinzolamide** are topical carbonic anhydrase inhibitors. They
are unlicensed in children but are used in those resistant to beta-blockers or those

in whom beta-blockers are contra-indicated. They are used alone or as an adjunct to a topical beta-blocker. Systemic absorption can rarely cause sulphonamide-like side-effects and may require discontinuation if severe.

The **osmotic diuretics**, intravenous hypertonic **mannitol** (section 2.2.5) or **glycerol** by mouth, are useful short-term ocular hypotensive drugs.

ACETAZOLAMIDE

Cautions not generally recommended for prolonged use but if given monitor blood count and plasma electrolyte concentration; pulmonary obstruction (risk of acidosis); avoid extravasation at injection site (risk of necrosis); **interactions:** Appendix 1 (diuretics)

Contra-indications hypokalaemia, hyponatraemia, hyperchloraemic acidosis; sulphonamide hypersensitivity

Hepatic impairment manufacturer advises avoid

Renal impairment avoid; metabolic acidosis

Pregnancy manufacturer advises avoid, especially in first trimester (toxicity in *animal* studies)

Breast-feeding amount too small to be harmful

Side-effects nausea, vomiting, diarrhoea, taste disturbance; loss of appetite, paraesthesia, flushing, headache, dizziness, fatigue, irritability, depression; thirst, polyuria; metabolic acidosis and electrolyte disturbances on long-term therapy; occasionally, drowsiness, confusion, hearing disturbances, urticaria, melaena, glycosuria, haematuria, abnormal liver function, renal calculi, blood disorders including agranulocytosis and thrombocytopenia, rashes including Stevens-Johnson syndrome and toxic epidermal necrolysis; rarely, photosensitivity, liver damage, flaccid paralysis, convulsions; transient myopia reported

Licensed use not licensed for use in children for treatment of glaucoma

Indication and dose

> Reduction of intra-ocular pressure in open-angle glaucoma, secondary glaucoma, perioperatively in angle-closure glaucoma
> • By mouth or by intravenous injection
>   **Child 1 month–12 years** 5 mg/kg 2–4 times daily, adjusted according to response, max. 750 mg daily
>   **Child 12–18 years** 250 mg 2–4 times daily

> Epilepsy
> • By mouth or slow intravenous injection
>   **Neonate** initially 2.5 mg/kg 2–3 times daily, followed by 5–7 mg/kg 2–3 times daily (maintenance dose)
>
>   **Child 1 month–12 years** initially 2.5 mg/kg 2–3 times daily, followed by 5–7 mg/kg 2–3 times daily, max. 750 mg daily (maintenance dose)
>   **Child 12–18 years** 250 mg 2–4 times daily

> Raised intracranial pressure
> • By mouth or slow intravenous injection
>   **Child 1 month–12 years** initially 8 mg/kg 3 times daily, increased as necessary to max. 100 mg/kg daily

Diamox® (Goldshield) ⓅⓄⓂ
Tablets, acetazolamide 250 mg. Net price 112-tab pack = £12.68. Label: 3

Sodium Parenteral (= injection), powder for reconstitution, acetazolamide (as sodium salt). Net price 500-mg vial = £14.76

◢ Modified release
Diamox® SR (Goldshield) ⓅⓄⓂ
Capsules, m/r, orange, enclosing orange f/c pellets, acetazolamide 250 mg. Net price 30-cap pack = £13.88. Label: 3, 25

Dose
> **Child 12–18 years** glaucoma, 1–2 capsules daily

◢ Extemporaneous formulations available see Extemporaneous Preparations, p. 8

BRINZOLAMIDE

Cautions systemic absorption follows topical application; neonates and infants with immature renal tubules—risk of metabolic acidosis; **interactions:** Appendix 1 (brinzolamide)

Contra-indications hyperchloraemic acidosis

Hepatic impairment manufacturer advises avoid

Renal impairment see Cautions above; also avoid if estimated glomerular filtration rate less than 30 mL/minute/1.73 m²

Pregnancy manufacturer advises avoid unless essential—toxicity in *animal* studies

Breast-feeding manufacturer advises avoid

Side-effects local irritation, taste disturbance; less commonly nausea, dyspepsia, dry mouth, chest pain, epistaxis, haemoptysis, dyspnoea, rhinitis, pharyngitis, bronchitis, paraesthesia, depression, dizziness, headache, dermatitis, alopecia, corneal erosion

Licensed use not licensed for use in children

Indication and dose

> Adjunct to beta-blockers or used alone in raised intra-ocular pressure in ocular hypertension and in open-angle glaucoma if beta-blocker alone inadequate or inappropriate
>
>   Apply twice daily increased to 3 times daily if necessary

Azopt® (Alcon) ⓅⓄⓂ
Eye drops, brinzolamide 10 mg/mL, net price 5 mL = £6.69
Excipients include benzalkonium chloride, disodium edetate

11

Eye

644

11.6 Treatment of glaucoma

BNFC 2010–2011

DORZOLAMIDE

Cautions systemic absorption follows topical application; history of renal calculi; neonates and infants with immature renal tubules—risk of metabolic acidosis; chronic corneal defects, history of intra-ocular surgery; **interactions:** Appendix 1 (dorzolamide)

Contra-indications hyperchloraemic acidosis

Hepatic impairment manufacturer advises caution—no information available

Renal impairment see Cautions above; also avoid if estimated glomerular filtration rate less than 30 mL/minute/1.73 m²

Pregnancy manufacturer advises avoid—toxicity in *animal* studies

Breast-feeding manufacturer advises avoid—no information available

Side-effects nausea, bitter taste; headache, asthenia; ocular irritation, blurred vision, lacrimation, conjunctivitis, superficial punctuate keratitis, eyelid inflammation; *less commonly* iridocyclitis; *rarely* hypersensitivity reactions (including urticaria, angioedema, bronchospasm), dizziness, paraesthesia, urolithiasis, eyelid crusting, transient myopia, corneal oedema, epistaxis, dry mouth, throat irritation; also reported metabolic acidosis

Licensed use not licensed for use in children

Indication and dose

Raised intra-ocular pressure in ocular hypertension, open-angle glaucoma, pseudo-exfoliative glaucoma *either* as adjunct to beta-blocker *or* used alone in patients unresponsive to beta-blockers or if beta-blockers contra-indicated

Used alone, apply 3 times daily; with topical beta-blocker, apply twice daily

Trusopt® (MSD) PoM
Ophthalmic solution (= eye drops), in *Ocumeter® Plus* metered-dose unit, dorzolamide (as hydrochloride) 2%, net price 5 mL = £6.33
Excipients include benzalkonium chloride

Unit dose eye drops, dorzolamide (as hydrochloride) 2%, net price 60 × 0.2 mL = £24.18

With timolol
For prescribing information on timolol, see section 11.6, Beta-blockers

Cosopt® (MSD) PoM
Ophthalmic solution (= eye drops), dorzolamide (as hydrochloride) 2%, timolol (as maleate) 0.5%, net price 5 mL = £10.05
Excipients include benzalkonium chloride

Unit dose eye drops, dorzolamide (as hydrochloride) 2%, timolol (as maleate) 0.5%, net price 60 × 0.2 mL = £28.59

Dose
Raised intra-ocular pressure in open-angle glaucoma, or pseudoexfoliative glaucoma when beta-blockers alone not adequate

Apply twice daily

Miotics

Pilocarpine is a miotic used in the management of raised intra-ocular pressure. The small pupil is an unfortunate side-effect of these drugs (except when pilocarpine is used temporarily before an operation for angle-closure glaucoma). Miotics act by opening up the inefficient drainage channels in the trabecular meshwork which may be occluded by contraction or spasm of the ciliary muscle.

Cautions A darkly pigmented iris may require higher concentration of the miotic or more frequent administration and care should be taken to avoid overdosage. Retinal detachment has occurred in susceptible individuals and those with retinal disease; therefore fundus examination is advised before starting treatment with a miotic. Care is also required in conjunctival or corneal damage. Intra-ocular pressure and visual fields should be monitored in those with chronic simple glaucoma and those receiving long-term treatment with a miotic. Miotics should be used with caution in cardiac disease, hypertension, asthma, peptic ulceration and urinary-tract obstruction.

Counselling Blurred vision may affect performance of skilled tasks (e.g. driving) particularly at night or in reduced lighting

Contra-indications Miotics are contra-indicated in conditions where pupillary constriction is undesirable such as acute iritis, anterior uveitis and some forms of secondary glaucoma. They should be avoided in acute inflammatory disease of the anterior segment.

Side-effects Ciliary spasm leads to headache and browache which may be more severe in the initial 2–4 weeks of treatment. Ocular side-effects include burning, itching, smarting, blurred vision, conjunctival vascular congestion, myopia, lens changes with chronic use, vitreous haemorrhage, and pupillary block. Systemic side-effects are rare following application to the eye.

◢ PILOCARPINE

Cautions see notes above
Contra-indications see notes above
Side-effects see notes above
Licensed use not licensed for use in children

Indication and dose
See also notes above

> Raised intra-ocular pressure in ocular hypertension and open-angle glaucoma
>
> **Child 1 month–2 years** 1 drop of 0.5% or 1% solution 3 times daily
>
> **Child 2–18 years** 1 drop 4 times daily

> Pre-operatively in goniotomy and trabeculotomy
>
> **Child 1 month–18 years** apply 1% or 2% solution once daily

> Dry mouth (section 12.3.5)

Pilocarpine Hydrochloride (Non-proprietary) PoM
Eye drops, pilocarpine hydrochloride 0.5%, net price 10 mL = £1.66; 1%, 10 mL = £2.70; 2%, 10 mL = £2.58; 3%, 10 mL = £2.03; 4%, 10 mL = £3.45

◢ Single use
Minims® Pilocarpine Nitrate (Bausch & Lomb) PoM
Eye drops, pilocarpine nitrate 2%, net price 20 × 0.5 mL = £9.84

11.7 Local anaesthetics

Oxybuprocaine and **tetracaine** are widely used topical local anaesthetics. **Proxymetacaine** causes less initial stinging and is particularly useful for children. Oxybuprocaine or a combined preparation of lidocaine (lignocaine) and fluorescein is used for tonometry. Tetracaine produces more profound anaesthesia and is suitable for use before minor surgical procedures, such as the removal of corneal sutures. It has a temporary disruptive effect on the corneal epithelium. **Lidocaine**, with or without adrenaline (epinephrine), is injected into the eyelids for minor surgery, while retrobulbar or peribulbar injections are used for surgery of the globe itself. Local anaesthetics should never be used for the management of ocular symptoms.

Caution   Local anaesthetic eye drops should be avoided in preterm neonates because of the immaturity of the metabolising enzyme system.

◢ LIDOCAINE HYDROCHLORIDE
(Lignocaine hydrochloride)
Contra-indications avoid in preterm neonates

Indication and dose
Local anaesthetic
Use as required

Minims® Lidocaine and Fluorescein (Bausch & Lomb) PoM
Eye drops, lidocaine hydrochloride 4%, fluorescein sodium 0.25%. Net price 20 × 0.5 mL = £10.40

◢ OXYBUPROCAINE HYDROCHLORIDE
(Benoxinate hydrochloride)
Contra-indications avoid in preterm neonates

Indication and dose
Local anaesthetic
Use as required

Minims® Oxybuprocaine Hydrochloride (Bausch & Lomb) PoM
Eye drops, oxybuprocaine hydrochloride 0.4%. Net price 20 × 0.5 mL = £8.61

◢ PROXYMETACAINE HYDROCHLORIDE
Contra-indications avoid in preterm neonates
Indication and dose
Local anaesthetic
Use as required

Minims® Proxymetacaine (Bausch & Lomb) PoM
Eye drops, proxymetacaine hydrochloride 0.5%.
Net price 20 × 0.5 mL = £9.04

◢ With fluorescein
Minims® Proxymetacaine and Fluorescein (Bausch & Lomb) PoM
Eye drops, proxymetacaine hydrochloride 0.5%, fluorescein sodium 0.25%. Net price 20 × 0.5 mL = £10.34

11
Eye

◼ TETRACAINE HYDROCHLORIDE

(Amethocaine hydrochloride)

Contra-indications avoid in preterm neonates

Indication and dose

Local anaesthetic

Use as required

Minims® Tetracaine Hydrochloride (Bausch & Lomb) PoM

Eye drops, tetracaine hydrochloride 0.5% and 1%. Net price 20 × 0.5 mL (both) = £8.63

11.8 Miscellaneous ophthalmic preparations

Certain eye drops, e.g. amphotericin, ceftazidime, cefuroxime, colistin, desferrioxamine, dexamethasone, gentamicin, and vancomycin, can be prepared aseptically in a specialist manufacturing unit from material supplied for injection.

Preparations may also be available from Moorfields Eye Hospital as manufactured specials, see also 'special-order' manufacturers or specialist importing companies, p. 957.

11.8.1 Tear deficiency, ocular lubricants, and astringents

Chronic soreness of the eyes associated with reduced or abnormal tear secretion often responds to tear replacement therapy. The severity of the condition and the child's preference will often guide the choice of preparation.

Hypromellose is the traditional choice of treatment for tear deficiency. It may need to be instilled frequently (e.g. hourly) for adequate relief. Ocular surface mucin is often abnormal in tear deficiency and the combination of hypromellose with a mucolytic such as **acetylcysteine** can be helpful.

The ability of **carbomers** to cling to the eye surface may help reduce frequency of application to 4 times daily.

Polyvinyl alcohol increases the persistence of the tear film and is useful when the ocular surface mucin is reduced.

Sodium hyaluronate eye drops are also used in the management of tear deficiency.

Sodium chloride 0.9% drops are sometimes useful in tear deficiency, and can be used as 'comfort drops' by contact lens wearers, and to facilitate lens removal. Special presentations of sodium chloride 0.9% and other irrigation solutions are used routinely for intra-ocular surgery and in first-aid for removal of harmful substances.

Eye ointments containing a **paraffin** can be used to lubricate the eye surface, especially in cases of recurrent corneal epithelial erosion. They may cause temporary visual disturbance and are best suited for application before sleep. Ointments should not be used during contact lens wear.

◼ ACETYLCYSTEINE

Indication and dose

Tear deficiency, impaired or abnormal mucus production

Apply 3–4 times daily

Ilube® (Alcon) PoM

Eye drops, acetylcysteine 5%, hypromellose 0.35%. Net price 10 mL = £4.49

Excipients include benzalkonium chloride, disodium edetate

◼ CARBOMERS

(Polyacrylic acid)

Synthetic high molecular weight polymers of acrylic acid cross-linked with either allyl ethers of sucrose or allyl ethers of pentaerithrityl

Licensed use some preparations not licensed for use in children

Indication and dose

Dry eyes including keratoconjunctivitis sicca, unstable tear film

Apply 3–4 times daily or as required

GelTears® (Chauvin)

Gel (= eye drops), carbomer 980 (polyacrylic acid) 0.2%, net price 10 g = £2.80

Excipients include benzalkonium chloride

Liposic® (Bausch & Lomb)

Gel (= eye drops), carbomer 980 (polyacrylic acid) 0.2%, net price 10 g = £2.96

Excipients include cetrimide

◁ **CARBOMERS** (*continued*)

Viscotears® (Novartis)
Liquid gel (= eye drops), carbomer 980 (polyacrylic acid) 0.2%, net price 10 g = £3.00
Excipients include cetrimide

Liquid gel (= eye drops), carbomer 980 (polyacrylic acid) 0.2%, net price 30 × 0.6-mL single-dose units = £5.53

CARMELLOSE SODIUM

Indication and dose

Dry eye conditions

Apply as required

Optive® (Allergan)
Eye drops, carmellose sodium 0.5%, glycerol, net price 10 mL = £7.49

◂Single use
Celluvisc® (Allergan)
Eye drops, carmellose sodium 0.5%, net price 30 × 0.4 mL = £5.75, 90 × 0.4 mL = £15.53; 1%, 30 × 0.4 mL = £3.00, 60 × 0.4 mL = £10.99

HYDROXYETHYLCELLULOSE

Indication and dose

Tear deficiency

Apply as required

Minims® **Artificial Tears** (Bausch & Lomb)
Eye drops, hydroxyethylcellulose 0.44%, sodium chloride 0.35%. Net price 20 × 0.5 mL = £7.48

HYDROXYPROPYL GUAR

Indication and dose

Dry eye conditions

Apply as required

Systane® (Alcon)
Eye drops, hydroxypropyl guar, net price 10 mL = £4.66

◂Single use
Systane® (Alcon)
Eye drops, hydroxypropyl guar, net price 28 × 0.8 mL = £4.66

HYPROMELLOSE

Indication and dose

Tear deficiency

Apply as required
Note The Royal Pharmaceutical Society of Great Britain has stated that where it is not possible to ascertain the strength of hypromellose prescribed, the prescriber should be contacted to clarify the strength intended.

Hypromellose (Non-proprietary)
Eye drops, hypromellose 0.3%, net price 10 mL = £1.68
Brands include *Artelac*®

Isopto Alkaline® (Alcon)
Eye drops, hypromellose 1%, net price 10 mL = 96p
Excipients include benzalkonium chloride

Isopto Plain® (Alcon)
Eye drops, hypromellose 0.5%, net price 10 mL = 82p
Excipients include benzalkonium chloride

Tears Naturale® (Alcon)
Eye drops, dextran '70' 0.1%, hypromellose 0.3%, net price 15 mL = £1.63
Excipients include benzalkonium chloride, disodium edetate

◂Single use
Hypromellose (Non-proprietary)
Eye drops, hypromellose 0.3%, net price 30 × 0.4 mL = £5.75
Brands include *Hydromoor*®

Artelac® **SDU** (Pharma-Global)
Eye drops, hypromellose 0.32%, net price 30 × 0.5 mL = £16.95

LIQUID PARAFFIN

Indication and dose

Dry eye conditions

Apply as required

Lacri-Lube® (Allergan)
Eye ointment, white soft paraffin 57.3%, liquid paraffin 42.5%, wool alcohols 0.2%. Net price 3.5 g = £2.28, 5 g = £3.32

11

Eye

PARAFFIN, YELLOW, SOFT

Indication and dose

See notes above

Apply 2 hourly as required

Simple Eye Ointment
Ointment, liquid paraffin 10%, wool fat 10%, in yellow soft paraffin. Net price 4 g = £2.80

POLYVINYL ALCOHOL

Indication and dose

Tear deficiency

Apply as required

Liquifilm Tears® (Allergan)
Ophthalmic solution (= eye drops), polyvinyl alcohol 1.4%. Net price 15 mL = £1.93
Excipients include benzalkonium chloride, disodium edetate

Ophthalmic solution (= eye drops), polyvinyl alcohol 1.4%, povidone 0.6%. Net price 30 × 0.4 mL = £5.35

Sno Tears® (Chauvin)
Eye drops, polyvinyl alcohol 1.4%. Net price 10 mL = £1.06
Excipients include benzalkonium chloride, disodium edetate

SODIUM CHLORIDE

Indication and dose

Irrigation, including first-aid removal of harmful substances

Use as required

Sodium Chloride 0.9% Solutions
See section 13.11.1

Balanced Salt Solution
Solution (sterile), sodium chloride 0.64%, sodium acetate 0.39%, sodium citrate 0.17%, calcium

chloride 0.048%, magnesium chloride 0.03%, potassium chloride 0.075%
For intra-ocular or topical irrigation during surgical procedures
Brands include *Iocare®*

◢Single use
Minims® Saline (Bausch & Lomb)
Eye drops, sodium chloride 0.9%. Net price 20 × 0.5 mL = £6.40

SODIUM HYALURONATE

Indication and dose

Dry eye conditions

Apply as required

Hylo-Forte® (Scope Opthalmics)
Eye drops, sodium hyaluronate 0.2%, net price 10 mL = £10.80

Hylo-Tear® (Scope Opthalmics)
Eye drops, sodium hyaluronate 0.1%, net price 10 mL = £9.80

Oxyal® (Kestrel Ophthalmics)
Eye drops, sodium hyaluronate 0.15%, net price 10 ml = £4.15

Vismed® Multi (TRB Chemedica)
Eye drops, sodium hyaluronate 0.18%, net price 10 mL = £6.81

◢Single use
Clinitas® (Altacor)
Eye drops, sodium hyaluronate 0.4%, net price 30 × 0.5 mL = £5.70

Ocusan® (Agepha)
Eye drops, sodium hyaluronate 0.2%, net price 20 × 0.5 mL = £5.25

Vismed® (TRB Chemedica)
Eye drops, sodium hyaluronate 0.18%, net price 20 × 0.3 mL = £5.10

11.8.2 Ocular diagnostic and peri-operative preparations

Ocular diagnostic preparations

Fluorescein sodium is used in diagnostic procedures and for locating damaged areas of the cornea due to injury or disease.

FLUORESCEIN SODIUM

Indication and dose

Detection of lesions and foreign bodies

Sufficient to stain damaged areas

Minims® Fluorescein Sodium (Bausch & Lomb)
Eye drops, fluorescein sodium 1% or 2%. Net price 20 × 0.5 mL (both) = £7.38

◢With local anaesthetic
Section 11.7

Ocular peri-operative drugs

Drugs used to prepare the eye for surgery and drugs that are injected into the anterior chamber at the time of surgery are included here.

Sodium hyaluronate is used during surgical procedures on the eye.

Apraclonidine, an alpha$_2$-adrenoceptor agonist, reduces intra-ocular pressure possibly by reducing the production of aqueous humour. It is used for short-term treatment only.

Balanced Salt Solution is used routinely in intra-ocular surgery (section 11.8.1).

ACETYLCHOLINE CHLORIDE

Licensed use not licensed for use in children

Indication and dose

Cataract surgery, penetrating keratoplasty, iridectomy, other anterior segment surgery requiring rapid complete miosis

Consult product literature

Miochol-E® (Novartis) PoM
Solution for intra-ocular irrigation, acetylcholine chloride 1%, mannitol 3% when reconstituted. Net price 2 mL-vial = £9.10

APRACLONIDINE

Note Apraclonidine is a derivative of clonidine

Cautions history of angina, severe coronary insufficiency, recent myocardial infarction, heart failure, cerebrovascular disease, vasovagal attack, chronic renal failure; depression; pregnancy and breast-feeding; monitor intra-ocular pressure and visual fields; loss of effect may occur over time; suspend treatment if reduction in vision occurs in end-stage glaucoma; monitor for excessive reduction in intra-ocular pressure following peri-operative use; **interactions:** Appendix 1 (alpha$_2$-adrenoceptor stimulants)

Skilled tasks Drowsiness may affect performance of skilled tasks (e.g. driving)

Contra-indications history of severe or unstable and uncontrolled cardiovascular disease

Side-effects dry mouth, taste disturbance; hyperaemia, ocular pruritus, discomfort and lacrimation (withdraw if ocular intolerance including oedema of lids and conjunctiva); headache, asthenia, dry nose; lid retraction, conjunctival blanching and mydriasis reported after peri-operative use; since absorption may follow topical application systemic effects (see Clonidine Hydrochloride, section 2.5.2) may occur

Licensed use 0.5% drops not licensed for use in children under 12 years; 1% drops not licensed for use in children

Indication and dose

See preparations below

Iopidine® (Alcon) PoM
Ophthalmic solution (= eye drops), apraclonidine 1% (as hydrochloride). Net price 12 × 2 single use 0.25-mL units = £79.36
Dose

Control or prevention of postoperative elevation of intra-ocular pressure after anterior segment laser surgery

Apply 1 drop 1 hour before laser procedure then 1 drop immediately after completion of procedure

Ophthalmic solution (= eye drops), apraclonidine 0.5% (as hydrochloride). Net price 5 mL = £11.10
Excipients include benzalkonium chloride
Dose

Short-term adjunctive treatment of chronic glaucoma in patients not adequately controlled by another drug (see note below)

Child 12–18 years apply 1 drop 3 times daily usually for max. 1 month
Note May not provide additional benefit if patient already using two drugs that suppress the production of aqueous humour

DICLOFENAC SODIUM

Licensed use not licensed for use in children

Indication and dose

Inhibition of intra-operative miosis during cataract surgery (but does not possess intrinsic mydriatic properties), postoperative inflammation in cataract surgery, strabismus surgery, argon laser trabeculoplasty

Consult product literature

Voltarol® Ophtha Multidose (Novartis) PoM
Eye drops, diclofenac sodium 0.1%, net price 5 mL = £6.68
Excipients include benzalkonium chloride, disodium edetate, propylene glycol

◢ **Single use**
Voltarol® Ophtha (Novartis) PoM
Eye drops, diclofenac sodium 0.1%. Net price pack of 5 single-dose units = £4.00, 40 single-dose units = £32.00

11 Eye

■ FLURBIPROFEN SODIUM

Licensed use not licensed for use in children

Indication and dose

Inhibition of intra-operative miosis (but does not possess intrinsic mydriatic properties), control of postoperative and post-laser trabeculoplasty inflammation (if corticosteroids contra-indicated)

Consult product literature

Ocufen® (Allergan) PoM
Ophthalmic solution (= eye drops), flurbiprofen sodium 0.03%, polyvinyl alcohol (*Liquifilm*®) 1.4%. Net price 40 × 0.4 mL = £37.15

■ KETOROLAC TROMETAMOL

Licensed use not licensed for use in children

Indication and dose

Prophylaxis and reduction of inflammation and associated symptoms following ocular surgery

Consult product literature

Acular® (Allergan) PoM
Eye drops, ketorolac trometamol 0.5%. Net price 5 mL = £3.00
Excipients include benzalkonium chloride, disodium edetate

11.9 Contact lenses

Some children and adolescents prefer to wear contact lenses rather than spectacles for both cosmetic and medical reasons. Visual defects are corrected by either rigid ('hard' or gas permeable) lenses or soft (hydrogel) lenses; soft lenses are the most popular type, because they are the most comfortable, but they may not give the best vision. Lenses should usually be worn for a specified number of hours each day. Continuous (extended) wear involves much greater risks to eye health and is not recommended except where medically indicated.

Contact lenses require meticulous care. Poor compliance with directions for use, and with daily cleaning and disinfection, can result in complications including ulcerative keratitis and conjunctival problems (such as purulent or papillary conjunctivitis). One-day disposable lenses, which are worn only once and therefore require no maintenance or storage, are becoming increasingly popular.

Acanthamoeba keratitis, a sight-threatening condition, is associated with ineffective lens cleaning and disinfection or the use of contaminated lens cases. The condition is especially associated with the use of soft lenses (including frequently replaced lenses) and should be treated by specialists.

Contact lenses and drug treatment   Special care is required in prescribing eye preparations for contact lens users. Some drugs and preservatives in eye preparations can accumulate in hydrogel lenses and can cause adverse reactions. Therefore, unless medically indicated, the lenses should be removed before instillation and not worn during the period of treatment. Alternatively, unpreserved drops can be used. Eye drops may, however, be instilled over rigid corneal contact lenses. Ointment preparations should never be used in conjunction with contact lens wear; oily eye drops should also be avoided.

Many drugs given systemically can also have adverse effects on contact lens wear. These include oral contraceptives (particularly those with a higher oestrogen content), drugs which reduce blink rate (e.g. anxiolytics, hypnotics, antihistamines, and muscle relaxants), drugs which reduce lacrimation (e.g. antihistamines, antimuscarinics, phenothiazines and related drugs, some beta-blockers, diuretics, and tricyclic antidepressants), and drugs which increase lacrimation (including ephedrine and hydralazine). Other drugs that can affect contact lens wear are isotretinoin (can cause conjunctival inflammation), aspirin (salicylic acid appears in tears and can be absorbed by contact lenses—leading to irritation), and rifampicin and sulfasalazine (can discolour lenses).

12 Ear, nose, and oropharynx

This chapter also includes advice on the drug management of the following:
allergic rhinitis, p. 657
nasal polyps, p. 657
oropharyngeal infections, p. 665
periodontitis, p. 663

12.1 Drugs acting on the ear

12.1.1 Otitis externa
12.1.2 Otitis media
12.1.3 Removal of ear wax

12.1.1 Otitis externa

Otitis externa is an inflammatory reaction of the lining of the ear canal usually associated with an underlying seborrhoeic dermatitis or eczema; it is important to exclude an underlying chronic otitis media before treatment is commenced. Many cases recover after thorough cleansing of the external ear canal by suction or dry mopping.

A frequent problem in resistant cases is the difficulty in applying lotions and ointments satisfactorily to the relatively inaccessible affected skin. The most effective method is to introduce a ribbon gauze dressing or sponge wick soaked with **corticosteroid** ear drops or with an astringent such as **aluminium acetate** solution. When this is not practical, the ear should be gently cleansed with a probe covered in cotton wool and the patient encouraged to lie with the affected ear uppermost for ten minutes after the canal has been filled with a liberal quantity of the appropriate solution.

Secondary infection in otitis externa may be of bacterial, fungal, or viral origin. If infection is present, a topical anti-infective which is not used systemically (such as **neomycin** or **clioquinol**) may be used, but for only about a week because excessive use may result in fungal infections that are difficult to treat. Sensitivity to the anti-infective or solvent may occur and resistance to antibacterials is a possibility with prolonged use. **Aluminium acetate** ear drops are also effective against bacterial infection and inflammation of the ear. **Chloramphenicol** may be used, but the ear drops contain propylene glycol and cause hypersensitivity reactions in about 10% of patients. Solutions containing an anti-infective and a corticosteroid (such as *Locorten-Vioform®*) are used for treating children when infection is present with inflammation and eczema. **Clotrimazole** 1% solution is used topically to treat fungal infection in otitis externa.

In view of reports of ototoxicity in patients with a perforated tympanic membrane (eardrum), the CSM has stated that treatment with a topical aminoglycoside antibiotic is contra-indicated in those with a tympanic perforation. However, many specialists do use these drops cautiously in the presence of a perforation in children with otitis media (section 12.1.2) and when other measures have failed for otitis externa.

A solution of **acetic acid** 2% acts as an antifungal and antibacterial in the external ear canal and may be used to treat mild otitis externa. More severe cases require treatment with an anti-inflammatory preparation with or without an anti-infective drug. A proprietary preparation containing acetic acid 2% (*EarCalm®* spray) is on sale to the public for children over 12 years.

For severe pain associated with otitis externa, a simple analgesic, such as **paracetamol** (section 4.7.1) or **ibuprofen** (section 10.1.1), can be used. A systemic antibacterial (Table 1, section 5.1) can be used if there is spreading cellulitis or if the child is systemically unwell. When a resistant staphylococcal infection (a boil) is present in the external auditory canal, oral **flucloxacillin** (section 5.1.1.2) is the drug of choice; oral **ciprofloxacin** (section 5.1.12) or a systemic aminoglycoside may be needed for pseudomonal infections, particularly in children with diabetes or compromised immunity.

The skin of the pinna adjacent to the ear canal is often affected by eczema. A topical corticosteroid (section 13.4) cream or ointment is then required, but prolonged use should be avoided.

Administration To administer ear drops, lay the child down with the head turned to one side; for an infant pull the earlobe back and down, for an older child pull the earlobe back and up.

Astringent preparations

ALUMINIUM ACETATE

Licensed use not licensed

Indication and dose

Inflammation in otitis externa (see notes above)

Insert into meatus or apply on a ribbon gauze dressing or sponge wick which should be kept saturated with the ear drops

Aluminium Acetate (Non-proprietary)
Ear drops 13%, aluminium sulphate 2.25 g, calcium carbonate 1 g, tartaric acid 450 mg, acetic acid (33%) 2.5 mL, purified water 7.5 mL
Available as manufactured special

Ear drops 8%, dilute 8 parts aluminium acetate ear drops (13%) with 5 parts purified water. Must be freshly prepared

Anti-inflammatory preparations

Corticosteroids

Topical corticosteroids are used to treat inflammation and eczema in otitis externa.

Cautions Prolonged use of topical corticosteroid ear preparations should be avoided.

Contra-indications Corticosteroid ear preparations should be avoided in the presence of an untreated ear infection. If infection is present, the corticosteroid should be used in combination with a suitable anti-infective (see notes above).

Side-effects Local sensitivity reactions may occur.

BETAMETHASONE SODIUM PHOSPHATE

Cautions see notes above
Contra-indications see notes above
Side-effects see notes above
Licensed use licensed for use in children (age range not specified by manufacturers)

Indication and dose

> Eczematous inflammation in otitis externa (see notes above); for dose, see under preparations

> Eye section 11.4.1

> Nose section 12.2.1 and section 12.2.3

Betnesol® (UCB Pharma) [PoM]
> Drops (for ear, eye, or nose), betamethasone sodium phosphate 0.1%. Net price 10 mL = £2.23
> **Excipients** include benzalkonium chloride, disodium edetate

Dose
> *Ear*, instil 2–3 drops every 2–3 hours; reduce frequency when relief obtained

Vistamethasone® (Martindale) [PoM]
> Drops (for ear, eye, or nose), betamethasone sodium phosphate 0.1%. Net price 5 mL = £1.02; 10 mL = £1.16
> **Excipients** include benzalkonium chloride, disodium edetate

Dose
> *Ear*, instil 2–3 drops every 3–4 hours; reduce frequency when relief obtained

◢**With antibacterial**
Betnesol-N® (UCB Pharma) [PoM]
> Drops (for ear, eye, or nose), betamethasone sodium phosphate 0.1%, neomycin sulphate 0.5%. Net price 10 mL = £2.30
> **Excipients** include benzalkonium chloride, disodium edetate

Dose
> *Ear*, instil 2–3 drops 3–4 times daily

DEXAMETHASONE

Cautions see notes above
Contra-indications see notes above
Side-effects see notes above
Licensed use licensed for use in children (age range not specified by manufacturers)

Indication and dose

> Eczematous inflammation in otitis externa (see notes above); for dose, see under preparations

◢**With antibacterial**
Otomize® (GSK Consumer Healthcare) [PoM]
> Ear spray, dexamethasone 0.1%, neomycin sulphate 3250 units/mL, glacial acetic acid 2%. Net price 5-mL pump-action aerosol unit = £3.79
> **Excipients** include hydroxybenzoates (parabens)

Dose
> *Ear*, apply 1 metered spray 3 times daily

Sofradex® (Sanofi-Aventis) [PoM] ◢
> Drops (for ear or eye), dexamethasone (as sodium metasulphobenzoate) 0.05%, framycetin sulphate 0.5%, gramicidin 0.005%. Net price 10 mL = £6.25
> **Excipients** include polysorbate 80

Dose
> *Ear*, instil 2–3 drops 3–4 times daily; *eye*, section 11.4.1

FLUMETASONE PIVALATE
(Flumethasone Pivalate)
Cautions see notes above
Contra-indications see notes above
Side-effects see notes above

Indication and dose

> Eczematous inflammation in otitis externa (see notes above); for dose, see under preparation

◢**With antibacterial**
Locorten-Vioform® (Amdipharm) [PoM]
> Ear drops, flumetasone pivalate 0.02%, clioquinol 1%. Net price 7.5 mL = £1.76
> **Contra-indications** iodine sensitivity

Dose
> **Child 2–18 years** instil 2–3 drops into the ear twice daily for 7–10 days

> **Note** Clioquinol stains skin and clothing

HYDROCORTISONE

Cautions see notes above

Contra-indications see notes above

Side-effects see notes above

Licensed use *Otosporin®* not licensed for use in children under 3 years; *other preparations* licensed for use in children (age range not specified by manufacturers)

Indication and dose

> Eczematous inflammation in otitis externa (see notes above); for dose, see under preparations

12 Ear, nose, and oropharynx

◻ HYDROCORTISONE (*continued*)

◢With antibacterial

Gentisone® HC (Amdipharm) [PoM]
Ear drops, hydrocortisone acetate 1%, gentamicin 0.3% (as sulphate). Net price 10 mL = £3.69
Excipients include benzalkonium chloride, disodium edetate

Dose
Ear, instil 2–4 drops 3–4 times daily and at night

Otosporin® (GSK) [PoM] ◢
Ear drops, hydrocortisone 1%, neomycin sulphate 3400 units, polymyxin B sulphate 10 000 units/mL. Net price 5 mL = £2.00; 10 mL = £4.00
Excipients include cetostearyl alcohol, hydroxybenzoates (parabens), polysorbate 20

Dose
Child 3–18 years instil 3 drops into the ear 3–4 times daily

PREDNISOLONE SODIUM PHOSPHATE

Cautions see notes above
Contra-indications see notes above
Side-effects see notes above
Licensed use licensed for use in children (age range not specified by manufacturers)

Indication and dose
Eczematous inflammation in otitis externa (see notes above); for dose, see under preparations

Eye section 11.4.1

Predsol® (UCB Pharma) [PoM]
Drops (for ear or eye), prednisolone sodium phosphate 0.5%. Net price 10 mL = £1.92
Excipients include benzalkonium chloride, disodium edetate

Dose
Ear, instil 2–3 drops every 2–3 hours; reduce frequency when relief obtained

◢With antibacterial

Predsol-N® (UCB Pharma) [PoM]
Drops (for ear or eye), prednisolone sodium phosphate 0.5%, neomycin sulphate 0.5%. Net price 10 mL = £2.27
Excipients include benzalkonium chloride, disodium edetate

Dose
Ear, instil 2–3 drops 3–4 times daily

Anti-infective preparations

CHLORAMPHENICOL ◢

Cautions avoid prolonged use (see notes above)
Side-effects high incidence of sensitivity reactions to vehicle
Licensed use licensed for use in children (age range not specified by manufacturers)

Indication and dose
Bacterial infection in otitis externa (but see notes above); for dose, see under preparation

Chloramphenicol (Non-proprietary) [PoM] ◢
Ear drops, chloramphenicol in propylene glycol, net price 5%, 10 mL = £1.78; 10%, 10 mL = £5.62
Excipients include propylene glycol

Dose
Ear, instil 2–3 drops 2–3 times daily

CLOTRIMAZOLE

Side-effects occasional local irritation or sensitivity
Licensed use licensed for use in children (age range not specified by manufacturer)

Indication and dose
Fungal infection in otitis externa (see notes above); for dose, see under preparation

Canesten® (Bayer Consumer Care)
Solution, clotrimazole 1% in polyethylene glycol 400 (macrogol 400). Net price 20 mL = £2.43

Dose
Ear, apply 2–3 times daily continuing for at least 14 days after disappearance of infection

FRAMYCETIN SULPHATE

Cautions avoid prolonged use (see notes above)
Contra-indications perforated tympanic membrane (see p. 652)
Side-effects local sensitivity

Indication and dose
Bacterial infection in otitis externa (see notes above)

Eye section 11.3.1

◢With corticosteroid
Sofradex®
see Dexamethasone, p. 653

GENTAMICIN

Cautions avoid prolonged use (see notes above)

Contra-indications perforated tympanic membrane (but see p. 652 and section 12.1.2)

Side-effects local sensitivity

Licensed use licensed for use in children (age range not specified by manufacturer)

Indication and dose

> Bacterial infection in otitis externa (see notes above); for dose, see under preparations

Genticin® (Amdipharm) [PoM]

> Drops (for ear or eye), gentamicin 0.3% (as sulphate). Net price 10 mL = £2.13
> **Excipients** include benzalkonium chloride

Dose

> *Ear*, instil 2–3 drops 3–4 times daily and at night; *eye*, section 11.3.1

◀With corticosteroid

Gentisone® HC

> see Hydrocortisone, p. 654

NEOMYCIN SULPHATE

Cautions avoid prolonged use (see notes above)

Contra-indications perforated tympanic membrane (see p. 652)

Side-effects local sensitivity

Indication and dose

> Bacterial infection in otitis externa (see notes above)

◀With corticosteroid

Betnesol-N® [PoM]

> see Betamethasone, p. 653

Otomize®

> see Dexamethasone, p. 653

Otosporin®

> see Hydrocortisone, p. 654

Predsol-N®

> see Prednisolone, p. 654

12.1.2 Otitis media

Acute otitis media   Acute otitis media is the commonest cause of severe aural pain in young children and may occur with even minor upper respiratory tract infections. Children diagnosed with acute otitis media should not be prescribed antibacterials routinely as many infections, especially those accompanying coryza, are caused by viruses. Most uncomplicated cases resolve without antibacterial treatment and a **simple analgesic**, such as paracetamol, may be sufficient. In children without systemic features, a **systemic antibacterial** (Table 1, section 5.1) may be started after 72 hours if there is no improvement, or earlier if there is deterioration, if the child is systemically unwell, if the child is at high risk of serious complications (e.g. in immunosuppression, cystic fibrosis), if mastoiditis is present, or in children under 2 years of age with bilateral otitis media. Perforation of the tympanic membrane in children with *acute otitis media* usually heals spontaneously without treatment; if there is no improvement, e.g. pain or discharge persists, a systemic antibacterial (Table 1, section 5.1) can be given. Topical antibacterial treatment of acute otitis media is ineffective and there is no place for ear drops containing a local anaesthetic.

Otitis media with effusion   Otitis media with effusion ('glue ear') occurs in about 10% of children and in 90% of children with cleft palates. Antimicrobials, corticosteroids, decongestants, and antihistamines have little place in the routine management of otitis media with effusion. If 'glue ear' persists for more than a month or two, the child should be referred for assessment and follow up because of the risk of long-term hearing impairment which can delay language development. Untreated or resistant glue ear may be responsible for some types of *chronic otitis media.*

Chronic otitis media   Opportunistic organisms are often present in the debris, keratin, and necrotic bone of the middle ear and mastoid in children with chronic otitis media. The mainstay of treatment is thorough cleansing with aural microsuction, which may completely resolve long-standing infection. Cleansing may be followed by topical treatment as for otitis externa (section 12.1.1); this is particularly beneficial for discharging ears or infections of the mastoid cavity. Acute exacerbations of chronic infection may require treatment with an oral antibacterial (Table 1, section 5.1); a swab should be taken to identify infecting organisms and antibacterial sensitivity. Parenteral antibacterial treatment is required if *Pseudomonas aeruginosa* or *Proteus spp.* are present.

12

Ear, nose, and oropharynx

The CSM has stated that topical treatment with ototoxic antibacterials is contra-indicated in the presence of a perforation (section 12.1.1). However, many specialists use ear drops containing **aminoglycosides** (e.g. neomycin) or **polymyxins** if the otitis media has failed to settle with systemic antibacterials; it is considered that the pus in the middle ear associated with otitis media carries a higher risk of ototoxicity than the drops themselves. **Ciprofloxacin** or **ofloxacin** ear drops (available from specialist importing companies) or eye drops used in the ear [unlicensed indication] are an effective alternative to aminoglycoside ear drops for chronic otitis media in patients with perforation of the tympanic membrane.

12.1.3 Removal of ear wax

Ear wax (cerumen) is a normal bodily secretion which provides a protective film on the meatal skin and need only be removed if it causes hearing loss or interferes with a proper view of the ear drum.

Ear wax causing discomfort or impaired hearing may be softened with simple remedies such as **olive oil** ear drops or **almond oil** ear drops; **sodium bicarbonate** ear drops are also effective, but may cause dryness of the ear canal. If the wax is hard and impacted, the drops may be used twice daily for several days. The child should lie with the affected ear uppermost for 5 to 10 minutes after a generous amount of the softening remedy has been introduced into the ear. Proprietary preparations containing organic solvents can irritate the meatal skin, and in most cases the simple remedies indicated above are just as effective and less likely to cause irritation. Docusate sodium or urea hydrogen peroxide are ingredients in a number of proprietary preparations for softening ear wax.

If necessary, wax may be removed by irrigation with water (warmed to body temperature). Ear irrigation is generally best avoided in young children, in children who have had otitis media in the last 6 weeks, in otitis externa, and in children with learning disabilities, cleft palate, a history of ear drum perforation, or previous ear surgery. A child who has hearing in one ear only should not have that ear irrigated because even a very slight risk of damage is unacceptable in this situation.

For administration of ear drops, see p. 652.

Almond Oil (Non-proprietary)
Ear drops, almond oil in a suitable container
Allow to warm to room temperature before use

Olive Oil (Non-proprietary)
Ear drops, olive oil in a suitable container
Allow to warm to room temperature before use

Sodium Bicarbonate (Non-proprietary)
Ear drops, sodium bicarbonate 5%, net price 10 mL = £1.25

Cerumol® (Thornton & Ross)
Ear drops, chlorobutanol 5%, arachis (peanut) oil 57.3%. Net price 11 mL = £1.76

Exterol® (Dermal)
Ear drops, urea–hydrogen peroxide complex 5% in glycerol. Net price 8 mL = £1.77

Molcer® (Wallace Mfg)
Ear drops, docusate sodium 5%. Net price 15 mL = £5.60
Excipients include propylene glycol

Otex® (DDD)
Ear drops, urea–hydrogen peroxide 5%. Net price 8 mL = £2.64

Waxsol® (Norgine)
Ear drops, docusate sodium 0.5%. Net price 10 mL = £1.21

12.2 Drugs acting on the nose

12.2.1 Drugs used in nasal allergy
12.2.2 Topical nasal decongestants
12.2.3 Nasal preparations for infection

Rhinitis is often self-limiting but bacterial sinusitis may require treatment with antibacterials (Table 1, section 5.1). Many nasal preparations contain sympathomimetic drugs (section 12.2.2) which can give rise to rebound congestion (*rhinitis medicamentosa*) and may damage the nasal cilia. **Sodium chloride 0.9%** solution may be used as a douche or 'sniff' following endonasal surgery.

Administration   To administer nasal drops, lay the child face-upward with the neck extended, instil the drops, then sit the child up and tilt the head forward.

Nasal polyps   Short-term use of corticosteroid nasal drops helps to shrink nasal polyps; to be effective, the drops must be administered with the child in the 'head down' position. A short course of a systemic corticosteroid (section 6.3.2) may be required initially to shrink large polyps. A corticosteroid nasal spray can be used to maintain the reduction in swelling and also for the initial treatment of small polyps.

12.2.1 Drugs used in nasal allergy

Mild allergic rhinitis is controlled by **antihistamines** (see also section 3.4.1) or topical **nasal corticosteroids**; systemic nasal decongestants (section 3.10) are not recommended for use in children. Topical nasal decongestants can be used for a short period to relieve congestion and allow penetration of a topical nasal corticosteroid.

More persistent symptoms can be relieved by topical nasal **corticosteroids** or **cromoglicate**; the topical antihistamine, **azelastine**, is useful for controlling breakthrough symptoms in allergic rhinitis. Azelastine is less effective than nasal corticosteroids, but probably more effective than sodium cromoglicate. In seasonal allergic rhinitis (e.g. hay fever), treatment should begin 2 to 3 weeks before the season commences and may have to be continued for several months; continuous long-term treatment may be required in perennial rhinitis.

Montelukast (section 3.3.2) is less effective than topical nasal corticosteroids; montelukast can be used in children with seasonal allergic rhinitis (unresponsive to other treatments) and concomitant asthma.

Children with disabling symptoms of seasonal rhinitis (e.g. students taking important examinations), may be treated with oral **corticosteroids** (section 6.3.2) for short periods. Oral corticosteroids may also be used at the beginning of a course of treatment with a corticosteroid spray to relieve severe mucosal oedema and allow the spray to penetrate the nasal mucosa.

Sometimes allergic rhinitis is accompanied by vasomotor rhinitis. In this situation, the addition of topical nasal **ipratropium bromide** (section 12.2.2) can reduce watery rhinorrhoea.

Pregnancy   If a pregnant woman cannot tolerate the symptoms of allergic rhinitis, treatment with nasal beclometasone, budesonide, fluticasone propionate, or sodium cromoglicate may be considered.

Antihistamines

AZELASTINE HYDROCHLORIDE

Side-effects   irritation of nasal mucosa; bitter taste (if applied incorrectly)

Indication and dose

Treatment of allergic rhinitis for dose, see under preparation

Rhinolast® (Meda) [PoM]
Nasal spray, azelastine hydrochloride 140 micrograms (0.14 mL)/metered spray. Net price 22 mL (157-spray unit with metered pump) = £8.57
Excipients include sodium edetate

Dose

Child 5–18 years apply 140 micrograms (1 spray) into each nostril twice daily

Note Preparations of azelastine hydrochloride can be sold to the public for nasal administration in aqueous form (other than by aerosol) for the treatment of seasonal allergic rhinitis or perennial allergic rhinitis in children over 5 years, subject to max. single dose of 140 micrograms per nostril, max. daily dose of 280 micrograms per nostril, and a pack size limit of 36 doses

Corticosteroids

Nasal preparations containing corticosteroids have a useful role in the prophylaxis and treatment of allergic rhinitis (see notes above).

Cautions   Corticosteroid nasal preparations should be avoided in the presence of untreated nasal infections, and also after nasal surgery (until healing has occurred); they should also be avoided in pulmonary tuberculosis. Systemic absorption may follow nasal administration particularly if high doses are used or if treatment is prolonged; for cautions and side-effects of systemic corticosteroids, see section 6.3.2. The risk of systemic effects may be greater with nasal drops than with nasal sprays; drops are administered incorrectly more often than sprays. The CSM recommends that the height of children receiving prolonged treatment with nasal corticosteroids is monitored; if growth is slowed, referral to a paediatrician should be considered.

Side-effects Local side-effects include dryness, irritation of nose and throat, and epistaxis. Nasal ulceration has been reported, and occurs commonly with nasal preparations containing fluticasone furoate or mometasone furoate. Nasal septal perforation (usually following nasal surgery) occurs very rarely. Raised intra-ocular pressure or glaucoma may occur rarely. Headache, smell and taste disturbances may also occur. Hypersensitivity reactions, including bronchospasm, have been reported.

BECLOMETASONE DIPROPIONATE
(Beclomethasone Dipropionate)

Cautions see notes above
Side-effects see notes above

Indication and dose
Prophylaxis and treatment of allergic and vasomotor rhinitis

Child 6–18 years apply 100 micrograms (2 sprays) into each nostril twice daily; max. total 400 micrograms (8 sprays) daily; when symptoms controlled, dose reduced to 50 micrograms (1 spray) into each nostril twice daily

Beclometasone (Non-proprietary) [PoM]
Nasal spray, beclometasone dipropionate 50 micrograms/metered spray. Net price 200-spray unit = £3.06
Brands include *Nasobec Aqueous*®

Beconase® (A&H) [PoM]
Nasal spray (aqueous suspension), beclometasone dipropionate 50 micrograms/metered spray. Net price 200-spray unit with applicator = £2.19
Excipients include benzalkonium chloride, polysorbate 80

BETAMETHASONE SODIUM PHOSPHATE

Cautions see notes above
Side-effects see notes above
Licensed use licensed for use in children (age range not specified by manufacturer)

Indication and dose
Non-infected inflammatory conditions of nose
for dose, see under preparations

Eye section 11.4.1

Ear section 12.1.1

Betnesol® (UCB Pharma) [PoM]
Drops (for ear, eye, or nose), betamethasone sodium phosphate 0.1%, net price 10 mL = £2.23
Excipients include benzalkonium chloride, disodium edetate
Dose
Nose, instil 2–3 drops into each nostril 2–3 times daily

Vistamethasone® (Martindale) [PoM]
Drops (for ear, eye, or nose), betamethasone sodium phosphate 0.1%. Net price 5 mL = £1.02, 10 mL = £1.16
Excipients include benzalkonium chloride, disodium edetate
Dose
Nose, instil 2–3 drops into each nostril twice daily

BUDESONIDE

Cautions see notes above; **interactions**: Appendix 1 (corticosteroids)
Side-effects see notes above

Indication and dose
See under preparations

Budesonide (Non-proprietary) [PoM]
Nasal spray, budesonide 100 micrograms/metered spray, net price 100-spray unit = £5.90
Dose
Prophylaxis and treatment of allergic and vasomotor rhinitis

Child 12–18 years apply 200 micrograms (2 sprays) into each nostril once daily in the morning or 100 micrograms (1 spray) into each nostril twice daily; when control achieved reduce to 100 micrograms (1 spray) into each nostril once daily

Nasal polyps
Child 12–18 years apply 100 micrograms (1 spray) into each nostril twice daily for up to 3 months

Rhinocort Aqua® (AstraZeneca) [PoM]
Nasal spray, budesonide 64 micrograms/metered spray. Net price 120-spray unit = £4.49
Excipients include disodium edetate, polysorbate 80, potassium sorbate
Dose
Rhinitis
Child 12–18 years 128 micrograms (2 sprays) into each nostril once daily in the morning or 64 micrograms (1 spray) into each nostril twice daily; when control achieved reduce to 64 micrograms (1 spray) into each nostril once daily; max. duration of treatment 3 months

◻ **BUDESONIDE** *(continued)*

Nasal polyps
Child 12–18 years 64 micrograms (1 spray) into each nostril twice daily for up to 3 months

---

◼ FLUNISOLIDE

Cautions see notes above
Side-effects see notes above

Indication and dose

Prophylaxis and treatment of allergic rhinitis

Child 5–14 years initially 25 micrograms (1 spray) into each nostril up to 3 times daily then reduced for maintenance

Child 14–18 years 50 micrograms (2 sprays) into each nostril twice daily, increased if neces-sary to max. 3 times daily then reduced for maintenance

Syntaris® (IVAX) [PoM]
Aqueous nasal spray, flunisolide 25 micrograms/metered spray. Net price 240-spray unit with pump and applicator = £5.05
Excipients include benzalkonium chloride, butylated hydroxy-toluene, disodium edetate, polysorbate 20, propylene glycol

---

◼ FLUTICASONE PROPIONATE

Cautions see notes above; **interactions:** Appendix 1 (corticosteroids)
Side-effects see notes above

Indication and dose

Prophylaxis and treatment of allergic rhinitis

Child 4–12 years 50 micrograms (1 spray) into each nostril once daily, preferably in the morning, increased to max. twice daily if required

Child 12–18 years 100 micrograms (2 sprays) into each nostril once daily, preferably in the morning, increased to max. twice daily if required; when control achieved reduce to 50 micrograms (1 spray) into each nostril once daily

Nasal polyps see *Flixonase Nasule®* below

Flixonase® (A&H) [PoM]
Aqueous nasal spray, fluticasone propionate 50 micrograms/metered spray. Net price 150-spray unit with applicator = £11.23
Excipients include benzalkonium chloride, polysorbate 80

Flixonase Nasule® (A&H) [PoM]
Nasal drops, fluticasone propionate 400 micrograms/unit dose, net price 28 × 0.4-mL units = £13.25
Excipients include polysorbate 20

Dose
Nasal polyps
Child 16–18 years instil 200 micrograms (approx. 6 drops) into each nostril once or twice daily; consider alternative treatment if no improvement after 4–6 weeks

Nasofan® (IVAX) [PoM]
Aqueous nasal spray, fluticasone propionate 50 micrograms/metered spray. Net price 150–spray unit = £8.41
Excipients include benzalkonium chloride, polysorbate 80

◢ Fluticasone furoate
Avamys® (GSK) ▼ [PoM]
Nasal spray, fluticasone furoate 27.5 micrograms/metered spray, net price 120-spray unit = £6.44
Excipients include benzalkonium chloride, disodium edetate, polysorbate 80

Dose
Prophylaxis and treatment of allergic rhinitis
Child 6–12 years 27.5 micrograms (1 spray) into each nostril once daily, increased if necessary to 55 micrograms (2 sprays) into each nostril once daily; when control achieved reduce to 27.5 micrograms (1 spray) into each nostril once daily
Child 12–18 years 55 micrograms (2 sprays) into each nostril once daily; when control achieved reduce to minimum effective dose, 27.5 micrograms (1 spray) into each nostril once daily may be sufficient

---

◼ MOMETASONE FUROATE

Cautions see notes above
Side-effects see notes above

Indication and dose

See under preparation

Nasonex® (Schering-Plough) [PoM]
Nasal spray, mometasone furoate 50 micrograms/metered spray. Net price 140-spray unit = £7.68
Excipients include benzalkonium chloride, polysorbate 80

Dose
Prophylaxis and treatment of allergic rhinitis
Child 6–12 years 50 micrograms (1 spray) into each nostril once daily
Child 12–18 years 100 micrograms (2 sprays) into each nostril once daily, increased to max. 200 micrograms (4 sprays) into each nostril once daily; when control achieved reduce to 50 micrograms (1 spray) into each nostril once daily

◢ TRIAMCINOLONE ACETONIDE

Cautions see notes above

Side-effects see notes above

Licensed use not licensed for use in children under 6 years

Indication and dose

> **Treatment of allergic rhinitis**
>
> **Child 2–6 years** 55 micrograms (1 spray) into each nostril once daily; max. duration of treatment 4 weeks
>
> **Child 6–12 years** 55 micrograms (1 spray) into each nostril once daily, increased if necessary to 110 micrograms (2 sprays) into each nostril once daily; when control achieved reduce to 55 micrograms (1 spray) into each nostril once daily; max. duration of treatment 3 months
>
> **Child 12–18 years** 110 micrograms (2 sprays) into each nostril once daily; when control achieved, reduce to 55 micrograms (1 spray) into each nostril once daily

Nasacort® (Sanofi-Aventis) [PoM]

Aqueous nasal spray, triamcinolone acetonide 55 micrograms/metered spray. Net price 120-spray unit = £7.39

Excipients include benzalkonium chloride, disodium edetate, polysorbate 80

◢ Cromoglicate

◢ SODIUM CROMOGLICATE

(Sodium Cromoglycate)

Side-effects local irritation; rarely transient bronchospasm

Licensed use licensed for use in children (age range not specified by manufacturers)

Indication and dose

> **Prophylaxis of allergic rhinitis** for dose, see under preparations

Rynacrom® (Sanofi-Aventis)

4% aqueous nasal spray, sodium cromoglicate 4% (5.2 mg/spray). Net price 22 mL (150-spray unit with pump) = £17.07

Excipients include benzalkonium chloride, disodium edetate

Dose

Nose, 1 spray into each nostril 2–4 times daily

Vividrin® (Pharma-Global)

Nasal spray, sodium cromoglicate 2%. Net price 15 mL (approx. 110-spray unit) = £11.60

Excipients include benzalkonium chloride, edetic acid, polysorbate 80

Dose

Nose, 1 spray into each nostril 4–6 times daily

12.2.2 Topical nasal decongestants

Sodium chloride 0.9% given as nasal drops or spray may relieve nasal congestion by helping to liquefy mucous secretions in children with rhinitis. In infants, 1–2 drops of sodium chloride 0.9% solution in each nostril before feeds will help relieve congestion and allow more effective suckling.

Inhalation of **warm moist air** is useful in the treatment of symptoms of acute nasal congestion in infants and children, but the use of boiling water for steam inhalation is dangerous for children and should **not** be recommended. Volatile substances (section 3.8) such as menthol and eucalyptus may encourage inhalation of warm moist air.

Topical nasal decongestants containing sympathomimetics can cause rebound congestion (*rhinitis medicamentosa*) following prolonged use (more than 7 days), and are therefore of limited value in the treatment of nasal congestion.

Ephedrine nasal drops is the least likely of the sympathomimetic nasal decongestants to cause rebound congestion and can provide relief for several hours. The more potent sympathomimetic drugs **oxymetazoline** and **xylometazoline** are more likely to cause a rebound effect.

The CHM/MHRA has stated that non-prescription cough and cold medicines containing ephedrine, oxymetazoline, or xylometazoline can be considered for up to 5 days' treatment in children aged 6–12 years after basic principals of best care have been tried; these medicines should not be used in children under 6 years of age (section 3.9.1).

Non-allergic watery rhinorrhoea often responds well to treatment with the antimuscarinic **ipratropium bromide**.

Recurrent, persistent bleeding may respond to the use of a sympathomimetic nasal spray; if infection is present, chlorhexidine and neomycin (*Naseptin*®) cream (section 12.2.3) may be effective.

Systemic nasal decongestants—see section 3.10.

Sinusitis and oral pain   Sinusitis affecting the maxillary antrum can cause pain in the upper jaw. Where this is associated with blockage of the opening from the sinus into the nasal cavity, it may be helpful to relieve the congestion with inhalation of warm moist air (section 3.8) or with **ephedrine nasal drops** (see above). For antibacterial treatment of sinusitis, see Table 1, section 5.1.

Sympathomimetics

EPHEDRINE HYDROCHLORIDE

Cautions   see notes above; also avoid excessive or prolonged use; hyperthyroidism; diabetes mellitus; cardiovascular disease (including hypertension); **interactions:** Appendix 1 (sympathomimetics)

Pregnancy   avoid

Breast-feeding   avoid

Side-effects   local irritation, nausea, headache; after excessive use tolerance with diminished effect, rebound congestion; cardiovascular effects also reported

Licensed use   not licensed for use in children under 12 years

Indication and dose

> Nasal congestion (see notes above)
>
> > **Child 6–18 years** (on a specialist's advice only for child 6–12 years) instil 1–2 drops (0.5% strength) into each nostril up to 3 or 4 times daily; max. duration 5 days (7 days in child over 12 years of age)

¹**Ephedrine** (Non-proprietary)
Nasal drops, ephedrine hydrochloride 0.5%, net price 10 mL = £1.30; 1%, 10 mL = £1.56

Note The BP directs that if no strength is specified 0.5% drops should be supplied

Dental prescribing on NHS Ephedrine nasal drops may be prescribed

1. Can be sold to the public provided no more than 180 mg of ephedrine base (or salts) are supplied at one time, and pseudoephedrine salts are not supplied at the same time; for conditions that apply to supplies made at the request of a patient, see *Medicines, Ethics and Practice*, No. 33, London, Pharmaceutical Press, 2009 (and subsequent editions)

XYLOMETAZOLINE HYDROCHLORIDE

Cautions   see under Ephedrine Hydrochloride and notes above; also avoid excessive or prolonged use

Pregnancy   avoid

Side-effects   see under Ephedrine Hydrochloride and notes above; in small children, also restlessness, sleep disturbances, and hallucinations (discontinue treatment)

Indication and dose

> Nasal congestion for dose, see under preparations

Xylometazoline (Non-proprietary)
Nasal drops, xylometazoline hydrochloride 0.1%, net price 10 mL = £1.91

Dose

> **Child 12–18 years** instil 2–3 drops into each nostril 2–3 times daily when required; max. duration 7 days

Brands include *Otradrops*®, *Otrivine*® ᴺᴴˢ

Paediatric nasal drops, xylometazoline hydrochloride 0.05%, net price 10 mL = £1.59

Dose

> **Child 6–12 years** instil 1–2 drops into each nostril 1–2 times daily when required; max. duration 5 days

Brands include *Otradrops*®, *Otrivine*® ᴺᴴˢ

Nasal spray, xylometazoline hydrochloride 0.1%, net price 10 mL = £1.91

Dose

> **Child 12–18 years** apply 1 spray into each nostril 2–3 times daily when required; max. duration 7 days

Brands include *Otraspray*®, *Otrivine*® ᴺᴴˢ

Antimuscarinic

IPRATROPIUM BROMIDE

Cautions   see section 3.1.2; avoid spraying near eyes

Side-effects   epistaxis, nasal dryness, and irritation; less frequently nausea, headache, and pharyngitis; *very rarely* antimuscarinic effects such as gastro-intestinal motility disturbances, palpitations, and urinary retention

Indication and dose

> Rhinorrhoea associated with allergic and non-allergic rhinitis
>
> > **Child 12–18 years** apply 42 micrograms (2 sprays) into each nostril 2–3 times daily

12

Ear, nose, and oropharynx

◁ **IPRATROPIUM BROMIDE** *(continued)*

Asthma and reversible airways obstruction
section 3.1.2

Rinatec® (Boehringer Ingelheim) [PoM]
Nasal spray 0.03%, ipratropium bromide 21 micrograms/metered spray. Net price 180-dose unit = £3.99
Excipients include benzalkonium chloride, disodium edetate

12.2.3 Nasal preparations for infection

There is **no** evidence that topical anti-infective nasal preparations have any therapeutic value in rhinitis or sinusitis; for elimination of nasal staphylococci, see below. Acute complications such as periorbital cellulitis require hospital treatment. For systemic treatment of sinusitis, see Table 1, section 5.1.

Betnesol-N® (UCB Pharma) [PoM] ◢
Drops (for ear, eye, or nose), betamethasone sodium phosphate 0.1%, neomycin sulphate 0.5%. Net price 10 mL = £2.30
Excipients include benzalkonium chloride, disodium edetate

Dose

Nose, instil 2–3 drops into each nostril 2–3 times daily

Note *Betnesol-N®* licensed for use in children (age range not specified by manufacturer)

Nasal staphylococci

Elimination of organisms such as staphylococci from the nasal vestibule can be achieved by the use of a cream containing **chlorhexidine** and **neomycin** (*Naseptin®*), but re-colonisation frequently occurs. Coagulase-positive staphylococci are present in the noses of 40% of the population. A nasal ointment containing **mupirocin** is also available; it should probably be held in reserve for resistant infections. In hospitals or in care establishments, mupirocin nasal ointment should be reserved for the *eradication* (in both patients and staff) of nasal carriage of meticillin-resistant *Staphylococcus aureus* (MRSA). The ointment should be applied 3 times daily for 5 days and a sample taken 2 days after treatment to confirm eradication. The course may be repeated if the sample is positive (and the throat is not colonised). To avoid the development of resistance, the treatment course should not exceed 7 days and the course should not be repeated on more than one occasion. If the MRSA strain is mupirocin-resistant or does not respond after 2 courses, consider alternative products such as chlorhexidine and neomycin cream. For eradication of MRSA also consult local infection control policy. See section 13.10.1 for treatment of MRSA-infected open wounds. See section 5.1.1.2 for *treatment* of children with MRSA-positive throat swabs or systemic MRSA infection.

Bactroban Nasal® (GSK) [PoM]
Nasal ointment, mupirocin 2% (as calcium salt) in white soft paraffin basis. Net price 3 g = £5.80
Dose

For eradication of nasal carriage of staphylococci, including meticillin-resistant *Staphylococcus aureus* (MRSA)
Apply 2–3 times daily to the inner surface of each nostril (see notes above)

Naseptin® (Alliance) [PoM]
Cream, chlorhexidine hydrochloride 0.1%, neomycin sulphate 0.5%, net price 15 g = £1.90
Excipients include arachis (peanut) oil, cetostearyl alcohol

Dose

For eradication of nasal carriage of staphylococci
Apply to nostrils 4 times daily for 10 days

For preventing nasal carriage of staphylococci
Apply to nostrils twice daily

12.3 Drugs acting on the oropharynx

12.3.1 Drugs for oral ulceration and inflammation

Ulceration of the oral mucosa may be caused by trauma (physical or chemical), recurrent aphthous ulcers, infections, carcinoma, dermatological disorders, nutritional deficiencies, gastro-intestinal disease, haematopoietic disorders, and drug therapy. It is important to establish the diagnosis in each case as the majority of

12 Ear, nose, and oropharynx

these lesions require specific management in addition to local treatment. Local treatment aims to protect the ulcerated area, to relieve pain, to reduce inflammation, or to control secondary infection. Children with an unexplained mouth ulcer of more than 3 weeks' duration require urgent referral to hospital to exclude secondary causes such as leukaemia.

Simple mouthwashes   A **saline** mouthwash (section 12.3.4) may relieve the pain of traumatic ulceration. The mouthwash is made up with warm water and used at frequent intervals until the discomfort and swelling subsides.

Antiseptic mouthwashes   Secondary bacterial infection may be a feature of any mucosal ulceration; it can increase discomfort and delay healing. Use of **chlorhexidine** mouthwash (section 12.3.4) is often beneficial and may accelerate healing of recurrent aphthous ulcers.

Mechanical protection   **Carmellose gelatin paste** may relieve some discomfort arising from ulceration by protecting the ulcer site. As the paste adheres to dry mucosa, it is difficult to apply effectively to the tongue and oropharynx.

Corticosteroids   Topical corticosteroid therapy may be used for some forms of oral ulceration; for aphthous ulcers it is most effective if applied in the 'prodromal' phase. Thrush or other types of candidiasis are recognised complications of corticosteroid treatment.

Hydrocortisone oromucosal tablets are useful in recurrent aphthous ulcers and erosive lichenoid lesions.

Beclometasone dipropionate inhaler (p. 188) 50–100 micrograms sprayed twice daily on the oral mucosa is used to manage oral ulceration [unlicensed indication]. Alternatively, **betamethasone** soluble tablets dissolved in water, can be used as a mouthwash to treat oral ulceration.

Systemic corticosteroid therapy (section 6.3.2) is reserved for severe conditions such as pemphigus vulgaris.

Local analgesics   Local analgesics have a limited role in the management of oral ulceration. When applied topically their action is of a relatively short duration and analgesia cannot be maintained continuously throughout the day. When local anaesthetics are used in the mouth, care must be taken not to produce anaesthesia of the pharynx before meals as this might lead to choking.

Benzydamine mouthwash or spray may be useful in reducing the discomfort associated with a variety of ulcerative conditions. It has also been found to be effective in reducing the discomfort of tonsillectomy and post-irradiation mucositis. Some children find the full-strength mouthwash causes some stinging and, for them, it should be diluted with an equal volume of water.

Flurbiprofen lozenges are licensed for the relief of sore throat in adolescents.

Choline salicylate dental gel has some analgesic action and may provide relief for recurrent aphthous ulcers in children over 16 years of age.

Periodontitis   Low-dose **doxycycline** (*Periostat®*) is licensed as an adjunct to scaling and root planing for the treatment of periodontitis in children over 12 years; a low dose of doxycycline reduces collagenase activity without inhibiting bacteria associated with periodontitis. For anti-infectives used in the treatment of destructive (refractory) forms of periodontal disease, see section 12.3.2 and Table 1, section 5.1. For mouthwashes used for oral hygiene and plaque inhibition, see section 12.3.4.

▌ BENZYDAMINE HYDROCHLORIDE

Side-effects occasional numbness or stinging; rarely hypersensitivity reactions

Licensed use *Difflam® Spray* licensed for use in children (age range not specified by manufacturer)

Indication and dose

Painful inflammatory conditions of oropharynx
for dose, see under preparations

Difflam® (3M)

Oral rinse, green, benzydamine hydrochloride 0.15%, net price 200 mL (*Difflam® Sore Throat Rinse*) = £2.50; 300 mL = £3.81

Dose

Child 12–18 years rinse or gargle, using 15 mL (dilute with an equal volume of water if stinging occurs) every 1½–3 hours as required, usually for not more than 7 days

Dental prescribing on NHS May be prescribed as Benzydamine Mouthwash 0.15%

◻ **BENZYDAMINE HYDROCHLORIDE** (*continued*)

Spray, benzydamine hydrochloride 0.15%. Net price 30-mL unit = £3.01

Dose

Child under 6 years 1 puff per 4 kg body-weight to max. 4 puffs onto affected area every 1½–3 hours

Child 6–12 years 4 puffs onto affected area every 1½–3 hours

Child 12–18 years 4–8 puffs onto affected area every 1½–3 hours

Dental prescribing on NHS May be prescribed as Benzydamine Oromucosal Spray 0.15%

CARMELLOSE SODIUM

Licensed use licensed for use in children (age range not specified by manufacturer)

Indication and dose

Mechanical protection of oral and perioral lesions for dose, see under preparation

Orabase® (ConvaTec)
Protective paste (= oral paste), carmellose sodium 16.7%, pectin 16.7%, gelatin 16.7%, in *Plastibase®*. Net price 30 g = £2.02; 100 g = £4.48

Dose

Apply a thin layer when necessary after meals

Dental prescribing on NHS May be prescribed as Carmellose Gelatin Paste

---

CORTICOSTEROIDS

Contra-indications untreated oral infection

Side-effects occasional exacerbation of local infection; thrush or other candidal infections

Licensed use *Corlan® Pellets* licensed for use in children (under 12 years—on medical advice only)

Indication and dose

Oral and perioral lesions for dose, see under preparations

Betnesol® (UCB Pharma) [PoM]
Soluble tablets, pink, scored, betamethasone 500 micrograms (as sodium phosphate), net price 100-tab pack = £4.97. Label: 10, steroid card, 13, 21

Dose
Oral ulceration

Child 12–18 years 500 micrograms dissolved in 20 ml water and rinsed around the mouth 4 times daily; not to be swallowed

Dental prescribing on NHS May be prescribed as Betamethasone Soluble Tablets 500 micrograms

Corlan® (UCB Pharma)
Pellets (= oromucosal tablets), hydrocortisone 2.5 mg (as sodium succinate). Net price 20 = £2.03

Dose

1 lozenge 4 times daily, allowed to dissolve slowly in the mouth in contact with the ulcer

Dental prescribing on NHS May be prescribed as Hydrocortisone Oromucosal Tablets

---

DOXYCYCLINE

Cautions section 5.1.3; monitor for superficial fungal infection, particularly if predisposition to oral candidiasis

Contra-indications section 5.1.3

Hepatic impairment section 5.1.3

Renal impairment section 5.1.3

Pregnancy section 5.1.3

Breast-feeding section 5.1.3

Side-effects section 5.1.3; fungal superinfection

Indication and dose

See under preparations

Oral herpes section 12.3.2

Other indications section 5.1.3

Periostat® (Alliance) [PoM]
Tablets, f/c, doxycycline (as hyclate) 20 mg, net price 56-tab pack = £16.50. Label: 6, 11, 27, counselling, posture

Dose
Periodontitis (as an adjunct to gingival scaling and root planing)

Child 12–18 years 20 mg twice daily for 3 months

Counselling Tablets should be swallowed whole with plenty of fluid, while sitting or standing

Dental prescribing on NHS May be prescribed as Doxycycline Tablets 20 mg

◢**Local application**
For severe recurrent aphthous ulceration, the contents of a 100 mg doxycycline capsule can be stirred into a small amount of water then rinsed around the mouth for 2–3 minutes 4 times daily usually for 3 days; it should preferably not be swallowed [unlicensed indication].

Note Doxycycline stains teeth; avoid in children under 12 years of age

FLURBIPROFEN

Cautions section 10.1.1
Contra-indications section 10.1.1
Hepatic impairment section 10.1.1
Renal impairment section 10.1.1
Pregnancy section 10.1.1
Breast-feeding section 10.1.1
Side-effects taste disturbance, mouth ulcers (move lozenge around mouth); see also section 10.1.1

Indication and dose

Relief of sore throat for dose, see under preparation

Strefen® (Reckitt Benckiser)
Lozenges, flurbiprofen 8.75 mg, net price 16 = £2.24
Dose

Child 12–18 years allow 1 lozenge to dissolve slowly in the mouth every 3–6 hours, max. 5 lozenges in 24 hours, for max. 3 days

SALICYLATES

Cautions frequent application, especially in children, may give rise to salicylate poisoning
Contra-indications children under 16 years
Reye's syndrome The CHM has advised that topical oral pain relief products containing salicylate salts should not be used in children under 16 years, as a cautionary measure due to the theoretical risk of Reye's syndrome

Indication and dose

Mild oral and perioral lesions for dose, see under preparations

◢Choline salicylate
Choline Salicylate Dental Gel, BP
Oral gel, choline salicylate 8.7% in a flavoured gel basis, net price 15 g = £1.89
Brands include *Bonjela®* (sugar-free)
Dose

Child 16–18 years apply ½-inch of gel with gentle massage not more often than every 3 hours

Dental prescribing on NHS Choline Salicylate Dental Gel may be prescribed

◢Salicylic acid
Pyralvex® (Norgine)
Oral paint, brown, rhubarb extract (anthraquinone glycosides 0.5%), salicylic acid 1%. Net price 10 mL with brush = £3.25
Dose

Child 16–18 years apply 3–4 times daily

12.3.2 Oropharyngeal anti-infective drugs

Sore throat is usually a self-limiting condition often caused by viral infection which does not benefit from anti-infective treatment. Adequate analgesia may be all that is required. Systemic **antibacterials** (Table 1, section 5.1) should only be used in severe cases where there is concern for the child's overall clinical condition. Acute ulcerative gingivitis (Vincent's infection) requires treatment with oral **metronidazole** (section 5.1.11).

Benzydamine (section 12.3.1) may be beneficial in relieving pain and dysphagia in children, especially after tonsillectomy or the use of a nasogastric tube.

Oropharyngeal viral infections

Children with varicella–zoster infection often develop painful lesions in the mouth and throat. **Benzydamine** (section 12.3.1) may be used to provide local analgesia. **Chlorhexidine** mouthwash or gel (section 12.3.4) will control plaque accumulation if toothbrushing is painful and will also help to control secondary infection in general.

In severe herpetic stomatitis systemic **aciclovir** or **valaciclovir** (section 5.3.2.1) may be used for oral lesions associated with herpes zoster. Aciclovir and valaciclovir are also used to prevent frequently recurring herpes simplex lesions of the mouth particularly when associated with the initiation of erythema multiforme. For the treatment of labial herpes simplex infections, see section 13.10.3.

Herpes infections of the mouth in children aged over 12 years may also respond to rinsing the mouth with **doxycycline** (section 12.3.1).

Oropharyngeal fungal infections

Fungal infections of the mouth are usually caused by *Candida* spp. (candidiasis or candidosis). Different types of oropharyngeal candidiasis are managed as follows:

Thrush   Acute pseudomembranous candidiasis (thrush), is usually an acute infection but it may persist for months in patients receiving inhaled corticoster-

12

Ear, nose, and oropharynx

oids, cytotoxics, or broad-spectrum antibacterials. Thrush also occurs in patients with serious systemic disease associated with reduced immunity such as leukaemia, other malignancies, and HIV infection. Any predisposing condition should be managed appropriately. When thrush is associated with corticosteroid inhalers, rinsing the mouth with water (or cleaning a child's teeth) immediately after using the inhaler may avoid the problem. Treatment with **nystatin** or **miconazole** may be needed. **Fluconazole** (section 5.2) is effective for unresponsive infections or if a topical antifungal drug cannot be used. Topical therapy may not be adequate in immunocompromised children and an oral triazole antifungal is preferred (section 5.2).

Acute erythematous candidiasis   Acute erythematous (atrophic) candidiasis is a relatively uncommon condition associated with corticosteroid and broad-spectrum antibacterial use and with HIV disease. It is usually treated with **fluconazole** (section 5.2).

Angular cheilitis   Angular cheilitis (angular stomatitis) is characterised by soreness, erythema and fissuring at the angles of the mouth. It may represent a nutritional deficiency or it may be related to orofacial granulomatosis or HIV infection. Both yeasts (*Candida* spp.) and bacteria (*Staphylococcus aureus* and beta-haemolytic streptococci) are commonly involved as interacting, infective factors. While the underlying cause is being identified and treated, it is often helpful to apply **miconazole** cream (see p. 719) or **sodium fusidate** ointment (p. 717); if the angular cheilitis is unresponsive to treatment, **miconazole** and **hydrocortisone** cream or ointment (see p. 682) can be used.

Immunocompromised patients   For advice on prevention of fungal infections in immunocompromised children see p. 369.

For the role of antiseptic mouthwashes in the prevention of oral candidiasis in immunocompromised children, see section 12.3.4.

Drugs used in oropharyngeal candidiasis   Nystatin is not absorbed from the gastro-intestinal tract and is applied locally (as suspension) to the mouth for treating local fungal infections. **Miconazole** is used by local application (as an oral gel) in the mouth but it is also absorbed to the extent that potential interactions need to be considered. Miconazole also has some activity against Gram-positive bacteria including streptococci and staphylococci. In neonates, nystatin oral suspension or miconazole oral gel is used for the treatment of oropharyngeal candidiasis; to prevent re-infection it is important to ensure that the mother's breast nipples and the teats of feeding bottles are cleaned adequately.

Fluconazole (section 5.2) given by mouth is reliably absorbed; it is used for infections that do not respond to topical therapy or when topical therapy cannot be used. **Itraconazole** (section 5.2) can be used for fluconazole-resistant infections.

If candidal infection fails to respond after 1 to 2 weeks of treatment with antifungal drugs the child should be sent for investigation to eliminate the possibility of underlying disease. Persistent infection may also be caused by re-infection from the genito-urinary or gastro-intestinal tract.

MICONAZOLE

Cautions   avoid in acute porphyria (section 9.8.2); **interactions:** Appendix 1 (antifungals, imidazole)

Contra-indications   impaired swallowing reflex

Hepatic impairment   avoid

Pregnancy   manufacturer advises avoid if possible—toxicity at high doses in *animal* studies

Breast-feeding   manufacturer advises caution—no information available

Side-effects   nausea and vomiting, *very rarely* diarrhoea (usually on long-term treatment), hepatitis, rash, toxic epidermal necrolysis, and Stevens-Johnson syndrome

Licensed use   not licensed for use in children under 4 months of age or during first 5–6 months of life of an infant born pre-term

Indication and dose

Prevention and treatment of oral and intestinal fungal infections
- By mouth

Neonate (oral fungal infections only) 1 mL 2–4 times daily smeared around the mouth after feeds

Child 1 month–2 years 2.5 mL twice daily smeared around the mouth after food

◁ **MICONAZOLE** (*continued*)

Child 2–6 years 5 mL twice daily after food; retain near lesions before swallowing

Child 6–12 years 5 mL 4 times daily after food; retain near lesions before swallowing

Child 12–18 years 5–10 mL 4 times daily after food; retain near lesions before swallowing
Note Treatment should be continued for 48 hours after lesions have healed

Localised lesions

Child 2–18 years smear small amount on affected area with clean finger 4 times daily for

5–7 days (orthodontic appliances should be removed at night and brushed with gel); continue treatment for 48 hours after lesions have healed

[1] **Daktarin®** (Janssen-Cilag) [PoM]
Oral gel, sugar-free, orange-flavoured, miconazole 24 mg/mL (20 mg/g). Net price 15-g tube = £2.85, 80-g tube = £4.47. Label: 9, counselling, hold in mouth, after food
Dental prescribing on NHS May be prescribed as Miconazole Oromucosal Gel
1. 15-g tube can be sold to the public

▮ NYSTATIN

Side-effects oral irritation and sensitisation, nausea reported; see also section 5.2
Licensed use *suspension* not licensed for use in neonates for the treatment of candidiasis
Indication and dose

Oral and perioral fungal infections

Neonate 100 000 units 4 times daily after feeds

Child 1 month–18 years 100 000 units 4 times daily after food

Note Treatment is usually given for 7 days, and continued for 48 hours after lesions have healed.
Intestinal fungal infections section 5.2

Skin infections section 13.10.2

Nystan® (Squibb) [PoM]
Oral suspension, yellow, nystatin 100 000 units/mL. Net price 30 mL with pipette = £1.91. Label: 9, counselling, use of pipette, hold in mouth, after food
Dental prescribing on NHS May be prescribed as Nystatin Oral Suspension

---

▐ 12.3.3 ▏ Lozenges and sprays

There is no convincing evidence that antiseptic lozenges and sprays have a beneficial action and they sometimes irritate and cause sore tongue and sore lips. Some preparations also contain local anaesthetics which relieve pain but may cause sensitisation.

▐ 12.3.4 ▏ Mouthwashes and gargles

Superficial infections of the mouth are often helped by warm mouthwashes which have a mechanical cleansing effect and cause some local hyperaemia. However, to be effective, they must be used frequently and vigorously. Mouthwashes may not be suitable for children under 7 years (risk of the solution being swallowed); the mouthwash or dental gel may be applied using a cotton bud.

A warm saline mouthwash is ideal for its cleansing effect and can be prepared either by dissolving half a teaspoonful of salt in a glassful of warm water or by diluting **compound sodium chloride mouthwash** with an equal volume of warm water. **Mouthwash solution-tablets** containing thymol are used to remove unpleasant tastes.

Mouthwashes containing an oxidising agent, such as **hydrogen peroxide**, may be useful in the treatment of acute ulcerative gingivitis (Vincent's infection). Hydrogen peroxide solution has also a mechanical cleansing effect arising from frothing when in contact with oral debris, but in concentrations greater than 1.5% may cause ulceration and tissue damage.

Chlorhexidine is an effective antiseptic which has the advantage of inhibiting plaque formation on the teeth. It does not, however, completely control plaque deposition and is not a substitute for effective toothbrushing. Moreover, chlorhexidine preparations do not penetrate significantly into stagnation areas and are therefore of little value in the control of dental caries or of periodontal disease once pocketing has developed. Chlorhexidine preparations are of little value in the control of acute necrotising ulcerative gingivitis. With prolonged use, chlorhexidine causes reversible brown staining of teeth and tongue. Chlorhexidine may

12

Ear, nose, and oropharynx

be incompatible with some ingredients in toothpaste, causing an unpleasant taste in the mouth; allow at least 30 minutes between using the mouthwash and toothpaste.

Chlorhexidine can be used as a mouthwash, spray or gel for secondary infection in mucosal ulceration and for controlling gingivitis, as an adjunct to other oral hygiene measures. These preparations may also be used instead of toothbrushing where there is a painful periodontal condition (e.g. primary herpetic stomatitis) or if the child has a haemorrhagic disorder, or is disabled. Chlorhexidine mouthwash is used in the prevention of oral candidiasis in immunocompromised patients. Chlorhexidine mouthwash reduces the incidence of alveolar osteitis following tooth extraction. Chlorhexidine mouthwash should not be used for the prevention of endocarditis in children undergoing dental procedures.

CHLORHEXIDINE GLUCONATE

Side-effects mucosal irritation (if desquamation occurs, discontinue treatment or dilute mouthwash with an equal volume of water); taste disturbance; reversible brown staining of teeth, and of silicate or composite restorations; tongue discoloration; parotid gland swelling reported

Note Chlorhexidine gluconate may be incompatible with some ingredients in toothpaste; leave an interval of at least 30 minutes between using mouthwash and toothpaste

Licensed use licensed for use in children (age range not specified by manufacturer); *Corsodyl*® not licesned for use in children under 12 years (unless on the advice of a healthcare professional)

Indication and dose

See under preparations below

Chlorhexidine (Non-proprietary)
Mouthwash, chlorhexidine gluconate 0.2%, net price 300 mL = £1.99

Dose

> **Oral hygiene and plaque inhibition, oral candidiasis, gingivitis, and management of aphthous ulcers**
> Rinse mouth with 10 mL for about 1 minute twice daily

> **Dental prescribing on NHS** Chlorhexidine Mouthwash may be prescribed

Chlorohex® (Colgate-Palmolive)
Chlorohex 1200® mouthwash, chlorhexidine gluconate 0.12% (mint-flavoured). Net price 300 mL = £2.00

Dose

> **Oral hygiene and plaque inhibition**
> Rinse mouth with 15 mL for about 30 seconds twice daily

Corsodyl® (GSK Consumer Healthcare)
Dental gel, chlorhexidine gluconate 1%. Net price 50 g = £1.21

Dose

> **Oral hygiene and plaque inhibition and gingivitis**
> Brush on the teeth once or twice daily

> **Oral candidiasis and management of aphthous ulcers**
> Apply to affected areas once or twice daily

> **Dental prescribing on NHS** May be prescribed as Chlorhexidine Gluconate Gel

Mouthwash, chlorhexidine gluconate 0.2%. Net price 300 mL (original or mint) = £1.93, 600 mL (mint) = £3.85

Dose

> **Oral hygiene and plaque inhibition, oral candidiasis, gingivitis, and management of aphthous ulcers**
> Rinse mouth with 10 mL for about 1 minute twice daily

Oral spray, chlorhexidine gluconate 0.2% (mint-flavoured). Net price 60 mL = £4.10

Dose

> **Oral hygiene and plaque inhibition, oral candidiasis, gingivitis, and management of aphthous ulcers**
> Apply as required to tooth, gingival, or ulcer surfaces using up to 12 actuations (approx. 0.14 mL/actuation) twice daily

> **Dental prescribing on NHS** May be prescribed as Chlorhexidine Oral Spray

Periogard® (Colgate-Palmolive)
Oromucosal solution, alcohol-free, chlorhexidine gluconate 0.2%, net price 300 mL = £1.97

Dose

> **Short-term treatment of inflammation of gingival and oral mucosa**
> **Child 6–18 years** rinse mouth with 10 mL for about 1 minute twice daily, usually for up to 7 days

> **Dental prescribing on NHS** May be prescribed as Chlorhexidine Oromucosal Solution, Alcohol-free, 0.2%

◀**With chlorobutanol**
Eludril® (Fabre)
Mouthwash or gargle, chlorhexidine gluconate 0.1%, chlorobutanol 0.5% (mint-flavoured), net price 90 mL = £1.36, 250 mL = £2.83, 500 mL = £5.06

Dose

> **Oral hygiene and plaque inhibition**
> Use 10–15 mL (diluted with warm water in measuring cup provided) 2–3 times daily

HEXETIDINE

Side-effects local irritation; *very rarely* taste disturbance and transient anaesthesia

Indication and dose

> **Oral hygiene** for dose, see preparation below

Oraldene® (McNeil)
Mouthwash or gargle, red or blue-green (mint-flavoured), hexetidine 0.1%. Net price 100 mL = £1.31; 200 mL = £2.02

Dose

> **Child 6–18 years** use 15 mL (undiluted) 2–3 times daily

◢ HYDROGEN PEROXIDE

Side-effects hypertrophy of papillae of tongue on prolonged use

Indication and dose

> **Oral hygiene** (see notes above); for dose, see under preparations

Hydrogen Peroxide Mouthwash, BP

Mouthwash, consists of Hydrogen Peroxide Solution 6% (= approx. 20 volume) BP

Dose
> Rinse the mouth for 2–3 minutes with 15 mL diluted in half a tumblerful of warm water 2–3 times daily (see notes above)

Dental prescribing on NHS Hydrogen Peroxide Mouthwash may be prescribed

Peroxyl® (Colgate-Palmolive)
Mouthwash, hydrogen peroxide 1.5%, net price 300 mL = £3.26

Dose
> **Child 6–18 years,** rinse the mouth with 10 mL for about 1 minute 3 times daily (after meals and at bedtime) for max. 7 days

◢ SODIUM CHLORIDE

Indication and dose

> **Oral hygiene** (see notes above); for dose, see under preparation

Sodium Chloride Mouthwash, Compound, BP

Mouthwash, sodium bicarbonate 1%, sodium chloride 1.5% in a suitable vehicle with a peppermint flavour

Dose
> Extemporaneous preparations should be prepared according to the following formula: sodium chloride 1.5 g, sodium bicarbonate 1 g, concentrated peppermint emulsion 2.5 mL, double-strength chloroform water 50 mL, water to 100 mL
>
> To be diluted with an equal volume of warm water

Dental prescribing on NHS Compound Sodium Chloride Mouthwash may be prescribed

◢ THYMOL

Indication and dose

> **Oral hygiene** (see notes above); for dose, see under preparation

Mouthwash Solution-tablets

Consist of tablets which may contain antimicrobial, colouring, and flavouring agents in a suitable soluble effervescent basis to make a mouthwash suitable for dental purposes. Net price 100-tab pack = £15.09

Dose
> Dissolve 1 tablet in a tumblerful of warm water

Note Mouthwash Solution-tablets may contain ingredients such as thymol

Dental prescribing on NHS Mouthwash Solution-tablets may be prescribed

12.3.5 Treatment of dry mouth

Dry mouth (xerostomia) may be caused by drugs with antimuscarinic (anticholinergic) side-effects (e.g. antispasmodics and sedating antihistamines), by irradiation of the head and neck region or by damage to or disease of the salivary glands. Children with a persistently dry mouth may develop a burning or scalded sensation and have poor oral hygiene; they may develop dental caries, periodontal disease, and oral infections (particularly candidiasis). Dry mouth may be relieved in many patients by simple measures such as frequent sips of cool drinks or sucking pieces of ice or sugar-free fruit pastilles. Sugar-free chewing gum stimulates salivation in patients with residual salivary function.

Artificial saliva can provide useful relief of dry mouth. A properly balanced artificial saliva should be of a neutral pH and contain electrolytes (including fluoride) to correspond approximately to the composition of saliva. The acidic pH of some artificial saliva products may be inappropriate.

Local treatment

Artificial saliva products with **ACBS approval** may be prescribed for children with dry mouth as a result of having (or having undergone) radiotherapy, or sicca syndrome. SST tablets and *Salinum*® liquid may also be prescribed on the NHS.

AS Saliva Orthana® (AS Pharma)

Oral spray, gastric mucin (porcine) 3.5%, xylitol 2%, sodium fluoride 4.2 mg/litre, with preservatives and flavouring agents, pH neutral, net price 50-mL bottle = £4.92; 450-mL refill = £34.27

Dose

(ACBS) spray 2–3 times onto oral and pharyngeal mucosa, when required

Dental prescribing on NHS *AS Saliva Orthana*® Oral Spray may be prescribed

Lozenges, mucin 65 mg, xylitol 59 mg, in a sorbitol basis, pH neutral, net price 30-lozenge pack = £3.50

Note *AS Saliva Orthana*® lozenges do not contain fluoride

Dental prescribing on NHS *AS Saliva Orthana*® Lozenges may be prescribed

Biotène Oralbalance® (GSK)

Saliva replacement gel, lactoperoxidase, lactoferrin, lysozyme, glucose oxidase, xylitol in a gel basis, net price 50-g tube = £4.10; 24 × 12.4 mL tube = £30.40 (for hospital use)

Dose

(ACBS) apply to gums and tongue as required

Note Avoid use with toothpastes containing detergents (including foaming agents)

Dental prescribing on NHS *Biotène Oralbalance*® Saliva Replacement Gel may be prescribed

BioXtra® (RIS Products)

Gel, lactoperoxidase, lactoferrin, lysozyme, whey colostrum, xylitol and other ingredients, net price 40-mL tube = £3.94, 50-mL spray = £3.94

Dose

(ACBS) apply to oral mucosa as required

Dental prescribing on NHS *BioXtra*® Gel may be prescribed

Glandosane® (Fresenius Kabi)

Aerosol spray, carmellose sodium 500 mg, sorbitol 1.5 g, potassium chloride 60 mg, sodium chloride 42.2 mg, magnesium chloride 2.6 mg, calcium chloride 7.3 mg, and dipotassium hydrogen phosphate 17.1 mg/50 g, pH 5.75, net price 50-mL unit (neutral, lemon or peppermint flavoured) = £4.70

Dose

(ACBS) spray onto oral and pharyngeal mucosa as required

Dental prescribing on NHS *Glandosane*® Aerosol Spray may be prescribed

Salinum® (Crawford)

Liquid sugar free, linseed extract (containing polysaccharides), with dipotassium phosphate buffer and preservatives, pH 6–7, net price 300-mL bottle = £13.50

Dose

Symptomatic treatment of dry mouth

Approx. 2 mL rinsed around the mouth and then swallowed, when required

Dental prescribing on NHS *Salinum*® Liquid may be prescribed as Artificial Saliva Liquid

Saliveze® (Wyvern)

Oral spray, carmellose sodium (sodium carboxymethylcellulose), calcium chloride, magnesium chloride, potassium chloride, sodium chloride, and dibasic sodium phosphate, pH neutral, net price 50-mL bottle (mint-flavoured) = £3.50

Dose

(ACBS) 1 spray onto oral mucosa as required

Dental prescribing on NHS *Saliveze*® Oral Spray may be prescribed

Salivix® (Galen)

Pastilles, sugar-free, reddish-amber, acacia, malic acid and other ingredients. Net price 50-pastille pack = £3.50

Dose

(ACBS) suck 1 pastille when required

Dental prescribing on NHS *Salivix*® Pastilles may be prescribed

SST (Medac)

Tablets, sugar-free, citric acid, malic acid and other ingredients in a sorbitol base, net price 100-tab pack = £4.86

Dose

Symptomatic treatment of dry mouth in patients with impaired salivary gland function and patent salivary ducts

Allow 1 tablet to dissolve slowly in the mouth when required

Dental prescribing on NHS May be prescribed as Saliva Stimulating Tablets

Xerotin® (SpePharm)

Oral spray, sugar-free, water, sorbitol, carmellose (carboxymethylcellulose), potassium chloride, sodium chloride, potassium phosphate, magnesium chloride, calcium chloride and other ingredients, pH neutral. Net price 100-mL unit = £6.86

Dose

Symptomatic treatment of dry mouth

Spray as required

Dental prescribing on NHS *Xerotin*® Oral Spray may be prescribed as Artificial Saliva Oral Spray

13 Skin

13 Skin

This chapter also includes advice on the management of the following:
candidiasis, p. 719
dermatophytoses, p. 719
head lice, p. 724
nappy rash, p. 678
pityriasis versicolor, p. 719
scabies, p. 724

The British Association of Dermatologists' list of preferred unlicensed dermatological preparations (specials) is available at http://www.bad.org.uk/site/495/default.aspx

13.1 Management of skin conditions

When prescribing topical preparations for the treatment of skin conditions in children, the site of application, the condition being treated, and the child's (and carer's) preference for a particular vehicle all need to be taken into consideration.

Neonates Caution is required when prescribing topical preparations for neonates—their large body surface area in relation to body mass increases susceptibility to toxicity from systemic absorption of substances applied to the skin. Topical preparations containing potentially sensitising substances such as corticosteroids, aminoglycosides, iodine, and parasiticidal drugs should be avoided. Preparations containing alcohol should be avoided because they can dehydrate the skin, cause pain if applied to raw areas, and the alcohol can cause necrosis.

In *preterm neonates*, the skin is more fragile and offers a poor barrier, especially in the first fortnight after birth. Preterm infants, especially if below 32 weeks postmenstrual age, may also require special measures to maintain skin hydration.

13.1.1 Vehicles

The vehicle in topical preparations for the skin affects the degree of hydration, has a mild anti-inflammatory effect, and aids the penetration of the active drug. Therefore, the vehicle, as well as the active drug, should be chosen on the basis of their suitability for the child's skin condition.

Applications are usually viscous solutions, emulsions, or suspensions for application to the skin (including the scalp) or nails.

Collodions are painted on the skin and allowed to dry to leave a flexible film over the site of application.

Creams are emulsions of oil and water and are generally well absorbed into the skin. They may contain an antimicrobial preservative unless the active ingredient or basis is intrinsically bactericidal and fungicidal. Generally, creams are cosmetically more acceptable than ointments because they are less greasy and easier to apply.

Gels consist of active ingredients in suitable hydrophilic or hydrophobic bases; they generally have a high water content. Gels are particularly suitable for application to the face and scalp.

Lotions have a cooling effect and may be preferred to ointments or creams for application over a hairy area. Lotions in alcoholic basis can sting if used on broken skin. *Shake lotions* (such as calamine lotion) contain insoluble powders which leave a deposit on the skin surface.

Ointments are greasy preparations which are normally anhydrous and insoluble in water, and are more occlusive than creams. They are particularly suitable for chronic, dry lesions. The most commonly used ointment bases consist of soft paraffin or a combination of soft, liquid and hard paraffin. Some ointment bases have both *hydrophilic* and *lipophilic* properties; they may have occlusive properties on the skin surface, encourage hydration, and also be miscible with water; they often have a mild anti-inflammatory effect. *Water-soluble ointments* contain macrogols which are freely soluble in water and are therefore readily washed off; they have a limited but useful role where ready removal is desirable.

Pastes are stiff preparations containing a high proportion of finely powdered solids such as zinc oxide and starch suspended in an ointment. They are used for circumscribed lesions such as those which occur in lichen simplex, chronic eczema, or psoriasis. They are less occlusive than ointments and can be used to protect inflamed, lichenified, or excoriated skin.

Dusting powders are used only rarely. They reduce friction between opposing skin surfaces. Dusting powders should not be applied to moist areas because they can cake and abrade the skin. Talc is a lubricant but it does not absorb moisture; it can cause respiratory irritation. Starch is less lubricant but absorbs water.

Dilution The BP directs that creams and ointments should **not** normally be diluted but that should dilution be necessary care should be taken, in particular, to prevent microbial contamination. The appropriate diluent should be used and heating should be avoided during mixing; excessive dilution may affect the stability of some creams. Diluted creams should normally be used within 2 weeks of their preparation.

13.1.2 Suitable quantities for prescribing

Suitable quantities of dermatological preparations to be prescribed for specific areas of the body

Area of the body	Creams and Ointments	Lotions
Face	15–30 g	100 mL
Both hands	25–50 g	200 mL
Scalp	50–100 g	200 mL
Both arms or both legs	100–200 g	200 mL
Trunk	400 g	500 mL
Groins and genitalia	15–25 g	100 mL

The amounts shown above are usually suitable for children 12–18 years for twice daily application for 1 week; smaller quantities will be required for children under 12 years. These recommendations **do not apply** to corticosteroid preparations.

13.1.3 Excipients and sensitisation

Excipients in topical products rarely cause problems. If a patch test indicates allergy to an excipient, then products containing the substance should be avoided (see also Anaphylaxis, p. 202). The following excipients in topical preparations may rarely be associated with sensitisation; the presence of these excipients is indicated in the entries for topical products. See also Excipients, under General Guidance, p. 3.

Beeswax	Imidurea
Benzyl alcohol	Isopropyl palmitate
Butylated hydroxyanisole	N-(3-Chloroallyl)hexaminium chloride (quaternium 15)
Butylated hydroxytoluene	
Cetostearyl alcohol (including cetyl and stearyl alcohol)	Polysorbates
Chlorocresol	Propylene glycol
Edetic acid (EDTA)	Sodium metabisulphite
Ethylenediamine	Sorbic acid
Fragrances	Wool fat and related substances including lanolin[1]
Hydroxybenzoates (parabens)	

1. Purified versions of wool fat have reduced the problem

13.2 Emollient and barrier preparations

13.2.1 Emollients
13.2.2 Barrier preparations

Borderline substances The preparations marked 'ACBS' are regarded as drugs when prescribed in accordance with the advice of the Advisory Committee on Borderline Substances for the clinical conditions listed. Prescriptions issued in accordance with this advice and endorsed 'ACBS' will normally not be investigated. See Appendix 2 for listing by clinical condition.

13.2.1 Emollients

Emollients hydrate the skin, soften the skin, act as barrier to water and external irritants, and are indicated for all dry or scaling disorders. Their effects are short-lived and they should be applied frequently even after improvement occurs. They are useful in dry and eczematous disorders, and to a lesser extent in psoriasis (section 13.5.2); they should be applied immediately after washing or bathing to maximise the effect of skin hydration. Light emollients, such as **aqueous cream**, are suitable for many dry skin conditions but more greasy preparations, such as **white soft paraffin**, **emulsifying ointment**, and **liquid and white soft paraffin ointment**, are often more effective. The severity of the condition, the child's (or carer's) preference, and the site of application will often guide the choice of emollient. Some ingredients rarely cause sensitisation (section 13.1.3) and this should be suspected if an eczematous reaction occurs. Ointments may exacerbate acne and folliculitis.

> **Fire hazard with paraffin-based emollients**
> Emulsifying ointment or 50% Liquid Paraffin and 50% White Soft Paraffin Ointment in contact with dressings and clothing is easily ignited by a naked flame. The risk is greater when these preparations are applied to large areas of the body, and clothing or dressings become soaked with the ointment. Patients should be told to keep away from fire or flames, and not to smoke when using these preparations. The risk of fire should be considered when using large quantities of any paraffin-based emollient.

Preparations such as **aqueous cream** and **emulsifying ointment** can be used as soap substitutes; the preparation is rubbed on the skin before rinsing off completely. The addition of a bath oil (section 13.2.1.1) may also be helpful.

In the *neonate*, a preservative-free paraffin-based emollient hydrates the skin without affecting the normal skin flora; substances such as olive oil are also used. The development of blisters (epidermolysis bullosa) or ichthyosis may be alleviated by applying liquid and white soft paraffin ointment while awaiting dermatological investigation.

Preparations containing an antibacterial (section 13.10.1) should be avoided unless infection is present or is a frequent complication of the dry skin condition.

Urea is a keratin softener used in the treatment of dry, scaling conditions (including ichthyosis). It is occasionally used with other topical agents such as corticosteroids to enhance penetration of the skin.

◀**Non-proprietary emollient preparations**

Aqueous Cream, BP
Cream, emulsifying ointment 30%, [1]phenoxyethanol 1% in freshly boiled and cooled purified water, net price 100 g = £1.36, 500 g = £1.86
Excipients include cetostearyl alcohol
1. The BP permits use of alternative antimicrobials provided their identity and concentration are stated on the label

Emulsifying Ointment, BP
Ointment, emulsifying wax 30%, white soft paraffin 50%, liquid paraffin 20%, net price 500 g = £2.36
Excipients include cetostearyl alcohol

Hydrous Ointment, BP
Ointment, (oily cream), dried magnesium sulphate 0.5%, phenoxyethanol 1%, wool alcohols ointment 50%, in freshly boiled and cooled purified water, net price 500 g = £2.16

Liquid and White Soft Paraffin Ointment, NPF
Ointment, liquid paraffin 50%, white soft paraffin 50%, net price 500 g = £4.13

Paraffin, White Soft, BP
White petroleum jelly, net price 100 g = 46p

Paraffin, Yellow Soft, BP
Yellow petroleum jelly, net price 100 g = 38p

◢Proprietary emollient preparations

Aveeno® (J&J)
Cream, colloidal oatmeal in emollient basis, net price 100 mL = £3.78, 300-mL pump pack = £6.80
Excipients include benzyl alcohol, cetyl alcohol, isopropyl palmitate
ACBS: For endogenous and exogenous eczema, xeroderma, and ichthyosis

Lotion, colloidal oatmeal in emollient basis, net price 400 mL = £6.42
Excipients include benzyl alcohol, cetyl alcohol, isopropyl palmitate
ACBS: as for *Aveeno®* Cream

Cetraben® (Genus)
Emollient cream, white soft paraffin 13.2%, light liquid paraffin 10.5%, net price 50-g pump pack = £1.17, 150-g pump pack = £2.88, 500-g pump pack = £5.39, 1.05-kg pump pack = £11.11
Excipients include cetostearyl alcohol, hydroxybenzoates (parabens)

Dermamist® (Alliance)
Spray application, white soft paraffin 10% in a basis containing liquid paraffin, fractionated coconut oil, net price 250-mL pressurised aerosol unit = £6.45
Excipients none as listed in section 13.1.3
Note Flammable

Diprobase® (Schering-Plough)
Cream, cetomacrogol 2.25%, cetostearyl alcohol 7.2%, liquid paraffin 6%, white soft paraffin 15%, water-miscible basis used for *Diprosone®* cream, net price 50 g = £1.30; 500-g pump pack = £6.58
Excipients include cetostearyl alcohol, chlorocresol

Ointment, liquid paraffin 5%, white soft paraffin 95%, basis used for *Diprosone®* ointment, net price 50 g = £1.30
Excipients none as listed in section 13.1.3

Doublebase® (Dermal)
Emollient shower gel, isopropyl myristate 15%, liquid paraffin 15%, net price 200 g = £5.29
Excipients none as listed in section 13.1.3
Note Also available as *Doublebase® Emollient Wash Gel*

Gel, isopropyl myristate 15%, liquid paraffin 15%, net price 100 g = £2.69, 500 g = £5.92
Excipients none as listed in section 13.1.3

E45® (Reckitt Benckiser)
Cream, light liquid paraffin 12.6%, white soft paraffin 14.5%, hypoallergenic anhydrous wool fat (hypoallergenic lanolin) 1% in self-emulsifying monostearin, net price 50 g = £1.40, 125 g = £2.55, 350 g = £4.46, 500-g pump pack = £5.39
Excipients include cetyl alcohol, hydroxybenzoates (parabens)

Emollient Wash Cream, soap substitute, zinc oxide 5% in an emollient basis, net price 250-mL pump pack = £3.19
Excipients none as listed in section 13.1.3
ACBS: for endogenous and exogenous eczema, xeroderma, and ichthyosis

Lotion, light liquid paraffin 4%, cetomacrogol, white soft paraffin 10%, hypoallergenic anhydrous wool fat (hypoallergenic lanolin) 1% in glyceryl monostearate, net price 200 mL = £2.40, 500-mL pump pack = £4.50
Excipients include isopropyl palmitate, hydroxybenzoates (parabens), benzyl alcohol
ACBS: for symptomatic relief of dry skin conditions, such as those associated with atopic eczema and contact dermatitis

Emollin® (C D Medical)
Spray, liquid paraffin 50%, white soft paraffin 50% in aerosol basis, net price 150 mL = £3.74, 240 mL = £5.98
Excipients none as listed in section 13.1.3

Epaderm® (Mölnlycke)
Cream, yellow soft paraffin 15%, liquid paraffin 10%, emulsifying wax 5%, net price 50-g pump pack = £1.59, 500-g pump pack = £6.50
Excipients include cetostearyl alcohol; chlorocresol

Ointment, emulsifying wax 30%, yellow soft paraffin 30%, liquid paraffin 40%, net price 125 g = £3.69, 500 g = £6.26, 1 kg = £11.53
Excipients include cetostearyl alcohol

Hewletts® (Kestrel)
Cream, hydrous wool fat 4%, zinc oxide 8%, arachis (peanut) oil, oleic acid, white soft paraffin, net price 35 g = £1.43, 400 g = £6.69
Excipients include fragrance

Hydromol® (Alliance)
Cream, sodium pidolate 2.5%, liquid paraffin 13.8%, net price 50 g = £2.04, 100 g = £3.80, 500 g = £11.09
Excipients include cetostearyl alcohol, hydroxybenzoates (parabens)

Ointment, yellow soft paraffin 30%, emulsifying wax 30%, liquid paraffin 40%, net price 125 g = £2.79, 500 g = £4.74, 1 kg = £8.81
Excipients include cetostearyl alcohol

Linola® Gamma (Linderma)
Cream, evening primrose oil 20%, net price 50 g = £2.83, 250 g = £8.20
Excipients include beeswax, hydroxybenzoates (parabens), propylene glycol
Cautions epilepsy (but hazard unlikely with topical preparations)

Lipobase® (Astellas)
Cream, fatty cream basis used for *Locoid Lipocream®*, net price 50 g = £2.08
Excipients include cetostearyl alcohol, hydroxybenzoates (parabens)
For dry skin conditions, also for use during treatment with topical corticosteroid and as diluent for *Locoid Lipocream®*

Oilatum® (Stiefel)
Cream, light liquid paraffin 6%, white soft paraffin 15%, net price 40 g = £1.30, 150 g = £2.46, 500-mL pump pack = £4.99, 1.05-litre pump pack = £9.98; *Oilatum® Junior* 150 g = £3.38, 350-mL pump pack = £4.65, 500-mL pump pack = £6.35, 1.05-litre pump pack = £9.98
Excipients include benzyl alcohol, cetostearyl alcohol

Shower emollient (gel), light liquid paraffin 70%, net price (with fragrance or fragrance–free) 150 g = £5.15

QV® (Crawford)
Cream, glycerol 10%, light liquid paraffin 10%, white soft paraffin 5%, net price 100 g = £1.95, 500 g = £5.60
Excipients include cetostearyl alcohol, hydroxybenzoates (parabens)

Lotion, white soft paraffin 5%, net price 250 mL = £3.00
Excipients include cetostearyl alcohol, hydroxybenzoates (parabens)

Wash, glycerol 10%, net price 200 mL = £2.50
Excipients include hydroxybenzoates (parabens)

13 Skin

Ultrabase® (Valeant)

Cream, water-miscible, containing liquid paraffin and white soft paraffin, net price 50 g = £1.58, 500-g pump pack = £16.23

Excipients include fragrance, hydroxybenzoates (parabens), disodium edetate, stearyl alcohol

Unguentum M® (Almirall)

Cream, containing saturated neutral oil, liquid paraffin, white soft paraffin, net price 50 g = £1.41, 100 g = £2.78, 200-mL pump pack = £5.50, 500 g = £8.48

Excipients include cetostearyl alcohol, polysorbate 40, propylene glycol, sorbic acid

Zerobase® (Zeroderma)

Cream, liquid paraffin 11%, net price 500 g pump pack = £5.26

Excipients include cetostearyl alcohol, chlorocresol

◀ **Preparations containing urea**

Aquadrate® (Alliance)

Cream, urea 10%, net price 100 g = £4.37

Excipients none as listed in section 13.1.3

Dose

Apply thinly and rub into area when required

Balneum® (Almirall)

Cream, urea 5%, ceramide 0.1%, net price 50-g pump pack = £2.80, 500-g pump pack = £9.80

Excipients include cetostearyl alcohol, polysorbates, propylene glycol

Dose

Apply twice daily

Balneum® Plus Cream, urea 5%, lauromacrogols 3%, net price 100 g = £3.29, 175-g pump pack = £8.33, 500-g pump pack = £16.42

Excipients include benzyl alcohol, polysorbates

Dose

Apply twice daily

Calmurid® (Galderma)

Cream, urea 10%, lactic acid 5%, net price 100 g = £5.70, 500-g pump pack = £27.42

Excipients none as listed in section 13.1.3

Dose

Apply a thick layer for 3–5 minutes, massage into area, and remove excess, usually twice daily. Use half-strength cream for 1 week if stinging occurs

Note Can be diluted with aqueous cream (life of diluted cream 14 days)

E45® Itch Relief Cream (Reckitt Benckiser)

Cream, urea 5%, macrogol lauryl ether 3%, net price 50 g = £2.55, 100 g = £3.47, 500-g pump pack = £17.09

Excipients include benzyl alcohol, polysorbates

Dose

Apply twice daily

Eucerin® Intensive (Beiersdorf)

Cream, urea 10%, net price 100 mL = £7.59

Excipients include benzyl alcohol, isopropyl palmitate, wool fat

Dose

Apply thinly and rub into area twice daily

Lotion, urea 10%, net price 250 mL = £7.93

Excipients include benzyl alcohol, isopropyl palmitate

Dose

Apply sparingly and rub into area twice daily

Hydromol® Intensive (Alliance)

Cream, urea 10 %, net price 30 g = £1.64, 100 g = £4.37

Excipients none as listed in section 13.1.3

Dose

Apply thinly twice daily

Nutraplus® (Galderma)

Cream, urea 10%, net price 100 g = £4.37

Excipients include hydroxybenzoates (parabens), propylene glycol

Dose

Apply 2–3 times daily

◀ **With antimicrobials**

Dermol® (Dermal)

Cream, benzalkonium chloride 0.1%, chlorhexidine hydrochloride 0.1%, isopropyl myristate 10%, liquid paraffin 10%, net price 100-g tube = £2.90, 500-g pump pack = £6.72

Excipients include cetostearyl alcohol

Dose

Apply to skin or use as soap substitute

Dermol® 500 Lotion, benzalkonium chloride 0.1%, chlorhexidine hydrochloride 0.1%, liquid paraffin 2.5%, isopropyl myristate 2.5%, net price 500-mL pump pack = £6.13

Excipients include cetostearyl alcohol

Dose

Apply to skin or use as soap substitute

Dermol® 200 Shower Emollient, benzalkonium chloride 0.1%, chlorhexidine hydrochloride 0.1%, liquid paraffin 2.5%, isopropyl myristate 2.5%, net price 200 mL = £3.61

Excipients include cetostearyl alcohol

Dose

Apply to skin or use as soap substitute

13.2.1.1   Emollient bath additives

Emollient bath additives should be added to bath water; some can be applied to wet skin undiluted and rinsed off. Hydration can be improved by soaking in the bath for 10–20 minutes. In dry skin conditions soap should be avoided (see section 13.2.1 for soap substitutes).

The quantities of bath additives recommended for older children are suitable for an adult-size bath. Proportionately less should be used for a child-size bath or a washbasin; recommended bath additive quantities for younger children reflect this.

Skin

13

> These preparations make skin and surfaces slippery—particular care is
> needed when bathing a child.

Aveeno® (J&J)

Bath oil, colloidal oatmeal, white oat fraction in emollient basis, net price 250 mL = £4.28
Excipients include beeswax, fragrance
ACBS: for endogenous and exogenous eczema, xeroderma, and ichthyosis

Dose

> **Child 2–18 years** add 20–30 mL to bath water or apply to wet skin and rinse

Colloidal® bath additive, oatmeal, white oat fraction in emollient basis, net price 10 × 50-g sachets = £7.33; *Baby Bath Additive*®, 10 × 15-g sachets = £4.39
Excipients none as listed in section 13.1.3
ACBS: as for *Aveeno*® Bath oil

Dose

> **Child 1 month–12 years** add 15 g to bath water
>
> **Child 12–18 years** add 50 g to bath water

Balneum® (Almirall)

Balneum® bath oil, soya oil 84.75%, net price 200 mL = £2.48, 500 mL = £5.38, 1 litre = £10.39
Excipients include butylated hydroxytoluene, propylene glycol, fragrance

Dose

> **Neonate** add 5–15 mL to bath water; do not use undiluted
>
> **Child 1 month–2 years** add 5–15 mL to bath water; do not use undiluted
>
> **Child 2–18 years** add 20–60 mL to bath water; do not use undiluted

Balneum Plus® bath oil, soya oil 82.95%, mixed lauromacrogols 15%, net price 500 mL = £6.66
Excipients include butylated hydroxytoluene, propylene glycol, fragrance

Dose

> **Neonate** add 5 mL to bath water or apply to wet skin and rinse
>
> **Child 1 month–2 years** add 5 mL to bath water or apply to wet skin and rinse
>
> **Child 2–18 years** add 10–20 mL to bath water or apply to wet skin and rinse

Cetraben® (Genus)

Emollient bath additive, light liquid paraffin 82.8%, net price 500 mL = £5.25

Dose

> **Neonate** add ½ capful to bath water or apply to wet skin and rinse
>
> **Child 1 month–12 years** add ½–1 capful to bath water or apply to wet skin and rinse
>
> **Child 12–18 years** add 1–2 capfuls to bath water or apply to wet skin and rinse

Dermalo® (Dermal)

Bath emollient, acetylated wool alcohols 5%, liquid paraffin 65%, net price 500 mL = £3.50
Excipients none as listed in section 13.1.3

Dose

> **Neonate** add 5 mL to bath water or apply to wet skin and rinse
>
> **Child 1 month–12 years** add 5–10 mL to bath water or apply to wet skin and rinse
>
> **Child 12–18 years** add 15–20 mL to bath water or apply to wet skin and rinse

Diprobath® (Schering-Plough)

Bath additive, isopropyl myristate 39%, light liquid paraffin 46%, net price 500 mL = £6.84
Excipients none as listed in section 13.1.3

Dose

> **Neonate** add 5 mL to bath water; do not use undiluted
>
> **Child 1 month–12 years** add 10 mL to bath water; do not use undiluted
>
> **Child 12–18 years** add 25–50 mL to bath water; do not use undiluted

Doublebase® (Dermal)

Emollient bath additive, liquid paraffin 65%, net price 500 mL = £5.54
Excipients include cetostearyl alcohol

Dose

> **Neonate** add 5–10 mL to bath water
>
> **Child 1 month–12 years** add 5–10 mL to bath water
>
> **Child 12–18 years** add 15–20 mL to bath water

E45® (Reckitt Benckiser)

Emollient bath oil, cetyl dimeticone 5%, liquid paraffin 91%, net price 250 mL = £3.19, 500 mL = £5.11
Excipients none as listed in section 13.1.3
ACBS: for endogenous and exogenous eczema, xeroderma, and ichthyosis

Dose

> **Neonate** add 5 mL to bath water or apply to wet skin and rinse
>
> **Child 1 month–12 years** add 5–10 mL to bath water or apply to wet skin and rinse
>
> **Child 12–18 years** add 15 mL to bath water or apply to wet skin and rinse

Hydromol® (Alliance)

Bath and Shower Emollient, isopropyl myristate 13%, light liquid paraffin 37.8%, net price 350 mL = £3.61, 500 mL = £4.11, 1 litre = £8.19
Excipients none as listed in section 13.1.3

Dose

> **Neonate** add ½ capful to bath water or apply to wet skin and rinse
>
> **Child 1 month–12 years** add ½–2 capfuls to bath water or apply to wet skin and rinse
>
> **Child 12–18 years** add 1–3 capfuls to bath water or apply to wet skin and rinse

13

Skin

Oilatum® (Stiefel)
Emollient bath additive (emulsion), acetylated wool alcohols 5%, liquid paraffin 63.4%, net price 250 mL = £2.75, 500 mL = £4.57
Excipients include isopropyl palmitate, fragrance
Dose

> **Neonate** add ½ capful to bath water or apply to wet skin and rinse
>
> **Child 1 month–12 years** add ½–2 capfuls to bath water or apply to wet skin and rinse
>
> **Child 12–18 years** add 1–3 capfuls to bath water or apply to wet skin and rinse

Junior emollient bath additive, light liquid paraffin 63.4%, net price 150 mL = £2.82, 250 mL = £3.25, 300 mL = £5.10, 600 mL = £5.89
Excipients include wool fat, isopropyl palmitate
Dose

> **Neonate** add ½ capful to bath water or apply to wet skin and rinse
>
> **Child 1 month–12 years** add ½–2 capfuls to bath water or apply to wet skin and rinse
>
> **Child 12–18 years** add 1–3 capfuls to bath water or apply to wet skin and rinse

QV® (Crawford)
Bath oil, light liquid paraffin 85.09%, net price 200 mL = £2.20, 500 mL = £4.50
Excipients include hydroxybenzoates (parabens)
Dose

> **Child 1 month–1 year** add 4 mL to bath water or apply to wet skin and rinse
>
> **Child 1–12 years** add 7 mL to bath water or apply to wet skin and rinse
>
> **Child 12–18 years** add 10 mL to bath water or apply to wet skin and rinse

◢With antimicrobials
Dermol® 600 (Dermal)
Bath emollient, benzalkonium chloride 0.5%, liquid paraffin 25%, isopropyl myristate 25%, net price 600 mL = £7.67
Excipients include polysorbate 60
Dose

> **Child 1 month–2 years** add 5–15 mL to bath water; do not use undiluted
>
> **Child 2–18 years** add 15–30 mL to bath water; do not use undiluted

Emulsiderm® (Dermal)
Liquid emulsion, liquid paraffin 25%, isopropyl myristate 25%, benzalkonium chloride 0.5%, net price 300 mL (with 15-mL measure) = £3.92, 1 litre (with 30-mL measure) = £12.18
Excipients include polysorbate 60
Dose

> **Child 1 month–2 years** add 5–10 mL to bath water or rub into dry skin until absorbed
>
> **Child 2–18 years** add 10–30 mL to bath water or rub into dry skin until absorbed

Oilatum® Plus (Stiefel)
Bath additive, benzalkonium chloride 6%, triclosan 2%, light liquid paraffin 52.5%, net price 500 mL = £6.98
Excipients include wool fat, isopropyl palmitate
Dose

> **Child 6 months–1 year** add 1 mL to bath water; do not use undiluted
>
> **Child 1–18 years** add 1–2 capfuls to bath water; do not use undiluted

◢With tar
Section 13.5.2

13.2.2 Barrier preparations

Barrier preparations often contain water-repellent substances such as **dimeticone** (dimethicone), natural oils, and paraffins, to help protect the skin from abrasion and irritation; they are used to protect intact skin around stomas and pressure sores, and as a barrier against nappy rash. In neonates, barrier preparations which do not contain potentially sensitising excipients (section 13.1.3) are preferred. Where the skin has broken down, barrier preparations have a limited role in protecting adjacent skin. **Zinc ointments** or barrier creams with zinc oxide or titanium salts, are used to aid healing of uninfected, excoriated skin.

Nappy rash (dermatitis) The first line of treatment is to ensure that nappies are changed frequently and that tightly fitting water-proof pants are avoided. The rash may clear when left exposed to the air and a barrier preparation can be helpful. If the rash is associated with a yeast or fungal infection, an antifungal cream such as clotrimazole cream (section 13.10.2) is useful. A mild corticosteroid such as hydrocortisone 1% is useful in moderate to severe inflammation, but it should be avoided in neonates. The barrier preparation is applied after the corticosteroid preparation to prevent further damage. Hydrocortisone may be used in combination with antifungal and antibacterial drugs (section 13.4) if there is considerable inflammation, erosion, and infection. Preparations containing hydrocortisone should be applied for no more than a week; the hydrocortisone should be discontinued as soon as the inflammation subsides. The occlusive effect of nappies and water-proof pants may increase absorption of corticosteroid (for cautions, see section 13.4).

Non-proprietary barrier preparations

Zinc Cream, BP
Cream, zinc oxide 32%, arachis (peanut) oil 32%, calcium hydroxide 0.045%, oleic acid 0.5%, wool fat 8%, in freshly boiled and cooled purified water, net price 50 g = 50p

Zinc Ointment, BP
Ointment, zinc oxide 15%, in Simple Ointment BP 1988 (which contains wool fat 5%, hard paraffin 5%, cetostearyl alcohol 5%, white soft paraffin 85%), net price 25 g = 22p

Zinc and Castor Oil Ointment, BP
Ointment, zinc oxide 7.5%, castor oil 50%, arachis (peanut) oil 30.5%, white beeswax 10%, cetostearyl alcohol 2%, net price 500 g = £2.86

Proprietary barrier preparations

Conotrane® (Astellas)
Cream, benzalkonium chloride 0.1%, dimeticone 22%, net price 100 g = 88p, 500 g = £3.51
Excipients include cetostearyl alcohol, fragrance

Drapolene® (Chefaro UK)
Cream, benzalkonium chloride 0.01%, cetrimide 0.2% in a basis containing white soft paraffin, cetyl alcohol and wool fat, net price 100 g = £1.54, 200 g = £2.50, 350 g = £3.75
Excipients include cetyl alcohol, chlorocresol, wool fat

Medicaid® (LPC)
Cream, cetrimide 0.5% in a basis containing light liquid paraffin, white soft paraffin, cetostearyl alcohol, glyceryl monostearate, net price 50 g = £1.69
Excipients include cetostearyl alcohol, fragrance, hydroxybenzoates (parabens), wool fat

Metanium® (Ransom)
Ointment, titanium dioxide 20%, titanium peroxide 5%, titanium salicylate 3% in a basis containing dimeticone, light liquid paraffin, white soft paraffin, and benzoin tincture, net price 30 g = £2.01
Excipients none as listed in section 13.1.3

Morhulin® (Actavis)
Ointment, cod-liver oil 11.4%, zinc oxide 38%, in a basis containing liquid paraffin and yellow soft paraffin, net price 50 g = £1.91
Excipients include wool fat derivative

Siopel® (Centrapharm)
Barrier cream, dimeticone '1000' 10%, cetrimide 0.3%, arachis (peanut) oil, net price 50 g = £2.15
Excipients include butylated hydroxytoluene, cetostearyl alcohol, hydroxybenzoates (parabens)

Sprilon® (Ayrton Saunders)
Spray application, dimeticone 1.04%, zinc oxide 12.5%, in a basis containing wool alcohols, cetostearyl alcohol, dextran, white soft paraffin, liquid paraffin, propellants, net price 115-g pressurised aerosol unit = £3.54
Excipients include cetostearyl alcohol, hydroxybenzoates (parabens), wool fat
Note Flammable

Sudocrem® (Forest)
Cream, benzyl alcohol 0.39%, benzyl benzoate 1.01%, benzyl cinnamate 0.15%, hydrous wool fat (hypoallergenic lanolin) 4%, zinc oxide 15.25%, net price 30 g = £1.13, 60 g = £1.25, 125 g = £1.84, 250 g = £3.09, 400 g = £4.34
Excipients include beeswax (synthetic), propylene glycol, fragrance

Vasogen® (Forest)
Barrier cream, dimeticone 20%, calamine 1.5%, zinc oxide 7.5%, net price 50 g = 80p, 100 g = £1.36
Excipients include hydroxybenzoates (parabens), wool fat

13.3 Topical antipruritics

Pruritus may be caused by systemic disease (such as drug hypersensitivity, obstructive jaundice, endocrine disease, chronic renal disease, and certain malignant diseases), skin disease (such as eczema, psoriasis, urticaria, and scabies) or as a side-effect of opioid analgesics. Where possible the underlying cause should be treated. For the treatment of pruritus in palliative care, see Prescribing in Palliative Care, p. 27. Pruritus caused by cholestasis generally requires a bile acid sequestrant (section 1.9.2).

An **emollient** (section 13.2.1) may be of value where the pruritus is associated with dry skin. Preparations containing **calamine** or **crotamiton** are sometimes used but are of uncertain value.

A topical preparation containing **doxepin 5%** is licensed for the relief of pruritus in eczema in children over 12 years; it can cause drowsiness and there may be a risk of sensitisation.

Topical antihistamines and local anaesthetics (section 15.2) are only marginally effective and occasionally cause sensitisation. For *insect stings* and *insect bites*, a short course of a topical corticosteroid is appropriate. Short-term treatment with a **sedating antihistamine** (section 3.4.1) may help in insect stings and in intractable pruritus where sedation is desirable. Calamine preparations are of little value for the treatment of insect stings or bites.

In *pruritus ani*, the underlying cause such as faecal soiling, eczema, psoriasis, or helminth infection should be treated; for preparations used to relieve pruritus ani, see section 1.7.

CALAMINE

Indication and dose

Pruritus but see notes above

Calamine (Non-proprietary)
Aqueous cream, calamine 4%, zinc oxide 3%, liquid paraffin 20%, self-emulsifying glyceryl monostearate 5%, cetomacrogol emulsifying wax 5%, phenoxyethanol 0.5%, freshly boiled and cooled purified water 62.5%, net price 100 mL = 84p

Lotion (= cutaneous suspension), calamine 15%, zinc oxide 5%, glycerol 5%, bentonite 3%, sodium citrate 0.5%, liquefied phenol 0.5%, in freshly boiled and cooled purified water, net price 200 mL = 63p

Oily lotion (BP 1980), calamine 5%, arachis (peanut) oil 50%, oleic acid 0.5%, wool fat 1%, in calcium hydroxide solution, net price 200 mL = £1.57

CROTAMITON

Cautions avoid use near eyes and broken skin; use on doctor's advice for children under 3 years
Contra-indications acute exudative dermatoses

Indication and dose

Pruritus (including pruritus after scabies—section 13.10.4) see notes above

Apply 2–3 times daily (for pruritus after scabies in children under 3 years apply once daily only)

Eurax® (Novartis Consumer Health)
Cream, crotamiton 10%, net price 30 g = £2.27, 100 g = £3.95
Excipients include beeswax, fragrance, hydroxybenzoates (parabens), stearyl alcohol

Lotion, crotamiton 10%, net price 100 mL = £2.99
Excipients include cetyl alcohol, fragrance, propylene glycol, sorbic acid, stearyl alcohol

DOXEPIN HYDROCHLORIDE

Cautions susceptibility to angle-closure glaucoma, urinary retention, mania; avoid application to large areas; **interactions:** Appendix 1 (antidepressants, tricyclic)
Skilled tasks Drowsiness may affect performance of skilled tasks (e.g. driving); effects of alcohol enhanced
Hepatic impairment manufacturer advises caution in severe liver disease
Pregnancy manufacturer advises use only if potential benefit outweighs risk
Breast-feeding manufacturer advises use only if potential benefit outweighs risk
Side-effects drowsiness; local burning, stinging, irritation, tingling and rash; systemic side-effects such as antimuscarinic affects, headache, fever,

dizziness, gastro-intestinal disturbances also reported

Indication and dose

Pruritus in eczema

Child 12–18 years apply thinly 3–4 times daily; usual max. 3 g per application; usual total max. 12 g daily; coverage should be less than 10% of body surface area

Depressive illness section 4.3.1

Xepin® (CHS) [PoM]
Cream, doxepin hydrochloride 5%, net price 30 g = £11.70. Label: 2, 10, patient information leaflet
Excipients include benzyl alcohol

13 Skin

13.4 Topical corticosteroids

Topical corticosteroids are used for the treatment of inflammatory conditions of the skin (other than those arising from an infection), particularly eczema (section 13.5.1), contact dermatitis, insect stings (p. 48), and eczema of scabies (section 13.10.4). Corticosteroids suppress the inflammatory reaction during use; they are not curative and on discontinuation a rebound exacerbation of the condition may occur. They are generally used to relieve symptoms and suppress signs of the disorder when other measures such as emollients are ineffective.

Children, especially infants, are particularly susceptible to side-effects. However, concern about the safety of topical corticosteroids in children should not result in the child being undertreated. The aim is to control the condition as well as possible; inadequate treatment will perpetuate the condition. Carers of young children should be advised that treatment should **not** necessarily be reserved to 'treat only the worst areas' and they may need to be advised that patient information leaflets may contain inappropriate advice for the child's condition.

In an acute flare-up of atopic eczema, it may be appropriate to use more potent formulations of topical corticosteroids for a short period to regain control of the condition. Continuous daily application of a mild corticosteroid such as hydrocortisone 1% is equivalent to a potent corticosteroid such as betamethasone 0.1% applied intermittently.

Topical corticosteroids are of no value in the treatment of *urticaria*. They may worsen ulcerated or secondarily infected lesions. They should not be used indiscriminately in *pruritus* (where they will only benefit if inflammation is causing the itch) and are **not** recommended for *acne vulgaris*.

Systemic or potent topical corticosteroids should be avoided or given only under specialist supervision in *psoriasis* because, although they may suppress the psoriasis in the short term, relapse or vigorous rebound occurs on withdrawal (sometimes precipitating severe pustular psoriasis). Topical use of potent corticosteroids on widespread psoriasis can lead to systemic as well as to local side-effects. It is reasonable, however, to prescribe a mild to moderate topical corticosteroid for a short period (2–4 weeks) for *flexural* and *facial psoriasis*, and to use a more potent corticosteroid such as betamethasone or fluocinonide for *psoriasis* of the *scalp*, *palms*, or *soles* (see below for cautions in psoriasis).

In general, the most potent topical corticosteroids should be reserved for recalcitrant dermatoses such as *chronic discoid lupus erythematosus*, *lichen simplex chronicus*, *hypertrophic lichen planus*, and *palmoplantar pustulosis*. Potent corticosteroids should generally be avoided on the face and skin flexures, but specialists occasionally prescribe them for use on these areas in certain circumstances.

When topical treatment has failed, intralesional corticosteroid injections (section 10.1.2.2) may be used. These are more effective than the very potent topical corticosteroid preparations and should be reserved for severe cases where there are localised lesions such as *keloid scars*, *hypertrophic lichen planus*, or *localised alopecia areata*.

Choice   Water-miscible corticosteroid *creams* are suitable for moist or weeping lesions whereas *ointments* are generally chosen for dry, lichenified or scaly lesions or where a more occlusive effect is required. *Lotions* may be useful when minimal application to a large or hair-bearing area is required or for the treatment of exudative lesions. *Occlusive polythene or hydrocolloid dressings* increase absorption, but also increase the risk of side-effects; they are therefore used only under supervision on a short-term basis for areas of very thick skin (such as the palms and soles). Disposable nappies and tight fitting pants also increase the risk of side-effects by increasing absorption of the corticosteroid. The inclusion of urea or salicylic acid also increases the penetration of the corticosteroid.

'Wet-wrap bandaging' (section 13.5.1) increases absorption into the skin, but should be initiated only by a dermatologist and application supervised by a healthcare professional trained in the technique.

In the *BNF for Children*, topical corticosteroids for the skin are categorised as 'mild', 'moderately potent', 'potent' or 'very potent' (see p. 683); the **least potent** preparation which is effective should be chosen but dilution should be avoided whenever possible.

Topical hydrocortisone is usually used in children under 1 year of age. Moderately potent and potent topical corticosteroids should be used with great care in children and for short periods (1–2 weeks) only. A very potent corticosteroid should be initiated under the supervision of a specialist.

Appropriate topical corticosteroids for specific conditions are:

- *insect bites and stings*—mild corticosteroid such as hydrocortisone 1% cream;
- *severely inflamed nappy rash* in infant over 1 month (section 13.2.2)—mild corticosteroid such as hydrocortisone 0.5 or 1% for 5–7 days (combined with antimicrobial if infected);
- *mild to moderate eczema, flexural and facial eczema or psoriasis*—mild corticosteroid such as hydrocortisone 1%;
- *severe eczema of the face and neck*—moderately potent corticosteroid for 3–5 days only, if not controlled by a mild corticosteroid;
- *severe eczema on the trunk and limbs*—moderately potent or potent corticosteroid for 1–2 weeks only, switching to a less potent preparation as the condition improves;
- *eczema affecting area with thickened skin* (e.g. soles of feet)—potent topical corticosteroid in combination with urea or salicylic acid (to increase penetration of corticosteroid).

Perioral lesions **Hydrocortisone** cream 1% can be used for up to 7 days to treat uninfected inflammatory lesions on the lips and on the skin surrounding the mouth. **Hydrocortisone and miconazole** cream or ointment is useful where infection by susceptible organisms and inflammation co-exist, particularly for initial treatment (up to 7 days) e.g. in angular cheilitis (see also p. 666). Organisms susceptible to miconazole include *Candida* spp. and many Gram-positive bacteria including streptococci and staphylococci.

Cautions Avoid prolonged use of a topical corticosteroid particularly on the face (and keep away from eyes). Use potent or very potent corticosteroids under specialist supervision; extreme caution is required in dermatoses of infancy including nappy rash—treatment should be limited to 5–7 days.

Psoriasis The use of potent or very potent corticosteroids in psoriasis can result in rebound relapse, development of generalised pustular psoriasis, and local and systemic toxicity, see notes above.

Contra-indications Topical corticosteroids are contra-indicated in untreated bacterial, fungal, or viral skin lesions, in acne, and in perioral dermatitis; potent corticosteroids are contra-indicated in widespread plaque psoriasis (see notes above).

Side-effects *Mild* and *moderately potent* topical corticosteroids are associated with few side-effects but particular care is required when treating neonates and infants, and in the use of *potent* and *very potent* corticosteroids. Absorption through the skin can rarely cause adrenal suppression and even Cushing's syndrome (section 6.3.2), depending on the area of the body being treated and the duration of treatment. Absorption of corticosteroid is greatest from severely inflamed skin, thin skin (especially on the face or genital area), from flexural sites (e.g. axillae groins), and in infants where skin surface area is higher in relation to body-weight; absorption is increased by occlusion.

Local side-effects include: spread and worsening of untreated infection; thinning of the skin which may be restored over a period after stopping treatment but the original structure may never return; irreversible striae atrophicae and telan-giectasia; contact dermatitis; perioral dermatitis; acne, or worsening of acne or rosacea; mild depigmentation which may be reversible; hypertrichosis also reported.

Children and their carers should be reassured that side effects such as skin thinning and systemic effects rarely occur when topical corticosteroids are used appropriately.

> **Safe Practice**
> In order to minimise the side-effects of a topical corticosteroid, it is important to apply it **thinly** to affected areas **only**, no more frequently than **twice daily**, and to use the least potent formulation which is fully effective.

Application Topical corticosteroid preparations should be applied no more frequently than twice daily; once daily is often sufficient.

Topical corticosteroids are spread thinly on the skin; the length of cream or ointment expelled from a tube may be used to specify the quantity to be applied to a given area of skin. This length can be measured in terms of a *fingertip unit* (the distance from the tip of the adult index finger to the first crease). One fingertip unit (approximately 500 mg) is sufficient to cover an area that is twice that of the flat adult palm.

If a child is using topical corticosteroids of different potencies, the child and their carers should be told when to use each corticosteroid. The potency of each topical corticosteroid (see Topical Corticosteroid Preparation Potencies, p. 683) should be included on the label with the directions for use. The label should be attached to the container (for example, the tube) rather than the outer packaging.

Mixing topical preparations on the skin should be avoided where possible; several minutes should elapse between application of different preparations.

Compound preparations The advantages of including other substances (such as antibacterials or antifungals) with corticosteroids in topical preparations are uncertain, but such combinations may have a place where inflammatory skin conditions are associated with bacterial or fungal infection, such as infected eczema. In these cases the antimicrobial drug should be chosen according to the sensitivity of the infecting organism and used regularly for a short period (typically twice daily for 1 week). Longer use increases the likelihood of resistance and of sensitisation.

The keratolytic effect of salicylic acid facilitates the absorption of topical corticosteroids; however, excessive and prolonged use of topical preparations containing salicylic acid may result in symptoms of salicylism.

Topical corticosteroid potencies

Potency of a topical corticosteroid preparation depends upon the formulation as well as the corticosteroid. Therefore, proprietary names are shown below.

Mild

Hydrocortisone 0.1–2.5%, *Dioderm, Mildison, Synalar 1 in 10 Dilution*

Mild with antimicrobials *Canesten HC, Daktacort, Econacort, Fucidin H, Nystaform-HC, Timodine*

Mild with crotamiton *Eurax-Hydrocortisone*

Moderate

Betnovate-RD, Eumovate, Haelan, Modrasone, Synalar 1 in 4 Dilution, Ultralanum Plain

Moderate with antimicrobials *Trimovate*

Moderate with urea *Alphaderm, Calmurid HC*

Potent

Betamethasone valerate 0.1%, *Betacap, Bettamousse, Betnovate, Cutivate, Diprosone, Elocon,* Hydrocortisone butyrate, *Locoid, Locoid Crelo, Metosyn, Nerisone, Synalar*

Potent with antimicrobials *Aureocort, Betnovate-C, Betnovate-N, Fucibet, Lotriderm, Synalar C, Synalar N*

Potent with salicylic acid *Diprosalic*

Very potent

Dermovate, Nerisone Forte

Very potent with antimicrobials *Dermovate-NN*

◢ HYDROCORTISONE

Cautions see notes above

Contra-indications see notes above

Side-effects see notes above

Indication and dose

> **Mild inflammatory skin disorders such as eczemas (but for over-the-counter preparations, see below)**
>
> Apply thinly 1–2 times daily

> **Nappy rash** see notes above and section 13.2.2

◢ Over-the-counter hydrocortisone preparations

Skin creams and ointments containing hydrocortisone (alone or with other ingredients) can be sold to the public for the treatment of allergic contact dermatitis, irritant dermatitis, insect bite reactions and mild to moderate eczema in children over 10 years, to be applied sparingly over the affected area 1–2 times daily for max. 1 week. Over-the-counter hydrocortisone preparations should not be sold without medical advice for children under 10 years or for pregnant women; they should **not** be sold for application to the face, anogenital region, broken or infected skin (including cold sores, acne, and athlete's foot); over-the-counter hydrocortisone preparations containing clotrimazole or miconazole nitrate can be sold to the public for treatment of athlete's foot and candidal intertrigo

Hydrocortisone (Non-proprietary) ℞

Cream, hydrocortisone 0.5%, net price, 15 g = £2.23, 30 g = £5.19; 1%, 15 g = £1.66, 30 g = £2.10, 50 g = £6.28; 2.5%, 15 g = £17.82. Label: 28, counselling, application, see p. 682. Potency: mild

Dental prescribing on NHS Hydrocortisone Cream 1% 15 g may be prescribed

Ointment, hydrocortisone 0.5%, net price 15 g = £2.73, 30 g = £5.23; 1%, 15 g = £1.79, 30 g = £2.38, 50 g = £7.86; 2.5%, 15 g = £21.32. Label: 28, counselling, application, see p. 682. Potency: mild
When hydrocortisone cream or ointment is prescribed and no strength is stated, the 1% strength should be supplied

◢ Proprietary hydrocortisone preparations

Dioderm® (Dermal) ℞

Cream, hydrocortisone 0.1%, net price 30 g = £2.43. Label: 28, counselling, application, see p. 682. Potency: mild

Excipients include cetostearyl alcohol, propylene glycol

Note Although this contains only 0.1% hydrocortisone, the formulation is designed to provide a clinical activity comparable to that of Hydrocortisone Cream 1% BP

Mildison® (Astellas) ℞

Lipocream, hydrocortisone 1%, net price 30 g = £2.45. Label: 28, counselling, application, see p. 682. Potency: mild

Excipients include cetostearyl alcohol, hydroxybenzoates (parabens)

△ HYDROCORTISONE (*continued*)

◢Compound preparations

Compound preparations with coal tar see section 13.5.2

Alphaderm® (Alliance) PoM

Cream, hydrocortisone 1%, urea 10%, net price 30 g = £2.38; 100 g = £7.03. Label: 28, counselling, application, see p. 682. Potency: moderate
Excipients none as listed in section 13.1.3

Calmurid HC® (Galderma) PoM

Cream, hydrocortisone 1%, urea 10%, lactic acid 5%, net price 30 g = £2.80, 50 g = £4.67. Label: 28, counselling, application, see p. 682. Potency: moderate
Excipients none as listed in section 13.1.3

Note If stinging occurs, manufacturer advises dilute to half-strength with aqueous cream for 1 week then transfer to undiluted preparation (but see section 13.1.1 for advice to avoid dilution where possible)

¹**Eurax-Hydrocortisone®** (Novartis Consumer Health) PoM

Cream, hydrocortisone 0.25%, crotamiton 10%, net price 30 g = 87p. Label: 28, counselling, application, see p. 682. Potency: mild
Excipients include fragrance, hydroxybenzoates (parabens), propylene glycol, stearyl alcohol

1. A 15-g tube is on sale to the public for treatment of contact dermatitis and insect bites in children 10–18 years.

◢With antimicrobials

See notes above for comment on compound preparations

¹**Canesten HC®** (Bayer Consumer Care) PoM

Cream, hydrocortisone 1%, clotrimazole 1%, net price 30 g = £2.42. Label: 28, counselling, application, see p. 682. Potency: mild
Excipients include benzyl alcohol, cetostearyl alcohol

1. A 15-g tube is on sale to the public for the treatment of athlete's foot and fungal infection of skin folds with associated inflammation in children 10–18 years.

Daktacort® (Janssen-Cilag) PoM

Cream, hydrocortisone 1%, miconazole nitrate 2%, net price 30 g = £1.83. Label: 28, counselling, application, see p. 682. Potency: mild
Excipients include butylated hydroxyanisole, disodium edetate

Dental prescribing on NHS May be prescribed as Miconazole and Hydrocortisone Cream for max. 7 days

Note A 15-g tube is on sale to the public for the treatment of athlete's foot and candidal intertrigo in children 10–18 years

Ointment, hydrocortisone 1%, miconazole nitrate 2%, net price 30 g = £2.01. Label: 28, counselling, application, see p. 682. Potency: mild
Excipients none as listed in section 13.1.3

Dental prescribing on NHS May be prescribed as Miconazole and Hydrocortisone Ointment for max. 7 days

Fucidin H® (LEO) PoM

Cream, hydrocortisone acetate 1%, fusidic acid 2%, net price 30 g = £5.09, 60 g = £10.18. Label: 28, counselling, application, see p. 682. Potency: mild
Excipients include butylated hydroxyanisole, cetyl alcohol, polysorbate 60, potassium sorbate

Nystaform-HC® (Typharm) PoM

Cream, hydrocortisone 0.5%, nystatin 100 000 units/g, chlorhexidine hydrochloride 1%, net price 30 g = £2.66. Label: 28, counselling, application, see p. 682. Potency: mild
Excipients include benzyl alcohol, cetostearyl alcohol, polysorbate '60'

Ointment, hydrocortisone 1%, nystatin 100 000 units/g, chlorhexidine acetate 1%, net price 30 g = £2.66. Label: 28, counselling, application, see p. 682. Potency: mild
Excipients none as listed in section 13.1.3

Timodine® (Alliance) PoM

Cream, hydrocortisone 0.5%, nystatin 100 000 units/g, benzalkonium chloride solution 0.2%, dimeticone '350' 10%, net price 30 g = £2.03. Label: 28, counselling, application, see p. 682. Potency: mild
Excipients include butylated hydroxyanisole, cetostearyl alcohol, hydroxybenzoates (parabens), sodium metabisulphite, sorbic acid

---

◢ **HYDROCORTISONE BUTYRATE**

Cautions see notes above
Contra-indications see notes above
Side-effects see notes above

Indication and dose

Severe inflammatory skin disorders such as eczemas unresponsive to less potent corticosteroids, psoriasis see notes above

Child 1–18 years apply thinly 1–2 times daily

Locoid® (Astellas) PoM

Cream, hydrocortisone butyrate 0.1%, net price 30 g = £2.29, 100 g = £7.05. Label: 28, counselling, application, see p. 682. Potency: potent
Excipients include cetostearyl alcohol, hydroxybenzoates (parabens)

Lipocream, hydrocortisone butyrate 0.1%, net price 30 g = £2.41, 100 g = £7.38. Label: 28, counselling, application, see p. 682. Potency: potent
Excipients include benzyl alcohol, cetostearyl alcohol, hydroxybenzoates (parabens)

Note For bland cream basis see *Lipobase®*, section 13.2.1

Ointment, hydrocortisone butyrate 0.1%, net price 30 g = £2.29, 100 g = £7.05. Label: 28, counselling, application, see p. 682. Potency: potent
Excipients none as listed in section 13.1.3

Scalp lotion, hydrocortisone butyrate 0.1%, in an aqueous isopropyl alcohol basis, net price 100 mL = £9.76. Label: 15, 28, counselling, application, see p. 682. Potency: potent
Excipients none as listed in section 13.1.3

Locoid Crelo® (Astellas) PoM

Lotion (topical emulsion), hydrocortisone butyrate 0.1% in a water-miscible basis, net price 100 g (with

◁ **HYDROCORTISONE BUTYRATE (*continued*)**

applicator nozzle) = £8.44. Label: 28, counselling,
application, see p. 682. Potency: potent
Excipients include butylated hydroxytoluene, cetostearyl
alcohol, hydroxybenzoates (parabens), propylene glycol

ALCLOMETASONE DIPROPIONATE

Cautions see notes above

Contra-indications see notes above

Side-effects see notes above

Licensed use licensed for use in children (age
range not specified by manufacturer)

Indication and dose

Inflammatory skin disorders such as eczemas

Apply thinly 1–2 times daily

Modrasone® (TEVA UK) (PoM)
Cream, alclometasone dipropionate 0.05%, net
price 50 g = £2.68. Label: 28, counselling, application, see p. 682. Potency: moderate
Excipients include cetostearyl alcohol, chlorocresol, propylene glycol

Ointment, alclometasone dipropionate 0.05%, net
price 50 g = £2.68. Label: 28, counselling, application, see p. 682. Potency: moderate
Excipients include beeswax, propylene glycol

BETAMETHASONE ESTERS

Cautions see notes above; use of more than 100 g
per week of 0.1% preparation likely to cause
adrenal suppression

Contra-indications see notes above

Side-effects see notes above

Licensed use *Betacap®*, *Betnovate®*, *Betnovate-C®*,
and *Betnovate-RD®* not licensed for use in
children under 1 year; *Bettamousse®* and *Fucibet®*
Lipid Cream not licensed for use in children under
6 years; *Betnovate-N®* not licensed for use in
children under 2 years; *Lotriderm®* not licensed
for use in children under 12 years; *all other
preparations* licensed for use in children (age
range not specified by manufacturer)

Indication and dose

Severe inflammatory skin disorders such as
eczemas unresponsive to less potent corticosteroids, psoriasis see notes above

Apply thinly 1–2 times daily

Betamethasone Valerate (Non-proprietary) (PoM)
Cream, betamethasone (as valerate) 0.1%, net price
30 g = £2.52, 100 g = £5.63. Label: 28, counselling,
application, see p. 682. Potency: potent

Ointment, betamethasone (as valerate) 0.1%, net
price 30 g = £2.51, 100 g = £4.07. Label: 28, counselling, application, see p. 682. Potency: potent

Betacap® (Dermal) (PoM)
Scalp application, betamethasone (as valerate)
0.1% in a water-miscible basis containing coconut
oil derivative, net price 100 mL = £3.81. Label: 15,
28, counselling, application, see p. 682. Potency:
potent
Excipients none as listed in section 13.1.3

Betnovate® (GSK) (PoM)
Cream, betamethasone (as valerate) 0.1% in a
water-miscible basis, net price 30 g = £1.43, 100 g =
£4.05. Label: 28, counselling, application, see
p. 682. Potency: potent
Excipients include cetostearyl alcohol, chlorocresol

Ointment, betamethasone (as valerate) 0.1% in an
anhydrous paraffin basis, net price 30 g = £1.43,
100 g = £4.05. Label: 28, counselling, application,
see p. 682. Potency: potent
Excipients none as listed in section 13.1.3

Lotion, betamethasone (as valerate) 0.1%, net price
100 mL = £4.67. Label: 28, counselling, application,
see p. 682. Potency: potent
Excipients include cetostearyl alcohol, hydroxybenzoates
(parabens)

Scalp application, betamethasone (as valerate)
0.1% in a water-miscible basis, net price 100 mL =
£5.09. Label: 15, 28, counselling, application, see
p. 682. Potency: potent
Excipients none as listed in section 13.1.3

Betnovate-RD® (GSK) (PoM)
Cream, betamethasone (as valerate) 0.025% in a
water-miscible basis (1 in 4 dilution of *Betnovate®*
cream), net price 100 g = £3.21. Label: 28, counselling, application, see p. 682. Potency: moderate
Excipients include cetostearyl alcohol, chlorocresol

Ointment, betamethasone (as valerate) 0.025% in
an anhydrous paraffin basis (1 in 4 dilution of
Betnovate® ointment), net price 100 g = £3.21.
Label: 28, counselling, application, see p. 682.
Potency: moderate
Excipients none as listed in section 13.1.3

Bettamousse® (UCB Pharma) (PoM)
Foam (= scalp application), betamethasone valerate 0.12% (≡ betamethasone 0.1%), net price 100 g
= £9.37. Label: 28, counselling, application, see
p. 682. Potency: potent
Excipients include cetyl alcohol, polysorbate 60, propylene
glycol, stearyl alcohol

Note Flammable

Diprosone® (Schering-Plough) (PoM)
Cream, betamethasone (as dipropionate) 0.05%,
net price 30 g = £2.20, 100 g = £6.24. Label: 28,
counselling, application, see p. 682. Potency: potent
Excipients include cetostearyl alcohol, chlorocresol

Ointment, betamethasone (as dipropionate) 0.05%,
net price 30 g = £2.20, 100 g = £6.24. Label: 28,
counselling, application, see p. 682. Potency: potent
Excipients none as listed in section 13.1.3

Lotion, betamethasone (as dipropionate) 0.05%, net
price 30 mL = £2.78, 100 mL = £7.95. Label: 28,
counselling, application, see p. 682. Potency: potent
Excipients none as listed in section 13.1.3

13

Skin

△ **BETAMETHASONE ESTERS** (*continued*)

▰**With salicylic acid**
See notes above for comment on compound preparations
For prescribing information on salicylic acid, see p. 697

Diprosalic® (Schering-Plough) (PoM)
Ointment, betamethasone (as dipropionate) 0.05%, salicylic acid 3%, net price 30 g = £3.24, 100 g = £9.32. Label: 28, counselling, application, see p. 682. Potency: potent
Excipients none as listed in section 13.1.3

Dose
Apply thinly 1–2 times daily; max. 60 g per week

Scalp application, betamethasone (as dipropionate) 0.05%, salicylic acid 2%, in an alcoholic basis, net price 100 mL = £10.30. Label: 28, counselling, application, see p. 682. Potency: potent
Excipients include disodium edetate

Dose
Apply a few drops 1–2 times daily

▰**With antimicrobials**
See notes above for comment on compound preparations

Betnovate-C® (Chemidex) (PoM)
Cream, betamethasone (as valerate) 0.1%, clioquinol 3%, net price 30 g = £1.76. Label: 28, counselling, application, see p. 682. Potency: potent
Excipients include cetostearyl alcohol, chlorocresol

Note Stains clothing

Ointment, betamethasone (as valerate) 0.1%, clioquinol 3%, net price 30 g = £1.76. Label: 28, counselling, application, see p. 682. Potency: potent
Excipients none as listed in section 13.1.3

Note Stains clothing

Betnovate-N® (Chemidex) (PoM)
Cream, betamethasone (as valerate) 0.1%, neomycin sulphate 0.5%, net price 30 g = £1.76, 100 g = £4.88. Label: 28, counselling, application, see p. 682. Potency: potent
Excipients include cetostearyl alcohol, chlorocresol

Ointment, betamethasone (as valerate) 0.1%, neomycin sulphate 0.5%, net price 30 g = £1.76, 100 g = £4.88. Label: 28, counselling, application, see p. 682. Potency: potent
Excipients none as listed in section 13.1.3

Fucibet® (LEO) (PoM)
Cream, betamethasone (as valerate) 0.1%, fusidic acid 2%, net price 30 g = £5.40, 60 g = £10.79. Label: 28, counselling, application, see p. 682. Potency: potent
Excipients include cetostearyl alcohol, chlorocresol

Lipid cream, betamethasone (as valerate) 0.1%, fusidic acid 2%, net price 30 g = £5.62. Label: 28, counselling, application, see p. 682. Potency: potent
Excipients include cetostearyl alcohol, hydroxybenzoates (parabens)

Lotriderm® (TEVA UK) (PoM)
Cream, betamethasone dipropionate 0.064% (≡ betamethasone 0.05%), clotrimazole 1%, net price 30 g = £6.34. Label: 28, counselling, application, see p. 682. Potency: potent
Excipients include benzyl alcohol, cetostearyl alcohol, propylene glycol

CLOBETASOL PROPIONATE

Cautions see notes above

Contra-indications see notes above

Side-effects see notes above

Licensed use *Dermovate®* not licensed for use in children under 1 year; *Dermovate-NN®* not licensed for use in children under 2 years

Indication and dose

Short-term treatment only of severe resistant inflammatory skin disorders such as recalcitrant eczemas unresponsive to less potent corticosteroids, psoriasis see notes above

Apply thinly 1–2 times daily for up to 4 weeks; max. 50 g of 0.05% preparation per week

Dermovate® (GSK) (PoM)
Cream, clobetasol propionate 0.05%, net price 30 g = £2.75, 100 g = £8.06. Label: 28, counselling, application, see p. 682. Potency: very potent
Excipients include beeswax (or beeswax substitute), cetostearyl alcohol, chlorocresol, propylene glycol

Ointment, clobetasol propionate 0.05%, net price 30 g = £2.75, 100 g = £8.06. Label: 28, counselling, application, see p. 682. Potency: very potent
Excipients include propylene glycol

Scalp application, clobetasol propionate 0.05%, in a thickened alcoholic basis, net price 30 mL = £3.13, 100 mL = £10.63. Label: 15, 28, counselling, application, see p. 682. Potency: very potent
Excipients none as listed in section 13.1.3

▰**With antimicrobials**
See notes above for comment on compound preparations

Dermovate-NN® (Chemidex) (PoM)
Cream, clobetasol propionate 0.05%, neomycin sulphate 0.5%, nystatin 100 000 units/g, net price 30 g = £3.91. Label: 28, counselling, application, see p. 682. Potency: very potent
Excipients include arachis (peanut) oil, beeswax or beeswax substitute

Ointment, clobetasol propionate 0.05%, neomycin sulphate 0.5%, nystatin 100 000 units/g, in a paraffin basis, net price 30 g = £3.91. Label: 28, counselling, application, see p. 682. Potency: very potent
Excipients none as listed in section 13.1.3

CLOBETASONE BUTYRATE

Cautions see notes above

Contra-indications see notes above

Side-effects see notes above

Licensed use licensed for use in children (age range not specified by manufacturer)

13 Skin

◻ **CLOBETASONE BUTYRATE** *(continued)*

Indication and dose

Eczemas and dermatitis of all types; maintenance between courses of more potent corticosteroids

> Apply thinly 1–2 times daily

¹**Eumovate®** (GSK) PoM

Cream, clobetasone butyrate 0.05%, net price 30 g = £1.89, 100 g = £5.54. Label: 28, counselling, application, see p. 682. Potency: moderate
Excipients include beeswax substitute, cetostearyl alcohol, chlorocresol

Ointment, clobetasone butyrate 0.05%, net price 30 g = £1.89, 100 g = £5.54. Label: 28, counselling, application, see p. 682. Potency: moderate
Excipients none as listed in section 13.1.3

1. Cream can be sold to the public for short-term symptomatic treatment and control of patches of eczema and dermatitis (but not seborrhoeic dermatitis) in children over 12 years provided pack does not contain more than 15 g

◀**With antimicrobials**
See notes above for comment on compound preparations

Trimovate® (GSK) PoM

Cream, clobetasone butyrate 0.05%, oxytetracycline 3% (as calcium salt), nystatin 100 000 units/g, net price 30 g = £3.35. Label: 28, counselling, application, see p. 682. Potency: moderate
Excipients include cetostearyl alcohol, chlorocresol, sodium metabisulphite

Note Stains clothing

◼ **DIFLUCORTOLONE VALERATE**

Cautions see notes above
Contra-indications see notes above
Side-effects see notes above
Licensed use *Nerisone®* licensed for use in children (age range not specified by manufacturer); *Nerisone Forte®* not licensed for use in children under 4 years

Indication and dose

Severe inflammatory skin disorders such as eczemas unresponsive to less potent corticosteroids; high strength (0.3%), short-term treatment of severe exacerbations, psoriasis see notes above

> Apply thinly 1–2 times daily for up to 4 weeks (0.1% preparations) or 2 weeks (0.3% preparations), reducing strength as condition responds; max. 60 g of 0.3% per week

Nerisone® (Meadow) PoM

Cream, diflucortolone valerate 0.1%, net price 30 g = £1.59. Label: 28, counselling, application, see p. 682. Potency: potent
Excipients include disodium edetate, hydroxybenzoates (parabens), stearyl alcohol

Oily cream, diflucortolone valerate 0.1%, net price 30 g = £2.56. Label: 28, counselling, application, see p. 682. Potency: potent
Excipients include beeswax

Ointment, diflucortolone valerate 0.1%, net price 30 g = £1.59. Label: 28, counselling, application, see p. 682. Potency: potent
Excipients none as listed in section 13.1.3

Nerisone Forte® (Meadow) PoM

Oily cream, diflucortolone valerate 0.3%, net price 15 g = £2.09. Label: 28, counselling, application, see p. 682. Potency: very potent
Excipients include beeswax

Ointment, diflucortolone valerate 0.3%, net price 15 g = £2.09. Label: 28, counselling, application, see p. 682. Potency: very potent
Excipients none as listed in section 13.1.3

13
Skin

◼ **FLUDROXYCORTIDE**
(Flurandrenolone)
Cautions see notes above
Contra-indications see notes above
Side-effects see notes above
Licensed use licensed for use in children (age range not specified by manufacturer)

Indication and dose

Inflammatory skin disorders such as eczemas

> Apply thinly 1–2 times daily

Haelan® (Typharm) PoM

Cream, fludroxycortide 0.0125%, net price 60 g = £3.26. Label: 28, counselling, application, see p. 682. Potency: moderate
Excipients include cetyl alcohol, propylene glycol

Ointment, fludroxycortide 0.0125%, net price 60 g = £3.26. Label: 28, counselling, application, see p. 682. Potency: moderate
Excipients include beeswax, cetyl alcohol, polysorbate

Tape, polythene adhesive film impregnated with fludroxycortide 4 micrograms /cm², net price 7.5 cm × 50 cm = £9.27, 7.5 cm × 200 cm = £24.95

Dose

Chronic localised recalcitrant dermatoses (but not acute or weeping)

> Cut tape to fit lesion, apply to clean, dry skin shorn of hair, usually for 12 hours daily

■ FLUOCINOLONE ACETONIDE

Cautions see notes above

Contra-indications see notes above

Side-effects see notes above

Licensed use not licensed for use in children under 1 year

Indication and dose

> Severe inflammatory skin disorders such as eczemas, psoriasis see notes above
>
> Apply thinly 1–2 times daily, reducing strength as condition responds

Synalar® (GP Pharma) PoM
> Cream, fluocinolone acetonide 0.025%, net price 30 g = £3.76, 100 g = £10.68. Label: 28, counselling, application, see p. 682. Potency: potent
> Excipients include benzyl alcohol, cetostearyl alcohol, polysorbates, propylene glycol

> Gel, fluocinolone acetonide 0.025%, net price 30 g = £5.56. For use on scalp and other hairy areas. Label: 28, counselling, application, see p. 682. Potency: potent
> Excipients include hydroxybenzoates (parabens), propylene glycol

> Ointment, fluocinolone acetonide 0.025%, net price 30 g = £3.76, 100 g = £10.68. Label: 28, counselling, application, see p. 682. Potency: potent
> Excipients include propylene glycol, wool fat

Synalar 1 in 4 Dilution® (GP Pharma) PoM
> Cream, fluocinolone acetonide 0.00625%, net price 50 g = £4.40. Label: 28, counselling, application, see p. 682. Potency: moderate
> Excipients include benzyl alcohol, cetostearyl alcohol, polysorbates, propylene glycol

> Ointment, fluocinolone acetonide 0.00625%, net price 50 g = £4.40. Label: 28, counselling, application, see p. 682. Potency: moderate
> Excipients include propylene glycol, wool fat

Synalar 1 in 10 Dilution® (GP Pharma) PoM
> Cream, fluocinolone acetonide 0.0025%, net price 50 g = £4.16. Label: 28, counselling, application, see p. 682. Potency: mild
> Excipients include benzyl alcohol, cetostearyl alcohol, polysorbates, propylene glycol

■ With antibacterials
See notes above for comment on compound preparations

Synalar C® (GP Pharma) PoM
> Cream, fluocinolone acetonide 0.025%, clioquinol 3%, net price 15 g = £2.42. Label: 28, counselling, application, see p. 682. Potency: potent
> Excipients include cetostearyl alcohol, disodium edetate, hydroxybenzoates (parabens), polysorbates, propylene glycol

> Ointment, fluocinolone acetonide 0.025%, clioquinol 3%, net price 15 g = £2.42. Label: 28, counselling, application, see p. 682. Potency: potent.
>
> **Note** stains clothing
> Excipients include propylene glycol, wool fat

Synalar N® (GP Pharma) PoM
> Cream, fluocinolone acetonide 0.025%, neomycin sulphate 0.5%, net price 30 g = £3.96. Label: 28, counselling, application, see p. 682. Potency: potent
> Excipients include cetostearyl alcohol, hydroxybenzoates (parabens), polysorbates, propylene glycol

> Ointment, fluocinolone acetonide 0.025%, neomycin sulphate 0.5%, in a greasy basis, net price 30 g = £3.96. Label: 28, counselling, application, see p. 682. Potency: potent
> Excipients include propylene glycol, wool fat

■ FLUOCINONIDE

Cautions see notes above

Contra-indications see notes above

Side-effects see notes above

Licensed use not licensed for use in children under 1 year

Indication and dose

> Severe inflammatory skin disorders such as eczemas unresponsive to less potent corticosteroids, psoriasis see notes above
>
> Apply thinly 1–2 times daily

Metosyn® (GP Pharma) PoM
> FAPG cream, fluocinonide 0.05%, net price 25 g = £3.30, 100 g = £11.12. Label: 28, counselling, application, see p. 682. Potency: potent
> Excipients include propylene glycol

> Ointment, fluocinonide 0.05%, net price 25 g = £2.92, 100 g = £10.96. Label: 28, counselling, application, see p. 682. Potency: potent
> Excipients include propylene glycol, wool fat

■ FLUOCORTOLONE

Cautions see notes above

Contra-indications see notes above

Side-effects see notes above

Licensed use licensed for use in children (age range not specified by manufacturer)

Indication and dose

> Severe inflammatory skin disorders such as eczemas unresponsive to less potent corticosteroids, psoriasis see notes above
>
> Apply thinly 1–2 times daily

Ultralanum Plain® (Meadow) PoM
> Cream, fluocortolone caproate 0.25%, fluocortolone pivalate 0.25%, net price 50 g = £2.95. Label: 28, counselling, application, see p. 682. Potency: moderate
> Excipients include disodium edetate, fragrance, hydroxybenzoates (parabens), stearyl alcohol

> Ointment, fluocortolone 0.25%, fluocortolone caproate 0.25%, net price 50 g = £2.95. Label: 28, counselling, application, see p. 682. Potency: moderate
> Excipients include wool fat, fragrance

13 Skin

FLUTICASONE PROPIONATE

Cautions see notes above
Contra-indications see notes above
Side-effects see notes above
Licensed use not licensed for use in children under 3 months

Indication and dose

Inflammatory skin disorders such as dermatitis and eczemas unresponsive to less potent corticosteroids, psoriasis see notes above

Apply thinly 1–2 times daily

Cutivate® (GSK) [PoM]
Cream, fluticasone propionate 0.05%, net price 15 g = £2.32, 30 g = £4.50. Label: 28, counselling, application, see p. 682. Potency: potent
Excipients include cetostearyl alcohol, imidurea, propylene glycol

Ointment, fluticasone propionate 0.005%, net price 15 g = £2.32, 30 g = £4.50. Label: 28, counselling, application, see p. 682. Potency: potent
Excipients include propylene glycol

MOMETASONE FUROATE

Cautions see notes above
Contra-indications see notes above
Side-effects see notes above
Licensed use licensed for use in children (age range not specified by manufacturer)

Indication and dose

Severe inflammatory skin disorders such as eczemas unresponsive to less potent corticosteroids, psoriasis see notes above

Apply thinly once daily (to scalp in case of lotion)

Elocon® (Schering-Plough) [PoM]
Cream, mometasone furoate 0.1%, net price 30 g = £4.45, 100 g = £12.82. Label: 28, counselling, application, see p. 682. Potency: potent
Excipients include propylene glycol, stearyl alcohol

Ointment, mometasone furoate 0.1%, net price 30 g = £4.45, 100 g = £12.82. Label: 28, counselling, application, see p. 682. Potency: potent
Excipients include propylene glycol

Scalp lotion, mometasone furoate 0.1% in an aqueous isopropyl alcohol basis, net price 30 mL = £4.45. Label: 28, counselling, application, see p. 682. Potency: potent
Excipients include propylene glycol

TRIAMCINOLONE ACETONIDE

Cautions see notes above
Contra-indications see notes above
Side-effects see notes above
Licensed use *Aureocort®* not licensed for use in children under 8 years

Indication and dose

Severe inflammatory skin disorders such as eczemas unresponsive to less potent corticosteroids, psoriasis see notes above

Apply thinly 1–2 times daily

◢**With antimicrobials**
See notes above for comment on compound preparations

Aureocort® (Goldshield) [PoM]
Ointment, triamcinolone acetonide 0.1%, chlortetracycline hydrochloride 3%, in an anhydrous greasy basis containing wool fat and white soft paraffin, net price 15 g = £2.70. Label: 28, counselling, application, see p. 682. Potency: potent
Excipients include wool fat
Note Stains clothing

13 Skin

13.5   Preparations for eczema and psoriasis

13.5.1   Preparations for eczema

The main types of eczema (dermatitis) in children are atopic, irritant and allergic contact; different types may co-exist. *Atopic eczema* is the most common type and it usually involves dry skin as well as infection and lichenification caused by scratching and rubbing. *Seborrhoeic dermatitis* (see below) is also common in infants.

Management of eczema involves the removal or treatment of contributory factors; known or suspected irritants and contact allergens should be avoided. Rarely, ingredients in topical medicinal products may sensitise the skin (section

13.1.3); *BNF for Children* lists active ingredients together with excipients that have been associated with skin sensitisation.

Skin dryness and the consequent irritant eczema requires **emollients** (section 13.2.1) applied regularly and liberally to the affected area; this can be supplemented with bath or shower emollients. The use of emollients should continue even if the eczema improves or if other treatment is being used.

Topical corticosteroids (section 13.4) are also required in the management of eczema; the potency of the corticosteroid should be appropriate to the severity and site of the condition, and the age of the child. Mild corticosteroids are generally used on the face and on flexures; the more potent corticosteroids are generally required for use on lichenified areas of eczema or for severe eczema on the scalp, limbs, and trunk. Treatment should be reviewed regularly, especially if a potent corticosteroid is required. In children with frequent flares (2–3 per month), a topical corticosteroid can be applied on 2 consecutive days each week to prevent further flares.

Bandages (including those containing **zinc** and **ichthammol**) are sometimes applied over topical corticosteroids or emollients to treat eczema of the limbs. Wet elasticated viscose stockinette is used for 'wet-wrap' bandaging over topical corticosteroids or emollients to cool the skin and relieve itching, but there is an increased risk of infection and excessive absorption of the corticosteroid; 'wet-wrap' bandaging should be used under specialist supervision.

For details of elasticated viscose stockinette tubular bandages and garments, and silk clothing, see BNF section A8.8.3

For the role of topical **pimecrolimus** and **tacrolimus** in atopic eczema, see section 13.5.3.

Infection Bacterial infection (commonly with *Staphylococcus aureus* and occasionally with *Streptococcus pyogenes*) can exacerbate eczema. A topical antibacterial such as fusidic acid (section 13.10.1) may be used for small areas of mild infection; treatment should be limited to a short course (typically 1 week) to reduce the risk of drug resistance or skin sensitisation. Associated eczema is treated simultaneously with a moderately potent or potent topical corticosteroid which can be combined with an antimicrobial such as clioquinol.

Eczema involving moderate to severe, widespread, or recurrent infection requires the use of a systemic antibacterial (section 5.1, table 1) that is active against the infecting organism. Preparations that combine an antiseptic with an emollient application (section 13.2.1) and with a bath emollient (section 13.2.1.1) can also be used; antiseptic shampoos (section 13.9) can be used on the scalp.

Intertriginous eczema commonly involves candida and bacteria; it is best treated with a mild or moderately potent topical corticosteroid combined with a suitable antimicrobial drug. For the treatment of nappy rash, see section 13.2.2.

Widespread *herpes simplex infection* may complicate atopic eczema (eczema herpeticum) and treatment under specialist supervision with a systemic antiviral drug (section 5.3.2.1) is indicated. Secondary bacterial infection often exacerbates eczema herpeticum.

The management of *seborrhoeic dermatitis* is described below.

Management of other features of eczema *Lichenification*, which results from repeated scratching, is treated initially with a potent corticosteroid. Bandages containing **ichthammol** (to reduce pruritus) and other substances such as **zinc oxide** can be applied over the corticosteroid or emollient. **Coal tar** (section 13.5.2) and ichthammol can be useful in some cases of *chronic eczema*. *Discoid eczema*, with thickened plaques in chronic atopic eczema, is usually treated with a topical antiseptic preparation, a potent topical corticosteroid, and paste bandages containing zinc oxide and ichthammol.

A *non-sedating* antihistamine (section 3.4.1) may be of some value in relieving severe itching or urticaria associated with eczema. A *sedating* antihistamine (section 3.4.1) can be used at night if itching causes sleep disturbance, but a large dose may be needed and drowsiness may persist on the following day.

Exudative ('*weeping*') *eczema* requires a potent corticosteroid initially; infection may also be present and require specific treatment (see above). **Potassium permanganate** solution (1 in 10 000) can be used as a soak in exudating eczema for its antiseptic and astringent effects; treatment should be stopped when exudation stops.

Severe refractory eczema is best managed under specialist supervision; it may require phototherapy or drugs that act on the immune system (section 13.5.3).

Seborrhoeic dermatitis   *Seborrhoeic dermatitis* (*seborrhoeic eczema*) is associated with species of the yeast *Malassezia*. *Infantile seborrhoeic dermatitis* affects particularly the body folds, nappy area and scalp; it is treated with emollients and mild topical corticosteroids with suitable antimicrobials. Infantile seborrhoeic dermatitis affecting the scalp (*cradle cap*) is treated by hydrating the scalp using natural oils and the use of mild shampoo (section 13.9).

In older children, seborrhoeic dermatitis affects the scalp, paranasal areas, and eyebrows. Shampoos active against the yeast (including those containing ketoconazole and coal tar, section 13.9) and combinations of mild topical corticosteroids with suitable antimicrobials (section 13.4) are used to treat older children.

ICHTHAMMOL

Side-effects skin irritation
Licensed use no information available

Indication and dose

Chronic lichenified eczema

  Child 1–18 years apply 1–3 times daily

Ichthammol Ointment, BP 1980
Ointment, ichthammol 10%, yellow soft paraffin 45%, wool fat 45%

Zinc and Ichthammol Cream, BP
Cream, ichthammol 5%, cetostearyl alcohol 3%, wool fat 10%, in zinc cream

Medicated bandages

Zinc paste bandages are also used with **coal tar** or **ichthammol** in chronic lichenified skin conditions such as chronic eczema (ichthammol often being preferred since its action is considered to be milder). They are also used with **calamine** in milder eczematous skin conditions (but the inclusion of **clioquinol** may lead to irritation in susceptible children).

Zinc Paste Bandage, BP 1993
Cotton fabric, plain weave, impregnated with suitable paste containing zinc oxide; requires additional bandaging. Net price 6 m × 7.5 cm = £3.24 (Mölnlycke—*Steripaste*® (15%), *excipients: include* polysorbate 80); £3.23 (S&N Hlth—*Viscopaste PB7*® (10%), *excipients: include* cetostearyl alcohol, hydroxybenzoates)

Zinc Paste and Calamine Bandage
(Drug Tariff specification 5). Cotton fabric, plain weave, impregnated with suitable paste containing calamine and zinc oxide; requires additional bandaging. Net price 6 m × 7.5 cm = £3.33 (Mölnlycke—*Calaband*®)

Zinc Paste, Calamine, and Clioquinol Bandage, BP 1993
Cotton fabric, plain weave, impregnated with suitable paste containing calamine, clioquinol, and zinc oxide;

requires additional bandaging. Net price 6 m × 7.5 cm = £3.33 (Mölnlycke—*Quinaband*®, *excipients: include* hydroxybenzoates)

Zinc Paste and Ichthammol Bandage, BP 1993
Cotton fabric, plain weave, impregnated with suitable paste containing zinc oxide and ichthammol; requires additional bandaging. Net price 6 m × 7.5 cm = £3.45 (S&N Hlth—*Ichthopaste*® (6/2%), *excipients: include* cetostearyl alcohol)

◀Medicated stocking
Zipzoc® (S&N Hlth.)
Sterile rayon stocking impregnated with ointment containing zinc oxide 20%. 4-pouch carton = £12.52; 10-pouch carton = £31.30

13
Skin

13.5.2 Preparations for psoriasis

Psoriasis is characterised by epidermal thickening and scaling. It commonly affects extensor surfaces and the scalp. For mild psoriasis, reassurance and treatment with an emollient may be all that is necessary. *Guttate psoriasis* is a distinctive form of psoriasis that characteristically occurs in children and young adults, often following a streptococcal throat infection or tonsillitis.

Occasionally psoriasis is provoked or exacerbated by drugs such as lithium, chloroquine and hydroxychloroquine, beta-blockers, non-steroidal anti-inflammatory drugs, and ACE inhibitors. Psoriasis may not occur until the drug has been taken for weeks or months.

Emollients (section 13.2.1), in addition to their effects on dryness, scaling and cracking, may have an antiproliferative effect in psoriasis. They are particularly useful in *inflammatory psoriasis* and in *chronic stable plaque psoriasis*.

For *chronic stable plaque psoriasis* on extensor surfaces of trunk and limbs preparations containing **coal tar** are moderately effective, but the smell is unacceptable to some children. **Vitamin D** and its analogues are effective and cosmetically acceptable alternatives to preparations containing coal tar or dithranol. **Dithranol** is the most effective topical antipsoriatic agent but it irritates and stains the skin and it should be used only under specialist supervision. Adverse effects of dithranol are minimised by using a 'short-contact technique' (see below) and by starting with low concentration preparations. **Tazarotene**, a topical retinoid for the treatment of mild to moderate plaque psoriasis, is not recommended for use in children under 18 years. These medications can irritate the skin particularly in the flexures and they are not suitable for the more inflammatory forms of psoriasis; their use should be suspended during an inflammatory phase of psoriasis. The efficacy and the irritancy of each substance varies between patients. If a substance irritates significantly, it should be stopped or the concentration reduced; if it is tolerated, its effects should be assessed after 4 to 6 weeks and treatment continued if it is effective.

Widespread *unstable psoriasis* of erythrodermic or generalised pustular type requires urgent specialist assessment. Initial topical treatment should be limited to using emollients frequently and generously. More localised acute or subacute *inflammatory psoriasis* with hot, spreading or itchy lesions, should be treated topically with emollients or with a corticosteroid of moderate potency.

Scalp psoriasis is usually scaly, and the scale may be thick and adherent. This requires softening with an emollient ointment, cream, or oil and usually combined with **salicylic acid** as a keratolytic.

Some preparations for psoriasis affecting the scalp combine salicylic acid with coal tar or **sulphur**. The preparation should be applied generously and left on for at least an hour, often more conveniently overnight, before washing it off. If a corticosteroid lotion or gel is required (e.g. for itch), it can be used in the morning.

Calcipotriol and **tacalcitol** are analogues of vitamin D that affect cell division and differentiation. **Calcitriol** is an active form of vitamin D. Vitamin D and its analogues are used as first-line treatment for plaque psoriasis; they do not smell or stain and they may be more acceptable than tar or dithranol products. Of the vitamin D analogues, tacalcitol and calcitriol are less likely to irritate.

Coal tar has anti-inflammatory properties that are useful in chronic plaque psoriasis; it also has antiscaling properties. Contact of coal tar products with normal skin is not normally harmful and preparations containing coal tar can be used for widespread small lesions; however, irritation, contact allergy, and sterile folliculitis can occur. Preparations containing up to 6% coal tar may be used on children 1 month to 2 years; preparations containing coal tar 10% may be used on children over 2 years with more severe psoriasis. For shampoo preparations containing coal tar, see section 13.9.

Dithranol is effective for chronic plaque psoriasis. Its major disadvantages are irritation (for which individual susceptibility varies) and staining of skin and of clothing. It should be applied to chronic extensor plaques only, carefully avoiding normal skin. Dithranol is not generally suitable for widespread small lesions nor should it be used in the flexures or on the face. Treatment should be started with a low concentration such as dithranol 0.1%, and the strength increased gradually every few days up to 3%, according to tolerance. Proprietary preparations are more suitable for home use; they are usually washed off after 20–30 minutes ('short contact' technique). Specialist nurses may apply intensive treatment with dithranol paste which is covered by stockinette dressings and usually retained overnight. Dithranol should be discontinued if even a low concentration causes acute inflammation; continued use can result in the psoriasis becoming unstable. When applying dithranol, hands should be protected by gloves or they should be washed thoroughly afterwards.

A topical **corticosteroid** (section 13.4) is not generally suitable as the sole treatment of extensive chronic plaque psoriasis; any early improvement is not usually maintained and there is a risk of the condition deteriorating or of precipitating an unstable form of psoriasis (e.g. erythrodermic psoriasis or generalised pustular psoriasis). However, it may be appropriate to treat psoriasis in specific sites such as the face and flexures usually with a mild corticosteroid, and psoriasis of the scalp, palms and soles with a potent corticosteroid.

Combining the use of a corticosteroid with another specific topical treatment may be beneficial in chronic plaque psoriasis; the drugs may be used separately at different times of the day or used together in a single formulation. *Eczema* co-existing with psoriasis may be treated with a corticosteroid, or coal tar, or both. Systemic or potent topical corticosteroids should be avoided or used only under specialist supervision; although corticosteroids may suppress psoriasis in the short term, relapse or vigorous rebound occurs on withdrawal.

Phototherapy Phototherapy is available in specialist centres under the supervision of a dermatologist. Narrow band ultraviolet B (UVB) radiation is usually effective for *chronic stable psoriasis* and for *guttate psoriasis*. It can be considered for children with moderately severe psoriasis in whom topical treatment has failed, but it may irritate inflammatory psoriasis. The use of phototherapy and photochemotherapy in children is limited by concerns over carcinogenicity and premature ageing.

Photochemotherapy combining long-wave ultraviolet A radiation with a psoralen (PUVA) is available in specialist centres under the supervision of a dermatologist. The psoralen, which enhances the effect of irradiation, is administered either by mouth or topically. PUVA is effective in most forms of psoriasis, including the *localised palmoplantar pustular psoriasis*. Early adverse effects include phototoxicity and pruritus. Higher cumulative doses exaggerate skin ageing, increase the risk of dysplastic and neoplastic skin lesions especially squamous cancer, and pose a theoretical risk of cataracts.

Phototherapy combined with coal tar, dithranol, topical vitamin D or vitamin D analogues, or oral acitretin, allows reduction of the cumulative dose of phototherapy required to treat psoriasis.

Systemic treatment Systemic treatment is required for severe, resistant, unstable or complicated forms of psoriasis, and it should be initiated only under specialist supervision. Systemic drugs for psoriasis include acitretin and drugs that affect the immune response (section 13.5.3).

Acitretin, a metabolite of etretinate, is a retinoid (vitamin A derivative); it is prescribed by specialists. The main indication of acitretin is severe psoriasis resistant to other forms of therapy. It is also used in disorders of keratinisation such as severe *Darier's disease* (keratosis follicularis), and some forms of *ichthyosis*. Although a minority of cases of psoriasis respond well to acitretin alone, it is only moderately effective in many cases; adverse effects are a limiting factor. A therapeutic effect occurs after 2 to 4 weeks and the maximum benefit after 4 to 6 weeks or longer. Continuous treatment for longer than 6 months is not usually necessary in psoriasis. However, some patients, particularly those with severe ichthyosis, may benefit from longer treatment, provided that the lowest effective dose is used, patients are monitored carefully for adverse effects, and the need for treatment is reviewed regularly. Topical preparations containing keratolytics should normally be stopped before administration of acitretin. Liberal use of emollients should be encouraged and topical corticosteroids can be continued if necessary.

Acitretin is teratogenic; in females of child-bearing age, the possibility of pregnancy must be excluded before treatment and effective contraception must be used during treatment and for at least 3 years afterwards (oral progestogen-only contraceptives not considered effective). Common side-effects derive from its widespread but reversible effects on epithelia, such as dry and cracking lips, dry skin and mucosal surfaces, hair thinning, paronychia, and soft and sticky palms and soles. Liver function and blood-lipid concentration should be monitored before starting treatment, after 1 month, and then 3-monthly during treatment. Musculoskeletal development should also be monitored closely.

13

Skin

Topical preparations for psoriasis

Vitamin D and analogues

Calcipotriol, **calcitriol**, and **tacalcitol** are used for the management of *plaque psoriasis*. They should be avoided by those with calcium metabolism disorders, and used with caution in *generalised pustular* or *erythrodermic exfoliative psoriasis* (enhanced risk of hypercalcaemia). Local skin reactions (itching, erythema, burning, paraesthesia, dermatitis) are common. Hands should be washed thoroughly after application to avoid inadvertent transfer to other body areas. Aggravation of psoriasis has also been reported.

CALCIPOTRIOL

Cautions see notes above; avoid use on face; avoid excessive exposure to sunlight and sun-lamps

Contra-indications see notes above

Pregnancy manufacturer advises avoid if possible

Breast-feeding no information available

Side-effects see notes above; also photosensitivity; rarely facial or perioral dermatitis, skin atrophy

Licensed use Calcipotriol ointment and scalp solution, *Dovonex® Scalp Solution*, *Dovobet®*, and *Xamiol®* not licensed for use in children

Indication and dose

> **Plaque psoriasis**
>
> **Child 6–18 years** apply cream *or* ointment twice daily; 6–12 years max. 50 g weekly, over 12 years max. 75 g weekly (less with scalp solution, see below)
> **Note** Patient information leaflet for *Dovonex®* cream advises liberal application (but note max. recommended weekly dose, above)

> **Scalp psoriasis (specialist use only)**
>
> **Child 6–12 years** apply scalp solution twice daily; max. 30 mL weekly (less when used with cream or ointment, see below)
>
> **Child 12–18 years** apply scalp solution twice daily; max. 45 mL weekly (less when used with cream or ointment, see below)

Note When preparations used together max. total calcipotriol 2.5 mg in any one week for child 6–12 years (e.g. scalp solution 20 mL with cream or ointment 30 g); max. 3.75 mg in any one week for child 12–18 years (e.g. scalp solution 30 mL with cream or ointment 45 g)

Calcipotriol (Non-proprietary) [PoM]
Ointment, calcipotriol 50 micrograms/g, net price 120 g = £24.43

Scalp solution, calcipotriol 50 micrograms/mL, net price 60 mL = £12.53, 120 mL = £26.07
Excipients include propylene glycol

Dovonex® (LEO) [PoM]
Cream, calcipotriol 50 micrograms/g, net price 60 g = £11.55, 120 g = £23.10
Excipients include cetostearyl alcohol, disodium edetate

Scalp solution, calcipotriol 50 micrograms/mL, net price 60 mL = £12.53, 120 mL = £26.07
Excipients include propylene glycol

With betamethasone

For prescribing information, and for comment on the limited role of corticosteroids in psoriasis, see section 13.4.

Dovobet® (LEO) [PoM]
Ointment, betamethasone 0.05% (as dipropionate), calcipotriol 50 micrograms/g, net price 60 g = £33.63, 120 g = £62.46. Label: 28
Excipients none as listed in section 13.1.3

Dose

> **Stable plaque psoriasis (specialist use only)**
>
> **Child 12–18 years** apply once daily to max. 30% of body surface for up to 4 weeks; max. 75 g weekly; subsequent courses repeated after an interval of at least 4 weeks

Note When different preparations containing calcipotriol used together, max. total calcipotriol 3.75 mg in any one week for child 12–18 years

Xamiol® (LEO) [PoM]
Scalp gel, betamethasone 0.05% (as dipropionate), calcipotriol 50 micrograms/g, net price 60 g = £36.50. Label: 28
Excipients include butylated hydroxytoluene

Dose

> **Scalp psoriasis (specialist use only)**
>
> **Child 12–18 years** apply 1–4 g to scalp once daily, shampoo off after leaving on scalp overnight or during day; usual duration of therapy, 4 weeks

Note When different preparations containing calcipotriol used together, max. total calcipotriol 3.75 mg in any one week for child 12–18 years

CALCITRIOL

(1,25-Dihydroxycholecalciferol)

Cautions see notes above

Contra-indications see notes above; do not apply under occlusion

Hepatic impairment manufacturer advises avoid—no information available

Renal impairment manufacturer advises avoid—no information available

Pregnancy avoid; use in restricted amounts if clearly necessary (significant systemic absorption); monitor urine- and plasma-calcium concentration

Breast-feeding manufacturer advises avoid

Side-effects see notes above

Indication and dose

> **Mild to moderate plaque psoriasis**
>
> **Child 12–18 years** apply twice daily; not more than 35% of body surface to be treated daily, max. 30 g daily

Silkis® (Galderma) [PoM]
Ointment, calcitriol 3 micrograms/g, net price 100 g = £13.87
Excipients none as listed in section 13.1.3

TACALCITOL

Cautions see notes above; avoid eyes; monitor serum-calcium concentration if risk of hypercalcaemia; if used in conjunction with UV treatment, UV radiation should be given in the morning and tacalcitol applied at bedtime

Contra-indications see notes above

Renal impairment monitor serum-calcium concentration

Pregnancy manufacturer advises avoid unless no safer alternative—no information available

Breast-feeding manufacturer advises avoid application to breast area; no information available on presence in milk

◻ **TACALCITOL** (*continued*)

Side-effects see notes above

Indication and dose

> Plaque psoriasis
>
> > **Child 12–18 years** apply once daily preferably at bedtime; max. 10 g *ointment* or 10 mL *lotion* daily
> > **Note** When lotion and ointment used together, max. total tacalcitol 280 micrograms in any one week (e.g. lotion 30 mL with ointment 40 g)

Curatoderm® (Almirall) ᴾᵒᴹ
Lotion, tacalcitol (as monohydrate) 4 micrograms/ g, net price 30 mL = £12.73
Excipients include disodium edetate, propylene glycol

Ointment, tacalcitol (as monohydrate) 4 micrograms/g, net price 30 g = £13.40, 60 g = £23.14, 100 g = £30.86
Excipients none as listed in section 13.1.3

Tars

TARS

Cautions avoid eyes, mucosa, genital or rectal areas, and broken or inflamed skin; use suitable chemical protection gloves for extemporaneous preparation

Contra-indications not for use in sore, acute, or pustular psoriasis or in presence of infection

Pregnancy no adverse effects reported

Breast-feeding no adverse effects reported

Side-effects skin irritation and acne-like eruptions, photosensitivity; stains skin, hair, and fabric

Indication and dose

> Psoriasis and occasionally chronic atopic eczema
>
> > Apply 1–3 times daily starting with low-strength preparations; proprietary preparations, see individual entries below
> > **Note** For shampoo preparations see section 13.9

◢ **Non-proprietary preparations**
May be difficult to obtain. Patients may find newer proprietary preparations more acceptable

Coal Tar Paste, BP
Paste, strong coal tar solution 7.5%, in compound zinc paste

Zinc and Coal Tar Paste, BP
Paste, zinc oxide 6%, coal tar 6%, emulsifying wax 5%, starch 38%, yellow soft paraffin 45%
Excipients include cetostearyl alcohol

◢ **Proprietary preparations**

Carbo-Dome® (Sandoz)
Cream, coal tar solution 10%, in a water-miscible basis, net price 30 g = £4.77, 100 g = £16.38
Excipients include beeswax, hydroxybenzoates (parabens)

Dose
> Psoriasis
> > Apply to skin 2–3 times daily

Cocois® (UCB Pharma)
Scalp ointment, coal tar solution 12%, salicylic acid 2%, precipitated sulphur 4%, in a coconut oil emollient basis, net price 40 g (with applicator nozzle) = £5.98, 100 g = £11.23
Excipients include cetostearyl alcohol

Dose
> Scaly scalp disorders including psoriasis, eczema, seborrhoeic dermatitis and dandruff
> > **Child 6–12 years** medical supervision required

> > **Child 12–18 years** apply to scalp once weekly as necessary (if severe use daily for first 3–7 days), shampoo off after 1 hour

Exorex® (Forest)
Lotion, prepared coal tar 1% in an emollient basis, net price 100 mL = £8.11, 250 mL = £16.24
Excipients include hydroxybenzoates (parabens), polysorbate 80

Dose
> Psoriasis
> > Apply to skin or scalp 2–3 times daily; product can be diluted with a few drops of water before applying

Psoriderm® (Dermal)
Cream, coal tar 6%, lecithin 0.4%, net price 225 mL = £9.57
Excipients include isopropyl palmitate, propylene glycol

Dose
> Psoriasis
> > Apply to skin or scalp 1–2 times daily

Scalp lotion—section 13.9

Sebco® (Centrapharm)
Scalp ointment, coal tar solution 12%, salicylic acid 2%, precipitated sulphur 4%, in a coconut oil emollient basis, net price 40 g = £4.54, 100 g = £8.52
Excipients include cetostearyl alcohol

Dose
> Scaly scalp disorders including psoriasis, eczema, seborrhoeic dermatitis and dandruff
> > **Child 6–12 years** medical supervision required

> > **Child 12–18 years** apply to scalp as necessary (if severe use daily for first 3–7 days), shampoo off after 1 hour

◢ **Bath preparations**

Coal Tar Solution, BP
Solution, coal tar 20%, polysorbate '80' 5%, in alcohol (96%), net price 500 mL = £7.25. Label: 15
Excipients include polysorbates

Dose
> Use 100 mL in an adult-size bath, and proportionally less for a child's bath

Note Strong Coal Tar Solution BP contains coal tar 40%

13
Skin

▢ TARS *(continued)*

Pinetarsol® (Crawford)
Bath oil, tar 2.3% in a light liquid paraffin basis, net price 200 mL = £4.75, 500 mL = £7.95
Excipients include fragrance

Dose
> **Eczema and psoriasis**
> Use 15–30 mL in adult-size bath *or* apply directly to wet skin and rinse after a few minutes; can be used as a soap substitute

Gel, tar 1.6%, net price 100 g = £4.95

Dose
> **Eczema and psoriasis**
> Apply directly to wet skin and rinse after a few minutes; can be used as a soap substitute

Solution, tar 2.3%, net price 200 mL = £4.45, 500 mL = £7.45

Dose
> **Eczema and psoriasis**
> Use 15–30 mL in adult-size bath *or* dilute 15 mL with 3 litres of water and apply to affected areas *or* apply solution directly to wet skin and rinse after a few minutes; can be used as a soap substitute

Polytar Emollient® (Stiefel)
Bath additive, coal tar solution 2.5%, arachis (peanut) oil extract of coal tar 7.5%, tar 7.5%, cade oil 7.5%, liquid paraffin 35%, net price 500 mL = £5.78
Excipients include isopropyl palmitate

Dose
> **Psoriasis, eczema, atopic and pruritic dermatoses**
> Use 2–4 capfuls (15–30 mL) in adult-size bath and proportionally less for a child's bath; soak for 20 minutes

Psoriderm® (Dermal)
Bath emulsion, coal tar 40%, net price 200 mL = £2.79
Excipients include polysorbate 20

Dose
> **Psoriasis**
> Use 30 mL in adult-size bath, and proportionally less for a child's bath; soak for 5 minutes

◢ With corticosteroids
Alphosyl HC® (GSK Consumer Healthcare) [PoM]
Cream, coal tar extract 5%, hydrocortisone 0.5%, allantoin 2%, net price 100 g = £3.16. Label: 28. Potency: mild
Excipients include beeswax, cetyl alcohol, hydroxybenzoates (parabens), isopropyl palmitate, wool fat

Dose
> **Psoriasis**
> **Child 5–18 years** apply thinly twice daily

Dithranol

◢ DITHRANOL
(Anthralin)

Cautions avoid use near eyes and sensitive areas of skin; see also notes above

Contra-indications hypersensitivity; acute and pustular psoriasis

Pregnancy no adverse effects reported

Breast-feeding no adverse effects reported

Side-effects local burning sensation and irritation; stains skin, hair, and fabrics

Licensed use *Dithrocream®* and *Psorin®* licensed for use in children (age range not specified by manufacturer); *Micanol®* licensed for use in children, but not recommended for infants or young children (age range not specified by manufacturer)

Indication and dose
> **Subacute and chronic psoriasis**
> See notes above and under preparations
> **Note** Some of these dithranol preparations also contain coal tar or salicylic acid—for prescribing information see under Tars or under Salicylic Acid

◢ Non-proprietary preparations
¹Dithranol Ointment, BP [PoM]
Ointment, dithranol, in yellow soft paraffin; usual strengths 0.1–2%. Part of basis may be replaced by hard paraffin if a stiffer preparation is required. Label: 28
1. [PoM] if dithranol content more than 1%, otherwise may be sold to the public

Dithranol Paste, BP
Paste, dithranol in zinc and salicylic acid (Lassar's) paste. Usual strengths 0.1–1% of dithranol. Label: 28

◢ Proprietary preparations
Dithrocream® (Dermal)
Cream, dithranol 0.1%, net price 50 g = £3.83; 0.25%, 50 g = £4.10; 0.5%, 50 g = £4.73; 1%, 50 g = £5.51; [PoM] 2%, 50 g = £6.89. Label: 28
Excipients include cetostearyl alcohol, chlorocresol

Dose
> For application to skin or scalp; 0.1–0.5% cream suitable for overnight treatment, 1–2% cream for max. 1 hour

Micanol® (GP Pharma)
Cream, dithranol 1% in a lipid-stabilised basis, net price 50 g = £13.48; [PoM] 3%, 50 g = £16.79. Label: 28
Excipients none as listed in section 13.1.3

Dose
> For application to skin or scalp, apply 1% cream for up to 30 minutes once daily, if necessary 3% cream can be used under medical supervision

Note At the end of contact time, use plenty of lukewarm (not hot) water to rinse off cream; soap may be used *after* the cream has been rinsed off; use shampoo before applying cream to scalp and if necessary after cream has been rinsed off

⌐ **DITHRANOL (continued)**

Psorin® (LPC)
Ointment, dithranol 0.11%, coal tar 1%, salicylic acid 1.6%, net price 50 g = £9.22, 100 g = £18.44. Label: 28
Excipients include beeswax, wool fat

Dose
> For application to skin up to twice daily

Scalp gel, dithranol 0.25%, salicylic acid 1.6% in gel basis containing methyl salicylate, net price 50 g = £7.03. Label: 28
Excipients none as listed in section 13.1.3

Dose
> For application to scalp, initially apply on alternate days for 10–20 minutes; may be increased to daily application for max. 1 hour and then wash off

Salicylic acid

SALICYLIC ACID

For coal tar preparations containing salicylic acid, see under Tars p.695; for dithranol preparations containing salicylic acid see under Dithranol, above

Cautions see notes above; avoid broken or inflamed skin
Salicylate toxicity Salicylate toxicity may occur particularly if applied on large areas of skin or on neonatal skin

Side-effects sensitivity, excessive drying, irritation, systemic effects after widespread use (see under Cautions)

Indication and dose

Hyperkeratotic skin disorders see under preparation

Acne section 13.6.1

Warts and calluses section 13.7

Scalp conditions section 13.9

Fungal nail infections section 13.10.2

Zinc and Salicylic Acid Paste, BP
Paste, (Lassar's Paste), zinc oxide 24%, salicylic acid 2%, starch 24%, white soft paraffin 50%, net price 25 g = 17p

Dose
> **Child 1 month–18 years** apply twice daily

Oral retinoids for psoriasis

ACITRETIN

Note Acitretin is a metabolite of etretinate

Cautions in children use only in exceptional circumstances (premature epiphyseal closure reported); in females of childbearing age exclude pregnancy before starting (test for pregnancy within 2 weeks before treatment and monthly thereafter; start treatment on day 2 or 3 of menstrual cycle)—females of childbearing age (including those with history of infertility) should avoid pregnancy and use effective contraception for at least 1 month before, during, and for at least 3 years after treatment (oral progestogen-only contraceptives not considered effective); patients should avoid concomitant tetracycline or methotrexate, high doses of vitamin A (more than 4000–5000 units daily) and use of keratolytics, and should not donate blood during or for at least 1 year after stopping therapy (teratogenic risk); check liver function at start, after 1 month, then every 3 months; monitor plasma lipids; diabetes (can alter glucose tolerance—initial frequent blood glucose checks); radiographic assessment on long-term treatment; investigate atypical musculoskeletal symptoms; avoid excessive exposure to sunlight and unsupervised use of sunlamps; **interactions:** Appendix 1 (retinoids)

Contra-indications hyperlipidaemia

Hepatic impairment avoid—further impairment may occur

Renal impairment avoid; increased risk of toxicity

Pregnancy avoid—teratogenic; effective contraception must be used—see Cautions above

Breast-feeding avoid

Side-effects dryness of mucous membranes (sometimes erosion), of skin (sometimes scaling, thinning, erythema especially of face, and pruritus), and of conjunctiva (sometimes conjunctivitis and decreased tolerance of contact lenses); sticky skin, dermatitis; other side-effects reported include palmoplantar exfoliation, epistaxis, epidermal and nail fragility, oedema, paronychia, granulomatous lesions, bullous eruptions, reversible hair thinning and alopecia, myalgia and arthralgia, occasional nausea, headache, malaise, drowsiness, rhinitis, sweating, taste disturbance, and gingivitis; benign intracranial hypertension (discontinue if severe headache, vomiting, diarrhoea, abdominal pain, and visual disturbance occur; **avoid** concomitant tetracyclines); photosensitivity, corneal ulceration, raised liver enzymes, rarely jaundice and hepatitis (**avoid** concomitant methotrexate); raised serum triglycerides or cholesterol; decreased night vision reported; skeletal hyperostosis and extraosseous calcification reported following long-term administration of etretinate (and premature epiphyseal closure in children, see Cautions)

13
Skin

◁ **ACITRETIN (continued)**

Indication and dose

Harlequin ichthyosis (under expert supervision only)

• By mouth

Neonate 500 micrograms/kg once daily with food or milk (occasionally up to 1 mg/kg daily) with careful monitoring of musculoskeletal development

Severe extensive psoriasis resistant to other forms of therapy, palmoplantar pustular psoriasis, severe congenital ichthyosis, severe Darier's disease (keratosis follicularis) (all under expert supervision **only**)

• By mouth

Child 1 month–12 years 500 micrograms/kg once daily with food or milk (occasionally up to 1 mg/kg daily) to max. 35 mg daily with careful monitoring of musculoskeletal development (see also p. 693)

Child 12–18 years initially 25–30 mg daily (Darier's disease 10 mg daily) for 2–4 weeks, then adjusted according to response, usual range 25–50 mg daily; up to 75 mg daily for short periods in psoriasis and ichthyosis (see also p. 693)

Neotigason® (Actavis) (PoM)
Capsules, acitretin 10 mg (brown/white), net price 60-cap pack = £24.27; 25 mg (brown/yellow), 60-cap pack = £56.30. Label: 10, patient information leaflet, 21

◢Extemporaneous formulations available see Extemporaneous Preparations, p. 8

13.5.3   Drugs affecting the immune response

Drugs affecting the immune response are used for eczema or psoriasis.

Pimecrolimus by topical application is licensed for *mild to moderate atopic eczema*. **Tacrolimus** is licensed for topical use in *moderate to severe atopic eczema*. Both are drugs whose long-term safety is still being evaluated and they should not usually be considered first-line treatment unless there is a specific reason to avoid or reduce the use of topical corticosteroids. Treatment with topical pimecrolimus or topical tacrolimus should be initiated only by prescribers experienced in treating atopic eczema.

> **NICE guidance**
>
> **Tacrolimus and pimecrolimus for atopic eczema (August 2004)**
> Topical pimecrolimus and tacrolimus are options for atopic eczema not controlled by maximal topical corticosteroid treatment or if there is a risk of important corticosteroid side-effects (particularly skin atrophy).
>
> Topical pimecrolimus is recommended for moderate atopic eczema on the face and neck of children aged 2–16 years and topical tacrolimus is recommended for moderate to severe atopic eczema in children over 2 years. Pimecrolimus and tacrolimus should be used within their licensed indications.

For the role of topical corticosteroids in eczema, see section 13.5.1, and for comment on their limited role in psoriasis, see section 13.4. A systemic corticosteroid (section 6.3.2) such as prednisolone may be used in *severe* refractory eczema.

Systemic drugs acting on the immune system are generally used by **specialists** in a hospital setting.

Ciclosporin (cyclosporin) by mouth can be used for *severe psoriasis* and for *severe eczema*. **Azathioprine** (section 8.2.1) or **mycophenolate mofetil** (section 8.2.1) are also used for severe refractory eczema in children.

Methotrexate can be used for *severe resistant psoriasis*; the dose is given **once weekly** and adjusted according to severity of the condition and haematological and biochemical measurements. Folic acid (section 9.1.2) should be given to reduce the possibility of methotrexate toxicity. Folic acid can be given at a dose of 5 mg once weekly; alternative regimens may be used in some settings.

Etanercept (a cytokine modulator) is licensed in children over 8 years of age for the treatment of *severe plaque psoriasis* that is inadequately controlled by other systemic treatments and photochemotherapy, or when these other treatments cannot be used because of intolerance or contra-indications.

CICLOSPORIN
(Cyclosporin)

Cautions section 8.2.2

Additional cautions in atopic dermatitis and psoriasis *Contra-indicated* in abnormal renal function, uncontrolled hypertension (see also below), infections not under control, and malignancy (see also below). Dermatological and physical examination, including blood pressure and renal function measurements required at least twice before starting. During treatment, monitor serum creatinine every 2 weeks for first 3 months then every month; reduce dose by 25–50% if serum creatinine increases more than 30% above baseline (even if within normal range) and discontinue if reduction not successful within one month. Discontinue if hypertension develops that cannot be controlled by dose reduction or antihypertensive therapy. Avoid excessive exposure to sunlight and avoid use of UVB or PUVA. *In atopic dermatitis,* also allow herpes simplex infections to clear before starting (if they occur during treatment withdraw if severe); *Staphylococcus aureus* skin infections not absolute contra-indication providing controlled (but avoid erythromycin unless no other alternative—see also **interactions**: Appendix 1 (ciclosporin)); investigate lymphadenopathy that persists despite improvement in atopic dermatitis. *In psoriasis,* also exclude malignancies (including those of skin and cervix) before starting (biopsy any lesions not typical of psoriasis) and treat patients with pre-malignant or pre-malignant conditions of skin only after appropriate treatment (and if no other option); discontinue if lymphoproliferative disorder develops

Hepatic impairment section 8.2.2

Renal impairment see Cautions above

Pregnancy section 8.2.2

Breast-feeding section 8.2.2

Side-effects section 8.2.2

Licensed use not licensed for use in children under 16 years for atopic eczema (dermatitis) or psoriasis

Indication and dose

> **Short-term treatment (usually max. 8 weeks but may be used for longer by specialists) of severe atopic dermatitis where conventional therapy ineffective or inappropriate**
> - By mouth, administered in accordance with expert advice
>
>   Child 1 month–18 years initially 1.25 mg/kg twice daily, if good initial response not achieved within 2 weeks, increase rapidly to max. 2.5 mg/kg twice daily; initial dose of 2.5 mg/kg twice daily if very severe

> **Severe psoriasis where conventional therapy ineffective or inappropriate**
> - By mouth, administered in accordance with expert advice
>
>   Child 1 month–18 years initially 1.25 mg/kg twice daily, increased gradually to max. 2.5 mg/kg twice daily if no improvement within 1 month (discontinue if response still insufficient after 6 weeks); initial dose of 2.5 mg/kg twice daily justified if condition requires rapid improvement
>
> Important For preparations and counselling and for advice on conversion between the preparations, see section 8.2.2

> **Refractory ulcerative colitis** section 1.5.3

> **Transplantation and graft-versus-host disease** section 8.2.2

◢Preparations
Section 8.2.2

METHOTREXATE

Cautions see section 8.1.3, also photosensitivity—psoriasis lesions aggravated by UV radiation (skin ulceration reported)

Contra-indications section 8.1.3

Hepatic impairment avoid—dose-related toxicity

Renal impairment section 8.1.3

Pregnancy section 8.1.3

Breast-feeding section 8.1.3

Side-effects section 8.1.3

Licensed use not licensed for use in children with psoriasis

Indication and dose

> **Severe uncontrolled psoriasis unresponsive to conventional therapy (specialist use only)**
> - By mouth
>
>   Child 2–18 years initially 200 micrograms/kg (max. 10 mg) once **weekly** increased according to response to 400 micrograms/kg (max. 25 mg) once **weekly**

> Safe Practice Note that the above dose is a **weekly** dose. To avoid error with low-dose methotrexate, it is recommended that:
> - the child or their carer is carefully advised of the **dose** and **frequency** and the reason for taking methotrexate and any other prescribed medicine (e.g. folic acid);
> - only one strength of methotrexate tablet (usually 2.5 mg) is prescribed and dispensed;
> - the prescription and the dispensing label clearly show the dose and frequency of methotrexate administration;
> - the child or their carer is warned to report immediately the onset of any feature of blood disorders (e.g. sore throat, bruising, and mouth ulcers), liver toxicity (e.g. nausea, vomiting, abdominal discomfort, and dark urine), and respiratory effects (e.g. shortness of breath).

> **Malignant disease** section 8.1.3

> **Rheumatoid arthritis** section 10.1.3

> **Severe Crohn's disease** section 1.5.3

◢Preparations
Section 10.1.3

13

Skin

PIMECROLIMUS

Cautions UV light (avoid excessive exposure to sunlight and sunlamps), avoid other topical treatments except emollients at treatment site; alcohol consumption (risk of facial flushing and skin irritation)

Contra-indications contact with eyes and mucous membranes, application under occlusion, infection at treatment site; congenital epidermal barrier defects; generalised erythroderma; immunodeficiency; concomitant use with drugs that cause immunosuppression (may be prescribed in exceptional circumstances by specialists); application to malignant or potentially malignant skin lesions

Side-effects burning sensation, pruritus, erythema, skin infections (including folliculitis and *less commonly* impetigo, herpes simplex and zoster, molluscum contagiosum); *rarely* papilloma, skin

discoloration, local reactions including pain, paraesthesia, peeling, dryness, oedema, and worsening of eczema; skin malignancy reported

Indication and dose

> Short-term treatment of mild to moderate atopic eczema (including flares) when topical corticosteroids cannot be used; see also notes above
>
> > **Child 2–18 years** apply twice daily until symptoms resolve (stop treatment if eczema worsens or no response after 6 weeks)

Elidel® (Novartis) PoM
Cream, pimecrolimus 1%, net price 30 g = £19.69, 60 g = £37.41, 100 g = £59.07. Label: 4, 28
Excipients include benzyl alcohol, cetyl alcohol, propylene glycol, stearyl alcohol

TACROLIMUS

Cautions infection at treatment site, UV light (avoid excessive exposure to sunlight and sunlamps); alcohol consumption (risk of facial flushing and skin irritation)

Contra-indications hypersensitivity to macrolides; congenital epidermal barrier defects; generalised erythroderma; immunodeficiency; concomitant use with drugs that cause immunosuppression (may be prescribed in exceptional circumstances by specialists); application to malignant or potentially malignant skin lesions; application under occlusion; avoid contact with eyes and mucous membranes

Pregnancy manufacturer advises avoid unless essential; toxicity in *animal* studies following systemic administration

Breast-feeding manufacturer advises avoid—present in milk following systemic administration

Side-effects application-site reactions including rash, irritation, pain, and paraesthesia; herpes simplex infection, Kaposi's varicelliform eruption; application-site infections (with preventative therapy); *less commonly* acne; rosacea, and skin malignancy also reported

Indication and dose

> Short-term treatment of moderate to severe atopic eczema (including flares) either unresponsive to, or in children intolerant of conventional therapy; see also notes above
>
> > **Child 2–16 years** initially apply 0.03% ointment thinly twice daily for up to 3 weeks (consider other treatment if eczema worsens or if no

improvement after 2 weeks) then reduce to once daily until lesion clears

> > **Child 16–18 years** initially apply 0.1% ointment thinly twice daily until lesion clears (consider other treatment if eczema worsens or if no improvement after 2 weeks); reduce to once daily or switch to 0.03% ointment if clinical condition allows

> Prevention of flares in children with moderate to severe atopic eczema and 4 or more flares a year, who have responded to initial treatment with topical tacrolimus
>
> > **Child 2–16 years** apply 0.03% ointment thinly twice weekly (with an interval of 2–3 days between applications); use short-term treatment regimen during an acute flare; interrupt preventative therapy after 1 year to reassess condition

> > **Child 16–18 years** apply 0.1% ointment thinly twice weekly (with an interval of 2–3 days between applications); use short-term treatment regimen during an acute flare; review need for preventative therapy after 1 year

Other indications section 8.2.2

Protopic® (Astellas) PoM
Ointment, tacrolimus (as monohydrate) 0.03%, net price 30 g = £19.44, 60 g = £36.94; 0.1%, 30 g = £21.60, 60 g = £41.04. Label: 4, 11, 28
Excipients include beeswax

Cytokine modulators

ETANERCEPT

Cautions section 10.1.3; monitor for non-melanoma skin cancer before and during treatment

Contra-indications section 10.1.3
Hepatic impairment section 10.1.3
Pregnancy section 10.1.3

Breast-feeding section 10.1.3
Side-effects section 10.1.3

13 Skin

◻ **ETANERCEPT** (*continued*)

Indication and dose

Severe plaque psoriasis
- **By subcutaneous injection**

  Child 8–18 years 800 micrograms/kg (max. 50 mg) once weekly; max. treatment duration 24 weeks; discontinue if no response after 12 weeks

Polyarticular-course juvenile idiopathic arthritis

section 10.1.3

◢**Preparations**
Section 10.1.3

13.6 Acne and rosacea

13.6.1 Topical preparations for acne
13.6.2 Oral preparations for acne

Acne vulgaris   Acne vulgaris commonly affects children around puberty and occasionally affects infants. Treatment of acne should be commenced early to prevent scarring; lesions may worsen before improving. The choice of treatment depends on age, severity, and whether the acne is predominantly inflammatory or comedonal.

Mild to moderate acne is generally treated with topical preparations, such as benzoyl peroxide, azelaic acid, and retinoids, (section 13.6.1).

For *moderate to severe inflammatory acne* or where topical preparations are not tolerated or are ineffective or where application to the site is difficult, systemic treatment (section 13.6.2) with oral antibacterials may be effective. **Co-cyprindiol** (cyproterone acetate with ethinylestradiol) has anti-androgenic properties and may be useful in young women with acne refractory to other treatments.

Severe acne, acne unresponsive to prolonged courses of oral antibacterials, acne with scarring, or acne associated with psychological problems calls for early referral to a consultant dermatologist who may prescribe oral **isotretinoin** (section 13.6.2).

Neonatal and infantile acne   Inflammatory papules, pustules, and occasionally comedones may develop at birth or within the first month; most neonates with acne do not require treatment. Acne developing at 3–6 months of age may be more severe and persistent; lesions are usually confined to the face. Topical preparations containing benzoyl peroxide (at the lowest strength possible to avoid irritation), azelaic acid, adapalene, or tretinoin may be used if treatment for infantile acne is necessary. In infants with inflammatory acne, oral **erythromycin** (section 5.1.5) is used because topical preparations for acne are not well tolerated. In cases of erythromycin-resistant acne, oral isotretinoin (section 13.6.2) can be given on the advice of a consultant dermatologist.

Rosacea   The adult form of rosacea rarely occurs in children. Persistent or repeated use of potent topical corticosteroids may cause periorificial rosacea (steroid acne). The pustules and papules of rosacea may be treated for at least 6 weeks with a topical **metronidazole** preparation (section 13.10.1.2), or a systemic antibacterial such as **erythromycin** (section 5.1.5), or for a child over 12 years, **oxytetracycline** (section 5.1.3). Tetracyclines are **contra-indicated** in children under 12 years of age.

13.6.1 Topical preparations for acne

In mild to moderate acne, comedones and inflamed lesions respond well to benzoyl peroxide (see below) or topical retinoids (see p. 703). Alternatively, topical application of an antibacterial such as erythromycin or clindamycin may be effective for inflammatory acne. However, topical antibacterials are probably no more effective than benzoyl peroxide and may promote the emergence of resistant organisms. If topical preparations prove inadequate oral preparations may be needed (section 13.6.2). The choice of product and formulation (gel, solution, lotion, or cream) is largely determined by skin type, patient preference, and previous usage of acne products.

13

Skin

Benzoyl peroxide and azelaic acid

Benzoyl peroxide is effective in mild to moderate acne. Both comedones and inflamed lesions respond well to benzoyl peroxide. The lower concentrations seem to be as effective as higher concentrations in reducing inflammation. It is usual to start with a lower strength and to increase the concentration of benzoyl peroxide gradually. Adverse effects include local skin irritation, particularly when therapy is initiated, but the scaling and redness often subside with a reduction in benzoyl peroxide concentration, frequency, and area of application. If the acne does not respond after 2 months then use of a topical antibacterial should be considered.

Azelaic acid has antimicrobial and anticomedonal properties. It may be used as an alternative to benzoyl peroxide or to a topical retinoid for treating mild to moderate comedonal acne, particularly of the face; azelaic acid is less likely to cause local irritation than benzoyl peroxide.

BENZOYL PEROXIDE

Cautions avoid contact with eyes, mouth, and mucous membranes; may bleach fabrics and hair; avoid excessive exposure to sunlight

Side-effects skin irritation (reduce frequency or suspend use until irritation subsides and re-introduce at reduced frequency)

Licensed use *Quinoderm*® is licensed for use in children; *all other preparations*, not licensed for use in treatment of infantile acne

Indication and dose

> **Acne vulgaris**
>
> > **Child 12–18 years** apply 1–2 times daily preferably after washing with soap and water, start treatment with lower-strength preparations
> > **Note** May bleach clothing

> **Infantile acne**
>
> > **Neonate** apply 1–2 times daily; start treatment with lower-strength preparations
> >
> > **Child 1 month–2 years** apply 1–2 times daily; start treatment with lower-strength preparations

Acnecide® (Galderma)
Gel, benzoyl peroxide 5% in an aqueous gel basis, net price 60 g = £4.17
Excipients include propylene glycol

Brevoxyl® (Stiefel)
Cream, benzoyl peroxide 4% in an aqueous basis, net price 40 g = £3.30
Excipients include cetyl alcohol, fragrance, stearyl alcohol

PanOxyl® (Stiefel)
Aquagel (= aqueous gel), benzoyl peroxide 2.5%, net price 40 g = £1.76; 5%, 40 g = £1.92; 10%, 40 g = £2.13
Excipients include propylene glycol

Cream, benzoyl peroxide 5% in a non-greasy basis, net price 40 g = £1.89
Excipients include isopropyl palmitate, propylene glycol

Gel, benzoyl peroxide 5% in an aqueous alcoholic basis, net price 40 g = £1.51; 10%, 40 g = £1.69
Excipients include fragrance

Wash, benzoyl peroxide 10% in a detergent basis, net price 150 mL = £4.00
Excipients include imidurea

◢**With antimicrobials**

Duac® **Once Daily** (Stiefel) [PoM]
Gel, benzoyl peroxide 5%, clindamycin 1% (as phosphate) in an aqueous basis, net price 25 g = £9.95, 50 g = £19.90
Excipients include disodium edetate

Dose
> **Acne vulgaris**
> > **Child 12–18 years** apply once daily in the evening

Quinoderm® (Ferndale)
Cream, benzoyl peroxide 5%, potassium hydroxyquinoline sulphate 0.5%, in an astringent vanishing-cream basis, net price 50 g = £2.21
Excipients include cetostearyl alcohol, edetic acid (EDTA)

Cream, benzoyl peroxide 10%, potassium hydroxyquinoline sulphate 0.5%, in an astringent vanishing-cream basis, net price 25 g = £1.30, 50 g = £2.49
Excipients include cetostearyl alcohol, edetic acid (EDTA)

Dose
> **Infantile acne, acne vulgaris, acneform eruptions, impetigo, folliculitis**
> > Apply 2–3 times daily

AZELAIC ACID

Cautions avoid contact with eyes, mouth, and mucous membranes

Side-effects local irritation (reduce frequency or discontinue temporarily); *less commonly* skin discoloration; *very rarely* photosensitisation

Licensed use not licensed for use in infantile acne

Indication and dose

> See under preparations

Finacea® (Meda) [PoM]
Gel, azelaic acid 15%, net price 30 g = £7.48
Excipients include disodium edetate, polysorbate 80, propylene glycol

Dose
> **Facial acne vulgaris**
> > **Child 12–18 years** apply twice daily; discontinue if no improvement after 1 month

13 Skin

◻ **AZELAIC ACID (continued)**

Skinoren® (Meda) [PoM]
  Cream, azelaic acid 20%, net price 30 g = £3.74
  Excipients include propylene glycol

Dose
  Acne vulgaris, infantile acne
    Apply twice daily (sensitive skin, once daily for first week). Extended treatment may be required but manufacturer advises period of treatment should not exceed 6 months

Topical antibacterials for acne

In the treatment of mild to moderate inflammatory acne, topical antibacterials may be no more effective than topical benzoyl peroxide or tretinoin. Topical antibacterials are probably best reserved for children who wish to avoid oral antibacterials or who cannot tolerate them.

Topical preparations of **erythromycin** and **clindamycin** may be used to treat *inflamed lesions* in mild to moderate acne when topical benzoyl peroxide or tretinoin is ineffective or poorly tolerated. Topical benzoyl peroxide, azelaic acid, or retinoids used in combination with an antibacterial (topical or systemic) may be more effective than an antibacterial used alone. Topical antibacterials can produce mild irritation of the skin, and on rare occasions cause sensitisation.

Antibacterial resistance of *Propionibacterium acnes* is increasing; there is cross-resistance between erythromycin and clindamycin. To avoid development of resistance:

- when possible use non-antibiotic antimicrobials (such as benzoyl peroxide or azelaic acid);
- avoid concomitant treatment with different oral and topical antibacterials;
- if a particular antibacterial is effective, use it for repeat courses if needed (short intervening courses of benzoyl peroxide or azelaic acid may eliminate any resistant propionibacteria);
- do not continue treatment for longer than necessary (but treatment with a topical preparation should be continued for at least 6 months).

ANTIBACTERIALS

Cautions some manufacturers advise preparations containing alcohol are not suitable for use with benzoyl peroxide

Indication and dose
  Acne vulgaris for dose, see under preparations

Dalacin T® (Pharmacia) [PoM]
  Topical solution, clindamycin 1% (as phosphate), in an aqueous alcoholic basis, net price (both with applicator) 30 mL = £4.34, 50 mL = £7.23
  Excipients include propylene glycol

Dose
  Apply twice daily

  Lotion, clindamycin 1% (as phosphate) in an aqueous basis, net price 30 mL = £5.08, 50 mL = £8.47
  Excipients include cetostearyl alcohol, hydroxybenzoates (parabens)

Dose
  Apply twice daily

Stiemycin® (Stiefel) [PoM]
  Solution, erythromycin 2% in an alcoholic basis, net price 50 mL = £7.69
  Excipients include propylene glycol

Dose
  Apply twice daily

Zindaclin® (Crawford) [PoM]
  Gel, clindamycin 1% (as phosphate), net price 30 g = £8.66
  Excipients include propylene glycol

Dose
  Child 12–18 years apply once daily

Zineryt® (Astellas) [PoM]
  Topical solution, powder for reconstitution, erythromycin 40 mg, zinc acetate 12 mg/mL when reconstituted with solvent containing ethanol, net price per pack of powder and solvent to provide 30 mL = £7.71, 90 mL = £22.24
  Excipients none as listed in section 13.1.3

Dose
  Apply twice daily

Topical retinoids and related preparations for acne

Topical **tretinoin** and its isomer **isotretinoin** are useful for treating comedones and inflammatory lesions in mild to moderate acne. Patients should be warned that some redness and skin peeling may occur initially but settles with time. Several months of treatment may be needed to achieve an optimal response and the treatment should be continued until no new lesions develop.

13 Skin

Tretinoin is used under specialist supervision to treat infantile acne, see Neonatal and Infantile Acne, p. 701.

Adapalene, a retinoid-like drug, is used for mild to moderate acne vulgaris and may also be used to treat infantile acne. It is less irritant than topical retinoids.

Cautions Topical retinoids should be avoided in severe acne involving large areas. Contact with eyes, nostrils, mouth and mucous membranes, eczematous, broken or sunburned skin should be avoided. Topical retinoids should be used with caution on sensitive areas such as the neck, and accumulation in angles of the nose should be avoided. Exposure to UV light (including sunlight, solariums) should be avoided; if sun exposure is unavoidable, an appropriate sunscreen (section 13.8.1) or protective clothing should be used. Use of retinoids with abrasive cleaners, comedogenic or astringent cosmetics should be avoided. Allow peeling (e.g. resulting from use of benzoyl peroxide) to subside before using a topical retinoid; alternating a preparation that causes peeling with a topical retinoid may give rise to contact dermatitis (reduce frequency of retinoid application).

Pregnancy Topical retinoids are contra-indicated in pregnancy; females of child-bearing age must use effective contraception (oral progestogen-only contraceptives not considered effective).

Side-effects Local reactions include burning, erythema, stinging, pruritus, dry or peeling skin (discontinue if severe). Increased sensitivity to UVB light or sunlight occurs. Temporary changes of skin pigmentation have been reported. Eye irritation and oedema, and blistering or crusting of skin have been reported rarely.

ADAPALENE

Cautions see notes above

Pregnancy see notes above

Breast-feeding amount of drug in breast milk probably too small to be harmful; avoid application to mother's chest; ensure infant does not come in contact with treated areas

Side-effects see notes above

Licensed use not licensed for use in infantile acne

Indication and dose

Infantile acne

Neonate apply thinly once daily at night

Child 1 month–2 years apply thinly once daily at night

Mild to moderate acne vulgaris

Apply thinly once daily before retiring

Differin® (Galderma) [PoM]
Cream, adapalene 0.1%, net price 45 g = £11.40.
Label: 11
Excipients include disodium edetate, hydroxybenzoates (parabens)

Gel, adapalene 0.1%, net price 45 g = £11.40.
Label: 11
Excipients include disodium edetate, hydroxybenzoates (parabens), propylene glycol

ISOTRETINOIN

Note Isotretinoin is an isomer of tretinoin
Important For prescribing information on isotretinoin when given by mouth, see p. 707

Cautions (*topical application* only) see notes above; also personal or familial history of cutaneous epithelioma

Contra-indications (*topical application* only) rosacea; perioral dermatitis

Pregnancy (*topical application* only) see notes above

Breast-feeding avoid

Side-effects (*topical application* only) see notes above

Indication and dose

Acne vulgaris

Apply thinly 1–2 times daily

Isotrex® (Stiefel) [PoM]
Gel, isotretinoin 0.05%, net price 30 g = £5.94.
Label: 11
Excipients include butylated hydroxytoluene

◢With antibacterial
Isotrexin® (Stiefel) [PoM]
Gel, isotretinoin 0.05%, erythromycin 2% in ethanolic basis, net price 30 g = £7.47. Label: 11
Excipients include butylated hydroxytoluene

TRETINOIN

Note Tretinoin is the acid form of vitamin A
Cautions see notes above

Contra-indications personal or familial history of cutaneous epithelioma; rosacea; perioral dermatitis

13 Skin

◁ TRETINOIN (*continued*)

Pregnancy see notes above

Breast-feeding amount of drug in milk after topical application probably too small to be harmful; ensure infant does not come into contact with treated areas

Side-effects see notes above

Licensed use *Retin-A*® not licensed for use in infantile acne

Indication and dose

See under preparations

Malignant disease section 8.1.5

Retin-A® (Janssen-Cilag) [PoM]
Gel, tretinoin 0.01%, net price 60 g = £5.39; 0.025%, 60 g = £5.39. Label: 11
Excipients include butylated hydroxytoluene

Dose

Infantile acne
Apply 0.01% gel thinly 1–2 times daily; increase to 0.025% gel if necessary

Acne vulgaris, particularly that associated with oily skin
Apply thinly 1–2 times daily

◢With antibacterial

Aknemycin Plus® (Almirall) [PoM]
Solution, tretinoin 0.025%, erythromycin 4% in an alcoholic basis, net price 25 mL = £7.05. Label: 11
Excipients none as listed in section 13.1.3

Dose

Acne (all forms), particularly that associated with oily skin
Apply thinly 1–2 times daily

Other topical preparations for acne

Salicylic acid is available in various preparations for sale direct to the public for the treatment of mild acne. Other products are more suitable for acne; salicylic acid is used mainly for its keratolytic effect.

Preparations containing **sulphur** and **abrasive agents** are not considered beneficial in acne.

Topical **corticosteroids** should **not** be used in acne.

A topical preparation of **nicotinamide** is available for inflammatory acne.

◢ NICOTINAMIDE

Cautions avoid contact with eyes and mucous membranes (including nose and mouth); reduce frequency of application if excessive dryness, irritation or peeling

Side-effects dryness of skin; also pruritus, erythema, burning and irritation

Licensed use licensed for use in children (age range not specified by manufacturer)

Indication and dose

Inflammatory acne vulgaris see under preparations below

Nicam® (Dermal)
Gel, nicotinamide 4%, net price 60 g = £7.20
Excipients none as listed in section 13.1.3

Dose

Apply twice daily; reduce to once daily or on alternate days if irritation occurs

---

◢ SALICYLIC ACID

Cautions risk of significant systemic absorption in neonates; avoid contact with mouth, eyes, mucous membranes; systemic effects after excessive use

Salicylate toxicity Salicylate toxicity can occur particularly if applied on large areas of skin or on neonatal skin

Side-effects local irritation

Licensed use licensed for use in children (age range not specified by manufacturer)

Indication and dose

Acne vulgaris see under preparation

Psoriasis section 13.5.2

Warts and calluses section 13.7

Fungal nail infections section 13.10.2

Acnisal® (Alliance)
Topical solution, salicylic acid 2% in a detergent and emollient basis, net price 177 mL = £3.39.
Excipients include benzyl alcohol

Dose

Apply up to 3 times daily

13

Skin

13.6.2 Oral preparations for acne

Oral antibacterials for acne

Oral antibacterials may be used in *moderate to severe inflammatory acne* when topical treatment is not adequately effective or is inappropriate. Concomitant anticomedonal treatment with topical benzoyl peroxide or azelaic acid may also be required (section 13.6.1).

Tetracyclines should not be given to children under 12 years. In children over 12 years, either **oxytetracycline** or **tetracycline** (section 5.1.3) is usually given for acne in a dose of 500 mg twice daily. If there is no improvement after the first 3 months another oral antibacterial should be used. Maximum improvement usually occurs after 4 to 6 months but in more severe cases treatment may need to be continued for 2 years or longer.

Doxycycline and **lymecycline** (section 5.1.3) are alternatives to tetracycline in children over 12 years. Doxycycline can be used in a dose of 100 mg daily. Lymecycline is given in a dose of 408 mg daily.

Although **minocycline** is as effective as other tetracyclines for acne, it is associated with a greater risk of lupus erythematosus-like syndrome. Minocycline sometimes causes irreversible pigmentation; it is given in a dose of 100 mg once daily or 50 mg twice daily.

Erythromycin (section 5.1.5) in a dose of 500 mg twice daily for children over 12 years is an alternative for the management of moderate to severe acne with inflamed lesions, but propionibacteria strains resistant to erythromycin are becoming widespread and this may explain poor response. Infants with acne requiring oral treatment with erythromycin should be given 250 mg once daily *or* 125 mg twice daily; in cases of erythromycin-resistant *P. acnes* in infants, oral isotretinoin may be used on the advice of a consultant dermatologist.

Concomitant use of different topical and systemic antibacterials is undesirable owing to the increased likelihood of the development of bacterial resistance.

Hormone treatment for acne

Co-cyprindiol (cyproterone acetate with ethinylestradiol) contains an anti-androgen. It is no more effective than an oral broad-spectrum antibacterial but is useful in females of childbearing age who also wish to receive oral contraception.

Improvement of acne with co-cyprindiol probably occurs because of decreased sebum secretion which is under androgen control. Some females with moderately severe hirsutism may also benefit because hair growth is also androgen-dependent. Contra-indications of co-cyprindiol include pregnancy and a predisposition to thrombosis.

> **CSM advice**
> Venous thromboembolism occurs more frequently in women taking co-cyprindiol than those taking a low-dose combined oral contraceptive. The CSM has reminded prescribers that co-cyprindiol is licensed for use in women with severe acne which has not responded to oral antibacterials and for moderately severe hirsutism; it should not be used solely for contraception. It is contra-indicated in those with a personal or close family history of venous thromboembolism. Women with severe acne or hirsutism may have an inherently increased risk of cardiovascular disease.

13 Skin

CO-CYPRINDIOL

A mixture of cyproterone acetate and ethinylestradiol in the mass proportions 2000 parts to 35 parts, respectively

Cautions see under Combined Hormonal Contraceptives, section 7.3.1

Contra-indications see under Combined Hormonal Contraceptives, section 7.3.1

Hepatic impairment see under Combined Hormonal Contraceptives, section 7.3.1

Pregnancy avoid—risk of feminisation of male fetus with cyproterone

Breast-feeding manufacturer advises avoid; possibility of anti-androgen effects in neonate with cyproterone

Side-effects see under Combined Hormonal Contraceptives, section 7.3.1

Licensed use licensed for use in females of childbearing age

◁ CO-CYPRINDIOL (*continued*)

Indication and dose

Severe acne in females of childbearing age refractory to prolonged oral antibacterial therapy (but see notes above), moderately severe hirsutism

- By mouth

  1 Tablet daily for 21 days starting on day 1 of menstrual cycle and repeated after a 7-day interval, usually for several months; withdraw 3–4 months after acne or hirsutism completely resolved (repeat courses may be given if recurrence); long-term treatment may be necessary for severe symptoms

Co-cyprindiol (Non-proprietary) PoM
Tablets, co-cyprindiol 2000/35 (cyproterone acetate 2 mg, ethinylestradiol 35 micrograms), net price 63-tab pack = £3.95
Brands include *Acnocin®, Cicafem®, Clairette®*

Dianette® (Bayer Schering) PoM
Tablets, beige, s/c, co-cyprindiol 2000/35 (cyproterone acetate 2 mg, ethinylestradiol 35 micrograms), net price 21-tab pack = £2.92

Oral retinoid for acne

The retinoid **isotretinoin** reduces sebum secretion. It is used for the systemic treatment of nodulo-cystic and conglobate acne, severe acne, acne with scarring, or for acne which has not responded to an adequate course of a systemic antibacterial. Isotretinoin is used for the treatment of severe infantile acne resistant to erythromycin.

Isotretinoin is a toxic drug that should be prescribed **only** by, or under the supervision of, a consultant dermatologist. It is given for at least 16 weeks; repeat courses are not normally required.

Side-effects of isotretinoin include severe dryness of the skin and mucous membranes, nose bleeds, and joint pains. The drug is **teratogenic** and must **not** be given to females of child-bearing age unless they practise effective contraception (oral progestogen-only contraceptives not considered effective) and then only after detailed assessment and explanation by the physician. They must also be registered with a pregnancy prevention programme (see under Cautions below).

Although a causal link between isotretinoin use and psychiatric changes (including suicidal ideation) has not been established, the possibility should be considered before initiating treatment; if psychiatric changes occur during treatment, isotretinoin should be stopped, the prescriber informed, and specialist psychiatric advice should be sought.

ISOTRETINOIN

Note Isotretinoin is an isomer of tretinoin

Cautions avoid blood donation during treatment and for at least 1 month after treatment; history of depression—monitor all patients for depression; measure hepatic function and serum lipids before treatment, 1 month after starting and then every 3 months (reduce dose or discontinue if transaminase or serum lipids persistently raised); discontinue if uncontrolled hypertriglyceridaemia or pancreatitis; diabetes; dry eye syndrome (associated with risk of keratitis); avoid keratolytics; interactions: Appendix 1 (retinoids)

Pregnancy prevention In women of child-bearing potential, exclude pregnancy up to 3 days before treatment (start treatment on day 2 or 3 of menstrual cycle), every month during treatment (unless there are compelling reasons to indicate that there is no risk of pregnancy), and 5 weeks after stopping treatment—perform pregnancy test in the first 3 days of the menstrual cycle. Women must practise effective contraception for at least 1 month before starting treatment, during treatment, and for at least 1 month after stopping treatment. Women should be advised to use at least 1 method of contraception, but ideally they should use 2 methods of contraception. Oral progestogen-only contraceptives are not considered effective. Barrier methods should not be used alone, but can be used in conjunction with other contraceptive methods. Each prescription for isotretinoin should be limited to a supply of up to 30 days' treatment and

dispensed within 7 days of the date stated on the prescription. Women should be advised to discontinue treatment and to seek prompt medical attention if they become pregnant during treatment or within 1 month of stopping treatment.

Counselling Warn patient to avoid wax epilation (risk of epidermal stripping), dermabrasion, and laser skin treatments (risk of scarring) during treatment and for at least 6 months after stopping; patient should avoid exposure to UV light (including sunlight) and use sunscreen and emollient (including lip balm) preparations from the start of treatment

Contra-indications hypervitaminosis A, hyperlipidaemia

Hepatic impairment avoid—further impairment may occur

Renal impairment in severe impairment, reduce initial dose and increase gradually, if necessary, up to 1 mg/kg daily as tolerated

Pregnancy avoid—teratogenic; effective contraception must be used—see Pregnancy Prevention above

Breast-feeding avoid

Side-effects dryness of skin (with dermatitis, scaling, thinning, erythema, pruritus), epidermal fragility (trauma may cause blistering), dryness of lips (sometimes cheilitis), dryness of eyes (with

◻ **ISOTRETINOIN** (*continued*)

blepharitis and conjunctivitis), dryness of pharyngeal mucosa (with hoarseness), dryness of nasal mucosa (with epistaxis), headache, myalgia and arthralgia, raised plasma concentration of triglycerides, of glucose, of serum transaminases, and of cholesterol (risk of pancreatitis if triglycerides above 9 mmol/litre), haematuria and proteinuria, thrombocytopenia, thrombocytosis, neutropenia and anaemia; *rarely* mood changes (depression, suicidal ideation, aggressive behaviour, anxiety)—expert referral required, exacerbation of acne, acne fulminans, allergic skin reactions, and hypersensitivity, alopecia; *very rarely* nausea, inflammatory bowel disease, diarrhoea (discontinue if severe) benign intracranial hypertension (avoid concomitant tetracyclines) convulsions, malaise, drowsiness, dizziness, lymphadenopathy, increased sweating, hyperuricaemia, raised serum creatinine concentration and glomerulonephritis, hepatitis, tendinitis, bone changes (including reduced bone density, early epiphyseal closure, and skeletal hyperstosis following long-term administration), visual disturbances (papilloedema, corneal opacities, cataracts, decreased night vision, photophobia, blurred vision, colour blindness)—expert referral required and consider withdrawal, decreased tolerance to contact lenses and keratitis, impaired hearing, Gram-positive infections of skin and mucous membranes, allergic vasculitis and granulomatous lesions, paronychia, hirsutism, nail dystrophy, skin hyperpigmentation, photosensitivity

Indication and dose

> **Acne vulgaris** under supervision of consultant dermatologist, see notes above
>
> • **By mouth**
>
>> **Child 12–18 years** 500 micrograms/kg once daily increased if necessary to 1 mg/kg (in 1–2 divided doses) for 16–24 weeks (repeat treatment course after a period of at least 8 weeks if failure or relapse after first course); max. cumulative dose 150 mg/kg per course

> **Severe infantile acne** under supervision of a consultant dermatologist, see p. 701
>
> • **By mouth**
>
>> **Child 1 month–2 years** 200 micrograms/kg once daily increased if necessary to 1 mg/kg daily (in 1–2 divided doses) for 16–24 weeks; max. cumulative dose 150 mg/kg per course

Isotretinoin (Non-proprietary) ℗ℴℳ
Capsules, isotretinoin 5 mg, net price 56-cap pack = £14.99; 20 mg, 56-cap pack = £39.99. Label: 10, patient information leaflet, 11, 21

Roaccutane® (Roche) ℗ℴℳ
Capsules, isotretinoin 10 mg (brown-red), net price 30-cap pack = £17.46; 20 mg (brown-red/white), 30-cap pack = £24.04. Label: 10, patient information card, 11, 21

◢Extemporaneous formulations available see Extemporaneous Preparations, p. 8

13.7 Preparations for warts and calluses

Warts (verruca vulgaris) are common, benign, self-limiting, and usually asymptomatic. They are caused by a human papillomavirus, which most frequently affects the hands, feet (plantar warts), and the anogenital region (see below); treatment usually relies on local tissue destruction and is required only if the warts are painful, unsightly, persistent, or cause distress. In immunocompromised children, warts may be more difficult to eradicate.

Preparations of **salicylic acid, formaldehyde, gluteraldehyde** or **silver nitrate** are used for the removal of warts on hands and feet. **Salicylic acid** is a useful keratolytic which may be considered first-line in the treatment of warts; it is also suitable for the removal of *corns and calluses*. Preparations of salicylic acid in a collodion basis are available but some children may develop an allergy to colophony in the formulation; collodion should be avoided in children allergic to elastic adhesive plaster. An ointment combining **salicylic acid** with **podophyllum resin** (*Posalfilin®*) is available for treating plantar warts; severe systemic toxicity including gastro-intestinal, renal, haematological, and CNS effects may occur with excessive application of preparations containing podophyllin. Cryotherapy causes pain, swelling, and blistering and may be no more effective than topical salicylic acid in the treatment of warts.

◢ **SALICYLIC ACID**

Cautions significant peripheral neuropathy, patients with diabetes at risk of neuropathic ulcers; protect surrounding skin and avoid broken skin; not suitable for application to face, anogenital region, or large areas

Side-effects skin irritation, see notes above

Licensed use not licensed for use in children under 2 years

Indication and dose

> **Warts on hands and feet (plantar)**
>
> For dose see preparations; apply carefully to wart and protect surrounding skin (e.g. with soft paraffin or specially designed plaster); rub wart surface gently with file or pumice stone once weekly; treatment may need to be continued for up to 3 months

▱ **SALICYLIC ACID** (*continued*)

Psoriasis section 13.5.2

Acne section 13.6.1

Fungal nail infections section 13.10.2

Cuplex® (Crawford)
Gel, salicylic acid 11%, lactic acid 4%, in a collodion basis, net price 5 g = £2.23. Label: 15

Dose

Apply twice daily

Note Contains colophony (see notes above)

Duofilm® (Stiefel)
Paint, salicylic acid 16.7%, lactic acid 16.7%, in flexible collodion, net price 15 mL (with applicator) = £2.25. Label: 15

Dose

Apply daily

Occlusal® (Alliance)
Cutaneous solution, salicylic acid 26% in polyacrylic solution, net price 10 mL (with applicator) = £3.56. Label: 15

Dose

Apply daily

Salactol® (Dermal)
Paint, salicylic acid 16.7%, lactic acid 16.7%, in flexible collodion, net price 10 mL (with applicator) = £1.74. Label: 15

Dose

Apply daily

Note Contains colophony (see notes above)

Salatac® (Dermal)
Gel, salicylic acid 12%, lactic acid 4% in a collodion basis, net price 8 g (with applicator) = £3.03. Label: 15

Dose

Apply daily

Verrugon® (Ransom)
Ointment, salicylic acid 50% in a paraffin basis, net price 6 g = £3.00

Dose

Apply daily

◢**With podophyllum**

Posalfilin® (Norgine)
Ointment, podophyllum resin 20%, salicylic acid 25%, net price 10 g = £3.37

Dose

Plantar warts

Apply daily

Note Owing to the salicylic acid content, not suitable for anogenital warts; owing to the podophyllum content also contra-indicated in pregnancy and breast-feeding

▰ **FORMALDEHYDE**

Cautions see under Salicylic Acid
Side-effects see under Salicylic Acid
Licensed use licensed for use in children (age range not specified by manufacturer)

Indication and dose

Warts, particularly plantar warts for dose see preparation below

Veracur® (Typharm)
Gel, formaldehyde 0.75% in a water-miscible gel basis, net price 15 g = £2.41.

Dose

Apply twice daily

▰ **GLUTARALDEHYDE**

Cautions protect surrounding skin; not for application to face, mucosa, or anogenital areas
Side-effects rashes, skin irritation (discontinue if severe); stains skin brown
Licensed use licensed for use in children (age range not specified by manufacturer)

Indication and dose

Warts, particularly plantar warts

Apply twice daily

Glutarol® (Dermal)
Solution (= application), glutaraldehyde 10%, net price 10 mL (with applicator) = £2.10

▰ **SILVER NITRATE**

Cautions protect surrounding skin and avoid broken skin; not suitable for application to face, anogenital region, or large areas
Side-effects chemical burns on surrounding skin; stains skin and fabric
Licensed use no age range specified by manufacturer

Indication and dose

Common warts and verrucas

Apply moistened caustic pencil tip for 1–2 minutes; repeat after 24 hours up to max. 3 applications for warts *or* max. 6 applications for verrucas

Instructions in proprietary packs generally incorporate advice to remove dead skin before use by gentle filing and to cover with adhesive dressing after application

13

Skin

◻ **SILVER NITRATE** (*continued*)

Umbilical granulomas

Apply moistened caustic pencil tip (usually containing silver nitrate 40%) for 1–2 minutes while protecting surrounding skin with soft paraffin

Silver nitrate (Non-proprietary)
Caustic pencil, tip containing silver nitrate 40%, potassium nitrate 60%, net price = 93p

AVOCA® (Bray)
Caustic pencil, tip containing silver nitrate 95%, potassium nitrate 5%, net price, treatment pack (including emery file, 6 adhesive dressings and protector pads) = £1.94.

Anogenital warts

Anogenital warts (condylomata acuminata) in children are often asymptomatic and require only a simple barrier preparation. If treatment is required it should be supervised by a hospital specialist. Persistent warts on genital skin may require treatment with cryotherapy or other forms of physical ablation under general anaesthesia.

Podophyllotoxin (the major active ingredient of podophyllum), or imiquimod are used to treat external anogenital warts; these preparations can cause considerable irritation of the treated area and are therefore suitable only for children who are able to cooperate with the treatment.

IMIQUIMOD

Cautions avoid normal or broken skin and open wounds; not suitable for internal genital warts; uncircumcised males (risk of phimosis or stricture of foreskin); autoimmune disease; immunosuppressed patients

Pregnancy no evidence of teratogenicity or toxicity in *animal* studies; manufacturer advises caution

Breast-feeding no information available

Side-effects local reactions (including itching, burning sensation, erythema, erosion, oedema, excoriation, and scabbing); headache; influenza-like symptoms; myalgia; *less commonly* local ulceration and alopecia; *rarely* Stevens-Johnson syndrome and cutaneous lupus erythematosus-like effect; *very rarely* dysuria in females; permanent hypopigmentation or hyperpigmentation reported

Licensed use not licensed for use in children

Indication and dose

External genital and perianal warts (for use under specialist supervision only)

Apply thinly 3 times a week at night until lesions resolve (max. 16 weeks)

Important Should be rubbed in and allowed to stay on the treated area for 6–10 hours then washed off with mild soap and water (uncircumcised males treating warts under foreskin should wash the area daily). The cream should be washed off before sexual contact

Aldara® (Meda) ℞
Cream, imiquimod 5%, net price 12-sachet pack = £51.32. Label: 10, patient information leaflet
Excipients include benzyl alcohol, cetyl alcohol, hydroxybenzoates (parabens), polysorbate 60, stearyl alcohol
Condoms may damage latex condoms and diaphragms

PODOPHYLLOTOXIN

Cautions see notes above; avoid normal skin and open wounds; keep away from face; very irritant to eyes

Pregnancy avoid

Breast-feeding avoid

Side-effects local irritation

Licensed use not licensed for use in children

Indication and dose

See under preparations (for use under specialist supervision only)

Condyline® (Ardern) ℞
Solution, podophyllotoxin 0.5% in alcoholic basis, net price 3.5 mL (with applicators) = £14.49.
Label: 15

Dose

Condylomata acuminata affecting the penis or the female external genitalia
Child 2–18 years (see notes above) apply twice daily for 3 consecutive days; treatment may be repeated at

weekly intervals if necessary for a total of five 3-day treatment courses; direct medical supervision for lesions in the female and for lesions greater than 4 cm² in the male; max. 50 single applications ('loops') per session (consult product literature)

Warticon® (Stiefel) ℞
Cream, podophyllotoxin 0.15%, net price 5 g (with mirror) = £14.86
Excipients include butylated hydroxyanisole, cetyl alcohol, hydroxybenzoates (parabens), sorbic acid, stearyl alcohol

Dose

Condylomata acuminata affecting the penis or the female external genitalia
Child 2–18 years (see notes above) apply twice daily for 3 consecutive days; treatment may be repeated at weekly intervals if necessary for a total of four 3-day treatment courses; direct medical supervision for lesions greater than 4 cm²

◁ **PODOPHYLLOTOXIN (continued)**

Solution, blue, podophyllotoxin 0.5% in alcoholic basis, net price 3 mL (with applicators) = £12.38. Label: 15

Dose

Condylomata acuminata affecting the penis or the female external genitalia

Child 2–18 years (see notes above) apply twice daily for 3 consecutive days; treatment may be repeated at weekly intervals if necessary for a total of four 3-day treatment courses; direct medical supervision for lesions greater than 4 cm²; max. 50 single applications ('loops') per session (consult product literature)

13.8 Sunscreens and camouflagers

13.8.1 Sunscreen preparations
13.8.2 Camouflagers

13.8.1 Sunscreen preparations

Solar ultraviolet irradiation can be harmful to the skin. It is responsible for disorders such as *polymorphic light eruption, solar urticaria,* and it provokes the various *cutaneous porphyrias.* It also provokes (or at least aggravates) skin lesions of *lupus erythematosus* and may aggravate some other *dermatoses.* Certain drugs, such as demeclocycline, phenothiazines, or amiodarone, can cause photosensitivity. All these conditions (as well as *sunburn*) may occur after relatively short periods of exposure to the sun. Solar ultraviolet irradiation may provoke attacks of recurrent herpes labialis (but it is not known whether the effect of sunlight exposure is local or systemic).

The effects of exposure over longer periods include *ageing changes* and more importantly the initiation of *skin cancer.*

Solar ultraviolet radiation is approximately 200–400 nm in wavelength. The medium wavelengths (290–320 nm, known as UVB) cause *sunburn.* The long wavelengths (320–400 nm, known as UVA) are responsible for many *photosensitivity reactions* and *photodermatoses.* Both UVA and UVB contribute to long-term *photodamage* and to the changes responsible for *skin cancer* and ageing.

Sunscreen preparations contain substances that protect the skin against UVA and UVB radiation, but they are no substitute for covering the skin and avoiding sunlight. Protective clothing and sun avoidance (rather than the use of sunscreen preparations) are recommended for children under 6 months of age.

The sun protection factor (SPF, usually indicated in the preparation title) provides guidance on the degree of protection offered against UVB; it indicates the multiples of protection provided against burning, compared with unprotected skin; for example, an SPF of 8 should enable a child to remain 8 times longer in the sun without burning. However, in practice users do not apply sufficient sunscreen product and the protection is lower than that found in experimental studies. Some manufacturers use a star rating system to indicate the protection against UVA relative to protection against UVB for sunscreen products. However, the usefulness of the star rating system remains controversial. The EU Commission (September 2006) has recommended that the UVA protection factor for a sunscreen should be at least one-third of the sun protection factor (SPF); products that achieve this requirement will be labelled with a UVA logo alongside the SPF classification. Preparations that also contain reflective substances, such as titanium dioxide, provide the most effective protection against UVA.

Sunscreen preparations may rarely cause allergic reactions.

> For optimum photoprotection, sunscreen preparations should be applied **thickly** and **frequently** (approximately 2 hourly). In photodermatoses, they should be used from spring to autumn. As maximum protection from sunlight is desirable, preparations with the highest SPF should be prescribed.

Borderline substances   The preparations marked 'ACBS' cannot be prescribed on the NHS except for skin protection against ultraviolet radiation in abnormal cutaneous photosensitivity resulting from genetic disorders or photodermatoses, including vitiligo and those resulting from radiotherapy; chronic or recurrent

13 Skin

herpes simplex labialis. Preparations with SPF less than 30 should not normally be prescribed. See also Appendix 2.

Delph® (Fenton)
Lotion, (UVA and UVB protection; UVB-SPF 30), avobenzone 4%, octinoxate 4.8%, oxybenzone 1.5%, titanium dioxide 2.5%, net price 200 mL = £3.53. ACBS
Excipients include cetostearyl alcohol, fragrance, hydroxybenzoates (parabens), imidurea

SpectraBan® (Stiefel)
Ultra lotion (UVA and UVB protection; UVB-SPF 28), water resistant, avobenzone 2%, oxybenzone 3%, padimate-O 8%, titanium dioxide 2%, net price 150 mL = £6.54. ACBS
Excipients include benzyl alcohol, disodium edetate, sorbic acid, fragrance

Sunsense® Ultra (Crawford)
Lotion (UVA and UVB protection; UVB-SPF 50+), octinoxate 7.5%, oxybenzone 3%, titanium dioxide 3.5%, net price 50-mL bottle with roll-on applicator = £4.11, 125 mL = £6.86, 500 mL = £15.54. ACBS
Excipients include butylated hydroxytoluene, cetyl alcohol, fragrance, hydroxybenzoates (parabens), propylene glycol

Uvistat® (LPC)
Cream (UVA and UVB protection; UVB-SPF 30), avobenzone 5%, bisoctrizole 1.5%, octinoxate 7.5%, octocrilene 4%, titanium dioxide 5.2%, net price 125 mL = £7.45. ACBS
Excipients include disodium edetate, hydroxybenzoates (parabens), propylene glycol

Cream (UVA and UVB protection; UVB-SPF 50), amiloxate 2%, avobenzone 5%, bisoctrizole 6%, octinoxate 10%, octocrilene 4%, titanium dioxide 4.8%, net price 125 mL = £8.45. ACBS
Excipients include disodium edetate, polysorbate 60, propylene glycol

Lipscreen (UVA and UVB protection; UVB-SPF 50), avobenzone 5%, bemotrizinol 3%, octinoxate 10%, octocrilene 4%, titanium dioxide 3%, net price 5 g = £2.99. ACBS
Excipients include butylated hydroxytoluene, hydroxybenzoates (parabens)

Photodamage

Actinic keratoses occur very rarely in healthy children; *actinic cheilitis* may occur on the lips of adolescents following excessive sun exposure.

Diclofenac gel (*Solaraze®*) and **fluorouracil** cream are licensed for the treatment of actinic keratoses but they are not licensed for use in children.

In children with photosensitivity disorders, such as erythropoietic protoporphyria, specialists may use **betacarotene**, **mepacrine**, **chloroquine** or **hydroxychloroquine** (section 10.1.3) to reduce skin reactions.

BETACAROTENE

Note Betacarotene is a precursor to vitamin A

Cautions monitor vitamin A intake; **interactions:** Appendix 1 (vitamins)

Hepatic impairment avoid

Renal impairment use with caution

Pregnancy partially converted to vitamin A, but does not give rise to abnormally high serum concentration; manufacturer advises use only if potential benefit outweighs risk

Breast-feeding use with caution—present in milk

Side-effects loose stools; yellow discoloration of skin; *rarely*, bruising, arthralgia

Licensed use not licensed for use in UK

Indication and dose

Management of photosensitivity reactions in erythropoietic protoporphyria (specialist use only)

- By mouth

    Child 1–5 years 60–90 mg daily in single or divided doses

    Child 5–9 years 90–120 mg daily in single or divided doses

    Child 9–12 years 120–150 mg daily in single or divided doses

    Child 12–16 years 150–180 mg daily in single or divided doses

    Child 16–18 years 180–300 mg daily in single or divided doses

Note Protection not total—avoid strong sunlight and use sunscreen preparations; generally 2–6 weeks of treatment (resulting in yellow coloration of palms and soles) necessary before increasing exposure to sunlight; dose should be adjusted according to level of exposure to sunlight

Betacarotene (Non-proprietary)
Capsules, 15 mg, 25 mg are available from 'special-order' manufacturers or specialist importing companies, see p. 957. Label: 21

13.8.2 Camouflagers

Disfigurement of the skin can be very distressing and may have a marked psychological effect, especially in children. Cosmetic preparations may be used to camouflage unsightly scars, skin deformities, and pigment abnormalities, such as vitiligo and birthmarks.

Opaque cover foundation or cream is used to mask skin pigment abnormalities; careful application using a combination of dark- and light-coloured cover creams set with powder helps to minimise the appearance of skin deformities.

Borderline substances The preparations marked 'ACBS' cannot be prescribed on the NHS for postoperative scars and other deformities except as adjunctive therapy in the relief of emotional disturbances due to disfiguring skin disease, such as vitiligo.

Covermark® (Skin Camouflage Co.)
Classic foundation (masking cream), net price 15 mL (10 shades) = £11.32. ACBS
Excipients include beeswax, hydroxybenzoates (parabens), fragrance
Finishing powder, net price 25 g = £11.32. ACBS
Excipients include beeswax, hydroxybenzoates (parabens), fragrance

Dermacolor® (Fox)
Camouflage creme, (100 shades), net price 25 g = £9.96. ACBS
Excipients include beeswax, butylated hydroxytoluene, fragrance, propylene glycol, stearyl alcohol, wool fat
Fixing powder, (7 shades), net price 60 g = £8.45. ACBS
Excipients include fragrance

Keromask® (Lornamead)
Masking cream, (9 shades), net price 15 mL = £5.68. ACBS
Excipients include butylated hydroxyanisole, hydroxybenzoates (parabens), wool fat, propylene glycol
Finishing powder, net price 20 g = £5.68. ACBS
Excipients include butylated hydroxytoluene, hydroxybenzoates (parabens)

Veil® (Thomas Blake)
Cover cream (40 shades), net price 19 g = £19.65, 44 g = £29.22, 70 g = £36.90. ACBS
Excipients include hydroxybenzoates (parabens), wool fat derivative
Finishing powder, translucent, net price 35 g = £21.55. ACBS
Excipients include butylated hydroxyanisole, hydroxybenzoates (parabens)

13.9 Shampoos and other preparations for scalp conditions

The detergent action of shampoo removes grease (sebum) from hair. Prepubertal children produce very little grease and require shampoo less frequently than adults. Shampoos can be used as vehicles for medicinal products, but their usefulness is limited by the short time the product is in contact with the scalp and by their irritant nature.

Oils and ointments are very useful for scaly, dry scalp conditions; if a greasy appearance is cosmetically unacceptable, the preparation may be applied at night and washed out in the morning. Alcohol-based lotions are rarely used in children; alcohol causes painful stinging on broken skin and the fumes may exacerbate asthma.

Itchy, inflammatory, eczematous scalp conditions may be relieved by a simple emollient oil such as **olive oil** or **coconut oil** (arachis oil (ground nut oil, peanut oil) is best avoided in children under 5 years). In more severe cases a topical **corticosteroid** (section 13.4) may be required. Preparations containing **coal tar** are used for the common scaly scalp conditions of childhood including seborrhoeic dermatitis, dandruff (a mild form of seborrhoeic dermatitis), and psoriasis (section 13.5.2); **salicylic acid** is used as a keratolytic in some scalp preparations.

Shampoos containing antimicrobials such as **selenium sulphide** or **ketoconazole** are used for seborrhoeic dermatitis and dandruff in which yeast infection has been implicated, and for tinea capitis (ringworm of the scalp, section 13.10.2). Bacterial infection affecting the scalp (usually secondary to eczema, head lice, or ringworm) may be treated with shampoos containing antimicrobials such as **pyrithione zinc**, **cetrimide**, or **povidone–iodine**.

In neonates and infants, *cradle cap* (which is also a form of seborrhoeic eczema) can be treated by massaging **coconut oil** or **olive oil** into the scalp; a bland emollient such as **emulsifying ointment** can be rubbed onto the affected area once or twice daily before bathing and a mild shampoo used.

◀**Shampoos**
[1]**Ketoconazole** (Non-proprietary) PoM
Cream—section 13.10.2
Shampoo, ketoconazole 2%, net price 120 mL = £3.02
Excipients include imidurea
Brands include *Dandrazol® 2% Shampoo*, *Nizoral®*

Dose

Seborrhoeic dermatitis and dandruff
Treatment, apply twice weekly for 2–4 weeks; prophylaxis, apply once every 1–2 weeks

Pityriasis versicolor
Treatment, apply once daily for max. 5 days; prophylaxis, apply once daily for up to 3 days before sun exposure; leave preparation on for 3–5 minutes before rinsing

1. Can be sold to the public for the prevention and treatment of dandruff and seborrhoeic dermatitis of the scalp as a shampoo formulation containing ketoconazole max. 2%, in a pack containing max. 120 mL and labelled to show a max. frequency of application of once every 3 days

Alphosyl 2 in 1® (GSK Consumer Healthcare)

Shampoo, alcoholic coal tar extract 5%, net price 125 mL = £1.81, 250 mL = £3.43
Excipients include hydroxybenzoates (parabens), fragrance

Dose

Dandruff

Use once or twice weekly as necessary

Psoriasis, seborrhoeic dermatitis, scaling and itching

Use every 2–3 days

Capasal® (Dermal)

Shampoo, coal tar 1%, coconut oil 1%, salicylic acid 0.5%, net price 250 mL = £4.78
Excipients none as listed in section 13.1.3

Dose

Scaly scalp disorders including psoriasis, seborrhoeic dermatitis, dandruff, and cradle cap

Apply daily as necessary

Ceanel Concentrate® (Ferndale)

Shampoo, cetrimide 10%, undecenoic acid 1%, phenylethyl alcohol 7.5%, net price 150 mL = £3.40, 500 mL = £9.80
Excipients none as listed in section 13.1.3

Dose

Scalp psoriasis, seborrhoeic dermatitis, dandruff

Apply 3 times in first week then twice weekly

Dermax® (Dermal)

Shampoo, benzalkonium chloride 0.5%, net price 250 mL = £5.78
Excipients none as listed in section 13.1.3

Dose

Seborrhoeic scalp conditions associated with dandruff and scaling

Apply as necessary

Meted® (Alliance)

Shampoo, salicylic acid 3%, sulphur 5%, net price 120 mL = £3.80
Excipients include fragrance

Dose

Scaly scalp disorders including psoriasis, seborrhoeic dermatitis, and dandruff

Apply at least twice weekly

Pentrax® (Alliance)

Shampoo, coal tar 4.3%, net price 120 mL = £3.80
Excipients none as listed in section 13.1.3

Dose

Scaly scalp disorders including psoriasis, seborrhoeic dermatitis, and dandruff

Apply at least twice weekly

Polytar AF® (Stiefel)

Shampoo, arachis (peanut) oil extract of coal tar 0.3%, cade oil 0.3%, coal tar solution 0.1%, pine tar 0.3%, pyrithione zinc 1%, net price 250 mL = £6.52
Excipients include fragrance, imidurea

Dose

Scaly scalp disorders including psoriasis, seborrhoeic dermatitis, and dandruff

Apply 2–3 times weekly for at least 3 weeks

Psoriderm® (Dermal)

Scalp lotion (= shampoo), coal tar 2.5%, lecithin 0.3%, net price 250 mL = £4.81
Excipients include disodium edetate

Dose

Scalp psoriasis

Use as necessary

Selsun® (Chattem UK)

Shampoo, selenium sulphide 2.5%, net price 50 mL = £1.44, 100 mL = £1.96, 150 mL = £2.75
Excipients include fragrance

Cautions avoid using 48 hours before or after applying hair colouring, straightening or waving preparations

Dose

Seborrhoeic dermatitis and dandruff

Child 5–18 years apply twice weekly for 2 weeks then once weekly for 2 weeks and then as necessary

Pityriasis versicolor [unlicensed indication]

Child 5–18 years dilute shampoo with water and apply to affected area, leave on for at least 30 minutes; apply 2–7 times over a two-week period; repeat course as necessary

T/Gel® (J&J)

Shampoo, coal tar extract 2%, net price 125 mL = £3.18, 250 mL = £4.78
Excipients include fragrance, hydroxybenzoates (parabens), imidurea, tetrasodium edetate

Dose

Scalp psoriasis, seborrhoeic dermatitis, dandruff

Apply 2–3 times weekly

◄**Other scalp preparations**

Cocois®

Section 13.5.2

Polytar® (Stiefel)

Liquid, arachis (peanut) oil extract of coal tar 0.3%, cade oil 0.3%, coal tar solution 0.1%, oleyl alcohol 1%, tar 0.3%, net price 250 mL = £2.23
Excipients include fragrance, imidurea, polysorbate 80

Dose

Scalp disorders including psoriasis, seborrhoea, eczema, pruritus, and dandruff

Apply 1–2 times weekly

Polytar Plus® (Stiefel)

Liquid, ingredients as *Polytar®* liquid with hydrolysed animal protein 3%, net price 500 mL = £3.91
Excipients include fragrance, imidurea, polysorbate 80

Dose

Scalp disorders including psoriasis, seborrhoea, eczema, pruritus, and dandruff

Apply 1–2 times weekly

13 Skin

13.10 Anti-infective skin preparations

13.10.1 Antibacterial preparations
13.10.2 Antifungal preparations
13.10.3 Antiviral preparations
13.10.4 Parasiticidal preparations
13.10.5 Preparations for minor cuts and abrasions

13.10.1 Antibacterial preparations

Topical antibacterial preparations are used to treat localised bacterial skin infections caused by Gram-positive organisms (particularly by staphylococci or streptococci). Systemic antibacterial treatment (Table 1, section 5.1) is more appropriate for deep-seated skin infections.

Problems associated with the use of topical antibacterials include bacterial resistance, contact sensitisation, and superinfection. In order to minimise the development of resistance, antibacterials used systemically (e.g. fusidic acid) should not generally be chosen for topical use. *Resistant organisms* are more common in hospitals, and whenever possible swabs should be taken for bacteriological examination before beginning treatment.

Neomycin applied topically may cause sensitisation and cross-sensitivity with other aminoglycoside antibacterials such as gentamicin may occur. Topical antibacterials applied over large areas can cause systemic toxicity; ototoxicity with neomycin and with **polymyxins** is a particular risk for neonates and children with renal impairment.

Superficial bacterial infection of the skin may be treated with a topical antiseptic such as **povidine–iodine** (section 13.11.4) which also softens crusts.

Bacterial infections such as *impetigo* and *folliculitis* can be treated with a short course of topical **fusidic acid**; **mupirocin** should be used only to treat meticillin-resistant *Staphylococcus aureus*.

For extensive or long-standing impetigo, an oral antibacterial such as **flucloxacillin** (or **clarithromycin** in children with penicillin-allergy), Table 1, section 5.1, should be used. A mild antiseptic may help to soften crusts. Mild antiseptics may be useful in reducing the spread of infection, but there is little evidence to support the use of topical antiseptics alone in the treatment of impetigo.

Cellulitis, a rapidly spreading deeply seated inflammation of the skin and subcutaneous tissue, requires systemic antibacterial treatment (see Table 1, section 5.1). Lower leg infections or infections spreading around wounds are almost always cellulitis. *Erysipelas*, a superficial infection with clearly defined edges (and often affecting the face), is also treated with a systemic antibacterial (see Table 1, section 5.1). Both infections can be caused by streptococci or staphylococci, or both organisms.

Staphylococcal scalded-skin syndrome requires urgent treatment with a systemic antibacterial, such as flucloxacillin (see Table 1, section 5.1).

Mupirocin is not related to any other antibacterial in use; it is effective for skin infections, particularly those due to Gram-positive organisms but it is not indicated for pseudomonal infection. Although *Staphylococcus aureus* strains with low-level resistance to mupirocin are emerging, it is generally useful in infections resistant to other antibacterials. To avoid the development of resistance, mupirocin or fusidic acid should not be used for longer than 10 days and local microbiology advice should be sought before using it in hospital. In the presence of mupirocin-resistant MRSA infection, a topical antiseptic, such as povidone–iodine, chlorhexidine, or alcohol, can be used (section 13.11); their use should be discussed with the local microbiologist.

Mupirocin ointment contains macrogol; extensive absorption of macrogol through the mucous membranes or through application to thin or damaged skin may result in renal toxicity, especially in neonates. Mupirocin nasal ointment is formulated in a paraffin base and may be more suitable for the treatment of MRSA-infected open wound in neonates.

Metronidazole gel is used topically in children to reduce the odour associated with anaerobic infections and for the treatment of periorificial rosacea (section

13

Skin

13.6); oral metronidazole (section 5.1.11) is used to treat wounds infected with anaerobic bacteria.

Retapamulin can be used for impetigo and other superficial bacterial skin infections caused by *Staphylococcus aureus* and *Streptococcus pyogenes* that are resistant to first-line topical antibacterials. However, it is not effective against MRSA. The *Scottish Medicines Consortium* (p. 4) has advised (March 2008) that retapamulin (*Altargo*®) is **not** recommended for use within NHS Scotland for the treatment of superficial skin infections.

Silver sulfadiazine (silver sulphadiazine) is licensed for the prevention and treatment of infection in burns but the use of appropriate dressings may be more effective. Systemic effects may occur following extensive application of silver sulfadiazine; its use is not recommended in neonates.

13.10.1.1 Antibacterial preparations only used topically

MUPIROCIN

Renal impairment manufacturer advises caution when *Bactroban*® ointment used in moderate or severe impairment because it contains macrogol

Pregnancy manufacturer advises avoid unless potential benefit outweighs risk—no information available

Breast-feeding no information available

Side-effects local reactions including urticaria, pruritus, burning sensation, rash

Licensed use *Bactroban*® *ointment* licensed for use in children (age range not specified by manufacturer); *Bactroban*® *cream* not recommended for use in children under 1 year

Indication and dose

> **Bacterial skin infections** (see also notes above)
>
> **Child 1 month–18 years** apply up to 3 times daily for up to 10 days

Bactroban® (GSK) [PoM]
Cream, mupirocin (as mupirocin calcium) 2%, net price 15 g = £4.38
Excipients include benzyl alcohol, cetyl alcohol, stearyl alcohol

Ointment, mupirocin 2%, net price 15 g = £4.38
Excipients none as listed in section 13.1.3

Nasal ointment—section 12.2.3

NEOMYCIN SULPHATE

Cautions large areas—if large areas of skin are being treated ototoxicity may be a hazard in children, particularly in those with renal impairment

Contra-indications neonates

Renal impairment see Cautions above

Side-effects sensitisation (see also notes above)

Licensed use *Neomycin Cream BPC*—no information available

Indication and dose

> **Bacterial skin infections** see under preparation

Neomycin Cream BPC [PoM]
Cream, neomycin sulphate 0.5%, cetomacrogol emulsifying ointment 30%, chlorocresol 0.1%, disodium edetate 0.01%, in freshly boiled and cooled purified water, net price 15 g = £2.17
Excipients include cetostearyl alcohol, edetic acid (EDTA)
Dose
> Apply up to 3 times daily (short-term use)

POLYMYXINS

Cautions large areas—if large areas of skin are being treated nephrotoxicity and neurotoxicity may be a hazard, particularly in children with renal impairment

Renal impairment see Cautions above

Side-effects sensitisation (see also notes above)

Licensed use licensed for use in children (age range not specified by manufacturer)

Indication and dose

> **Bacterial skin infections** see under preparation

Polyfax® (TEVA UK) [PoM]
Ointment, polymyxin B sulphate 10 000 units, bacitracin zinc 500 units/g, net price 4 g = £3.26, 20 g = £4.62
Excipients none as listed in section 13.1.3
Dose
> Apply twice daily or more frequently if required

13 Skin

RETAPAMULIN

Contra-indications contact with eyes and mucous membranes

Side-effects local reactions including irritation, erythema, pain, and pruritus

Indication and dose

> **Superficial bacterial skin infections** (but see also notes above)
>
> > **Child 9 months–18 years** apply thinly twice daily for 5 days; review treatment if no response within 2–3 days

Altargo® (GSK) ▼ PoM
    Ointment, retapamulin 1%, net price 5 g = £7.89.
    Label: 28
    Excipients include butylated hydroxytoluene

SILVER SULFADIAZINE

(Silver sulphadiazine)

Cautions G6PD deficiency; may inactivate enzymatic debriding agents—concomitant use may be inappropriate; **interactions:** Appendix 1 (sulphonamides)

Large areas Plasma-sulfadiazine concentrations may approach therapeutic levels with *side-effects* and *interactions* as for sulphonamides (see section 5.1.8) if large areas of skin are treated. Owing to the association of sulphonamides with severe blood and skin disorders treatment should be stopped immediately if blood disorders or rashes develop—but leucopenia developing 2–3 days after starting treatment of burns patients is reported usually to be self-limiting and silver sulfadiazine need not usually be discontinued provided blood counts are monitored carefully to ensure return to baseline within a few days. Argyria may also occur if large areas of skin are treated (or if application is prolonged).

Contra-indications sensitivity to sulphonamides; not recommended for neonates

Hepatic impairment manufacturer advises caution if significant impairment; see also Large areas, above

Renal impairment manufacturer advises caution if significant impairment; see also Large areas, above

Pregnancy risk of neonatal haemolysis and methaemoglobinaemia in third trimester

Breast-feeding small risk of kernicterus in jaundiced infants and of haemolysis in G6PD deficient infants

Side-effects allergic reactions including burning, itching and rashes; argyria reported following prolonged use; leucopenia reported (monitor blood count)

Licensed use no age range specified by manufacturer but see contra-indications, above

Indication and dose

> **Prophylaxis and treatment of infection in burn wounds, for conservative management of finger-tip injuries** see under preparation below

> **Adjunct to short-term treatment of infection in pressure sores, adjunct to prophylaxis of infection in skin graft donor sites and extensive abrasions** consult product literature for details

Flamazine® (S&N Hlth.) PoM
    Cream, silver sulfadiazine 1%, net price 20 g = £2.91, 50 g = £3.85, 250 g = £10.32, 500 g = £18.27
    Excipients include cetyl alcohol, polysorbates, propylene glycol

Dose

> **Burns**
>
> > **Child 1 month–18 years** apply daily or more frequently if very exudative

> **Finger-tip injuries**
>
> > **Child 1 month–18 years** apply every 2–3 days

Note apply with sterile applicator

13.10.1.2 Antibacterial preparations also used systemically

Sodium fusidate is a narrow-spectrum antibacterial used for staphylococcal infections. For the role of sodium fusidate in the treatment of impetigo see p. 715.

Metronidazole is used topically to treat rosacea and to reduce the odour associated with anaerobic infections; oral metronidazole (section 5.1.11) is used to treat wounds infected with anaerobic bacteria.

Angular cheilitis An ointment containing sodium fusidate is used in the fissures of angular cheilitis when associated with staphylococcal infection. For further information on angular cheilitis, see p. 666.

FUSIDIC ACID

Cautions see notes above; avoid contact with eyes

Side-effects rarely hypersensitivity reactions

Licensed use licensed for use in children (age range not specified by manufacturer)

Indication and dose

> **Staphylococcal skin infections**
>
> > Apply 3–4 times daily, usually for 7 days

◁ **FUSIDIC ACID** (*continued*)

Penicillin-resistant staphylococcal infections
Section 5.1.7

Staphylococcal eye infections
Section 11.3.1

Fucidin® (LEO) [PoM]
Cream, fusidic acid 2%, net price 15 g = £1.92, 30 g
= £3.64
Excipients include butylated hydroxyanisole, cetyl alcohol

Ointment, sodium fusidate 2%, net price 15 g =
£2.23, 30 g = £3.79
Excipients include cetyl alcohol, wool fat

Dental prescribing on NHS May be prescribed as Sodium
Fusidate ointment

▌ METRONIDAZOLE

Cautions avoid exposure to strong sunlight or UV
light

Side-effects skin irritation

Licensed use *Metrotop®* licensed for use in children (age range not specified by manufacturer);
Acea® and *Anabact®* not licensed for use in
children under 12 years; *Noritate®* not licensed for
use in children under 16 years; *Metrogel®*,
Metrosa®, *Rosiced®*, *Rozex®*, and *Zyomet®* not
licensed for use in children

Indication and dose

Malodorous tumours and wounds
For dose see preparations

Rosacea (see also section 13.6)
For dose see preparations

***Helicobacter pylori* eradication**
Section 1.3

Anaerobic infections
Section 5.1.11 and section 7.2.2

Protozoal infections
Section 5.4.2

Acea® (Ferndale) [PoM]
Gel, metronidazole 0.75%, net price 40 g = £9.95
Excipients include disodium edetate, hydroxybenzoates
(parabens)
Dose

Acute inflammatory exacerbations of rosacea
Child 1–18 years apply thinly twice daily

Anabact® (CHS) [PoM]
Gel, metronidazole 0.75%, net price 15 g = £4.47,
30 g = £7.89
Excipients include hydroxybenzoates (parabens), propylene
glycol
Dose

Malodorous fungating tumours and skin ulcers
Apply to clean wound 1–2 times daily and cover with non-adherent dressing

Metrogel® (Galderma) [PoM]
Gel, metronidazole 0.75%, net price 40 g = £9.95
Excipients include hydroxybenzoates (parabens), propylene
glycol
Dose

Acute inflammatory exacerbations of rosacea
Child 1–18 years apply thinly twice daily

Malodorous fungating tumours
Apply to clean wound 1–2 times daily and cover with non-adherant dressing

Metrosa® (Linderma) [PoM]
Gel, metronidazole 0.75%, net price 40 g = £19.90
Excipients include propylene glycol
Dose

Acute exacerbation of rosacea
Child 1–18 years apply thinly twice daily

Metrotop® (Mölnlycke) [PoM]
Gel, metronidazole 0.8%, net price 15 g = £4.59,
30 g = £8.10, 60 g = £14.30
Excipients none as listed in section 13.1.3
Dose

Malodorous fungating tumours and skin ulcers
Apply to clean wound 1–2 times daily and cover (flat wounds, apply liberally; cavities, smear gel on paraffin gauze and pack loosely)

Rosiced® (Fabre) [PoM]
Cream, metronidazole 0.75%, net price 30 g = £7.50
Excipients include propylene glycol
Dose

Inflammatory papules and pustules of rosacea
Child 1–18 years apply twice daily for 6 weeks (longer if necessary)

Rozex® (Galderma) [PoM]
Cream, metronidazole 0.75%, net price 40 g = £9.95
Excipients include benzyl alcohol, isopropyl palmitate
Gel, metronidazole 0.75%, net price 40 g = £9.95
Excipients include disodium edetate, hydroxybenzoates
(parabens), propylene glycol
Dose

Inflammatory papules, pustules and erythema of rosacea
Child 1–18 years apply twice daily

Zyomet® (Goldshield) [PoM]
Gel, metronidazole 0.75%, net price 30 g = £12.00
Excipients include benzyl alcohol, disodium edetate, propy-
lene glycol
Dose

Acute inflammatory exacerbations of rosacea
Child 1–18 years apply thinly twice daily

13 Skin

13.10.2 Antifungal preparations

Most localised fungal infections are treated with topical preparations. To prevent relapse, local antifungal treatment should be continued for 1–2 weeks after the disappearance of all signs of infection. Systemic therapy (section 5.2) is necessary for nail or scalp infection or if the skin infection is widespread, disseminated or intractable. Specimens of scale, nail or hair should be sent for mycological examination before starting treatment, unless the diagnosis is certain.

Dermatophytoses   Ringworm infection can affect the scalp (tinea capitis), body (tinea corporis), groin (tinea cruris), hand (tinea manuum), foot (tinea pedis, athlete's foot), or nail (tinea unguium, onychomycosis). Tinea capitis is a common childhood infection that requires systemic treatment with an oral antifungal (section 5.2); additional application of a topical antifungal, during the early stages of treatment, may reduce the risk of transmission. A topical antifungal can also be used to treat asymptomatic carriers of scalp ringworm.

Tinea corporis and tinea pedis infections in children respond to treatment with a topical **imidazole** (clotrimazole, econazole, ketoconazole, miconazole, or sulconazole) or **terbinafine** cream. Nystatin is less effective against tinea.

Compound benzoic acid ointment (Whitfield's ointment) has been used for ringworm infections but it is cosmetically less acceptable than proprietary preparations. Antifungal dusting powders are of little therapeutic value in the treatment of fungal skin infections and may cause skin irritation; they may have some role in preventing re-infection.

Antifungal treatment may not be necessary in asymptomatic children with tinea infection of the nails. If treatment is necessary, a systemic antifungal (section 5.2) is more effective than topical therapy. However, topical application of **amorolfine** or **tioconazole** may be useful for treating early onychomycosis when involvement is limited to mild distal disease in up to 2 nails, or for superficial white onychomycosis, or where there are contra-indications to systemic therapy. Chronic paronychia on the fingers (usually due to a candidal infection) should be treated with topical clotrimazole or nystatin, but these preparations should be used with caution in children who suck their fingers. Chronic paronychia of the toes (usually due to dermatophyte infection) can be treated with topical terbinafine.

Pityriasis versicolor   Pityriasis (tinea) versicolor can be treated with **ketoconazole** shampoo or **selenium sulphide** shampoo (section 13.9). Topical imidazole antifungals, **clotrimazole, econazole, ketoconazole, miconazole**, and **sulconazole**, and topical **terbinafine** are alternatives, but large quantities may be required.

If topical therapy fails, or if the infection is widespread, pityriasis versicolor is treated systemically with an azole antifungal (section 5.2). Relapse is common, especially in the immunocompromised.

Candidiasis   Candidal skin infections can be treated with topical imidazole antifungals **clotrimazole, econazole, ketoconazole, miconazole**, or **sulconazole**; topical terbinafine is an alternative. Topical application of **nystatin** is also effective for candidiasis but it is ineffective against dermatophytosis. Refractory candidiasis requires systemic treatment (section 5.2) generally with a triazole such as fluconazole; systemic treatment with griseofulvin or terbinafine is **not appropriate** for refractory candidiasis. For the treatment of oral candiasis see section 12.3.2 and for the management of nappy rash see section 13.2.2.

Angular cheilitis   Miconazole cream is used in the fissures of angular cheilitis when associated with *Candida*. For further information on angular cheilitis, see p. 666.

Cautions   Contact with eyes and mucous membranes should be avoided.

Side-effects   Occasional local irritation and hypersensitivity reactions include mild burning sensation, erythema, and itching. Treatment should be discontinued if symptoms are severe.

Compound topical preparations   Combination of an imidazole and a mild corticosteroid (such as hydrocortisone 1%) (section 13.4) may be of value in the treatment of eczematous intertrigo and, in the first few days only, of a severely inflamed patch of ringworm. Combination of a mild corticosteroid with either an imidazole or nystatin may be of use in the treatment of *intertriginous eczema* associated with candida.

AMOROLFINE

Cautions see notes above; also avoid contact with ears

Pregnancy systemic absorption very low, but manufacturer advises avoid—no information available

Breast-feeding manufacturer advises avoid—no information available

Side-effects see notes above

Licensed use not licensed for use in children under 12 years

Indication and dose

See under preparations

Loceryl® (Galderma) [PoM]
Cream, amorolfine (as hydrochloride) 0.25%, net price 20 g = £3.52. Label: 10, patient information leaflet
Excipients include cetostearyl alcohol, disodium edetate

Dose

Fungal skin infections

Apply once daily after cleansing in the evening for at least 2–3 weeks (up to 6 weeks for foot infection) continuing for 3–5 days after lesions have healed

Nail lacquer, amorolfine (as hydrochloride) 5%, net price 5-mL pack (with nail files, spatulas and cleansing swabs) = £18.17. Label: 10, patient information leaflet
Excipients none as listed in section 13.1.3

Dose

Fungal nail infections

Apply to infected nails 1–2 times weekly after filing and cleansing; allow to dry (approx. 3 minutes); treat finger nails for 6 months, toe nails for 9–12 months (review at intervals of 3 months); avoid nail varnish or artificial nails during treatment

Note Use with caution in child likely to suck affected digits

BENZOIC ACID

Licensed use licensed for use in children (age range not specified by manufacturer)

Indication and dose

Ringworm (tinea) but see notes above; dose under preparation

◢With salicylic acid
For prescribing information on salicylic acid, see p. 697

Benzoic Acid Ointment, Compound, BP (Whitfield's ointment)
Ointment, benzoic acid 6%, salicylic acid 3%, in emulsifying ointment
Excipients include cetostearyl alcohol

Dose

Child 1 month–18 years apply twice daily

CLOTRIMAZOLE

Cautions see notes above

Pregnancy minimal absorption from skin; not known to be harmful

Side-effects see notes above

Licensed use licensed for use in children (age range not specified by manufacturer)

Indication and dose

Fungal skin infections

Apply 2–3 times daily

Vaginal candidiasis section 7.2.2

Otitis externa section 12.1.1

Clotrimazole (Non-proprietary)
Cream, clotrimazole 1%, net price 20 g = £1.77

Canesten® (Bayer Consumer Care)
Cream, clotrimazole 1%, net price 20 g = £2.14, 50 g = £3.80
Excipients include benzyl alcohol, cetostearyl alcohol, polysorbate 60

Solution, clotrimazole 1% in macrogol 400 (polyethylene glycol 400), net price 20 mL = £2.43. For hairy areas
Excipients none as listed in section 13.1.3

Spray, clotrimazole 1%, in 30% isopropyl alcohol, net price 40-mL atomiser = £4.99. Label: 15. For large or hairy areas
Excipients include propylene glycol

ECONAZOLE NITRATE

Cautions see notes above

Pregnancy minimal absorption from skin; not known to be harmful

Side-effects see notes above

Licensed use *Pevaryl®*, no age range specified by manufacturer

Indication and dose

Fungal skin infections

Apply twice daily

Fungal nail infections

Apply once daily under occlusive dressing

Vaginal candidiasis section 7.2.2

◁ **ECONAZOLE NITRATE** (*continued*)

Pevaryl® (Janssen-Cilag)
Cream, econazole nitrate 1%, net price 30 g = £2.65
Excipients include butylated hydroxyanisole, fragrance

▰ KETOCONAZOLE

Cautions see notes above; do **not** use within 2 weeks of a potent topical corticosteroid for seborrhoeic dermatitis—risk of skin sensitisation
Side-effects see notes above

Indication and dose

Tinea pedis

Apply twice daily

Other fungal infections

Apply 1–2 times daily

Systemic or resistant fungal infections section 5.2

Vulval candidiasis section 7.2.2

Nizoral® (Janssen-Cilag) [PoM]
¹Cream, ketoconazole 2%, net price 30 g = £3.40
Excipients include cetyl alcohol, polysorbates, propylene glycol, stearyl alcohol
Note A 15-g tube is available for sale to the public for the treatment of tinea pedis, tinea cruris, and candidal intertrigo

Shampoo—section 13.9
1. [NHS] except for seborrhoeic dermatitis and pityriasis versicolor and endorsed 'SLS'

▰ MICONAZOLE NITRATE

Cautions see notes above
Side-effects see notes above
Licensed use Licensed for use in children (age range not specified by manufacturer)

Indication and dose

Fungal skin infections

Neonate apply twice daily continuing for 10 days after lesions have healed

Child 1 month–18 years apply twice daily continuing for 10 days after lesions have healed

Fungal nail infections

Apply 1–2 times daily

Oral and intestinal fungal infections section 12.3.2

Vaginal candidiasis section 7.2.2

Miconazole (Non-proprietary)
Cream, miconazole nitrate 2%, net price 20 g = £2.05, 45 g = £1.97
Dental prescribing on NHS Miconazole cream may be prescribed

Daktarin® (Janssen-Cilag)
Cream, miconazole nitrate 2%, net price 30 g = £1.85
Excipients include butylated hydroxyanisole

▰ NYSTATIN

Cautions see notes above
Side-effects see notes above
Licensed use licensed for use in children (age range not specified by manufacturer)

Indication and dose

Skin infections due to *Candida* spp. for dose, see preparation

Intestinal candidiasis section 5.2

Oral fungal infections section 12.3.2

Nystaform® (Typharm) [PoM]
Cream, nystatin 100 000 units/g, chlorhexidine hydrochloride 1%, net price 30 g = £2.62
Excipients include benzyl alcohol, cetostearyl alcohol, polysorbate 60
Dose
Apply 2–3 times daily continuing for 7 days after lesions have healed.

▰ SALICYLIC ACID

Cautions avoid broken or inflamed skin
Salicylate toxicity Salicylate toxicity can occur particularly if applied on large areas of skin
Side-effects see notes above

Indication and dose

Fungal nail infections, particularly tinea

Child 5–18 years apply twice daily and after washing
Note Use with caution in child likely to suck affected digits

Hyperkeratotic skin disorders section 13.5.2

13

Skin

◁ **SALICYLIC ACID (continued)**

Acne vulgaris section 13.6.1

Warts and calluses section 13.7

Phytex® (Wynlit) ◢
Paint, salicylic acid 1.46% (total combined), tannic acid 4.89% and boric acid 3.12% (as borotannic complex), in a vehicle containing alcohol and ethyl acetate, net price 25 mL (with brush) = £2.81
Excipients none as listed in section 13.1.3
Note Flammable

SULCONAZOLE NITRATE

Cautions see notes above
Side-effects see notes above; also blistering

Indication and dose

Fungal skin infections
Apply 1–2 times daily continuing for 2–3 weeks after lesions have healed

Exelderm® (Centrapharm)
Cream, sulconazole nitrate 1%, net price 30 g = £3.90
Excipients include cetyl alcohol, polysorbates, propylene glycol, stearyl alcohol

TERBINAFINE

Cautions avoid contact with eyes
Pregnancy manufacturer advises use only if potential benefit outweighs risk—*animal* studies suggest no adverse effects
Breast-feeding manufacturer advises avoid—present in milk, but less than 5% of the dose is absorbed after topical application of terbinafine; avoid application to mother's chest
Side-effects see notes above
Licensed use not licensed for use in children

Indication and dose

Fungal skin infections
Apply thinly 1–2 times daily for up to 1 week in tinea pedis, 1–2 weeks in tinea corporis and tinea cruris, 2 weeks in cutaneous candidiasis and pityriasis versicolor; review after 2 weeks

Systemic therapy section 5.2

[1]**Terbinafine** (Non-proprietary) PoM
Cream, terbinafine hydrochloride 1%, net price 15 g = £4.59, 30 g = £3.36
1. Can be sold to the public for external use in children over 16 years for the treatment of tinea pedis and tinea cruris as a cream containing terbinafine hydrochloride max. 1% in a pack containing max. 15 g; also for the treatment of tinea pedis, tinea cruris, and tinea corporis as a spray containing terbinafine hydrochloride max. 1% in a pack containing max. 30 mL or as a gel containing terbinafine hydrochloride max. 1% in a pack containing max. 30 g

Lamisil® (Novartis Consumer Health) PoM
Cream, terbinafine hydrochloride 1%, net price 15 g = £4.86, 30 g = £8.76
Excipients include benzyl alcohol, cetyl alcohol, polysorbate 60, stearyl alcohol

TIOCONAZOLE

Cautions see notes above
Pregnancy manufacturer advises avoid
Side-effects see notes above; also local oedema, dry skin, nail discoloration, periungual inflammation, nail pain, rash, exfoliation
Licensed use licensed for use in children (age range not specified by manufacturer)

Indication and dose

Fungal nail infections
Apply to nails and surrounding skin twice daily for up to 6 months (may be extended to 12 months)

Trosyl® (Pfizer) PoM
Cutaneous solution, tioconazole 28%, net price 12 mL (with applicator brush) = £27.38
Excipients none as listed in section 13.1.3
Note Use with caution in child likely to suck affected digits

UNDECENOATES

Side-effects see notes above
Licensed use *Monphytol®* not licensed for use in children under 12 years; *Mycota®* licensed for use in children (age range not specified by manufacturer)

Indication and dose

See under preparations

Mycota® (Thornton & Ross)
Cream, zinc undecenoate 20%, undecenoic acid 5%, net price 25 g = £1.49
Excipients include fragrance
Dose

Treatment of athlete's foot
Apply twice daily continuing for 7 days after lesions have healed

Prevention of athlete's foot
Apply once daily

13 Skin

⌂ **UNDECENOATES** (*continued*)

Powder, zinc undecenoate 20%, undecenoic acid 2%, net price 70 g = £2.07
Excipients include fragrance

Dose

Treatment of athlete's foot

Apply twice daily continuing for 7 days after lesions have healed

Prevention of athlete's foot

Apply once daily

Spray application, undecenoic acid 3.9%, dichlorophen 0.4% (pressurised aerosol pack), net price 100 mL = £2.19
Excipients include fragrance

Dose

Treatment of athlete's foot

Apply twice daily continuing for 7 days after lesions have healed

Prevention of athlete's foot

Apply once daily

13.10.3 Antiviral preparations

See section 12.3.2 for drugs used in *herpetic stomatitis*, section 13.5.1 for *eczema herpeticum*, and section 11.3.3 for viral infections of the *eye*.

Aciclovir cream is used for the treatment of initial and recurrent labial, cutaneous, and genital *herpes simplex infections* in children; treatment should begin as early as possible. Systemic treatment is necessary for buccal or vaginal infections or if cold sores recur frequently (for details of systemic use see section 5.3.2.1).

Herpes labialis Aciclovir cream can be used for the treatment of initial and recurrent labial herpes simplex infections (cold sores). It is best applied at the earliest possible stage, usually when prodromal changes of sensation are felt in the lip and before vesicles appear.

Penciclovir cream is also licensed for the treatment of herpes labialis; it needs to be applied more frequently than aciclovir cream. These creams should not be used in the mouth.

ACICLOVIR
(Acyclovir)

Cautions avoid contact with eyes and mucous membranes

Pregnancy not known to be harmful—manufacturers advise use only when potential benefit outweighs risk; limited absorption from topical aciclovir preparations

Side-effects transient stinging or burning; occasionally erythema, itching or drying of the skin

Licensed use licensed for use in children (age range not specified by manufacturer)

Indication and dose

Herpes simplex infections

Apply to lesions every 4 hours (5 times daily) for 5–10 days, starting at first sign of attack

Herpes simplex and varicella–zoster infections section 5.3.2.1

Eye infections section 11.3.3

[1] **Aciclovir** (Non-proprietary) PoM
Cream, aciclovir 5%, net price 2 g = £1.16, 10 g = £2.09
Excipients include propylene glycol
Brands include *Zuvogen®* (*excipients* include cetyl alcohol, propylene glycol)
Dental prescribing on NHS Aciclovir Cream may be prescribed
1. A 2-g tube and a pump pack are on sale to the public for the treatment of cold sores

Zovirax® (GSK) PoM
Cream, aciclovir 5%, net price 2 g = £4.73, 10 g = £14.24
Excipients include cetostearyl alcohol, propylene glycol

PENCICLOVIR

Cautions avoid contact with eyes and mucous membranes

Side-effects transient stinging, burning, numbness; hypersensitivity reactions also reported

Licensed use not licensed for use in children under 12 years

Vectavir® (Novartis Consumer Health) PoM
Cream, penciclovir 1%, net price 2 g = £4.20
Excipients include cetostearyl alcohol, propylene glycol

Dose

Herpes labialis

Apply to lesions every 2 hours during waking hours for 4 days, starting at first sign of attack

Dental prescribing on NHS May be prescribed as Penciclovir Cream

13 Skin

13.10.4 Parasiticidal preparations

Suitable quantities of parasiticidal preparations

	Skin creams	Lotions	Cream rinses
Scalp (head lice)	—	50–100 mL	50–100 mL
Body (scabies)	30–60 g	100 mL	—
Body (crab lice)	30–60 g	100 mL	—

These amounts are usually suitable for a child 12–18 years for single application

Scabies

Permethrin is used for the treatment of *scabies* (*Sarcoptes scabiei*); **malathion** can be used if permethrin is inappropriate.

Benzyl benzoate is an irritant and should be avoided in children; it is less effective than malathion and permethrin.

Ivermectin (available from 'special-order' manufacturers or specialist importing companies, see p. 957), is used in combination with topical drugs, for the treatment of hyperkeratotic (crusted or 'Norwegian') scabies that does not respond to topical treatment alone.

Application   Although acaricides have traditionally been applied after a hot bath, this is **not** necessary and there is even evidence that a hot bath may increase absorption into the blood, removing them from their site of action on the skin.

All members of the affected household should be treated simultaneously. Treatment should be applied to the whole body including the scalp, neck, face, and ears. Particular attention should be paid to the webs of the fingers and toes and lotion brushed under the ends of nails. Malathion and permethrin should be applied twice, one week apart. It is important to warn users to reapply treatment to the hands if they are washed. Children with hyperkeratotic scabies may require 2 or 3 applications of acaricide on consecutive days to ensure that enough penetrates the skin crusts to kill all the mites.

Itching   The *itch* and *eczema* of scabies persists for some weeks after the infestation has been eliminated and treatment for pruritus and eczema (section 13.5.1) may be required. Application of **crotamiton** can be used to control itching after treatment with more effective acaricides. A topical **corticosteroid** (section 13.4) may help to reduce itch and inflammation after scabies has been treated successfully; however, persistent symptoms suggest failure of scabies eradication. Oral administration of a **sedating antihistamine** (section 3.4.1) at night may also be useful.

Head lice

Dimeticone is effective against head lice (*Pediculus humanus capitis*) and acts on the surface of the organism. **Malathion**, an organophosphorous insecticide, is an alternative but resistance has been reported. Benzyl benzoate is licensed for the treatment of head lice but it is not recommended for use in children.

Head lice infestation (pediculosis) should be treated using lotion or liquid formulations only if live lice are present. Shampoos are diluted too much in use to be effective. A contact time of 8–12 hours or overnight treatment is recommended for lotions and liquids; a 2-hour treatment is not sufficient to kill eggs.

In general, a course of treatment for head lice should be 2 applications of a parasiticidal product 7 days apart to kill lice emerging from any eggs that survive the first application. All affected individuals in a household should be treated at the same time.

Wet combing methods   Head lice can be mechanically removed by combing wet hair meticulously with a plastic detection comb (probably for at least 30 minutes each time) over the whole scalp at 4-day intervals for a minimum of 2 weeks and continued until no lice are found on 3 consecutive sessions; hair conditioner or vegetable oil can be used to facilitate the process. Several products are available and some are prescribable on the NHS.

13 Skin

Crab lice

Permethrin and **malathion** are used to eliminate *crab lice* (*Pthirus pubis*); permethrin is not licensed for treatment of crab lice in children under 18 years. An aqueous preparation should be applied, allowed to dry naturally and washed off after 12 hours; a second treatment is needed after 7 days to kill lice emerging from surviving eggs. All surfaces of the body should be treated, including the scalp, neck, and face (paying particular attention to the eyebrows and other facial hair). A different insecticide should be used if a course of treatment fails.

Parasiticidal preparations

Dimeticone coats head lice and interferes with water balance in lice by preventing excretion of water; it is less active against eggs and treatment should be repeated after 7 days.

Malathion is recommended for *scabies*, *head lice* and *crab lice* (see notes above). The risk of systemic effects associated with 1–2 applications of malathion is considered to be very low; however, except in the treatment of hyperkeratotic scabies (see notes above), applications of malathion liquid repeated at intervals of less than 1 week *or* application for more than 3 consecutive weeks should be **avoided** since the likelihood of eradication of lice is not increased.

Permethrin is effective for *scabies*. It is active against *head lice* but the formulation and licensed methods of application of the current products make them unsuitable for the treatment of head lice. Permethrin is also effective against *crab lice* but it is not licensed for this purpose in children under 18 years.

DIMETICONE

Cautions avoid contact with eyes

Side-effects skin irritation

Licensed use not licensed for use in children under 6 months except under medical supervision

Indication and dose

Head lice

Rub into dry hair and scalp, allow to dry naturally, shampoo after 8 hours (or overnight); repeat application after 7 days

Hedrin® (Thornton & Ross)

Lotion, dimeticone 4%, net price 50 mL = £2.98, 120-mL spray pack = £7.13, 150 mL = £6.83

Note Patients should be told to keep their hair away from fire and flames during treatment

MALATHION

Cautions avoid contact with eyes; do not use on broken or secondarily infected skin; do not use lotion more than once a week for 3 consecutive weeks; alcoholic lotions **not** recommended for head lice in children with severe eczema or asthma, or for scabies or crab lice (see notes above)

Side-effects skin irritation and hypersensitivity reactions; chemical burns also reported

Licensed use not licensed for use in children under 6 months except under medical supervision

Indication and dose

See notes above and under preparations

Head lice

Rub into dry hair and scalp, allow to dry naturally, remove by washing after 12 hours; repeat application after 7 days (see also notes above)

Crab lice

Apply over whole body, allow to dry naturally, wash off after 12 hours or overnight; repeat application after 7 days

Scabies

Apply over whole body, and wash off after 24 hours; if hands are washed with soap within 24 hours, they should be retreated; see also notes above; repeat application after 7 days

Note For scabies, manufacturer recommends application to the body but not necessarily to the head and neck. However, application should be extended to the scalp, neck, face, and ears

Derbac-M® (SSL)

Liquid, malathion 0.5% in an aqueous basis, net price 50 mL = £2.37, 200 mL = £5.93

Excipients include cetostearyl alcohol, fragrance, hydroxybenzoates (parabens)

For crab lice, head lice, and scabies

◢ PERMETHRIN

Cautions avoid contact with eyes; do not use on broken or secondarily infected skin

Side-effects pruritus, erythema, and stinging; rarely rashes and oedema

Licensed use *Dermal Cream* (scabies), not licensed for use in children under 2 months; children aged 2 months–2 years, medical supervison required; not licensed for treatment of crab lice in children under 18 years; *Creme Rinse* (head lice) not licensed for use in children under 6 months except under medical supervision

Indication and dose

See notes above

Scabies

Apply 5% preparation over whole body including face, neck, scalp and ears; wash off after 8–12 hours; if hands washed with soap within 8 hours of application, they should be treated

again with cream (see notes above); repeat application after 7 days

Note Manufacturer recommends application to the body but to exclude head and neck. However, application should be extended to the scalp, neck, face, and ears

Permethrin (Non-proprietary)
Cream, permethrin 5%, net price 30 g = £5.51

Lyclear® Creme Rinse (Chefaro UK) ◢
Cream rinse, permethrin 1% in basis containing isopropyl alcohol 20%, net price 59 mL = £2.38, 2 × 59-mL pack = £4.32
Excipients include cetyl alcohol

Note Use not recommended, therefore no dose stated (product too diluted in use and insufficient contact time)

Lyclear® Dermal Cream (Chefaro UK)
Dermal cream, permethrin 5%, net price 30 g = £5.71. Label: 10, patient information leaflet
Excipients include butylated hydroxytoluene, wool fat derivative

13.10.5 Preparations for minor cuts and abrasions

Cetrimide cream is used to treat minor cuts and abrasions. **Proflavine** cream may be used to treat infected wounds or burns, but has now been largely superseded by other antiseptics or suitable antibacterials.

Cetrimide Cream, BP
Cream, cetrimide 0.5% in a suitable water-miscible basis such as cetostearyl alcohol 5%, liquid paraffin 50% in freshly boiled and cooled purified water, net price 50 g = £1.11

Proflavine Cream, BPC
Cream, proflavine hemisulphate 0.1%, yellow beeswax 2.5%, chlorocresol 0.1%, liquid paraffin 67.3%, freshly boiled and cooled purified water 25%, wool fat 5%, net price 100 mL = 68p
Excipients include beeswax, wool fat

Note Stains clothing

Collodion

Flexible collodion may be used to seal minor cuts and wounds that have partially healed.

Collodion, Flexible, BP
Collodion, castor oil 2.5%, colophony 2.5% in a collodion basis, prepared by dissolving pyroxylin (10%) in a mixture of 3 volumes of ether and 1

volume of alcohol (90%), net price 10 mL = 25p. Label: 15
Contra-indications allergy to colophony in elastic adhesive plasters and tape

Skin tissue adhesive

Tissue adhesives are used for closure of minor skin wounds and for additional suture support. They should be applied by an appropriately trained healthcare professional. Skin tissue adhesives may cause skin sensitisation.

Dermabond ProPen® (Ethicon)
Topical skin adhesive, sterile, octyl 2-cyanoacrylate, net price 0.5 mL = £18.38

Epiglu® (Schuco)
Tissue adhesive, sterile, ethyl-2-cyanoacrylate 954.5 mg/g, polymethylmethacrylate, net price 4 × 3-g vials = £149.50 (with dispensing pipettes and pallete)

Histoacryl® (Braun)
Tissue adhesive, sterile, enbucrilate, net price 5 × 200-mg unit (blue) = £32.00, 10 × 200-mg unit (blue) = £67.20, 5 × 500-mg unit (clear or blue) = £34.65, 10 × 500-mg unit (blue) = £69.30

LiquiBand® (MedLogic)
Tissue adhesive, sterile, enbucrilate, net price 0.5-g amp = £5.50

13.11 Skin cleansers, antiseptics, and preparations for promotion of wound healing

Soap or detergent is used with water to cleanse intact skin but they can irritate infantile skin; emollient preparations such as aqueous cream or emulsifying ointment (section 13.2.1) that do not irritate the skin are best used in place of soap or detergent for cleansing dry or irritated skin.

An antiseptic is used for skin that is infected or that is susceptible to recurrent infection. Detergent preparations containing **chlorhexidine** or **povidone–iodine**, which should be thoroughly rinsed off, are used. Emollients may also contain antiseptics (section 13.2.1).

Antiseptics such as **chlorhexidine** or **povidone–iodine** are used on intact skin before surgical procedures; their antiseptic effect is enhanced by an alcoholic solvent. Antiseptic solutions containing **cetrimide** can be used if a detergent effect is also required. On neonatal skin, regular use of povidone–iodine and of preparations containing alcohol should be avoided.

For irrigating ulcers or wounds, lukewarm sterile **sodium chloride 0.9% solution** is used but tap water is often appropriate.

Potassium permanganate solution 1 in 10 000, a mild antiseptic with astringent properties, can be used as a soak for exudative eczematous areas (section 13.5.1); treatment should be stopped when the skin becomes dry. Potassium permanganate can stain skin and nails especially with prolonged use.

13.11.1 Alcohols and saline

ALCOHOL

Cautions flammable; avoid broken skin; patients have suffered severe burns when diathermy has been preceded by application of alcoholic skin disinfectants

Contra-indications neonates, see section 13.1

Indication and dose

Skin preparation before injection

Apply to skin as necessary

SODIUM CHLORIDE

Indication and dose

See notes above

Nebuliser diluent section 3.1.5

Sodium depletion section 9.2.1.2

Electrolyte imbalance section 9.2.2.1

Eye section 11.8.1

Oral hygiene section 12.3.4

Sodium Chloride (Non-proprietary)
Solution (sterile), sodium chloride 0.9%, net price 25 × 20-mL unit = £5.50, 200–mL can = £2.65, 1 litre = 97p

Industrial Methylated Spirit, BP
Solution, 19 volumes of ethanol and 1 volume approved wood naphtha, net price '66 OP' (containing 95% by volume alcohol) 100 mL = 39p; '74 OP' (containing 99% by volume alcohol) 100 mL = 39p. Label: 15

Surgical Spirit, BP
Spirit, methyl salicylate 0.5 mL, diethyl phthalate 2%, castor oil 2.5%, in industrial methylated spirit, net price 100 mL = 20p. Label: 15

Flowfusor® (Fresenius Kabi)
Solution (sterile), sodium chloride 0.9%, net price 120-mL Bellows Pack = £1.53

Irriclens® (ConvaTec)
Solution in aerosol can (sterile), sodium chloride 0.9%, net price 240-mL can = £3.27

Irripod® (C D Medical)
Solution (sterile), sodium chloride 0.9%, net price 25 × 20-mL sachet = £5.50

Miniversol® (Aguettant)
Solution (sterile), sodium chloride 0.9%, net price 30 × 45-mL unit = £13.20; 30 × 100-mL unit = £19.50

Normasol® (Mölnlycke)
Solution (sterile), sodium chloride 0.9%, net price 25 × 25-mL sachet = £6.10; 10 × 100-mL sachet = £7.41

13

Skin

◻ **SODIUM CHLORIDE** (*continued*)

Stericlens® (C D Medical)
Solution in aerosol can (sterile), sodium chloride 0.9%, net price 100-mL can = £1.94, 240-mL can = £2.95

Steripod® Sodium Chloride (Medlock)
Solution (sterile), sodium chloride 0.9%, net price 25 × 20-mL sachet = £7.51

13.11.2 Chlorhexidine salts

CHLORHEXIDINE

Cautions avoid contact with eyes, brain, meninges and middle ear; not for use in body cavities; alcoholic solutions not suitable before diathermy or for use on neonatal skin
Side-effects occasional sensitivity

Indication and dose
See under preparations

Bladder irrigation and catheter patency solutions section 7.4.4

Chlorhexidine 0.05% (Baxter)
2000 Solution (sterile), pink, chlorhexidine acetate 0.05%, net price 500 mL = 72p, 1000 mL = 77p
For cleansing and disinfecting wounds and burns

Cepton® (LPC)
Skin wash (= solution), red, chlorhexidine gluconate 1%, net price 150 mL = £2.48
For use as skin wash in acne

Lotion, blue, chlorhexidine gluconate 0.1%, net price 150 mL = £2.48
For skin disinfection in acne

ChloraPrep® (Enturia)
Cutaneous solution, sterile, chlorhexidine gluconate 2% in isopropyl alcohol 70%, net price (single applicator) 0.67 mL = 30p, 1.5 mL = 55p, 3 mL = 85p, 10.5 mL = £2.92, 26 mL = £6.50; (single applicator, with tint) 3 mL = 89p, 10.5 mL = £3.07, 26 mL = £6.83
For skin disinfection before invasive procedures; Child under 2 months not recommended
Note Flammable

CX Antiseptic Dusting Powder® (Ecolab)
Dusting powder, sterile, chlorhexidine acetate 1%, net price 15 g = £2.68
For skin disinfection

Hibiscrub® (Mölnlycke)
Cleansing solution, red, chlorhexidine gluconate 4%, perfumed, in a surfactant solution, net price 250 mL = £4.25, 500 mL = £5.25, 5 litres = £16.20
Excipients include fragrance
Use instead of soap for pre-operative hand and skin preparation and for general hand and skin disinfection

Hibi® Liquid Hand Rub (Mölnlycke)
Solution, chlorhexidine gluconate 0.5%, in isopropyl alcohol 70% with emollients, net price 500 mL = £5.25
To be used undiluted for hand and skin disinfection

Hibitane Obstetric® (Centrapharm)
Cream, chlorhexidine gluconate solution 5% (≡ 1% chlorhexidine gluconate), in a pourable water-miscible basis, net price 250 mL = £4.44
For use in obstetrics and gynaecology as an antiseptic and lubricant (for application to skin around vulva and perineum and to hands of midwife or doctor)

Hydrex® (Ecolab)
Solution, chlorhexidine gluconate solution 2.5% (≡ chlorhexidine gluconate 0.5%), in an alcoholic solution, net price 600 mL (clear) = £2.06; 600 mL (pink) = £2.06, 200-mL spray = £1.77, 500-mL spray = £3.01; 600 mL (blue) = £2.26
Note Flammable
For pre-operative skin disinfection

Surgical scrub, chlorhexidine gluconate 4% in a surfactant solution, net price 250 mL = £1.93, 500 mL = £2.05
For pre-operative hand and skin preparation and for general hand disinfection

Unisept® (Medlock)
Solution (sterile), pink, chlorhexidine gluconate 0.05%, net price 25 × 25-mL sachet = £5.40; 10 × 100-mL sachet = £6.67
For cleansing and disinfecting wounds and burns and swabbing in obstetrics

◀ **With cetrimide**

Tisept® (Medlock)
Solution (sterile), yellow, chlorhexidine gluconate 0.015%, cetrimide 0.15%, net price 25 × 25-mL sachet = £5.20; 10 × 100-mL sachet = £6.68
To be used undiluted for general skin disinfection and wound cleansing

Travasept 100® (Baxter)
Solution (sterile), yellow, chlorhexidine acetate 0.015%, cetrimide 0.15%, net price 500 mL = 72p, 1 litre = 77p
To be used undiluted in skin disinfection such as wound cleansing and obstetrics

Concentrates

Hibitane® Plus 5% Concentrate (Mölnlycke)
Solution, red, chlorhexidine gluconate 5%, in a perfumed aqueous solution, net price 5 litres = £14.50

Dose

Pre-operative skin preparation
Dilute 1 in 10 (0.5%) with alcohol 70%

General skin disinfection
Dilute 1 in 100 (0.05%) with water

Note Alcoholic solutions not suitable for use before diathermy (see Alcohol, p. 727) or on neonatal skin

13 **Skin**

13.11.3 Cationic surfactants and soaps

CETRIMIDE

Cautions avoid contact with eyes; avoid use in body cavities

Side-effects skin irritation and occasionally sensitisation

Indication and dose

Skin disinfection

◀Preparations

Ingredient of *Tisept®* and *Travasept® 100*, see above

13.11.4 Iodine

POVIDONE–IODINE

Cautions broken skin (see below)

Large open wounds The application of povidone–iodine to large wounds or severe burns may produce systemic adverse effects such as metabolic acidosis, hypernatraemia, and impairment of renal function

Contra-indications preterm neonate gestational age under 32 weeks; infants body-weight under 1.5 kg; regular use in neonates; thyroid disorders; concomitant lithium treatment

Renal impairment avoid regular application to inflamed or broken skin or mucosa

Pregnancy sufficient iodine may be absorbed to affect the fetal thyroid in the second and third trimester

Breast-feeding avoid regular or excessive use

Side-effects rarely sensitivity; may interfere with thyroid function tests

Indication and dose

Skin disinfection see preparations

Betadine® (Mölnlycke)

Dry powder spray, povidone–iodine 2.5% in a pressurised aerosol unit, net price 150-g unit = £2.63

For skin disinfection, particularly minor wounds and infections; child under 2 years not recommended

Note Not for use in serous cavities

Savlon® Dry (Novartis Consumer Health)

Powder spray, povidone–iodine 1.14% in a pressurised aerosol unit, net price 50-mL unit = £2.39

For minor wounds

Videne® (Ecolab)

Alcoholic tincture, povidone–iodine 10%, net price 500 mL = £2.50

Dose

Apply undiluted in pre-operative skin disinfection

Note Flammable—caution in procedures involving hot wire cautery and diathermy; avoid use in neonates

Antiseptic solution, povidone–iodine 10% in aqueous solution, net price 500 mL = £2.50

Dose

Apply undiluted in pre-operative skin disinfection and general antisepsis

Surgical scrub, povidone–iodine 7.5% in aqueous solution, net price 500 mL = £2.50

Dose

Use as a pre-operative scrub for hand and skin disinfection

13.11.5 Phenolics

Triclosan has been used for disinfection of the hands and wounds, and for disinfection of the skin before surgery.

13.11.6 Oxidisers and dyes

HYDROGEN PEROXIDE

Cautions large or deep wounds; avoid on healthy skin and eyes; bleaches fabric; incompatible with products containing iodine or potassium permanganate

Licensed use licensed for use in children (age range not specified by manufacturer)

Indication and dose

Superficial bacterial skin infection see under preparation below

Crystacide® (GP Pharma)

Cream, hydrogen peroxide 1%, net price 10 g = £4.82, 25 g = £8.07, 40 g = £11.62

Dose

Superficial bacterial skin infection

Apply 2–3 times daily for up to 3 weeks

Excipients include edetic acid (EDTA), propylene glycol

13

Skin

POTASSIUM PERMANGANATE

Cautions irritant to mucous membranes

Indication and dose

Cleansing and deodorising suppurating eczematous reactions (section 13.5.1) and wounds

For wet dressings or baths, use approx. 0.01% (1 in 10 000) solution
Note Stains skin and clothing

Potassium Permanganate Solution
Solution, potassium permanganate 0.1% (1 in 1000) in water

Note to be diluted 1 in 10 to provide a 0.01% (1 in 10 000) solution

Permitabs® (Alliance)
Solution tablets, for preparation of topical solution, potassium permanganate 400 mg, net price 30-tab pack = £9.85

Note 1 tablet dissolved in 4 litres of water provides a 0.01% (1 in 10 000) solution

13.11.7 Preparations for promotion of wound healing

Desloughing agents Alginate, hydrogel, and hydrocolloid dressings (BNF Appendix 8) are effective in wound debridement. Sterile larvae (maggots) (*LarvE®*, Zoobiotic) are also used for managing sloughing wounds and are prescribable on the NHS.

Desloughing solutions and creams are of little clinical value. Substances applied to an open area are easily absorbed and perilesional skin is easily sensitised.

Growth factor A topical preparation of **becaplermin** (recombinant human platelet-derived growth factor) is used as an adjunct treatment of full-thickness, neuropathic, diabetic ulcers. It enhances the formulation of granulation tissue, thereby promoting wound healing.

For further information on wound management products and elastic hosiery, see BNF Appendix 8.

BECAPLERMIN

(Recombinant human platelet-derived growth factor)

Cautions avoid on sites with infection or peripheral arteriopathy

Contra-indications malignant disease

Side-effects pain; infections including cellulitis and osteomyelitis, local reactions including erythema; *rarely* bullous eruption, oedema, and hypertrophic granulation

Licensed use not licensed for use in children

Indication and dose

Full-thickness, neuropathic, diabetic ulcers (no larger than 5 cm²)

Apply thin layer daily and cover with gauze dressing moistened with physiological saline; max. duration of treatment 20 weeks (reassess if no healing after first 10 weeks)

Regranex® (Janssen-Cilag) [PoM]
Gel, becaplermin (recombinant human platelet-derived growth factor) 0.01%, net price 15 g = £245.78
Excipients include hydroxybenzoates (parabens)

13.12 Antiperspirants

Aluminium chloride is a potent antiperspirant used in the treatment of axillary, palmar, and plantar hyperhidrosis. Aluminium salts are also incorporated in preparations used for minor fungal skin infections associated with hyperhidrosis.

In more severe cases specialists use tap water or **glycopyrronium bromide** (as a 0.05% solution) in the iontophoretic treatment of hyperhidrosis of palms and soles.

Botulinum A toxin-haemagglutinin complex (section 4.9.3) is available for use intradermally for severe hyperhidrosis of the axillae unresponsive to topical antiperspirant or other antihidrotic treatment; intradermal treatment is unlikely to be tolerated by most children and should be administered under hospital specialist supervision.

◼ ALUMINIUM SALTS

Cautions avoid contact with eyes or mucous membranes; avoid use on broken or irritated skin; do not shave axillae or use depilatories within 12 hours of application; avoid contact with clothing

Side-effects skin irritation

Licensed use licensed for use in children (age range not specified by manufacturer)

Indication and dose

> **Hyperhidrosis affecting axillae, hands or feet**
>
> Apply liquid formulation at night to dry skin, wash off the following morning, initially apply daily then reduce frequency as condition improves—do not bathe immediately before use

> **Hyperhidrosis, bromidrosis, intertrigo, and prevention of tinea pedis and related conditions**
>
> Apply powder to dry skin

Anhydrol® Forte (Dermal)
Solution (= application), aluminium chloride hexahydrate 20% in an alcoholic basis, net price 60-mL bottle with roll-on applicator = £2.54. Label: 15
Excipients none as listed in section 13.1.3

¹ Driclor® (Stiefel)
Application, aluminium chloride hexahydrate 20% in an alcoholic basis, net price 60-mL bottle with roll-on applicator = £2.82. Label: 15
Excipients none as listed in section 13.1.3
1. A 30-mL pack is on sale to the public

ZeaSORB® (Stiefel)
Dusting powder, aldioxa 0.22%, chloroxylenol 0.5%, net price 50 g = £2.61
Excipients include fragrance

◼ GLYCOPYRRONIUM BROMIDE

Cautions see section 15.1.3 (but poorly absorbed and systemic effects unlikely)

Contra-indications see section 15.1.3 (but poorly absorbed and systemic effects unlikely), infections affecting the treatment site

Side-effects see section 15.1.3 (but poorly absorbed and systemic effects unlikely), tingling at administration site

Licensed use licensed for use in children (age range not specified by manufacturer)

Indication and dose

> **Iontophoretic treatment of hyperhidrosis**
>
> Consult product literature; only 1 site to be treated at a time, max. 2 sites treated in any 24 hours, treatment not to be repeated within 7 days

Other indications section 15.1.3

Robinul® (Anpharm) [PoM]
Powder, glycopyrronium bromide, net price 3 g = £110.00

13.13 Topical circulatory preparations

These preparations are used to improve circulation in conditions such as bruising and superficial thrombophlebitis but are of little value. First aid measures such as rest, ice, compression, and elevation should be used. Topical preparations containing heparinoids should not be used on large areas of skin, broken or sensitive skin, or mucous membranes. Chilblains are best managed by avoidance of exposure to cold; neither systemic nor topical vasodilator therapy is established as being effective.

Hirudoid® (Genus)
Cream, heparinoid 0.3% in a vanishing-cream basis, net price 50 g = £3.99
Excipients include cetostearyl alcohol, hydroxybenzoates (parabens)

Dose
Superficial thrombophlebitis, bruising, and haematoma
> **Child 5–18 years** apply up to 4 times daily

Gel, heparinoid 0.3%, net price 50 g = £3.99
Excipients include propylene glycol, fragrance

Dose
Superficial thrombophlebitis, bruising, and haematoma
> **Child 5–18 years** apply up to 4 times daily

13

Skin

14 Immunological products and vaccines

14.1 Active immunity

Active immunity can be acquired by natural disease or by vaccination. **Vaccines** stimulate production of antibodies and other components of the immune mechanism; they consist of either:

1. a *live attenuated* form of a virus (e.g. measles, mumps, and rubella vaccine) or bacteria (e.g. BCG vaccine), or
2. *inactivated* preparations of a virus (e.g. influenza vaccine) or bacteria, or
3. *detoxified* exotoxins produced by a micro-organism (e.g. tetanus vaccine), or
4. *extracts of* a micro-organism, which may be derived from the organism (e.g. pneumococcal vaccine) or produced by recombinant DNA technology (e.g. hepatitis B vaccine).

Live attenuated vaccines usually produce durable immunity but not always as long-lasting as that resulting from natural infection.

Inactivated vaccines may require a primary series of injections of vaccine to produce an adequate antibody response, and in most cases booster (reinforcing) injections are required; the duration of immunity varies from months to many years. Some inactivated vaccines are adsorbed onto an adjuvant (such as aluminium hydroxide) to enhance the antibody response.

> Advice in this chapter reflects that in the handbook *Immunisation against Infectious Disease* (2006), which in turn reflects the guidance of the Joint Committee on Vaccination and Immunisation (JCVI).
>
> Chapters from the handbook are available at www.dh.gov.uk
>
> The advice in this chapter also incorporates changes announced by the Chief Medical Officer and Health Department Updates.

Cautions Most children can safely receive the majority of vaccines. Vaccination may be postponed if the child is suffering from an acute illness; however, it is not necessary to postpone immunisation in children with minor illnesses without fever or systemic upset. See also Predisposition to Neurological Problems, below. For individuals with bleeding disorders, see Route of Administration, below. If alcohol or disinfectant is used for cleansing the skin it should be allowed to evaporate before vaccination to prevent possible inactivation of live vaccines.

When two live virus vaccines are required (and are not available as a combined preparation) they should be given either simultaneously at different sites or separated by an interval of at least 4 weeks. For **interactions** see Appendix 1 (vaccines).

See also Cautions under individual vaccines.

Contra-indications Vaccines are contra-indicated in children who have a confirmed anaphylactic reaction to a preceding dose of a vaccine containing the same antigens or vaccine component (such as antibacterials in viral vaccines). The presence of the following excipients in vaccines and immunological products has been noted under the relevant entries:

Gelatin	Neomycin	Streptomycin
Gentamicin	Penicillins	Thiomersal
Kanamycin	Polymyxin B	

Hypersensitivity to egg with evidence of previous anaphylactic reaction, contra-indicates influenza vaccine (prepared in hens' eggs), tick-borne encephalitis vaccine, and yellow fever vaccine. See also Cautions under MMR vaccine.

See also Vaccines and HIV infection, below.

Live vaccines may be contra-indicated temporarily in children who are:

● immunosuppressed (see Impaired Immune Response, below);

● pregnant (see Pregnancy and Breast-feeding, below).

See also Contra-indications under individual vaccines.

Impaired immune response Immune response to vaccines may be reduced in immunosuppressed children and there is also a risk of generalised infection with live vaccines. Severely immunosuppressed children should not be given live vaccines (including those with severe primary immunodeficiency). Specialist advice should be sought for children being treated with high doses of corticosteroids (dose equivalents of prednisolone: **children**, 2 mg/kg (or more than 40 mg) daily for at least 1 week or 1 mg/kg daily for 1 month), or other immunosuppressive drugs[1], and for children with malignant conditions undergoing chemotherapy or generalised radiotherapy[1,2]. For special reference to *HIV infection*, see below.

The Royal College of Paediatrics and Child Health has produced a statement, *Immunisation of the Immunocompromised Child (2002)* (available at www.rcpch.ac.uk).

Pregnancy Live vaccines should not be administered routinely during pregnancy because of the theoretical risk of fetal infection but where there is a significant risk of exposure to disease (e.g. to yellow fever), the need for vaccination usually outweighs any possible risk to the fetus. Termination of pregnancy following inadvertent immunisation is not recommended. There is no evidence of risk from vaccinating pregnant women with inactivated viral or bacterial vaccines or toxoids. For use of specific vaccines during pregnancy, see under individual vaccines.

Breast-feeding Although there is a theoretical risk of live vaccine being present in breast milk, vaccination is not contra-indicated for women who are breast-feeding when there is significant risk of exposure to disease. There is no evidence of risk from vaccinating women who are breast-feeding, with inactivated viral or bacterial vaccines or toxoids. For use of specific vaccines during breast-feeding, see under individual vaccines.

Side-effects Injection of a vaccine may be followed by local reactions such as pain, inflammation, redness, and lymphangitis. An induration or sterile abscess may develop at the injection site. Gastro-intestinal disturbances, fever, headache, irritability, loss of appetite, fatigue, myalgia, and malaise are among the most commonly reported side-effects. Other side-effects include influenza-like symptoms, dizziness, paraesthesia, asthenia, drowsiness, arthralgia, rash, and lymphadenopathy. Hypersensitivity reactions, such as bronchospasm, angioedema, urticaria, and anaphylaxis, are very rare but can be fatal (see section 3.4.3 for management of allergic emergencies).

Oral vaccines, such as cholera, live poliomyelitis, rotavirus, and live typhoid, can also cause gastro-intestinal disturbances such as nausea, vomiting, abdominal pain and cramps, and diarrhoea.

See also Predisposition to Neurological Problems, below.

Some vaccines (e.g. poliomyelitis) produce very few reactions, while others (e.g. measles, mumps and rubella) may cause a very mild form of the disease. Occasionally more serious adverse reactions can occur—these should always be reported to the CHM (see Adverse Reactions to Drugs, p. 15).

There is no evidence that premature babies are at increased risk of adverse reactions to vaccines, see also Preterm birth, below.

> **Predisposition to neurological problems**
> When there is a personal or family history of *febrile* convulsions, there is an increased risk of these occurring during fever from any cause including immunisation, but this is not a contra-indication to immunisation. In children who have had a seizure associated with fever without neurological deterioration, immunisation is *recommended*; advice on the *prevention of fever* (see Post-immunisation Pyrexia in Infants, below) should be given before immunisation. When a child has had a convulsion not associated with fever, and the neurological condition is not deteriorating, immunisation is *recommended*.
>
> Children with stable neurological disorders (e.g. spina bifida, congenital brain abnormality, and peri-natal hypoxic-ischaemic encephalopathy) should be immunised according to the recommended schedule.
>
> When there is a *still evolving neurological problem*, including poorly controlled epilepsy, immunisation should be deferred and the child referred to a specialist. Immunisation is recommended if a cause for the neurological disorder is identified. If a cause is not identified, immunisation should be deferred until the condition is stable.

> **Post-immunisation pyrexia in infants**
> The parent should be advised that if pyrexia develops after childhood immunisation and the infant seems distressed, a dose of paracetamol can be given and, if necessary, a second dose can be given 6 hours later; ibuprofen may be used if paracetamol is unsuitable. The parent should be warned to seek medical advice if the pyrexia persists.
>
> For post-immunisation pyrexia in an infant aged 2–3 months, the dose of paracetamol is 60 mg; the dose of ibuprofen is 50 mg (on a doctor's advice). An oral syringe can be obtained from any pharmacy to give the small volume required.

Further information on adverse effects associated with specific vaccines can be found under individual vaccines.

Vaccines and HIV infection   HIV-positive children with or without symptoms can receive the following live vaccines:

> MMR (but avoid if immunity significantly impaired), varicella-zoster (but avoid if immunity significantly impaired—consult product literature);[1]

and the following inactivated vaccines:

> anthrax, cholera (oral), diphtheria, haemophilus influenzae type b, hepatitis A, hepatitis B, human papilloma virus, influenza, meningococcal, pertussis, pneumococcal, poliomyelitis[2], rabies, tetanus, tick-borne encephalitis, typhoid (injection).

HIV-positive children should **not** receive:

> BCG, typhoid (oral), yellow fever[3]

Note The above advice differs from that for other immunocompromised children; Immunisation of HIV-infected Children issued by Children's HIV Association (CHIVA) are available at www.chiva.org.uk

1. Use of normal immunoglobulin should be considered after exposure to measles (see p. 764) and varicella–zoster immunoglobulin considered after exposure to chickenpox or herpes zoster (see p. 767).
2. Inactivated poliomyelitis vaccine is now used instead of oral poliomyelitis vaccine for routine immunisation of children.
3. If yellow fever risk is unavoidable, specialist advice should be sought.

Immunisation schedule

Vaccines for the childhood immunisation schedule should be obtained from **local health organisations** or **direct from Movianto**—not to be prescribed on FP10 (HS21 in Northern Ireland; GP10 in Scotland; WP10 in Wales).

> **Preterm birth**
>
> Babies born preterm should receive all routine immunisations based on their actual date of birth. The risk of apnoea following vaccination is increased in preterm babies, particularly in those born at or before 28 weeks postmenstrual age. If babies at risk of apnoea are in hospital at the time of their first immunisation, they should be monitored for 48 hours after immunisation. If a baby develops apnoea, bradycardia, or desaturation after the first immunisation, the second immunisation should also be given in hospital with similar monitoring. Seroconversion may be unreliable in babies born earlier than 28 weeks' gestation or in babies treated with corticosteroids for chronic lung disease; consideration should be given to testing for antibodies against *Haemophilus influenzae* (type b), meningococcal C, and hepatitis B after primary immunisation.

When to immunise (for preterm infants—see note above)	Vaccine given and dose schedule (for details of dose, see under individual vaccines)
Neonates at risk only	• **BCG Vaccine** See section 14.4, BCG Vaccines • **Hepatitis B Vaccine** See section 14.4, Hepatitis B Vaccine
2 months	• **Diphtheria, Tetanus, Pertussis (Acellular, Component), Poliomyelitis (Inactivated), and Haemophilus Type b Conjugate Vaccine (Adsorbed)** First dose • **Pneumococcal Polysaccharide Conjugate Vaccine (Adsorbed)** First dose
3 months	• **Diphtheria, Tetanus, Pertussis (Acellular, Component), Poliomyelitis (Inactivated), and Haemophilus Type b Conjugate Vaccine (Adsorbed)** Second dose • **Meningococcal Group C Conjugate Vaccine** First dose
4 months	• **Diphtheria, Tetanus, Pertussis (Acellular, Component), Poliomyelitis (Inactivated), and Haemophilus Type b Conjugate Vaccine (Adsorbed)** Third dose • **Meningococcal Group C Conjugate Vaccine** Second dose • **Pneumococcal Polysaccharide Conjugate Vaccine (Adsorbed)** Second dose
12 months[1]	• **Haemophilus Type b Conjugate Vaccine and Meningococcal Group C Conjugate Vaccine** Single booster dose
13 months[1]	• **Measles, Mumps and Rubella Vaccine, Live (MMR)** First dose • **Pneumococcal Polysaccharide Conjugate Vaccine (Adsorbed)** Single booster dose
Between 3 years and 4 months, and 5 years	• **Adsorbed Diphtheria [low dose], Tetanus, Pertussis (Acellular, Component) and Poliomyelitis (Inactivated) Vaccine** *or* **Adsorbed Diphtheria, Tetanus, Pertussis (Acellular, Component) and Poliomyelitis (Inactivated) Vaccine** *or* **Diphtheria, Tetanus, Pertussis (Acellular, Component) Poliomyelitis (Inactivated) and Haemophilus Type b Conjugate Vaccine (Adsorbed)** Single booster dose **Note:** Preferably allow interval of at least 3 years after completing primary course; can be given at same session as MMR Vaccine but use separate syringe and needle, and give in different limb • **Measles, Mumps and Rubella Vaccine, Live (MMR)** Second dose
12–13 years (females only)	• **Human Papilloma Virus Vaccine** 3 doses; second dose 1–2 months, and third dose 6 months after first dose[2]
13–18 years	• **Adsorbed Diphtheria [low dose], Tetanus, and Poliomyelitis (Inactivated) Vaccine** Single booster dose
During adult life, women of child-bearing age susceptible to rubella	• **Measles, Mumps and Rubella Vaccine, Live (MMR)** Women of child-bearing age who have not received 2 doses of a rubella-containing vaccine or who do not have a positive antibody test for rubella should be offered rubella immunisation (using the MMR vaccine)—exclude pregnancy before immunisation, but see also section 14.4, Measles, Mumps and Rubella Vaccine
During adult life, if not previously immunised	• **Adsorbed Diphtheria [low dose], Tetanus, and Poliomyelitis (Inactivated) Vaccine** 3 doses at intervals of 1 month Booster dose at least 1 year after primary course and again 5–10 years later

14 Immunological products and vaccines

---

1. Alternatively, the vaccines recommended at 12 months and 13 months can be given together at either 12 or 13 months of age
2. The two human papilloma virus vaccines are not interchangeable and one vaccine product should be used for the entire course; however, Department of Health (November 2008) states for individuals with previous incomplete vaccination with *Gardasil*®, who are eligible for HPV vaccination under the national programme, *Cervarix*® can be used to complete the vaccination course if necessary; the individual must be informed that *Cervarix*® does not protect against genital warts.

Vaccines and asplenia The following vaccines are recommended for asplenic children or those with splenic dysfunction:

haemophilus influenzae type b, influenza, meningococcal group C, pneumococcal.

For antibiotic prophylaxis in asplenia see p. 312.

Route of administration Vaccines should not be given intravenously. Most vaccines are given by the intramuscular route; some vaccines are given by other routes—the intradermal route for BCG vaccine, deep subcutaneous route for Japanese encephalitis and varicella vaccines, and the oral route for cholera, live poliomyelitis, rotavirus, and live typhoid vaccines. The intramuscular route should not be used in children with **bleeding disorders** such as haemophilia or thrombocytopenia; vaccines usually given by the intramuscular route should be given by deep subcutaneous injection instead.

Note The Department of Health has advised *against the use of jet guns* for vaccination owing to the risk of transmitting blood-borne infections, such as HIV.

High-risk groups

For information on high-risk groups, see section 14.4 under individual vaccines

BCG Vaccines, p. 737

Hepatitis A Vaccine, p. 743

Hepatitis B Vaccine, p. 745

Influenza Vaccine, p. 748

Pneumococcal Vaccines, p. 754

Tetanus Vaccines, p. 758

Children with unknown or incomplete immunisation history

For children born in the UK who present with an inadequate or unknown immunisation history, investigation into immunisations received should be carried out. Outstanding doses should be administered where the routine childhood immunisation schedule has not been completed.

For advice on the immunisation of children coming to the UK, consult the handbook *Immunisation against Infectious Disease* (2006) (available at www.dh.gov.uk)

14.2 Passive immunity

Immunity with immediate protection against certain infective organisms can be obtained by injecting preparations made from the plasma of immune individuals with adequate levels of antibody to the disease for which protection is sought (see under Immunoglobulins, section 14.5). The duration of this passive immunity varies according to the dose and the type of immunoglobulin. Passive immunity may last only a few weeks; when necessary, passive immunisation can be repeated.

Antibodies of human origin are usually termed *immunoglobulins*. The term *antiserum* is applied to material prepared in animals. Because of serum sickness and other allergic-type reactions that may follow injections of antisera, this therapy has been replaced whenever possible by the use of immunoglobulins. Reactions are theoretically possible after injection of human immunoglobulins, but reports of such reactions are very rare.

14.3 Storage and use

Care must be taken to store all vaccines and other immunological products under the conditions recommended in the product literature, otherwise the preparation may become ineffective. **Refrigerated storage** is usually necessary; many vaccines and immunoglobulins need to be stored at 2–8°C and not allowed to freeze.

Vaccines and immunoglobulins should be protected from light. Reconstituted vaccines and opened multi-dose vials must be used within the period recommended in the product literature. Unused vaccines should be disposed of by incineration at a registered disposal contractor.

Particular attention must be paid to instructions on the use of diluents. Vaccines which are liquid suspensions or are reconstituted before use should be adequately mixed to ensure uniformity of the material to be injected.

14.4 Vaccines and antisera

Availability   Anthrax and yellow fever vaccines, botulism antitoxin, diphtheria antitoxin, and snake and spider venom antitoxins are available from local designated holding centres.

For antivenom, see Emergency Treatment of Poisoning, p. 47.

Enquiries for vaccines not available commercially can also be made to:

Immunisation Policy, Monitoring and Surveillance
Department of Health
Wellington House
133–155 Waterloo Road
London, SE1 8UG.
Tel: (020) 7972 4047

In Scotland information about availability of vaccines can be obtained from a Specialist in Pharmaceutical Public Health. In Wales enquiries for vaccines not commercially available should be directed to:

Welsh Medicines Information Centre
University Hospital of Wales
Cardiff, CF14 4XW.
Tel: (029) 2074 2979

and in Northern Ireland:

Regional Pharmacist (procurement co-ordination)
United Hospitals Trust Pharmacy Dept
Whiteabbey Hospital
Doagh Road
Newtownabbey, BT37 9RH.
Tel: (028) 9086 5181 ext 2386

For further details of availability, see under individual vaccines.

Anthrax vaccine

Anthrax vaccine is rarely required for children. For further information see BNF section 14.4.

BCG vaccines

BCG (Bacillus Calmette-Guérin) is a live attenuated strain derived from *Mycobacterium bovis* which stimulates the development of hypersensitivity to *M. tuberculosis*. BCG vaccine should be given intradermally by operators skilled in the technique (see below).

The expected reaction to successful BCG vaccination is induration at the site of injection followed by a local lesion which starts as a papule 2 or more weeks after vaccination; the lesion may ulcerate then subside over several weeks or months, leaving a small flat scar. A dry dressing may be used if the ulcer discharges, but air should **not** be excluded.

All children of 6 years and over being considered for BCG immunisation must first be given a skin test for hypersensitivity to tuberculoprotein (see under Diagnostic agents, below). A skin test is not necessary for a child under 6 years, provided that the child has not stayed for longer than 3 months in a country with an incidence[1] of tuberculosis greater than 40 per 100 000, the child has not had contact with a

1. List of countries or primary care trusts where the incidence of tuberculosis is greater than 40 cases per 100 000 is available at www.hpa.org.uk

person with tuberculosis, and there is no family history of tuberculosis within the last 5 years.

BCG is recommended for the following groups of children if BCG immunisation has not previously been carried out and they are negative for tuberculoprotein hypersensitivity:

- all neonates and infants (0–12 months) born in areas where the incidence[1] of tuberculosis is greater than 40 per 100 000;

- neonates, infants, and children under 16 years with a parent or grandparent born in a country with an incidence[1] of tuberculosis greater than 40 per 100 000;

- new immigrants aged under 16 years who were born in, or lived for more than 3 months in a country with an incidence[1] of tuberculosis greater than 40 per 100 000;

- new immigrants aged 16–18 years from Sub-Saharan Africa or a country[1] with an incidence of tuberculosis greater than 500 per 100 000;

- contacts of those with active respiratory tuberculosis;

- children under 16 years intending to live with local people for more than 3 months in a country with an incidence[1] of tuberculosis greater than 40 per 100 000 (section 14.6).

BCG vaccine can be given simultaneously with another live vaccine (see also section 14.1), but if they are not given at the same time, an interval of 4 weeks should normally be allowed between them. When BCG is given to infants, there is no need to delay routine primary immunisations. No further vaccination should be given in the arm used for BCG vaccination for at least 3 months because of the risk of regional lymphadenitis.

For advice on chemoprophylaxis against tuberculosis, see section 5.1.9; for treatment of infection following vaccination, seek expert advice.

BACILLUS CALMETTE-GUÉRIN VACCINE

BCG vaccine

Cautions see section 14.1; **interactions:** Appendix 1 (vaccines)

Contra-indications see section 14.1; also neonate in household contact with known or suspected case of active tuberculosis; generalised septic skin conditions (for children with eczema, lesion-free site should be used)

Pregnancy see p. 733

Breast-feeding see p. 733

Side-effects see section 14.1 and notes above; *also* at the injection-site, subcutaneous abscess, prolonged ulceration; *rarely* disseminated complications such as osteitis or osteomyelitis

Indication and dose

Immunisation against tuberculosis
- By intradermal injection

Neonate 0.05 mL

Child 1 month–1 year 0.05 mL

Child 1–18 years 0.1 mL

Intradermal injection technique Skin is stretched between thumb and forefinger and needle (size 25G or 26G) inserted (bevel upwards) for about 3 mm into superficial layers of dermis (almost parallel with surface). Needle should be short with short bevel (can usually be seen through epidermis during insertion). Tense raised blanched bleb showing tips of hair follicles is sign of correct injection; 7 mm bleb ≡ 0.1 mL injection, 3 mm bleb ≡ 0.05 mL injection; if considerable resistance not felt, needle is too deep and should be removed and reinserted before giving more vaccine.
To be injected at insertion of deltoid muscle onto humerus (keloid formation more likely with sites higher on arm); tip of shoulder should be **avoided**.

◢ Intradermal

Bacillus Calmette-Guérin Vaccine [PoM]
BCG Vaccine, Dried/Tub/BCG
Injection, (powder for suspension), freeze-dried preparation of live bacteria of a strain derived from the bacillus of Calmette and Guérin
Available from health organisations or direct from Moviano (SSI brand, multidose vial with diluent)

Diagnostic agents

The *Mantoux test* is recommended for tuberculin skin testing, but no licensed preparation is currently available. Guidance for healthcare professionals is available at www.immunisation.nhs.uk.

In the Mantoux test, the diagnostic dose is administered by intradermal injection of Tuberculin Purified Protein Derivative (PPD).

---

1. List of countries or primary care trusts where the incidence of tuberculosis is greater than 40 cases per 100 000 is available at www.hpa.org.uk

The *Heaf test* (involving the use of multiple-puncture apparatus) is no longer available.

Note Response to tuberculin may be suppressed by live viral vaccines, viral infection, sarcoidosis, corticosteroid therapy, or immunosuppression due to disease or treatment. Tuberculin testing should not be carried out within 4 weeks of receiving a live viral vaccine

Two interferon gamma release assay (IGRA) tests are also available as an aid in the diagnosis of tuberculosis infection: *QuantiFERON®-TB Gold* and *T-SPOT®.TB*. Both tests measure T-cell mediated immune response to synthetic antigens. For further information on the use of interferon gamma release assay tests for tuberculosis, see www.hpa.org.uk.

Tuberculin Purified Protein Derivative PoM
(Tuberculin PPD)

Injection, heat-treated products of growth and lysis of appropriate *Mycobacterium* spp. 20 units/mL (2 units/0.1-mL dose) (for routine use), 1.5-mL vial; 100 units/mL (10 units/0.1-mL dose), 1.5-mL vial

Dose

Mantoux test
* **By intradermal injection**

2 units (0.1 mL of 20 units/mL strength) for routine Mantoux test; if first test is negative and a further test

is considered appropriate 10 units (0.1 mL of 100 units/mL strength)

Available from Movianto (SSI brand)
Important The strength of tuberculin PPD in this product may be different to the strengths of products used previously for the Mantoux test; care is required to select the correct strength

---

Botulism antitoxin

A polyvalent botulism antitoxin is available for the post-exposure prophylaxis of botulism and for the treatment of children thought to be suffering from botulism. It specifically neutralises the toxins produced by *Clostridium botulinum* types A, B, and E. It is not effective against infantile botulism as the toxin (type A) is seldom, if ever, found in the blood in this type of infection.

Hypersensitivity reactions are a problem. It is essential to read the contra-indications, warnings, and details of sensitivity tests on the package insert. Prior to treatment checks should be made regarding previous administration of any antitoxin and history of any allergic condition, e.g. asthma, hay fever, etc. All children should be tested for sensitivity (diluting the antitoxin if history of allergy).

Botulism Antitoxin PoM

A preparation containing the specific antitoxic globulins that have the power of neutralising the toxins formed by types A, B, and E of *Clostridium botulinum*.

Note The BP title Botulinum Antitoxin is not used because the preparation currently in use may have a different specification

Dose

Prophylaxis
Consult product literature

Available from local designated centres, for details see TOXBASE (requires registration) www.toxbase.org. For

supplies outside working hours apply to other designated centres or to the duty doctor at the Health Protection Agency (Tel (020) 8200 6868). For major incidents, obtain supplies from the local blood bank

---

Cholera vaccine

Cholera vaccine (oral) contains inactivated Inaba (including El-Tor biotype) and Ogawa strains of *Vibrio cholerae*, serotype O1 together with recombinant B-subunit of the cholera toxin produced in Inaba strains of *V.cholerae*, serotype O1.

Oral cholera vaccine is licensed for travellers to endemic or epidemic areas on the basis of current recommendations (see also section 14.6). Immunisation should be completed at least 1 week before potential exposure. However, there is no requirement for cholera vaccination for international travel.

Immunisation with cholera vaccine does not provide complete protection and all travellers to a country where cholera exists should be warned that scrupulous attention to food, water, and personal hygiene is **essential**.

Injectable cholera vaccine provides unreliable protection and is no longer available in the UK.

14

Immunological products and vaccines

CHOLERA VACCINE

Cautions see section 14.1 and notes above

Contra-indications see section 14.1

Pregnancy see p. 733

Breast-feeding see p. 733

Side-effects see section 14.1; also *rarely* respiratory symptoms such as rhinitis and cough; *very rarely* sore throat, insomnia

Indication and dose

See notes above

• By mouth

Child 2–6 years 3 doses each separated by an interval of 1–6 weeks

Child 6–18 years 2 doses separated by an interval of 1–6 weeks

Note If more than 6 weeks have elapsed between doses, the primary course should be restarted

A single booster dose can be given 2 years after primary course for children 6–18 years, and 6 months after primary course for children 2–6 years. If more than 2 years have elapsed since the last vaccination, the primary course should be repeated

Administration Dissolve effervescent sodium bicarbonate granules in a glassful of water (approximately 150 mL). For child over 6 years, add vaccine suspension to make one dose. For child 2–6 years, discard half (approximately 75 mL) of the solution, then add vaccine suspension to make one dose. Drink within 2 hours. Food, drink and other oral medicines should be avoided for 1 hour before and after vaccination

Dukoral® (Crucell) (PoM)
Oral suspension, for dilution with solution of effervescent sodium bicarbonate granules, heat- and formaldehyde-inactivated Inaba (including El-Tor biotype) and Ogawa strains of *Vibrio cholerae* bacteria and recombinant cholera toxin B-subunit produced in *V. cholerae*, net price 2-dose pack = £23.42. Counselling, administration

---

Diphtheria Vaccines

Diphtheria vaccines are prepared from the toxin of *Corynebacterium diphtheriae* and adsorption on aluminium hydroxide or aluminium phosphate improves antigenicity. The vaccine stimulates the production of the protective antitoxin. The quantity of diphtheria toxoid in a preparation determines whether the vaccine is defined as 'high dose' or 'low dose'. Vaccines containing the higher dose of diphtheria toxoid are used for primary immunisation of children under 10 years of age. Vaccines containing the lower dose of diphtheria toxoid are used for primary immunisation in children over 10 years. Single-antigen diphtheria vaccine is not available and adsorbed diphtheria vaccine is given as a combination product containing other vaccines.

For primary immunisation *of children aged between 2 months and 10 years* vaccination is recommended usually in the form of 3 doses (separated by 1-month intervals) of **diphtheria, tetanus, pertussis (acellular, component), poliomyelitis (inactivated) and haemophilus type b conjugate vaccine (adsorbed)** (see Immunisation schedule, section 14.1). In unimmunised children aged *over 10 years* the primary course comprises of 3 doses of **adsorbed diphtheria** [low dose], **tetanus and poliomyelitis (inactivated) vaccine**.

A booster dose should be given 3 years after the primary course (this interval can be reduced to a minimum of 1 year if the primary course was delayed). Children *under 10 years* should receive *either* **adsorbed diphtheria, tetanus, pertussis (acellular, component) and poliomyelitis (inactivated) vaccine** *or* **adsorbed diphtheria** [low dose], **tetanus, pertussis (acellular, component) and poliomyelitis (inactivated) vaccine**. Children aged *over 10 years* should receive **adsorbed diphtheria** [low dose], **tetanus, and poliomyelitis (inactivated) vaccine**.

A second booster dose, of adsorbed diphtheria [low dose], tetanus and poliomyelitis (inactivated) vaccine, should be given 10 years after the previous booster dose (this interval can be reduced to a minimum of 5 years if previous doses were delayed). For children who have been vaccinated following a tetanus-prone wound, see Tetanus vaccines, p. 758.

Travel Children travelling to areas with a risk of diphtheria infection should be fully immunised according to the UK schedule (see also section 14.6). If more than 10 years have lapsed since completion of the UK schedule, a dose of **adsorbed diphtheria** [low dose], **tetanus and poliomyelitis (inactivated) vaccine** should be administered.

Contacts Advice on the management of cases of diphtheria, carriers, contacts and outbreaks must be sought from health protection units. The immunisation history of infected children and their contacts should be determined; those who have been incompletely immunised should complete their immunisation and fully immunised individuals should receive a reinforcing dose. For advice on antibacterial treatment to prevent a secondary case of diphtheria in a non-immune child, see Table 2, section 5.1.

◢ DIPHTHERIA-CONTAINING VACCINES

Cautions see section 14.1; see also individual components of vaccines

Contra-indications see section 14.1; see also individual components of vaccines

Pregnancy see p. 733

Breast-feeding see p. 733

Side-effects see section 14.1; also restlessness, sleep disturbances, and unusual crying in infants;

Licensed use *Infanrix-IPV + Hib*® not licensed for use in children over 36 months; *Pediacel*® not licensed in children over 4 years but Department of Health recommends that these be used for children up to 10 years

Indication and dose

See notes above and under preparations

◢ **Diphtheria-containing vaccines for children under 10 years**

Important Not recommended for children *aged 10 years or over* (see Diphtheria vaccines for children over 10)

Diphtheria, Tetanus, Pertussis (Acellular, Component), Poliomyelitis (Inactivated) and Haemophilus Type b Conjugate Vaccine (Adsorbed) ꞏPoMꞏ
Injection, suspension of diphtheria toxoid, tetanus toxoid, acellular pertussis, inactivated poliomyelitis and *Haemophilus influenzae* type b (conjugated to tetanus protein), net price 0.5-mL prefilled syringe = £19.94
Excipients may include neomycin, polymyxin B and streptomycin

Dose
> Primary immunisation
> • By intramuscular injection
> **Child 2 months–10 years** 3 doses each of 0.5 mL separated by intervals of 1 month; *see also* notes on booster doses, above

Available as part of childhood immunisation schedule, from health organisations or Movianto
Brands include *Infanrix-IPV+Hib*®, *Pediacel*®

Adsorbed Diphtheria, Tetanus, Pertussis (Acellular, Component) and Poliomyelitis (Inactivated) Vaccine ꞏPoMꞏ
Injection, suspension of diphtheria toxoid, tetanus toxoid, acellular pertussis and inactivated poliomyelitis vaccine components adsorbed on a mineral carrier, net price 0.5-mL prefilled syringe = £17.56
Excipients may include neomycin and polymyxin B

Dose
> First booster dose
> • By intramuscular injection
> **Child 3–10 years** 0.5 mL 3 years after primary immunisation; *see also* notes on booster doses, above

Available as part of childhood immunisation schedule, from health organisations or Movianto
Brands include *Infanrix-IPV*®

Adsorbed Diphtheria [low dose], Tetanus, Pertussis (Acellular, Component) and Poliomyelitis (Inactivated) Vaccine ꞏPoMꞏ
Injection, suspension of diphtheria toxoid [low dose], tetanus toxoid, acellular pertussis and inactivated poliomyelitis vaccine components adsorbed on a mineral carrier, net price 0.5-mL prefilled syringe = £11.98
Excipients may include neomycin, polymyxin B and streptomycin

Dose
> First booster dose
> • By intramuscular injection
> **Child 3–10 years** 0.5 mL 3 years after primary immunisation; *see also* notes on booster doses, above

Available as part of childhood immunisation schedule, from health organisations or Movianto
Brands include *Repevax*®

◢ **Diphtheria-containing vaccines for children over 10 years**

A low dose of diphtheria toxoid is sufficient to recall immunity in older children previously immunised against diphtheria but whose immunity may have diminished with time; it is insufficient to cause serious reactions in a child who is already immune. Preparations containing low dose diphtheria should be used for children *over 10 years*, both for primary immunisation and booster doses.

Adsorbed Diphtheria [low dose], Tetanus and Poliomyelitis (Inactivated) Vaccine ꞏPoMꞏ
Injection, suspension of diphtheria toxoid [low dose], tetanus toxoid and inactivated poliomyelitis vaccine components adsorbed on a mineral carrier, net price 0.5-mL prefilled syringe = £6.48
Excipients may include neomycin, polymyxin B and streptomycin

Dose
> Primary immunisation
> • By intramuscular injection
> **Child 10–18 years** 3 doses each of 0.5 mL separated by intervals of 1 month; second booster dose, 0.5 mL given 10 years after first booster dose (may also be used as first booster dose in those over 10 years who have received only 3 previous doses of a diphtheria-containing vaccine); *see also* notes on booster doses, above

Available as part of childhood schedule, from health organisations or Movianto
Brands include *Revaxis*®

◢ **Diphtheria antitoxin**

Diphtheria antitoxin is used for passive immunisation in suspected cases of diphtheria only (without waiting for bacteriological confirmation); tests for hypersensitivity should be first carried out. It is derived from horse serum, and reactions are com-

▢ **DIPHTHERIA-CONTAINING VACCINES (*continued*)**

mon after administration; resuscitation facilities should be available immediately.

It is no longer used for prophylaxis because of the risk of hypersensitivity; unimmunised contacts should be promptly investigated and given antibacterial prophylaxis (Table 2, section 5.1) and vaccine (see Contacts above, p. 741).

Diphtheria Antitoxin PoM
Dip/Ser

Dose
Prophylaxis

Not recommended therefore no dose stated (see notes above)

Treatment

Consult product literature

Available from Centre for Infections (Tel (020) 8200 6868) or in Northern Ireland from Public Health Laboratory, Belfast City Hospital (Tel (028) 9032 9241).

Haemophilus type B conjugate vaccine

Haemophilus influenzae type b (Hib) vaccine is made from capsular polysaccharide; it is conjugated with a protein such as tetanus toxoid to increase immunogenicity, especially in young children. Haemophilus influenzae type b vaccine is given in combination with diphtheria, tetanus, pertussis (acellular, component) and poliomyelitis (inactivated) vaccine, (see under Diphtheria containing Vaccines) as a component of the primary course of childhood immunisation (see Immunisation schedule, section 14.1). For infants under 1 year, the course consists of 3 doses of a vaccine containing haemophilus influenzae type b component, with an interval of 1 month between doses. A booster dose of haemophilus influenzae type b vaccine (combined with meningococcal group C conjugate vaccine) should be given at around 12–13 months of age.

Children 1–10 years who have not been immunised against *Haemophilus influenzae type b* need to receive only 1 dose of the vaccine (combined with meningococcal group C conjugate vaccine). However, if a primary course of immunisation has not been completed, these children should be given 3 doses of diphtheria, tetanus, pertussis (acellular, component), poliomyelitis (inactivated) and haemophilus type b conjugate vaccine (adsorbed). The risk of infection falls sharply in older children and the vaccine is not normally required for children over 10 years.

Haemophilus influenzae type b vaccine may be given to those over 10 years who are considered to be at increased risk of invasive *H. influenzae* type b disease (such as those with sickle-cell disease and those receiving treatment for malignancy).

For use of rifampicin in the prevention of secondary cases of Haemophilus influenza type b disease, see Table 2, section 5.1

Asplenia or splenic dysfunction Haemophilus influenzae type b vaccine is recommended for children with asplenia or splenic dysfunction. Immunised children over 1 year, who develop splenic dysfunction, should be given 1 additional dose of haemophilus influenzae type b vaccine combined with meningococcal group C conjugate vaccine). For elective splenectomy, the vaccine should ideally be given at least 2 weeks before surgery. Children over 1 year, who are not immunised against *Haemophilus influenzae* type b, should be given 2 doses of haemophilus influenzae type b vaccine (combined with meningococcal group C conjugate vaccine) with an interval of 2 months between doses. However, children under 10 years, who are not immunised against diphtheria, tetanus, pertussis, poliomyelitis, and *Haemophilus influenzae* type b should be given 3 doses (with an interval of 1 month between doses) of combined diphtheria, tetanus, pertussis (acellular component), poliomyelitis (inactivated) and haemophilus type b conjugate vaccine.

◤ HAEMOPHILUS TYPE B CONJUGATE VACCINE

Cautions see section 14.1

Contra-indications see section 14.1

Pregnancy see p. 733

Breast-feeding see p. 733

Side-effects see section 14.1; also, atopic dermatitis, hypotonia

Licensed use *Menitorix®* is not licensed for use in children over 2 years

Indication and dose

See notes above and under preparation

Primary immunisation, see under Diphtheria-containing vaccines

Menitorix® (GSK) PoM
Injection, powder for reconstitution, capsular polysaccharide of *Haemophilus influenzae* type b and capsular polysaccharide of *Neisseria meningiti-*

◻ **HAEMOPHILUS TYPE B CONJUGATE VACCINE (*continued*)**

dis group C (both conjugated to tetanus protein), net price single dose vial (with syringe containing 0.5 mL diluent) = £39.87

Dose

- By intramuscular injection
  CHILD 1 –10 years , 0.5 mL

CHILD over 1 year , with asplenia or splenic dysfunction (see notes above), 0.5 mL

Available as part of the childhood immunisation schedule from Moviano

◢**Combined vaccines**
  See also Diphtheria-containing vaccines

Hepatitis A vaccine

Hepatitis A vaccine is prepared from formaldehyde-inactivated hepatitis A virus grown in human diploid cells.

Immunisation is recommended for:

- residents of homes for those with severe learning difficulties;
- children with haemophilia treated with plasma-derived clotting factors;
- children with severe liver disease;
- children travelling to high-risk areas (see p. 769);
- adolescents who are at risk due to their sexual behaviour;
- parenteral drug abusers.

Immunisation should be considered for:

- children with chronic liver disease including chronic hepatitis B or chronic hepatitis C;
- prevention of secondary cases in close contacts of confirmed cases of hepatitis A, within 7 days of onset of disease in the primary case.

A booster dose of hepatitis A vaccine is usually given 6–12 months after the initial dose. A second booster dose can be given 20 years after the previous booster dose to those who continue to be at risk. Specialist advice should be sought on re-immunisation of immunocompromised individuals.

In children under 16 years, a single dose of the combined vaccine *Ambirix*® can be used to provide rapid protection against hepatitis A.

Intramuscular **normal immunoglobulin** (section 14.5.1) is recommended for use in addition to Hepatitis A vaccine, for contacts of patients with delayed confirmation of hepatitis A infection, or for individuals at high-risk of severe disease.

◢ HEPATITIS A VACCINE

Cautions section 14.1
Contra-indications section 14.1
Pregnancy see p. 733
Breast-feeding see p. 733
Side-effects section 14.1; for combination vaccines, see also Typhoid vaccines, p. 760

Indication and dose

Immunisation against hepatitis A infection
  for dose, see under preparations

◢**Single component**
Avaxim® (Sanofi Pasteur) ᴘᴏᴹ
  Injection, suspension of formaldehyde-inactivated hepatitis A virus (GBM grown in human diploid cells) 320 antigen units/mL adsorbed onto aluminium hydroxide, net price 0.5-mL prefilled syringe = £18.60
  Excipients include neomycin

Dose

- By intramuscular injection
  (See note below)

  Child 16–18 years 0.5 mL as a single dose; booster dose 0.5 mL 6–12 months after initial dose
  Note Booster dose may be delayed by up to 3 years if not given after recommended interval following primary dose with *Avaxim*®. The deltoid region is the

preferred site of injection; not to be injected into the buttock (vaccine efficacy reduced). The subcutaneous route may be used for children with bleeding disorders

Epaxal® (Crucell) ᴘᴏᴹ
  Injection, suspension of formaldehyde-inactivated hepatitis A virus (RG-SB grown in human diploid cells) at least 48 units/mL, net price 0.5-mL pre-filled syringe = £23.81

Dose

- By intramuscular injection
  (See note below)

  Child 1–18 years 0.5 mL as a single dose; booster dose 0.5 mL 6–12 months after initial dose (1–6 months if splenectomised)
  Note Booster dose may be delayed by up to 4 years if not given after recommended interval following primary dose. The deltoid region is the preferred site of injection. The subcutaneous route may be used for children with bleeding disorders

Important *Epaxal*® contains influenza virus haemagglutinin grown in the allantoic cavity of chick embryos, and is therefore contra-indicated in those hypersensitive to eggs or chicken protein.

Havrix Monodose® (GSK) ᴘᴏᴹ
  Injection, suspension of formaldehyde-inactivated hepatitis A virus (HM 175 grown in human diploid cells) 1440 ELISA units/mL adsorbed onto alu-

14

Immunological products and vaccines

☐ **HEPATITIS A VACCINE (continued)**

minium hydroxide, net price 1-mL prefilled syringe = £22.14, 0.5-mL (720 ELISA units) prefilled syringe (*Havrix Junior Monodose®*) = £16.77
Excipients include neomycin

Dose
- **By intramuscular injection**
  (See note below)

  Child 1–15 years 0.5 mL as a single dose; booster dose 0.5 mL 6–12 months after initial dose

  Child 16–18 years 1 mL as a single dose; booster dose 1 mL 6–12 months after initial dose

  Note Booster dose may be delayed by up to 3 years if not given after recommended interval following primary dose with *Havrix Monodose®*. The deltoid region is the preferred site of injection. The subcutaneous route may be used for children with bleeding disorders

Vaqta® Paediatric (Sanofi Pasteur) ⓅⓄⓂ
Injection, suspension of formaldehyde-inactivated hepatitis A virus (grown in human diploid cells) 50 antigen units/mL adsorbed onto aluminium hydroxyphosphate sulphate, net price 0.5-mL prefilled syringe = £15.04
Excipients include neomycin

Dose
- **By intramuscular injection**
  (See note below)

  Child 1–18 years 0.5 mL as a single dose; booster dose 0.5 mL 6–18 months after initial dose

  Note The deltoid region is the preferred site of injection. The subcutaneous route may be used for children with bleeding disorders (but immune response may be reduced)

◢**With hepatitis B vaccine**
Ambirix® (GSK) ▼ ⓅⓄⓂ
Injection, suspension of inactivated hepatitis A virus (grown in human diploid cells) 720 ELISA units/mL adsorbed onto aluminium hydroxide, and recombinant (DNA) hepatitis B surface antigen (grown in yeast cells) 20 micrograms/mL adsorbed onto aluminium hydroxide and aluminium phosphate, net price 1-mL prefilled syringe = £31.18
Excipients include neomycin

Dose
- **By intramuscular injection**
  (See note below)

  Child 1–15 years primary course, 2 doses of 1 mL, the second 6–12 months after initial dose

  Note Primary course should be completed with *Ambirix®* (single component vaccines given at appropriate intervals may be used for booster dose); the deltoid region is the preferred site of injection in older children; anterolateral thigh is the preferred site in infants; not to be injected into the buttock (vaccine efficacy reduced); subcutaneous route used for children with bleeding disorders (but immune response may be reduced)

  Important *Ambirix®* not recommended for post-exposure prophylaxis following percutaneous (needle-stick), ocular, or mucous membrane exposure to hepatitis B virus

Twinrix® (GSK) ⓅⓄⓂ
Injection, inactivated hepatitis A virus (grown in human diploid cells) 720 ELISA units/mL adsorbed onto aluminium hydroxide, and recombinant (DNA) hepatitis B surface antigen (grown in yeast cells) 20 micrograms/mL adsorbed onto aluminium phosphate, net price 1-mL prefilled syringe

(*Twinrix® Adult*) = £27.76, 0.5-mL prefilled syringe (*Twinrix® Paediatric*) = £20.79
Excipients include neomycin

Dose
- **By intramuscular injection**
  (See note below)

  Child 1–15 years primary course 3 doses of 0.5 mL (*Twinrix® Paediatric*), the second 1 month and the third 6 months after first dose

  Child 16–18 years primary course, 3 doses of 1 mL (*Twinrix® Adult*), the second 1 month and the third 6 months after first dose

  Accelerated schedule (e.g. for travellers departing within 1 month) for child over 16 years, second dose given 7 days after first dose, third dose after further 14 days and fourth dose 12 months after the first dose

  Note Primary course should be completed with *Twinrix®* (single component vaccines given at appropriate intervals may be used for booster dose); the deltoid region is the preferred site of injection in older children; anterolateral thigh is the preferred site in infants; not to be injected into the buttock (vaccine efficacy reduced); subcutaneous route used for children with bleeding disorders (but immune response may be reduced).

  Important *Twinrix®* not recommended for post-exposure prophylaxis following percutaneous (needle-stick), ocular or mucous membrane exposure to hepatitis B virus.

◢**With typhoid vaccine**
Hepatyrix® (GSK) ⓅⓄⓂ
Injection, suspension of inactivated hepatitis A virus (grown in human diploid cells) 1440 ELISA units/mL adsorbed onto aluminium hydroxide, combined with typhoid vaccine containing 25 micrograms/mL virulence polysaccharide antigen of *Salmonella typhi*, net price 1-mL prefilled syringe = £32.08
Excipients include neomycin

Dose
- **By intramuscular injection**
  (See note below)

  Child 15–18 years 1 mL as a single dose; booster doses, see under single component hepatitis A vaccine (above) and under polysaccharide typhoid vaccine, p. 760

  Note The deltoid region is the preferred site of injection; not to be injected into the buttock (vaccine efficacy reduced). The subcutaneous route may be used for children with bleeding disorders

ViATIM® (Sanofi Pasteur) ⓅⓄⓂ
Injection, suspension of inactivated hepatitis A virus (grown in human diploid cells) 160 antigen units/mL adsorbed onto aluminium hydroxide, combined with typhoid vaccine containing 25 micrograms/mL virulence polysaccharide antigen of *Salmonella typhi*, net price 1-mL prefilled syringe = £29.80

Dose
- **By intramuscular injection**
  (See note below)

  Child 16–18 years 1 mL as a single dose; booster doses, see under single component hepatitis A vaccine (above) and under polysaccharide typhoid vaccine, p. 760

  Note The deltoid region is the preferred site of injection; not to be injected into the buttock (vaccine efficacy reduced). The subcutaneous route may be used for children with bleeding disorders

Hepatitis B vaccine

Hepatitis B vaccine contains inactivated hepatitis B virus surface antigen (HBsAg) adsorbed on to aluminium hydroxide adjuvant. It is made biosynthetically using recombinant DNA technology. The vaccine is used in individuals at high risk of contracting hepatitis B.

In the UK, high-risk groups include:

- parenteral drug misusers, their sexual partners, and household contacts; other drug misusers who are likely to 'progress' to injecting;
- adolescents who are at risk from their sexual behaviour,
- close family contacts of an individual with chronic hepatitis B infection;
- babies whose mothers have had acute hepatitis B during pregnancy *or* are positive for hepatitis B surface antigen (regardless of e-antigen markers); hepatitis B vaccination is started immediately on delivery and *hepatitis B immunoglobulin* (see p. 766) given at the same time (but at a different site). Babies whose mothers are positive for hepatitis B surface antigen and for e-antigen antibody should receive the vaccine only (but babies weighing 1.5 kg or less should also receive the immunoglobulin regardless of the mother's e-antigen antibody status);
- children with haemophilia, those receiving regular blood transfusions or blood products, and carers responsible for the administration of such products;
- children with chronic renal failure including those on haemodialysis. Children receiving haemodialysis should be monitored for antibodies annually and re-immunised if necessary. Home carers (of dialysis patients) should be vaccinated;
- children with chronic liver disease;
- patients of day-care or residential accommodation for those with severe learning difficulties;
- children in custodial institutions;
- children travelling to areas of high or intermediate prevalence who are at increased risk or who plan to remain there for lengthy periods (see p. 769);
- families adopting children from countries with a high or intermediate prevalence of hepatitis B;
- foster carers and their families.

Different immunisation schedules for hepatitis B vaccine are recommended for specific circumstances (see under individual preparations); an 'accelerated schedule' is recommended for pre-exposure prophylaxis in high–risk groups where rapid protection is required, and for post-exposure prophylaxis (see below). Generally, three or four doses are required for primary immunisation. Immunisation may take up to 6 months to confer adequate protection; the duration of immunity is not known precisely, but a single booster 5 years after the primary course may be sufficient to maintain immunity for those who continue to be at risk.

Immunisation does not eliminate the need for commonsense precautions for avoiding the risk of infection from known carriers by the routes of infection which have been clearly established, consult *Guidance for Clinical Health Care Workers: Protection against Infection with Blood-borne Viruses* (available at www.dh.gov.uk). Accidental inoculation of hepatitis B virus-infected blood into a wound, incision, needle-prick, or abrasion may lead to infection, whereas it is unlikely that indirect exposure to a carrier will do so.

Following significant exposure to hepatis B, an accelerated schedule, with the second dose given 1 month, and the third dose 2 months after the initial dose, is recommended. For those at continued risk, a fourth dose should be given 12 months after the first dose. More detailed guidance is given in the *Immunisation against Infectious Disease* handbook, see p. 732

Specific **hepatitis B immunoglobulin** ('HBIG') is available for use with the vaccine in those accidentally inoculated and in neonates at special risk of infection (section 14.5.2).

A combined hepatitis A and hepatitis B vaccine is also available.

14

Immunological products and vaccines

◢ HEPATITIS B VACCINE

Cautions section 14.1

Contra-indications section 14.1

Pregnancy see p. 733

Breast-feeding see p. 733

Side-effects section 14.1

Indication and dose

Immunisation against hepatitis B infection

For dose see under preparations

◢**Single component**

Engerix B® (GSK) [PoM]

Injection, suspension of hepatitis B surface antigen (prepared from yeast cells by recombinant DNA technique) 20 micrograms/mL adsorbed onto aluminium hydroxide, net price 0.5-mL (paediatric) prefilled syringe = £9.67, 1-mL vial = £12.34, 1-mL prefilled syringe = £12.99

Dose

- **By intramuscular injection**
  (See note below)

  Neonate (except if born to hepatitis B surface antigen-positive mother, see below), 3 doses of 10 micrograms, second dose 1 month and third dose 6 months after first dose

  Child 1 month–16 years 3 doses of 10 micrograms, second dose 1 month and third dose 6 months after first dose

  Child 16–18 years 3 doses of 20 micrograms, second dose 1 month and third dose 6 months after first dose
  Accelerated schedule (all age groups), second dose 1 month after first dose, third dose 2 months after first dose and fourth dose 12 months after first dose
  Alternative schedule for Child 11–15 years, 2 doses of 20 micrograms, the second dose 6 months after the first dose (this schedule not suitable if high risk of infection between doses or if compliance with second dose uncertain)

Infant born to hepatitis B surface antigen-positive mother (see also notes above)
- **By intramuscular injection**
  (See note below)

  Neonate 4 doses of 10 micrograms, first dose at birth with hepatitis B immunoglobulin injection (separate site) the second 1 month, the third 2 months and the fourth 12 months after first dose

Renal insufficiency (including haemodialysis patients)
- **By intramuscular injection**
  (See note below)

  Neonate (except if born to hepatitis B surface antigen positive mother, see above), 3 doses of 10 micrograms, second dose 1 month and third dose 6 months after first dose *or* accelerated schedule, 4 doses of 10 micrograms, second dose 1 month, third dose 2 months, and fourth dose 12 months after first dose; immunisation schedule and booster doses may need to be adjusted in those with low antibody concentration

  Child 1 month–16 years 3 doses of 10 micrograms, second dose 1 month and third dose 6 months after first dose *or* accelerated schedule, 4 doses of 10 micrograms, second dose 1 month, third dose 2 months, and fourth dose 12 months after first dose; immunisation schedule and booster doses may need to be adjusted in those with low antibody concentration

  Child 16–18 years 4 doses of 40 micrograms, the second 1 month, the third 2 months and the fourth 6 months after the first dose; immunisation schedule and booster doses may need to be adjusted in those with low antibody concentration

Note Deltoid muscle is preferred site of injection in older children; anterolateral thigh is preferred site in neonates, infants and young children; not to be injected into the buttock (vaccine efficacy reduced)

Fendrix® (GSK) [PoM]

Injection, suspension of hepatitis B surface antigen (prepared from yeast cells by recombinant DNA technique) 40 micrograms/mL adsorbed onto aluminium phosphate, net price 0.5-mL prefilled syringe = £38.10

Excipients include traces of thiomersal

Dose

Renal insufficiency patients (including pre-haemo-dialysis and haemodialysis patients)
- **By intramuscular injection**
  (See below)

  Child 15–18 years 4 doses of 20 micrograms, the second 1 month, the third 2 months and the fourth 6 months after the first dose; immunisation schedule and booster doses may need to be adjusted in those with low antibody concentration

Note Deltoid muscle is preferred site of injection; not to be injected into the buttock (vaccine efficacy reduced)

HBvaxPRO® (Sanofi Pasteur) [PoM]

Injection, suspension of hepatitis B surface antigen (prepared from yeast cells by recombinant DNA technique) 10 micrograms/mL adsorbed onto aluminium hydroxyphosphate sulphate, net price 0.5-mL (5-microgram) prefilled syringe = £9.13, 1-mL (10-microgram) prefilled syringe = £12.44; 40 micrograms/mL, 1-mL (40-microgram) vial = £28.16

Dose

- **By intramuscular injection**
  (See note below)

  Neonate (except if born to hepatitis B surface antigen-positive mother, see below), 3 doses of 5 micrograms, second dose 1 month and third dose 6 months after first dose

  Child 1 month–16 years 3 doses of 5 micrograms, second dose 1 month and third dose 6 months after first dose

  Child 16–18 years 3 doses of 10 micrograms, second dose 1 month and third dose 6 months after first dose
  Accelerated schedule (all age groups), second dose 1 month after first dose, third dose 2 months after first dose with fourth dose at 12 months
  Booster doses may be required in immunocompromised patients with low antibody concentration

Infant born to hepatitis B surface antigen-positive mother (see also notes above)
- **By intramuscular injection**
  (See note below)

  Neonate 5 micrograms, first dose at birth with hepatitis B immunoglobulin injection (separate site), the second 1 month, the third 2 months and the fourth 12 months after the first dose

△ **HEPATITIS B VACCINE (continued)**

Chronic haemodialysis patients
• **By intramuscular injection**
(See note below)

Child 16–18 years 3 doses of 40 micrograms, second dose 1 month and third dose 6 months after first dose; booster doses may be required in those with low antibody concentration

Note Deltoid muscle is preferred site of injection in older children; anterolateral thigh is preferred site in neonates

and infants; not to be injected into the buttock (vaccine efficacy reduced)

◀**With hepatitis A vaccine**
See Hepatitis A Vaccine

Human papilloma virus vaccines

Human papilloma virus vaccine is available as a bivalent vaccine (*Cervarix®*) or a quadrivalent vaccine (*Gardasil®*). *Cervarix®* is licensed for use in females for the prevention of cervical cancer and other pre-cancerous lesions caused by human papilloma virus types 16 and 18. *Gardasil®* is licensed for use in females for the prevention of cervical cancer, genital warts and pre-cancerous lesions caused by human papilloma virus types 6, 11, 16 and 18. The two vaccines are not interchangeable and one vaccine product should be used for an entire course. However, the Department of Health (November 2008) states for individuals with previous incomplete vaccination with *Gardasil®*, who are eligible for HPV vaccination under the national programme, *Cervarix®* can be used to complete the vaccination course if necessary; the individual must be informed that *Cervarix®* does not protect against genital warts.

Human papilloma virus vaccine will be most effective if given before sexual activity starts. The first dose is given to females aged 12 to 13 years, the second and third doses are given 1–2 and 6 months after the first dose (see Immunisation schedule, section 14.1); all 3 doses should be given within a 12-month period. If the course is interrupted, it should be resumed but not repeated, allowing the appropriate interval between the remaining doses. Where there are significant challenges in scheduling vaccination, or a high likelihood that the third dose will not be given, the third dose of *Cervarix®* can be given 3 months after the second dose. Under the national programme in England, females remain eligible to receive the vaccine up to the age of 18 years if they did not receive the vaccine when scheduled. Where appropriate, immunisation with human papillomavirus vaccine should be offered to females coming into the UK as they may not have been offered protection in their country of origin. The duration of protection has not been established, but current studies suggest that protection is maintained for at least 6 years after completion of the primary course.

◢ HUMAN PAPILLOMA VIRUS VACCINES

Cautions see section 14.1

Contra-indications see section 14.1

Pregnancy not known to be harmful, but vaccination should be postponed until completion of pregnancy

Breast-feeding see p. 733

Side-effects see section 14.1

Indication and dose
see notes above and under preparations
Note To avoid confusion, prescribers should specify the brand to be dispensed

Cervarix® (GSK) ▼ PoM
Injection, suspension of virus-like particles of human papilloma virus type 16 (40 micrograms/mL), type 18 (40 micrograms/mL) capsid protein (prepared by recombinant DNA technique using a Baculovirus expression system) in monophosphoryl lipid A adjuvant adsorbed onto aluminium

hydroxide, net price 0.5-mL prefilled syringe = £80.50

Note To avoid confusion, prescribers should specify the brand to be dispensed

Dose
Prevention of premalignant genital lesions and cervical cancer (see notes above)
• **By intramuscular injection into deltoid region**
Child 10–18 years 3 doses of 0.5 mL, the second 1 month and the third 6 months after the first dose

Gardasil® (Sanofi Pasteur) ▼ PoM
Injection, suspension of virus-like particles of human papilloma virus type 6 (40 micrograms/mL), type 11 (80 micrograms/mL), type 16 (80 micrograms/mL), type 18 (40 micrograms/mL) capsid protein (prepared from yeast cells by recombinant DNA technique) adsorbed onto alu-

14

Immunological products and vaccines

◻ **HUMAN PAPILLOMA VIRUS VACCINES (continued)**

minium hydroxyphosphate sulphate, net price 0.5-mL prefilled syringe = £88.50

Note To avoid confusion, prescribers should specify the brand to be dispensed

Dose

Prevention of premalignant genital lesions, cervical cancer and genital warts (see notes above)

• By intramuscular injection preferably into deltoid region or higher anterolateral thigh

Child 9–18 years 3 doses of 0.5 mL, the second 2 months and the third 6 months after the first dose

Alternative schedule for Child 9–18 years, 3 doses of 0.5 mL, the second at least 1 month and the third at least 4 months after the first dose; schedule should be completed within 12 months

Influenza vaccine

While most viruses are antigenically stable, the influenza viruses A and B (especially A) are constantly altering their antigenic structure as indicated by changes in the haemagglutinins (H) and neuraminidases (N) on the surface of the viruses. It is essential that influenza vaccines in use contain the H and N components of the prevalent strain or strains recommended each year by the World Health Organization.

Seasonal influenza vaccines   Seasonal influenza vaccines will not control epidemics — immunisation is recommended *only for persons at high risk*. Annual immunisation is strongly recommended for children (including infants that were preterm or low birth-weight) aged over 6 months with the following conditions:

• chronic respiratory disease (includes asthma treated with continuous or repeated use of inhaled or systemic corticosteroids or asthma with previous exacerbations requiring hospital admission);

• chronic heart disease;

• chronic liver disease;

• chronic renal disease;

• chronic neurological disease;

• diabetes mellitus;

• immunosuppression because of disease (including asplenia or splenic dysfunction) or treatment (including chemotherapy and prolonged corticosteroid treatment);

• HIV infection (regardless of immune status).

Influenza immunisation is also recommended for children living in long-stay facilities, and for carers of children whose welfare may be at risk if the carer falls ill. Influenza immunisation should also be considered for household contacts of immunocompromised individuals.

Pandemic influenza a(h1n1)v vaccines   *Pandemrix®* and *Celvapan®* are licensed for the prevention of influenza A(H1N1)v (swine flu) during a pandemic. The individuals prioritised for vaccination against this strain are similar to those for seasonal influenza. Vaccination against influenza A(H1N1)v is also recommended in pregnant women and all children aged 6 months–5 years. *Pandemrix®* is the preferred vaccine in children under 18 years of age and pregnant women. Seasonal influenza vaccine should continue to be offered as normal.

Further information on pandemic influenza, avian influenza and swine influenza may be found at www.dh.gov.uk/pandemicflu and at www.hpa.org.uk.

INFLUENZA VACCINES

Cautions see section 14.1; **interactions:** Appendix 1 (vaccines)

Contra-indications see section 14.1

Pregnancy not known to be harmful

Breast-feeding not known to be harmful

Side-effects see section 14.1; also reported, febrile convulsions and trasient thrombocytopenia

Licensed use Inactivated Influenza Vaccine (Surface Antigen) and *Fluvirin®* are not licensed for use in children under 4 years

Immunological products and vaccines

14

◁ **INFLUENZA VACCINES (continued)**

Indication and dose

Annual immunisation against seasonal influenza

• By intramuscular injection

Child 6 months–3 years 0.25–0.5 mL (repeated after 4–6 weeks in children not previously vaccinated)

Child 3–13 years 0.5 mL (repeated after 4–6 weeks in children not previously vaccinated)

Child 13–18 years 0.5 mL as a single dose

Pandemic influenza A(H1N1)v

See under *Celvapan®* and *Pandemrix®* below

◢ **Seasonal influenza vaccines**

Inactivated Influenza Vaccine (Split Virion) (PoM)

Flu

Injection, suspension of formaldehyde-inactivated influenza virus (split virion) grown in fertilised hens' eggs, net price 0.25-mL prefilled syringe = £6.29, 0.5-mL prefilled syringe = £6.29

Excipients may include neomycin and polymyxin

Available from Sanofi Pasteur

Inactivated Influenza Vaccine (Surface Antigen) (PoM)

Flu or Flu(adj)

Injection, suspension of propiolactone-inactivated influenza virus (surface antigen) grown in fertilised hens' eggs, net price 0.5-mL prefilled syringe = £4.15

Excipients may include neomycin, polymyxin B and traces of thiomersal

Available from Novartis Vaccines

Agrippal® (Novartis Vaccines) (PoM)

Injection, suspension of formaldehyde-inactivated influenza virus (surface antigen) grown in fertilised hens' eggs, net price 0.5-mL prefilled syringe = £5.85

Excipients include kanamycin and neomycin

Begrivac® (Novartis Vaccines) (PoM)

Injection, suspension of formaldehyde-inactivated influenza virus (split virion) grown in fertilised hens' eggs, net price 0.5-mL prefilled syringe = £5.85

Excipients include polymyxin B

Enzira® (Wyeth) (PoM)

Injection, suspension of inactivated influenza virus (split virion) grown in fertilised hens' eggs, net price 0.5-mL prefilled syringe = £6.33

Excipients include neomycin and polymyxin

Fluarix® (GSK) (PoM)

Injection, suspension of formaldehyde-inactivated influenza virus (split virion) grown in fertilised hens' eggs, net price 0.5-mL prefilled syringe = £4.49

Excipients include gentamicin

Fluvirin® (Novartis Vaccines) (PoM)

Injection, suspension of formaldehyde-inactivated influenza virus (surface antigen) grown in fertilised hens' eggs, net price 0.5 mL prefilled syringe = £5.55

Excipients include neomycin, polymyxin B, and traces of thiomersal

Imuvac® (Solvay) (PoM)

Injection, suspension of formaldehyde-inactivated influenza virus (surface antigen) grown in fertilised hens' eggs, net price 0.5-mL prefilled syringe = £6.59

Excipients include gentamicin

Influvac Sub-unit® (Solvay) (PoM)

Injection, suspension of formaldehyde-inactivated influenza virus (surface antigen) grown in fertilised hens' eggs, net price 0.5-mL prefilled syringe = £5.22

Excipients include gentamicin

Mastaflu® (MASTA) (PoM)

Injection, suspension of formaldehyde-inactivated influenza virus (surface antigen) grown in fertilised hens' eggs, net price 0.5-mL prefilled syringe = £6.50

Excipients include gentamicin

Viroflu® (Sanofi Pasteur) (PoM)

Injection, suspension of inactivated influenza virus (surface antigen, virosome) grown in fertilised hens' eggs, net price 0.5-mL prefilled syringe = £6.33

Excipients include neomycin and polymyxin B

◢ **Pandemic influenza A(H1N1)v vaccines**

Celvapan® (Baxter) ▼ (PoM)

Injection, suspension of formaldehyde-inactivated influenza A(H1N1)v virus (whole virion, grown in vero cells), 15 micrograms/mL, 5-mL multidose vial contains 10 doses of 0.5 mL

Dose

Prevention of influenza during a pandemic

• By intramuscular injection

Child 6 months–18 years 2 doses each of 0.5 mL separated by an interval of at least 3 weeks

Note *Celvapan®* is not interchangeable with *Pandemrix®*

Pandemrix® (GSK) ▼ (PoM)

Injection, suspension of inactivated influenza A(H1N1)v virus (split virion, grown in fertilised hens' eggs) 7.5 micrograms/mL when mixed with emulsion of adjuvant, 5 mL of mixed multidose vial contains 10 doses of 0.5 mL

Excipients include gentamicin and thiomersal

Dose

Prevention of influenza during a pandemic

• By intramuscular injection

Child 6 months–10 years 0.25 mL as a single dose; in immunocompromised, repeat dose after an interval of at least 3 weeks

Child 10–18 years 0.5 mL as a single dose; in immunocompromised, repeat dose after an interval of at least 3 weeks

Note *Pandemrix®* is not interchangeable with *Celvapan®*

14

Immunological products and vaccines

Measles vaccine

Measles vaccine has been replaced by a combined live measles, mumps and rubella vaccine (MMR vaccine).

MMR vaccine may be used in the control of outbreaks of measles (see under MMR Vaccine).

◢**Single antigen vaccine**
No longer available in the UK

◢**Combined vaccines**
See MMR vaccine, below

Measles, Mumps and Rubella (MMR) vaccine

A combined live **measles, mumps, and rubella vaccine** (MMR vaccine) aims to eliminate measles, mumps and rubella (and congenital rubella syndrome). Every child should receive two doses of MMR vaccine by entry to primary school, unless there is a valid contra-indication (see section 14.1). MMR vaccine should be given irrespective of previous measles, mumps, or rubella infection or vaccination.

The first dose of MMR vaccine is given to children aged 12–13 months. A second dose is given before starting school at 3–5 years of age (see Immunisation schedule, section 14.1).

When protection against measles is required urgently (e.g. during a measles outbreak), the second dose of MMR vaccine can be given 1 month after the first dose; if the second dose is given before 18 months of age, then children should still receive the routine dose before starting school at 3–5 years of age.

Children presenting for pre-school booster who have not received the first dose of MMR vaccine should be given a dose of MMR vaccine followed 3 months later by a second dose. At school-leaving age or at entry into further education, MMR immunisation should be offered to individuals of both sexes who have not received 2 doses during childhood. In a young adult who has received only a single dose of MMR in childhood, a second dose is recommended to achieve full protection. If 2 doses of MMR vaccine are required, the second dose should be given one month after the initial dose.

MMR vaccine should be used to protect against rubella in *seronegative females of child-bearing age* (see Immunisation schedule, section 14.1). MMR vaccine may also be offered to previously *unimmunised and seronegative post-partum* mothers— vaccination a few days after delivery is important because about 60% of congenital abnormalities from rubella infection occur in babies of mothers who have borne more than one child. Immigrants arriving after the age of school immunisation are particularly likely to require immunisation.

Contacts   MMR vaccine may also be used in the control of outbreaks of measles and should be offered to susceptible children including babies aged over 6 months who are contacts of a case, within 3 days of exposure to infection; these children should still receive routine MMR vaccinations at the recommended ages. Children aged under 9 months for whom avoidance of measles infection is particularly important (such as those with history of recent severe illness) can be given normal immunoglobulin (section 14.5, p. 763) after exposure to measles; routine MMR immunisation should then be given after at least 3 months at the appropriate age.

MMR vaccine is **not suitable** for prophylaxis following exposure to mumps or rubella since the antibody response to the mumps and rubella components is too slow for effective prophylaxis.

Children with impaired immune response should not receive live vaccines (for advice on HIV see section 14.1). If they have been exposed to measles infection they should be given normal immunoglobulin (section 14.5).

Travel   Unimmunised children over 6 months of age travelling to areas where measles is endemic or epidemic should receive MMR vaccine. Children immunised before 12 months of age should still receive two doses of MMR at the recommended ages. If one dose of MMR has already been given to a child, then the second dose should be brought forward to at least one month after the first, to ensure complete protection. If the child is under 18 months of age and the second dose is given within 3 months of the first, then the routine dose, before starting school at 3–5 years, should still be given.

Side-effects   See section 14.1. Also malaise, fever, or a rash can occur after the first dose of MMR vaccine, most commonly about a week after vaccination and lasting about 2 to 3 days. Leaflets are available for parents on advice for reducing fever (including the use of paracetamol). Febrile seizures occur less commonly 6 to 11 days after MMR vaccination; the incidence of febrile seizures is lower than that following measles infection. Parotid swelling occurs occasionally, usually in the third week, and rarely, arthropathy 2 to 3 weeks after immunisation. Adverse reactions are considerably less frequent after the second dose of MMR vaccine than after the first dose.

Idiopathic thrombocytopenic purpura has occurred rarely following MMR vaccination, usually within 6 weeks of the first dose. The risk of idiopathic thrombocytopenic purpura after MMR vaccine is much less than the risk after infection with wild measles or rubella virus. The CSM has recommended that children who develop idiopathic thrombocytopenic purpura within 6 weeks of the first dose of MMR should undergo serological testing before the second dose is due; if the results suggest incomplete immunity against measles, mumps or rubella then a second dose of MMR is recommended. The Specialist and Reference Microbiology Division, Health Protection Agency offers free serological testing for children who develop idiopathic thrombocytopenic purpura *within 6 weeks* of the first dose of MMR.

Post-vaccination aseptic meningitis was reported (rarely and with complete recovery) following vaccination with MMR vaccine containing Urabe mumps vaccine, which has now been discontinued; no cases have been confirmed in association with the currently used Jeryl Lynn mumps vaccine. Children with post-vaccination symptoms are not infectious.

> Reviews undertaken on behalf of the CSM, the Medical Research Council, and the Cochrane Collaboration, have not found any evidence of a link between MMR vaccination and bowel disease or autism. The Chief Medical Officers have advised that the MMR vaccine is the safest and best way to protect children against measles, mumps, and rubella. Information (including fact sheets and a list of references) may be obtained from:
> www.immunisation.nhs.uk/Vaccines/MMR

MEASLES, MUMPS AND RUBELLA VACCINE, LIVE

Cautions   see section 14.1; also after immunoglobulin administration or blood transfusion, leave an interval of at least 3 months before MMR immunisation as antibody response to measles component may be reduced; **interactions:** Appendix 1 (vaccines)

Hypersensitivity to egg There is increasing evidence that MMR vaccine can be given safely even when the child has had an anaphylactic reaction to food containing egg (dislike of egg or refusal to eat egg is not a contra-indication). For children with a confirmed anaphylactic reaction to egg-containing food, MMR vaccine should be administered in a hospital setting.

Contra-indications   see section 14.1

Pregnancy   avoid pregnancy for at least 1 month after vaccination; see also, p. 733

Breast-feeding   see p. 733

Side-effects   see section 14.1 and notes above; also *less commonly* sleep disturbance, unusual crying in infants, also reported peripheral and optic neuritis.

Licensed use   *Priorix*® not licensed for use in children under 9 months, and *MMRvaxPro*® not licensed for use in children under 1 year

Indication and dose

Immunisation against measles, mumps, and rubella

- By intramuscular or deep subcutaneous injection

   CHILD 6 months–18 years primary immunisation, 2 doses each of 0.5 mL, see Immunisation schedule, section 14.1, p. 735; see also notes above for use in outbreaks, for contacts of cases, and for travel

◀Combined vaccines

MMRvaxPro® (Sanofi Pasteur) ▼ PoM
Injection, powder for reconstitution, live attenuated, measles virus (Enders' Edmonston strain) and mumps virus (Jeryl Lynn [Level B] strain) prepared in chick embryo cells, and rubella virus (Wistar RA 27/3 strain); single-dose vial (with syringe containing solvent)
Excipients include gelatin and neomycin
Only available as part of childhood immunisation schedule from health organisations or Moviato

Priorix® (GSK) PoM
Injection, powder for reconstitution, live attenuated, measles virus (Schwarz strain) and mumps virus (RIT 4385 strain) prepared in chick embryo cells, and rubella virus (Wistar RA 27/3 strain), net

14

Immunological products and vaccines

◁ **MEASLES, MUMPS AND RUBELLA VACCINE, LIVE (*continued*)**

price single-dose vial (with syringe containing solvent) = £6.37
Excipients include neomycin
Also available as part of childhood immunisation schedule
from health organisations or Movianto

Meningococcal vaccines

Almost all childhood meningococcal disease in the UK is caused by *Neisseria meningitidis* serogroups B and C. **Meningococcal Group C conjugate vaccine** protects only against infection by serogroup C. The risk of meningococcal disease declines with age—immunisation is not generally recommended after the age of 25 years.

Childhood immunisation   Meningococcal Group C conjugate vaccine provides long-term protection against infection by serogroup C of *Neisseria meningitidis*. Immunisation consists of 2 doses given at 3 months and 4 months of age; a booster dose should be given at 12–13 months of age, usually combined with haemophilus influenzae type b vaccine (see Immunisation Schedule, section 14.1, p. 735).

It is recommended that meningococcal group C conjugate vaccine be given to anyone aged under 25 years who has not been vaccinated previously with this vaccine; those over 1 year receive a single dose. Children with confirmed serogroup C disease, who have previously been immunised with meningococcal group C vaccine, should be offered meningococcal group C conjugate vaccine before discharge from hospital.

Meningococcal group C conjugate vaccine in patients with asplenia or splenic dysfunction   Meningococcal group C conjugate vaccine is recommended for children with asplenia or splenic dysfunction. Children under 1 year should be vaccinated according to the Immunisation Schedule (section 14.1). Unimmunised children over 1 year should be given 2 doses of meningococcal group C conjugate vaccine (usually combined with haemophilus influenzae type b vaccine) with an interval of 2 months between doses. Immunised children who develop splenic dysfunction should be given 1 additional dose of meningococcal group C conjugate vaccine (usually combined with haemophilus influenzae type b vaccine).

Travel   Children travelling to countries of risk (see below) should be immunised with a meningococcal vaccine that covers serotypes A, C, W135 and Y, even if they have previously received meningitis C conjugate vaccine. If the child has recently received meningococcal group C conjugate vaccine an interval of at least 2 weeks should be allowed before administration of the tetravalent (A, C, W135, and Y) vaccine. The antibody response to serotype C in unconjugated meningococcal polysaccharide vaccines in children under 18 months may be suboptimal.

Vaccination is particularly important for those living with local people or visiting an area of risk during outbreaks.

Immunisation recommendations and requirements for visa entry for individual countries should be checked before travelling, particularly to countries in Sub-Saharan Africa, Asia, and the Indian sub-continent where outbreaks and epidemics of meningococcal infection are reported. Country-by-country information is available from the National Travel Health Network and Centre (www.nathnac.org). Proof of vaccination with the tetravalent (A, C, W135 and Y) meningococcal vaccine is required for those travelling to Saudi Arabia during the Hajj and Umrah pilgrimages (where outbreaks of the W135 strain have occurred).

Contacts   For advice on the immunisation of *laboratory workers and close contacts* of cases of meningococcal disease in the UK and on the role of the vaccine in the control of *local outbreaks*, consult Guidelines for Public Health Management of Meningococcal Disease in the UK at www.hpa.org.uk. See Table 2, section 5.1 for antibacterial prophylaxis for prevention of secondary cases of meningococcal meningitis.

MENINGOCOCCAL VACCINES

Cautions see section 14.1
Contra-indications see section 14.1
Pregnancy see p. 733
Breast-feeding see p. 733
Side-effects see section 14.1; also *rarely* symptoms of meningitis reported (but no evidence that vaccine causes meningococcal C meningitis)
Licensed use *ACWYVax* not licensed in children under 2 years

Indication and dose

Immunisation against *Neisseria meningitidis*
for dose, see under preparations

◢Meningococcal Group C conjugate vaccine
Meningitec® (Wyeth) (PoM)
Injection, suspension of capsular polysaccharide antigen of *Neisseria meningitidis* group C (conjugated to *Corynebacterium diphtheriae* protein), adsorbed onto aluminium phosphate, net price 0.5-mL prefilled syringe = £7.50

Dose
• By intramuscular injection
Child 2 months–1 year for routine immunisation, 0.5 mL, see notes above and Immunisation schedule, section 14.1

Child 1–18 years 0.5 mL as a single dose
Note Subcutaneous route used for children with bleeding disorders

Available as part of childhood immunisation schedule from Movianto

Menjugate Kit® (Sanofi Pasteur) (PoM)
Injection, powder for reconstitution, capsular polysaccharide antigen of *Neisseria meningitidis* group C (conjugated to *Corynebacterium diphtheriae* protein), adsorbed onto aluminium hydroxide, single-dose vials

Dose
• By intramuscular injection
Child 2 months–1 year for routine immunisation, 0.5 mL, see notes above and Immunisation schedule, section 14.1

Child 1–18 years 0.5 mL as a single dose
Note Subcutaneous route used for children with bleeding disorders

NeisVac-C® (Baxter) (PoM)
Injection, suspension of polysaccharide antigen of *Neisseria meningitidis* group C (conjugated to tetanus toxoid protein), adsorbed onto aluminium hydroxide, 0.5-mL prefilled syringe

Dose
• By intramuscular injection
Child 2 months–1 year for routine immunisation, 0.5 mL, see notes above and Immunisation schedule, section 14.1

Child 1–18 years 0.5 mL as a single dose

Available from Movianto

◢Meningococcal Group C conjugate vaccine with Haemophilus Influenzae type B vaccine
See *Haemophilus Influenzae* type B vaccine

◢Meningococcal A, C, W135, and Y conjugate vaccine
Menveo® (Novartis Vaccines) ▼ (PoM)
Injection, powder for reconstitution, capsular oligosaccharide antigens of *Neisseria meningitidis* groups A, C, W135, and Y (conjugated to *Corynebacterium diphtheriae* protein), net price single-dose vial (with syringe containing diluent) = £40.01

Dose
• By intramuscular injection preferably into deltoid region
Child 11–18 years 0.5 mL as a single dose

◢Meningococcal polysaccharide A, C, W135 and Y vaccine
ACWY Vax® (GSK) ▼ (PoM)
Injection, powder for reconstitution, capsular polysaccharide antigens of *Neisseria meningitidis* groups A, C, W135 and Y, net price single-dose vial (with syringe containing diluent) = £16.73

Dose
• By deep subcutaneous injection
Child 3 months–2 years 2 doses (each of 0.5 mL) separated by an interval of 3 months; antibody response may be suboptimal in this age group

Child 2–18 years 0.5 mL as a single dose; booster dose for those at continued risk, 0.5 mL 5 years after initial dose (children under 5 years when first vaccinated, should be given a booster dose after 2–3 years)

Mumps vaccine

◢Single antigen vaccine
No longer available in the UK

◢Combined vaccines
See MMR Vaccine, p. 750

Pertussis vaccine

Pertussis vaccine is given as a combination preparation containing other vaccines (see Diphtheria Vaccines). Acellular vaccines are derived from highly purified components of *Bordetella pertussis*. Primary immunisation against pertussis (whooping cough) requires 3 doses of an acellular pertussis-containing vaccine (see Immunisation schedule, section 14.1, p. 735), given at intervals of 1 month from the age of 2 months.

A booster dose of an acellular pertussis-containing vaccine should be given 3 years after the primary course.

All children up to the age of 10 years should receive primary immunisation with diphtheria, tetanus, pertussis (acellular, component), poliomyelitis (inactivated) and haemophilus type b conjugate vaccine (adsorbed).

Children aged 1–10 years who have not received a *pertussis-containing* vaccine as part of their primary immunisation schedule should be offered 1 dose of a suitable pertussis-containing vaccine; after an interval of at least 1 year, a booster dose of a suitable pertussis-containing vaccine should be given. Immunisation against pertussis is not currently recommended in individuals over 10 years of age.

Cautions   Section 14.1

Contra-indications   Section 14.1

Pregnancy   see p. 733

Breast-feeding   see p. 733

Side effects   See also section 14.1. The incidence of local and systemic effects is generally lower with vaccines containing acellular pertussis components than with the whole-cell pertussis vaccine used. However, compared with primary vaccination, booster doses with vaccines containing acellular pertussis are reported to increase the risk of injection-site reactions (some of which affect the entire limb); local reactions do not contra-indicate further doses (see below).

The vaccine should not be withheld from children with a history to a preceding dose of:

- fever, irrespective of severity;
- persistent crying or screaming for more than 3 hours;
- severe local reaction, irrespective of extent.

◢ **Combined vaccines**
Combined vaccines, see under Diphtheria vaccines

Pneumococcal vaccines

Pneumococcal vaccines protect against infection with *Streptococcus pneumoniae* (pneumococcus); the vaccines contain polysaccharide from capsular pneumococci, **Pneumococcal polysaccharide vaccine** contains purified polysaccharide from 23 capsular types of pneumococci, whereas **pneumococcal polysaccharide conjugate vaccine** (adsorbed) contains polysaccharide from either 10 capsular types (*Synflorix®*) or 13 capsular types (*Prevenar* 13®) with the polysaccharide being conjugated to protein.

The 13-valent conjugate vaccine is used for childhood immunisation. The recommended schedule consists of 3 doses, the first at 2 months of age, the second at 4 months, and the third at 12–13 months (see Immunisation Schedule, section 14.1).

Pneumococcal vaccination is recommended for individuals at increased risk of pneumococcal infection as follows:

- child under 5 years with a history of invasive pneumococcal disease;
- asplenia or splenic dysfunction (including homozygous sickle cell disease and coeliac disease which could lead to splenic dysfunction);
- chronic respiratory disease (includes asthma treated with continuous or frequent use of a systemic corticosteroid);
- chronic heart disease;
- chronic renal disease;
- chronic liver disease;
- diabetes mellitus;
- immune deficiency because of disease (e.g. HIV infection) or treatment (including prolonged systemic corticosteroid treatment);
- presence of cochlear implant;
- conditions where leakage of cerebrospinal fluid could occur.

Where possible, the vaccine should be given at least 2 weeks before splenectomy, cochlear implant surgery, and chemotherapy; children and carers should be given advice about increased risk of pneumococcal infection. Prophylactic antibacterial therapy against pneumococcal infection (Table 2, section 5.1, p. 312) should not be stopped after immunisation. A patient card and information leaflet for patients with asplenia are available from the Department of Health or in Scotland from the Scottish Executive, Public Health Division 1 (Tel (0131) 244 2501).

Choice of vaccine   Children under 2 years at increased risk of pneumococcal infection (see list above) should receive the 13-valent pneumococcal polysaccharide conjugate vaccine (adsorbed) at the recommended ages, followed by a single dose of the 23-valent pneumococcal polysaccharide vaccine after their second birthday (see below). Children at increased risk of pneumococcal infection presenting late for vaccination should receive 2 doses (separated by at least 1 month) of the 13-valent pneumococcal polysaccharide conjugate vaccine (adsorbed) before the age of 12 months, and a third dose at 13 months. Children over 12 months and under 5 years (who have not been vaccinated or not completed the primary course) should receive a single dose of 13-valent pneumococcal polysaccharide conjugate vaccine (adsorbed) (2 doses separated by an interval of 2 months in the immunocompromised or those with asplenia or splenic dysfunction). All children under 5 years at increased risk of pneumococcal infection should receive a single dose of the 23-valent pneumococcal polysaccharide vaccine after their second birthday and at least 2 months after the final dose of the 13-valent pneumococcal polysaccharide conjugate vaccine (adsorbed).

Children over 5 years who are at increased risk of pneumococcal disease should receive a single dose of the 23-valent unconjugated pneumococcal polysaccharide vaccine.

Revaccination   In individuals with higher concentrations of antibodies to pneumococcal polysaccharides, revaccination with the 23-valent pneumococcal polysaccharide vaccine more commonly produces adverse reactions. Revaccination is therefore not recommended, except every 5 years in individuals in whom the antibody concentration is likely to decline rapidly (e.g. asplenia, splenic dysfunction and nephrotic syndrome). If there is doubt, the need for revaccination should be discussed with a haematologist, immunologist, or microbiologist.

◢ PNEUMOCOCCAL VACCINES

Cautions see section 14.1
Contra-indications see section 14.1
Pregnancy see p. 733
Breast-feeding see p. 733
Side-effects see section 14.1; *also* Revaccination, above

Indication and dose

Immunisation against pneumococcal infection
   for dose see under preparations

◢ Pneumococcal polysaccharide vaccines
Pneumovax® II (Sanofi Pasteur) [PoM]
   Injection, polysaccharide from each of 23 capsular types of pneumococcus, net price 0.5-mL vial = £8.49

Dose
• By subcutaneous or intramuscular injection
   Child 2–18 years 0.5 mL; revaccination, see notes above

◢ Pneumococcal polysaccharide conjugate vaccine (adsorbed)
Prevenar 13® (Wyeth) ▼ [PoM]
   Injection, polysaccharide from each of 13 capsular types of pneumococcus (conjugated to carrier protein) adsorbed onto aluminium phosphate, net price 0.5-mL prefilled syringe = £49.10

Dose
• By intramuscular injection
   Child 2 months–5 years 0.5 mL (see notes above and Immunisation schedule, section 14.1)
   Note Deltoid muscle is preferred site of injection in young children; anterolateral thigh is preferred site in infants
   The dose in *BNF for Children* may differ from that in product literature

Synflorix® (GSK) ▼ [PoM]
   Injection, polysaccharide from each of 10 capsular types of pneumococcus (conjugated to carrier proteins) adsorbed onto aluminium phosphate, net price 0.5-mL prefilled syringe = £27.60

Dose
• By intramuscular injection
   Child 6 weeks–2 years consult product literature

Note Deltoid muscle is preferred site of injection in young children; anterolateral thigh is preferred site in infants

▌ Poliomyelitis vaccines

Two types of poliomyelitis vaccine (containing strains of poliovirus types 1, 2, and 3) are available, inactivated poliomyelitis vaccine (for injection) and live (oral) poliomyelitis vaccine. **Inactivated poliomyelitis vaccine**, only available in combined preparation (see under Diphtheria vaccines, combined), is recommended for routine immunisation; it is given by injection and contains inactivated strains of human poliovirus types 1, 2 and 3.

A course of primary immunisation consists of 3 doses of a combined preparation containing inactivated poliomyelitis vaccine starting at 2 months of age with intervals of 1 month between doses (see Immunisation schedule, section 14.1). A course of 3 doses should also be given to all unimmunised children; no child should remain unimmunised against poliomyelitis.

Two booster doses of a preparation containing inactivated poliomyelitis vaccine are recommended, the first before school entry and the second before leaving school (see Immunisation schedule, section 14.1). Further booster doses should be given every 10 years only to individuals at special risk.

Preparations containing inactivated poliomyelitis vaccine can be used to complete an immunisation course initiated with the live (oral) poliomyelitis vaccine. **Live (oral) poliomyelitis vaccine** is available only for use during outbreaks. The live (oral) vaccine poses a very rare risk of vaccine-associated paralytic polio because the attenuated strain of the virus can revert to a virulent form. For this reason the live (oral) vaccine must **not** be used for immunosuppressed individuals or their household contacts. The use of inactivated poliomyelitis vaccine removes the risk of vaccine-associated paralytic polio altogether.

Travel Unimmunised travellers to areas with a high incidence of poliomyelitis should receive a full 3–dose course of a preparation containing inactivated poliomyelitis vaccine. Those who have not been vaccinated in the last 10 years should receive a booster dose of **adsorbed diphtheria [low dose], tetanus and poliomyelitis (inactivated) vaccine**. Information about countries with a high incidence of poliomyelitis can be obtained from www.travax.nhs.uk or from the National Travel Health Network and Centre, p. 770 (www.nathnac.org).

POLIOMYELITIS VACCINES

Cautions see section 14.1; *also for live vaccine*, interactions: Appendix 1 (vaccines)

Contra-indications see notes above and section 14.1

Pregnancy see p. 733

Breast-feeding see p. 733

Side-effects see notes above and section 14.1

Indication and dose
See under preparations

◢**Combined vaccines**
See under Diphtheria-containing Vaccines

◢**Inactivated (Salk) Vaccine**
See under Diphtheria-containing Vaccines

◢Live (oral) (Sabin) vaccine
Poliomyelitis Vaccine, Live (Oral) (GSK) (PoM)
OPV

A suspension of suitable live attenuated strains of poliomyelitis virus, types 1, 2, and 3. Available in single-dose and 10-dose containers
Excipients include neomycin and polymyxin B

Dose

Control of outbreaks
• By mouth
  Child 1 month–18 years 3 drops; may be given on a lump of sugar; not to be given with foods which contain preservatives

Note Live poliomyelitis vaccine loses potency once the container has been opened—any vaccine remaining at the end of an immunisation session should be discarded; whenever possible sessions should be arranged to avoid undue wastage.

Rabies vaccine

Rabies vaccine contains inactivated rabies virus cultivated in either human diploid cells or purified chick embryo cells; vaccines are used for pre- and post-exposure prophylaxis.

Pre-exposure prophylaxis Immunisation should be offered to children at high risk of exposure to rabies—where there is limited access to prompt medical care for those living in areas where rabies is enzootic, for those travelling to such areas for longer than 1 month, and for those on shorter visits who may be exposed to unusual risk. Transmission of rabies by humans has not been recorded but it is advised that those caring for children with the disease should be vaccinated.

Immunisation against rabies is indicated during pregnancy if there is substantial risk of exposure to rabies and rapid access to post-exposure prophylaxis is likely to be limited.

Up-to-date country-by-country information on the incidence of rabies can be obtained from the National Travel Health Network and Centre (www.nathnac.org) and, in Scotland, from Health Protection Scotland (www.hps.scot.nhs.uk).

Immunisation against rabies requires 3 doses of rabies vaccine, with further booster doses for those who remain at continued risk.

Post-exposure management Following potential exposure to rabies, the wound or site of exposure (e.g. mucous membrane) should be cleansed under running water and washed for several minutes with soapy water as soon as possible after exposure. Disinfectant and a simple dressing can be applied, but suturing should be delayed because it may increase the risk of introducing rabies virus into the nerves.

Post-exposure prophylaxis against rabies depends on the level of risk in the country, the nature of exposure, and the individual's immunity. In each case, expert risk assessment and advice on appropriate management should be obtained from the Health Protection Agency Virus Reference Department, Colindale, London (tel. (020) 8200 4400) or the Centre for Infections (tel. (020) 8200 6868), in Scotland from Health Protection Scotland (tel. (0141) 300 1100), in Northern Ireland from the Public Health Laboratory, Belfast City Hospital (tel. (028) 9032 9241).

There are no specific contra-indications to the use of rabies vaccine for post-exposure prophylaxis and its use should be considered whenever a child has been attacked by an animal in a country where rabies is enzootic, even if there is no direct evidence of rabies in the attacking animal. Because of the potential consequences of untreated rabies exposure and because rabies vaccination has not been associated with fetal abnormalities, pregnancy is not considered a contra-indication to post-exposure prophylaxis.

For post-exposure prophylaxis of *fully immunised* individuals (who have previously received pre-exposure or post-exposure prophylaxis with cell-derived rabies vaccine), 2 doses of cell-derived vaccine, given on day 0 and day 3, are likely to be sufficient. Rabies immunoglobulin is not necessary in such cases.

Post-exposure treatment for *unimmunised individuals* (or those whose prophylaxis is possibly incomplete) comprises 5 doses of rabies vaccine given over 1 month (on days 0, 3, 7, 14, and 30); also, depending on the level of risk (determined by factors such as the nature of the bite and the country where it was sustained), rabies immunoglobulin (section 14.5.2) is given on day 0. The immunisation course can be discontinued if it is proved that the child was not at risk.

RABIES VACCINE

Cautions see section 14.1
Contra-indications see section 14.1; but see also Post-exposure Management in notes above
Pregnancy see p. 733
Breast-feeding see p. 733
Side-effects see section 14.1; also reported paresis

Indication and dose

Pre-exposure immunisation against rabies
• By intramuscular injection in deltoid region or anterolateral thigh in infants

Child 1 month–18 years 1 mL on days 0, 7, and 21 or 28; for those at continued risk give a single reinforcing dose 1 year after the primary course is completed and booster doses every 3–5 years; for those at intermittent risk give booster doses every 2–5 years

Post-exposure immunisation against rabies
• By intramuscular injection in deltoid region or anterolateral thigh in infants

Child 1 month–18 years 1 mL (see notes above)

Rabies Vaccine (Sanofi Pasteur) PoM
Rab
Injection, powder for reconstitution, freeze-dried inactivated Wistar rabies virus strain PM/WI 38 1503-3M cultivated in human diploid cells, net price single-dose vial with syringe containing diluent = £24.40
Excipients include neomycin

Rabipur® (Novartis Vaccines) PoM
Injection, powder for reconstitution, freeze-dried inactivated Flury LEP rabies virus strain cultivated in chick embryo cells, net price single-dose vial = £24.40
Excipients include neomycin

Rotavirus vaccine

Rotavirus vaccine is a live, oral vaccine licensed for immunisation of infants over 6 weeks of age for protection against gastro-enteritis caused by rotavirus infection. The vaccine is not included in the childhood immunisation schedule.

The rotavirus vaccine virus is excreted in the stool and may be transmitted to close contacts; the vaccine should be used with caution in those with immunosuppressed close contacts. Carers of a recently vaccinated baby should be advised of the need to wash their hands after changing the baby's nappies.

◢ ROTAVIRUS VACCINE

Cautions see section 14.1; *also* diarrhoea or vomiting (postpone vaccination); immunosuppressed close contacts (see notes above); **interactions**: Appendix 1 (vaccines)

Contra-indications see section 14.1; also predisposition to, or history of, intussusception

Side-effects see section 14.1

Indication and dose

Immunisation against gastro-enteritis caused by rotavirus infection

• By mouth

Child over 6 weeks 2 doses of 1 mL, separated by an interval of at least 4 weeks; course should

be completed before 24 weeks of age (preferably before 16 weeks)

Rotarix® (GSK) ▼ PoM
Oral suspension, powder for reconstitution, live attenuated rotavirus RIX4414 strain, net price single-dose vial (with oral syringe containing diluent) = £41.38

Rubella vaccine

A combined measles, mumps and rubella vaccine (MMR vaccine) aims to eliminate rubella (German measles) and congenital rubella syndrome. MMR vaccine is used for childhood vaccination as well as for vaccinating adults (including women of child-bearing age) who do not have immunity against rubella the combined live measles, mumps and rubella vaccine is a suitable alternative.

◢ **Single antigen vaccine**
No longer available in the UK; see MMR vaccine, p. 750

◢ **Combined vaccines**
see MMR vaccine

Smallpox vaccine

Limited supplies of **smallpox vaccine** are held at the Specialist and Reference Microbiology Division, Health Protection Agency (Tel. (020) 8200 4400) for the exclusive use of workers in laboratories where pox viruses (such as vaccinia) are handled.

If a wider use of the vaccine is being considered, *Guidelines for smallpox response and management in the post-eradication era* should be consulted at www.dh.gov.uk

---

Tetanus vaccines

Tetanus vaccine contains a cell-free purified toxin of *Clostridium tetani* adsorbed on aluminium hydroxide or aluminium phosphate to improve antigenicity.

Primary immunisation for children under 10 years consists of 3 doses of a combined preparation containing adsorbed tetanus vaccine (see Diphtheria-containing Vaccines), with an interval of 1 month between doses. Following routine childhood vaccination, 2 booster doses of a preparation containing adsorbed tetanus vaccine are recommended, the first before school entry and the second before leaving school. (see Immunisation schedule, section 14.1).

The recommended schedule of tetanus vaccination not only gives protection against tetanus in childhood but also gives the basic immunity for subsequent booster doses. In most circumstances, a total number of 5 doses of tetanus vaccine is considered sufficient for long-term protection.

For primary immunisation of children over 10 years previously unimmunised against tetanus, 3 doses of **adsorbed diphtheria [low dose], tetanus and poliomyelitis (inactivated) vaccine** are given with an interval of 1 month between doses (see Diphtheria-containing Vaccines).

Cautions See also Section 14.1. When a child presents for a booster dose but has been vaccinated following a tetanus-prone wound, the vaccine preparation administered at the time of injury should be determined. If this is not possible, the booster should still be given to ensure adequate protection against all antigens in the booster vaccine.

Very rarely, tetanus has developed after abdominal surgery; carers of children awaiting elective surgery should be asked about the child's tetanus immunisation status and the child should be immunised if necessary.

Parenteral drug abuse is also associated with tetanus; those abusing drugs by injection should be vaccinated if unimmunised—booster doses should be given if there is any doubt about their immunisation status.

Travel recommendations see section 14.6.

Contra-indications   See section 14.1

Pregnancy   see p. 733

Breast-feeding   see p. 733

Side-effects   See section 14.1

Wounds   Wounds are considered to be tetanus-prone if they are sustained more than 6 hours before surgical treatment *or* at any interval after injury and are puncture-type (particularly if contaminated with soil or manure) *or* show much devitalised tissue *or* are septic *or* are compound fractures *or* contain foreign bodies. All wounds should receive thorough cleansing.

- For *clean wounds*: fully immunised individuals (those who have received a total of 5 doses of a tetanus-containing vaccine at appropriate intervals) and those whose primary immunisation is complete (with boosters up to date), do not require tetanus vaccine; individuals whose primary immunisation is incomplete or whose boosters are not up to date require a reinforcing dose of a tetanus-containing vaccine (followed by further doses as required to complete the schedule); non-immunised individuals (or those whose immunisation status is not known or who have been fully immunised but are now immuno-compromised) should be given a dose of the appropriate tetanus-containing vaccine immediately (followed by completion of the full course of the vaccine if records confirm the need).

- For *tetanus-prone wounds*: management is as for clean wounds with the addition of a dose of tetanus immunoglobulin (section 14.5.2) given at a different site; in fully immunised individuals and those whose primary immunisation is complete (with boosters up to date) the immunoglobulin is needed only if the risk of infection is especially high (e.g. contamination with manure). Antibacterial prophylaxis (with benzylpenicillin, co-amoxiclav, or metronidazole) may also be required for tetanus-prone wounds.

◢**Combined vaccines**

See Diphtheria-containing Vaccines

Tick-borne encephalitis vaccine

Tick-borne encephalitis vaccine contains inactivated tick-bourne encephalitis virus cultivated in chick embryo cells. It is recommended for immunisation of those living in or visiting high-risk areas (see International Travel, section 14.6). Children walking or camping in warm forested areas of Central and Eastern Europe and Scandinavia, particularly from April to October when ticks are most prevalent, are at greatest risk of tick-borne encephalitis. For full protection, 3 doses of the vaccine are required; booster doses are required every 3–5 years for those still at risk. Ideally, immunisation should be completed at least one month before travel.

◢ TICK-BORNE ENCEPHALITIS VACCINE, INACTIVATED

Cautions see section 14.1
Contra-indications see section 14.1
Pregnancy see p. 733
Breast-feeding see p. 733
Side-effects see section 14.1

Indication and dose

Immunisation against tick-borne encephalitis
- By intramuscular injection in deltoid region or anterolateral thigh in infants

  Child 1–16 years initial immunisation, 3 doses of 0.25 mL, second dose after 1–3 months and third dose after a further 5–12 months

⌒ TICK-BORNE ENCEPHALITIS VACCINE, INACTIVATED (*continued*)

Child 16–18 years 3 doses each of 0.5 mL, second dose after 1–3 months and third dose after further 5–12 months

Immunocompromised (including those receiving immunosuppressants), antibody concentration may be measured 4 weeks after second dose and dose repeated if protective levels not achieved

Note To achieve more rapid protection, second dose may be given 14 days after first dose.

Booster doses, give first dose within 3 years after initial course, then every 3–5 years

TicoVac® (MASTA) PoM

Injection, suspension, formaldehyde-inactivated Neudörfl tick-borne encephalitis virus strain, (cultivated in chick embryo cells) adsorbed onto hydrated aluminium hydroxide, net price 0.25-mL prefilled syringe (*TicoVac Junior®*) = £28.00, 0.5-mL prefilled syringe = £32.00

Excipients include gentamicin and neomycin

Typhoid vaccines

Typhoid vaccine is available as Vi capsular polysaccharide injectable vaccine (from *Salmonella typhi*) for injection; and as live attenuated *Salmonella typhi* vaccine for oral use.

Typhoid immunisation is advised for children travelling to:

- areas where typhoid is endemic, especially if staying with or visiting local people
- endemic areas where frequent or prolonged exposure to poor sanitation and poor food hygiene is likely

Typhoid vaccination is not a substitute for scrupulous personal hygiene (see p. 769).

Capsular **polysaccharide typhoid vaccine** is usually given by *intramuscular* injection. Children under 2 years may respond suboptimally to the vaccine, but children aged between 1–2 years should be immunised if the risk of typhoid fever is considered high (immunisation is not recommended for infants under 12 months). Booster doses are needed every 3 years on continued exposure.

Oral typhoid vaccine is a **live attenuated** vaccine contained in an enteric-coated capsule. One capsule taken on alternate days for a total of 3 doses, provides protection 7–10 days after the last dose. Protection may persist for up to 3 years in those constantly (or repeatedly) exposed to *Salmonella typhi*, but occasional travellers require further courses at intervals of 1 year.

Interactions   Oral typhoid vaccine is inactivated by concomitant administration of antibacterials or antimalarials:

- Antibacterials should be avoided for 3 days before and after oral typhoid vaccination;
- Mefloquine should be avoided for at least 12 hours before or after oral typhoid;
- For other antimalarials, vaccination with oral typhoid vaccine should be completed at least 3 days before the first dose of the antimalarial (except proguanil hydrochloride with atovaquone, which may be given concomitantly).

TYPHOID VACCINE

Cautions section 14.1; **interactions**: see above and Appendix 1 (vaccines)

Contra-indications section 14.1; also for *oral* vaccine, acute gastro-intestinal illness

Pregnancy see p. 733

Breast-feeding see p. 733

Side-effects section 14.1

Indication and dose

Immunisation against typhoid fever
  for dose see under preparations

◀Typhoid polysaccharide vaccine for injection

Typherix® (GSK) PoM

Injection, Vi capsular polysaccharide typhoid vaccine, 50 micrograms/mL virulence polysaccharide antigen of *Salmonella typhi*, net price 0.5-mL prefilled syringe = £9.93

Dose

- By intramuscular injection

   Child under 2 years [unlicensed use], 0.5 mL, at least 2 weeks before potential exposure to typhoid infection; response may be suboptimal (see notes above)

   Child 2–18 years 0.5 mL, at least 2 weeks before potential exposure to typhoid infection

◻ **TYPHOID VACCINE** (*continued*)

Typhim Vi® (Sanofi Pasteur) PoM
Injection, Vi capsular polysaccharide typhoid
vaccine, 50 micrograms/mL virulence polysaccharide antigen of formaldehyde-inactivated
Salmonella typhi, net price 0.5-mL prefilled syringe
= £9.30

Dose
- **By intramuscular injection**
  Child under 2 years [unlicensed use], 0.5 mL, at least 2
  weeks before potential exposure to typhoid infection;
  response may be suboptimal (see notes above)

  Child 2–18 years 0.5 mL, at least 2 weeks before
  potential exposure to typhoid infection

◀ **Polysaccharide vaccine with hepatitis A vaccine**
See Hepatitis A Vaccine

◀ **Typhoid vaccine, live (oral)**
Vivotif® (Crucell) PoM
Capsules, e/c, live attenuated *Salmonella typhi*
(Ty21a), net price 3-cap pack = £14.77. Label: 23,
25, counselling, administration

Dose
- **By mouth**
  Child 6–18 years 1 capsule on days 1, 3, and 5
  Counselling Swallow as soon as possible after placing
  in mouth with a cold or lukewarm drink; it is important
  to store capsules in a refrigerator

Varicella–zoster vaccine

Varicella–zoster vaccine (live) is licensed for immunisation against varicella in
seronegative individuals. It is not recommended for routine use in children but
can be given to seronegative healthy children over 1 year who come into close
contact with individuals at high risk of severe varicella infections.

Rarely, the varicella–zoster vaccine virus has been transmitted from the vaccinated individual to close contacts. Therefore, contact with the following should be
avoided if a vaccine-related cutaneous rash develops within 4–6 weeks of the first
or second dose:

- varicella-susceptible pregnant females;
- individuals at high risk of severe varicella, including those with immunodeficiency or those receiving immunosuppressive therapy.

Varicella–zoster immunoglobulin is used to protect susceptible children at
increased risk of varicella infection, see p. 767.

VARICELLA–ZOSTER VACCINES

Cautions see section 14.1; also post-vaccination
close-contact with susceptible individuals (see
notes above): **interactions**: Appendix 1 (vaccines)

Contra-indications see section 14.1

Pregnancy avoid pregnancy for 3 months after
vaccination; see also p. 733

Breast-feeding see p. 733

Side-effects see section 14.1; *also* varicella-like
rash; *rarely* thrombocytopenia

Indication and dose

Immunisation against varicella infection (see
notes above)

For dose, see under preparations

Varilrix® (GSK) ▼ PoM
Injection, powder for reconstitution, live attenuated
varicella–zoster virus (Oka strain) propagated in

human diploid cells, net price 0.5-mL vial (with
diluent) = £27.31
Excipients include neomycin

Dose
- **By subcutaneous injection preferably into deltoid
  region**
  Child 1–18 years (see notes above), 2 doses of 0.5 mL
  separated by an interval of at least 6 weeks (minimum
  4 weeks)

Varivax® (Sanofi Pasteur) ▼ PoM
Injection powder for reconstitution, live attenuated
varicella-zoster virus (Oka/Merck strain) propagated in human diploid cells, net price 0.5-mL vial
(with diluent) = £30.89
Excipients include gelatin and neomycin

Dose
- **By intramuscular or subcutaneous injection into
  deltoid region (or higher anterolateral thigh in young
  children)**
  Child 1–13 years (see notes above) 2 doses of 0.5 mL
  separated by an interval of at least 4 weeks (2 doses
  separated by 12 weeks in children with asymptomatic
  HIV infection)

  Child 13–18 years 2 doses of 0.5 mL separated by 4–8
  weeks

Yellow fever vaccine

Live yellow fever vaccine is indicated for those travelling to or living in areas
where infection is endemic (see p. 768). Infants under 6 months of age should not
be vaccinated because there is a small risk of encephalitis; infants aged 6–9
months should be vaccinated only if the risk of yellow fever is high and unavoid-

14

Immunological products and vaccines

able (seek expert advice). The immunity which probably lasts for life is officially accepted for 10 years starting from 10 days after primary immunisation and for a further 10 years immediately after revaccination.

Very rarely vaccine-associated adverse effects have been reported, such as viscerotropic disease (yellow fever vaccine-associated viscerotropic disease, YEL-AVD), a syndrome which may include metabolic acidosis, muscle and liver cytolysis, and multi-organ failure. Neurological disorders (yellow fever vaccine-associated neurotropic disease, YEL-AND) such as encephalitis have also been reported. These *very rare* adverse effects have usually occured after the first dose of yellow fever vaccine in those with no previous immunity.

Pregnancy   Live yellow fever vaccine should not be given during pregnancy, but if a significant risk of exposure cannot be avoided then vaccination should be delayed to the third trimester if possible (but the need for immunisation usually outweighs risk to the fetus).

Breast-feeding   Vaccination should be considered in breast-feeding women when there is a real risk to the mother from yellow fever disease.

YELLOW FEVER VACCINE

Cautions see section 14.1; also see **interactions:** Appendix 1 (vaccines)

Contra-indications see section 14.1 and notes above; also children under 6 months; history of thymus dysfunction

Pregnancy see notes above

Breast-feeding see notes above

Side-effects see section 14.1; *also* reported neurotropic disease, and viscerotropic disease (see notes above)

Indication and dose

Immunisation against yellow fever

• By deep subcutaneous injection

Child 9 months–18 years 0.5 mL (see also notes above)

Yellow Fever Vaccine, Live PoM
Yel(live)
Injection, powder for reconstitution, live, attenuated 17D-204 strain of yellow fever virus, cultivated in chick embryos; single dose vial with syringe containing 0.5 mL diluent
Available (only to designated Yellow Fever Vaccination centres) as *Stamaril*®

14.5 Immunoglobulins

14.5.1   Normal Immunoglobulin
14.5.2   Disease-specific immunoglobulins
14.5.3   Anti-D (Rh₀) immunoglobulin

Two types of human immunoglobulin preparation are available, **normal immunoglobulin** and **disease-specific immunoglobulins**.

Human immunoglobulin is a sterile preparation of concentrated antibodies (immune globulins) recovered from pooled human plasma or serum obtained from outside the UK, tested and found non-reactive for hepatitis B surface antigen and for antibodies against hepatitis C virus and human immunodeficiency virus (types 1 and 2). A global shortage of human immunoglobulin and the rapidly increasing range of clinical indications for treatment with immunoglobulins has resulted in the need for a Demand Management programme in the UK (for further information consult www.ivig.nhs.uk and *Clinical Guidelines for Immunoglobulin Use*, www.dh.gov.uk.

Immunoglobulins of animal origin (antisera) were frequently associated with hypersensitivity reactions and are no longer used.

Further information on the use of immunoglobulins is included in the Health Protection Agency's *Immunoglobulin Handbook*: www.hpa.org.uk and in the Department of Health's publication, *Immunisation against Infectious Disease*, www.dh.gov.uk.

Availability   **Normal immunoglobulin** for intramuscular administration is available from some regional Health Protection Agencies and microbiology laboratories for protection of contacts and the control of outbreaks of hepatitis A, measles, and rubella only. For other indications, subcutaneous or intravenous normal immunoglobulin should be purchased from the manufacturer.

Disease-specific immunoglobulins (section 14.5.2) are available from some regional Health Protection Agencies and microbiology laboratories with the exception of **tetanus immunoglobulin** which is available from BPL, hospital pharmacies, or blood transfusion departments. **Rabies immunoglobulin** is available from the Specialist and Reference Microbiology Division, Health Protection Agency. **Hepatitis B immunoglobulin** required by transplant centres should be obtained commercially.

In Scotland all immunoglobulins are available from the *Blood Transfusion Service*.

14.5.1 Normal Immunoglobulin

Human **normal immunoglobulin** ('HNIG') is prepared from pools of at least 1000 donations of human plasma; it contains immunoglobulin G (IgG) and antibodies to hepatitis A, measles, mumps, rubella, varicella, and other viruses that are currently prevalent in the general population.

Normal immunoglobulin may **interfere with the immune response to live virus vaccines** which should therefore only be given **at least 3 weeks before or 3 months after** an injection of normal immunoglobulin (this does not apply to yellow fever vaccine since normal immunoglobulin does not contain antibody to this virus).

Uses   Normal immunoglobulin (containing 10–18% protein) is administered by *intramuscular injection* for the protection of susceptible contacts against **hepatitis A** virus (infectious hepatitis), **measles** and, to a lesser extent, **rubella**. Injection of immunoglobulin produces immediate protection lasting for several weeks.

Normal immunoglobulin (containing 3–12% protein) for *intravenous administration* is used as *replacement therapy* for children with congenital agammaglobulinaemia and hypogammaglobulinaemia, and for the short-term treatment of idiopathic thrombocytopenic purpura and Kawasaki syndrome; it is also used for the prophylaxis of infection following bone-marrow transplantation and in children with symptomatic HIV infection who have recurrent bacterial infections. Normal immunoglobulin for replacement therapy may also be given intramuscularly or subcutaneously, but intravenous formulations are normally preferred. Intravenous immunoglobulin is also used in the treatment of Guillain-Barré syndrome as an alternative to plasma exchange.

The dose of normal immunoglobulin used as replacement therapy in patients with immunodeficiencies is **not the same** as the dose required for treatment of acute conditions. For Kawasaki syndrome a single dose of 2 g/kg by intravenous infusion should be given with concomitant aspirin (see section 2.9) within 10 days of onset of symptoms (but children with a delayed diagnosis may also benefit).

For guidance on the use of intravenous normal immunoglobulins and alternative therapies for other conditions, consult *Clinical Guidelines for Immunoglobulin Use* (www.dh.gov.uk).

Hepatitis A   Hepatitis A vaccine is preferred for children at risk of infection (see p. 743) including those visiting areas where the disease is highly endemic (all countries excluding Northern and Western Europe, North America, Japan, Australia, and New Zealand). In unimmunised children, transmission of hepatitis A is reduced by good hygiene. Intramuscular normal immunoglobulin is no longer recommended for routine prophylaxis in travellers but it may be indicated for immunocompromised patients if their antibody response to the vaccine is unlikely to be adequate.

Intramuscular normal immunoglobulin is of value in the prevention of infection in close contacts of confirmed cases of hepatitis A where there has been a delay of more than 7 days in identifying contacts, or for close contacts at high risk of

14

Immunological products and vaccines

severe disease. Hepatitis A vaccine may be given at the same time, but it should be given at a separate injection site.

Measles   Intramuscular normal immunoglobulin may be given to prevent or attenuate an attack of measles in children with compromised immunity. Children with compromised immunity who have come into contact with measles should receive intramuscular normal immunoglobulin as soon as possible after exposure. It is most effective if given within 72 hours but can be effective if given within 6 days. For children receiving intravenous immunoglobulin for treatment of other conditions (see above), 100 mg/kg given within 3 weeks before measles exposure should prevent measles.

Intramuscular normal immunoglobulin should also be considered for the following individuals if they have been in contact with a confirmed case of measles or with a person associated with a local outbreak:

- non-immune pregnant women
- infants under 9 months

Further advice should be sought from the Centre for Infections, Health Protection Agency (tel. (020) 8200 6868).

Children with normal immunity who are not in the above categories and who have not been fully immunised against measles, can be given MMR vaccine (section 14.4) for prophylaxis following exposure to measles.

Rubella   Intramuscular immunoglobulin after exposure to rubella does **not** prevent infection in non-immune contacts and is **not** recommended for protection of pregnant females exposed to rubella. It may, however, reduce the likelihood of a clinical attack which may possibly reduce the risk to the fetus. Risk of intrauterine transmission is greatest in the first 11 weeks of pregnancy, between 16 and 20 weeks there is a minimal risk of deafness only, after 20 weeks there is no increased risk. Intramuscular normal immunoglobulin should be used only if termination of pregnancy would be unacceptable to the pregnant individual—it should be given as soon as possible after exposure. Serological follow-up of recipients is essential.

For routine prophylaxis, see MMR vaccine (p. 750).

NORMAL IMMUNOGLOBULIN

Cautions hypo- or agammaglobulinaemia with or without IgA deficiency; interference with live virus vaccines—see p. 763

 Intravenous use Thrombophilic disorders, or risk factors for arterial or venous thromboembolic events; obesity; ensure adequate hydration, renal insufficiency

Contra-indications patients with selective IgA deficiency who have known antibody against IgA

Renal impairment monitor for acute renal failure (intravenous preparations with added sucrose have been associated with cases of renal dysfunction and acute renal failure)

Side-effects nausea, chills, fever, headache, arthralgia, low back pain; *rarely* hypotension, anaphylaxis, cutaneous skin reactions; also reported with *intravenous use* aseptic meningitis, acute renal failure, haemolytic anaemia, thromboembolic events (including myocardial infarction, stroke, pulmonary embolism, and deep vein thrombosis)

 Note Adverse reactions are more likely to occur in patients receiving normal immunoglobulin for the first time, or following a prolonged period between treatments, or when a different brand of normal immunoglobulin is administered

Indication and dose

 See under preparations

 Note Antibody titres can vary widely between normal immunoglobulin preparations from different manufacturers—formulations are **not interchangeable**; patients should be maintained on the same formulation throughout long-term treatment to avoid adverse effects

◢**For intramuscular use**

Normal Immunoglobulin [PoM]

 Normal immunoglobulin injection. 250-mg vial; 750-mg vial

Dose

> **To control outbreaks of hepatitis A** (see notes above)
> - By deep intramuscular injection
>   **Child under 10 years** 250 mg
>   **Child 10–18 years** 500 mg

> **Measles prophylaxis or to attenuate an attack**
> - By deep intramuscular injection
>   **Child under 1 year** 250 mg
>   **Child 1–3 years** 500 mg
>   **Child 3–18 years** 750 mg

14   Immunological products and vaccines

◁ **NORMAL IMMUNOGLOBULIN (continued)**

Rubella in pregnancy, prevention of clinical attack
- By deep intramuscular injection
  750 mg

Available from the Centre for Infections and other regional Health Protection Agency offices (for contacts and control of outbreaks only, see above)

◀**For subcutaneous use**
Note Preparations for subcutaneous use may be administered by intramuscular injection if subcutaneous route not possible; intramuscular route not recommended for patients with thrombocytopenia or other bleeding disorders

Subcuvia® (Baxter) PoM
Normal immunoglobulin (protein 16%) injection, net price 5-mL vial = £32.56, 10-mL vial = £65.12
Dose
Antibody deficiency syndromes
- By subcutaneous injection
  Consult product literature (not licensed for use in children under 12 years)

Subgam® (BPL) PoM
Normal immunoglobulin (protein 14–18%) injection, net price 250-mg vial = £11.20, 750-mg vial = £28.50, 1.5-g vial = £57.00
Dose
Antibody deficiency syndromes
- By subcutaneous injection
  Consult product literature

Hepatitis A prophylaxis (see also notes above)
- By intramuscular injection
  Child under 10 years 500 mg
  Child 10–18 years 750 mg

Measles prophylaxis
- By intramuscular injection
  Child under 1 year 250 mg
  Child 1–3 years 500 mg
  Child 3–18 years 750 mg

Rubella prophylaxis in pregnancy (see also notes above)
- By intramuscular injection
  750 mg

Tetanus prophylaxis (see also p. 767)
- By intramuscular injection
  250 units

Note *Subgam®* is not licensed for prophylactic use, but due to difficulty in obtaining suitable immunoglobulin products, the Health Protection Agency recommends intramuscular use for prophylaxis against Hepatitis A, measles, or rubella

Vivaglobin® (CSL Behring) PoM
Normal immunoglobulin (protein 16%) injection, net price 3-mL vial £17.76, 10-mL vial = £59.20, 20-mL vial = £118.40
Dose
Antibody deficiency syndromes
- By subcutaneous injection
  Consult product literature

◀**For intravenous use**
Note Dose recommendation for Kawasaki Sydrome, see section 14.5.1; other indications—consult product literature for dosage regimens

Flebogamma® (Grifols) PoM
Intravenous infusion, human normal immunoglobulin (protein 5%), net price 0.5 g (10 mL) = £20.00, 2.5 g (50 mL) = £100.00, 5 g (100 mL) = £200.00, 10 g (200 mL) = £400.00
Note Contains sorbitol 50 mg/mL; contra-indicated in patients with hereditary fructose intolerance

Gammagard S/D® (Baxter) PoM
Intravenous infusion, powder for reconstitution, human normal immunoglobulin (providing protein 5% or 10%), net price 0.5 g (with diluent) = £20.05, 2.5 g (with diluent) = £100.25, 5 g (with diluent) = £200.50, 10 g (with diluent) = £401.00

Intratect® (Biotest UK) PoM
Intravenous infusion, human normal immunoglobulin (protein 5%), net price 1 g (20 mL) = £45.00, 2.5 g (50 mL) = £112.50, 5 g (100 mL) = £225.00, 10 g (200 mL) = £450.00

Kiovig® (Baxter) PoM
Intravenous infusion, human normal immunoglobulin (protein 10%), net price 1 g (10 mL) = £49.00, 2.5 g (25 mL) = £122.50, 5 g (50 mL) = £245.00, 10 g (100 mL) = £490.00, 20 g (200 mL) = £980.00
Note Use Glucose 5% intravenous infusion, if dilution prior to administration is required

Octagam® (Octapharma) ▼ PoM
Intravenous infusion, human normal immunoglobulin (protein 5%), net price 2.5 g (50 mL) = £120.00, 5 g (100 mL) = £240.00, 10 g (200 mL) = £480.00, (protein 10%), 5 g (50 mL) = £345.00, 10 g (100 mL) = £690.00,
Note Contains maltose (may cause falsely elevated results with blood glucose testing systems)

Privigen® (CSL Behring) ▼ PoM
Intravenous infusion, human normal immunoglobulin (protein 10%), net price 2.5 g (25 mL) = £135.00, 5 g (50 mL) = £270.00, 10 g (100 mL) = £540.00, 20 g (200 mL) = £1080.00
Note Contains L-proline; contra-indicated in patients with hyperprolinaemia

Vigam® (BPL) ▼ PoM
Intravenous infusion, human normal immunoglobulin (protein 5%), net price 2.5 g (50 mL) = £95.00, 5 g (100 mL) = £190.00, 10 g (200 mL) = £380.00
Note Contains sucrose (see Renal Impairment above)

14 Immunological products and vaccines

14.5.2 Disease-specific immunoglobulins

Specific immunoglobulins are prepared by pooling the plasma of selected human donors with high levels of the specific antibody required. For further information, see *Immunoglobulin Handbook* (www.hpa.org.uk).

There are no specific immunoglobulins for hepatitis A, measles, or rubella—normal immunoglobulin, section 14.5.1 is used in certain circumstances. There is no specific immunoglobulin for mumps; neither normal immunoglobulin nor MMR vaccine is effective as post-exposure prophylaxis.

Hepatitis B

Disease-specific **hepatitis B immunoglobulin** ('HBIG') is available for use in association with hepatitis B vaccine for the prevention of infection in infants born to mothers who have become infected with this virus in pregnancy or who are high-risk carriers (see Hepatitis B Vaccine, p. 745). Hepatitis B immunoglobulin will not inhibit the antibody response when given at the same time as hepatitis B vaccine, but should be given in different sites.

HEPATITIS B IMMUNOGLOBULIN

Cautions IgA deficiency; interference with live virus vaccines—see under Normal Immunoglobulin, p. 763

Side-effects injection site swelling and pain, arthralgia; *rarely* anaphylaxis chest tightness, dyspnoea; also reported tremor, dizziness, facial oedema, glossitis, and buccal ulceration; for side-effects associated with *intravenous* immunoglobulins, see section 14.5.1

Indication and dose

See under preparations and see also notes above

Hepatitis B Immunoglobulin [PoM]
Injection, hepatitis B-specific immunoglobulin, 100 units/mL. Vials containing 200 units or 500 units, available from selected Health Protection Agency and NHS laboratories (except for Transplant Centres, see p. 763), also available from BPL

Note Hepatitis B immunoglobulin for *intravenous* use is available from BPL on a named-patient basis.

Dose
Prophylaxis against hepatitis B infection
• By intramuscular injection
(As soon as possible after exposure; ideally within 48 hours, but no later than 7 days after exposure)

Child 1 month–5 years 200 units

Child 5–10 years 300 units

Child 10–18 years 500 units

Prevention of transmitted infection at birth
• By intramuscular injection

Neonate 200 units as soon as possible after birth; for full details consult *Immunisation against Infectious Disease* (www.dh.gov.uk)

Heptatect® CP (Biotest UK) ▼ [PoM]
Intravenous infusion, hepatitis B-specific immunoglobulin 50 units/mL, net price 500 units (10 mL) = £300.00, 2000 units (40 mL) = £1100.00

Dose
Following exposure to hepatitis B virus-contaminated material (as soon as possible after exposure, but no later than 72 hours)
• By intravenous infusion

Child 2–18 years 8–10 units/kg; repeat dose after 2 months if necessary, infuse at initial rate of 0.1 mL/kg/hour for 10 minutes, then increase rate gradually to max. 1 mL/kg/hour

Prevention of transmitted infection at birth
• By intravenous infusion

Neonate 20–50 units/kg (minimum dose 100 units) given at a rate of 2 mL over 5–15 minutes

Prophylaxis against re-infection of transplanted liver
Consult product literature

Rabies

Following exposure of an unimmunised child to an animal in or from a country where the risk of rabies is high, the site of the bite should be washed with soapy water and specific **rabies immunoglobulin** of human origin should be administered. All of the dose should be injected around the site of the wound; if this is difficult or the wound has completely healed it can be given in the anterolateral thigh (remote from the site used for vaccination). Rabies vaccine should also be given intramuscularly at a different site (for details see Rabies Vaccine, p. 756).

RABIES IMMUNOGLOBULIN

Cautions IgA deficiency; interference with live virus vaccines—see p. 763 under Normal Immunoglobulin

Side-effects injection site swelling and pain; *rarely* anaphylaxis; buccal ulceration, glossitis,

14 Immunological products and vaccines

◁ **RABIES IMMUNOGLOBULIN** (*continued*)

chest tightness, dyspnoea, tremor, dizziness, arthralgia, and facial oedema also reported

Indication and dose

Post-exposure prophylaxis against rabies infection

• **By intramuscular injection**

20 units/kg, *by infiltration* in and around the cleansed wound; if the wound not visible or healed or if infiltration of whole volume not possible, give remainder *by intramuscular injection* into anterolateral thigh (remote from vaccination site)

Note The potency of individual batches of rabies immunoglobulin from the manufacturer may vary;

potency may also be described differently by different manufacturers. It is therefore essential to know the potency of the batch to be used and the weight of the patient in order to calculate the specific volume required to provide the necessary dose

Rabies Immunoglobulin PoM
(Antirabies Immunoglobulin Injection)

See notes above

Available from Specialist and Reference Microbiology Division, Health Protection Agency (see section 14.5 under Availability) (also from BPL)

Tetanus

Tetanus immunoglobulin, together with metronidazole (section 5.1.11) and wound cleansing, should also be used for the treatment of established cases of tetanus.

For the management of tetanus-prone wounds, **tetanus immunoglobulin** of human origin should be used in addition to wound cleansing and, where appropriate, antibacterial prophylaxis and a tetanus-containing vaccine (see Diphtheria-containing Vaccines, section 14.4).

Where intramuscular tetanus immunoglobulin is in short supply, normal immunoglobulin (section 14.5.1) may be used as an alternative for both treatment and prophylaxis; see www.hpa.org.uk for further details

TETANUS IMMUNOGLOBULIN

Cautions IgA deficiency; interference with live virus vaccines—see, p. 763

Side-effects injection site swelling and pain; *rarely* anaphylaxis; buccal ulceration; glossitis, chest tightness, dyspnoea, tremor, dizziness, arthralgia, and facial oedema also reported

Indication and dose

Post-exposure prophylaxis

• **By intramuscular injection**

250 units, increased to 500 units if more than 24 hours have elapsed or there is risk of heavy contamination or following burns

Treatment of tetanus infection

• **By intramuscular injection**

150 units/kg (multiple sites)

Tetanus Immunoglobulin PoM
(Antitetanus Immunoglobulin Injection)
Available from BPL

Note May be difficult to obtain

Varicella–zoster

Varicella–zoster immunoglobulin (VZIG) is recommended for individuals who are at increased risk of severe varicella *and* who have no antibodies to varicella–zoster virus *and* who have significant exposure to chickenpox or herpes zoster. Those at increased risk include:

• neonates whose mothers develop chickenpox in the period 7 days before to 7 days after delivery;

• susceptible neonates exposed in the first 7 days of life;

• susceptible neonates or infants exposed whilst requiring intensive or prolonged special care nursing;

• susceptible women exposed at any stage of pregnancy (but when supplies of VZIG are short, may only be issued to those exposed in the first 20 weeks' gestation or to those near term) providing VZIG is given within 10 days of contact;

14

Immunological products and vaccines

- immunocompromised individuals including those who have received corticosteroids in the previous 3 months at the following dose equivalents of prednisolone: *children* 2 mg/kg daily (or more than 40 mg) for at least 1 week or 1 mg/kg daily for 1 month.

Important: for full details consult *Immunisation against Infectious Disease.* **Varicella–zoster vaccine** is available—see section 14.4.

For treatment of varicella–zoster infections and attenuation of infection if varicella–zoster immunoglobulin not indicated, see section 5.3.2.1

VARICELLA–ZOSTER IMMUNOGLOBULIN

Cautions IgA deficiency; interference with live virus vaccines—see p. 763 under Normal Immunoglobulins

Side-effects injection site swelling and pain; *rarely* anaphylaxis

Indication and dose

Prophylaxis against varicella infection (as soon as possible—not later than 10 days after exposure)

- By deep intramuscular injection

  Neonate 250 mg

  Child 1 month–6 years 250 mg

  Child 6–11 years 500 mg

  Child 11–15 years 750 mg

  Child 15–18 years 1 g

  Give second dose if further exposure occurs more than 3 weeks after first dose

  Note No evidence that effective in treatment of severe disease.
  Normal immunoglobulin for intravenous use (section 14.5.1) may be used in those unable to receive intramuscular injection.

Varicella–Zoster Immunoglobulin [PoM]
(Antivaricella–zoster Immunoglobulin)
Available from selected Health Protection Agency and NHS laboratories (see section 14.5 under Availability) (also from BPL)

14.5.3 Anti-D (Rh$_0$) immunoglobulin

This section is not included in *BNF for Children*. See BNF for use of Anti-D (Rh$_0$) immunoglobulin

14.6 International travel

Note For advice on **malaria chemoprophylaxis**, see section 5.4.1.

No special immunisation is required for travellers to the United States, Europe, Australia, or New Zealand although all travellers should have immunity to tetanus and poliomyelitis (and childhood immunisations should be up to date); see also Tick-borne Encephalitis, p. 759. Certain precautions are required in Non-European areas surrounding the Mediterranean, in Africa, the Middle East, Asia, and South America.

Travellers to areas that have a high incidence of **poliomyelitis** or **tuberculosis** should be immunised with the appropriate vaccine; in the case of poliomyelitis previously immunised adults may be given a booster dose of a preparation containing inactivated poliomyelitis vaccine. BCG immunisation is recommended for travellers aged under 16 years proposing to stay for longer than 3 months (or in close contact with the local population) in countries with an incidence[1] of tuberculosis greater than 40 per 100 000; it should preferably be given three months or more before departure.

Pandemic influenza vaccine A(H1N1)v (see p. 749) can be offered to travellers visiting countries in the southern hemisphere during their influenza season.

Yellow fever immunisation is recommended for travel to the endemic zones of Africa and South America. Many countries require an International Certificate of Vaccination from individuals arriving from, or who have been travelling through, endemic areas, whilst other countries require a certificate from all entering

---

1. List of countries where the incidence of tuberculosis is greater than 40 cases per 100 000 is available at www.hpa.org.uk

travellers (consult the Department of Health handbook, *Health Information for Overseas Travel*, www.dh.gov.uk).

Immunisation against **meningococcal meningitis** is recommended for a number of areas of the world (for details, see p. 752).

Protection against **hepatitis A** is recommended for travellers to high-risk areas outside Northern and Western Europe, North America, Japan, Australia and New Zealand. Hepatitis A vaccine (see p. 743) is preferred and it is likely to be effective even if given shortly before departure; normal immunoglobulin is no longer given routinely but may be indicated in the immunocompromised (see p. 763). Special care must also be taken with food hygiene (see below).

Hepatitis B vaccine (see p. 745) is recommended for those travelling to areas of high prevalence who plan to remain there for lengthy periods and who may therefore be at increased risk of acquiring infection as the result of medical or dental procedures carried out in those countries. Short-term tourists are not generally at increased risk of infection but may place themselves at risk by their sexual behaviour when abroad.

Prophylactic immunisation against **rabies** (see p. 756) is recommended for travellers to enzootic areas on long journeys or to areas out of reach of immediate medical attention.

Travellers who have not had a **tetanus** booster in the last 10 years and are visiting areas where medical attention may not be accessible should receive a booster dose of adsorbed diphtheria [low dose], tetanus and inactivated poliomyelitis vaccine (see p. 740), even if they have received 5 doses of a tetanus-containing vaccine previously.

Typhoid vaccine is indicated for travellers to countries where typhoid is endemic, but the vaccine is no substitute for personal precautions (see below).

There is no requirement for cholera vaccination as a condition for entry into any country, but **oral cholera vaccine** (see p. 739) should be considered for backpackers and those travelling to situations where the risk is greatest (e.g. refugee camps). Regardless of vaccination, travellers to areas where cholera is endemic should take special care with food hygiene (see below).

Advice on **diphtheria**, on **Japanese encephalitis**[1] (vaccine available on named-patient basis from MASTA) and on **tick-borne encephalitis** is included in *Health Information for Overseas Travel*, see below.

Food hygiene   In areas where sanitation is poor, good food hygiene is important to help prevent hepatitis A, typhoid, cholera, and other diarrhoeal diseases (including travellers' diarrhoea). Food should be freshly prepared and hot, and uncooked vegetables (including green salads) should be avoided; only fruits which can be peeled should be eaten. Only suitable bottled water, or tap water that has been boiled, or treated with sterilising tablets should be used for drinking.

Information on health advice for travellers

The Department of Health handbook, *Health Information for Overseas Travel* (2001), which draws together essential information *for healthcare professionals* regarding health advice for travellers, can be obtained from

The Stationery Office

PO Box 29, Norwich NR3 1GN

Telephone orders, 0870 600 5522

Fax: 0870 600 5533

www.tso.co.uk

Health professionals and travellers can find the latest information on immunisation requirements and precautions for avoiding disease while travelling from www.nathnac.org

---

14

Immunological products and vaccines

---

1. Japanese encephalitis vaccine not prescribable on the NHS; health authorities may investigate circumstances under which vaccine prescribed

Immunisation requirements change from time to time, and information on the current requirements for any particular country may be obtained from the embassy or legation of the appropriate country or from:

National Travel Health Network and Centre
Hospital for Tropical Diseases
Mortimer Market Centre
Capper Street, off Tottenham Court Road
London, WC1E 6AU.
Tel: 0845 602 6712
(9 a.m.–noon, 2–4.30 p.m. weekdays for healthcare professionals **only**)
www.nathnac.org

Travel Medicine Team
Health Protection Scotland
Clifton House
Clifton Place
Glasgow, G3 7LN.
Tel: (0141) 300 1100
(2 p.m.–4 p.m. weekdays)
www.travax.nhs.uk (registration required. Annual fee may be payable for users outside NHS Scotland)

Welsh Medicines Information Centre
University Hospital of Wales
Cardiff, CF14 4XW.
Tel: (029) 2074 2979
(08.30 a.m.–5 p.m. weekdays for health professionals in Wales **only**)

Department of Health and Social Services
Castle Buildings
Stormont
Belfast, BT4 3PP.
Tel: (028) 9052 0000

15 Anaesthesia

15.1 General anaesthesia

15.1.1 Intravenous anaesthetics
15.1.2 Inhalational anaesthetics
15.1.3 Antimuscarinic drugs
15.1.4 Sedative and analgesic peri-operative drugs
15.1.5 Neuromuscular blocking drugs
15.1.6 Drugs for reversal of neuromuscular blockade
15.1.7 Antagonists for central and respiratory depression
15.1.8 Drugs for malignant hyperthermia

> **Important**
> The drugs in section 15.1 should be used only by experienced personnel and where adequate resuscitation equipment is available.

Several different types of drug are given together during general anaesthesia. Anaesthesia is induced with either a volatile drug given by inhalation (section 15.1.2) or with an intravenously administered drug (section 15.1.1); anaesthesia is maintained with an intravenous or inhalational anaesthetic. Analgesics (section 15.1.4), usually short-acting opioids, are also used. The use of neuromuscular blocking drugs (section 15.1.5) necessitates intermittent positive-pressure ventilation. Following surgery, anticholinesterases (section 15.1.6) can be given to reverse the effects of neuromuscular blocking drugs; specific antagonists (section 15.1.7) can be used to reverse central and respiratory depression caused by some drugs used in surgery. A topical local anaesthetic (section 15.2) can be used to reduce pain at the injection site.

Individual requirements vary considerably and the recommended doses are only a guide. Smaller doses are indicated in ill, shocked, or debilitated children and in significant hepatic impairment, while robust individuals may require larger doses. The required dose of induction agent may be less if the patient has been premedicated with a sedative agent (section 15.1.4) or if an opioid analgesic has been used.

Surgery and long-term medication The risk of losing disease control on stopping long-term medication before surgery is often greater than the risk posed by continuing it during surgery. It is vital that the anaesthetist knows about **all** drugs that a child is (or has been) taking.

Children with adrenal atrophy resulting from long-term corticosteroid use (section 6.3.2) may suffer a precipitous fall in blood pressure unless corticosteroid cover is provided during anaesthesia and in the immediate postoperative period. Anaesthetists must therefore know whether a child is, or has been, receiving corticosteroids (including high-dose inhaled corticosteroids).

15
Anaesthesia

Other drugs that should normally not be stopped before surgery include drugs for epilepsy, asthma, immunosuppression, and metabolic, endocrine and cardiovascular disorders (but see potassium sparing diuretics, below). Expert advice is required for children receiving antivirals for HIV infection. For general advice on surgery in children with diabetes, see section 6.1.1.

Children taking antiplatelet medication or an oral anticoagulant present an increased risk for surgery. In these circumstances, the anaesthetist and surgeon should assess the relative risks and decide jointly whether the antiplatelet or the anticoagulant drug should be stopped or replaced with unfractionated or low molecular weight heparin therapy.

Drugs that should be stopped before surgery include combined oral contraceptives (see Surgery, section 7.3.1 for details). If antidepressants need to be stopped, they should be withdrawn gradually to avoid withdrawal symptoms. Tricyclic antidepressants need not be stopped, but there may be an increased risk of arrhythmias and hypotension (and dangerous interactions with vasopressor drugs); therefore, the anaesthetist should be informed if they are not stopped. Lithium should be stopped 24 hours before major surgery but the normal dose can be continued for minor surgery (with careful monitoring of fluids and electrolytes). Potassium-sparing diuretics may need to be withheld on the morning of surgery because hyperkalaemia may develop if renal perfusion is impaired or if there is tissue damage.

Anaesthesia and skilled tasks   Children and their carers should be very carefully warned about the risk of undertaking skilled tasks after the use of sedatives and analgesics during minor outpatient procedures. For intravenous benzodiazepines and for a short general anaesthetic the risk extends to **at least 24 hours** after administration. Responsible persons should be available to take children home. The dangers of taking **alcohol** should also be emphasised.

Prophylaxis of acid aspiration   Regurgitation and aspiration of gastric contents (Mendelson's syndrome) can be a complication of general anaesthesia, particularly in obstetrics and in gastro-oesophageal reflux disease; prophylaxis against acid aspiration is not routinely used in children but may be required in high-risk cases.

An H_2-receptor antagonist (section 1.3.1) or a **proton pump inhibitor** (section 1.3.5), such as omeprazole, can be used before surgery to increase the pH and reduce the volume of gastric fluid. They do not affect the pH of fluid already in the stomach and this limits their value in emergency procedures; oral H_2-receptor antagonists can be given 1–2 hours before the procedure, but omeprazole must be given at least 12 hours earlier.

Anaesthesia, sedation, and resuscitation in dental practice

For details see *A Conscious Decision: A review of the use of general anaesthesia and conscious sedation in primary dental care*; report by a group chaired by the Chief Medical Officer and Chief Dental Officer, July 2000 and associated documents. Further details can also be found in *Conscious Sedation in the Provision of Dental Care*; report of an Expert Group on Sedation for Dentistry (commissioned by the Department of Health), 2003. Both documents are available at www.dh.gov.uk.

Guidance is also included in *Standards for Dental Professionals*, London, General Dental Council, May 2005 (and as amended subsequently) and *Conscious Sedation in Dentistry: Dental Clinical Guidance*, Scottish Dental Clinical Effectiveness Programme, May 2006.

Gas cylinders

Each gas cylinder bears a label with the name of the gas contained in the cylinder. The name or chemical symbol of the gas appears on the shoulder of the cylinder and is also clearly and indelibly stamped on the cylinder valve.

The colours on the valve end of the cylinder extend down to the shoulder; in the case of mixed gases the colours for the individual gases are applied in four segments, two for each colour.

Gas cylinders should be stored in a cool well-ventilated room, free from flammable materials.

No lubricant of any description should be used on the cylinder valves.

15.1.1 Intravenous anaesthetics

Intravenous anaesthetics may be used either to induce anaesthesia or for maintenance of anaesthesia throughout surgery. Intravenous anaesthetics nearly all produce their effect in one arm-brain circulation time and can cause apnoea and hypotension, and so adequate resuscitative facilities **must** be available. They are **contra-indicated** if the anaesthetist is not confident of being able to maintain the airway. Extreme care is required in surgery of the mouth, pharynx, or larynx and in children with acute circulatory failure (shock) or fixed cardiac output.

To facilitate tracheal intubation, induction is usually followed by a neuromuscular blocking drug (section 15.1.5) or a short-acting opioid (section 15.1.4.3).

The doses of all intravenous anaesthetic drugs should be titrated according to response (except when using 'rapid sequence induction'). The doses and rates of administration should be reduced in those with hypovolaemia or cardiovascular disease; reduced doses may also be required in premedicated children.

Total intravenous anaesthesia   This is a technique in which surgery is carried out with all drugs given intravenously. Respiration can be spontaneous, or controlled with oxygen-enriched air. Neuromuscular blocking drugs can be used to provide relaxation and prevent reflex muscle movements. The main problem to be overcome is the assessment of depth of anaesthesia. Target Controlled Infusion (TCI) systems can be used to titrate intravenous anaesthetic infusions to predicted plasma-drug concentrations; specific models with paediatric pharmacokinetic data should be used for children.

Anaesthesia and skilled tasks   See section 15.1.

Drugs used for intravenous anaesthesia   **Propofol**, the most widely used intravenous anaesthetic, can be used for induction or maintenance of anaesthesia in children, but it is not commonly used in neonates.

Propofol is associated with rapid recovery and less hangover effect than other intravenous anaesthetics. It causes pain on intravenous injection which can be reduced by intravenous lidocaine. Significant extraneous muscle movements can occur. Rarely, convulsions, anaphylaxis, and delayed recovery from anaesthesia can occur after propofol administration; the onset of convulsions can be delayed. Propofol is associated with bradycardia, occasionally profound; intravenous administration of an antimuscarinic drug is used to treat this.

Propofol is contra-indicated in children under 17 years receiving intensive care because of the risk of potentially fatal effects, including metabolic acidosis, cardiac failure, rhabdomyolysis, hyperlipidaemia, and hepatomegaly.

Thiopental sodium (thiopentone sodium) is a barbiturate that is used widely for induction of anaesthesia, but it has no analgesic properties. Induction is generally smooth and rapid, but dose-related cardiorespiratory depression can occur. Awakening from a moderate dose of thiopental is rapid because the drug redistributes into other tissues, particularly fat. However, metabolism is slow and sedative effects can persist for 24 hours. Repeated doses have a cumulative effect particularly in neonates, and recovery is much slower.

Etomidate is an intravenous agent associated with rapid recovery without a hangover effect. Etomidate causes less hypotension than thiopental and propofol during induction. It produces a high incidence of extraneous muscle movements, which can be minimised by an opioid analgesic or a short-acting benzodiazepine given just before induction. Pain on injection can be reduced by injecting into a larger vein or by giving an opioid analgesic just before induction. Etomidate suppresses adrenocortical function, particularly on continuous administration, and it should not be used for maintenance of anaesthesia.

Ketamine has good analgesic properties at sub-anaesthetic dosage and it causes less hypotension than thiopental and propofol during induction. It is often used in children requiring repeat anaesthesia (such as for serial burns dressings), however recovery is relatively slow and there is a high incidence of extraneous muscle

15

Anaesthesia

movements. The main disadvantage of ketamine is the high incidence of hallucinations, nightmares, and other transient psychotic effects; these can be reduced by a benzodiazepine, such as diazepam or midazolam. Ketamine also has abuse potential and may lead to dependence.

ETOMIDATE

Cautions see notes above; avoid in acute porphyria (section 9.8.2); **interactions:** Appendix 1 (anaesthetics, general)

Contra-indications see notes above

Hepatic impairment reduce dose in liver cirrhosis

Pregnancy depresses neonatal respiration if used during delivery

Breast-feeding avoid for 24 hours after administration

Side-effects see notes above; also coughing, hiccups, shivering, allergic reactions (including bronchospasm and anaphylaxis); respiratory depression, arrhythmias, and convulsions also reported

Indication and dose

See under preparations

Etomidate-Lipuro® (Braun) PoM
Injection (emulsion), etomidate 2 mg/mL, net price 10-mL amp = £1.53

Dose
> **Induction of anaesthesia**
> • By slow intravenous injection
> **Child 1 month–18 years** 150–300 micrograms/kg; child under 10 years may need up to 400 micrograms/kg

Hypnomidate® (Janssen-Cilag) PoM
Injection, etomidate 2 mg/mL, net price 10-mL amp = £1.41
Excipients include propylene glycol (see Excipients, p. 3)

Dose
> **Induction of anaesthesia**
> • By slow intravenous injection
> **Child 1 month–18 years** 300 micrograms/kg; max. total dose 60 mg

KETAMINE

Cautions see notes above; increased cerebrospinal fluid pressure; predisposition to hallucinations or nightmares; **interactions:** Appendix 1 (anaesthetics, general)

Contra-indications see notes above; hypertension, pre-eclampsia or eclampsia, severe cardiac disease, stroke; raised intracranial pressure; head trauma; acute porphyria (section 9.8.2)

Pregnancy depresses neonatal respiration if used during delivery

Side-effects see notes above; also tachycardia, hypertension, arrhythmias, hypotension, bradycardia; increased salivation, laryngospasm; anxiety, insomnia, diplopia, nystagmus, raised intra-ocular pressure; rashes, injection-site reactions; anaphylaxis also reported

Indication and dose

Premedication prior to invasive or painful procedures
• By intravenous injection
Child 1 month–18 years 1–2 mg/kg as a single dose

Induction and maintenance of anaesthesia (short procedures)
• By intravenous injection over at least 60 seconds
Neonate 1–2 mg/kg produces 5–10 minutes of surgical anaesthesia, adjusted according to response

Child 1 month–12 years 1–2 mg/kg produces 5–10 minutes of surgical anaesthesia, adjusted according to response

Child 12–18 years 1–4.5 mg/kg (usually 2 mg/kg) produces 5–10 minutes of surgical anaesthesia, adjusted according to response

• By intramuscular injection
Neonate 4 mg/kg usually produces 15 minutes of surgical anaesthesia, adjusted according to response

Child 1 month–18 years 4–13 mg/kg (4 mg/kg sufficient for some diagnostic procedures), adjusted according to response; 10 mg/kg usually produces 12–25 minutes of surgical anaesthesia

Induction and maintenance of anaesthesia (longer procedures)
• By intravenous administration
Neonate initially 0.5–2 mg/kg by *intravenous injection*, followed by a *continuous intravenous infusion* of 8 micrograms/kg/minute adjusted according to response; up to 30 micrograms/kg/minute may be used to produce deep anaesthesia

Child 1 month–18 years initially 0.5–2 mg/kg by *intravenous injection* followed by a *continuous intravenous infusion* of 10–45 micrograms/kg/minute adjusted according to response

Administration for *continuous intravenous infusion*, dilute to a concentration of 1 mg/mL with Glucose 5% *or* Sodium Chloride 0.9%; use microdrip infusion for maintenance of anaesthesia
For *intravenous injection*, dilute 100 mg/mL strength to a concentration of not more than 50 mg/mL with Glucose 5% *or* Sodium Chloride 0.9% *or* Water for Injections

Ketalar® (Pfizer) PoM
Injection, ketamine (as hydrochloride) 10 mg/mL, net price 20-mL vial = £5.06; 50 mg/mL, 10-mL vial = £8.77; 100 mg/mL, 10-mL vial = £16.10

PROPOFOL

Cautions see notes above; cardiac impairment; respiratory impairment; hypovolaemia; epilepsy; hypotension; raised intracranial pressure; monitor blood-lipid concentration if risk of fat overload or if sedation longer than 3 days; **interactions:** Appendix 1 (anaesthetics, general)

Contra-indications see notes above

Hepatic impairment use with caution

Renal impairment use with caution

Pregnancy depresses neonatal respiration if used during delivery; max. dose for maintenance of anaesthesia, 6 mg/kg/hour

Breast-feeding present in milk but amount probably too small to be harmful

Side-effects see notes above; also hypotension, tachycardia, flushing; transient apnoea, hyperventilation, coughing, and hiccup during induction; headache; *less commonly* thrombosis, phlebitis; *rarely* arrhythmia, headache, vertigo, shivering, euphoria; *very rarely* pancreatitis, pulmonary oedema, sexual disinhibition, and discoloration of urine; serious and sometimes fatal side-effects reported with prolonged infusion of doses exceeding 5 mg/kg/hour, including metabolic acidosis, rhabdomyolysis, hyperkalaemia, and cardiac failure, dystonia and dyskinesia also reported

Licensed use *Diprivan®* 2%, *Propofol-Lipuro®* 2%, and *Propoven®* 2% not licensed for use in children under 3 years; *Diprofusor® TCI* ('target controlled infusion') system not licensed for use in children

Indication and dose

Induction of anaesthesia using 0.5% *or* 1% injection
- By intravenous injection or by intravenous infusion

    Child 1 month–12 years 2.5–4 mg/kg administered slowly until response

    Child 12–18 years 1.5–2.5 mg/kg at a rate of 20–40 mg every 10 seconds until response

Induction of anaesthesia using 2% injection
- By intravenous infusion

    Child 3–12 years 2.5–4 mg/kg administered slowly until response

    Child 12–18 years 1.5–2.5 mg/kg at a rate of 20–40 mg every 10 seconds until response

Maintenance of anaesthesia using 1% injection
- By continuous intravenous infusion

    Child 1 month–12 years 9–15 mg/kg/hour, adjusted according to response

    Child 12–18 years 4–12 mg/kg/hour, adjusted according to response

Maintenance of anaesthesia using 2% injection
- By continuous intravenous infusion

    Child 3–12 years 9–15 mg/kg/hour, adjusted according to response

    Child 12–18 years 4–12 mg/kg/hour, adjusted according to response

Sedation of ventilated children in intensive care using 1% *or* 2% injection
- By continuous intravenous infusion

    Child 17–18 years 0.3–4 mg/kg/hour, adjusted according to response

Induction of sedation for surgical and diagnostic procedures using 0.5% *or* 1% injection
- By intravenous injection over 1–5 minutes

    Child 17–18 years 0.5–1 mg/kg

Maintenance of sedation for surgical and diagnostic procedures using 0.5%, 1%, *or* 2% injection
- By intravenous infusion

    Child 17–18 years 1.5–4.5 mg/kg/hour (additionally if rapid increase in sedation required, *by intravenous injection* using 0.5% *or* 1% injection, 10–20 mg)

Administration for *continuous intravenous infusion*; microbiological filter not recommended; **0.5% *or* 1% emulsion** may be infused undiluted using a suitable infusion pump; may also be administered via a Y-piece close to injection site co-administered with Glucose 5% *or* Sodium Chloride 0.9%; *alternatively* dilute to a concentration not less than 2 mg/mL (1 mg/mL for 0.5% injection) with Glucose 5% (*or* Sodium Chloride 0.9% for *Propofol-Lipuro®*, *Propoven®*, Braun, and Fresenius Kabi brands); use glass or PVC containers (if PVC bag used, it should be full—withdraw volume of infusion fluid equal to that of propofol to be added); give within 6 hours of preparation

2% emulsion do not dilute; may be administered via a Y-piece close to injection site co-administered with Glucose 5% *or* Sodium Chloride 0.9%

Propofol (Non-proprietary) ▣PoM
0.5% injection (emulsion), propofol 5 mg/mL, net price 20-mL amp = £3.46
Brands include *Propofol-Lipuro®*

1% injection (emulsion), propofol 10 mg/mL, net price 20-mL amp = £4.18, 50-mL bottle = £10.10, 100-mL bottle = £19.40
Brands include *Propofol-Lipuro®*, *Propoven®*

2% injection (emulsion), propofol 20 mg/mL, net price 50-mL vial = £21.30
Brands include *Propofol-Lipuro®*, *Propoven®*

Diprivan® (AstraZeneca) ▣PoM
1% injection (emulsion), propofol 10 mg/mL, net price 20-mL amp = £1.07, 50-mL prefilled syringe (for use with *Diprifusor® TCI* system) = £4.72

2% injection (emulsion), propofol 20 mg/mL, net price 50-mL prefilled syringe (for use with *Diprifusor® TCI* system) = £5.27

◼ THIOPENTAL SODIUM
(Thiopentone sodium)

Cautions see notes above; cardiovascular disease; reconstituted solution is highly alkaline—extravasation causes tissue necrosis and severe pain; avoid intra-arterial injection; **interactions:** Appendix 1 (anaesthetics, general)

Contra-indications see notes above; acute porphyria (section 9.8.2); myotonic dystrophy

Hepatic impairment reduce induction dose in severe liver disease

Pregnancy depresses neonatal respiration if used during delivery; dose should not exceed 250 mg

Breast-feeding present in milk—avoid

Side-effects hypotension, arrhythmias, myocardial depression, laryngeal spasm, cough, sneezing; hypersensitivity reactions; rash, injection-site reactions; excessive doses associated with hypothermia and profound reduction in cerebral function

Licensed use not licensed for use in status epilepticus; not licensed for use by intravenous infusion

Indication and dose

Induction of anaesthesia
- By slow intravenous injection

Neonate initially up to 2 mg/kg, then 1 mg/kg repeated as necessary (max. total dose 4 mg/kg)

Child 1 month–18 years initially up to 4 mg/kg, then 1 mg/kg repeated as necessary (max. total dose 7 mg/kg)

Prolonged status epilepticus
- By slow intravenous injection and intravenous infusion

Neonate initially up to 2 mg/kg by intravenous injection, then up to 8 mg/kg/hour by continuous intravenous infusion, adjusted according to response

Child 1 month–18 years initially up to 4 mg/kg by intravenous injection, then up to 8 mg/kg/hour by continuous intravenous infusion, adjusted according to response

Administration For *intravenous injection*, dilute to a concentration of 25 mg/mL with Water for Injections, and give over at least 10–15 seconds; for *intravenous infusion* dilute to a concentration of 2.5 mg/mL with Sodium Chloride 0.9%

Thiopental (Link) PoM
Injection, powder for reconstitution, thiopental sodium, net price 500-mg vial = £3.06

15.1.2 Inhalational anaesthetics

Inhalational anaesthetics include gases and volatile liquids. *Gaseous anaesthetics* require suitable equipment for storage and administration. They may be supplied via hospital pipelines or from metal cylinders (section 15.1). *Volatile liquid anaesthetics* are administered using calibrated vaporisers, using air, oxygen, or nitrous oxide-oxygen mixtures as the carrier gas. To prevent hypoxia, the inspired gas mixture should contain a minimum of 25% oxygen at all times. Higher concentrations of oxygen (greater than 30%) are usually required during inhalational anaesthesia with nitrous oxide, see Nitrous Oxide, p. 778.

Anaesthesia and skilled tasks See section 15.1.

Volatile liquid anaesthetics

Volatile liquid anaesthetics can be used for induction and maintenance of anaesthesia, and following induction with an intravenous anaesthetic (section 15.1.1).

Volatile liquid anaesthetics can trigger malignant hyperthermia (section 15.1.8) and are contra-indicated in those susceptible to malignant hyperthermia. They can increase cerebrospinal pressure and should be used with caution in those with raised intracranial pressure. They can also cause hepatotoxicity in those who are sensitised to halogenated anaesthetics; halothane has been associated with severe hepatotoxicity (**important**: see below). In children with neuromuscular disease, inhalational anaesthetics are very rarely associated with hyperkalaemia, resulting in cardiac arrhythmias and death. Cardiorespiratory depression, hypotension, and arrhythmias are common side-effects of volatile liquid anaesthetics.

Isoflurane is a volatile liquid anaesthetic. Heart rhythm is generally stable during isoflurane anaesthesia, but heart-rate can rise. Systemic arterial pressure and cardiac output can fall, owing to a decrease in systemic vascular resistance. Muscle relaxation occurs and the effects of muscle relaxant drugs are potentiated. Isoflurane can irritate mucous membranes, causing cough, breath-holding, and laryngospasm.

Desflurane is a rapid-acting volatile liquid anaesthetic; it is reported to have about one-fifth the potency of isoflurane. Emergence and recovery from anaesthesia are particularly rapid because of its low solubility. Desflurane is not

15 Anaesthesia

recommended for induction of anaesthesia as it is irritant to the upper respiratory tract; cough, breath-holding, apnoea, laryngospasm, and increased secretions can occur.

Sevoflurane is a rapid-acting volatile liquid anaesthetic and is more potent than desflurane. Emergence and recovery are particularly rapid but slower than desflurane. Sevoflurane is non-irritant and is therefore used for inhalational induction of anaesthesia. Sevoflurane can interact with carbon dioxide absorbents to form compound A, a potentially nephrotoxic vinyl ether. However, in spite of extensive use, no cases of sevoflurane-induced permanent renal injury have been reported and the carbon dioxide absorbents used in the UK produce very low concentrations of compound A, even in low-flow anaesthetic systems.

Halothane is a volatile liquid anaesthetic that has largely been superseded by newer agents, but is used occasionally by very specialised paediatric anaesthetists to manage difficult airways (with careful monitoring for cardiorespiratory depression and arrhythmias). Its advantages are that it is potent, induction is smooth, and the vapour is non-irritant and seldom induces coughing or breath-holding.

Halothane hepatotoxicity

Severe hepatotoxicity can follow halothane anaesthesia. It occurs more frequently after repeated exposure to halothane and has a high mortality. The risk of severe hepatotoxicity appears to be increased by repeated exposures within a short time interval, but even after a long interval (sometimes of several years), susceptible patients have been reported to develop jaundice. Since there is no reliable way of identifying patients at risk, the following precautions are recommended before the use of halothane:

- a careful anaesthetic history should be taken to determine previous exposure and previous reactions to halothane;

- repeated exposure to halothane within a period of **at least** 3 months should be **avoided** unless there are **overriding** clinical circumstances;

- a history of unexplained jaundice or pyrexia in a patient following exposure to halothane is an absolute **contra-indication** to its future use in that patient.

DESFLURANE

Cautions see notes above; **interactions:** Appendix 1 (anaesthetics, general)

Contra-indications see notes above

Pregnancy depresses neonatal respiration if used during delivery

Breast-feeding avoid—no information available

Side-effects see notes above

Indication and dose

Induction of anaesthesia

- By inhalation through specifically calibrated vaporiser

  Child 12–18 years 4–11%, but **not** recommended (see notes above)

Maintenance of anaesthesia

- By inhalation through specifically calibrated vaporiser

  Neonate 2–6% in nitrous oxide-oxygen; 2.5–8.5% in oxygen or oxygen-enriched air

  Child 1 month–18 years 2–6% in nitrous oxide-oxygen; 2.5–8.5% in oxygen or oxygen-enriched air

Suprane® (Baxter) (PoM)
Desflurane, net price 240 mL = £63.31

HALOTHANE

Cautions see notes above (**important:** see Halothane Hepatotoxicity above); avoid for dental procedures in those under 18 years unless treated in hospital (high risk of arrhythmia); avoid in acute porphyria (section 9.8.2); **interactions:** Appendix 1 (anaesthetics, general)

Contra-indications see notes above

Hepatic impairment avoid if history of unexplained pyrexia or jaundice following previous exposure to halothane

Pregnancy depresses neonatal respiration if used during delivery

Breast-feeding present in milk—withhold for 24 hours after termination of anaesthesia

Side-effects see notes above

◁ **HALOTHANE** (*continued*)

Indication and dose

Induction of anaesthesia
• By inhalation through specifically calibrated vaporiser

  Child 1 month–18 years initially 0.5% then increased gradually according to response to 2–5% in oxygen or nitrous oxide-oxygen

Maintenance of anaesthesia
• By inhalation through specifically calibrated vaporiser

  Child 1 month–18 years 0.5–2% in oxygen, or oxygen-air, or nitrous oxide-oxygen

Halothane (Non-proprietary) PoM
Available from 'special-order' manufacturers or specialist importing companies, see p. 957

ISOFLURANE

Cautions see notes above; **interactions:** Appendix 1 (anaesthetics, general)

Contra-indications see notes above

Pregnancy depresses neonatal respiration if used during delivery

Breast-feeding avoid—withhold for at least 12 hours after termination of anaesthesia

Side-effects see notes above

Indication and dose

Induction of anaesthesia
• By inhalation through specifically calibrated vaporiser

  Neonate increased gradually according to response from 0.5–3% in oxygen or nitrous oxide-oxygen

  Child 1 month–18 years increased gradually according to response from 0.5–3% in oxygen or nitrous oxide-oxygen

Maintenance of anaesthesia
• By inhalation through specifically calibrated vaporiser

  Neonate 1–2.5% in nitrous oxide-oxygen; additional 0.5–1% may be required if given with oxygen alone

  Child 1 month–18 years 1–2.5% in nitrous oxide-oxygen; additional 0.5–1% may be required if given with oxygen alone; caesarean section, 0.5–0.75% in nitrous oxide-oxygen

Isoflurane (Abbott)
Isoflurane, net price 250 mL = £47.50

AErrane® (Baxter)
Isoflurane, net price 250 mL = £27.00

SEVOFLURANE

Cautions see notes above; **interactions:** Appendix 1 (anaesthetics, general)

Contra-indications see notes above

Renal impairment use with caution

Pregnancy depresses neonatal respiration if used during delivery

Breast-feeding use with caution—no information available

Side-effects see notes above; also urinary retention, leucopenia, agitation; dystonia, rash, and seizures also reported

Indication and dose

Induction of anaesthesia
• By inhalation through specifically calibrated vaporiser

  Neonate up to 4% in oxygen or nitrous oxide-oxygen, according to response

  Child 1 month–18 years initially 0.5–1% then increased gradually up to 8% in oxygen or nitrous oxide-oxygen, according to response

Maintenance of anaesthesia
• By inhalation through specifically calibrated vaporiser

  Neonate 0.5–2% in oxygen or nitrous oxide-oxygen, according to response

  Child 1 month–18 years 0.5–3% in oxygen or nitrous oxide-oxygen, according to response

Sevoflurane (Non-proprietary) PoM
Sevoflurane, net price 250 mL = £123.00

Nitrous oxide

Nitrous oxide is used for maintenance of anaesthesia and, in sub-anaesthetic concentrations, for analgesia. For *anaesthesia* it is commonly used in a concentration of 50 to 66% in oxygen as part of a balanced technique in association with other inhalational or intravenous agents. Nitrous oxide is unsatisfactory as a sole anaesthetic owing to lack of potency, but is useful as part of a combination of drugs since it allows a significant reduction in dosage.

For *analgesia* (without loss of consciousness) a mixture of nitrous oxide and oxygen containing 50% of each gas (*Entonox®*, *Equanox®*) is used. Self-administration using a demand valve may be used in children who are able to self-regulate their intake (usually over 5 years of age) for painful dressing changes, as an aid to postoperative physiotherapy, for wound debridement and in emergency ambulances.

Nitrous oxide may have a deleterious effect if used in children with an air-containing closed space since nitrous oxide diffuses into such a space with a resulting increase in pressure. This effect may be dangerous in the presence of a pneumothorax, which may enlarge to compromise respiration, or in the presence of intracranial air after head injury. Hypoxia can occur immediately following the administration of nitrous oxide; additional oxygen should always be given for several minutes after stopping the flow of nitrous oxide.

Exposure of children to nitrous oxide for prolonged periods, either by continuous or by intermittent administration, may result in megaloblastic anaemia owing to interference with the action of vitamin B_{12}; neurological toxic effects can occur without preceding overt haematological changes. For the same reason, exposure of theatre staff to nitrous oxide should be minimised. Depression of white cell formation may also occur.

Assessment of plasma-vitamin B_{12} concentration should be considered before nitrous oxide anaesthesia in children at risk of deficiency, including children who have a poor or vegetarian diet and children with a history of anaemia. Nitrous oxide should **not** be given continuously for longer than 24 hours or more frequently than every 4 days without close supervision and haematological monitoring.

◢ NITROUS OXIDE

Cautions see notes above; **interactions**: Appendix 1 (anaesthetics, general)

Contra-indications susceptibility to malignant hyperthermia

Pregnancy depresses neonatal respiration if used during delivery

Side-effects see notes above

Indication and dose

Maintenance of light anaesthesia
- By inhalation using suitable anaesthetic apparatus

  Neonate up to 66% in oxygen

  Child 1 month–18 years up to 66% in oxygen

Analgesia
- By inhalation using suitable anaesthetic apparatus
  (see also notes above)

  Neonate up to 50% in oxygen, according to the child's needs

  Child 1 month–18 years up to 50% in oxygen, according to the child's needs

---

15.1.3 Antimuscarinic drugs

Antimuscarinic drugs are used (less commonly nowadays) as premedicants to dry bronchial and salivary secretions which are increased by intubation, upper airway surgery, or some inhalational anaesthetics, but they should not be used for this indication in children with cystic fibrosis. Antimuscarinics are also used before or with neostigmine (section 15.1.6) to prevent bradycardia, excessive salivation, and other muscarinic actions of neostigmine. They also prevent bradycardia and hypotension associated with drugs such as halothane, propofol, and suxamethonium.

Atropine sulphate is now rarely used for premedication but still has an emergency role in the treatment of vagotonic side-effects. For its role in cardiopulmonary resuscitation, see section 2.7.3.

Hyoscine hydrobromide reduces secretions and also provides a degree of amnesia, sedation and anti-emesis. Unlike atropine it may produce bradycardia rather than tachycardia. In some children hyoscine may cause the central anticholinergic syndrome (excitement, ataxia, hallucinations, behavioural abnormalities, and drowsiness).

Glycopyrronium bromide reduces salivary secretions. When given intravenously it produces less tachycardia than atropine. It is widely used with neostigmine for reversal of non-depolarising muscle relaxants (section 15.1.5).

Glycopyrronium or hyoscine hydrobromide are also used to control excessive secretions in upper airways or hypersalivation in palliative care and in children unable to control posture or with abnormal swallowing reflex; effective dose varies and tolerance may develop. The intramuscular route should be avoided if possible. Hyoscine transdermal patches may also be used (section 4.6).

ATROPINE SULPHATE

Cautions section 1.2
 Duration of action Since atropine has a shorter duration of action than neostigmine, late unopposed bradycardia may result; close monitoring of the patient is necessary

Contra-indications section 1.2

Pregnancy not known to be harmful; use with caution

Breast-feeding small amount present in milk—use with caution

Side-effects section 1.2

Licensed use not licensed for use by oral route; not licensed for use in children under 12 years for intra-operative bradycardia

Indication and dose

Premedication
• By mouth 1–2 hours before induction
 Neonate 20–40 micrograms/kg

 Child 1 month–18 years 20–40 micrograms/kg (max. 900 micrograms)

• By subcutaneous or intramuscular injection 30–60 minutes before induction
 Neonate 10–15 micrograms/kg (subcutaneous route recommended)

 Child 1 month–12 years 10–30 micrograms/kg (minimum 100 micrograms, max. 600 micrograms)
 Child 12–18 years 300–600 micrograms

Intra-operative bradycardia
• By intravenous injection
 Neonate 20 micrograms/kg

 Child 1 month–12 years 10–20 micrograms/kg
 Child 12–18 years 300–600 micrograms (larger doses in emergencies)

Control of muscarinic side-effects of neostigmine 50 micrograms/kg in reversal of competitive neuromuscular block
• By intravenous injection
 Neonate 20 micrograms/kg

 Child 1 month–12 years 20 micrograms/kg (max. 1.2 mg)
 Child 12–18 years 0.6–1.2 mg

Control of muscarinic side-effects of edrophonium in reversal of competitive neuromuscular block
• By intravenous injection
 Child 1 month–18 years 7 micrograms/kg (max. 600 micrograms)

Cycloplegia, anterior uveitis (section 11.5)

Administration for administration *by mouth*, injection solution may be given orally

[1]**Atropine** (Non-proprietary) PoM
Injection, atropine sulphate 600 micrograms/mL, net price 1-mL amp = 55p
Note Other strengths also available
Injection, prefilled disposable syringe, atropine sulphate 100 micrograms/mL, net price 5 mL = £4.58, 10 mL = £5.39, 30 mL = £8.95
Injection, prefilled disposable syringe, atropine sulphate 200 micrograms/mL, net price 5 mL = £5.90; 300 micrograms/mL, 10 mL = £5.91; 600 micrograms/mL, 1 mL = £5.91
Oral solution, atropine sulphate 100 micrograms/mL available from 'special-order' manufacturers or specialist importing companies, see p. 957
1. PoM restriction does not apply where administration is for saving life in emergency

[1]**Minijet® Atropine** (UCB Pharma) PoM
Injection, atropine sulphate 100 micrograms/mL, net price 5 mL = £5.04, 10 mL = £5.93, 30 mL = £9.85
1. PoM restriction does not apply where administration is for saving life in emergency

GLYCOPYRRONIUM BROMIDE
(Glycopyrrolate)

Cautions section 1.2
Contra-indications section 1.2
Side-effects section 1.2
Licensed use not licensed for use in control of upper airways secretion and hypersalivation

Indication and dose

Premedication at induction
• By intravenous or intramuscular injection
 Neonate 5 micrograms/kg

 Child 1 month–18 years 4–8 micrograms/kg (max. 200 micrograms)

◻ **GLYCOPYRRONIUM BROMIDE (continued)**

Intra-operative bradycardia
- By intravenous injection

  Neonate 10 micrograms/kg, repeated if necessary

  Child 1 month–18 years 4–8 micrograms/kg (max. 200 micrograms), repeated if necessary

Control of muscarinic side-effects of neostigmine in reversal of competitive neuromuscular block
- By intravenous injection

  Neonate 10 micrograms/kg

  Child 1 month–18 years 10 micrograms/kg (max. 500 micrograms)

Control of upper airways secretion and hypersalivation
- By mouth

  Child 1 month–18 years 40–100 micrograms/kg (max. 2 mg) 3–4 times daily, adjusted according to response

- By subcutaneous infusion

  Child 1 month–12 years 12–40 micrograms/kg/24 hours (max. 1.2 mg)

  Child 12–18 years 0.6–1.2 mg/24 hours

- By subcutaneous injection or intramuscular injection or intravenous injection (but see notes above)

  Child 1 month–12 years 4–10 micrograms/kg (max. 200 micrograms) 4 times a day when required

  Child 12–18 years 200 micrograms every 4 hours when required

Administration for administration *by mouth*, injection solution may be given or crushed tablets suspended in water

Glycopyrronium bromide (Non-proprietary)
Injection, glycopyrronium bromide 200 micrograms/mL, net price 1-mL amp = 54p, 3-mL amp = 91p

Tablets, glycopyrronium bromide 1 mg and 2 mg
Available on a named-patient basis from specialist importing companies, p. 957

◀**With neostigmine metilsulphate**
Section 15.1.6

▰ **HYOSCINE HYDROBROMIDE**
(Scopolamine hydrobromide)

Cautions see notes in section 1.2 and notes above; also epilepsy

Contra-indications see notes in section 1.2

Hepatic impairment see Hyoscine Hydrobromide, section 4.6

Renal impairment see Hyoscine Hydrobromide, section 4.6

Pregnancy see Hyoscine Hydrobromide, section 4.6

Breast-feeding see Hyoscine Hydrobromide, section 4.6

Side-effects see notes in section 1.2

Indication and dose
Premedication
- By subcutaneous or intramuscular injection 30–60 minutes before induction

  Child 1–12 years 15 micrograms/kg (max. 600 micrograms)

  Child 12–18 years 200–600 micrograms

  Note Same dose may be given by intravenous injection immediately before induction

Motion sickness, excessive respiratory secretions, hypersalivation associated with clozapine therapy section 4.6

Hyoscine (Non-proprietary) [PoM]
Injection, hyoscine hydrobromide 400 micrograms/mL, net price 1-mL amp = £2.88; 600 micrograms/mL, 1-mL amp = £2.67

◀**Preparations**
For transdermal and oral preparations see section 4.6

15 Anaesthesia

15.1.4 **Sedative and analgesic peri-operative drugs**

15.1.4.1 Anxiolytics and neuroleptics
15.1.4.2 Non-opioid analgesics
15.1.4.3 Opioid analgesics

Premedication These drugs are given to allay fear and anxiety in the pre-operative period (including the night before an operation), to relieve pain and discomfort when present, and to augment the action of subsequent anaesthetic agents. A number of the drugs used also provide some degree of pre-operative amnesia. The choice will vary with the individual child, the nature of the operative procedure, the anaesthetic to be used, and other prevailing circumstances such as outpatients, obstetrics, and recovery facilities. The choice also varies between elective and emergency operations. Oral administration is preferred where possible; the rectal route should only be used in exceptional circumstances.

The use of anxiolytic or sedative drugs as premedication in children is declining, but can be useful in selected cases. Sedative premedication should be avoided in children with a compromised airway, CNS depression, or a history of sleep apnoea.

Application of a local anaesthetic (section 15.2) to the injection site can help to prevent pain.

Sedation for clinical procedures Anxiety about a clinical procedure can be minimised by using a sedative drug, usually a benzodiazepine, for its anxiolytic and amnesic effect. The child should be **monitored carefully** as soon as the sedative is given until recovery after the procedure; concomitant use of sedatives potentiates the CNS depressant effects of analgesics. For a painful procedure, the sedative may be given with a local anaesthetic (administered topically, by infiltration or as a nerve block as appropriate) and an analgesic such as paracetamol or an NSAID.

Oral **midazolam** is the most common premedicant for children. Midazolam is suitable for sedating a child for a procedure lasting no longer than 20 minutes; it is given by mouth 30–60 minutes before the procedure. Alternatively, **temazepam** may be given by mouth 60–90 minutes before the procedure. If the procedure is likely to last 20–60 minutes, **chloral hydrate** or **triclofos** (section 4.1.1) by mouth are effective, especially in children of pre-school age; secobarbital (quinalbarbitone) can be used in older children but the risk of excessive sedation and cardiorespiratory depression is greater. The antihistamine **alimemazine** (trimeprazine, section 3.4.1) is occasionally used orally as a premedicant, but when given alone it may cause postoperative restlessness in the presence of pain. Alimemazine also has antiemetic properties though it is rarely used for this indication.

If deep sedation is required a general anaesthetic (e.g. propofol or ketamine), or a potent opioid (e.g. fentanyl) can be used, however they should be used only under the supervision of a specialist experienced in the use of these drugs.

Dental procedures Anxiolytics diminish tension, anxiety and panic, and may benefit anxious children, however they should be used under specialist supervision only. Children and their carers should be carefully warned about the risk of undertaking skilled tasks (**important**: for general advice on anaesthesia and skilled tasks, see p. 772). For futher information on hypnotics and anxiolytics, see p. 215. For further information on hypnotics used for dental procedures, see p. 216.

Anaesthesia and skilled tasks See section 15.1.

15.1.4.1 Anxiolytics and neuroleptics

Benzodiazepines

Benzodiazepines possess useful properties for premedication including relief of anxiety, sedation, and amnesia; short-acting benzodiazepines taken by mouth are the most common premedicants. They have no analgesic effect so an opioid analgesic may sometimes be required for pain.

Benzodiazepines can alleviate anxiety at doses that do not necessarily cause excessive sedation and they are of particular value during short procedures or during operations under local anaesthesia (including dentistry). Amnesia reduces the likelihood of any unpleasant memories of the procedure (although benzodiazepines, particularly when used for more profound sedation, can sometimes induce sexual fantasies in adolescents). Benzodiazepines are also used in intensive care units for sedation, particularly in those receiving assisted ventilation.

Benzodiazepines may occasionally cause marked respiratory depression and facilities for its treatment are essential; flumazenil (section 15.1.7) is used to antagonise the effects of benzodiazepines. They are best avoided in myasthenia gravis, especially peri-operatively.

Diazepam is used to produce mild sedation with amnesia. It is a long-acting drug with active metabolites and a second period of drowsiness can occur several hours after its administration. Peri-operative use of diazepam is not generally recommended; its effect and timing of response are unreliable and paradoxical effects may occur.

Diazepam is relatively insoluble in water and preparations formulated in organic solvents are painful on intravenous injection and give rise to a high incidence of venous thrombosis (which may not be noticed for several days after the injection). Intramuscular injection of diazepam is also painful and absorption is erratic; administration by the intramuscular route is not recommended. An emulsion formulated for intravenous injection is less irritant and reduces the risk of venous thrombosis; it is not suitable for intramuscular injection. Diazepam is also available as a rectal solution.

Temazepam is given by mouth in older children and has a shorter duration of action and a more rapid onset than diazepam given by mouth. It has been used as a premedicant in inpatient and day-case surgery; anxiolytic and sedative effects last about 90 minutes although there may be residual drowsiness.

Lorazepam produces more prolonged sedation than temazepam and it has marked amnesic effects. It is used as a premedicant the night before major surgery; a further, smaller dose may be required the following morning if any delay in starting surgery is anticipated. Alternatively the first dose may be given early in the morning on the day of operation.

Midazolam is a water-soluble benzodiazepine that is often used by intravenous injection in preference to intravenous diazepam; it has a quick onset of action and recovery is faster than from diazepam, making it suitable for day cases. Recovery may be longer in children with a low cardiac output, or after repeated dosing. Midazolam can be given by mouth, but its bitter acidic taste may need to be disguised. It can also be given buccally or intranasally; use of the intranasal route is limited by nasal discomfort and is not recommended. Midazolam is associated with profound sedation when high doses are given or when it is used with certain other drugs. It can cause severe disinhibition and restlessness in some children. Midazolam is not recommended for prolonged sedation in neonates; drug accumulation is likely to occur.

Overdosage with midazolam
There have been reports of overdosage in adults when high strength midazolam injection has been used for conscious sedation. The use of high strength midazolam (5 mg/mL in 2 mL and 10 mL ampoules, or 2 mg/mL in 5 mL ampoules) should be restricted to general anaesthesia, intensive care, palliative care, or other situations where the risk has been assessed. It is advised that flumazenil (section 15.1.7) is available where midazolam is used, to reverse the effects if necessary.

◣ DIAZEPAM

Cautions see notes above and section 4.8.2

Contra-indications see section 4.8.2

Hepatic impairment see Benzodiazepines, section 4.8.1

Renal impairment see Benzodiazepines, section 4.8.1

Pregnancy see Benzodiazepines, section 4.8.1

Breast-feeding see Benzodiazepines, section 4.8.1

Side-effects see notes above and section 4.8.2

Indication and dose

Premedication and sedation for clinical procedures (but see notes above)

• By mouth 45–60 minutes before procedure
  Child 1 month–12 years 200–300 micrograms/kg (max. 10 mg)

Child 12–18 years 200–300 micrograms/kg (max. 20 mg)

• By intravenous injection over 2–4 minutes into large vein (specialist use only); emulsion preparation preferred
  Child 1 month–12 years 100–200 micrograms/kg (max. 5 mg) immediately before procedure
  Child 12–18 years 100–200 micrograms/kg (max. 20 mg) immediately before procedure

• By rectum (as rectal solution) approximately 30 minutes before procedure
  Child 1–3 years 5 mg
  Child 3–12 years 5–10 mg
  Child 12–18 years 10 mg

Status epilepticus section 4.8.2

◻ **DIAZEPAM** (*continued*)

Febrile convulsions section 4.8.3

Muscle spasm section 10.2.2

Diazepam (Non-proprietary) PoM
Tablets, diazepam 2 mg, net price 28 = 98p; 5 mg, 28 = £1.01; 10 mg, 28 = £1.02. Label: 2 or 19
Brands include *Rimapam®* ⱼₕₛ, *Tensium®* ⱼₕₛ
Dental prescribing on NHS Diazepam Tablets may be prescribed

Oral solution, diazepam 2 mg/5 mL, net price 100 mL = £6.08. Label: 2 or 19
Brands include *Dialar®* ⱼₕₛ
Dental prescribing on NHS Diazepam Oral Solution 2 mg/5 mL may be prescribed

Strong oral solution, diazepam 5 mg/5 mL, net price 100-mL pack = £6.38. Label: 2 or 19 ⱼₕₛ
Brands include *Dialar®* ⱼₕₛ

◢**Parenteral preparations and rectal solution**
Section 4.8.2

LORAZEPAM

Cautions see notes above and section 4.8.2; **interactions:** Appendix 1 (anxiolytics and hypnotics)

Contra-indications see Diazepam, section 4.8.2

Hepatic impairment see Benzodiazepines, section 4.8.1

Renal impairment see Benzodiazepines, section 4.8.1

Pregnancy see Benzodiazepines, section 4.8.1

Breast-feeding see Benzodiazepines, section 4.8.1

Side-effects see notes above and Diazepam, section 4.8.2

Licensed use not licensed for use in children under 5 years by mouth; not licensed for use in children under 12 years by intravenous injection

Indication and dose
Premedication
• **By mouth**
Child 1 month–12 years 50–100 micrograms/kg (max. 4 mg) at least 1 hour before surgery
Child 12–18 years 1–4 mg at least 1 hour before surgery
Note Same dose may be given the night before surgery in addition to, or to replace, dose before surgery

• **By intravenous injection**
Child 1 month–18 years 50–100 micrograms/kg (max. 4 mg)
Note Give intravenous injection 30–45 minutes before surgery

Status epilepticus section 4.8.2

Administration for *intravenous injection*, dilute injection solution with an equal volume of Sodium Chloride 0.9% *or* Water for Injections; give over 3–5 minutes; max. rate 50 micrograms/kg over 3 minutes

Lorazepam (Non-proprietary) PoM
Tablets, lorazepam 1 mg, net price 28-tab pack = £6.80; 2.5 mg, 28-tab pack = £10.25. Label: 2 or 19

Injection, lorazepam 4 mg/mL, net price 1-mL amp = 35p
Excipients include benzyl alcohol (avoid in neonates see Excipients, p. 3), propylene glycol
Brands include *Ativan®*

◢Extemporaneous formulations available see Extemporaneous Preparations, p. 8

MIDAZOLAM

Cautions see notes above; cardiac disease; respiratory disease; myasthenia gravis; neonates; history of drug or alcohol abuse; reduce dose if debilitated; risk of severe hypotension in children with hypovolaemia, vasoconstriction, hypothermia; avoid prolonged use (and abrupt withdrawal thereafter); **interactions:** Appendix 1 (anxiolytics and hypnotics)

Contra-indications marked neuromuscular respiratory weakness including unstable myasthenia gravis; severe respiratory depression; acute pulmonary insufficiency

Hepatic impairment use with caution; can precipitate coma

Renal impairment start with small doses in severe impairment; increased cerebral sensitivity

Pregnancy avoid regular use (risk of neonatal withdrawal symptoms); use only if clear indication such as seizure control (high doses during late pregnancy or labour may cause neonatal hypothermia, hypotonia, and respiratory depression)

Breast-feeding present in milk—avoid breast-feeding for 24 hours after administration

Side-effects see notes above; gastro-intestinal disturbances, increased appetite, jaundice; hypotension, cardiac arrest, heart rate changes, anaphylaxis, thrombosis; laryngospasm, bronchospasm, respiratory depression and respiratory arrest (particularly with high doses or on rapid injection); drowsiness, confusion, ataxia, amnesia, headache, euphoria, hallucinations, convulsions (more common in neonates), fatigue, dizziness, vertigo, involuntary movements, paradoxical excitement and aggression, dysarthria; urinary retention, incontinence; blood disorders; muscle weakness; visual disturbances; salivation changes; skin reactions; injection-site reactions; with *intranasal administration* burning sensation, lacrimation, and severe irritation of nasal mucosa

◻ **MIDAZOLAM** (continued)

Licensed use not licensed for use in children under 6 months for premedication and conscious sedation; not licensed for use by mouth, or by buccal administration

Indication and dose

Conscious sedation for procedures (but see notes above)

• **By mouth**

Child 1 month–18 years 500 micrograms/kg (max. 20 mg) 30–60 minutes before procedure

• **By buccal administration**

Child 6 months–10 years 200–300 micrograms/kg (max. 5 mg)

Child 10–18 years 6–7 mg (max. 8 mg if 70 kg or over)

• **By rectum**

Child 6 months–12 years 300–500 micrograms/kg 15–30 minutes before procedure

• **By intravenous injection over 2–3 minutes 5–10 minutes before procedure**

Child 1 month–6 years initially 25–50 micrograms/kg, increased if necessary in small steps (max. total dose 6 mg)

Child 6–12 years initially 25–50 micrograms/kg, increased if necessary in small steps (max. total dose 10 mg)

Child 12–18 years initially 25–50 micrograms/kg, increased if necessary in small steps (max. total dose 7.5 mg)

Premedication (but see notes above)

• **By mouth**

Child 1 month–18 years 500 micrograms/kg (max. 20 mg) 15–30 minutes before the procedure

• **By rectum**

Child 6 months–12 years 300–500 micrograms/kg 15–30 minutes before induction

Induction of anaesthesia (but rarely used)

• **By slow intravenous injection**

Child 7–18 years initially 150 micrograms/kg (max. 7.5 mg) given in steps of 50 micrograms/kg (max. 2.5 mg) over 2–5 minutes; wait for 2–5 minutes then give additional doses of 50 micrograms/kg (max. 2.5 mg) every 2 minutes if necessary; max. total dose 500 micrograms/kg (not exceeding 25 mg)

Sedation in intensive care

• **By intravenous injection and continuous intravenous infusion**

Neonate less than 32 weeks gestational age 30 micrograms/kg/hour by continuous intravenous infusion adjusted according to response

Neonate over 32 weeks gestational age 60 micrograms/kg/hour by continuous intravenous infusion adjusted according to response

Child 1–6 months 60 micrograms/kg/hour by continuous intravenous infusion adjusted according to response

Child 6 months–12 years initially 50–200 micrograms/kg by slow intravenous injection over at least 3 minutes followed by 30–120 micrograms/kg/hour by continuous intravenous infusion adjusted according to response

Child 12–18 years initially 30–300 micrograms/kg by slow intravenous injection given in steps of 1–2.5 mg every 2 minutes followed by 30–200 micrograms/kg/hour by continuous intravenous infusion adjusted according to response

Note Initial dose may not be required and lower maintenance doses needed if opioid analgesics also used; reduce dose (or reduce or omit initial dose) in hypovolaemia, vasoconstriction, or hypothermia

Status epilepticus section 4.8.2

Administration for administration by mouth, injection solution may be diluted with apple or black currant juice, chocolate sauce, or cola

For buccal administration, administer half of the dose between the upper lip and gum on each side of the mouth using an oral syringe; retain in the mouth for at least 5 minutes then swallow

For continuous intravenous infusion, dilute with Glucose 5% or Sodium Chloride 0.9%

Neonatal intensive care, dilute 15 mg/kg bodyweight to a final volume of 50 mL with infusion fluid; an intravenous infusion rate of 0.1 mL/hour provides a dose of 30 micrograms/kg/hour

For rectal administration of the injection solution, attach a plastic applicator onto the end of a syringe; if the volume to be given rectally is too small, dilute with Water for Injections

Midazolam (Non-proprietary) ⒸⒹ
Oral liquid, midazolam 2.5 mg/mL, 100 mL
Available from 'special-order' manufacturers or specialist importing companies, see p. 957

Buccal liquid, midazolam 10 mg/mL, 5 mL and 25 mL
Available from 'special-order' manufacturers or specialist importing companies, see p. 957

Injection, midazolam (as hydrochloride) 1 mg/mL, net price 2-mL amp = 50p, 5-mL amp = 60p, 50-mL vial = £7.87; 2 mg/mL, 5-mL amp = 65p; 5 mg/mL, 2-mL amp = 58p, 10-mL amp = £2.50

Hypnovel® (Roche) ⒸⒹ
Injection, midazolam (as hydrochloride) 2 mg/mL, net price 5-mL amp = 86p; 5 mg/mL, 2-mL amp = 73p

15

Anaesthesia

TEMAZEPAM

Cautions see notes above and Diazepam, section 4.8.2; **interactions**: Appendix 1 (anxiolytics and hypnotics)

Contra-indications see Diazepam, section 4.8.2

Hepatic impairment see Benzodiazepines, section 4.8.1

Renal impairment see Benzodiazepines, section 4.8.1

Pregnancy see Benzodiazepines, section 4.8.1

Breast-feeding see Benzodiazepines, section 4.8.1

Side-effects see notes above and Diazepam, section 4.8.2

Licensed use tablets not licensed for use in children

Indication and dose

> Premedication and sedation for clinical procedures
> * By mouth
>   **Child 1–12 years** 1 mg/kg (max. 30 mg) 1 hour before surgery

> **Child 12–18 years** 20–30 mg 1 hour before surgery

Temazepam (Non-proprietary) CD
Tablets, temazepam 10 mg, net price 28-tab pack = £4.88; 20 mg, 28-tab pack = £2.77. Label: 19

Dental prescribing on NHS Temazepam Tablets may be prescribed

Oral solution, temazepam 10 mg/5 mL, net price 300 mL = £25.57. Label: 19

Note Sugar-free versions are available and can be ordered by specifying 'sugar-free' on the prescription

Dental prescribing on NHS Temazepam Oral Solution may be prescribed

Note See p. 11 for prescribing requirements of controlled drugs

15.1.4.2 Non-opioid analgesics

Since non-steroidal anti-inflammatory drugs (NSAIDs) do not depress respiration, do not impair gastro-intestinal motility, and do not cause dependence, they may be useful alternatives or adjuncts to opioids for the relief of postoperative pain. NSAIDs may be inadequate for the relief of severe pain.

Diclofenac, **ibuprofen** (section 10.1.1), **paracetamol** (section 4.7.1), and **ketorolac** are used to relieve postoperative pain in children; diclofenac and paracetamol can be given parenterally and rectally as well as by mouth. Ketorolac is given by mouth or by intravenous injection.

KETOROLAC TROMETAMOL

Cautions section 10.1.1; avoid in acute porphyria (section 9.8.2); **interactions**: Appendix 1 (NSAIDs)

Contra-indications section 10.1.1; also complete or partial syndrome of nasal polyps; haemorrhagic diatheses (including coagulation disorders) and following operations with high risk of haemorrhage or incomplete haemostasis; confirmed or suspected cerebrovascular bleeding; hypovolaemia or dehydration

Hepatic impairment section 10.1.1

Renal impairment max. 60 mg daily by intramuscular or intravenous injection; avoid if serum creatinine greater than 160 micromol/litre; see also section 10.1.1

Pregnancy section 10.1.1

Breast-feeding amount too small to be harmful

Side-effects section 10.1.1; also gastro-intestinal disturbances, taste disturbances, dry mouth; flushing, bradycardia, palpitation, chest pain, hypertension, pallor; dyspnoea, asthma; malaise, euphoria, psychosis, paraesthesia, convulsions, abnormal dreams, hyperkinesia, confusion, hallucinations, urinary frequency, thirst, sweating; hyponatraemia, hyperkalaemia, myalgia; visual disturbances (including optic neuritis); purpura, pain at injection site

Licensed use not licensed for use in children under 16 years

Indication and dose

> Short-term management of moderate to severe acute postoperative pain only
> * By mouth
>   **Child 16–18 years** 10 mg every 4–6 hours as required; max. 40 mg daily; max. duration of treatment 7 days
>
> * By intravenous injection over at least 15 seconds
>   **Child 6 months–16 years** initially 0.5–1 mg/kg (max. 15 mg), then 500 micrograms/kg (max. 15 mg) every 6 hours as required; max. 60 mg daily; max. duration of treatment 2 days
>
> * By intramuscular injection *or* by intravenous injection over at least 15 seconds
>   **Child 16–18 years** initially 10 mg, then 10–30 mg every 4–6 hours as required (up to every 2 hours during initial postoperative period); max. 90 mg daily (children weighing less than 50 kg max. 60 mg daily); max. duration of treatment 2 days
>   **Note** When converting from parenteral to oral administration, total combined dose on the day of converting should not exceed 90 mg (60 mg in children weighing less than 50 kg) of which the oral component should not exceed 40 mg

◁ **KETOROLAC TROMETAMOL (continued)**

Ketorolac (Non-proprietary) (PoM)
Injection, ketorolac trometamol 30 mg/mL, net price 1-mL amp = £1.14

Injection, ketorolac trometamol 10 mg/mL, net price 1-mL amp = 91p; 30 mg/mL, 1-mL amp = £1.09

Toradol® (Roche) (PoM)
Tablets, ivory, f/c, ketorolac trometamol 10 mg, net price 20-tab pack = £5.56. Label: 17, 21

15.1.4.3 Opioid analgesics

Opioid analgesics are now rarely used as premedicants; they are more likely to be administered at induction. Pre-operative use of opioid analgesics is generally limited to children who require control of existing pain. The main side-effects of opioid analgesics are respiratory depression, cardiovascular depression, nausea, and vomiting; for general notes on opioid analgesics and their use in postoperative pain, see section 4.7.2.

For the management of opioid-induced respiratory depression, see section 15.1.7.

Intra-operative analgesia Opioid analgesics given in small doses before or with induction reduce the dose requirement of some drugs used during anaesthesia.

Alfentanil, **fentanyl**, and **remifentanil** are particularly useful because they act within 1–2 minutes and have short durations of action. The initial doses of alfentanil or fentanyl are followed either by successive intravenous injections or by an intravenous infusion; prolonged infusions increase the duration of effect. Repeated intra-operative doses of alfentanil or fentanyl should be given with care since the resulting respiratory depression can persist postoperatively and occasionally it may become apparent for the first time postoperatively when monitoring of the child might be less intensive. Alfentanil, fentanyl, and remifentanil can cause muscle rigidity, particularly of the chest wall muscle or jaw muscle, which can be managed by the use of neuromuscular blocking drugs.

In contrast to other opioids which are metabolised in the liver, remifentanil undergoes rapid metabolism by non-specific blood and tissue esterases; its short duration of action allows prolonged administration at high dosage, without accumulation, and with little risk of residual postoperative respiratory depression. Remifentanil should not be given by intravenous injection intra-operatively, but is well suited to continuous infusion; a supplementary analgesic is given before stopping the infusion of remifentanil.

Neonates The half-life of fentanyl and alfentanil is prolonged in neonates and accumulation is likely with prolonged use.

▌ ALFENTANIL

Cautions section 4.7.2 and notes above
Contra-indications section 4.7.2
Hepatic impairment section 4.7.2
Renal impairment section 4.7.2
Pregnancy section 4.7.2
Breast-feeding present in milk—withhold breast-feeding for 24 hours
Side-effects section 4.7.2 and notes above; also hypertension, myoclonic movements; less commonly arrhythmias, cough, hiccup, laryngospasm; also reported cardiac arrest, convulsions, and pyrexia

Indication and dose

To avoid excessive dosage in obese children, dose may need to be calculated on the basis of ideal weight for height

Analgesia especially during short procedures; enhancement of anaesthesia
• By intravenous injection over 30 seconds (with assisted ventilation)

Neonate initially 5–20 micrograms/kg; supplemental doses up to 10 micrograms/kg

Child 1 month–18 years initially 10–20 micrograms/kg; supplemental doses up to 10 micrograms/kg

• By intravenous infusion (with assisted ventilation)

Neonate initially 10–50 micrograms/kg over 10 minutes followed by 0.5–1 micrograms/kg/minute

Child 1 month–18 years initially 50–100 micrograms/kg over 10 minutes followed by 0.5–1 micrograms/kg/minute

Administration for continuous or intermittent intravenous infusion dilute in Glucose 5% or Sodium Chloride 0.9% or Compound Sodium Lactate

15
Anaesthesia

○ **ALFENTANIL** (*continued*)

Alfentanil (Non-proprietary) (CD)
Injection, alfentanil (as hydrochloride) 500 micrograms/mL, net price 2-mL amp = 70p, 10-mL amp = £3.20

Intensive care injection, alfentanil (as hydrochloride) 5 mg/mL, net price 1-mL amp = £2.50
Note To be diluted before use

Rapifen® (Janssen-Cilag) (CD)
Injection, alfentanil (as hydrochloride) 500 micrograms/mL, net price 2-mL amp = 65p; 10-mL amp = £2.96

Intensive care injection, alfentanil (as hydrochloride) 5 mg/mL, net price 1-mL amp = £2.37
Note To be diluted before use

◢ FENTANYL

Cautions see Fentanyl, section 4.7.2 and notes above

Contra-indications see notes in section 4.7.2

Hepatic impairment see notes in section 4.7.2

Renal impairment see notes in section 4.7.2

Pregnancy see notes in section 4.7.2

Breast-feeding see Fentanyl, section 4.7.2

Side-effects see Fentanyl, section 4.7.2 and notes above; also myoclonic movements; *less commonly* laryngospasm; *rarely* asystole, insomnia

Licensed use not licensed for use in children under 2 years

Indication and dose

> To avoid excessive dosage in obese children, dose may need to be calculated on the basis of ideal weight for height

> **Spontaneous respiration: analgesia during operation, enhancement of anaesthesia**
> • By intravenous injection over at least 30 seconds
>
> **Child 1 month–12 years** initially 1–3 micrograms/kg, then 1 microgram/kg as required
>
> **Child 12–18 years** initially 50–100 micrograms (max. 200 micrograms on specialist advice), then 25–50 micrograms as required

> **Assisted ventilation: analgesia during operation, enhancement of anaesthesia**
> • By intravenous injection over at least 30 seconds
>
> **Neonate** initially 1–5 micrograms/kg, then 1–3 micrograms/kg as required

> **Child 1 month–12 years** initially 1–5 micrograms/kg, then 1–3 micrograms/kg as required
>
> **Child 12–18 years** initially 1–5 micrograms/kg, then 50–200 micrograms as required

> **Assisted ventilation: analgesia and respiratory depression in intensive care**
> • By intravenous administration
>
> **Neonate** initially by *intravenous injection* 1–5 micrograms/kg, then by *intravenous infusion*, 1.5 micrograms/kg/hour adjusted according to response
>
> **Child 1 month–18 years** initially by *intravenous injection* 1–5 micrograms/kg, then by *intravenous infusion*, 1–6 micrograms/kg/hour adjusted according to response

Analgesia in other situations section 4.7.2

Administration for *intravenous infusion*, injection solution may be diluted in Glucose 5% *or* Sodium Chloride 0.9%

Fentanyl (Non-proprietary) (CD)
Injection, fentanyl (as citrate) 50 micrograms/mL, net price 2-mL amp = 30p, 10-mL amp = 64p

Sublimaze® (Janssen-Cilag) (CD)
Injection, fentanyl (as citrate) 50 micrograms/mL, net price 2-mL amp = 22p, 10-mL amp = £1.05

◢ REMIFENTANIL

Cautions section 4.7.2 and notes above

Contra-indications section 4.7.2 and notes above; left ventricular dysfunction

Hepatic impairment section 4.7.2

Pregnancy no information available; see also section 4.7.2

Breast-feeding use with caution—present in milk in *animal* studies

Side-effects section 4.7.2 and notes above; also hypertension, hypoxia; *very rarely* asystole and anaphylaxis

Indication and dose

> To avoid excessive dosage in obese children, dose should be calculated on the basis of ideal weight for height

> **Enhancement and maintenance of anaesthesia in ventilated patients**
> • By intravenous administration
>
> **Neonate** by *intravenous infusion* 0.4–1 microgram/kg/minute; additional doses of 1 microgram/kg can be given by *intravenous injection* during the intravenous infusion
>
> **Child 1–12 years** initially by *intravenous injection* 0.1–1 micrograms/kg over at least 30 seconds (omitted if not required) then by *intravenous infusion* 0.05–1.3 micrograms/kg/minute according to anaesthetic technique and adjusted according to response; additional doses can be given by *intravenous injection* during the intravenous infusion

◻ **REMIFENTANIL (continued)**

Child 12–18 years initially by *intravenous injection* 0.1–1 micrograms/kg over at least 30 seconds (omitted if not required) then by *intravenous infusion* 0.05–2 micrograms/kg/minute according to anaesthetic technique and adjusted according to response; additional doses can be given by *intravenous injection* during the intravenous infusion

Administration for *intravenous injection*, reconstitute to a concentration of 1 mg/mL; for *continuous intravenous infusion*, dilute further with Glu-

cose 5% *or* Sodium Chloride 0.9% *or* Water for Injections to a concentration of 20–25 micrograms/mL for Child 1–12 years or 20–250 micrograms/mL (usually 50 micrograms/mL) for Child 12–18 years

Ultiva® (GSK) ⒸⒹ
Injection, powder for reconstitution, remifentanil (as hydrochloride), net price 1-mg vial = £5.12; 2-mg vial = £10.23; 5-mg vial = £25.58

15.1.5 Neuromuscular blocking drugs

Neuromuscular blocking drugs used in anaesthesia are also known as **muscle relaxants**. By specific blockade of the neuromuscular junction they enable light anaesthesia to be used with adequate relaxation of the muscles of the abdomen and diaphragm. They also relax the vocal cords and allow the passage of a tracheal tube. Their action differs from the muscle relaxants used in musculo-skeletal disorders (section 10.2.2) that act on the spinal cord or brain.

Children who have received a neuromuscular blocking drug should **always** have their respiration assisted or controlled until the drug has been inactivated or antagonised (section 15.1.6). They should also receive sufficient concomitant inhalational or intravenous anaesthetic or sedative drugs to prevent awareness.

Non-depolarising neuromuscular blocking drugs

Non-depolarising neuromuscular blocking drugs (also known as competitive muscle relaxants) compete with acetylcholine for receptor sites at the neuromuscular junction and their action can be reversed with anticholinesterases, such as neostigmine (section 15.1.6). Non-depolarising neuromuscular blocking drugs can be divided into the **aminosteroid** group, comprising pancuronium, rocuronium, and vecuronium, and the **benzylisoquinolinium** group, which includes atracurium, cisatracurium, and mivacurium.

Non-depolarising neuromuscular blocking drugs have a slower onset of action than suxamethonium. These drugs can be classified by their duration of action as short-acting (15–30 minutes), intermediate-acting (30–40 minutes), and long-acting (60–120 minutes), although duration of action is dose-dependent. Drugs with a shorter or intermediate duration of action, such as atracurium and vecuronium, are more widely used than those with a longer duration of action, such as pancuronium.

Non-depolarising neuromuscular blocking drugs have no sedative or analgesic effects and are not considered to trigger malignant hyperthermia.

For children receiving intensive care and who require tracheal intubation and mechanical ventilation, a non-depolarising neuromuscular blocking drug is chosen according to its onset of effect, duration of action, and side-effects. Rocuronium, with a rapid onset of effect, may facilitate intubation. Atracurium or cisatracurium may be suitable for long-term neuromuscular blockade since their duration of action is not dependent on elimination by the liver or the kidneys.

Cautions Allergic cross-reactivity between neuromuscular blocking drugs has been reported; caution is advised in cases of hypersensitivity to these drugs. Their activity is prolonged in children with myasthenia gravis and in hypothermia, therefore lower doses are required. Non-depolarising neuromuscular blocking drugs should be used with great care in those with other neuromuscular disorders and those with fluid and electrolyte disturbances, as response in these children is unpredictable. Resistance may develop in children with burns who may require increased doses; low plasma cholinesterase activity in these children requires dose titration for mivacurium. **Interactions:** Appendix 1 (muscle relaxants).

Side-effects Benzylisoquinolinium non-depolarising neuromuscular blocking drugs (except cisatracurium) are associated with histamine release, which can cause skin flushing, hypotension, tachycardia, bronchospasm, and very rarely, anaphylactoid reactions. Most aminosteroid neuromuscular blocking drugs pro-

15

Anaesthesia

duce minimal histamine release. Drugs with vagolytic activity can counteract any bradycardia that occurs during surgery. Acute myopathy has also been reported after prolonged use in intensive care.

Atracurium, a mixture of 10 isomers, is a benzylisoquinolinium neuromuscular blocking drug with an intermediate duration of action. It undergoes non-enzymatic metabolism which is independent of liver and kidney function, thus allowing its use in children with hepatic or renal impairment. Cardiovascular effects are associated with significant histamine release. Neonates may be more sensitive to the effects of atracurium and lower doses may be required.

Cisatracurium is a single isomer of atracurium. It is more potent and has a slightly longer duration of action than atracurium and provides greater cardiovascular stability because cisatracurium lacks histamine-releasing effects. In children aged 1 month to 12 years, cisatracurium has a shorter duration of action and produces faster spontaneous recovery.

Mivacurium, a benzylisoquinolinium neuromuscular blocking drug, has a short duration of action. It is metabolised by plasma cholinesterase and muscle paralysis is prolonged in individuals deficient in this enzyme. It is not associated with vagolytic activity or ganglionic blockade although histamine release can occur, particularly with rapid injection. In children under 12 years mivacurium has a faster onset, shorter duration of action, and produces more rapid spontaneous recovery.

Pancuronium, an aminosteroid neuromuscular blocking drug, has a long duration of action and is often used in children receiving long-term mechanical ventilation in intensive care units. It lacks a histamine-releasing effect, but vagolytic and sympathomimetic effects can cause tachycardia and hypertension. The half-life of pancuronium in neonates is prolonged; neonates should receive postoperative intermittent positive pressure ventilation.

Rocuronium exerts an effect within 2 minutes and has the most rapid onset of any of the non-depolarising neuromuscular blocking drugs. It is an aminosteroid neuromuscular blocking drug with an intermediate duration of action. It is reported to have minimal cardiovascular effects; high doses produce mild vagolytic activity. In children under 12 years, rocuronium has a faster onset and shorter duration of action.

Vecuronium, an aminosteroid neuromuscular blocking drug, has an intermediate duration of action. It does not generally produce histamine release and lacks cardiovascular effects. In neonates and infants, vecuronium has a faster onset and a longer duration of action; recovery is longer in these children. Unexpected sustained neuromuscular blockade may occur in neonates.

15 Anaesthesia

ATRACURIUM BESILATE
(Atracurium besylate)

Cautions see notes above

Pregnancy does not cross placenta in significant amounts but manufacturer advises use only if potential benefit outweighs risk

Breast-feeding unlikely to be harmful following recovery from neuromuscular block; some manufacturers advise avoiding breast-feeding for 24 hours after administration

Side-effects see notes above; seizures also reported

Licensed use not licensed for use in neonates

Indication and dose

> To avoid excessive dosage in obese children, dose should be calculated on the basis of ideal weight for height

Neuromuscular blockade (short to intermediate duration) for surgery
• By intravenous administration

Neonate initially by *intravenous injection* 300–500 micrograms/kg followed *either* by *intra-venous injection*, 100–200 micrograms/kg repeated as necessary *or* by *intravenous infusion*, 300–400 micrograms/kg/hour adjusted according to response

Child 1 month–18 years initially by *intravenous injection* 300–600 micrograms/kg then 100–200 micrograms/kg repeated as necessary *or* initially by *intravenous injection* 200–600 micrograms/kg followed by *intravenous infusion*, 300–600 micrograms/kg/hour adjusted to response

Neuromuscular blockade during intensive care
• By intravenous administration

Neonate initially by *intravenous injection* 300–500 micrograms/kg followed *either* by *intravenous injection*, 100–200 micrograms/kg repeated as necessary *or* by *intravenous infusion*, 300–400 micrograms/kg/hour adjusted according to response; higher doses may be necessary

◁ ATRACURIUM BESILATE (continued)

Child 1 month–18 years initially by *intravenous injection* 300–600 micrograms/kg (optional) then by *intravenous infusion*, 270–1770 micrograms/kg/hour (usual dose 650–780 micrograms/kg/hour)

Administration for *continuous intravenous infusion*, dilute to a concentration of 0.5–5 mg/mL with Glucose 5% *or* Sodium Chloride 0.9% *or* Ringer's solution *or* Compound Sodium Lactate; stability varies with diluent.

Neonatal intensive care, dilute 60 mg/kg body-weight to a final volume of 50 mL with Glucose 5% or Sodium Chloride 0.9%; minimum concentration of 500 micrograms/mL, max. concentra-

tion of 5 mg/mL; an intravenous infusion rate of 0.1 mL/hour provides a dose of 120 micrograms/kg/hour

Atracurium (Non-proprietary) PoM
Injection, atracurium besilate 10 mg/mL, net price 2.5-mL amp = £1.85; 5-mL amp = £3.37; 25-mL vial = £14.45

Tracrium® (GSK) PoM
Injection, atracurium besilate 10 mg/mL, net price 2.5-mL amp = £1.66; 5-mL amp = £3.00; 25-mL vial = £12.91

■ CISATRACURIUM

Cautions see notes above
Pregnancy avoid—no information available
Breast-feeding no information available
Side-effects see notes above; also bradycardia

Indication and dose

To avoid excessive dosage in obese children, dose should be calculated on the basis of ideal weight for height

Neuromuscular blockade (intermediate duration) for intubation and during surgery
• By intravenous injection

Child 1 month–2 years initially 150 micrograms/kg, then 30 micrograms/kg repeated approx. every 20 minutes as necessary

Child 2–12 years initially 150 micrograms/kg (80–100 micrograms/kg if not for intubation), then 20 micrograms/kg repeated approx. every 10 minutes as necessary

Child 12–18 years initially 150 micrograms/kg, then 30 micrograms/kg repeated approx. every 20 minutes as necessary

• By intravenous infusion

Child 2–18 years initially 180 micrograms/kg/hour, reduced to 60–120 micrograms/kg/hour when stable; infusion rate may need to be reduced by up to 40% if used with isoflurane

Administration for *continuous intravenous infusion*, dilute to a concentration of 0.1–2 mg/mL with Glucose 5% *or* Sodium Chloride 0.9%; solutions of 2 mg/mL and 5 mg/mL may be infused undiluted

Nimbex® (GSK) PoM
Injection, cisatracurium (as besilate) 2 mg/mL, net price 10-mL amp = £7.55

Forte injection, cisatracurium (as besilate) 5 mg/mL, net price 30-mL vial = £31.09

■ MIVACURIUM

Cautions see notes above; low plasma cholinesterase activity
Hepatic impairment reduce dose in severe impairment
Renal impairment clinical effect prolonged in renal failure—reduce dose according to response
Pregnancy avoid—no information available
Side-effects see notes above

Indication and dose

To avoid excessive dosage in obese children, dose should be calculated on the basis of ideal weight for height

Neuromuscular blockade (short duration) during surgery
• By intravenous administration

Child 2–6 months by *intravenous injection* initially 150 micrograms/kg, then *either* by *intravenous injection* 100 micrograms/kg repeated every 6–9 minutes as necessary *or* by *intravenous infusion*, 8–10 micrograms/kg/minute, adjusted if necessary every 3 minutes by 1 microgram/kg/minute to usual dose 11–14 micrograms/kg/minute

Child 6 months–12 years by *intravenous injection* initially 200 micrograms/kg, then *either* by *intravenous injection* 100 micrograms/kg repeated every 6–9 minutes as necessary *or* by *intravenous infusion*, 8–10 micrograms/kg/minute, adjusted if necessary every 3 minutes by 1 microgram/kg/minute to usual dose 11–14 micrograms/kg/minute

Child 12–18 years by *intravenous injection* initially 70–250 micrograms/kg, then *either* by *intravenous injection* 100 micrograms/kg repeated every 15 minutes as necessary *or* by *intravenous infusion*, 8–10 micrograms/kg/minute, adjusted if necessary every 3 minutes by 1 microgram/kg/minute to usual dose of 6–7 micrograms/kg/minute

Administration for *intravenous injection*, give undiluted or dilute in Glucose 5% *or* Sodium Chloride 0.9%. Doses up to 150 micrograms/kg may be given over 5–15 seconds, higher doses should be given over 30 seconds. In asthma, cardiovascular disease or in those sensitive to reduced arterial blood pressure, give over 60 seconds.

15
Anaesthesia

◻ **MIVACURIUM (continued)**

Mivacron® (GSK) PoM
Injection, mivacurium (as chloride) 2 mg/mL, net price 5-mL amp = £2.79; 10-mL amp = £4.51

▰ PANCURONIUM BROMIDE

Cautions see notes above

Hepatic impairment possibly slower onset, higher dose requirement, and prolonged recovery time

Renal impairment use with caution; prolonged duration of block

Pregnancy avoid unless potential benefit outweighs risk—no information available

Breast-feeding avoid unless potential benefit outweighs risk—no information available

Side-effects see notes above

Indication and dose

> To avoid excessive dosage in obese children, dose should be calculated on the basis of ideal weight for height

Neuromuscular blockade (long duration) during surgery
• By intravenous injection

> **Neonate** initially 100 micrograms/kg, then 50 micrograms/kg repeated as necessary

> **Child 1 month–18 years** initially 100 micrograms/kg, then 20 micrograms/kg repeated as necessary

Administration for *intravenous injection*, give undiluted *or* dilute in Glucose 5% *or* Sodium Chloride 0.9%

Pancuronium (Non-proprietary) PoM
Injection, pancuronium bromide 2 mg/mL, net price 2-mL amp = £1.20

▰ ROCURONIUM BROMIDE

Cautions see notes above

Hepatic impairment reduce dose

Renal impairment reduce maintenance dose; prolonged paralysis

Pregnancy use with caution

Breast-feeding avoid unless potential benefit outweighs risk—present in milk in *animal* studies

Side-effects see notes above

Indication and dose

> To avoid excessive dosage in obese children, dose should be calculated on the basis of ideal weight for height

Neuromuscular blockade (intermediate duration) during surgery
• By intravenous administration

> **Child 1 month–18 years** initially by *intravenous injection* 600 micrograms/kg, then *either* by *intravenous injection*, 150 micrograms/kg repeated as required *or* by *intravenous infusion*, 300–600 micrograms/kg/hour adjusted according to response

Administration for *continuous intravenous infusion* or via drip tubing, may be diluted with Glucose 5% *or* Sodium Chloride 0.9%

Esmeron® (Organon) PoM
Injection, rocuronium bromide 10 mg/mL, net price 5-mL vial = £2.95, 10-mL vial = £5.90

▰ VECURONIUM BROMIDE

Cautions see notes above

Hepatic impairment caution in significant impairment

Renal impairment caution in renal failure

Pregnancy avoid unless potential benefit outweighs risk—no information available

Breast-feeding no information available

Side-effects see notes above

Licensed use not licensed for assisted ventilation in intensive care

Indication and dose

> To avoid excessive dosage in obese children, dose should be calculated on the basis of ideal weight for height

Neuromuscular blockade (intermediate duration) during surgery
• By intravenous administration

> **Neonate** by *intravenous injection* initially 80 micrograms/kg, then 30–50 micrograms/kg adjusted according to response

> **Child 1 month–18 years** by *intravenous injection* initially 80–100 micrograms/kg, then *either* by *intravenous injection*, 20–30 micrograms/kg repeated as required *or* by *intravenous infusion*, 0.8–1.4 micrograms/kg/minute, adjusted according to response

Assisted ventilation in intensive care
• By intravenous injection

> **Neonate** initially 80 micrograms/kg, then 30–50 micrograms/kg adjusted according to response

◻ **VECURONIUM BROMIDE** (*continued*)

• By intravenous administration

Neonate by *intravenous injection* 80 micrograms/
kg, then by *intravenous infusion*, 0.8–1.4 micr-
ograms/kg/minute, adjusted according to
response (risk of accumulation—consider interruption of infusion)

Administration reconstitute each vial with 5 mL
Water for Injections to give a 2 mg/mL solution;
alternatively reconstitute with up to 10 mL Glucose 5% *or* Sodium Chloride 0.9% *or* Water for
Injections *or* Ringer's solution—unsuitable for
further dilution if not reconstituted with Water for
Injections.

For *continuous intravenous infusion*, dilute reconstituted solution to a concentration up to
40 micrograms/mL with Glucose 5% *or* Sodium
Chloride 0.9% *or* Ringer's solution; reconstituted
solution can also be given via drip tubing.
Neonatal intensive care, reconstitute each vial with
5 mL Water for Injections to give a 2 mg/mL
solution. Dilute 5 mg/kg body-weight to a final
volume of 50 mL with Glucose 5% or Sodium
Chloride 0.9%; an intravenous infusion rate of
0.5 mL/hour provides a dose of 50 micrograms/
kg/hour; minimum concentration of 40 micr-
ograms/mL

Norcuron® (Organon) [PoM]
Injection, powder for reconstitution, vecuronium
bromide, net price 10-mg vial = £3.75 (with water
for injections)

Depolarising neuromuscular blocking drugs

Suxamethonium has the most rapid onset of action of any of the neuromuscular
blocking drugs and is ideal if fast onset and brief duration of action are required
e.g. with tracheal intubation. Neonates and young children are less sensitive to
suxamethonium and a higher dose may be required.

Suxamethonium acts by mimicking acetylcholine at the neuromuscular junction
but hydrolysis is much slower than for acetylcholine; depolarisation is therefore
prolonged, resulting in neuromuscular blockade. Unlike the non-depolarising
neuromuscular blocking drugs, its action cannot be reversed and recovery is
spontaneous; anticholinesterases such as neostigmine potentiate the neuromuscular block.

Suxamethonium should be given after anaesthetic induction because paralysis is
usually preceded by painful muscle fasciculations. Bradycardia may occur; premedication with atropine (section 15.1.3) reduces bradycardia as well as the
excessive salivation associated with suxamethonium use.

Prolonged paralysis may occur in **dual block**, which occurs with high or repeated
doses of suxamethonium and is caused by the development of a non-depolarising
block following the initial depolarising block; edrophonium (section 15.1.6) may
be used to confirm the diagnosis of dual block. Children with myasthenia gravis
are resistant to suxamethonium but can develop dual block resulting in delayed
recovery. Prolonged paralysis may also occur in those with low or atypical plasma
cholinesterase. Assisted ventilation should be continued until muscle function is
restored.

SUXAMETHONIUM CHLORIDE
(Succinylcholine chloride)

Cautions see notes above; hypersensitivity to
other neuromuscular blocking drugs; patients
with cardiac, respiratory or neuromuscular disease; raised intra-ocular pressure (avoid in
penetrating eye injury); severe sepsis (risk of
hyperkalaemia); **interactions:** Appendix 1
(muscle relaxants)

Contra-indications family history of malignant
hyperthermia, hyperkalaemia; major trauma,
severe burns, neurological disease involving
acute wasting of major muscle, prolonged
immobilisation—risk of hyperkalaemia; personal
or family history of congenital myotonic disease,
Duchenne muscular dystrophy; low plasma-
cholinesterase activity (including severe liver
disease, see below)

Hepatic impairment prolonged apnoea may
occur in severe liver disease because of reduced
hepatic synthesis of pseudocholinesterase

Pregnancy mildly prolonged maternal paralysis
may occur

Breast-feeding no information available

Side-effects see notes above; also increased gastric pressure; hyperkalaemia; postoperative
muscle pain, myoglobinuria, myoglobinaemia;
increased intraocular pressure; flushing, rash;
rarely arrhythmias, cardiac arrest; bronchospasm,
apnoea, prolonged respiratory depression; limited jaw mobility; *very rarely* anaphylactic reactions, malignant hyperthermia; *also reported*
hypertension, hypotension, rhabdomyolysis

Indication and dose

**Neuromuscular blockade (short duration) dur-
ing surgery**
• By intravenous injection

Neonate 2 mg/kg produces 5-10 minutes
paralysis

Child 1 month–1 year 2 mg/kg

Child 1–18 years 1 mg/kg

15 Anaesthesia

◻ **SUXAMETHONIUM CHLORIDE (*continued*)**

• By intramuscular injection

Neonate up to 4 mg/kg produces 10–30 minutes paralysis (after 2–3 minute delay)

Child 1 month–1 year up to 4–5 mg/kg (paralysis after 2–3 minute delay)

Child 1–12 years up to 4 mg/kg (paralysis after 2–3 minute delay); max. 150 mg

Administration for *intravenous injection*, give undiluted *or* dilute with Glucose 5% *or* Sodium Chloride 0.9%

Suxamethonium Chloride (Non-proprietary) PoM
Injection, suxamethonium chloride 50 mg/mL, net price 2-mL amp = 64p, 2-mL prefilled syringe = £8.45

Anectine® (GSK) PoM
Injection, suxamethonium chloride 50 mg/mL, net price 2-mL amp = 71p

---

15.1.6 Drugs for reversal of neuromuscular blockade

Anticholinesterases

Anticholinesterases reverse the effects of the non-depolarising (competitive) neuromuscular blocking drugs such as pancuronium, but they prolong the action of the depolarising neuromuscular blocking drug suxamethonium.

Edrophonium has a transient action and may be used in the diagnosis of suspected dual block due to suxamethonium. Atropine (section 15.1.3) is given before or with edrophonium to prevent muscarinic effects of edrophonium; it is also used in the diagnosis of myasthenia gravis (section 10.2.1).

Neostigmine has a longer duration of action than edrophonium and is used specifically for reversal of non-depolarising (competitive) blockade. It acts within one minute of intravenous injection and its effects last for 20 to 30 minutes; a second dose may then be necessary. Glycopyrronium or alternatively atropine (section 15.1.3), given before or with neostigmine, prevent bradycardia, excessive salivation, and other muscarinic effects of neostigmine.

▲ EDROPHONIUM CHLORIDE

Cautions section 10.2.1; atropine should also be given

Contra-indications section 10.2.1

Pregnancy section 10.2.1

Breast-feeding section 10.2.1

Side-effects section 10.2.1

Indication and dose

Brief reversal of non-depolarising neuromuscular blockade

• By intravenous injection over several minutes

Child 1 month–18 years 500–700 micrograms/kg (after or with atropine)

Myasthenia gravis section 10.2.1

Edrophonium (Non-proprietary) PoM
Injection, edrophonium chloride 10 mg/mL, net price 1-mL amp = £8.65

▲ NEOSTIGMINE METILSULFATE
(Neostigmine methylsulphate)

Cautions section 10.2.1; glycopyrronium or atropine should also be given

Contra-indications section 10.2.1

Renal impairment section 10.2.1

Pregnancy section 10.2.1

Breast-feeding section 10.2.1

Side-effects section 10.2.1

Indication and dose

Reversal of non-depolarising muscle block

• By intravenous injection over 1 minute

Neonate 50 micrograms/kg, after or with glycopyrronium or atropine; a further dose of 25 micrograms/kg may be required

Child 1 month–12 years 50 micrograms/kg (max. 2.5 mg) after or with glycopyrronium or atropine; a further dose of 25 micrograms/kg may be required

Child 12–18 years 50 micrograms/kg (max. 2.5 mg) after or with glycopyrronium or atropine; a further dose of 25 micrograms/kg (max. 2.5 mg) may be required

Myasthenia gravis section 10.2.1

Administration for *intravenous injection*, give undiluted *or* dilute with Glucose 5% *or* Sodium Chloride 0.9% *or* Water for Injections

◻ **NEOSTIGMINE METILSULFATE (continued)**

Neostigmine (Non-proprietary) [PoM]
Injection, neostigmine metilsulfate 2.5 mg/mL, net price 1-mL amp = 58p

◢**With glycopyrronium**

Glycopyrronium-Neostigmine (Non-proprietary) [PoM]
Injection, neostigmine metilsulfate 2.5 mg, glycopyrronium bromide 500 micrograms/mL, net price 1-mL amp = 91p

Dose

> Reversal of non-depolarising neuromuscular blockade
> • By intravenous injection over 10–30 seconds
>> **Child 1 month–18 years** 0.02 mL/kg (or 0.2 mL/kg of a 1 in 10 dilution), dose may be repeated if required (total max. 2 mL)
>
> **Administration** for *intravenous injection*, may be diluted with Sodium Chloride 0.9% or Water for Injections

Other drugs for reversal of neuromuscular blockade

Sugammadex is a modified gamma cyclodextrin used for reversal of neuromuscular blockade induced by rocuronium (section 15.1.5).

◢ SUGAMMADEX

Cautions recurrence of neuromuscular blockade—monitor respiratory function until fully recovered; recovery may be delayed in cardiovascular disease; wait 24 hours before re-administering rocuronium; **interactions:** Appendix 1 (sugammadex)

Renal impairment avoid if estimated glomerular filtration rate less then 30 mL/minute/1.73 m²

Pregnancy use with caution—no information available

Side-effects taste disturbances; *less commonly* allergic reactions; bronchospasm also reported

Indication and dose

> Routine reversal of neuromuscular blockade induced by rocuronium
> • By intravenous injection
>> **Child 2–18 years** 2 mg/kg (consult product literature)
>
> **Administration** for *intravenous injection* dose may be diluted to a concentration of 10 mg/mL with Sodium Chloride 0.9%

Bridion® (Schering-Plough) ▼ [PoM]
Injection, sugammadex (as sodium salt) 100 mg/mL, net price 2-mL amp = £59.64, 5-mL amp = £149.10
Electrolytes Na⁺ 0.42 mmol/mL

15.1.7 Antagonists for central and respiratory depression

Respiratory depression is a major concern with opioid analgesics and it may be treated by artificial ventilation or be reversed by an opioid antagonist. **Naloxone** given intravenously immediately reverses opioid-induced respiratory depression but the dose may have to be repeated because of its **short duration of action**. Intramuscular injection of naloxone produces a more gradual and prolonged effect but absorption may be erratic. Care is required in children requiring pain relief because naloxone also antagonises the analgesic effect of opioids.

Neonates Naloxone is used in newborn infants to reverse respiratory depression and sedation resulting from the use of opioids by the mother, usually for pain during labour. In neonates the effects of opioids may persist for up to 48 hours and in such cases naloxone is often given by intramuscular injection for its prolonged effect. In severe respiratory depression after birth, breathing should first be established (using artificial means if necessary) and naloxone administered only if use of opioids by the mother is thought to cause the respiratory depression; the infant should be monitored closely and further doses of naloxone administered as necessary.

Flumazenil is a benzodiazepine antagonist for the reversal of the central sedative effects of benzodiazepines after anaesthetic and similar procedures. Flumazenil has a shorter half-life and duration of action than diazepam and midazolam, so children may become resedated.

Doxapram (section 3.5.1) is a central and respiratory stimulant but is of limited value in anaesthesia.

15 Anaesthesia

FLUMAZENIL

Cautions short-acting (repeat doses may be necessary—benzodiazepine effects may persist for at least 24 hours); benzodiazepine dependence (may precipitate withdrawal symptoms); prolonged benzodiazepine therapy for epilepsy (risk of convulsions); history of panic disorders (risk of recurrence); ensure neuromuscular blockade cleared before giving; avoid rapid injection in high-risk or anxious children and following major surgery; head injury (rapid reversal of benzodiazepine sedation may cause convulsions)

Contra-indications life-threatening condition (e.g. raised intracranial pressure, status epilepticus) controlled by benzodiazepines

Hepatic impairment carefully titrate dose

Pregnancy may cross placenta in small amounts—avoid unless potential benefit outweighs risk

Breast-feeding avoid breast-feeding for 24 hours

Side-effects nausea, vomiting, and flushing; if wakening too rapid, agitation, anxiety, and fear; transient increase in blood pressure and heart-rate in intensive care patients; *very rarely* convulsions (particularly in those with epilepsy), hypersensitivity reactions including anaphylaxis

Licensed use not licensed for use in children

Indication and dose

> Reversal of sedative effects of benzodiazepines
> • **By intravenous injection over 15 seconds (question aetiology if no response to repeated injection)**
>
> > **Neonate** 10 micrograms/kg, repeat at 1-minute intervals if required

> **Child 1 month–12 years** 10 micrograms/kg (max. single dose 200 micrograms), repeated at 1-minute intervals if required; max. total dose of 40 micrograms/kg (1 mg) (2 mg in intensive care)

> **Child 12–18 years** 200 micrograms, repeated at 1-minute intervals if required; max. total dose 1 mg (2 mg in intensive care)

> • **By intravenous infusion, if drowsiness recurs after injection**
>
> > **Neonate** 2–10 micrograms/kg/hour, adjusted according to response

> > **Child 1 month–18 years** 2–10 micrograms/kg/ hour, adjusted according to response; max. 400 micrograms/hour

> **Overdosage with benzodiazepines** see Emergency Treatment of Poisoning p. 41

Administration for *continuous intravenous infusion*, dilute with Glucose 5% *or* Sodium Chloride 0.9%

Flumazenil (Non-proprietary) PoM
Injection, flumazenil 100 micrograms/mL, net price 5-mL amp = £14.49

Anexate® (Roche) PoM
Injection, flumazenil 100 micrograms/mL, net price 5-mL amp = £13.93

NALOXONE HYDROCHLORIDE

Cautions cardiovascular disease or those receiving cardiotoxic drugs (serious adverse cardiovascular effects reported); maternal physical dependence on opioids (may precipitate withdrawal in newborn); pain (see also under Titration of Dose, below); has short duration of action (see notes above)

Titration of dose In postoperative use, the dose should be titrated for each child in order to obtain sufficient respiratory response; however, naloxone antagonises analgesia

Pregnancy use only if potential benefit outweighs risk

Breast-feeding not orally bioavailable

Side-effects nausea, vomiting; hypotension, hypertension, ventricular tachycardia and fibrillation, cardiac arrest; hyperventilation, dyspnoea, pulmonary oedema; headache, dizziness; *less commonly* diarrhoea, dry mouth, agitation, excitement, paraesthesia, tremor, sweating; *very rarely* seizures and erythema multiforme

Indication and dose

> Reversal of respiratory and CNS depression in neonate following maternal opioid use during labour
> • **By intramuscular injection**
>
> > **Neonate** 200 micrograms (60 micrograms/kg) as a single dose at birth

> • **By intravenous or subcutaneous injection**
>
> > **Neonate** 10 micrograms/kg, repeated every 2–3 minutes if required

> Reversal of respiratory depression caused by medicinal use of opioids
> • **By intravenous injection**
>
> > **Neonate** 1 microgram/kg, repeated every 2–3 minutes if required

> > **Child 1 month–12 years** 1 microgram/kg, repeated every 2–3 minutes if required

> > **Child 12–18 years** 1.5–3 micrograms/kg; if response inadequate, give subsequent doses of 100 micrograms every 2 minutes

> **Overdosage with opioids** see Emergency Treatment of Poisoning p. 39

◄Preparation
See Emergency Treatment of Poisoning p. 40

15.1.8 Drugs for malignant hyperthermia

Malignant hyperthermia is a rare but potentially lethal complication of anaesthesia. It is characterised by a rapid rise in temperature, increased muscle rigidity, tachycardia, and acidosis. The most common triggers of malignant hyperthermia are the volatile anaesthetics. Suxamethonium has also been implicated, but malignant hyperthermia is more likely if it is given following a volatile anaesthetic. Volatile anaesthetics and suxamethonium should be avoided during anaesthesia in children at high risk of malignant hyperthermia.

Dantrolene is used in the treatment of malignant hyperthermia. It acts on skeletal muscle cells by interfering with calcium efflux, thereby stopping the contractile process.

DANTROLENE SODIUM

Cautions avoid extravasation (risk of tissue necrosis); **interactions:** Appendix 1 (muscle relaxants)

Pregnancy use only if potential benefit outweighs risk

Breast-feeding present in milk—use only if potential benefit outweighs risk

Side-effects hepatotoxicity, pulmonary oedema, dizziness, weakness, and injection-site reactions including erythema, rash, swelling, and thrombophlebitis

Indication and dose

Malignant hyperthermia
- By rapid intravenous injection

  Child 1 month–18 years initially 2–3 mg/kg, then 1 mg/kg repeated as required (total max. dose 10 mg/kg)

Chronic severe spasticity of voluntary muscle see section 10.2.2

Dantrium Intravenous® (SpePharm) PoM
Injection, powder for reconstitution, dantrolene sodium, net price 20-mg vial = £51.00 (hosp. only)

15.2 Local anaesthesia

The use of local anaesthetics by injection or by application to mucous membranes to produce local analgesia is discussed in this section.

See also section 1.7 (anus), section 11.7 (eye), section 12.3 (oropharynx), and section 13.3 (skin).

Use of local anaesthetics Local anaesthetic drugs act by causing a reversible block to conduction along nerve fibres. The drugs used vary widely in their potency, toxicity, duration of action, stability, solubility in water, and ability to penetrate mucous membranes. These variations determine their suitability for use by various routes, e.g. topical (surface), infiltration, peripheral nerve block, intravenous regional anaesthesia (Bier's block), plexus, epidural (extradural) or spinal block. Local anaesthetics may also be used for postoperative pain relief, thereby reducing the need for analgesics such as opioids.

Administration In estimating the safe dosage of these drugs it is important to take account of the rate at which they are absorbed and excreted as well as their potency. The child's age, weight, physique, and clinical condition, the degree of vascularity of the area to which the drug is to be applied, and the duration of administration are other factors which must be taken into account.

Local anaesthetics do not rely on the circulation to transport them to their sites of action, but uptake into the systemic circulation is important in terminating their action and producing toxicity. Following most regional anaesthetic procedures, maximum arterial plasma concentrations of anaesthetic develop within about 10 to 25 minutes, so **careful surveillance** for toxic effects is necessary during the first 30 minutes after injection. Great care must be taken to avoid accidental intravascular injection. Local anaesthesia around the oral cavity may impair swallowing and therefore increase the risk of aspiration.

Epidural anaesthesia is commonly used during surgery, often combined with general anaesthesia, because of its protective effect against the stress response of surgery. It is often used for major surgery in children, including orthopaedic and abdominal surgery.

Toxicity Toxic effects associated with local anaesthetics usually result from excessively high plasma concentrations; single application of topical lidocaine

15

Anaesthesia

preparations does not generally cause systemic side-effects. Effects initially include a feeling of inebriation and lightheadedness followed by sedation, circumoral paraesthesia and twitching; convulsions can occur in severe reactions. On intravenous injection convulsions and cardiovascular collapse may occur very rapidly. Hypersensitivity reactions occur mainly with the ester-type local anaesthetics such as benzocaine and tetracaine (amethocaine); reactions are less frequent with the amide types such as lidocaine (lignocaine), bupivacaine, levobupivacaine, prilocaine, and ropivacaine. Cross-sensitivity reactions may be avoided by using the alternative chemical type. Local anaesthetics may be associated with methaemoglobinaemia; prilocaine and benzocaine have been implicated.

When prolonged analgesia is required, a long-acting local anaesthetic is preferred to minimise the likelihood of cumulative systemic toxicity. Local anaesthetic injections should be given slowly in order to detect inadvertent intravascular administration. Local anaesthetics should **not** be injected into inflamed or infected tissues nor should they be applied to the traumatised urethra. In such cases absorption into the blood may increase the possibility of systemic side-effects. The local anaesthetic effect may also be reduced by the altered local pH. Local anaesthetics can be ototoxic and should **not** be applied to the middle ear.

Use of vasoconstrictors Most local anaesthetics cause dilation of blood vessels. The addition of a vasoconstrictor such as **adrenaline (epinephrine)** diminishes local blood flow, slows the rate of absorption of the local anaesthetic, and prolongs its local effect. Adrenaline must be used in a low concentration (e.g. 1 in 400 000–1 in 200 000) for this purpose and it is **not** advisable to give adrenaline with a local anaesthetic injection in digits or appendages because of the risk of ischaemic necrosis.

When adrenaline is included the final concentration should be no more than 1 in 200 000 (5 micrograms/mL), but see also Dental Anaesthesia, below. The total dose of adrenaline should **not** exceed 5 micrograms/kg (1 mL/kg of a 1 in 200 000 solution). Care must also be taken to calculate a safe maximum dose of local anaesthetic when using combination products. For general cautions associated with the use of adrenaline, see section 2.7.3. For drug interactions, see Appendix 1 (sympathomimetics).

Dental anaesthesia Lidocaine (lignocaine) is widely used in dental procedures; it is most often used in combination with **adrenaline** (epinephrine). Lidocaine 2% combined with adrenaline 1 in 80 000 (12.5 micrograms/mL) is a safe and effective preparation; there is no justification for using higher concentrations of adrenaline.

The local anaesthetics **articaine** (carticaine) and **mepivacaine** are also used in dentistry; they are available in cartridges suitable for dental use. Mepivacaine is available with or without adrenaline (as *Scandonest*®) and articaine is available with adrenaline (as *Septanest*®).

In children with severe hypertension or unstable cardiac rhythm, the use of adrenaline in a local anaesthetic may be hazardous. For these children mepivacaine may be used. Alternatively, **prilocaine** with or without felypressin can be used but there is no evidence that it is any safer.

Great care should be taken to avoid inadvertent intravenous administration of a preparation containing adrenaline.

Lidocaine

Lidocaine (lignocaine) is effectively absorbed from mucous membranes and is a useful surface anaesthetic in concentrations up to 10%. Except for surface anaesthesia and dental anaesthesia, solutions should not usually exceed 1% in strength. The duration of the block (with adrenaline) is about 90 minutes.

Application of a mixture of lidocaine and prilocaine (*EMLA*®) under an occlusive dressing provides surface anaesthesia for 1–2 hours. *EMLA*® does not appear to be effective in providing local anaesthesia for heel lancing in neonates.

▲ LIDOCAINE HYDROCHLORIDE
(Lignocaine hydrochloride)

Cautions see notes above; see section 2.3.2 for effects on heart; also epilepsy, respiratory impairment, impaired cardiac conduction, bradycardia, severe shock; acute porphyria (section 9.8.2); myasthenia gravis; reduce dose in debilitated; resuscitative equipment should be available; **interactions:** Appendix 1 (lidocaine)

Contra-indications see notes above; also hypovolaemia, complete heart block; do not use solutions containing adrenaline for anaesthesia in appendages

Hepatic impairment use with caution—increased risk of side-effects

Renal impairment possible accumulation of lidocaine and active metabolite; use with caution in severe impairment

Pregnancy large doses during delivery can cause neonatal respiratory depression, hypotonia, and bradycardia after paracervical or epidural block

Breast-feeding amount too small to be harmful

Side-effects see notes above and section 2.3.2; also CNS effects include confusion, respiratory depression and convulsions; hypotension and bradycardia (may lead to cardiac arrest); hypersensitivity reported

Licensed use *EMLA*® cream not licensed for use in children under 1 year

Indication and dose

Local anaesthesia
- **By local infiltration**
(see also Administration p. 797 and *Safe Practice* warning below)

> **Neonate** according to nature of procedure, up to 3 mg/kg (0.3 mL/kg of 1% solution), repeated not more often than every 4 hours

> **Child 1 month–12 years** according to nature of procedure, up to 3 mg/kg (0.3 mL/kg of 1% solution), repeated not more often than every 4 hours

> **Child 12–18 years** according to nature of procedure, up to 200 mg, repeated not more often than every 4 hours

> **Ventricular arrhythmias** section 2.3.2

> **Intravenous regional anaesthesia and nerve blocks** seek expert advice

> **Dental anaesthesia** seek expert advice

> **Safe Practice** The licensed doses stated above may not be appropriate in some settings and expert advice should be sought

▲ Lidocaine hydrochloride injections

Lidocaine (Non-proprietary) PoM
Injection 0.5%, lidocaine hydrochloride 5 mg/mL, net price 10-mL amp = 35p

Injection 1%, lidocaine hydrochloride 10 mg/mL, net price 2-mL amp = 21p; 5-mL amp = 26p; 10-mL amp = 39p; 10-mL prefilled syringe = £4.53; 20-mL amp = 78p

Injection 2%, lidocaine hydrochloride 20 mg/mL, net price 2-mL amp = 27p; 5-mL amp = 27p

Xylocaine® (AstraZeneca) PoM
Injection 1% with adrenaline 1 in 200 000, anhydrous lidocaine hydrochloride 10 mg/mL, adrenaline 1 in 200 000 (5 micrograms/mL), net price 20-mL vial = 99p

Injection 2% with adrenaline 1 in 200 000, anhydrous lidocaine hydrochloride 20 mg/mL, adrenaline 1 in 200 000 (5 micrograms/mL), net price 20-mL vial = £1.04

▲ Lidocaine injections for dental use

Note Consult expert dental sources for specific advice in relation to dose of lidocaine for dental anaesthesia

A variety of lidocaine injections with adrenaline are available in dental cartridges; brand names include *Lignospan Special*®, *Rexocaine*®, and *Xylocaine*®

▲ Lidocaine for surface anaesthesia

Important. Rapid and extensive absorption may result in systemic side-effects

Lidocaine (Non-proprietary)
Ointment, lidocaine hydrochloride 5%, net price 15 g = 88p

Dose
> **Dental practice**
> **Child** rub gently into dry gum

> **Pain relief (in anal fissures, haemorrhoids, pruritus ani, pruritus vulvae, herpes zoster)**
> **Child** 1–2 mL applied when necessary; avoid long-term use

Solution, lidocaine hydrochloride 4%, net price 25 mL = £1.35

Dose
> **Biopsy in mouth**
> **Child** up to 3 mg/kg with suitable spray *or* swab (with adrenaline if necessary); max. 5 mL

> **Puncture of maxillary sinus or polypectomy**
> **Child** up to 3 mg/kg; apply with swab for 2–3 minutes (with adrenaline)

> **Bronchoscopy and bronchography**
> **Child** up to 3 mg/kg; 2–3 mL with suitable spray

EMLA® (AstraZeneca)
Drug Tariff cream, lidocaine 2.5%, prilocaine 2.5%, net price 5-g tube = £1.73

Surgical pack cream, lidocaine 2.5%, prilocaine 2.5%, net price 30-g tube = £10.25

Premedication pack cream, lidocaine 2.5%, prilocaine 2.5%, net price 5 × 5-g tube with 12 occlusive dressings = £9.75

Cautions not for preterm neonates, children under 1 year receiving treatment with methaemoglobin-inducing agents, wounds, mucous membranes, or atopic dermatitis; avoid use near eyes or middle ear; although systemic absorption low, caution in anaemia, in congenital or acquired methaemoglobinaemia or in G6PD deficiency (see also Prilocaine, p. 801)

15
Anaesthesia

◁ **LIDOCAINE HYDROCHLORIDE** (continued)

Side-effects include administration site reactions such as transient paleness, redness, oedema, itching, burning sensation, and localised lesions

Dose

> **Anaesthesia before minor skin procedures including venepuncture**
>
> **Neonate** apply max. 1 g under occlusive dressing for max. 1 hour before procedure; max. 1 dose in 24 hours
>
> **Child 1–3 months or body-weight less than 5 kg** apply max. 1 g under occlusive dressing for max. 1 hour before procedure; max. 1 dose in 24 hours
>
> **Child 3 months–1 year and body weight over 5 kg** apply max. 2 g under occlusive dressing for max. 4 hours before procedure; max. 2 doses in 24 hours
>
> **Child 1–18 years** apply thick layer under occlusive dressing 1–5 hours before procedure (2–5 hours before procedures on large areas e.g. split skin grafting); max. 2 doses in 24 hours for child 1–12 years

Note Shorter application time of 15–30 minutes is recommended for children with atopic dermatitis

Instillagel® (CliniMed)
Gel, lidocaine hydrochloride 2%, chlorhexidine gluconate solution 0.25%, in a sterile lubricant basis in disposable syringe, net price 6-mL syringe = £1.41, 11-mL syringe = £1.58
Excipients include hydroxybenzoates (parabens)

Laryngojet® (UCB Pharma) PoM
Jet spray 4% (disposable kit for laryngotracheal anaesthesia), lidocaine hydrochloride 40 mg/mL, net price per unit (4-mL vial and disposable sterile cannula with cover and vial injector) = £5.10
Cautions may be rapidly and almost completely absorbed from respiratory tract and systemic side-effects may occur; extreme caution if mucosa has been traumatised or if sepsis present

Dose

> **Bronchoscopy, laryngoscopy, oesophagoscopy, endotracheal intubation, and biopsy**
>
> **Child** up to 0.075 mL/kg (3 mg/kg) as a single dose instilled as jet spray or applied with a swab; max. 5 mL (200 mg)

LMX 4® (Ferndale)
Cream lidocaine 4%, net price 5-g tube = £2.98; 5 × 5-g tube with 10 occlusive dressings = £16.90
Excipients include benzyl alcohol and propylene glycol
Cautions not for wounds, mucous membranes, or atopic dermatis; avoid use near eyes or middle ear; although

systemic absorption low, caution in acutely ill or debilitated children
Hepatic impairment although systemic absorption low, caution in severe impairment
Side-effects irritation and rash

Dose

> **Anaesthesia before venous cannulation or venepuncture**
>
> **Child 1 month–18 years** apply thick layer (1–2.5 g; child under 1 year max 1 g) to small area (2.5 cm × 2.5 cm) of non-irritated skin at least 30 minutes before procedure (max 60 minutes); remove cream with gauze and perform procedure after approximately 5 minutes

Rapydan® (EUSA Pharma) PoM
Medicated plasters, lidocaine 70 mg, tetracaine 70 mg, net price 25 = £98.00
Excipients include hydroxybenzoates (parabens)

Dose

> **Needle puncture**
>
> **Child 3–18 years** apply 1–2 plasters to intact skin 30 minutes before needle puncture; max. 2 plasters daily

The *Scottish Medicines Consortium* (p. 4) has advised (May 2008) that lidocaine 70 mg/tetracaine 70 mg medicated plaster (*Rapydan®*) is **not** recommended for use within NHS Scotland

Xylocaine® (AstraZeneca)
Spray (= pump spray), lidocaine 10% (100 mg/g) supplying 10 mg lidocaine/dose; 500 spray doses per container, net price 50-mL bottle = £3.13

Dose

> **Bronchoscopy, laryngoscopy, oesophagoscopy, endotracheal intubation**
>
> **Child up to 18 years** up to 3 mg/kg

Note Lidocaine can damage plastic cuffs of endotracheal tubes

◢ **Lidocaine for ear, nose, and oropharyngeal use**
For prescribing information on phenylephrine, see section 2.7.2

Lidocaine with Phenylephrine (Non-proprietary)
Topical solution, lidocaine hydrochloride 5%, phenylephrine hydrochloride 0.5%, net price 2.5 mL (with nasal applicator) = £9.60

> ### Bupivacaine
>
> The advantage of **bupivacaine** over other local anaesthetics is its longer duration of action (3–7 hours). It has a slow onset of action, taking up to 30 minutes for full effect. It is often used in lumbar epidural blockade and is particularly suitable for continuous epidural analgesia in labour or for postoperative pain relief. It is the principal drug used for spinal anaesthesia.

◣ BUPIVACAINE HYDROCHLORIDE

Cautions see under Lidocaine Hydrochloride and notes above; myocardial depression may be more severe and more resistant to treatment; **interactions**: Appendix 1 (bupivacaine)

Contra-indications see under Lidocaine Hydrochloride and notes above; intravenous regional anaesthesia (Bier's block)

Hepatic impairment use with caution in severe impairment

Renal impairment use with caution

Pregnancy large doses during delivery can cause neonatal respiratory depression, hypotonia, and bradycardia after paracervical or epidural block;

◻ BUPIVACAINE HYDROCHLORIDE (*continued*)

use lower doses for intrathecal use during late pregnancy

Breast-feeding amount too small to be harmful

Side-effects see under Lidocaine Hydrochloride and notes above

Indication and dose

> Adjusted according to child's physical status and nature of procedure, seek expert advice—
> **important**: see also under Administration, p. 797

Bupivacaine (Non-proprietary) PoM
Injection, anhydrous bupivacaine hydrochloride 2.5 mg/mL (0.25%), net price 10 mL = 82p; 5 mg/mL (0.5%), 10 mL = 94p

Note Bupivacaine hydrochloride injection 0.25% and 0.5% are available in glass or plastic ampoules, and sterile-wrapped glass ampoules

Infusion, anhydrous bupivacaine hydrochloride 1 mg/mL (0.1%), net price 100 mL = £8.41, 250 mL = £10.59; 1.25 mg/mL (0.125%), 250 mL = £10.80

Marcain® (AstraZeneca) PoM
Injection, anhydrous bupivacaine hydrochloride 2.5 mg/mL (*Marcain® 0.25%*), net price 10-mL *Polyamp®* = £1.06; 5 mg/mL (*Marcain® 0.5%*), 10-mL *Polyamp®* = £1.21

Marcain Heavy® (AstraZeneca) PoM
Injection, anhydrous bupivacaine hydrochloride 5 mg, glucose 80 mg/mL, net price 4-mL amp = £1.21

◢ With adrenaline
For prescribing information on adrenaline, see section 2.7.2

Bupivacaine and Adrenaline (Non-proprietary) PoM
Injection, anhydrous bupivacaine hydrochloride 2.5 mg/mL (0.25%), adrenaline 1 in 200 000 (5 micrograms/mL), net price 10-mL amp = £1.23
Injection, anhydrous bupivacaine hydrochloride 5 mg/mL (0.5%), adrenaline 1 in 200 000 (5 micrograms/mL), net price 10-mL amp = £1.40

Levobupivacaine

Levobupivacaine, an isomer of bupivacaine, has anaesthetic and analgesic properties similar to bupivacaine but is thought to have fewer adverse effects.

◢ LEVOBUPIVACAINE

Note Levobupivacaine is an isomer of bupivacaine

Cautions see under Lidocaine Hydrochloride and notes above; **interactions**: Appendix 1 (levobupivacaine)

Contra-indications see under Lidocaine Hydrochloride and notes above; intravenous regional anaesthesia (Bier's block); paracervical block in obstetrics

Hepatic impairment use with caution

Pregnancy large doses during delivery can cause neonatal respiratory depression, hypotonia, and bradycardia after paracervical or epidural block; avoid if possible in first trimester—toxicity in *animal* studies

Breast-feeding likely to be present in milk but risk to infant minimal

Side-effects see under Lidocaine Hydrochloride and notes above

Licensed use not licensed for use in children by epidural infusion

Indication and dose

> Adjusted according to child's physical status and nature of procedure, seek expert advice—
> **important**: see also under Administration, p. 797

Chirocaine® (Abbott) PoM
Injection, levobupivacaine (as hydrochloride) 2.5 mg/mL, net price 10-mL amp = £1.66; 5 mg/mL, 10-mL amp = £1.90; 7.5 mg/mL, 10-mL amp = £2.85

Infusion, levobupivacaine (as hydrochloride) 625 micrograms/mL, net price 100 mL = £7.80, 200 mL = £10.40; 1.25 mg/mL, net price 100 mL = £8.54, 200 mL = £12.20

Prilocaine

Prilocaine is a local anaesthetic of low toxicity which is similar to lidocaine (lignocaine). If used in high doses, methaemoglobinaemia may occur which can be treated with intravenous injection of methylthioninium chloride (methylene blue) 1% using a dose of 1 mg/kg. Neonates and infants under 6 months are particularly susceptible to methaemoglobinaemia.

◢ PRILOCAINE HYDROCHLORIDE

Cautions see under Lidocaine Hydrochloride and notes above; severe or untreated hypertension, severe heart disease; concomitant drugs which cause methaemoglobinaemia; **interactions**: Appendix 1 (prilocaine)

Contra-indications see under Lidocaine Hydrochloride and notes above; anaemia, or congenital or acquired methaemoglobinaemia

Hepatic impairment use with caution

Renal impairment use with caution

Pregnancy large doses during delivery can cause neonatal respiratory depression, hypotonia, and

◻ **PRILOCAINE HYDROCHLORIDE** *(continued)*

bradycardia after paracervical or epidural block; neonatal methaemoglobinaemia reported after paracervical block or pudendal block during delivery

Breast-feeding present in milk but not known to be harmful

Side-effects see under Lidocaine Hydrochloride and notes above; ocular toxicity (including blindness) reported with excessively high strengths used for ophthalmic procedures

Indication and dose

> **Infiltration anaesthesia (higher strengths for dental use only), nerve block**
>
> See under preparations below, seek expert advice—**important**: see also under Administration, p. 797

Citanest® (AstraZeneca) ℗

Injection 1%, prilocaine hydrochloride 10 mg/mL, net price 50-mL multidose vial = £2.01

Dose

> **Child 6 months–12 years** up to 5 mg/kg adjusted according to site of administration and response; max. 400 mg

Child 12–18 years 100–200 mg/minute, or in incremental doses, to max. total dose 400 mg (adjusted according to site of administration and response)

◢**With lidocaine**

EMLA®

See Lidocaine, p. 799

◢**For dental use**

Note Consult expert dental sources for specific advice in relation to dose of prilocaine for dental anaesthesia

Citanest® (Dentsply) ℗

Injection 4%, prilocaine hydrochloride 40 mg/mL, net price 2.2-mL cartridge = 17p

Citanest with Octapressin® (Dentsply) ℗

Injection 3%, prilocaine hydrochloride 30 mg/mL, felypressin 0.03 unit/mL, net price 1.8-mL cartridge and self-aspirating cartridge (both) = 15p

---

▰ **Ropivacaine**

Ropivacaine is an amide-type local anaesthetic agent similar to bupivacaine. It is less cardiotoxic than bupivacaine, but also less potent.

▰ ROPIVACAINE HYDROCHLORIDE

Cautions see under Lidocaine Hydrochloride and notes above; also acute porphyria (section 9.8.2); **interactions**: Appendix 1 (ropivacaine)

Contra-indications see under Lidocaine Hydrochloride and notes above; intravenous regional anaesthesia (Bier's block); paracervical block in obstetrics

Hepatic impairment use with caution in severe impairment

Renal impairment use with caution in chronic impairment

Pregnancy safety not established but not known to be harmful

Breast-feeding not known to be harmful

Side-effects see under Lidocaine Hydrochloride and notes above

Licensed use not licensed for use in children by epidural infusion

Indication and dose

> Adjust according to child's physical status and nature of procedure, seek expert advice—**important**: see also under Administration, p. 797

Naropin® (AstraZeneca) ℗

Injection, ropivacaine hydrochloride 2 mg/mL, net price 10-mL *Polyamp®* = £1.78; 7.5 mg/mL, 10-mL *Polyamp®* = £2.65; 10 mg/mL, 10-mL *Polyamp®* = £3.20

Epidural infusion, ropivacaine hydrochloride 2 mg/mL, net price 200-mL *Polybag®* = £14.45

▰ **Tetracaine**

Tetracaine (amethocaine) is an effective local anaesthetic for topical application; a 4% gel is indicated for anaesthesia prior to venepuncture or venous cannulation. Tetracaine remains effective for 4–6 hours after a single application in most children. It does not appear to be effective prior to neonatal heel lancing.

Tetracaine is rapidly absorbed from mucous membranes and should **never** be applied to inflamed, traumatised, or highly vascular surfaces. It should **never** be used to provide anaesthesia for bronchoscopy or cystoscopy, as lidocaine (lignocaine) is a safer alternative. It is used in ophthalmology (section 11.7) and in skin preparations (section 13.3).

15 Anaesthesia

TETRACAINE
(Amethocaine)

Cautions see notes above

Contra-indications see notes above

Side-effects see notes above; also erythema, oedema and pruritus; *very rarely* blistering
Important. Rapid and extensive absorption may result in systemic side-effects (see also notes above)

Licensed use not licensed for use in neonates

Ametop® (S&N Hlth.)
Gel, tetracaine 4%, net price 1.5-g tube = £1.08

Dose

> **Neonate** apply contents of tube (or appropriate proportion) to site of venepuncture or venous cannulation and cover with occlusive dressing; remove gel and dressing after 30 minutes for venepuncture and after 45 minutes for venous cannulation

> **Child 1 month–18 years** apply contents of tube (or appropriate proportion) to site of venepuncture or venous cannulation and cover with occlusive dressing; remove gel and dressing after 30 minutes for venepuncture and after 45 minutes for venous cannulation
> **Note** Child 5–18 years, contents of max. 5 tubes applied at separate sites at a single time, child 1 month–5 years, contents of max. 1 tube applied at separate sites at a single time

◀**With lidocaine**
Rapydan®
see Lidocaine, p. 800

A1 Interactions

Two or more drugs given at the same time may exert their effects independently or may interact. The interaction may be potentiation or antagonism of one drug by another, or occasionally some other effect. Adverse drug interactions should be reported to the CHM as for other adverse drug reactions.

Drug interactions may be **pharmacodynamic** or **pharmacokinetic**.

Pharmacodynamic interactions

These are interactions between drugs which have similar or antagonistic pharmacological effects or side-effects. They may be due to competition at receptor sites, or occur between drugs acting on the same physiological system. They are usually predictable from a knowledge of the pharmacology of the interacting drugs; in general, those demonstrated with one drug are likely to occur with related drugs. They occur to a greater or lesser extent in most patients who receive the interacting drugs.

Pharmacokinetic interactions

These occur when one drug alters the absorption, distribution, metabolism, or excretion of another, thus increasing or reducing the amount of drug available to produce its pharmacological effects. They are not easily predicted and many of them affect only a small proportion of patients taking the combination of drugs. Pharmacokinetic interactions occurring with one drug cannot be assumed to occur with related drugs unless their pharmacokinetic properties are known to be similar.

Pharmacokinetic interactions are of several types:

Affecting absorption The rate of absorption or the total amount absorbed can both be altered by drug interactions. Delayed absorption is rarely of clinical importance unless high peak plasma concentrations are required (e.g. when giving an analgesic). Reduction in the total amount absorbed, however, may result in ineffective therapy.

Due to changes in protein binding To a variable extent most drugs are loosely bound to plasma proteins. Protein-binding sites are non-specific and one drug can displace another thereby increasing its proportion free to diffuse from plasma to its site of action. This only produces a detectable increase in effect if it is an extensively bound drug (more than 90%) that is not widely distributed throughout the body. Even so displacement rarely produces more than transient potentiation because this increased concentration of free drug results in an increased rate of elimination.

Displacement from protein binding plays a part in the potentiation of warfarin by sulphonamides, and tolbutamide but the importance of these interactions is due mainly to the fact that warfarin metabolism is also inhibited.

Affecting metabolism Many drugs are metabolised in the liver. Induction of the hepatic microsomal enzyme system by one drug can gradually increase the rate of metabolism of another, resulting in lower plasma concentrations and a reduced effect. On withdrawal of the inducer plasma concentrations increase and toxicity may occur. Barbiturates, griseofulvin, many antiepileptics, and rifampicin are the most important enzyme inducers. Drugs affected include warfarin and the oral contraceptives.

Conversely when one drug inhibits the metabolism of another higher plasma concentrations are produced, rapidly resulting in an increased effect with risk of toxicity. Some drugs which potentiate warfarin and phenytoin do so by this mechanism.

Isoenzymes of the hepatic cytochrome P450 system interact with a wide range of drugs. Drugs may be substrates, inducers or inhibitors of the different isoenzymes. A great deal of *in-vitro* information is available on the effect of drugs on the isoenzymes; however, since drugs are eliminated by a number of different metabolic routes as well as renal excretion, the clinical effects of interactions cannot be predicted accurately from laboratory data on the cytochrome P450 isoenzymes. Except where a combination of drugs is specifically contra-indicated, the BNF presents only interactions that have been reported in clinical practice. In all cases the possibility of an interaction must be considered if toxic effects occur or if the activity of a drug diminishes.

Affecting renal excretion Drugs are eliminated through the kidney both by glomerular filtration and by active tubular secretion. Competition occurs between those which share active transport mechanisms in the proximal tubule. For example, salicylates and some other NSAIDs delay the excretion of methotrexate; serious methotrexate toxicity is possible.

Relative importance of interactions

Many drug interactions are harmless and many of those which are potentially harmful only occur in a small proportion of patients; moreover, the severity of an interaction varies from one patient to another. Drugs with a small therapeutic ratio (e.g. phenytoin) and those which require careful control of dosage (e.g. anti-coagulants, antihypertensives, and antidiabetics) are most often involved.

Patients at increased risk from drug interactions include those with impaired renal or liver function.

Hazardous interactions The symbol ● has been placed against interactions that are **potentially hazardous** and where combined administration of the drugs involved should be **avoided** (or only undertaken with caution and appropriate monitoring).

Interactions that have no symbol do not usually have serious consequences.

List of drug interactions

The following is an alphabetical list of drugs and their interactions; to avoid excessive cross-referencing each drug or group is listed twice: in the alphabetical list and also against the drug or group with which it interacts.
For explanation of symbol ● see above

Abacavir

Analgesics: abacavir possibly reduces plasma concentration of methadone

Antibacterials: plasma concentration of abacavir possibly reduced by rifampicin

Antiepileptics: plasma concentration of abacavir possibly reduced by phenytoin

● Antivirals: plasma concentration of abacavir reduced by ●tipranavir

Barbiturates: plasma concentration of abacavir possibly reduced by phenobarbital

Abatacept

Adalimumab: increased risk of side-effects when abatacept given with adalimumab

● Certolizumab pegol: avoid concomitant use of abatacept with ●certolizumab pegol

● Etanercept: avoid concomitant use of abatacept with ●etanercept

● Infliximab: avoid concomitant use of abatacept with ●infliximab

● Vaccines: avoid concomitant use of abatacept with live ●vaccines (see p. 733)

Acarbose *see* Antidiabetics

ACE Inhibitors

Alcohol: enhanced hypotensive effect when ACE inhibitors given with alcohol

Aldesleukin: enhanced hypotensive effect when ACE inhibitors given with aldesleukin

Allopurinol: increased risk of leucopenia and hypersensitivity reactions when ACE inhibitors given with allopurinol especially in renal impairment

Alpha-blockers: enhanced hypotensive effect when ACE inhibitors given with alpha-blockers

Anaesthetics, General: enhanced hypotensive effect when ACE inhibitors given with general anaesthetics

Analgesics: increased risk of renal impairment when ACE inhibitors given with NSAIDs, also hypotensive effect antagonised

Angiotensin-II Receptor Antagonists: increased risk of hyperkalaemia when ACE inhibitors given with angiotensin-II receptor antagonists

Antacids: absorption of ACE inhibitors possibly reduced by antacids; absorption of captopril, enalapril and fosinopril reduced by antacids

Antibacterials: plasma concentration of active metabolite of imidapril reduced by rifampicin (reduced antihypertensive effect); quinapril tablets reduce absorption of tetracyclines (quinapril tablets contain magnesium carbonate)

Anticoagulants: increased risk of hyperkalaemia when ACE inhibitors given with heparins

Antidepressants: hypotensive effect of ACE inhibitors possibly enhanced by MAOIs

Antidiabetics: ACE inhibitors possibly enhance hypoglycaemic effect of insulin, metformin and sulphonylureas

ACE Inhibitors (continued)

Antipsychotics: enhanced hypotensive effect when ACE inhibitors given with antipsychotics

Anxiolytics and Hypnotics: enhanced hypotensive effect when ACE inhibitors given with anxiolytics and hypnotics

Azathioprine: increased risk of anaemia or leucopenia when captopril given with azathioprine especially in renal impairment; increased risk of anaemia when enalapril given with azathioprine especially in renal impairment

Beta-blockers: enhanced hypotensive effect when ACE inhibitors given with beta-blockers

Calcium-channel Blockers: enhanced hypotensive effect when ACE inhibitors given with calcium-channel blockers

Cardiac Glycosides: captopril possibly increases plasma concentration of digoxin

• Ciclosporin: increased risk of hyperkalaemia when ACE inhibitors given with •ciclosporin

Clonidine: enhanced hypotensive effect when ACE inhibitors given with clonidine; antihypertensive effect of captopril possibly delayed by previous treatment with clonidine

Corticosteroids: hypotensive effect of ACE inhibitors antagonised by corticosteroids

Diazoxide: enhanced hypotensive effect when ACE inhibitors given with diazoxide

• Diuretics: enhanced hypotensive effect when ACE inhibitors given with •diuretics; increased risk of severe hyperkalaemia when ACE inhibitors given with •potassium-sparing diuretics and aldosterone antagonists (monitor potassium concentration with low-dose spironolactone in heart failure)

Dopaminergics: enhanced hypotensive effect when ACE inhibitors given with levodopa

• Lithium: ACE inhibitors reduce excretion of •lithium (increased plasma concentration)

Methyldopa: enhanced hypotensive effect when ACE inhibitors given with methyldopa

Moxisylyte: enhanced hypotensive effect when ACE inhibitors given with moxisylyte

Moxonidine: enhanced hypotensive effect when ACE inhibitors given with moxonidine

Muscle Relaxants: enhanced hypotensive effect when ACE inhibitors given with baclofen or tizanidine

Nitrates: enhanced hypotensive effect when ACE inhibitors given with nitrates

Oestrogens: hypotensive effect of ACE inhibitors antagonised by oestrogens

• Potassium Salts: increased risk of severe hyperkalaemia when ACE inhibitors given with •potassium salts

Probenecid: excretion of captopril reduced by probenecid

Prostaglandins: enhanced hypotensive effect when ACE inhibitors given with alprostadil

Vasodilator Antihypertensives: enhanced hypotensive effect when ACE inhibitors given with hydralazine, minoxidil or sodium nitroprusside

Acebutolol see Beta-blockers

Aceclofenac see NSAIDs

Acemetacin see NSAIDs

Acenocoumarol see Coumarins

Acetazolamide see Diuretics

Aciclovir

Note. Interactions do not apply to topical aciclovir preparations

Note. Valaciclovir interactions as for aciclovir

Ciclosporin: increased risk of nephrotoxicity when aciclovir given with ciclosporin

Mycophenolate: plasma concentration of aciclovir increased by mycophenolate, also plasma concentration of inactive metabolite of mycophenolate increased

Probenecid: excretion of aciclovir reduced by probenecid (increased plasma concentration)

Aciclovir (continued)

Tacrolimus: possible increased risk of nephrotoxicity when aciclovir given with tacrolimus

Theophylline: aciclovir possibly increases plasma concentration of theophylline

Acitretin see Retinoids

Acrivastine see Antihistamines

Adalimumab

Abatacept: increased risk of side-effects when adalimumab given with abatacept

• Anakinra: avoid concomitant use of adalimumab with •anakinra

• Vaccines: avoid concomitant use of adalimumab with live •vaccines (see p. 733)

Adefovir

Antivirals: avoidance of adefovir advised by manufacturer of tenofovir

Adenosine

Note. Possibility of interaction with drugs tending to impair myocardial conduction

Anaesthetics, Local: increased myocardial depression when anti-arrhythmics given with bupivacaine, levobupivacaine, prilocaine or ropivacaine

• Anti-arrhythmics: increased myocardial depression when anti-arrhythmics given with other •anti-arrhythmics

• Antipsychotics: increased risk of ventricular arrhythmias when anti-arrhythmics that prolong the QT interval given with •antipsychotics that prolong the QT interval

• Beta-blockers: increased myocardial depression when anti-arrhythmics given with •beta-blockers

• Dipyridamole: effect of adenosine enhanced and extended by •dipyridamole (important risk of toxicity)

Nicotine: effects of adenosine possibly enhanced by nicotine

Theophylline: anti-arrhythmic effect of adenosine antagonised by theophylline

Adrenaline (epinephrine) see Sympathomimetics

Adrenergic Neurone Blockers

Alcohol: enhanced hypotensive effect when adrenergic neurone blockers given with alcohol

Alpha-blockers: enhanced hypotensive effect when adrenergic neurone blockers given with alpha-blockers

• Anaesthetics, General: enhanced hypotensive effect when adrenergic neurone blockers given with •general anaesthetics

Analgesics: hypotensive effect of adrenergic neurone blockers antagonised by NSAIDs

Angiotensin-II Receptor Antagonists: enhanced hypotensive effect when adrenergic neurone blockers given with angiotensin-II receptor antagonists

Antidepressants: enhanced hypotensive effect when adrenergic neurone blockers given with MAOIs; hypotensive effect of adrenergic neurone blockers antagonised by tricyclics

Antipsychotics: hypotensive effect of adrenergic neurone blockers antagonised by haloperidol; hypotensive effect of adrenergic neurone blockers antagonised by higher doses of chlorpromazine; enhanced hypotensive effect when adrenergic neurone blockers given with phenothiazines

Anxiolytics and Hypnotics: enhanced hypotensive effect when adrenergic neurone blockers given with anxiolytics and hypnotics

Beta-blockers: enhanced hypotensive effect when adrenergic neurone blockers given with beta-blockers

Calcium-channel Blockers: enhanced hypotensive effect when adrenergic neurone blockers given with calcium-channel blockers

Clonidine: enhanced hypotensive effect when adrenergic neurone blockers given with clonidine

Adrenergic Neurone Blockers *(continued)*

Corticosteroids: hypotensive effect of adrenergic neurone blockers antagonised by corticosteroids

Diazoxide: enhanced hypotensive effect when adrenergic neurone blockers given with diazoxide

Diuretics: enhanced hypotensive effect when adrenergic neurone blockers given with diuretics

Dopaminergics: enhanced hypotensive effect when adrenergic neurone blockers given with levodopa

Methyldopa: enhanced hypotensive effect when adrenergic neurone blockers given with methyldopa

Moxisylyte: enhanced hypotensive effect when adrenergic neurone blockers given with moxisylyte

Moxonidine: enhanced hypotensive effect when adrenergic neurone blockers given with moxonidine

Muscle Relaxants: enhanced hypotensive effect when adrenergic neurone blockers given with baclofen or tizanidine

Nitrates: enhanced hypotensive effect when adrenergic neurone blockers given with nitrates

Oestrogens: hypotensive effect of adrenergic neurone blockers antagonised by oestrogens

Pizotifen: hypotensive effect of adrenergic neurone blockers antagonised by pizotifen

Prostaglandins: enhanced hypotensive effect when adrenergic neurone blockers given with alprostadil

• Sympathomimetics: hypotensive effect of guanethidine antagonised by ●dexamfetamine; hypotensive effect of adrenergic neurone blockers antagonised by ●ephedrine, ●isometheptene, ●metaraminol, ●methylphenidate, ●noradrenaline (norepinephrine), ●oxymetazoline, ●phenylephrine, ●pseudoephedrine and ●xylometazoline

Vasodilator Antihypertensives: enhanced hypotensive effect when adrenergic neurone blockers given with hydralazine, minoxidil or sodium nitroprusside

Adsorbents *see* Kaolin

Agalsidase Alfa and Beta

Anti-arrhythmics: effects of agalsidase alfa and beta possibly inhibited by amiodarone (manufacturers of agalsidase alfa and beta advise avoid concomitant use)

Antibacterials: effects of agalsidase alfa and beta possibly inhibited by gentamicin (manufacturers of agalsidase alfa and beta advise avoid concomitant use)

Antimalarials: effects of agalsidase alfa and beta possibly inhibited by chloroquine and hydroxychloroquine (manufacturers of agalsidase alfa and beta advise avoid concomitant use)

Agomelatine

• Antibacterials: manufacturer of agomelatine advises avoid concomitant use with ●ciprofloxacin

• Antidepressants: metabolism of agomelatine inhibited by ●fluvoxamine (increased plasma concentration)

• Antimalarials: avoidance of antidepressants advised by manufacturer of ●artemether/lumefantrine

Atomoxetine: possible increased risk of convulsions when antidepressants given with atomoxetine

Alcohol

ACE Inhibitors: enhanced hypotensive effect when alcohol given with ACE inhibitors

Adrenergic Neurone Blockers: enhanced hypotensive effect when alcohol given with adrenergic neurone blockers

Alpha-blockers: increased sedative effect when alcohol given with indoramin; enhanced hypotensive effect when alcohol given with alpha-blockers

Analgesics: enhanced hypotensive and sedative effects when alcohol given with opioid analgesics

Angiotensin-II Receptor Antagonists: enhanced hypotensive effect when alcohol given with angiotensin-II receptor antagonists

• Antibacterials: disulfiram-like reaction when alcohol given with metronidazole; possibility of disulfiram-like reaction when alcohol given with tinidazole;

Alcohol

• Antibacterials *(continued)*
increased risk of convulsions when alcohol given with ●cycloserine

• Anticoagulants: major changes in consumption of alcohol may affect anticoagulant control with ●coumarins or ●phenindione

• Antidepressants: some beverages containing alcohol and some dealcoholised beverages contain tyramine which interacts with ●MAOIs (hypertensive crisis)—if no tyramine, enhanced hypotensive effect; sedative effects possibly increased when alcohol given with SSRIs; increased sedative effect when alcohol given with ●mirtazapine, ●tricyclic-related antidepressants or ●tricyclics

Antidiabetics: alcohol enhances hypoglycaemic effect of antidiabetics; increased risk of lactic acidosis when alcohol given with metformin

Antiepileptics: alcohol possibly increases CNS side-effects of carbamazepine; increased sedative effect when alcohol given with primidone

Antifungals: effects of alcohol possibly enhanced by griseofulvin

Antihistamines: increased sedative effect when alcohol given with antihistamines (possibly less effect with non-sedating antihistamines)

Antimuscarinics: increased sedative effect when alcohol given with hyoscine

Antipsychotics: increased sedative effect when alcohol given with antipsychotics

Anxiolytics and Hypnotics: increased sedative effect when alcohol given with anxiolytics and hypnotics

Barbiturates: increased sedative effect when alcohol given with barbiturates

Beta-blockers: enhanced hypotensive effect when alcohol given with beta-blockers

Calcium-channel Blockers: enhanced hypotensive effect when alcohol given with calcium-channel blockers; plasma concentration of alcohol possibly increased by verapamil

Clonidine: enhanced hypotensive effect when alcohol given with clonidine

Cytotoxics: disulfiram-like reaction when alcohol given with procarbazine

Diazoxide: enhanced hypotensive effect when alcohol given with diazoxide

Disulfiram: disulfiram reaction when alcohol given with disulfiram (see BNF section 4.10)

Diuretics: enhanced hypotensive effect when alcohol given with diuretics

Dopaminergics: alcohol reduces tolerance to bromocriptine

Levamisole: possibility of disulfiram-like reaction when alcohol given with levamisole

Lofexidine: increased sedative effect when alcohol given with lofexidine

Methyldopa: enhanced hypotensive effect when alcohol given with methyldopa

Moxonidine: enhanced hypotensive effect when alcohol given with moxonidine

Muscle Relaxants: increased sedative effect when alcohol given with baclofen, methocarbamol or tizanidine

Nabilone: increased sedative effect when alcohol given with nabilone

Nicorandil: alcohol possibly enhances hypotensive effect of nicorandil

Nitrates: enhanced hypotensive effect when alcohol given with nitrates

• Paraldehyde: increased sedative effect when alcohol given with ●paraldehyde

• Retinoids: presence of alcohol causes etretinate to be formed from ●acitretin (increased risk of teratogenecity in women of child-bearing potential)

Sympathomimetics: alcohol possibly enhances effects of methylphenidate

Alcohol *(continued)*

Vasodilator Antihypertensives: enhanced hypotensive effect when alcohol given with hydralazine, minoxidil or sodium nitroprusside

Aldesleukin

ACE Inhibitors: enhanced hypotensive effect when aldesleukin given with ACE inhibitors

Alpha-blockers: enhanced hypotensive effect when aldesleukin given with alpha-blockers

Angiotensin-II Receptor Antagonists: enhanced hypotensive effect when aldesleukin given with angiotensin-II receptor antagonists

Antivirals: aldesleukin possibly increases plasma concentration of indinavir

Beta-blockers: enhanced hypotensive effect when aldesleukin given with beta-blockers

Calcium-channel Blockers: enhanced hypotensive effect when aldesleukin given with calcium-channel blockers

Clonidine: enhanced hypotensive effect when aldesleukin given with clonidine

• Corticosteroids: manufacturer of aldesleukin advises avoid concomitant use with ●corticosteroids

• Cytotoxics: manufacturer of aldesleukin advises avoid concomitant use with ●cisplatin, ●dacarbazine and ●vinblastine

Diazoxide: enhanced hypotensive effect when aldesleukin given with diazoxide

Diuretics: enhanced hypotensive effect when aldesleukin given with diuretics

Methyldopa: enhanced hypotensive effect when aldesleukin given with methyldopa

Moxonidine: enhanced hypotensive effect when aldesleukin given with moxonidine

Nitrates: enhanced hypotensive effect when aldesleukin given with nitrates

Vasodilator Antihypertensives: enhanced hypotensive effect when aldesleukin given with hydralazine, minoxidil or sodium nitroprusside

Alendronic Acid *see* Bisphosphonates

Alfentanil *see* Opioid Analgesics

Alfuzosin *see* Alpha-blockers

Alimemazine *see* Antihistamines

Aliskiren

Angiotensin-II Receptor Antagonists: plasma concentration of aliskiren possibly reduced by irbesartan

Anticoagulants: increased risk of hyperkalaemia when aliskiren given with heparins

Antifungals: plasma concentration of aliskiren increased by ketoconazole

Calcium-channel Blockers: manufacturer of aliskiren advises avoid concomitant use with verapamil

• Ciclosporin: plasma concentration of aliskiren increased by ●ciclosporin—avoid concomitant use

Diuretics: aliskiren reduces plasma concentration of furosemide; increased risk of hyperkalaemia when aliskiren given with potassium-sparing diuretics and aldosterone antagonists

Potassium Salts: increased risk of hyperkalaemia when aliskiren given with potassium salts

Alitretinoin *see* Retinoids

Alkylating Drugs *see* Busulfan, Carmustine, Cyclophosphamide, Estramustine, Ifosfamide, Lomustine, Melphalan, and Thiotepa

Allopurinol

ACE Inhibitors: increased risk of leucopenia and hypersensitivity reactions when allopurinol given with ACE inhibitors especially in renal impairment

Antibacterials: increased risk of rash when allopurinol given with amoxicillin or ampicillin

Anticoagulants: allopurinol possibly enhances anticoagulant effect of coumarins

• Antivirals: allopurinol increases plasma concentration of ●didanosine (risk of toxicity)—avoid concomitant use

Allopurinol *(continued)*

• Azathioprine: allopurinol enhances effects and increases toxicity of ●azathioprine (reduce dose of azathioprine to one quarter of usual dose)

Ciclosporin: allopurinol possibly increases plasma concentration of ciclosporin (risk of nephrotoxicity)

• Cytotoxics: allopurinol enhances effects and increases toxicity of ●mercaptopurine (reduce dose of mercaptopurine to one quarter of usual dose); avoidance of allopurinol advised by manufacturer of ●capecitabine

Diuretics: increased risk of hypersensitivity when allopurinol given with thiazides and related diuretics especially in renal impairment

Theophylline: allopurinol possibly increases plasma concentration of theophylline

Almotriptan *see* 5HT$_1$ Agonists

Alpha$_2$-adrenoceptor Stimulants *see* Apraclonidine, Brimonidine, Clonidine and Methyldopa

Alpha-blockers

ACE Inhibitors: enhanced hypotensive effect when alpha-blockers given with ACE inhibitors

Adrenergic Neurone Blockers: enhanced hypotensive effect when alpha-blockers given with adrenergic neurone blockers

Alcohol: enhanced hypotensive effect when alpha-blockers given with alcohol; increased sedative effect when indoramin given with alcohol

Aldesleukin: enhanced hypotensive effect when alpha-blockers given with aldesleukin

• Anaesthetics, General: enhanced hypotensive effect when alpha-blockers given with ●general anaesthetics

Analgesics: hypotensive effect of alpha-blockers antagonised by NSAIDs

Angiotensin-II Receptor Antagonists: enhanced hypotensive effect when alpha-blockers given with angiotensin-II receptor antagonists

• Antidepressants: enhanced hypotensive effect when alpha-blockers given with MAOIs; manufacturer of indoramin advises avoid concomitant use with ●MAOIs

Antifungals: plasma concentration of alfuzosin possibly increased by ketoconazole

Antipsychotics: enhanced hypotensive effect when alpha-blockers given with antipsychotics

• Antivirals: plasma concentration of alfuzosin possibly increased by ●ritonavir—avoid concomitant use

Anxiolytics and Hypnotics: enhanced hypotensive and sedative effects when alpha-blockers given with anxiolytics and hypnotics

• Beta-blockers: enhanced hypotensive effect when alpha-blockers given with ●beta-blockers, also increased risk of first-dose hypotension with post-synaptic alpha-blockers such as prazosin

• Calcium-channel Blockers: enhanced hypotensive effect when alpha-blockers given with ●calcium-channel blockers, also increased risk of first-dose hypotension with post-synaptic alpha-blockers such as prazosin

Cardiac Glycosides: prazosin increases plasma concentration of digoxin

Clonidine: enhanced hypotensive effect when alpha-blockers given with clonidine

Corticosteroids: hypotensive effect of alpha-blockers antagonised by corticosteroids

Diazoxide: enhanced hypotensive effect when alpha-blockers given with diazoxide

• Diuretics: enhanced hypotensive effect when alpha-blockers given with ●diuretics, also increased risk of first-dose hypotension with post-synaptic alpha-blockers such as prazosin

Dopaminergics: enhanced hypotensive effect when alpha-blockers given with levodopa

Methyldopa: enhanced hypotensive effect when alpha-blockers given with methyldopa

Alpha-blockers *(continued)*

- Moxisylyte: possible severe postural hypotension when alpha-blockers given with ●moxisylyte
  Moxonidine: enhanced hypotensive effect when alpha-blockers given with moxonidine
  Muscle Relaxants: enhanced hypotensive effect when alpha-blockers given with baclofen or tizanidine
  Nitrates: enhanced hypotensive effect when alpha-blockers given with nitrates
  Oestrogens: hypotensive effect of alpha-blockers antagonised by oestrogens
  Prostaglandins: enhanced hypotensive effect when alpha-blockers given with alprostadil
- Sildenafil: enhanced hypotensive effect when alpha-blockers given with ●sildenafil (avoid alpha-blockers for 4 hours after sildenafil)—see also
- Sympathomimetics: avoid concomitant use of tolazoline with ●adrenaline (epinephrine) or ●dopamine
- Tadalafil: enhanced hypotensive effect when alpha-blockers given with ●tadalafil—see also ; enhanced hypotensive effect when doxazosin given with ●tadalafil—manufacturer of tadalafil advises avoid concomitant use
- Ulcer-healing Drugs: effects of tolazoline antagonised by ●cimetidine and ●ranitidine
- Vardenafil: enhanced hypotensive effect when alpha-blockers (excludes tamsulosin) given with ●vardenafil—separate doses by 6 hours—see also
  Vasodilator Antihypertensives: enhanced hypotensive effect when alpha-blockers given with hydralazine, minoxidil or sodium nitroprusside

Alpha-blockers (post-synaptic) *see* Alpha-blockers

Alprazolam *see* Anxiolytics and Hypnotics

Alprostadil *see* Prostaglandins

Aluminium Hydroxide *see* Antacids

Amantadine

Antipsychotics: increased risk of extrapyramidal side-effects when amantadine given with antipsychotics
Bupropion: increased risk of side-effects when amantadine given with bupropion
- Memantine: increased risk of CNS toxicity when amantadine given with ●memantine (manufacturer of memantine advises avoid concomitant use); effects of dopaminergics possibly enhanced by memantine
  Methyldopa: increased risk of extrapyramidal side-effects when amantadine given with methyldopa; antiparkinsonian effect of dopaminergics antagonised by methyldopa
  Tetrabenazine: increased risk of extrapyramidal side-effects when amantadine given with tetrabenazine

Amikacin *see* Aminoglycosides

Amiloride *see* Diuretics

Aminoglycosides

Agalsidase Alfa and Beta: gentamicin possibly inhibits effects of agalsidase alfa and beta (manufacturers of agalsidase alfa and beta advise avoid concomitant use)
Analgesics: plasma concentration of amikacin and gentamicin in neonates possibly increased by indometacin
- Antibacterials: neomycin reduces absorption of phenoxymethylpenicillin; increased risk of nephrotoxicity when aminoglycosides given with colistin or polymyxins; increased risk of nephrotoxicity and ototoxicity when aminoglycosides given with capreomycin or ●vancomycin; possible increased risk of nephrotoxicity when aminoglycosides given with cephalosporins
- Anticoagulants: experience in anticoagulant clinics suggests that INR possibly altered when neomycin (given for local action on gut) is given with ●coumarins or ●phenindione
  Antidiabetics: neomycin possibly enhances hypoglycaemic effect of acarbose, also severity of gastro-intestinal effects increased

Aminoglycosides *(continued)*

Antifungals: increased risk of nephrotoxicity when aminoglycosides given with amphotericin
Bisphosphonates: increased risk of hypocalcaemia when aminoglycosides given with bisphosphonates
Cardiac Glycosides: gentamicin possibly increases plasma concentration of digoxin; neomycin reduces absorption of digoxin
- Ciclosporin: increased risk of nephrotoxicity when aminoglycosides given with ●ciclosporin
- Cytotoxics: neomycin possibly reduces absorption of methotrexate; neomycin reduces bioavailability of sorafenib; increased risk of nephrotoxicity and possibly of ototoxicity when aminoglycosides given with ●platinum compounds
- Diuretics: increased risk of ototoxicity when aminoglycosides given with ●loop diuretics
- Muscle Relaxants: aminoglycosides enhance effects of ●non-depolarising muscle relaxants and ●suxamethonium
  Oestrogens: antibacterials that do not induce liver enzymes possibly reduce contraceptive effect of oestrogens (risk probably small, see p. 486)
- Parasympathomimetics: aminoglycosides antagonise effects of ●neostigmine and ●pyridostigmine
- Tacrolimus: increased risk of nephrotoxicity when aminoglycosides given with ●tacrolimus
  Vaccines: antibacterials inactivate oral typhoid vaccine—see p. 760
  Vitamins: neomycin possibly reduces absorption of vitamin A

Aminophylline *see* Theophylline

Aminosalicylates

Azathioprine: possible increased risk of leucopenia when aminosalicylates given with azathioprine
Cardiac Glycosides: sulfasalazine possibly reduces absorption of digoxin
Cytotoxics: possible increased risk of leucopenia when aminosalicylates given with mercaptopurine
Folates: sulfasalazine possibly reduces absorption of folic acid

Amiodarone

Note. Amiodarone has a long half-life; there is a potential for drug interactions to occur for several weeks (or even months) after treatment with it has been stopped
Agalsidase Alfa and Beta: amiodarone possibly inhibits effects of agalsidase alfa and beta (manufacturers of agalsidase alfa and beta advise avoid concomitant use)
Anaesthetics, Local: increased myocardial depression when anti-arrhythmics given with bupivacaine, levobupivacaine, prilocaine or ropivacaine
- Anti-arrhythmics: increased myocardial depression when anti-arrhythmics given with other ●anti-arrhythmics; increased risk of ventricular arrhythmias when amiodarone given with ●disopyramide—avoid concomitant use; amiodarone increases plasma concentration of ●flecainide (halve dose of flecainide)
- Antibacterials: increased risk of ventricular arrhythmias when amiodarone given with *parenteral* ●erythromycin—avoid concomitant use; increased risk of ventricular arrhythmias when amiodarone given with ●levofloxacin or ●moxifloxacin—avoid concomitant use; increased risk of ventricular arrhythmias when amiodarone given with ●sulfamethoxazole and ●trimethoprim (as co-trimoxazole)—avoid concomitant use of co-trimoxazole
- Anticoagulants: amiodarone inhibits metabolism of ●coumarins and ●phenindione (enhanced anticoagulant effect); amiodarone increases plasma concentration of ●dabigatran etexilate (reduce dose of dabigatran etexilate)
- Antidepressants: increased risk of ventricular arrhythmias when amiodarone given with ●tricyclics—avoid concomitant use

Amiodarone *(continued)*

- Antiepileptics: amiodarone inhibits metabolism of ●phenytoin (increased plasma concentration)
- Antihistamines: increased risk of ventricular arrhythmias when amiodarone given with ●mizolastine—avoid concomitant use
- Antimalarials: avoidance of amiodarone advised by manufacturer of ●artemether/lumefantrine (risk of ventricular arrhythmias); increased risk of ventricular arrhythmias when amiodarone given with ●chloroquine and hydroxychloroquine, ●mefloquine or ●quinine—avoid concomitant use
- Antimuscarinics: increased risk of ventricular arrhythmias when amiodarone given with ●tolterodine
- Antipsychotics: increased risk of ventricular arrhythmias when anti-arrhythmics that prolong the QT interval given with ●antipsychotics that prolong the QT interval; increased risk of ventricular arrhythmias when amiodarone given with ●benperidol—manufacturer of benperidol advises avoid concomitant use; increased risk of ventricular arrhythmias when amiodarone given with ●amisulpride, ●droperidol, ●haloperidol, ●phenothiazines, ●pimozide, ●sertindole or ●zuclopenthixol—avoid concomitant use; increased risk of ventricular arrhythmias when amiodarone given with ●sulpiride
- Antivirals: plasma concentration of amiodarone possibly increased by ●atazanavir; plasma concentration of amiodarone possibly increased by ●fosamprenavir (increased risk of ventricular arrhythmias—avoid concomitant use); plasma concentration of amiodarone possibly increased by ●indinavir—avoid concomitant use; increased risk of ventricular arrhythmias when amiodarone given with ●nelfinavir—avoid concomitant use; plasma concentration of amiodarone increased by ●ritonavir (increased risk of ventricular arrhythmias—avoid concomitant use)
- Atomoxetine: increased risk of ventricular arrhythmias when amiodarone given with ●atomoxetine
- Beta-blockers: increased risk of bradycardia, AV block and myocardial depression when amiodarone given with ●beta-blockers; increased myocardial depression when anti-arrhythmics given with ●beta-blockers; increased risk of ventricular arrhythmias when amiodarone given with ●sotalol—avoid concomitant use
- Calcium-channel Blockers: increased risk of bradycardia, AV block and myocardial depression when amiodarone given with ●diltiazem or ●verapamil
- Cardiac Glycosides: amiodarone increases plasma concentration of ●digoxin (halve dose of digoxin)

  Ciclosporin: amiodarone possibly increases plasma concentration of ciclosporin
- Cytotoxics: increased risk of ventricular arrhythmias when amiodarone given with ●arsenic trioxide

  Diuretics: increased cardiac toxicity with amiodarone if hypokalaemia occurs with acetazolamide, loop diuretics or thiazides and related diuretics; amiodarone increases plasma concentration of eplerenone (reduce dose of eplerenone)

  Grapefruit Juice: plasma concentration of amiodarone increased by grapefruit juice
- Ivabradine: increased risk of ventricular arrhythmias when amiodarone given with ●ivabradine
- Lipid-regulating Drugs: increased risk of myopathy when amiodarone given with ●simvastatin
- Lithium: manufacturer of amiodarone advises avoid concomitant use with ●lithium (risk of ventricular arrhythmias)

  Orlistat: plasma concentration of amiodarone possibly reduced by orlistat
- Pentamidine Isetionate: increased risk of ventricular arrhythmias when amiodarone given with ●pentamidine isetionate—avoid concomitant use

Amiodarone *(continued)*

Thyroid Hormones: for concomitant use of amiodarone and thyroid hormones see p. 110

Ulcer-healing Drugs: plasma concentration of amiodarone increased by cimetidine

Amisulpride *see* Antipsychotics

Amitriptyline *see* Antidepressants, Tricyclic

Amlodipine *see* Calcium-channel Blockers

Amobarbital *see* Barbiturates

Amoxicillin *see* Penicillins

Amphotericin

Note. Close monitoring required with concomitant administration of nephrotoxic drugs or cytotoxics

Antibacterials: increased risk of nephrotoxicity when amphotericin given with aminoglycosides or polymyxins; possible increased risk of nephrotoxicity when amphotericin given with vancomycin

Antifungals: amphotericin reduces renal excretion and increases cellular uptake of flucytosine (toxicity possibly increased); effects of amphotericin possibly antagonised by imidazoles and triazoles

- Cardiac Glycosides: hypokalaemia caused by amphotericin increases cardiac toxicity with ●cardiac glycosides
- Ciclosporin: increased risk of nephrotoxicity when amphotericin given with ●ciclosporin
- Corticosteroids: increased risk of hypokalaemia when amphotericin given with ●corticosteroids—avoid concomitant use unless corticosteroids needed to control reactions
- Cytotoxics: increased risk of ventricular arrhythmias when amphotericin given with ●arsenic trioxide

  Diuretics: increased risk of hypokalaemia when amphotericin given with loop diuretics or thiazides and related diuretics

  Pentamidine Isetionate: possible increased risk of nephrotoxicity when amphotericin given with pentamidine isetionate
- Tacrolimus: increased risk of nephrotoxicity when amphotericin given with ●tacrolimus

Ampicillin *see* Penicillins

Anabolic Steroids

- Anticoagulants: anabolic steroids enhance anticoagulant effect of ●coumarins and ●phenindione

  Antidiabetics: anabolic steroids possibly enhance hypoglycaemic effect of antidiabetics

Anaesthetics, General

Note. See also Surgery and Long-term Medication, p. 771

ACE Inhibitors: enhanced hypotensive effect when general anaesthetics given with ACE inhibitors
- Adrenergic Neurone Blockers: enhanced hypotensive effect when general anaesthetics given with ●adrenergic neurone blockers
- Alpha-blockers: enhanced hypotensive effect when general anaesthetics given with ●alpha-blockers

  Analgesics: effects of thiopental possibly enhanced by aspirin; effects of intravenous general anaesthetics and volatile liquid general anaesthetics possibly enhanced by opioid analgesics

  Angiotensin-II Receptor Antagonists: enhanced hypotensive effect when general anaesthetics given with angiotensin-II receptor antagonists

  Antibacterials: effects of thiopental enhanced by sulphonamides; hypersensitivity-like reactions can occur when general anaesthetics given with *intravenous* vancomycin
- Antidepressants: Because of hazardous interactions between general anaesthetics and ●MAOIs, MAOIs should normally be stopped 2 weeks before surgery; increased risk of arrhythmias and hypotension when general anaesthetics given with tricyclics
- Antipsychotics: enhanced hypotensive effect when general anaesthetics given with ●antipsychotics; effects of thiopental enhanced by droperidol

Anaesthetics, General *(continued)*

Anxiolytics and Hypnotics: increased sedative effect when general anaesthetics given with anxiolytics and hypnotics

Beta-blockers: enhanced hypotensive effect when general anaesthetics given with beta-blockers

- Calcium-channel Blockers: enhanced hypotensive effect when general anaesthetics or isoflurane given with calcium-channel blockers; general anaesthetics enhance hypotensive effect of ●verapamil (also AV delay)

Clonidine: enhanced hypotensive effect when general anaesthetics given with clonidine

- Cytotoxics: nitrous oxide increases antifolate effect of ●methotrexate—avoid concomitant use

Diazoxide: enhanced hypotensive effect when general anaesthetics given with diazoxide

Diuretics: enhanced hypotensive effect when general anaesthetics given with diuretics

- Dopaminergics: increased risk of arrhythmias when volatile liquid general anaesthetics given with ●levodopa

Ergot Alkaloids: halothane reduces effects of ergometrine on the parturient uterus

- Memantine: increased risk of CNS toxicity when ketamine given with ●memantine (manufacturer of memantine advises avoid concomitant use)

Methyldopa: enhanced hypotensive effect when general anaesthetics given with methyldopa

Moxonidine: enhanced hypotensive effect when general anaesthetics given with moxonidine

- Muscle Relaxants: increased risk of myocardial depression and bradycardia when propofol given with ●suxamethonium; volatile liquid general anaesthetics enhance effects of non-depolarising muscle relaxants and suxamethonium; ketamine enhances effects of atracurium

Nitrates: enhanced hypotensive effect when general anaesthetics given with nitrates

Oxytocin: oxytocic effect possibly reduced, also enhanced hypotensive effect and risk of arrhythmias when volatile liquid general anaesthetics given with oxytocin

Probenecid: effects of thiopental possibly enhanced by probenecid

- Sympathomimetics: increased risk of arrhythmias when volatile liquid general anaesthetics given with ●adrenaline (epinephrine); increased risk of hypertension when volatile liquid general anaesthetics given with ●methylphenidate

Theophylline: increased risk of convulsions when ketamine given with theophylline; increased risk of arrhythmias when halothane given with theophylline

Vasodilator Antihypertensives: enhanced hypotensive effect when general anaesthetics given with hydralazine, minoxidil or sodium nitroprusside

Anaesthetics, General (intravenous) *see* Anaesthetics, General

Anaesthetics, General (volatile liquids) *see* Anaesthetics, General

Anaesthetics, Local *see* Bupivacaine, Levobupivacaine, Lidocaine, Prilocaine, and Ropivacaine

Anagrelide

- Cilostazol: manufacturer of anagrelide advises avoid concomitant use with ●cilostazol
- Phosphodiesterase Inhibitors: manufacturer of anagrelide advises avoid concomitant use with ●enoximone and ●milrinone

Anakinra

- Adalimumab: avoid concomitant use of anakinra with ●adalimumab
- Certolizumab pegol: avoid concomitant use of anakinra with ●certolizumab pegol
- Etanercept: avoid concomitant use of anakinra with ●etanercept

Anakinra *(continued)*

- Infliximab: avoid concomitant use of anakinra with ●infliximab
- Vaccines: avoid concomitant use of anakinra with live ●vaccines (see p. 733)

Analgesics *see* Aspirin, Nefopam, NSAIDs, Opioid Analgesics, and Paracetamol

Angiotensin-II Receptor Antagonists

ACE Inhibitors: increased risk of hyperkalaemia when angiotensin-II receptor antagonists given with ACE inhibitors

Adrenergic Neurone Blockers: enhanced hypotensive effect when angiotensin-II receptor antagonists given with adrenergic neurone blockers

Alcohol: enhanced hypotensive effect when angiotensin-II receptor antagonists given with alcohol

Aldesleukin: enhanced hypotensive effect when angiotensin-II receptor antagonists given with aldesleukin

Aliskiren: irbesartan possibly reduces plasma concentration of aliskiren

Alpha-blockers: enhanced hypotensive effect when angiotensin-II receptor antagonists given with alpha-blockers

Anaesthetics, General: enhanced hypotensive effect when angiotensin-II receptor antagonists given with general anaesthetics

Analgesics: increased risk of renal impairment when angiotensin-II receptor antagonists given with NSAIDs, also hypotensive effect antagonised

Antibacterials: plasma concentration of losartan and its active metabolite reduced by rifampicin

Anticoagulants: increased risk of hyperkalaemia when angiotensin-II receptor antagonists given with heparins

Antidepressants: hypotensive effect of angiotensin-II receptor antagonists possibly enhanced by MAOIs

Antipsychotics: enhanced hypotensive effect when angiotensin-II receptor antagonists given with antipsychotics

Anxiolytics and Hypnotics: enhanced hypotensive effect when angiotensin-II receptor antagonists given with anxiolytics and hypnotics

Beta-blockers: enhanced hypotensive effect when angiotensin-II receptor antagonists given with beta-blockers

Calcium-channel Blockers: enhanced hypotensive effect when angiotensin-II receptor antagonists given with calcium-channel blockers

- Ciclosporin: increased risk of hyperkalaemia when angiotensin-II receptor antagonists given with ●ciclosporin

Clonidine: enhanced hypotensive effect when angiotensin-II receptor antagonists given with clonidine

Corticosteroids: hypotensive effect of angiotensin-II receptor antagonists antagonised by corticosteroids

Diazoxide: enhanced hypotensive effect when angiotensin-II receptor antagonists given with diazoxide

- Diuretics: enhanced hypotensive effect when angiotensin-II receptor antagonists given with ●diuretics; increased risk of hyperkalaemia when angiotensin-II receptor antagonists given with ●potassium-sparing diuretics and aldosterone antagonists

Dopaminergics: enhanced hypotensive effect when angiotensin-II receptor antagonists given with levodopa

- Lithium: angiotensin-II receptor antagonists reduce excretion of ●lithium (increased plasma concentration)

Methyldopa: enhanced hypotensive effect when angiotensin-II receptor antagonists given with methyldopa

Moxisylyte: enhanced hypotensive effect when angiotensin-II receptor antagonists given with moxisylyte

Angiotensin-II Receptor Antagonists (continued)

Moxonidine: enhanced hypotensive effect when angiotensin-II receptor antagonists given with moxonidine

Muscle Relaxants: enhanced hypotensive effect when angiotensin-II receptor antagonists given with baclofen or tizanidine

Nitrates: enhanced hypotensive effect when angiotensin-II receptor antagonists given with nitrates

Oestrogens: hypotensive effect of angiotensin-II receptor antagonists antagonised by oestrogens

• Potassium Salts: increased risk of hyperkalaemia when angiotensin-II receptor antagonists given with ●potassium salts

Prostaglandins: enhanced hypotensive effect when angiotensin-II receptor antagonists given with alprostadil

Tacrolimus: increased risk of hyperkalaemia when angiotensin-II receptor antagonists given with tacrolimus

Vasodilator Antihypertensives: enhanced hypotensive effect when angiotensin-II receptor antagonists given with hydralazine, minoxidil or sodium nitroprusside

Antacids

Note. Antacids should preferably not be taken at the same time as other drugs since they may impair absorption

ACE Inhibitors: antacids possibly reduce absorption of ACE inhibitors; antacids reduce absorption of captopril, enalapril and fosinopril

Analgesics: alkaline urine due to some antacids increases excretion of aspirin

Antibacterials: antacids reduce absorption of azithromycin, cefaclor, cefpodoxime, ciprofloxacin, isoniazid, levofloxacin, moxifloxacin, norfloxacin, ofloxacin, rifampicin and tetracyclines; oral magnesium salts (as magnesium trisilicate) reduce absorption of nitrofurantoin

Antiepileptics: antacids reduce absorption of gabapentin and phenytoin

Antifungals: antacids reduce absorption of itraconazole and ketoconazole

Antihistamines: antacids reduce absorption of fexofenadine

Antimalarials: antacids reduce absorption of chloroquine and hydroxychloroquine; oral magnesium salts (as magnesium trisilicate) reduce absorption of proguanil

Antipsychotics: antacids reduce absorption of phenothiazines and sulpiride

Antivirals: antacids possibly reduce plasma concentration of atazanavir; antacids possibly reduce absorption of fosamprenavir; antacids reduce absorption of tipranavir

Bile Acids: antacids possibly reduce absorption of bile acids

Bisphosphonates: antacids reduce absorption of bisphosphonates

Cardiac Glycosides: antacids possibly reduce absorption of digoxin

Corticosteroids: antacids reduce absorption of deflazacort

Deferasirox: antacids containing aluminium possibly reduce absorption of deferasirox (manufacturer of deferasirox advises avoid concomitant use)

Dipyridamole: antacids possibly reduce absorption of dipyridamole

Iron: oral magnesium salts (as magnesium trisilicate) reduce absorption of *oral* iron

Lipid-regulating Drugs: antacids reduce absorption of rosuvastatin

Lithium: sodium bicarbonate increases excretion of lithium (reduced plasma concentration)

Mycophenolate: antacids reduce absorption of mycophenolate

Antacids (continued)

Penicillamine: antacids reduce absorption of penicillamine

Thyroid Hormones: antacids possibly reduce absorption of levothyroxine

Ulcer-healing Drugs: antacids possibly reduce absorption of lansoprazole

• Ulipristal: avoidance of antacids advised by manufacturer of ●ulipristal (plasma concentration of ulipristal possibly reduced)

Antazoline *see* Antihistamines

Anti-arrhythmics *see* Adenosine, Amiodarone, Disopyramide, Flecainide, Lidocaine, and Propafenone

Antibacterials *see* individual drugs

Antibiotics (cytotoxic) *see* Bleomycin, Doxorubicin, Epirubicin, Idarubicin, Mitomycin, and Mitoxantrone

Anticoagulants *see* Coumarins, Dabigatran etexilate, Heparins, Phenindione, and Rivaroxaban

Antidepressants *see* Agomelatine; Antidepressants, SSRI; Antidepressants, Tricyclic; Antidepressants, Tricyclic (related); MAOIs; Mirtazapine; Moclobemide; Reboxetine; St John's Wort; Tryptophan; Venlafaxine

Antidepressants, Noradrenaline Re-uptake Inhibitors *see* Reboxetine

Antidepressants, SSRI

Alcohol: sedative effects possibly increased when SSRIs given with alcohol

Anaesthetics, Local: fluvoxamine inhibits metabolism of ropivacaine—avoid prolonged administration of ropivacaine

• Analgesics: increased risk of bleeding when SSRIs given with ●NSAIDs or ●aspirin; fluoxetine, fluvoxamine, paroxetine and sertraline possibly increase plasma concentration of methadone; increased risk of CNS toxicity when SSRIs given with ●tramadol

Anti-arrhythmics: fluoxetine increases plasma concentration of flecainide; paroxetine possibly inhibits metabolism of propafenone (increased risk of toxicity)

• Anticoagulants: SSRIs possibly enhance anticoagulant effect of ●coumarins

• Antidepressants: avoidance of fluvoxamine advised by manufacturer of ●reboxetine; possible increased serotonergic effects when SSRIs given with duloxetine; fluvoxamine inhibits metabolism of ●duloxetine—avoid concomitant use; CNS effects of SSRIs increased by ●MAOIs (risk of serious toxicity); citalopram, escitalopram, fluvoxamine, paroxetine or sertraline should not be started until 2 weeks after stopping ●MAOIs, also MAOIs should not be started until at least 1 week after stopping citalopram, escitalopram, fluvoxamine, paroxetine or sertraline; fluoxetine should not be started until 2 weeks after stopping ●MAOIs, also MAOIs should not be started until at least 5 weeks after stopping fluoxetine; increased risk of CNS toxicity when escitalopram given with ●moclobemide, preferably avoid concomitant use; after stopping citalopram, escitalopram, fluvoxamine, paroxetine or sertraline do not start ●moclobemide for at least 1 week; after stopping fluoxetine do not start ●moclobemide for 5 weeks; increased serotonergic effects when SSRIs given with ●St John's wort—avoid concomitant use; fluvoxamine inhibits metabolism of ●agomelatine (increased plasma concentration); possible increased serotonergic effects when fluoxetine or fluvoxamine given with mirtazapine; SSRIs increase plasma concentration of some ●tricyclics; agitation and nausea may occur when SSRIs given with ●tryptophan

• Antiepileptics: SSRIs antagonise anticonvulsant effect of ●antiepileptics (convulsive threshold lowered); fluoxetine and fluvoxamine increase plasma concentration of ●carbamazepine; fluoxetine and fluvoxamine increase plasma concentration of ●phenytoin; plasma concentration of paroxetine reduced by phenytoin and primidone

Antidepressants, SSRI *(continued)*

Antihistamines: antidepressant effect of SSRIs possibly antagonised by cyproheptadine

• Antimalarials: avoidance of antidepressants advised by manufacturer of ●artemether/lumefantrine

Antimuscarinics: paroxetine increases plasma concentration of darifenacin and procyclidine

• Antipsychotics: avoidance of fluoxetine, fluvoxamine or sertraline advised by manufacturer of ●droperidol (risk of ventricular arrhythmias); fluoxetine increases plasma concentration of ●clozapine, ●haloperidol, risperidone, ●sertindole and ●zotepine; fluvoxamine possibly increases plasma concentration of haloperidol; paroxetine inhibits metabolism of perphenazine (reduce dose of perphenazine); fluoxetine and paroxetine possibly inhibit metabolism of ●aripiprazole (reduce dose of aripiprazole); citalopram possibly increases plasma concentration of clozapine (increased risk of toxicity); fluvoxamine, paroxetine and sertraline increase plasma concentration of ●clozapine; fluvoxamine increases plasma concentration of olanzapine; SSRIs possibly increase plasma concentration of ●pimozide (increased risk of ventricular arrhythmias—avoid concomitant use); paroxetine possibly increases plasma concentration of risperidone (increased risk of toxicity); paroxetine increases plasma concentration of ●sertindole

• Antivirals: plasma concentration of paroxetine and sertraline possibly reduced by darunavir; plasma concentration of SSRIs possibly increased by ●ritonavir; plasma concentration of paroxetine possibly reduced by ritonavir

• Anxiolytics and Hypnotics: fluoxetine increases plasma concentration of alprazolam; fluvoxamine increases plasma concentration of some benzodiazepines; fluvoxamine increases plasma concentration of ●melatonin—avoid concomitant use; sedative effects possibly increased when sertraline given with zolpidem

Atomoxetine: possible increased risk of convulsions when antidepressants given with atomoxetine; fluoxetine and paroxetine possibly inhibit metabolism of atomoxetine

Barbiturates: SSRIs antagonise anticonvulsant effect of barbiturates (convulsive threshold lowered); plasma concentration of paroxetine reduced by phenobarbital

Beta-blockers: citalopram and escitalopram increase plasma concentration of metoprolol; paroxetine possibly increases plasma concentration of metoprolol (enhanced effect); fluvoxamine increases plasma concentration of propranolol

Bupropion: plasma concentration of citalopram possibly increased by bupropion

Calcium-channel Blockers: fluoxetine possibly inhibits metabolism of nifedipine (increased plasma concentration)

• Clopidogrel: fluoxetine and fluvoxamine possibly reduce antiplatelet effect of ●clopidogrel

• Dopaminergics: caution with paroxetine advised by manufacturer of entacapone; fluoxetine should not be started until 2 weeks after stopping ●rasagiline, also rasagiline should not be started until at least 5 weeks after stopping fluoxetine; increased risk of CNS toxicity when SSRIs given with ●rasagiline; fluvoxamine should not be started until 2 weeks after stopping ●rasagiline; increased risk of hypertension and CNS excitation when fluvoxamine or sertraline given with ●selegiline (selegiline should not be started until 1 week after stopping fluvoxamine or sertraline, avoid fluvoxamine or sertraline for 2 weeks after stopping selegiline); increased risk of hypertension and CNS excitation when paroxetine given with ●selegiline (selegiline should not be started until 2 weeks after stopping paroxetine, avoid paroxetine for 2 weeks after stopping selegiline);

Antidepressants, SSRI

• Dopaminergics *(continued)*

increased risk of hypertension and CNS excitation when fluoxetine given with ●selegiline (selegiline should not be started until 5 weeks after stopping fluoxetine, avoid fluoxetine for 2 weeks after stopping selegiline); theoretical risk of serotonin syndrome if citalopram given with selegiline (especially if dose of selegiline exceeds 10 mg daily); manufacturer of escitalopram advises caution with selegiline

• Hormone Antagonists: fluoxetine and paroxetine possibly inhibit metabolism of ●tamoxifen to active metabolite (avoid concomitant use)

• 5HT₁ Agonists: fluvoxamine inhibits the metabolism of frovatriptan; increased risk of CNS toxicity when citalopram, escitalopram, fluoxetine, fluvoxamine or paroxetine given with ●sumatriptan; CNS toxicity reported when sertraline given with sumatriptan; fluvoxamine possibly inhibits metabolism of zolmitriptan (reduce dose of zolmitriptan)

• Lithium: Increased risk of CNS effects when SSRIs given with ●lithium (lithium toxicity reported)

• Muscle Relaxants: fluvoxamine increases plasma concentration of ●tizanidine (increased risk of toxicity)—avoid concomitant use

Parasympathomimetics: paroxetine increases plasma concentration of galantamine

Ranolazine: paroxetine increases plasma concentration of ranolazine

• Sibutramine: increased risk of CNS toxicity when SSRIs given with ●sibutramine (manufacturer of sibutramine advises avoid concomitant use)

Sympathomimetics: metabolism of SSRIs possibly inhibited by methylphenidate

• Theophylline: fluvoxamine increases plasma concentration of ●theophylline (concomitant use should usually be avoided, but where not possible halve theophylline dose and monitor plasma-theophylline concentration)

Ulcer-healing Drugs: plasma concentration of citalopram, escitalopram and sertraline increased by cimetidine; fluvoxamine possibly increases plasma concentration of lansoprazole; plasma concentration of escitalopram increased by omeprazole

Antidepressants, SSRI (related) *see* Duloxetine and Venlafaxine

Antidepressants, Tricyclic

Adrenergic Neurone Blockers: tricyclics antagonise hypotensive effect of adrenergic neurone blockers

• Alcohol: increased sedative effect when tricyclics given with ●alcohol

Alpha₂-adrenoceptor Stimulants: avoidance of tricyclics advised by manufacturer of apraclonidine and brimonidine

Anaesthetics, General: increased risk of arrhythmias and hypotension when tricyclics given with general anaesthetics

• Analgesics: increased risk of CNS toxicity when tricyclics given with ●tramadol; side-effects possibly increased when tricyclics given with nefopam; sedative effects possibly increased when tricyclics given with opioid analgesics

• Anti-arrhythmics: increased risk of ventricular arrhythmias when tricyclics given with ●amiodarone—avoid concomitant use; increased risk of ventricular arrhythmias when tricyclics given with ●disopyramide or ●flecainide; increased risk of arrhythmias when tricyclics given with ●propafenone

• Antibacterials: increased risk of ventricular arrhythmias when tricyclics given with ●moxifloxacin—avoid concomitant use

• Anticoagulants: tricyclics may enhance or reduce anticoagulant effect of ●coumarins

• Antidepressants: possible increased serotonergic effects when amitriptyline or clomipramine given

Antidepressants, Tricyclic

- Antidepressants *(continued)*
with duloxetine; increased risk of hypertension and CNS excitation when tricyclics given with ●MAOIs, tricyclics should not be started until 2 weeks after stopping MAOIs (3 weeks if starting clomipramine or imipramine), also MAOIs should not be started for at least 1–2 weeks after stopping tricyclics (3 weeks in the case of clomipramine or imipramine); after stopping tricyclics do not start ●moclobemide for at least 1 week; plasma concentration of some tricyclics increased by ●SSRIs; plasma concentration of ami-triptyline reduced by St John's wort
- Antiepileptics: tricyclics antagonise anticonvulsant effect of ●antiepileptics (convulsive threshold lowered); metabolism of tricyclics accelerated by ●carbamazepine (reduced plasma concentration and reduced effect); plasma concentration of tricyclics possibly reduced by ●phenytoin; tricyclics antago-nises anticonvulsant effect of ●primidone (convulsive threshold lowered), also metabolism of tricyclics possibly accelerated (reduced plasma concentration)
Antifungals: plasma concentration of imipramine and nortriptyline possibly increased by terbinafine
Antihistamines: increased antimuscarinic and sedative effects when tricyclics given with antihistamines
- Antimalarials: avoidance of antidepressants advised by manufacturer of ●artemether/lumefantrine
Antimuscarinics: increased risk of antimuscarinic side-effects when tricyclics given with antimuscarinics
- Antipsychotics: plasma concentration of tricyclics increased by ●antipsychotics—possibly increased risk of ventricular arrhythmias; avoidance of tricyc-lics advised by manufacturer of ●droperidol (risk of ventricular arrhythmias); possibly increased anti-muscarinic side-effects when tricyclics given with clozapine; increased risk of antimuscarinic side-effects when tricyclics given with phenothiazines; increased risk of ventricular arrhythmias when tricyclics given with ●pimozide—avoid concomitant use
- Antivirals: side-effects of tricyclics possibly increased by fosamprenavir; plasma concentration of tricyclics possibly increased by ●ritonavir
Anxiolytics and Hypnotics: increased sedative effect when tricyclics given with anxiolytics and hypnotics
- Atomoxetine: increased risk of ventricular arrhythmias when tricyclics given with ●atomoxetine; possible increased risk of convulsions when antidepressants given with atomoxetine
- Barbiturates: tricyclics antagonises anticonvulsant effect of ●barbiturates (convulsive threshold lowered), also metabolism of tricyclics possibly accelerated (reduced plasma concentration)
- Beta-blockers: plasma concentration of imipramine increased by labetalol and propranolol; increased risk of ventricular arrhythmias when tricyclics given with ●sotalol
Calcium-channel Blockers: plasma concentration of imipramine increased by diltiazem and verapamil; plasma concentration of tricyclics possibly increased by diltiazem and verapamil
- Clonidine: tricyclics antagonise hypotensive effect of ●clonidine, also increased risk of hypertension on clonidine withdrawal
- Cytotoxics: increased risk of ventricular arrhythmias when amitriptyline or clomipramine given with ●arsenic trioxide
Disulfiram: metabolism of tricyclics inhibited by disulfiram (increased plasma concentration); conco-mitant amitriptyline reported to increase disulfiram reaction with alcohol
Diuretics: increased risk of postural hypotension when tricyclics given with diuretics
- Dopaminergics: caution with tricyclics advised by manufacturer of entacapone; increased risk of CNS

Antidepressants, Tricyclic

- Dopaminergics *(continued)*
toxicity when tricyclics given with ●rasagiline; CNS toxicity reported when tricyclics given with ●selegiline
Lithium: risk of toxicity when tricyclics given with lithium
Muscle Relaxants: tricyclics enhance muscle relaxant effect of baclofen
Nicorandil: tricyclics possibly enhance hypotensive effect of nicorandil
Nitrates: tricyclics reduce effects of sublingual tablets of nitrates (failure to dissolve under tongue owing to dry mouth)
Oestrogens: antidepressant effect of tricyclics antag-onised by oestrogens (but side-effects of tricyclics possibly increased due to increased plasma con-centration)
- Pentamidine Isetionate: increased risk of ventricular arrhythmias when tricyclics given with ●pentamidine isetionate
- Sibutramine: increased risk of CNS toxicity when tricyclics given with ●sibutramine (manufacturer of sibutramine advises avoid concomitant use)
Sodium Oxybate: increased risk of side-effects when tricyclics given with sodium oxybate
- Sympathomimetics: increased risk of hypertension and arrhythmias when tricyclics given with ●adrenaline (epinephrine) (but local anaesthetics with adrenaline appear to be safe); metabolism of tricyclics possibly inhibited by methylphenidate; increased risk of hypertension and arrhythmias when tricyclics given with ●noradrenaline (norepinephrine)
Thyroid Hormones: effects of tricyclics possibly enhanced by thyroid hormones; effects of amitriptyline and imipramine enhanced by thyroid hormones
Ulcer-healing Drugs: plasma concentration of tricyclics possibly increased by cimetidine; metabolism of amitriptyline, doxepin, imipramine and nortriptyline inhibited by cimetidine (increased plasma concen-tration)

Antidepressants, Tricyclic (related)

- Alcohol: increased sedative effect when tricyclic-related antidepressants given with ●alcohol
Alpha$_2$-adrenoceptor Stimulants: avoidance of tri-cyclic-related antidepressants advised by manufac-turer of apraclonidine and brimonidine
Anticoagulants: trazodone may enhance or reduce anticoagulant effect of warfarin
- Antidepressants: tricyclic-related antidepressants should not be started until 2 weeks after stopping ●MAOIs, also MAOIs should not be started until at least 1–2 weeks after stopping tricyclic-related anti-depressants; after stopping tricyclic-related anti-depressants do not start ●moclobemide for at least 1 week
- Antiepileptics: tricyclic-related antidepressants possi-bly antagonise anticonvulsant effect of ●antiepileptics (convulsive threshold lowered); plasma concentration of mianserin reduced by ●carbamazepine and ●phenytoin; metabolism of mianserin accelerated by ●primidone (reduced plasma concentration)
Antihistamines: possible increased antimuscarinic and sedative effects when tricyclic-related antidepres-sants given with antihistamines
- Antimalarials: avoidance of antidepressants advised by manufacturer of ●artemether/lumefantrine
Antimuscarinics: possibly increased antimuscarinic side-effects when tricyclic-related antidepressants given with antimuscarinics
Antivirals: side-effects possibly increased when trazodone given with ritonavir

Antidepressants, Tricyclic (related) *(continued)*

Anxiolytics and Hypnotics: increased sedative effect when tricyclic-related antidepressants given with anxiolytics and hypnotics

Atomoxetine: possible increased risk of convulsions when antidepressants given with atomoxetine

● Barbiturates: tricyclic-related antidepressants possibly antagonise anticonvulsant effect of ●barbiturates (convulsive threshold lowered); metabolism of mianserin accelerated by ●phenobarbital (reduced plasma concentration)

Diazoxide: enhanced hypotensive effect when tricyclic-related antidepressants given with diazoxide

Nitrates: tricyclic-related antidepressants possibly reduce effects of sublingual tablets of nitrates (failure to dissolve under tongue owing to dry mouth)

● Sibutramine: increased risk of CNS toxicity when tricyclic-related antidepressants given with ●sibutramine (manufacturer of sibutramine advises avoid concomitant use)

Vasodilator Antihypertensives: enhanced hypotensive effect when tricyclic-related antidepressants given with hydralazine or sodium nitroprusside

Antidiabetics

Note. Other oral drugs may be taken at least 1 hour before or 4 hours after exenatide injection, or taken with a meal when exenatide is not administered, to minimise possible interference with absorption

ACE Inhibitors: hypoglycaemic effect of insulin, metformin and sulphonylureas possibly enhanced by ACE inhibitors

Alcohol: hypoglycaemic effect of antidiabetics enhanced by alcohol; increased risk of lactic acidosis when metformin given with alcohol

Anabolic Steroids: hypoglycaemic effect of antidiabetics possibly enhanced by anabolic steroids

● Analgesics: effects of sulphonylureas possibly enhanced by ●NSAIDs; effects of tolbutamide enhanced by ●azapropazone (avoid concomitant use)

Anti-arrhythmics: hypoglycaemic effect of gliclazide, insulin and metformin possibly enhanced by disopyramide

● Antibacterials: hypoglycaemic effect of acarbose possibly enhanced by neomycin, also severity of gastrointestinal effects increased; effects of repaglinide enhanced by clarithromycin; effects of glibenclamide possibly enhanced by ciprofloxacin and norfloxacin; plasma concentration of nateglinide reduced by rifampicin; hypoglycaemic effect of repaglinide possibly antagonised by rifampicin; plasma concentration of rosiglitazone reduced by ●rifampicin—consider increasing dose of rosiglitazone; effects of sulphonylureas enhanced by ●chloramphenicol; metabolism of tolbutamide accelerated by ●rifamycins (reduced effect); metabolism of sulphonylureas possibly accelerated by ●rifamycins (reduced effect); effects of sulphonylureas rarely enhanced by sulphonamides and trimethoprim; hypoglycaemic effect of sulphonylureas possibly enhanced by tetracyclines; hypoglycaemic effect of repaglinide possibly enhanced by trimethoprim—manufacturer advises avoid concomitant use

● Anticoagulants: exenatide possibly enhances anticoagulant effect of warfarin; hypoglycaemic effect of sulphonylureas possibly enhanced by ●coumarins, also possible changes to anticoagulant effect

Antidepressants: hypoglycaemic effect of antidiabetics possibly enhanced by MAOIs; hypoglycaemic effect of insulin, metformin and sulphonylureas enhanced by MAOIs

Antiepileptics: tolbutamide transiently increases plasma concentration of phenytoin (possibility of toxicity); plasma concentration of glibenclamide possibly reduced by topiramate

● Antifungals: plasma concentration of sulphonylureas increased by ●fluconazole and ●miconazole; hypoglycaemic effect of gliclazide and glipizide enhanced

Antidiabetics

● Antifungals *(continued)*

by ●miconazole—avoid concomitant use; hypoglycaemic effect of nateglinide possibly enhanced by fluconazole; hypoglycaemic effect of repaglinide possibly enhanced by itraconazole; hypoglycaemic effect of glipizide possibly enhanced by posaconazole; plasma concentration of sulphonylureas possibly increased by voriconazole

Antihistamines: thrombocyte count depressed when metformin given with ketotifen (manufacturer of ketotifen advises avoid concomitant use)

Antipsychotics: hypoglycaemic effect of sulphonylureas possibly antagonised by phenothiazines

Antivirals: plasma concentration of tolbutamide possibly increased by ritonavir

Aprepitant: plasma concentration of tolbutamide reduced by aprepitant

Beta-blockers: warning signs of hypoglycaemia (such as tremor) with antidiabetics may be masked when given with beta-blockers; hypoglycaemic effect of insulin enhanced by beta-blockers

● Bosentan: increased risk of hepatotoxicity when glibenclamide given with ●bosentan—avoid concomitant use

Calcium-channel Blockers: glucose tolerance occasionally impaired when insulin given with nifedipine

Cardiac Glycosides: acarbose possibly reduces plasma concentration of digoxin; sitagliptin increases plasma concentration of digoxin

Ciclosporin: hypoglycaemic effect of repaglinide possibly enhanced by ciclosporin

Corticosteroids: hypoglycaemic effect of antidiabetics antagonised by corticosteroids

● Cytotoxics: avoidance of repaglinide advised by manufacturer of ●lapatinib; metabolism of rosiglitazone possibly inhibited by paclitaxel

Deferasirox: plasma concentration of repaglinide increased by deferasirox

Diazoxide: hypoglycaemic effect of antidiabetics antagonised by diazoxide

Diuretics: hypoglycaemic effect of antidiabetics antagonised by loop diuretics and thiazides and related diuretics

Hormone Antagonists: requirements for insulin, metformin, repaglinide and sulphonylureas possibly reduced by lanreotide; requirements for insulin, metformin, repaglinide and sulphonylureas possibly reduced by octreotide

Leflunomide: hypoglycaemic effect of tolbutamide possibly enhanced by leflunomide

● Lipid-regulating Drugs: hypoglycaemic effect of acarbose possibly enhanced by colestyramine; hypoglycaemic effect of nateglinide possibly enhanced by gemfibrozil; increased risk of severe hypoglycaemia when repaglinide given with ●gemfibrozil—avoid concomitant use; plasma concentration of rosiglitazone increased by ●gemfibrozil (consider reducing dose of rosiglitazone); plasma concentration of glibenclamide possibly increased by fluvastatin; may be improved glucose tolerance and an additive effect when insulin or sulphonylureas given with fibrates

Oestrogens: hypoglycaemic effect of antidiabetics antagonised by oestrogens

Orlistat: avoidance of acarbose advised by manufacturer of orlistat

Pancreatin: hypoglycaemic effect of acarbose antagonised by pancreatin

Progestogens: hypoglycaemic effect of antidiabetics antagonised by progestogens

● Sulfinpyrazone: effects of sulphonylureas enhanced by ●sulfinpyrazone

Testosterone: hypoglycaemic effect of antidiabetics possibly enhanced by testosterone

Ulcer-healing Drugs: excretion of metformin reduced by cimetidine (increased plasma concentration);

Antidiabetics

Ulcer-healing Drugs *(continued)*
hypoglycaemic effect of sulphonylureas enhanced by cimetidine

Antiepileptics *see* Carbamazepine, Eslicarbazepine, Ethosuximide, Gabapentin, Lacosamide, Lamotrigine, Levetiracetam, Oxcarbazepine, Phenytoin, Primidone, Rufinamide, Stiripentol, Tiagabine, Topiramate, Valproate, Vigabatrin, and Zonisamide

Antifungals *see* Amphotericin; Antifungals, Imidazole; Antifungals, Triazole; Caspofungin; Flucytosine; Griseofulvin; Micafungin; Terbinafine

Antifungals, Imidazole

Aliskiren: ketoconazole increases plasma concentration of aliskiren

Alpha-blockers: ketoconazole possibly increases plasma concentration of alfuzosin

- Analgesics: ketoconazole inhibits metabolism of ●buprenorphine (reduce dose of buprenorphine)

Antacids: absorption of ketoconazole reduced by antacids

- Anti-arrhythmics: increased risk of ventricular arrhythmias when ketoconazole given with ●disopyramide—avoid concomitant use

- Antibacterials: metabolism of ketoconazole accelerated by ●rifampicin (reduced plasma concentration), also plasma concentration of rifampicin may be reduced by ketoconazole; plasma concentration of ketoconazole possibly reduced by isoniazid; avoidance of concomitant ketoconazole in severe renal and hepatic impairment advised by manufacturer of ●telithromycin

- Anticoagulants: ketoconazole enhances anticoagulant effect of ●coumarins; miconazole enhances anticoagulant effect of ●coumarins (miconazole oral gel and possibly vaginal formulations absorbed); ketoconazole increases plasma concentration of ●rivaroxaban—avoid concomitant use

- Antidepressants: avoidance of imidazoles advised by manufacturer of ●reboxetine; ketoconazole increases plasma concentration of mirtazapine

- Antidiabetics: miconazole enhances hypoglycaemic effect of ●gliclazide and ●glipizide—avoid concomitant use; miconazole increases plasma concentration of ●sulphonylureas

- Antiepileptics: ketoconazole and miconazole possibly increase plasma concentration of carbamazepine; miconazole enhances anticonvulsant effect of ●phenytoin (plasma concentration of phenytoin increased); plasma concentration of ketoconazole reduced by ●phenytoin

Antifungals: imidazoles possibly antagonise effects of amphotericin

- Antihistamines: manufacturer of loratadine advises ketoconazole possibly increases plasma concentration of loratadine; imidazoles possibly inhibit metabolism of ●mizolastine (avoid concomitant use); ketoconazole inhibits metabolism of ●mizolastine—avoid concomitant use; ketoconazole increases plasma concentration of rupatadine

- Antimalarials: avoidance of imidazoles advised by manufacturer of ●artemether/lumefantrine; ketoconazole increases plasma concentration of mefloquine

Antimuscarinics: absorption of ketoconazole reduced by antimuscarinics; ketoconazole increases plasma concentration of darifenacin—avoid concomitant use; manufacturer of fesoterodine advises dose reduction when ketoconazole given with fesoterodine—consult fesoterodine product literature; ketoconazole increases plasma concentration of solifenacin; avoidance of ketoconazole advised by manufacturer of tolterodine

- Antipsychotics: ketoconazole inhibits metabolism of ●aripiprazole (reduce dose of aripiprazole); increased risk of ventricular arrhythmias when imidazoles

Antifungals, Imidazole

- Antipsychotics *(continued)*
given with ●pimozide—avoid concomitant use; imidazoles possibly increase plasma concentration of quetiapine (reduce dose of quetiapine); possible increased risk of ventricular arrhythmias when imidazoles given with ●sertindole—avoid concomitant use; increased risk of ventricular arrhythmias when ketoconazole given with ●sertindole—avoid concomitant use

- Antivirals: plasma concentration of both drugs increased when ketoconazole given with darunavir; plasma concentration of ketoconazole increased by fosamprenavir; ketoconazole increases plasma concentration of ●indinavir and ●maraviroc (consider reducing dose of indinavir and maraviroc); plasma concentration of ketoconazole reduced by ●nevirapine—avoid concomitant use; combination of ketoconazole with ●ritonavir may increase plasma concentration of either drug (or both); imidazoles possibly increase plasma concentration of saquinavir; ketoconazole increases plasma concentration of saquinavir

- Anxiolytics and Hypnotics: ketoconazole increases plasma concentration of alprazolam; ketoconazole increases plasma concentration of ●midazolam (risk of prolonged sedation)

Aprepitant: ketoconazole increases plasma concentration of aprepitant

Bosentan: ketoconazole increases plasma concentration of bosentan

- Calcium-channel Blockers: ketoconazole inhibits metabolism of ●felodipine (increased plasma concentration); avoidance of ketoconazole advised by manufacturer of lercanidipine; ketoconazole possibly inhibits metabolism of dihydropyridines (increased plasma concentration)

- Ciclosporin: ketoconazole inhibits metabolism of ●ciclosporin (increased plasma concentration); miconazole possibly inhibits metabolism of ●ciclosporin (increased plasma concentration)

- Cilostazol: ketoconazole possibly increases plasma concentration of ●cilostazol—avoid concomitant use

Cinacalcet: ketoconazole inhibits metabolism of cinacalcet (increased plasma concentration)

- Clopidogrel: ketoconazole possibly reduces antiplatelet effect of ●clopidogrel

Corticosteroids: ketoconazole possibly inhibits metabolism of corticosteroids; ketoconazole increases plasma concentration of *inhaled* and *oral* budesonide; ketoconazole increases plasma concentration of active metabolite of ciclesonide; ketoconazole inhibits the metabolism of methylprednisolone; ketoconazole increases plasma concentration of *inhaled* mometasone

- Cytotoxics: ketoconazole possibly increases plasma concentration of dasatinib; ketoconazole inhibits metabolism of erlotinib and sunitinib (increased plasma concentration); ketoconazole increases plasma concentration of ●everolimus, ●lapatinib and ●nilotinib—avoid concomitant use; ketoconazole increases plasma concentration of bortezomib and imatinib; ketoconazole increases plasma concentration of active metabolite of ●temsirolimus—avoid concomitant use; *in vitro* studies suggest a possible interaction between ketoconazole and docetaxel (consult docetaxel product literature); ketoconazole reduces plasma concentration of ●irinotecan (but concentration of active metabolite of irinotecan increased)—avoid concomitant use

- Diuretics: ketoconazole increases plasma concentration of ●eplerenone—avoid concomitant use

- Domperidone: ketoconazole possibly increases risk of arrhythmias with ●domperidone

Antifungals, Imidazole *(continued)*

- Ergot Alkaloids: increased risk of ergotism when imidazoles given with ●ergotamine and methysergide—avoid concomitant use
- 5HT$_1$ Agonists: ketoconazole increases plasma concentration of almotriptan (increased risk of toxicity); ketoconazole increases plasma concentration of ●eletriptan (risk of toxicity)—avoid concomitant use
- Ivabradine: ketoconazole increases plasma concentration of ●ivabradine—avoid concomitant use
  Lanthanum: absorption of ketoconazole possibly reduced by lanthanum (give at least 2 hours apart)
- Lipid-regulating Drugs: possible increased risk of myopathy when imidazoles given with atorvastatin or simvastatin; increased risk of myopathy when ketoconazole given with ●simvastatin (avoid concomitant use); possible increased risk of myopathy when miconazole given with ●simvastatin—avoid concomitant use
  Oestrogens: anecdotal reports of contraceptive failure when imidazoles or ketoconazole given with oestrogens
  Parasympathomimetics: ketoconazole increases plasma concentration of galantamine
- Ranolazine: ketoconazole increases plasma concentration of ●ranolazine—avoid concomitant use
  Retinoids: ketoconazole increases plasma concentration of alitretinoin
  Sildenafil: ketoconazole increases plasma concentration of sildenafil—reduce initial dose of sildenafil
- Sirolimus: ketoconazole increases plasma concentration of ●sirolimus—avoid concomitant use; miconazole increases plasma concentration of ●sirolimus
- Tacrolimus: imidazoles possibly increase plasma concentration of ●tacrolimus; ketoconazole increases plasma concentration of ●tacrolimus
  Tadalafil: ketoconazole increases plasma concentration of tadalafil
- Theophylline: ketoconazole possibly increases plasma concentration of ●theophylline
  Tolvaptan: ketoconazole increases plasma concentration of tolvaptan
  Ulcer-healing Drugs: absorption of ketoconazole reduced by histamine H$_2$-antagonists, proton pump inhibitors and sucralfate
- Vardenafil: ketoconazole increases plasma concentration of ●vardenafil—avoid concomitant use
  Vitamins: ketoconazole possibly increases plasma concentration of paricalcitol

Antifungals, Polyene *see* Amphotericin

Antifungals, Triazole

Note. In general, fluconazole interactions relate to multiple-dose treatment

- Analgesics: fluconazole increases plasma concentration of celecoxib (halve dose of celecoxib); voriconazole increases plasma concentration of diclofenac and ibuprofen; fluconazole increases plasma concentration of parecoxib (reduce dose of parecoxib); voriconazole increases plasma concentration of ●alfentanil and ●methadone (consider reducing dose of alfentanil and methadone); fluconazole inhibits metabolism of alfentanil (risk of prolonged or delayed respiratory depression); itraconazole possibly inhibits metabolism of alfentanil; fluconazole and itraconazole possibly increase plasma concentration of fentanyl
  Antacids: absorption of itraconazole reduced by antacids
- Anti-arrhythmics: manufacturer of itraconazole advises avoid concomitant use with ●disopyramide
- Antibacterials: plasma concentration of itraconazole increased by clarithromycin; triazoles possibly increase plasma concentration of ●rifabutin (increased risk of uveitis—reduce rifabutin dose); posaconazole increases plasma concentration of ●rifabutin (also plasma concentration of posaconazole reduced); voriconazole increases plasma concentration of ●rifabutin, also rifabutin reduces plasma concentration of voriconazole (increase dose of voriconazole and also monitor for rifabutin toxicity); fluconazole increases plasma concentration of ●rifabutin (increased risk of uveitis—reduce rifabutin dose); plasma concentration of itraconazole reduced by ●rifabutin—avoid concomitant use; plasma concentration of posaconazole reduced by ●rifampicin; plasma concentration of voriconazole reduced by ●rifampicin—avoid concomitant use; metabolism of fluconazole and itraconazole accelerated by ●rifampicin (reduced plasma concentration)
- Anticoagulants: fluconazole, itraconazole and voriconazole enhance anticoagulant effect of ●coumarins; avoidance of itraconazole, posaconazole and voriconazole advised by manufacturer of rivaroxaban
- Antidepressants: avoidance of triazoles advised by manufacturer of ●reboxetine; plasma concentration of voriconazole reduced by ●St John's wort—avoid concomitant use
- Antidiabetics: posaconazole possibly enhances hypoglycaemic effect of glipizide; fluconazole possibly enhances hypoglycaemic effect of nateglinide; itraconazole possibly enhances hypoglycaemic effect of repaglinide; fluconazole increases plasma concentration of ●sulphonylureas; voriconazole possibly increases plasma concentration of sulphonylureas
- Antiepileptics: plasma concentration of itraconazole and posaconazole possibly reduced by ●carbamazepine; fluconazole possibly increases plasma concentration of carbamazepine; plasma concentration of voriconazole possibly reduced by ●carbamazepine and ●primidone—avoid concomitant use; plasma concentration of itraconazole reduced by ●phenytoin—avoid concomitant use; fluconazole increases plasma concentration of ●phenytoin (consider reducing dose of phenytoin); voriconazole increases plasma concentration of ●phenytoin, also phenytoin reduces plasma concentration of voriconazole (increase dose of voriconazole and also monitor for phenytoin toxicity); plasma concentration of posaconazole reduced by ●phenytoin; plasma concentration of posaconazole possibly reduced by ●primidone
  Antifungals: triazoles possibly antagonise effects of amphotericin; plasma concentration of itraconazole increased by micafungin (consider reducing dose of itraconazole)
- Antihistamines: itraconazole inhibits metabolism of ●mizolastine—avoid concomitant use
- Antimalarials: avoidance of triazoles advised by manufacturer of ●artemether/lumefantrine
  Antimuscarinics: avoidance of itraconazole advised by manufacturer of darifenacin and tolterodine; manufacturer of fesoterodine advises dose reduction when itraconazole given with fesoterodine—consult fesoterodine product literature; itraconazole increases plasma concentration of solifenacin
- Antipsychotics: itraconazole possibly increases plasma concentration of haloperidol; itraconazole possibly inhibits metabolism of ●aripiprazole (reduce dose of aripiprazole); increased risk of ventricular arrhythmias when triazoles given with ●pimozide—avoid concomitant use; triazoles possibly increase plasma concentration of quetiapine (reduce dose of quetiapine); possible increased risk of ventricular arrhythmias when triazoles given with ●sertindole—avoid concomitant use; increased risk of ventricular arrhythmias when itraconazole given with ●sertindole—avoid concomitant use
- Antivirals: posaconazole increases plasma concentration of ●atazanavir; plasma concentration of vorico-

Antifungals, Triazole

- Antibacterials *(continued)*
  zole reduced); voriconazole increases plasma concentration of ●rifabutin, also rifabutin reduces plasma concentration of voriconazole (increase dose of voriconazole and also monitor for rifabutin toxicity); fluconazole increases plasma concentration of ●rifabutin (increased risk of uveitis—reduce rifabutin dose); plasma concentration of itraconazole reduced by ●rifabutin—avoid concomitant use; plasma concentration of posaconazole reduced by ●rifampicin; plasma concentration of voriconazole reduced by ●rifampicin—avoid concomitant use; metabolism of fluconazole and itraconazole accelerated by ●rifampicin (reduced plasma concentration)

Antifungals, Triazole

- Antivirals *(continued)*
  nazole reduced by ●efavirenz, also plasma concentration of efavirenz increased (increase voriconazole dose and reduce efavirenz dose); plasma concentration of itraconazole and posaconazole reduced by ●efavirenz; plasma concentration of itraconazole possibly increased by fosamprenavir; itraconazole increases plasma concentration of ●indinavir (consider reducing dose of indinavir); fluconazole increases plasma concentration of ●nevirapine, ritonavir and tipranavir; plasma concentration of itraconazole possibly reduced by nevirapine—consider increasing dose of itraconazole; plasma concentration of voriconazole reduced by ●ritonavir—avoid concomitant use; combination of itraconazole with ●ritonavir may increase plasma concentration of either drug (or both); triazoles possibly increase plasma concentration of saquinavir; fluconazole increases plasma concentration of ●zidovudine (increased risk of toxicity)

- Anxiolytics and Hypnotics: itraconazole increases plasma concentration of alprazolam; posaconazole increases plasma concentration of ●midazolam; fluconazole and itraconazole increase plasma concentration of ●midazolam (risk of prolonged sedation); itraconazole increases plasma concentration of buspirone (reduce dose of buspirone)

- Barbiturates: plasma concentration of itraconazole and posaconazole possibly reduced by ●phenobarbital; plasma concentration of voriconazole possibly reduced by ●phenobarbital—avoid concomitant use

- Bosentan: fluconazole possibly increases plasma concentration of ●bosentan—avoid concomitant use; itraconazole possibly increases plasma concentration of bosentan

- Calcium-channel Blockers: negative inotropic effect possibly increased when itraconazole given with calcium-channel blockers; itraconazole inhibits metabolism of ●felodipine (increased plasma concentration); avoidance of itraconazole advised by manufacturer of lercanidipine; itraconazole possibly inhibits metabolism of dihydropyridines (increased plasma concentration)

- Cardiac Glycosides: itraconazole increases plasma concentration of ●digoxin

- Ciclosporin: fluconazole, itraconazole, posaconazole and voriconazole inhibit metabolism of ●ciclosporin (increased plasma concentration)

- Clopidogrel: fluconazole, itraconazole and voriconazole possibly reduce antiplatelet effect of ●clopidogrel

  Corticosteroids: itraconazole possibly inhibits metabolism of corticosteroids and methylprednisolone; itraconazole increases plasma concentration of *inhaled* budesonide

- Cytotoxics: itraconazole inhibits metabolism of busulfan (increased risk of toxicity); itraconazole possibly increases side-effects of cyclophosphamide; itraconazole, posaconazole and voriconazole possibly increase plasma concentration of ●everolimus—manufacturer of everolimus advises avoid concomitant use; itraconazole increases plasma concentration of gefitinib; avoidance of itraconazole, posaconazole and voriconazole advised by manufacturer of ●lapatinib; avoidance of itraconazole and voriconazole advised by manufacturer of ●nilotinib; posaconazole possibly inhibits metabolism of ●vinblastine and ●vincristine (increased risk of neurotoxicity); itraconazole possibly inhibits metabolism of ●vincristine and ●vinorelbine (increased risk of neurotoxicity)

- Diuretics: fluconazole increases plasma concentration of eplerenone (reduce dose of eplerenone); itraconazole increases plasma concentration of ●eplerenone—avoid concomitant use; plasma con-

Antifungals, Triazole

- Diuretics *(continued)*
  centration of fluconazole increased by hydrochlorothiazide

- Ergot Alkaloids: increased risk of ergotism when triazoles given with ●ergotamine and methysergide—avoid concomitant use

- 5HT$_1$ Agonists: itraconazole increases plasma concentration of ●eletriptan (risk of toxicity)—avoid concomitant use

- Ivabradine: fluconazole increases plasma concentration of ivabradine—reduce initial dose of ivabradine; itraconazole possibly increases plasma concentration of ●ivabradine—avoid concomitant use

- Lipid-regulating Drugs: possible increased risk of myopathy when triazoles given with atorvastatin or simvastatin; increased risk of myopathy when itraconazole or posaconazole given with ●atorvastatin (avoid concomitant use); fluconazole increases plasma concentration of fluvastatin; increased risk of myopathy when itraconazole or posaconazole given with ●simvastatin (avoid concomitant use)

  Oestrogens: anecdotal reports of contraceptive failure when fluconazole or itraconazole given with oestrogens

- Ranolazine: itraconazole, posaconazole and voriconazole possibly increase plasma concentration of ●ranolazine—manufacturer of ranolazine advises avoid concomitant use

  Sildenafil: itraconazole increases plasma concentration of sildenafil—reduce initial dose of sildenafil

- Sirolimus: posaconazole possibly increases plasma concentration of sirolimus; itraconazole and voriconazole increase plasma concentration of ●sirolimus—avoid concomitant use

- Tacrolimus: triazoles possibly increase plasma concentration of ●tacrolimus; posaconazole increases plasma concentration of ●tacrolimus (reduce dose of tacrolimus); fluconazole, itraconazole and voriconazole increase plasma concentration of ●tacrolimus

  Tadalafil: itraconazole possibly increases plasma concentration of tadalafil

- Theophylline: fluconazole possibly increases plasma concentration of ●theophylline

- Ulcer-healing Drugs: plasma concentration of posaconazole reduced by ●cimetidine; voriconazole possibly increases plasma concentration of esomeprazole; voriconazole increases plasma concentration of omeprazole (consider reducing dose of omeprazole); absorption of itraconazole reduced by histamine H$_2$-antagonists and proton pump inhibitors

- Vardenafil: itraconazole possibly increases plasma concentration of ●vardenafil—avoid concomitant use

Antihistamines

Note. Sedative interactions apply to a lesser extent to the non-sedating antihistamines. Interactions do not generally apply to antihistamines used for topical action (including inhalation)

  Alcohol: increased sedative effect when antihistamines given with alcohol (possibly less effect with non-sedating antihistamines)

- Analgesics: sedative effects possibly increased when sedating antihistamines given with ●opioid analgesics

  Antacids: absorption of fexofenadine reduced by antacids

- Anti-arrhythmics: increased risk of ventricular arrhythmias when mizolastine given with ●amiodarone, ●disopyramide, ●flecainide or ●propafenone—avoid concomitant use

- Antibacterials: plasma concentration of rupatadine increased by erythromycin; manufacturer of loratadine advises plasma concentration possibly increased by erythromycin; metabolism of mizolas-

Antihistamines
- Antibacterials *(continued)*
  tine inhibited by ●erythromycin—avoid concomitant use; increased risk of ventricular arrhythmias when mizolastine given with ●moxifloxacin—avoid concomitant use; metabolism of mizolastine possibly inhibited by ●macrolides (avoid concomitant use)

  Antidepressants: increased antimuscarinic and sedative effects when antihistamines given with MAOIs or tricyclics; cyproheptadine possibly antagonises antidepressant effect of SSRIs; possible increased antimuscarinic and sedative effects when antihistamines given with tricyclic-related antidepressants

  Antidiabetics: thrombocyte count depressed when ketotifen given with metformin (manufacturer of ketotifen advises avoid concomitant use)
- Antifungals: plasma concentration of rupatadine increased by ketoconazole; manufacturer of loratadine advises plasma concentration possibly increased by ketoconazole; metabolism of mizolastine inhibited by ●itraconazole or ●ketoconazole—avoid concomitant use; metabolism of mizolastine possibly inhibited by ●imidazoles (avoid concomitant use)

  Antimuscarinics: increased risk of antimuscarinic side-effects when antihistamines given with antimuscarinics

  Antivirals: plasma concentration of loratadine possibly increased by fosamprenavir; plasma concentration of chlorphenamine possibly increased by lopinavir; plasma concentration of non-sedating antihistamines possibly increased by ritonavir

  Anxiolytics and Hypnotics: increased sedative effect when antihistamines given with anxiolytics and hypnotics
- Beta-blockers: increased risk of ventricular arrhythmias when mizolastine given with ●sotalol—avoid concomitant use

  Betahistine: antihistamines theoretically antagonise effect of betahistine
- Grapefruit Juice: plasma concentration of rupatadine increased by ●grapefruit juice—avoid concomitant use

  Ulcer-healing Drugs: manufacturer of loratadine advises plasma concentration possibly increased by cimetidine

Antihistamines, Non-sedating *see* Antihistamines
Antihistamines, Sedating *see* Antihistamines
Antimalarials *see* Artemether with Lumefantrine, Chloroquine and Hydroxychloroquine, Mefloquine, Primaquine, Proguanil, and Quinine
Antimetabolites *see* Cytarabine, Fludarabine, Fluorouracil, Gemcitabine, Mercaptopurine, Methotrexate, Pemetrexed, Raltitrexed, and Tioguanine

Antimuscarinics
Note. Many drugs have antimuscarinic effects; concomitant use of two or more such drugs can increase side-effects such as dry mouth, urine retention, and constipation; concomitant use can also lead to confusion in the elderly. Interactions do not generally apply to antimuscarinics used by inhalation

  Alcohol: increased sedative effect when hyoscine given with alcohol

  Analgesics: increased risk of antimuscarinic side-effects when antimuscarinics given with nefopam
- Anti-arrhythmics: increased risk of ventricular arrhythmias when tolterodine given with ●amiodarone, ●disopyramide or ●flecainide; increased risk of antimuscarinic side-effects when antimuscarinics given with disopyramide

  Antibacterials: manufacturer of fesoterodine advises dose reduction when fesoterodine given with clarithromycin and telithromycin—consult fesoterodine product literature; manufacturer of tolterodine advises avoid concomitant use with clarithromycin and erythromycin; plasma concen-

Antimuscarinics
  Antibacterials *(continued)*
  tration of darifenacin possibly increased by erythromycin; plasma concentration of active metabolite of fesoterodine reduced by rifampicin

  Antidepressants: plasma concentration of darifenacin and procyclidine increased by paroxetine; increased risk of antimuscarinic side-effects when antimuscarinics given with MAOIs or tricyclics; possibly increased antimuscarinic side-effects when antimuscarinics given with tricyclic-related antidepressants

  Antifungals: antimuscarinics reduce absorption of ketoconazole; manufacturer of fesoterodine advises dose reduction when fesoterodine given with itraconazole and ketoconazole—consult fesoterodine product literature; plasma concentration of darifenacin increased by ketoconazole—avoid concomitant use; plasma concentration of solifenacin increased by itraconazole and ketoconazole; manufacturer of tolterodine advises avoid concomitant use with itraconazole and ketoconazole; manufacturer of darifenacin advises avoid concomitant use with itraconazole

  Antihistamines: increased risk of antimuscarinic side-effects when antimuscarinics given with antihistamines

  Antipsychotics: antimuscarinics possibly reduce effects of haloperidol; increased risk of antimuscarinic side-effects when antimuscarinics given with clozapine; antimuscarinics reduce plasma concentration of phenothiazines, but risk of antimuscarinic side-effects increased

  Antivirals: manufacturer of fesoterodine advises dose reduction when fesoterodine given with atazanavir, indinavir, nelfinavir, ritonavir and saquinavir—consult fesoterodine product literature; manufacturer of darifenacin advises avoid concomitant use with atazanavir, fosamprenavir, indinavir, lopinavir, nelfinavir, ritonavir, saquinavir and tipranavir; manufacturer of tolterodine advises avoid concomitant use with fosamprenavir, indinavir, lopinavir, nelfinavir, ritonavir and saquinavir; plasma concentration of solifenacin increased by nelfinavir and ritonavir
- Beta-blockers: increased risk of ventricular arrhythmias when tolterodine given with ●sotalol

  Calcium-channel Blockers: manufacturer of darifenacin advises avoid concomitant use with verapamil

  Cardiac Glycosides: darifenacin possibly increases plasma concentration of digoxin

  Ciclosporin: manufacturer of darifenacin advises avoid concomitant use with ciclosporin

  Domperidone: antimuscarinics antagonise effects of domperidone on gastro-intestinal activity

  Dopaminergics: antimuscarinics possibly reduce absorption of levodopa

  Memantine: effects of antimuscarinics possibly enhanced by memantine

  Metoclopramide: antimuscarinics antagonise effects of metoclopramide on gastro-intestinal activity

  Nitrates: antimuscarinics possibly reduce effects of sublingual tablets of nitrates (failure to dissolve under tongue owing to dry mouth)

  Parasympathomimetics: antimuscarinics antagonise effects of parasympathomimetics

Antipsychotics
Note. Increased risk of toxicity with myelosuppressive drugs
Note. Avoid concomitant use of clozapine with drugs that have a substantial potential for causing agranulocytosis

  ACE Inhibitors: enhanced hypotensive effect when antipsychotics given with ACE inhibitors

  Adrenergic Neurone Blockers: enhanced hypotensive effect when phenothiazines given with adrenergic neurone blockers; higher doses of chlorpromazine antagonise hypotensive effect of adrenergic neurone

Antipsychotics

Adrenergic Neurone Blockers *(continued)*
blockers; haloperidol antagonises hypotensive effect of adrenergic neurone blockers

Adsorbents: absorption of phenothiazines possibly reduced by kaolin

Alcohol: increased sedative effect when antipsychotics given with alcohol

Alpha-blockers: enhanced hypotensive effect when antipsychotics given with alpha-blockers

• Anaesthetics, General: droperidol enhances effects of thiopental; enhanced hypotensive effect when antipsychotics given with ●general anaesthetics

• Analgesics: avoid concomitant use of clozapine with ●azapropazone (increased risk of agranulocytosis); possible severe drowsiness when haloperidol given with indometacin; increased risk of ventricular arrhythmias when antipsychotics that prolong the QT interval given with ●methadone; increased risk of ventricular arrhythmias when amisulpride given with ●methadone—avoid concomitant use; increased risk of convulsions when antipsychotics given with tramadol; enhanced hypotensive and sedative effects when antipsychotics given with opioid analgesics

Angiotensin-II Receptor Antagonists: enhanced hypotensive effect when antipsychotics given with angiotensin-II receptor antagonists

Antacids: absorption of phenothiazines and sulpiride reduced by antacids

• Anti-arrhythmics: increased risk of ventricular arrhythmias when antipsychotics that prolong the QT interval given with ●anti-arrhythmics that prolong the QT interval; increased risk of ventricular arrhythmias when amisulpride, droperidol, haloperidol, phenothiazines, pimozide, sertindole or zuclopenthixol given with ●amiodarone—avoid concomitant use; increased risk of ventricular arrhythmias when benperidol given with ●amiodarone—manufacturer of benperidol advises avoid concomitant use; increased risk of ventricular arrhythmias when sulpiride given with ●amiodarone or ●disopyramide; increased risk of ventricular arrhythmias when amisulpride, droperidol, pimozide, sertindole or zuclopenthixol given with ●disopyramide—avoid concomitant use; possible increased risk of ventricular arrhythmias when haloperidol given with ●disopyramide—avoid concomitant use; increased risk of ventricular arrhythmias when phenothiazines given with ●disopyramide; increased risk of arrhythmias when clozapine given with ●flecainide

• Antibacterials: increased risk of ventricular arrhythmias when pimozide given with ●clarithromycin, ●moxifloxacin or ●telithromycin—avoid concomitant use; increased risk of ventricular arrhythmias when sertindole given with ●erythromycin or ●moxifloxacin—avoid concomitant use; increased risk of ventricular arrhythmias when amisulpride or zuclopenthixol given with *parenteral* ●erythromycin—avoid concomitant use; plasma concentration of clozapine possibly increased by ●erythromycin (possible increased risk of convulsions); possible increased risk of ventricular arrhythmias when pimozide given with ●erythromycin—avoid concomitant use; increased risk of ventricular arrhythmias when sulpiride given with *parenteral* ●erythromycin; plasma concentration of clozapine increased by ciprofloxacin; plasma concentration of olanzapine possibly increased by ciprofloxacin; increased risk of ventricular arrhythmias when droperidol, haloperidol, phenothiazines or zuclopenthixol given with ●moxifloxacin—avoid concomitant use; increased risk of ventricular arrhythmias when benperidol given with ●moxifloxacin—manufacturer of benperidol advises avoid concomitant use; plasma

Antipsychotics

• Antibacterials *(continued)*
concentration of aripiprazole possibly reduced by ●rifabutin and ●rifampicin—increase dose of aripiprazole; plasma concentration of clozapine possibly reduced by rifampicin; metabolism of haloperidol accelerated by ●rifampicin (reduced plasma concentration); avoid concomitant use of clozapine with ●chloramphenicol or ●sulphonamides (increased risk of agranulocytosis); manufacturer of droperidol advises avoid concomitant use with ●macrolides (risk of ventricular arrhythmias); plasma concentration of quetiapine possibly increased by macrolides (reduce dose of quetiapine); possible increased risk of ventricular arrhythmias when sertindole given with ●macrolides—avoid concomitant use

• Antidepressants: plasma concentration of clozapine possibly increased by citalopram (increased risk of toxicity); metabolism of aripiprazole possibly inhibited by ●fluoxetine and ●paroxetine (reduce dose of aripiprazole); plasma concentration of clozapine, haloperidol, risperidone, sertindole and zotepine increased by ●fluoxetine; manufacturer of droperidol advises avoid concomitant use with ●fluoxetine, ●fluvoxamine, ●sertraline or ●tricyclics (risk of ventricular arrhythmias); plasma concentration of clozapine and olanzapine increased by ●fluvoxamine; plasma concentration of haloperidol possibly increased by fluvoxamine; plasma concentration of clozapine and sertindole increased by ●paroxetine; plasma concentration of risperidone possibly increased by paroxetine (increased risk of toxicity); metabolism of perphenazine inhibited by paroxetine (reduce dose of perphenazine); plasma concentration of clozapine increased by ●sertraline and ●venlafaxine; plasma concentration of haloperidol increased by venlafaxine; clozapine possibly increases CNS effects of ●MAOIs; plasma concentration of pimozide possibly increased by ●SSRIs (increased risk of ventricular arrhythmias—avoid concomitant use); plasma concentration of aripiprazole possibly reduced by ●St John's wort—increase dose of aripiprazole; possibly increased antimuscarinic side-effects when clozapine given with tricyclics; antipsychotics increase plasma concentration of ●tricyclics—possibly increased risk of ventricular arrhythmias; increased risk of antimuscarinic side-effects when phenothiazines given with tricyclics; increased risk of ventricular arrhythmias when pimozide given with ●tricyclics—avoid concomitant use

Antidiabetics: phenothiazines possibly antagonise hypoglycaemic effect of sulphonylureas

• Antiepileptics: antipsychotics antagonise anticonvulsant effect of ●carbamazepine, ●ethosuximide, ●oxcarbazepine, ●phenytoin, ●primidone and ●valproate (convulsive threshold lowered); metabolism of haloperidol, olanzapine, quetiapine, risperidone and sertindole accelerated by carbamazepine (reduced plasma concentration); metabolism of clozapine accelerated by ●carbamazepine (reduced plasma concentration), also avoid concomitant use of drugs with substantial potential for causing agranulocytosis; plasma concentration of aripiprazole reduced by ●carbamazepine—increase dose of aripiprazole; plasma concentration of paliperidone reduced by carbamazepine; metabolism of clozapine, quetiapine and sertindole accelerated by phenytoin (reduced plasma concentration); plasma concentration of aripiprazole possibly reduced by ●phenytoin and ●primidone—increase dose of aripiprazole; metabolism of haloperidol accelerated by primidone (reduced plasma concentration); increased risk of neutropenia when olanzapine given with ●valproate

Antipsychotics *(continued)*

- Antifungals: metabolism of aripiprazole inhibited by ●ketoconazole (reduce dose of aripiprazole); increased risk of ventricular arrhythmias when sertindole given with ●itraconazole or ●ketoconazole—avoid concomitant use; metabolism of aripiprazole possibly inhibited by ●itraconazole (reduce dose of aripiprazole); plasma concentration of haloperidol possibly increased by itraconazole; increased risk of ventricular arrhythmias when pimozide given with ●imidazoles or ●triazoles—avoid concomitant use; possible increased risk of ventricular arrhythmias when sertindole given with ●imidazoles or ●triazoles—avoid concomitant use; plasma concentration of quetiapine possibly increased by imidazoles and triazoles (reduce dose of quetiapine)

- Antimalarials: avoidance of antipsychotics advised by manufacturer of ●artemether/lumefantrine; increased risk of ventricular arrhythmias when droperidol given with ●chloroquine and hydroxychloroquine or ●quinine—avoid concomitant use; increased risk of ventricular arrhythmias when pimozide given with ●mefloquine or ●quinine—avoid concomitant use; possible increased risk of ventricular arrhythmias when haloperidol given with ●mefloquine or ●quinine—avoid concomitant use

  Antimuscarinics: increased risk of antimuscarinic side-effects when clozapine given with antimuscarinics; plasma concentration of phenothiazines reduced by antimuscarinics, but risk of antimuscarinic side-effects increased; effects of haloperidol possibly reduced by antimuscarinics

- Antipsychotics: increased risk of ventricular arrhythmias when amisulpride, pimozide, sertindole or sulpiride given with ●droperidol—avoid concomitant use; increased risk of ventricular arrhythmias when phenothiazines that prolong the QT interval given with ●droperidol—avoid concomitant use; avoid concomitant use of clozapine with depot formulation of ●flupentixol, ●fluphenazine, ●haloperidol, ●pipotiazine, ●risperidone or ●zuclopenthixol as cannot be withdrawn quickly if neutropenia occurs; increased risk of ventricular arrhythmias when sulpiride given with ●haloperidol; chlorpromazine possibly increases plasma concentration of haloperidol; increased risk of ventricular arrhythmias when droperidol given with ●haloperidol—avoid concomitant use; increased risk of ventricular arrhythmias when sertindole given with ●amisulpride—avoid concomitant use; increased risk of ventricular arrhythmias when pimozide given with ●phenothiazines—avoid concomitant use; increased risk of ventricular arrhythmias when pimozide given with ●sulpiride

- Antivirals: plasma concentration of pimozide possibly increased by ●atazanavir—avoid concomitant use; metabolism of aripiprazole possibly inhibited by ●atazanavir, ●fosamprenavir, ●indinavir, ●lopinavir, ●nelfinavir, ●ritonavir and ●saquinavir (reduce dose of aripiprazole); plasma concentration of pimozide possibly increased by ●efavirenz, ●indinavir, ●nelfinavir and ●saquinavir (increased risk of ventricular arrhythmias—avoid concomitant use); plasma concentration of aripiprazole possibly reduced by ●efavirenz and ●nevirapine—increase dose of aripiprazole; plasma concentration of pimozide and sertindole increased by ●fosamprenavir (increased risk of ventricular arrhythmias—avoid concomitant use); plasma concentration of clozapine possibly increased by fosamprenavir; plasma concentration of sertindole increased by ●indinavir, ●lopinavir, ●nelfinavir, ●ritonavir and ●saquinavir (increased risk of ventricular arrhythmias—avoid concomitant use); plasma concentration of clozapine increased by ●ritonavir (increased risk of toxicity)—avoid con-

Antipsychotics

- Antivirals *(continued)*
  comitant use; plasma concentration of antipsychotics possibly increased by ●ritonavir; plasma concentration of pimozide increased by ●ritonavir (increased risk of ventricular arrhythmias—avoid concomitant use); plasma concentration of olanzapine reduced by ritonavir—consider increasing dose of olanzapine

- Anxiolytics and Hypnotics: increased sedative effect when antipsychotics given with anxiolytics and hypnotics; plasma concentration of zotepine increased by diazepam; serious adverse events reported with concomitant use of clozapine and ●lorazepam (causality not established); increased risk of hypotension, bradycardia and respiratory depression when *intramuscular* olanzapine given with *parenteral* ●benzodiazepines; plasma concentration of haloperidol increased by buspirone

- Aprepitant: avoidance of pimozide advised by manufacturer of ●aprepitant

- Atomoxetine: increased risk of ventricular arrhythmias when antipsychotics that prolong the QT interval given with ●atomoxetine

- Barbiturates: antipsychotics antagonise anticonvulsant effect of ●barbiturates (convulsive threshold lowered); plasma concentration of aripiprazole possibly reduced by ●phenobarbital—increase dose of aripiprazole; metabolism of haloperidol accelerated by phenobarbital (reduced plasma concentration); plasma concentration of both drugs reduced when chlorpromazine given with phenobarbital

- Beta-blockers: enhanced hypotensive effect when phenothiazines given with beta-blockers; plasma concentration of both drugs may increase when chlorpromazine given with ●propranolol; increased risk of ventricular arrhythmias when amisulpride, phenothiazines, pimozide, sertindole or sulpiride given with ●sotalol; increased risk of ventricular arrhythmias when droperidol or zuclopenthixol given with ●sotalol—avoid concomitant use; possible increased risk of ventricular arrhythmias when haloperidol given with ●sotalol—avoid concomitant use

  Calcium-channel Blockers: enhanced hypotensive effect when antipsychotics given with calcium-channel blockers

  Clonidine: enhanced hypotensive effect when phenothiazines given with clonidine

- Cytotoxics: avoid concomitant use of clozapine with ●cytotoxics (increased risk of agranulocytosis); avoidance of pimozide advised by manufacturer of ●lapatinib; increased risk of ventricular arrhythmias when antipsychotics that prolong the QT interval given with ●arsenic trioxide; increased risk of ventricular arrhythmias when haloperidol given with ●arsenic trioxide

  Desferrioxamine: manufacturer of levomepromazine advises avoid concomitant use with desferrioxamine; avoidance of prochlorperazine advised by manufacturer of desferrioxamine

  Diazoxide: enhanced hypotensive effect when phenothiazines given with diazoxide

- Diuretics: risk of ventricular arrhythmias with amisulpride or sertindole increased by hypokalaemia caused by ●diuretics; risk of ventricular arrhythmias with pimozide increased by hypokalaemia caused by ●diuretics (avoid concomitant use); enhanced hypotensive effect when phenothiazines given with diuretics

  Dopaminergics: increased risk of extrapyramidal side-effects when antipsychotics given with amantadine; antipsychotics antagonise effects of apomorphine, levodopa and pergolide; antipsychotics antagonise hypoprolactinaemic and antiparkinsonian effects of bromocriptine and cabergoline; manufacturer of

Antipsychotics

Dopaminergics *(continued)*
amisulpride advises avoid concomitant use of levo-dopa (antagonism of effect); avoidance of antipsychotics advised by manufacturer of pramipexole, ropinirole and rotigotine (antagonism of effect)

- Hormone Antagonists: manufacturer of droperidol advises avoid concomitant use with ●tamoxifen (risk of ventricular arrhythmias)

- Ivabradine: increased risk of ventricular arrhythmias when pimozide or sertindole given with ●ivabradine

- Lithium: increased risk of ventricular arrhythmias when sertindole given with ●lithium—avoid concomitant use; increased risk of extrapyramidal side-effects and possibly neurotoxicity when clozapine, flupentixol, haloperidol, phenothiazines or zuclopenthixol given with lithium; increased risk of extrapyramidal side-effects when sulpiride given with lithium

Memantine: effects of antipsychotics possibly reduced by memantine

Methyldopa: enhanced hypotensive effect when antipsychotics given with methyldopa (also increased risk of extrapyramidal effects)

Metoclopramide: increased risk of extrapyramidal side-effects when antipsychotics given with metoclopramide

Moxonidine: enhanced hypotensive effect when phenothiazines given with moxonidine

Muscle Relaxants: promazine possibly enhances effects of suxamethonium

Nitrates: enhanced hypotensive effect when phenothiazines given with nitrates

- Penicillamine: avoid concomitant use of clozapine with ●penicillamine (increased risk of agranulocytosis)

- Pentamidine Isetionate: increased risk of ventricular arrhythmias when amisulpride or droperidol given with ●pentamidine isetionate—avoid concomitant use; increased risk of ventricular arrhythmias when phenothiazines given with ●pentamidine isetionate

- Sibutramine: increased risk of CNS toxicity when antipsychotics given with ●sibutramine (manufacturer of sibutramine advises avoid concomitant use)

Sodium Benzoate: haloperidol possibly reduces effects of sodium benzoate

Sodium Oxybate: antipsychotics possibly enhance effects of sodium oxybate

Sodium Phenylbutyrate: haloperidol possibly reduces effects of sodium phenylbutyrate

Sympathomimetics: antipsychotics antagonise hypertensive effect of sympathomimetics; antipsychotic effects of chlorpromazine possibly antagonised by dexamfetamine; side-effects of risperidone possibly increased by methylphenidate

- Tacrolimus: manufacturer of droperidol advises avoid concomitant use with ●tacrolimus (risk of ventricular arrhythmias)

Tetrabenazine: increased risk of extrapyramidal side-effects when antipsychotics given with tetrabenazine

- Ulcer-healing Drugs: effects of antipsychotics, chlorpromazine and clozapine possibly enhanced by cimetidine; increased risk of ventricular arrhythmias when sertindole given with ●cimetidine—avoid concomitant use; plasma concentration of clozapine possibly reduced by omeprazole; absorption of sulpiride reduced by sucralfate

Vasodilator Antihypertensives: enhanced hypotensive effect when phenothiazines given with hydralazine, minoxidil or sodium nitroprusside

Antivirals *see* Abacavir, Aciclovir, Adefovir, Atazanavir, Cidofovir, Darunavir, Didanosine, Efavirenz, Emtricitabine, Etravirine, Famciclovir, Fosamprenavir, Foscarnet, Ganciclovir, Indinavir, Lamivudine, Lopinavir, Maraviroc, Nelfinavir, Nevirapine, Raltegravir, Ribavirin, Ritonavir, Saquinavir, Stavudine, Telbivudine, Tenofovir, Tipranavir, Valaciclovir, and Zidovudine

Anxiolytics and Hypnotics

ACE Inhibitors: enhanced hypotensive effect when anxiolytics and hypnotics given with ACE inhibitors

Adrenergic Neurone Blockers: enhanced hypotensive effect when anxiolytics and hypnotics given with adrenergic neurone blockers

Alcohol: increased sedative effect when anxiolytics and hypnotics given with alcohol

Alpha-blockers: enhanced hypotensive and sedative effects when anxiolytics and hypnotics given with alpha-blockers

Anaesthetics, General: increased sedative effect when anxiolytics and hypnotics given with general anaesthetics

Analgesics: increased sedative effect when anxiolytics and hypnotics given with opioid analgesics

Angiotensin-II Receptor Antagonists: enhanced hypotensive effect when anxiolytics and hypnotics given with angiotensin-II receptor antagonists

- Antibacterials: metabolism of midazolam inhibited by ●clarithromycin, ●erythromycin, ●quinupristin/dalfopristin and ●telithromycin (increased plasma concentration with increased sedation); plasma concentration of buspirone increased by erythromycin (reduce dose of buspirone); metabolism of zopiclone inhibited by erythromycin and quinupristin/dalfopristin; metabolism of benzodiazepines possibly accelerated by rifampicin (reduced plasma concentration); metabolism of diazepam accelerated by rifampicin (reduced plasma concentration); metabolism of buspirone and zaleplon possibly accelerated by rifampicin; metabolism of zolpidem accelerated by rifampicin (reduced plasma concentration and reduced effect); plasma concentration of zopiclone significantly reduced by rifampicin; metabolism of diazepam inhibited by isoniazid

Anticoagulants: chloral and triclofos may transiently enhance anticoagulant effect of coumarins

- Antidepressants: plasma concentration of alprazolam increased by fluoxetine; plasma concentration of melatonin increased by ●fluvoxamine—avoid concomitant use; plasma concentration of some benzodiazepines increased by fluvoxamine; sedative effects possibly increased when zolpidem given with sertraline; manufacturer of buspirone advises avoid concomitant use with MAOIs; plasma concentration of *oral* midazolam possibly reduced by St John's wort; increased sedative effect when anxiolytics and hypnotics given with mirtazapine, tricyclic-related antidepressants or tricyclics

Antiepileptics: plasma concentration of clonazepam often reduced by carbamazepine, phenytoin and primidone; plasma concentration of midazolam reduced by carbamazepine; diazepam increases or decreases plasma concentration of phenytoin; benzodiazepines possibly increase or decrease plasma concentration of phenytoin; plasma concentration of clobazam increased by stiripentol; increased risk of side-effects when clonazepam given with valproate; clobazam possibly increases plasma concentration of valproate; plasma concentration of diazepam and lorazepam possibly increased by valproate

- Antifungals: plasma concentration of alprazolam increased by itraconazole and ketoconazole; plasma concentration of midazolam increased by ●fluconazole, ●itraconazole and ●ketoconazole (risk of prolonged sedation); plasma concentration of buspirone increased by itraconazole (reduce dose of buspirone); plasma concentration of midazolam increased by ●posaconazole

Antihistamines: increased sedative effect when anxiolytics and hypnotics given with antihistamines

- Antipsychotics: increased sedative effect when anxiolytics and hypnotics given with antipsychotics; buspirone increases plasma concentration of

Anxiolytics and Hypnotics

- Antipsychotics *(continued)*
  haloperidol; serious adverse events reported with concomitant use of lorazepam and ●clozapine (causality not established); increased risk of hypotension, bradycardia and respiratory depression when *parenteral* benzodiazepines given with *intra-muscular* ●olanzapine; diazepam increases plasma concentration of zotepine

- Antivirals: plasma concentration of midazolam possibly increased by ●atazanavir—avoid concomitant use of *oral* midazolam; increased risk of prolonged sedation when midazolam given with ●efavirenz—avoid concomitant use; increased risk of prolonged sedation and respiratory depression when alprazolam, clonazepam, diazepam, flurazepam or midazolam given with ●fosamprenavir; plasma concentration of midazolam possibly increased by ●indinavir, ●nelfinavir and ●ritonavir (risk of prolonged sedation—avoid concomitant use of *oral* midazolam); increased risk of prolonged sedation when alprazolam given with ●indinavir—avoid concomitant use; plasma concentration of alprazolam, diazepam, flurazepam and zolpidem possibly increased by ●ritonavir (risk of extreme sedation and respiratory depression—avoid concomitant use); plasma concentration of anxiolytics and hypnotics possibly increased by ●ritonavir; plasma concentration of buspirone increased by ritonavir (increased risk of toxicity); plasma concentration of midazolam increased by ●saquinavir (risk of prolonged sedation—avoid concomitant use of *oral* midazolam)

  Aprepitant: plasma concentration of midazolam increased by aprepitant (risk of prolonged sedation)

  Barbiturates: plasma concentration of clonazepam often reduced by phenobarbital

  Beta-blockers: enhanced hypotensive effect when anxiolytics and hypnotics given with beta-blockers

  Calcium-channel Blockers: enhanced hypotensive effect when anxiolytics and hypnotics given with calcium-channel blockers; midazolam increases absorption of lercanidipine; metabolism of midazolam inhibited by diltiazem and verapamil (increased plasma concentration with increased sedation); plasma concentration of buspirone increased by diltiazem and verapamil (reduce dose of buspirone)

  Cardiac Glycosides: alprazolam increases plasma concentration of digoxin (increased risk of toxicity)

  Clonidine: enhanced hypotensive effect when anxiolytics and hypnotics given with clonidine

  Cytotoxics: plasma concentration of midazolam increased by nilotinib

  Deferasirox: plasma concentration of midazolam possibly reduced by deferasirox

  Diazoxide: enhanced hypotensive effect when anxiolytics and hypnotics given with diazoxide

  Disulfiram: metabolism of benzodiazepines inhibited by disulfiram (increased sedative effects); increased risk of temazepam toxicity when given with disulfiram

  Diuretics: enhanced hypotensive effect when anxiolytics and hypnotics given with diuretics; administration of chloral or triclofos with *parenteral* furosemide may displace thyroid hormone from binding sites

  Dopaminergics: benzodiazepines possibly antagonise effects of levodopa

  Grapefruit Juice: plasma concentration of buspirone increased by grapefruit juice

  Lofexidine: increased sedative effect when anxiolytics and hypnotics given with lofexidine

  Methyldopa: enhanced hypotensive effect when anxiolytics and hypnotics given with methyldopa

  Moxonidine: enhanced hypotensive effect when anxiolytics and hypnotics given with moxonidine;

Anxiolytics and Hypnotics

Moxonidine *(continued)*
  sedative effects possibly increased when benzodiazepines given with moxonidine

Muscle Relaxants: increased sedative effect when anxiolytics and hypnotics given with baclofen or tizanidine

Nabilone: increased sedative effect when anxiolytics and hypnotics given with nabilone

Nitrates: enhanced hypotensive effect when anxiolytics and hypnotics given with nitrates

Oestrogens: plasma concentration of melatonin increased by oestrogens

Probenecid: excretion of lorazepam reduced by probenecid (increased plasma concentration); excretion of nitrazepam possibly reduced by probenecid (increased plasma concentration)

- Sodium Oxybate: benzodiazepines enhance effects of ●sodium oxybate (avoid concomitant use)

Theophylline: effects of benzodiazepines possibly reduced by theophylline

Ulcer-healing Drugs: plasma concentration of melatonin increased by cimetidine; metabolism of benzodiazepines, clomethiazole and zaleplon inhibited by cimetidine (increased plasma concentration); metabolism of diazepam possibly inhibited by esomeprazole and omeprazole (increased plasma concentration)

Vasodilator Antihypertensives: enhanced hypotensive effect when anxiolytics and hypnotics given with hydralazine, minoxidil or sodium nitroprusside

Apomorphine

Antipsychotics: effects of apomorphine antagonised by antipsychotics

Dopaminergics: effects of apomorphine possibly enhanced by entacapone

Memantine: effects of dopaminergics possibly enhanced by memantine

Methyldopa: antiparkinsonian effect of dopaminergics antagonised by methyldopa

Apraclonidine

Antidepressants: manufacturer of apraclonidine advises avoid concomitant use with MAOIs, tricyclic-related antidepressants and tricyclics

Aprepitant

Note. Fosaprepitant is a prodrug of aprepitant

Antibacterials: plasma concentration of aprepitant possibly increased by clarithromycin and telithromycin; plasma concentration of aprepitant reduced by rifampicin

Anticoagulants: aprepitant possibly reduces anticoagulant effect of warfarin

- Antidepressants: manufacturer of aprepitant advises avoid concomitant use with ●St John's wort

Antidiabetics: aprepitant reduces plasma concentration of tolbutamide

Antiepileptics: plasma concentration of aprepitant possibly reduced by carbamazepine and phenytoin

Antifungals: plasma concentration of aprepitant increased by ketoconazole

- Antipsychotics: manufacturer of aprepitant advises avoid concomitant use with ●pimozide

Antivirals: plasma concentration of aprepitant possibly increased by ritonavir

Anxiolytics and Hypnotics: aprepitant increases plasma concentration of midazolam (risk of prolonged sedation)

Barbiturates: plasma concentration of aprepitant possibly reduced by phenobarbital

Calcium-channel Blockers: plasma concentration of both drugs may increase when aprepitant given with diltiazem

Corticosteroids: aprepitant inhibits metabolism of dexamethasone and methylprednisolone (reduce dose of dexamethasone and methylprednisolone)

Aprepitant *(continued)*

- Oestrogens: aprepitant possibly causes contraceptive failure of hormonal contraceptives containing ●oestrogens (alternative contraception recommended)
- Progestogens: aprepitant possibly causes contraceptive failure of hormonal contraceptives containing ●progestogens (alternative contraception recommended)

Aripiprazole *see* Antipsychotics

Arsenic Trioxide

- Anti-arrhythmics: increased risk of ventricular arrhythmias when arsenic trioxide given with ●amiodarone or ●disopyramide
- Antibacterials: increased risk of ventricular arrhythmias when arsenic trioxide given with ●erythromycin, ●levofloxacin or ●moxifloxacin
- Antidepressants: increased risk of ventricular arrhythmias when arsenic trioxide given with ●amitriptyline or ●clomipramine
  Antiepileptics: cytotoxics possibly reduce absorption of phenytoin
- Antifungals: increased risk of ventricular arrhythmias when arsenic trioxide given with ●amphotericin
- Antipsychotics: increased risk of ventricular arrhythmias when arsenic trioxide given with ●antipsychotics that prolong the QT interval; increased risk of ventricular arrhythmias when arsenic trioxide given with ●haloperidol; avoid concomitant use of cytotoxics with ●clozapine (increased risk of agranulocytosis)
- Beta-blockers: increased risk of ventricular arrhythmias when arsenic trioxide given with ●sotalol
  Cardiac Glycosides: cytotoxics reduce absorption of digoxin tablets
- Diuretics: risk of ventricular arrhythmias with arsenic trioxide increased by hypokalaemia caused by ●acetazolamide, ●loop diuretics or ●thiazides and related diuretics
- Lithium: increased risk of ventricular arrhythmias when arsenic trioxide given with ●lithium

Artemether with Lumefantrine

- Anti-arrhythmics: manufacturer of artemether/lumefantrine advises avoid concomitant use with ●amiodarone, ●disopyramide or ●flecainide (risk of ventricular arrhythmias)
- Antibacterials: manufacturer of artemether/lumefantrine advises avoid concomitant use with ●macrolides and ●quinolones
- Antidepressants: manufacturer of artemether/lumefantrine advises avoid concomitant use with ●antidepressants
- Antifungals: manufacturer of artemether/lumefantrine advises avoid concomitant use with ●imidazoles and ●triazoles
- Antimalarials: manufacturer of artemether/lumefantrine advises avoid concomitant use with ●antimalarials; increased risk of ventricular arrhythmias when artemether/lumefantrine given with ●quinine
- Antipsychotics: manufacturer of artemether/lumefantrine advises avoid concomitant use with ●antipsychotics
  Antivirals: manufacturer of artemether/lumefantrine advises caution with atazanavir, darunavir, fosamprenavir, indinavir, lopinavir, nelfinavir, ritonavir, saquinavir and tipranavir
- Beta-blockers: manufacturer of artemether/lumefantrine advises avoid concomitant use with ●metoprolol and atenolol
  Grapefruit Juice: plasma concentration of artemether/lumefantrine possibly increased by grapefruit juice
- Ulcer-healing Drugs: manufacturer of artemether/lumefantrine advises avoid concomitant use with ●cimetidine

Artemether with Lumefantrine *(continued)*
  Vaccines: antimalarials inactivate oral typhoid vaccine–see p. 760

Ascorbic acid *see* Vitamins

Aspirin

  Adsorbents: absorption of aspirin possibly reduced by kaolin
  Anaesthetics, General: aspirin possibly enhances effects of thiopental
- Analgesics: avoid concomitant use of aspirin with ●NSAIDs (increased side-effects); antiplatelet effect of aspirin possibly reduced by ibuprofen
  Antacids: excretion of aspirin increased by alkaline urine due to some antacids
- Anticoagulants: increased risk of bleeding when aspirin given with ●coumarins or ●phenindione (due to antiplatelet effect); aspirin enhances anticoagulant effect of ●heparins
- Antidepressants: increased risk of bleeding when aspirin given with ●SSRIs or ●venlafaxine
  Antiepileptics: aspirin enhances effects of phenytoin and valproate
  Cilostazol: manufacturer of cilostazol recommends dose of aspirin should not exceed 80 mg daily when given with cilostazol
  Clopidogrel: increased risk of bleeding when aspirin given with clopidogrel
  Corticosteroids: increased risk of gastro-intestinal bleeding and ulceration when aspirin given with corticosteroids, also corticosteroids reduce plasma concentration of salicylate
- Cytotoxics: aspirin reduces excretion of ●methotrexate (increased risk of toxicity)
  Diuretics: aspirin antagonises diuretic effect of spironolactone; increased risk of toxicity when high-dose aspirin given with carbonic anhydrase inhibitors
  Iloprost: increased risk of bleeding when aspirin given with iloprost
  Leukotriene Receptor Antagonists: aspirin increases plasma concentration of zafirlukast
  Metoclopramide: rate of absorption of aspirin increased by metoclopramide (enhanced effect)
  Probenecid: aspirin antagonises effects of probenecid
  Sibutramine: increased risk of bleeding when aspirin given with sibutramine
  Sulfinpyrazone: aspirin antagonises effects of sulfinpyrazone

Atazanavir

  Antacids: plasma concentration of atazanavir possibly reduced by antacids
- Anti-arrhythmics: atazanavir possibly increases plasma concentration of ●amiodarone and ●lidocaine
- Antibacterials: plasma concentration of both drugs increased when atazanavir given with clarithromycin; atazanavir increases plasma concentration of ●rifabutin (reduce dose of rifabutin); plasma concentration of atazanavir reduced by ●rifampicin—avoid concomitant use; avoidance of concomitant atazanavir in severe renal and hepatic impairment advised by manufacturer of ●telithromycin
  Anticoagulants: atazanavir may enhance or reduce anticoagulant effect of warfarin; avoidance of atazanavir advised by manufacturer of rivaroxaban
- Antidepressants: plasma concentration of atazanavir reduced by ●St John's wort—avoid concomitant use
- Antifungals: plasma concentration of atazanavir increased by ●posaconazole
  Antimalarials: caution with atazanavir advised by manufacturer of artemether/lumefantrine
  Antimuscarinics: avoidance of atazanavir advised by manufacturer of darifenacin; manufacturer of fesoterodine advises dose reduction when atazanavir given with fesoterodine—consult fesoterodine product literature

Atazanavir *(continued)*
- Antipsychotics: atazanavir possibly inhibits metabolism of ●aripiprazole (reduce dose of aripiprazole); atazanavir possibly increases plasma concentration of ●pimozide—avoid concomitant use
- Antivirals: manufacturer of atazanavir advises avoid concomitant use with ●efavirenz (plasma concentration of atazanavir reduced); avoid concomitant use of atazanavir with ●indinavir; atazanavir increases plasma concentration of ●maraviroc (consider reducing dose of maraviroc); plasma concentration of atazanavir possibly reduced by ●nevirapine—avoid concomitant use; atazanavir increases plasma concentration of saquinavir; plasma concentration of atazanavir reduced by tenofovir, also plasma concentration of tenofovir possibly increased; atazanavir increases plasma concentration of tipranavir (also plasma concentration of atazanavir reduced)
- Anxiolytics and Hypnotics: atazanavir possibly increases plasma concentration of ●midazolam—avoid concomitant use of *oral* midazolam
- Calcium-channel Blockers: atazanavir increases plasma concentration of ●diltiazem (reduce dose of diltiazem); atazanavir possibly increases plasma concentration of verapamil
- Ciclosporin: atazanavir possibly increases plasma concentration of ●ciclosporin
- Cytotoxics: atazanavir possibly increases plasma concentration of ●everolimus—manufacturer of everolimus advises avoid concomitant use; atazanavir possibly inhibits metabolism of ●irinotecan (increased risk of toxicity)
- Ergot Alkaloids: atazanavir possibly increases plasma concentration of ●ergot alkaloids—avoid concomitant use
- Lipid-regulating Drugs: possible increased risk of myopathy when atazanavir given with atorvastatin; possible increased risk of myopathy when atazanavir given with ●rosuvastatin—avoid concomitant use; increased risk of myopathy when atazanavir given with ●simvastatin (avoid concomitant use)
  Oestrogens: atazanavir increases plasma concentration of ethinylestradiol
- Ranolazine: atazanavir possibly increases plasma concentration of ●ranolazine—manufacturer of ranolazine advises avoid concomitant use
- Sildenafil: atazanavir possibly increases side-effects of ●sildenafil
- Sirolimus: atazanavir possibly increases plasma concentration of ●sirolimus
- Tacrolimus: atazanavir possibly increases plasma concentration of ●tacrolimus
- Ulcer-healing Drugs: plasma concentration of atazanavir possibly reduced by histamine H$_2$-antagonists; plasma concentration of atazanavir reduced by ●proton pump inhibitors

Atenolol *see* Beta-blockers
Atomoxetine
- Analgesics: increased risk of ventricular arrhythmias when atomoxetine given with ●methadone; possible increased risk of convulsions when atomoxetine given with tramadol
- Anti-arrhythmics: increased risk of ventricular arrhythmias when atomoxetine given with ●amiodarone or ●disopyramide
- Antibacterials: increased risk of ventricular arrhythmias when atomoxetine given with *parenteral* ●erythromycin; increased risk of ventricular arrhythmias when atomoxetine given with ●moxifloxacin
- Antidepressants: metabolism of atomoxetine possibly inhibited by fluoxetine and paroxetine; possible increased risk of convulsions when atomoxetine given with antidepressants; atomoxetine should not be started until 2 weeks after stopping ●MAOIs, also MAOIs should not be started until at least 2 weeks

Atomoxetine
- Antidepressants *(continued)*
  after stopping atomoxetine; increased risk of ventricular arrhythmias when atomoxetine given with ●tricyclics
- Antimalarials: increased risk of ventricular arrhythmias when atomoxetine given with ●mefloquine
- Antipsychotics: increased risk of ventricular arrhythmias when atomoxetine given with ●antipsychotics that prolong the QT interval
- Beta-blockers: increased risk of ventricular arrhythmias when atomoxetine given with ●sotalol
  Bupropion: possible increased risk of convulsions when atomoxetine given with bupropion
- Diuretics: risk of ventricular arrhythmias with atomoxetine increased by hypokalaemia caused by ●diuretics
  Sympathomimetics, Beta$_2$: Increased risk of cardiovascular side-effects when atomoxetine given with *parenteral* salbutamol

Atorvastatin *see* Statins
Atovaquone
- Antibacterials: plasma concentration of atovaquone reduced by ●rifabutin and ●rifampicin (possible therapeutic failure of atovaquone); plasma concentration of atovaquone reduced by tetracycline
  Antivirals: atovaquone possibly reduces plasma concentration of indinavir; atovaquone possibly inhibits metabolism of zidovudine (increased plasma concentration)
  Metoclopramide: plasma concentration of atovaquone reduced by metoclopramide

Atracurium *see* Muscle Relaxants
Atropine *see* Antimuscarinics
Azapropazone *see* NSAIDs
Azathioprine
  ACE Inhibitors: increased risk of anaemia or leucopenia when azathioprine given with captopril especially in renal impairment; increased risk of anaemia when azathioprine given with enalapril especially in renal impairment
- Allopurinol: enhanced effects and increased toxicity of azathioprine when given with ●allopurinol (reduce dose of azathioprine to one quarter of usual dose)
  Aminosalicylates: possible increased risk of leucopenia when azathioprine given with aminosalicylates
- Antibacterials: increased risk of haematological toxicity when azathioprine given with ●sulfamethoxazole (as co-trimoxazole); increased risk of haematological toxicity when azathioprine given with ●trimethoprim (also with co-trimoxazole)
- Anticoagulants: azathioprine possibly reduces anticoagulant effect of ●coumarins

Azithromycin *see* Macrolides
Aztreonam
- Anticoagulants: aztreonam possibly enhances anticoagulant effect of ●coumarins
  Oestrogens: antibacterials that do not induce liver enzymes possibly reduce contraceptive effect of oestrogens (risk probably small, see p. 486)
  Vaccines: antibacterials inactivate oral typhoid vaccine—see p. 760

Baclofen *see* Muscle Relaxants
Balsalazide *see* Aminosalicylates
Bambuterol *see* Sympathomimetics, Beta$_2$
Barbiturates
  Alcohol: increased sedative effect when barbiturates given with alcohol
  Analgesics: phenobarbital reduces plasma concentration of methadone; barbiturates possibly increase CNS effects of opioid analgesics
  Anti-arrhythmics: barbiturates accelerate metabolism of disopyramide (reduced plasma concentration)
- Antibacterials: barbiturates accelerate metabolism of ●chloramphenicol, doxycycline and metronidazole (reduced plasma concentration);

Barbiturates
- Antibacterials *(continued)*
  phenobarbital possibly reduces plasma concentration of rifampicin; phenobarbital reduces plasma concentration of ●telithromycin (avoid during and for 2 weeks after phenobarbital)
- Anticoagulants: barbiturates accelerate metabolism of ●coumarins (reduced anticoagulant effect)
- Antidepressants: phenobarbital reduces plasma concentration of paroxetine; phenobarbital accelerates metabolism of ●mianserin (reduced plasma concentration); anticonvulsant effect of barbiturates possibly antagonised by MAOIs and ●tricyclic-related antidepressants (convulsive threshold lowered); anticonvulsant effect of barbiturates antagonised by SSRIs (convulsive threshold lowered); avoid concomitant use of phenobarbital with ●St John's wort; anticonvulsant effect of barbiturates antagonised by ●tricyclics (convulsive threshold lowered), also metabolism of tricyclics possibly accelerated (reduced plasma concentration)
- Antiepileptics: phenobarbital reduces plasma concentration of carbamazepine, lamotrigine, tiagabine and zonisamide; phenobarbital possibly reduces plasma concentration of ethosuximide; plasma concentration of phenobarbital increased by oxcarbazepine, also plasma concentration of an active metabolite of oxcarbazepine reduced; plasma concentration of phenobarbital often increased by phenytoin, plasma concentration of phenytoin often reduced but may be increased; increased sedative effect when barbiturates given with primidone; plasma concentration of phenobarbital increased by ●stiripentol; plasma concentration of phenobarbital increased by valproate (also plasma concentration of valproate reduced); plasma concentration of phenobarbital possibly reduced by vigabatrin
- Antifungals: phenobarbital possibly reduces plasma concentration of itraconazole and ●posaconazole; phenobarbital possibly reduces plasma concentration of ●voriconazole—avoid concomitant use; phenobarbital reduces absorption of griseofulvin (reduced effect)
- Antipsychotics: anticonvulsant effect of barbiturates antagonised by ●antipsychotics (convulsive threshold lowered); phenobarbital accelerates metabolism of haloperidol (reduced plasma concentration); plasma concentration of both drugs reduced when phenobarbital given with chlorpromazine; phenobarbital possibly reduces plasma concentration of ●aripiprazole—increase dose of aripiprazole
- Antivirals: phenobarbital possibly reduces plasma concentration of abacavir, darunavir, fosamprenavir and ●lopinavir; avoidance of phenobarbital advised by manufacturer of etravirine; barbiturates possibly reduce plasma concentration of ●indinavir, ●nelfinavir and ●saquinavir; phenobarbital possibly reduces plasma concentration of ●indinavir, also plasma concentration of phenobarbital possibly increased
  Anxiolytics and Hypnotics: phenobarbital often reduces plasma concentration of clonazepam
  Aprepitant: phenobarbital possibly reduces plasma concentration of aprepitant
  Beta-blockers: barbiturates reduce plasma concentration of metoprolol and timolol; barbiturates possibly reduce plasma concentration of propranolol
- Calcium-channel Blockers: barbiturates reduce effects of ●felodipine and ●isradipine; barbiturates probably reduce effects of ●dihydropyridines, ●diltiazem and ●verapamil
  Cardiac Glycosides: barbiturates accelerate metabolism of digitoxin (reduced effect)
- Ciclosporin: barbiturates accelerate metabolism of ●ciclosporin (reduced effect)

Barbiturates *(continued)*
- Corticosteroids: barbiturates accelerate metabolism of ●corticosteroids (reduced effect)
  Cytotoxics: avoidance of barbiturates advised by manufacturer of gefitinib; phenobarbital possibly reduces plasma concentration of etoposide; phenobarbital reduces plasma concentration of irinotecan and its active metabolite
- Diuretics: phenobarbital reduces plasma concentration of ●eplerenone—avoid concomitant use; increased risk of osteomalacia when phenobarbital given with carbonic anhydrase inhibitors
  Folates: plasma concentration of phenobarbital possibly reduced by folates
  Hormone Antagonists: barbiturates possibly accelerate metabolism of toremifene (reduced plasma concentration)
  Leukotriene Receptor Antagonists: phenobarbital reduces plasma concentration of montelukast
  Lofexidine: increased sedative effect when barbiturates given with lofexidine
  Memantine: effects of barbiturates possibly reduced by memantine
- Oestrogens: barbiturates accelerate metabolism of ●oestrogens (reduced contraceptive effect—see p. 486)
- Progestogens: barbiturates accelerate metabolism of ●progestogens (reduced contraceptive effect—see p. 486)
- Sodium Oxybate: barbiturates enhance effects of ●sodium oxybate (avoid concomitant use)
  Sympathomimetics: plasma concentration of phenobarbital possibly increased by methylphenidate
- Tacrolimus: phenobarbital reduces plasma concentration of ●tacrolimus
  Theophylline: barbiturates accelerate metabolism of theophylline (reduced effect)
  Thyroid Hormones: barbiturates accelerate metabolism of thyroid hormones (may increase requirements for thyroid hormones in hypothyroidism)
  Tibolone: barbiturates accelerate metabolism of tibolone (reduced plasma concentration)
- Ulipristal: avoidance of phenobarbital advised by manufacturer of ●ulipristal (contraceptive effect of ulipristal possibly reduced)
  Vitamins: barbiturates possibly increase requirements for vitamin D

Beclometasone *see* Corticosteroids
Bemiparin *see* Heparins
Bendroflumethiazide *see* Diuretics
Benperidol *see* Antipsychotics
Benzodiazepines *see* Anxiolytics and Hypnotics
Benzthiazide *see* Diuretics
Benzylpenicillin *see* Penicillins
Beta-blockers
  Note. Since systemic absorption may follow topical application of beta-blockers to the eye the possibility of interactions, in particular, with drugs such as verapamil should be borne in mind
  ACE Inhibitors: enhanced hypotensive effect when beta-blockers given with ACE inhibitors
  Adrenergic Neurone Blockers: enhanced hypotensive effect when beta-blockers given with adrenergic neurone blockers
  Alcohol: enhanced hypotensive effect when beta-blockers given with alcohol
  Aldesleukin: enhanced hypotensive effect when beta-blockers given with aldesleukin
  Alpha-blockers: enhanced hypotensive effect when beta-blockers given with ●alpha-blockers, also increased risk of first-dose hypotension with post-synaptic alpha-blockers such as prazosin
  Anaesthetics, General: enhanced hypotensive effect when beta-blockers given with general anaesthetics
- Anaesthetics, Local: propranolol increases risk of ●bupivacaine toxicity

Beta-blockers *(continued)*

Analgesics: hypotensive effect of beta-blockers antagonised by NSAIDs; plasma concentration of esmolol possibly increased by morphine

Angiotensin-II Receptor Antagonists: enhanced hypotensive effect when beta-blockers given with angiotensin-II receptor antagonists

• Anti-arrhythmics: increased myocardial depression when beta-blockers given with ●anti-arrhythmics; increased risk of bradycardia, AV block and myocardial depression when beta-blockers given with ●amiodarone; increased risk of ventricular arrhythmias when sotalol given with ●amiodarone or ●disopyramide—avoid concomitant use; increased risk of myocardial depression and bradycardia when beta-blockers given with ●flecainide; propranolol increases risk of ●lidocaine toxicity; plasma concentration of metoprolol and propranolol increased by propafenone

• Antibacterials: increased risk of ventricular arrhythmias when sotalol given with ●moxifloxacin—avoid concomitant use; metabolism of bisoprolol and propranolol accelerated by rifampicin (plasma concentration significantly reduced); plasma concentration of carvedilol, celiprolol and metoprolol reduced by rifampicin

• Antidepressants: plasma concentration of metoprolol increased by citalopram and escitalopram; plasma concentration of propranolol increased by fluvoxamine; plasma concentration of metoprolol possibly increased by paroxetine (enhanced effect); labetalol and propranolol increase plasma concentration of imipramine; enhanced hypotensive effect when beta-blockers given with MAOIs; increased risk of ventricular arrhythmias when sotalol given with ●tricyclics

Antidiabetics: beta-blockers may mask warning signs of hypoglycaemia (such as tremor) with antidiabetics; beta-blockers enhance hypoglycaemic effect of insulin

• Antihistamines: increased risk of ventricular arrhythmias when sotalol given with ●mizolastine—avoid concomitant use

• Antimalarials: avoidance of metoprolol and sotalol advised by manufacturer of ●artemether/lumefantrine; increased risk of bradycardia when beta-blockers given with mefloquine

• Antimuscarinics: increased risk of ventricular arrhythmias when sotalol given with ●tolterodine

• Antipsychotics: increased risk of ventricular arrhythmias when sotalol given with ●droperidol or ●zuclopenthixol—avoid concomitant use; possible increased risk of ventricular arrhythmias when sotalol given with ●haloperidol—avoid concomitant use; plasma concentration of both drugs may increase when propranolol given with ●chlorpromazine; increased risk of ventricular arrhythmias when sotalol given with ●amisulpride, ●phenothiazines, ●pimozide, ●sertindole or ●sulpiride; enhanced hypotensive effect when beta-blockers given with phenothiazines

• Antivirals: avoidance of metoprolol for heart failure advised by manufacturer of ●tipranavir

Anxiolytics and Hypnotics: enhanced hypotensive effect when beta-blockers given with anxiolytics and hypnotics

• Atomoxetine: increased risk of ventricular arrhythmias when sotalol given with ●atomoxetine

Barbiturates: plasma concentration of metoprolol and timolol reduced by barbiturates; plasma concentration of propranolol possibly reduced by barbiturates

• Calcium-channel Blockers: enhanced hypotensive effect when beta-blockers given with calcium-channel blockers; possible severe hypotension and heart failure when beta-blockers given with ●nifedipine; increased risk of AV block and brady-

Beta-blockers

• Calcium-channel Blockers *(continued)*
cardia when beta-blockers given with ●diltiazem; asystole, severe hypotension and heart failure when beta-blockers given with ●verapamil (see p. 141)

Cardiac Glycosides: increased risk of AV block and bradycardia when beta-blockers given with cardiac glycosides

• Ciclosporin: carvedilol increases plasma concentration of ●ciclosporin

• Clonidine: increased risk of withdrawal hypertension when beta-blockers given with ●clonidine (withdraw beta-blockers several days before slowly withdrawing clonidine)

Corticosteroids: hypotensive effect of beta-blockers antagonised by corticosteroids

• Cytotoxics: increased risk of ventricular arrhythmias when sotalol given with ●arsenic trioxide

Diazoxide: enhanced hypotensive effect when beta-blockers given with diazoxide

• Diuretics: enhanced hypotensive effect when beta-blockers given with diuretics; risk of ventricular arrhythmias with sotalol increased by hypokalaemia caused by ●loop diuretics or ●thiazides and related diuretics

Dopaminergics: enhanced hypotensive effect when beta-blockers given with levodopa

Ergot Alkaloids: increased peripheral vasoconstriction when beta-blockers given with ergotamine and methysergide

5HT$_1$ Agonists: propranolol increases plasma concentration of rizatriptan (manufacturer of rizatriptan advises halve dose and avoid within 2 hours of propranolol)

• Ivabradine: increased risk of ventricular arrhythmias when sotalol given with ●ivabradine

Methyldopa: enhanced hypotensive effect when beta-blockers given with methyldopa

• Moxisylyte: possible severe postural hypotension when beta-blockers given with ●moxisylyte

Moxonidine: enhanced hypotensive effect when beta-blockers given with moxonidine

Muscle Relaxants: propranolol enhances effects of muscle relaxants; enhanced hypotensive effect when beta-blockers given with baclofen; possible enhanced hypotensive effect and bradycardia when beta-blockers given with tizanidine

Nitrates: enhanced hypotensive effect when beta-blockers given with nitrates

Oestrogens: hypotensive effect of beta-blockers antagonised by oestrogens

Parasympathomimetics: propranolol antagonises effects of neostigmine and pyridostigmine; increased risk of arrhythmias when beta-blockers given with pilocarpine

Prostaglandins: enhanced hypotensive effect when beta-blockers given with alprostadil

• Ranolazine: avoidance of sotalol advised by manufacturer of ●ranolazine

• Sympathomimetics: increased risk of severe hypertension and bradycardia when non-cardioselective beta-blockers given with ●adrenaline (epinephrine), also reponse to adrenaline (epinephrine) may be reduced; increased risk of severe hypertension and bradycardia when non-cardioselective beta-blockers given with ●dobutamine; possible increased risk of severe hypertension and bradycardia when non-cardioselective beta-blockers given with ●noradrenaline (norepinephrine)

Thyroid Hormones: metabolism of propranolol accelerated by levothyroxine

Ulcer-healing Drugs: plasma concentration of labetalol, metoprolol and propranolol increased by cimetidine

Vasodilator Antihypertensives: enhanced hypotensive effect when beta-blockers given with hydralazine, minoxidil or sodium nitroprusside

Betahistine

Antihistamines: effect of betahistine theoretically antagonised by antihistamines

Betamethasone *see* Corticosteroids

Betaxolol *see* Beta-blockers

Bethanechol *see* Parasympathomimetics

Bexarotene

Antiepileptics: cytotoxics possibly reduce absorption of phenytoin

• Antipsychotics: avoid concomitant use of cytotoxics with ●clozapine (increased risk of agranulocytosis)

Cardiac Glycosides: cytotoxics reduce absorption of digoxin tablets

• Lipid-regulating Drugs: plasma concentration of bexarotene increased by ●gemfibrozil—avoid concomitant use

Bezafibrate *see* Fibrates

Bicalutamide

Anticoagulants: bicalutamide possibly enhances anticoagulant effect of coumarins

Biguanides *see* Antidiabetics

Bile Acid Sequestrants *see* Colesevelam, Colestipol, and Colestyramine

Bile Acids *see* Ursodeoxycholic Acid

Bisoprolol *see* Beta-blockers

Bisphosphonates

Analgesics: bioavailability of tiludronic acid increased by indometacin

Antacids: absorption of bisphosphonates reduced by antacids

Antibacterials: increased risk of hypocalcaemia when bisphosphonates given with aminoglycosides

Calcium Salts: absorption of bisphosphonates reduced by calcium salts

• Cytotoxics: sodium clodronate increases plasma concentration of ●estramustine

Iron: absorption of bisphosphonates reduced by *oral* iron

Bleomycin

Antiepileptics: cytotoxics possibly reduce absorption of phenytoin

• Antipsychotics: avoid concomitant use of cytotoxics with ●clozapine (increased risk of agranulocytosis)

Cardiac Glycosides: cytotoxics reduce absorption of digoxin tablets

• Cytotoxics: increased pulmonary toxicity when bleomycin given with ●cisplatin

Bortezomib

Antiepileptics: cytotoxics possibly reduce absorption of phenytoin

Antifungals: plasma concentration of bortezomib increased by ketoconazole

• Antipsychotics: avoid concomitant use of cytotoxics with ●clozapine (increased risk of agranulocytosis)

Cardiac Glycosides: cytotoxics reduce absorption of digoxin tablets

Bosentan

• Antibacterials: plasma concentration of bosentan reduced by ●rifampicin—avoid concomitant use

Anticoagulants: manufacturer of bosentan recommends monitoring anticoagulant effect of coumarins

• Antidiabetics: increased risk of hepatotoxicity when bosentan given with ●glibenclamide—avoid concomitant use

• Antifungals: plasma concentration of bosentan increased by ketoconazole; plasma concentration of bosentan possibly increased by ●fluconazole—avoid concomitant use; plasma concentration of bosentan possibly increased by itraconazole

Antivirals: plasma concentration of bosentan possibly increased by ritonavir

• Ciclosporin: plasma concentration of bosentan increased by ●ciclosporin (also plasma concentration of ciclosporin reduced—avoid concomitant use)

Lipid-regulating Drugs: bosentan reduces plasma concentration of simvastatin

Bosentan *(continued)*

• Oestrogens: bosentan possibly causes contraceptive failure of hormonal contraceptives containing ●oestrogens (alternative contraception recommended)

• Progestogens: bosentan possibly causes contraceptive failure of hormonal contraceptives containing ●progestogens (alternative contraception recommended)

Sildenafil: bosentan reduces plasma concentration of sildenafil

Brimonidine

Antidepressants: manufacturer of brimonidine advises avoid concomitant use with MAOIs, tricyclic-related antidepressants and tricyclics

Brinzolamide *see* Diuretics

Bromocriptine

Alcohol: tolerance of bromocriptine reduced by alcohol

Antibacterials: plasma concentration of bromocriptine increased by erythromycin (increased risk of toxicity); plasma concentration of bromocriptine possibly increased by macrolides (increased risk of toxicity)

Antipsychotics: hypoprolactinaemic and antiparkinsonian effects of bromocriptine antagonised by antipsychotics

Domperidone: hypoprolactinaemic effect of bromocriptine possibly antagonised by domperidone

Hormone Antagonists: plasma concentration of bromocriptine increased by octreotide

Memantine: effects of dopaminergics possibly enhanced by memantine

Methyldopa: antiparkinsonian effect of dopaminergics antagonised by methyldopa

Metoclopramide: hypoprolactinaemic effect of bromocriptine antagonised by metoclopramide

• Sympathomimetics: risk of toxicity when bromocriptine given with ●isometheptene

Buclizine *see* Antihistamines

Budesonide *see* Corticosteroids

Bumetanide *see* Diuretics

Bupivacaine

Anti-arrhythmics: increased myocardial depression when bupivacaine given with anti-arrhythmics

• Beta-blockers: increased risk of bupivacaine toxicity when given with ●propranolol

Buprenorphine *see* Opioid Analgesics

Bupropion

Note. Bupropion should be administered with extreme caution to patients receiving other medication known to lower the seizure threshold—see CSM advice BNF section 4.10 and Cautions, Contra-indications and Side-effects of individual drugs

• Antidepressants: bupropion possibly increases plasma concentration of citalopram; manufacturer of bupropion advises avoid for 2 weeks after stopping ●MAOIs; manufacturer of bupropion advises avoid concomitant use with ●moclobemide

Antiepileptics: plasma concentration of bupropion reduced by carbamazepine and phenytoin; metabolism of bupropion inhibited by valproate

Antivirals: plasma concentration of bupropion reduced by ritonavir

Atomoxetine: possible increased risk of convulsions when bupropion given with atomoxetine

Dopaminergics: increased risk of side-effects when bupropion given with amantadine or levodopa

• Hormone Antagonists: bupropion possibly inhibits metabolism of ●tamoxifen to active metabolite (avoid concomitant use)

Buspirone *see* Anxiolytics and Hypnotics

Busulfan

Analgesics: metabolism of *intravenous* busulfan possibly inhibited by paracetamol (manufacturer of *intravenous* busulfan advises caution within 72 hours of paracetamol)

Busulfan *(continued)*
- Antibacterials: plasma concentration of busulfan increased by ●metronidazole (increased risk of toxicity)
  Antiepileptics: cytotoxics possibly reduce absorption of phenytoin; plasma concentration of busulfan possibly reduced by phenytoin
  Antifungals: metabolism of busulfan inhibited by itraconazole (increased risk of toxicity)
- Antipsychotics: avoid concomitant use of cytotoxics with ●clozapine (increased risk of agranulocytosis)
  Cardiac Glycosides: cytotoxics reduce absorption of digoxin tablets
  Cytotoxics: increased risk of hepatotoxicity when busulfan given with tioguanine

Butobarbital *see* Barbiturates

Butyrophenones *see* Antipsychotics

Cabergoline
  Antibacterials: plasma concentration of cabergoline increased by erythromycin (increased risk of toxicity); plasma concentration of cabergoline possibly increased by macrolides (increased risk of toxicity)
  Antipsychotics: hypoprolactinaemic and antiparkinsonian effects of cabergoline antagonised by antipsychotics
  Domperidone: hypoprolactinaemic effect of cabergoline possibly antagonised by domperidone
  Memantine: effects of dopaminergics possibly enhanced by memantine
  Methyldopa: antiparkinsonian effect of dopaminergics antagonised by methyldopa
  Metoclopramide: hypoprolactinaemic effect of cabergoline antagonised by metoclopramide

Calcium Salts
  Note. see also Antacids
  Antibacterials: calcium salts reduce absorption of ciprofloxacin and tetracycline
  Bisphosphonates: calcium salts reduce absorption of bisphosphonates
  Cardiac Glycosides: large *intravenous* doses of calcium salts can precipitate arrhythmias when given with cardiac glycosides
  Corticosteroids: absorption of calcium salts reduced by corticosteroids
  Diuretics: increased risk of hypercalcaemia when calcium salts given with thiazides and related diuretics
  Fluorides: calcium salts reduce absorption of fluorides
  Iron: calcium salts reduce absorption of *oral* iron
  Thyroid Hormones: calcium salts reduce absorption of levothyroxine
  Zinc: calcium salts reduce absorption of zinc

Calcium-channel Blockers
  Note. Dihydropyridine calcium-channel blockers include amlodipine, felodipine, isradipine, lacidipine, lercanidipine, nicardipine, nifedipine, and nimodipine
  ACE Inhibitors: enhanced hypotensive effect when calcium-channel blockers given with ACE inhibitors
  Adrenergic Neurone Blockers: enhanced hypotensive effect when calcium-channel blockers given with adrenergic neurone blockers
  Alcohol: enhanced hypotensive effect when calcium-channel blockers given with alcohol; verapamil possibly increases plasma concentration of alcohol
  Aldesleukin: enhanced hypotensive effect when calcium-channel blockers given with aldesleukin
  Aliskiren: avoidance of verapamil advised by manufacturer of aliskiren
- Alpha-blockers: enhanced hypotensive effect when calcium-channel blockers given with ●alpha-blockers, also increased risk of first-dose hypotension with post-synaptic alpha-blockers such as prazosin
- Anaesthetics, General: enhanced hypotensive effect when calcium-channel blockers given with general anaesthetics or isoflurane; hypotensive effect of verapamil enhanced by ●general anaesthetics (also AV delay)

Calcium-channel Blockers *(continued)*
  Analgesics: hypotensive effect of calcium-channel blockers antagonised by NSAIDs; diltiazem inhibits metabolism of alfentanil (risk of prolonged or delayed respiratory depression)
  Angiotensin-II Receptor Antagonists: enhanced hypotensive effect when calcium-channel blockers given with angiotensin-II receptor antagonists
- Anti-arrhythmics: increased risk of bradycardia, AV block and myocardial depression when diltiazem or verapamil given with ●amiodarone; increased risk of myocardial depression and asystole when verapamil given with ●disopyramide or ●flecainide
- Antibacterials: metabolism of verapamil possibly inhibited by ●clarithromycin and ●erythromycin (increased risk of toxicity); metabolism of felodipine possibly inhibited by erythromycin (increased plasma concentration); manufacturer of lercanidipine advises avoid concomitant use with erythromycin; metabolism of diltiazem, nifedipine, nimodipine and verapamil accelerated by ●rifampicin (plasma concentration significantly reduced); metabolism of isradipine and nicardipine possibly accelerated by ●rifampicin (possible significantly reduced plasma concentration); plasma concentration of nifedipine increased by ●quinupristin/dalfopristin
- Antidepressants: metabolism of nifedipine possibly inhibited by fluoxetine (increased plasma concentration); diltiazem and verapamil increase plasma concentration of imipramine; enhanced hypotensive effect when calcium-channel blockers given with MAOIs; plasma concentration of verapamil significantly reduced by ●St John's wort; plasma concentration of nifedipine reduced by St John's wort; plasma concentration of amlodipine possibly reduced by St John's wort; diltiazem and verapamil possibly increase plasma concentration of tricyclics
  Antidiabetics: glucose tolerance occasionally impaired when nifedipine given with insulin
- Antiepileptics: effects of dihydropyridines, nicardipine and nifedipine probably reduced by carbamazepine; effects of felodipine and isradipine reduced by carbamazepine; diltiazem and verapamil enhance effect of ●carbamazepine; effects of dihydropyridines, nicardipine and nifedipine probably reduced by ●phenytoin; effects of felodipine, isradipine and verapamil reduced by phenytoin; diltiazem increases plasma concentration of ●phenytoin but also effect of diltiazem reduced; effects of dihydropyridines, diltiazem and verapamil probably reduced by ●primidone; effects of felodipine and isradipine reduced by ●primidone
- Antifungals: metabolism of dihydropyridines possibly inhibited by itraconazole and ketoconazole (increased plasma concentration); metabolism of felodipine inhibited by ●itraconazole and ●ketoconazole (increased plasma concentration); manufacturer of lercanidipine advises avoid concomitant use with itraconazole and ketoconazole; negative inotropic effect possibly increased when calcium-channel blockers given with itraconazole; plasma concentration of nifedipine increased by micafungin
  Antimalarials: possible increased risk of bradycardia when calcium-channel blockers given with mefloquine
  Antimuscarinics: avoidance of verapamil advised by manufacturer of darifenacin
  Antipsychotics: enhanced hypotensive effect when calcium-channel blockers given with antipsychotics
- Antivirals: plasma concentration of diltiazem increased by ●atazanavir (reduce dose of diltiazem); plasma concentration of verapamil possibly increased by atazanavir; plasma concentration of diltiazem reduced by efavirenz; plasma concentration of

Calcium-channel Blockers

- Antivirals *(continued)*
  calcium-channel blockers possibly increased by
  ●ritonavir; manufacturer of lercanidipine advises
  avoid concomitant use with ritonavir

  Anxiolytics and Hypnotics: enhanced hypotensive
  effect when calcium-channel blockers given with
  anxiolytics and hypnotics; diltiazem and verapamil
  inhibit metabolism of midazolam (increased plasma
  concentration with increased sedation); absorption
  of lercanidipine increased by midazolam;
  diltiazem and verapamil increase plasma concentration of buspirone (reduce dose of buspirone)

  Aprepitant: plasma concentration of both drugs may
  increase when diltiazem given with aprepitant

- Barbiturates: effects of dihydropyridines, diltiazem and
  verapamil probably reduced by ●barbiturates; effects
  of felodipine and isradipine reduced by ●barbiturates

- Beta-blockers: enhanced hypotensive effect when
  calcium-channel blockers given with beta-blockers;
  increased risk of AV block and bradycardia when
  diltiazem given with ●beta-blockers; asystole, severe
  hypotension and heart failure when verapamil given
  with ●beta-blockers (see p. 141); possible severe
  hypotension and heart failure when nifedipine given
  with ●beta-blockers

  Calcium-channel Blockers: plasma concentration of
  both drugs may increase when diltiazem given with
  nifedipine

- Cardiac Glycosides: diltiazem, lercanidipine and nicardipine increase plasma concentration of ●digoxin;
  verapamil increases plasma concentration of
  ●digoxin, also increased risk of AV block and
  bradycardia; nifedipine possibly increases plasma
  concentration of ●digoxin

- Ciclosporin: diltiazem, nicardipine and verapamil
  increase plasma concentration of ●ciclosporin;
  combination of lercanidipine with ●ciclosporin may
  increase plasma concentration of either drug (or
  both)—avoid concomitant use; plasma concentration of nifedipine possibly increased by ciclosporin
  (increased risk of toxicity including gingival hyperplasia)

- Cilostazol: diltiazem increases plasma concentration of
  ●cilostazol—avoid concomitant use

  Clonidine: enhanced hypotensive effect when calcium-
  channel blockers given with clonidine

  Corticosteroids: hypotensive effect of calcium-channel
  blockers antagonised by corticosteroids

- Cytotoxics: plasma concentration of both drugs may
  increase when verapamil given with ●everolimus;
  nifedipine possibly inhibits metabolism of vincristine

  Diazoxide: enhanced hypotensive effect when calcium-
  channel blockers given with diazoxide

  Diuretics: enhanced hypotensive effect when calcium-
  channel blockers given with diuretics; diltiazem and
  verapamil increase plasma concentration of eplerenone (reduce dose of eplerenone)

  Dopaminergics: enhanced hypotensive effect when
  calcium-channel blockers given with levodopa

  Grapefruit Juice: plasma concentration of felodipine,
  isradipine, lacidipine, lercanidipine, nicardipine,
  nifedipine, nimodipine and verapamil increased by
  grapefruit juice

  Hormone Antagonists: diltiazem and verapamil
  increase plasma concentration of dutasteride

- Ivabradine: diltiazem and verapamil increase plasma
  concentration of ●ivabradine—avoid concomitant
  use

- Lipid-regulating Drugs: diltiazem increases plasma
  concentration of atorvastatin; possible increased risk
  of myopathy when diltiazem given with simvastatin;
  increased risk of myopathy when verapamil given
  with ●simvastatin

Calcium-channel Blockers *(continued)*

  Lithium: neurotoxicity may occur when diltiazem or
  verapamil given with lithium without increased
  plasma concentration of lithium

- Magnesium (parenteral): profound hypotension
  reported with concomitant use of nifedipine and
  ●parenteral magnesium in pre-eclampsia

  Methyldopa: enhanced hypotensive effect when
  calcium-channel blockers given with methyldopa

  Moxisylyte: enhanced hypotensive effect when
  calcium-channel blockers given with moxisylyte

  Moxonidine: enhanced hypotensive effect when
  calcium-channel blockers given with moxonidine

  Muscle Relaxants: verapamil enhances effects of non-
  depolarising muscle relaxants and suxamethonium;
  enhanced hypotensive effect when calcium-channel
  blockers given with baclofen or tizanidine; risk of
  arrhythmias when diltiazem given with *intravenous*
  dantrolene; hypotension, myocardial depression, and
  hyperkalaemia when verapamil given with *intravenous* dantrolene; calcium-channel blockers possibly enhance effects of non-depolarising muscle
  relaxants

  Nitrates: enhanced hypotensive effect when calcium-
  channel blockers given with nitrates

  Oestrogens: hypotensive effect of calcium-channel
  blockers antagonised by oestrogens

  Prostaglandins: enhanced hypotensive effect when
  calcium-channel blockers given with alprostadil

  Ranolazine: diltiazem and verapamil increase plasma
  concentration of ranolazine (consider reducing dose
  of ranolazine)

  Sildenafil: enhanced hypotensive effect when amlodipine given with sildenafil

- Sirolimus: diltiazem increases plasma concentration of
  ●sirolimus; plasma concentration of both drugs
  increased when verapamil given with ●sirolimus

- Tacrolimus: diltiazem and nifedipine increase plasma
  concentration of ●tacrolimus; felodipine,
  nicardipine and verapamil possibly increase plasma
  concentration of tacrolimus

- Theophylline: calcium-channel blockers possibly
  increase plasma concentration of ●theophylline
  (enhanced effect); diltiazem increases plasma concentration of theophylline; verapamil increases
  plasma concentration of ●theophylline (enhanced
  effect)

  Ulcer-healing Drugs: metabolism of calcium-channel
  blockers possibly inhibited by cimetidine (increased
  plasma concentration); plasma concentration of
  isradipine increased by cimetidine (halve dose of
  isradipine)

  Vardenafil: enhanced hypotensive effect when nifedipine given with vardenafil

  Vasodilator Antihypertensives: enhanced hypotensive
  effect when calcium-channel blockers given with
  hydralazine, minoxidil or sodium nitroprusside

Calcium-channel Blockers (dihydropyridines) *see*
  Calcium-channel Blockers

Candesartan *see* Angiotensin-II Receptor Antagonists

Capecitabine *see* Fluorouracil

Capreomycin

  Antibacterials: increased risk of nephrotoxicity when
  capreomycin given with colistin or polymyxins;
  increased risk of nephrotoxicity and ototoxicity when
  capreomycin given with aminoglycosides or vancomycin

  Cytotoxics: increased risk of nephrotoxicity and
  ototoxicity when capreomycin given with platinum
  compounds

  Oestrogens: antibacterials that do not induce liver
  enzymes possibly reduce contraceptive effect of
  oestrogens (risk probably small, see p. 486)

  Vaccines: antibacterials inactivate oral typhoid
  vaccine–see p. 760

Captopril *see* ACE Inhibitors

Carbamazepine

Alcohol: CNS side-effects of carbamazepine possibly increased by alcohol

- Analgesics: effects of carbamazepine enhanced by ●dextropropoxyphene; carbamazepine reduces plasma concentration of methadone; carbamazepine reduces effects of tramadol; carbamazepine possibly accelerates metabolism of paracetamol
- Antibacterials: plasma concentration of carbamazepine increased by ●clarithromycin and ●erythromycin; plasma concentration of carbamazepine reduced by ●rifabutin; carbamazepine accelerates metabolism of doxycycline (reduced effect); plasma concentration of carbamazepine increased by ●isoniazid (also possibly increased isoniazid hepatotoxicity); carbamazepine reduces plasma concentration of ●telithromycin (avoid during and for 2 weeks after carbamazepine)
- Anticoagulants: carbamazepine accelerates metabolism of ●coumarins (reduced anticoagulant effect)
- Antidepressants: plasma concentration of carbamazepine increased by ●fluoxetine and ●fluvoxamine; carbamazepine reduces plasma concentration of ●mianserin and mirtazapine; manufacturer of carbamazepine advises avoid for 2 weeks after stopping ●MAOIs, also antagonism of anticonvulsant effect; anticonvulsant effect of antiepileptics possibly antagonised by MAOIs and ●tricyclic-related antidepressants (convulsive threshold lowered); anticonvulsant effect of antiepileptics antagonised by ●SSRIs and ●tricyclics (convulsive threshold lowered); avoid concomitant use of antiepileptics with ●St John's wort; carbamazepine accelerates metabolism of ●tricyclics (reduced plasma concentration and reduced effect)
- Antiepileptics: plasma concentration of both drugs reduced when carbamazepine given with eslicarbazepine; carbamazepine possibly reduces plasma concentration of ●ethosuximide; carbamazepine often reduces plasma concentration of lamotrigine, also plasma concentration of an active metabolite of carbamazepine sometimes raised (but evidence is conflicting); possible increased risk of carbamazepine toxicity when given with levetiracetam; plasma concentration of carbamazepine sometimes reduced by oxcarbazepine (but concentration of an active metabolite of carbamazepine may be increased), also plasma concentration of an active metabolite of oxcarbazepine often reduced; plasma concentration of both drugs often reduced when carbamazepine given with phenytoin, also plasma concentration of phenytoin may be increased; plasma concentration of carbamazepine often reduced by primidone, also plasma concentration of primidone sometimes reduced (but concentration of an active metabolite of primidone often increased); plasma concentration of carbamazepine increased by ●stiripentol; carbamazepine reduces plasma concentration of tiagabine and zonisamide; carbamazepine often reduces plasma concentration of topiramate; carbamazepine reduces plasma concentration of valproate, also plasma concentration of active metabolite of carbamazepine increased
- Antifungals: plasma concentration of carbamazepine possibly increased by fluconazole, ketoconazole and miconazole; carbamazepine possibly reduces plasma concentration of itraconazole and ●posaconazole; carbamazepine possibly reduces plasma concentration of ●voriconazole—avoid concomitant use; carbamazepine possibly reduces plasma concentration of caspofungin—consider increasing dose of caspofungin
- Antimalarials: possible increased risk of convulsions when antiepileptics given with chloroquine and hydroxychloroquine; anticonvulsant effect of antiepileptics antagonised by ●mefloquine

Carbamazepine (continued)

- Antipsychotics: anticonvulsant effect of carbamazepine antagonised by ●antipsychotics (convulsive threshold lowered); carbamazepine accelerates metabolism of haloperidol, olanzapine, quetiapine, risperidone and sertindole (reduced plasma concentration); carbamazepine reduces plasma concentration of ●aripiprazole—increase dose of aripiprazole; carbamazepine accelerates metabolism of ●clozapine (reduced plasma concentration), also avoid concomitant use of drugs with substantial potential for causing agranulocytosis; carbamazepine reduces plasma concentration of paliperidone
- Antivirals: carbamazepine possibly reduces plasma concentration of darunavir, fosamprenavir, lopinavir, nelfinavir, saquinavir and tipranavir; plasma concentration of both drugs reduced when carbamazepine given with efavirenz; avoidance of carbamazepine advised by manufacturer of etravirine; carbamazepine possibly reduces plasma concentration of ●indinavir, also plasma concentration of carbamazepine possibly increased; plasma concentration of carbamazepine possibly increased by ●ritonavir

Anxiolytics and Hypnotics: carbamazepine often reduces plasma concentration of clonazepam; carbamazepine reduces plasma concentration of midazolam

Aprepitant: carbamazepine possibly reduces plasma concentration of aprepitant

Barbiturates: plasma concentration of carbamazepine reduced by phenobarbital

Bupropion: carbamazepine reduces plasma concentration of bupropion

- Calcium-channel Blockers: carbamazepine reduces effects of felodipine and isradipine; carbamazepine probably reduces effects of dihydropyridines, nicardipine and nifedipine; effects of carbamazepine enhanced by ●diltiazem and ●verapamil

Cardiac Glycosides: carbamazepine accelerates metabolism of digitoxin (reduced effect)

- Ciclosporin: carbamazepine accelerates metabolism of ●ciclosporin (reduced plasma concentration)
- Clopidogrel: carbamazepine possibly reduces antiplatelet effect of ●clopidogrel
- Corticosteroids: carbamazepine accelerates metabolism of ●corticosteroids (reduced effect)
- Cytotoxics: avoidance of carbamazepine advised by manufacturer of gefitinib; carbamazepine reduces plasma concentration of ●imatinib and ●lapatinib—avoid concomitant use; carbamazepine reduces plasma concentration of irinotecan and its active metabolite
- Diuretics: increased risk of hyponatraemia when carbamazepine given with diuretics; plasma concentration of carbamazepine increased by ●acetazolamide; carbamazepine reduces plasma concentration of ●eplerenone—avoid concomitant use
- Hormone Antagonists: metabolism of carbamazepine inhibited by ●danazol (increased risk of toxicity); carbamazepine possibly accelerates metabolism of toremifene (reduced plasma concentration)

$5HT_3$ Antagonists: carbamazepine accelerates metabolism of ondansetron (reduced effect)

- Lipid-regulating Drugs: carbamazepine reduces plasma concentration of ●simvastatin—consider increasing dose of simvastatin

Lithium: neurotoxicity may occur when carbamazepine given with lithium without increased plasma concentration of lithium

Muscle Relaxants: carbamazepine antagonises muscle relaxant effect of non-depolarising muscle relaxants (accelerated recovery from neuromuscular blockade)

Carbamazepine *(continued)*
- Oestrogens: carbamazepine accelerates metabolism of ●oestrogens (reduced contraceptive effect—see p. 486)
- Orlistat: possible increased risk of convulsions when antiepileptics given with ●orlistat
- Progestogens: carbamazepine accelerates metabolism of ●progestogens (reduced contraceptive effect—see p. 486)

Retinoids: plasma concentration of carbamazepine possibly reduced by isotretinoin

Theophylline: carbamazepine accelerates metabolism of theophylline (reduced effect)

Thyroid Hormones: carbamazepine accelerates metabolism of thyroid hormones (may increase requirements for thyroid hormones in hypothyroidism)

Tibolone: carbamazepine accelerates metabolism of tibolone (reduced plasma concentration)
- Ulcer-healing Drugs: metabolism of carbamazepine inhibited by ●cimetidine (increased plasma concentration)
- Ulipristal: avoidance of carbamazepine advised by manufacturer of ●ulipristal (contraceptive effect of ulipristal possibly reduced)

Vitamins: carbamazepine possibly increases requirements for vitamin D

Carbapenems *see* Doripenem, Ertapenem, Imipenem with Cilastatin, and Meropenem
Carbonic Anhydrase Inhibitors *see* Diuretics
Carboplatin *see* Platinum Compounds
Carboprost *see* Prostaglandins
Cardiac Glycosides

ACE Inhibitors: plasma concentration of digoxin possibly increased by captopril

Alpha-blockers: plasma concentration of digoxin increased by prazosin

Aminosalicylates: absorption of digoxin possibly reduced by sulfasalazine

Analgesics: plasma concentration of cardiac glycosides possibly increased by NSAIDs, also possible exacerbation of heart failure and reduction of renal function

Antacids: absorption of digoxin possibly reduced by antacids
- Anti-arrhythmics: plasma concentration of digoxin increased by ●amiodarone and ●propafenone (halve dose of digoxin)

Antibacterials: plasma concentration of digoxin possibly increased by gentamicin, telithromycin and trimethoprim; absorption of digoxin reduced by neomycin; plasma concentration of digoxin possibly reduced by rifampicin; plasma concentration of digoxin increased by macrolides (increased risk of toxicity); metabolism of digitoxin accelerated by rifamycins (reduced effect)
- Antidepressants: plasma concentration of digoxin reduced by ●St John's wort—avoid concomitant use

Antidiabetics: plasma concentration of digoxin possibly reduced by acarbose; plasma concentration of digoxin increased by sitagliptin

Antiepileptics: metabolism of digitoxin accelerated by carbamazepine, phenytoin and primidone (reduced effect); plasma concentration of digoxin possibly reduced by phenytoin
- Antifungals: increased cardiac toxicity with cardiac glycosides if hypokalaemia occurs with ●amphotericin; plasma concentration of digoxin increased by ●itraconazole
- Antimalarials: plasma concentration of digoxin possibly increased by ●chloroquine and hydroxychloroquine; possible increased risk of bradycardia when digoxin given with mefloquine; plasma concentration of digoxin increased by ●quinine

Antimuscarinics: plasma concentration of digoxin possibly increased by darifenacin

Cardiac Glycosides *(continued)*

Antivirals: plasma concentration of digoxin increased by etravirine; plasma concentration of digoxin possibly increased by ritonavir

Anxiolytics and Hypnotics: plasma concentration of digoxin increased by alprazolam (increased risk of toxicity)

Barbiturates: metabolism of digitoxin accelerated by barbiturates (reduced effect)

Beta-blockers: increased risk of AV block and bradycardia when cardiac glycosides given with beta-blockers

Calcium Salts: arrhythmias can be precipitated when cardiac glycosides given with large *intravenous* doses of calcium salts
- Calcium-channel Blockers: plasma concentration of digoxin increased by ●diltiazem, ●lercanidipine and ●nicardipine; plasma concentration of digoxin possibly increased by ●nifedipine; plasma concentration of digoxin increased by ●verapamil, also increased risk of AV block and bradycardia
- Ciclosporin: plasma concentration of digoxin increased by ●ciclosporin (increased risk of toxicity)

Corticosteroids: increased risk of hypokalaemia when cardiac glycosides given with corticosteroids

Cytotoxics: absorption of digoxin tablets reduced by cytotoxics
- Diuretics: increased cardiac toxicity with cardiac glycosides if hypokalaemia occurs with ●acetazolamide, ●loop diuretics or ●thiazides and related diuretics; plasma concentration of digoxin possibly increased by potassium canrenoate; plasma concentration of digitoxin possibly affected by spironolactone; plasma concentration of digoxin increased by ●spironolactone

Lenalidomide: plasma concentration of digoxin possibly increased by lenalidomide

Lipid-regulating Drugs: absorption of cardiac glycosides possibly reduced by colestipol and colestyramine; plasma concentration of digoxin possibly increased by atorvastatin

Muscle Relaxants: risk of ventricular arrhythmias when cardiac glycosides given with suxamethonium; possible increased risk of bradycardia when cardiac glycosides given with tizanidine

Penicillamine: plasma concentration of digoxin possibly reduced by penicillamine

Ranolazine: plasma concentration of digoxin increased by ranolazine

Sympathomimetics, Beta$_2$: plasma concentration of digoxin possibly reduced by salbutamol

Tolvaptan: plasma concentration of digoxin increased by tolvaptan (increased risk of toxicity)

Ulcer-healing Drugs: plasma concentration of digoxin possibly slightly increased by proton pump inhibitors; absorption of cardiac glycosides possibly reduced by sucralfate

Carmustine

Antiepileptics: cytotoxics possibly reduce absorption of phenytoin
- Antipsychotics: avoid concomitant use of cytotoxics with ●clozapine (increased risk of agranulocytosis)

Cardiac Glycosides: cytotoxics reduce absorption of digoxin tablets

Ulcer-healing Drugs: myelosuppressive effects of carmustine possibly enhanced by cimetidine

Carteolol *see* Beta-blockers
Carvedilol *see* Beta-blockers
Caspofungin

Antibacterials: plasma concentration of caspofungin initially increased and then reduced by rifampicin (consider increasing dose of caspofungin)

Antiepileptics: plasma concentration of caspofungin possibly reduced by carbamazepine and phenytoin—consider increasing dose of caspofungin

Caspofungin *(continued)*

Antivirals: plasma concentration of caspofungin possibly reduced by efavirenz and nevirapine—consider increasing dose of caspofungin

● Ciclosporin: plasma concentration of caspofungin increased by ●ciclosporin (manufacturer of caspofungin recommends monitoring liver enzymes)

Corticosteroids: plasma concentration of caspofungin possibly reduced by dexamethasone—consider increasing dose of caspofungin

● Tacrolimus: caspofungin reduces plasma concentration of ●tacrolimus

Cefaclor *see* Cephalosporins

Cefadroxil *see* Cephalosporins

Cefalexin *see* Cephalosporins

Cefixime *see* Cephalosporins

Cefotaxime *see* Cephalosporins

Cefpodoxime *see* Cephalosporins

Cefradine *see* Cephalosporins

Ceftazidime *see* Cephalosporins

Ceftriaxone *see* Cephalosporins

Cefuroxime *see* Cephalosporins

Celecoxib *see* NSAIDs

Celiprolol *see* Beta-blockers

Cephalosporins

Antacids: absorption of cefaclor and cefpodoxime reduced by antacids

Antibacterials: possible increased risk of nephrotoxicity when cephalosporins given with aminoglycosides

● Anticoagulants: cephalosporins possibly enhance anticoagulant effect of ●coumarins

Oestrogens: antibacterials that do not induce liver enzymes possibly reduce contraceptive effect of oestrogens (risk probably small, see p. 486)

Probenecid: excretion of cephalosporins reduced by probenecid (increased plasma concentration)

Ulcer-healing Drugs: absorption of cefpodoxime reduced by histamine H$_2$-antagonists

Vaccines: antibacterials inactivate oral typhoid vaccine–see p. 760

Certolizumab pegol

● Abatacept: avoid concomitant use of certolizumab pegol with ●abatacept

● Anakinra: avoid concomitant use of certolizumab pegol with ●anakinra

● Vaccines: avoid concomitant use of certolizumab pegol with live ●vaccines (see p. 733)

Cetirizine *see* Antihistamines

Chloral *see* Anxiolytics and Hypnotics

Chloramphenicol

Antibacterials: metabolism of chloramphenicol accelerated by rifampicin (reduced plasma concentration)

● Anticoagulants: chloramphenicol enhances anticoagulant effect of ●coumarins

● Antidiabetics: chloramphenicol enhances effects of ●sulphonylureas

● Antiepileptics: chloramphenicol increases plasma concentration of ●phenytoin (increased risk of toxicity); metabolism of chloramphenicol accelerated by ●primidone (reduced plasma concentration)

● Antipsychotics: avoid concomitant use of chloramphenicol with ●clozapine (increased risk of agranulocytosis)

● Barbiturates: metabolism of chloramphenicol accelerated by ●barbiturates (reduced plasma concentration)

● Ciclosporin: chloramphenicol possibly increases plasma concentration of ●ciclosporin

● Clopidogrel: chloramphenicol possibly reduces antiplatelet effect of ●clopidogrel

Hydroxocobalamin: chloramphenicol reduces response to hydroxocobalamin

Oestrogens: antibacterials that do not induce liver enzymes possibly reduce contraceptive effect of oestrogens (risk probably small, see p. 486)

Chloramphenicol *(continued)*

● Tacrolimus: chloramphenicol possibly increases plasma concentration of ●tacrolimus

Vaccines: antibacterials inactivate oral typhoid vaccine–see p. 760

Chlordiazepoxide *see* Anxiolytics and Hypnotics

Chloroquine and Hydroxychloroquine

Adsorbents: absorption of chloroquine and hydroxychloroquine reduced by kaolin

Agalsidase Alfa and Beta: chloroquine and hydroxychloroquine possibly inhibit effects of agalsidase alfa and beta (manufacturers of agalsidase alfa and beta advise avoid concomitant use)

Antacids: absorption of chloroquine and hydroxychloroquine reduced by antacids

● Anti-arrhythmics: increased risk of ventricular arrhythmias when chloroquine and hydroxychloroquine given with ●amiodarone—avoid concomitant use

● Antibacterials: increased risk of ventricular arrhythmias when chloroquine and hydroxychloroquine given with ●moxifloxacin—avoid concomitant use

Antiepileptics: possible increased risk of convulsions when chloroquine and hydroxychloroquine given with antiepileptics

● Antimalarials: avoidance of antimalarials advised by manufacturer of ●artemether/lumefantrine; increased risk of convulsions when chloroquine and hydroxychloroquine given with ●mefloquine

● Antipsychotics: increased risk of ventricular arrhythmias when chloroquine and hydroxychloroquine given with ●droperidol—avoid concomitant use

● Cardiac Glycosides: chloroquine and hydroxychloroquine possibly increase plasma concentration of ●digoxin

● Ciclosporin: chloroquine and hydroxychloroquine increase plasma concentration of ●ciclosporin (increased risk of toxicity)

Lanthanum: absorption of chloroquine and hydroxychloroquine possibly reduced by lanthanum (give at least 2 hours apart)

Laronidase: chloroquine and hydroxychloroquine possibly inhibit effects of laronidase (manufacturer of laronidase advises avoid concomitant use)

Parasympathomimetics: chloroquine and hydroxychloroquine have potential to increase symptoms of myasthenia gravis and thus diminish effect of neostigmine and pyridostigmine

Ulcer-healing Drugs: metabolism of chloroquine and hydroxychloroquine inhibited by cimetidine (increased plasma concentration)

Vaccines: antimalarials inactivate oral typhoid vaccine–see p. 760

Chlorothiazide *see* Diuretics

Chlorphenamine *see* Antihistamines

Chlorpromazine *see* Antipsychotics

Chlortalidone *see* Diuretics

Ciclesonide *see* Corticosteroids

Ciclosporin

● ACE Inhibitors: increased risk of hyperkalaemia when ciclosporin given with ●ACE inhibitors

● Aliskiren: ciclosporin increases plasma concentration of ●aliskiren—avoid concomitant use

Allopurinol: plasma concentration of ciclosporin possibly increased by allopurinol (risk of nephrotoxicity)

● Analgesics: increased risk of nephrotoxicity when ciclosporin given with ●NSAIDs; ciclosporin increases plasma concentration of ●diclofenac (halve dose of diclofenac)

● Angiotensin-II Receptor Antagonists: increased risk of hyperkalaemia when ciclosporin given with ●angiotensin-II receptor antagonists

Anti-arrhythmics: plasma concentration of ciclosporin possibly increased by amiodarone and propafenone

● Antibacterials: metabolism of ciclosporin inhibited by ●clarithromycin and ●erythromycin (increased plasma concentration); metabolism of ciclosporin

Ciclosporin

- **Antibacterials** *(continued)*
accelerated by ●rifampicin (reduced plasma concentration); plasma concentration of ciclosporin possibly reduced by ●sulfadiazine; plasma concentration of ciclosporin possibly increased by ●chloramphenicol, ●doxycycline and ●telithromycin; increased risk of nephrotoxicity when ciclosporin given with ●aminoglycosides, ●polymyxins, ●quinolones, ●sulphonamides or ●vancomycin; increased risk of myopathy when ciclosporin given with ●daptomycin (preferably avoid concomitant use); metabolism of ciclosporin possibly inhibited by ●macrolides (increased plasma concentration); plasma concentration of ciclosporin increased by ●quinupristin/dalfopristin; increased risk of nephrotoxicity when ciclosporin given with ●trimethoprim, also plasma concentration of ciclosporin reduced by *intravenous* trimethoprim
- **Antidepressants**: plasma concentration of ciclosporin reduced by ●St John's wort—avoid concomitant use
Antidiabetics: ciclosporin possibly enhances hypoglycaemic effect of repaglinide
- **Antiepileptics**: metabolism of ciclosporin accelerated by ●carbamazepine and ●phenytoin (reduced plasma concentration); plasma concentration of ciclosporin possibly reduced by oxcarbazepine; metabolism of ciclosporin accelerated by ●primidone (reduced effect)
- **Antifungals**: metabolism of ciclosporin inhibited by ●fluconazole, ●itraconazole, ●ketoconazole, ●posaconazole and ●voriconazole (increased plasma concentration); metabolism of ciclosporin possibly inhibited by ●miconazole (increased plasma concentration); increased risk of nephrotoxicity when ciclosporin given with ●amphotericin; ciclosporin increases plasma concentration of ●caspofungin (manufacturer of caspofungin recommends monitoring liver enzymes); plasma concentration of ciclosporin possibly reduced by griseofulvin and terbinafine; plasma concentration of ciclosporin possibly increased by micafungin
- **Antimalarials**: plasma concentration of ciclosporin increased by ●chloroquine and hydroxychloroquine (increased risk of toxicity)
Antimuscarinics: avoidance of ciclosporin advised by manufacturer of darifenacin
- **Antivirals**: increased risk of nephrotoxicity when ciclosporin given with aciclovir; plasma concentration of ciclosporin possibly increased by ●atazanavir, ●nelfinavir and ●ritonavir; plasma concentration of ciclosporin possibly reduced by ●efavirenz; plasma concentration of ciclosporin increased by ●indinavir; plasma concentration of both drugs increased when ciclosporin given with ●saquinavir
- **Barbiturates**: metabolism of ciclosporin accelerated by ●barbiturates (reduced effect)
- **Beta-blockers**: plasma concentration of ciclosporin increased by ●carvedilol
- **Bile Acids**: absorption of ciclosporin increased by ●ursodeoxycholic acid
- **Bosentan**: ciclosporin increases plasma concentration of ●bosentan (also plasma concentration of ciclosporin reduced—avoid concomitant use)
- **Calcium-channel Blockers**: combination of ciclosporin with ●lercanidipine may increase plasma concentration of either drug (or both)—avoid concomitant use; plasma concentration of ciclosporin increased by ●diltiazem, ●nicardipine and ●verapamil; ciclosporin possibly increases plasma concentration of nifedipine (increased risk of toxicity including gingival hyperplasia)
- **Cardiac Glycosides**: ciclosporin increases plasma concentration of ●digoxin (increased risk of toxicity)
- **Colchicine**: possible increased risk of nephrotoxicity and myotoxicity when ciclosporin given with

Ciclosporin

- **Colchicine** *(continued)*
●colchicine (increased plasma concentration of ciclosporin)
- **Corticosteroids**: plasma concentration of ciclosporin increased by high-dose ●methylprednisolone (risk of convulsions); ciclosporin increases plasma concentration of prednisolone
- **Cytotoxics**: increased risk of nephrotoxicity when ciclosporin given with ●melphalan; increased risk of neurotoxicity when ciclosporin given with ●doxorubicin; ciclosporin increases plasma concentration of ●epirubicin, ●everolimus and ●idarubicin; ciclosporin reduces excretion of mitoxantrone (increased plasma concentration); risk of toxicity when ciclosporin given with ●methotrexate; plasma concentration of ciclosporin possibly increased by imatinib; *in vitro* studies suggest a possible interaction between ciclosporin and docetaxel (consult docetaxel product literature); ciclosporin possibly increases plasma concentration of etoposide (increased risk of toxicity)
- **Diuretics**: increased risk of hyperkalaemia when ciclosporin given with ●potassium-sparing diuretics and aldosterone antagonists; increased risk of nephrotoxicity and possibly hypermagnesaemia when ciclosporin given with thiazides and related diuretics
- **Grapefruit Juice**: plasma concentration of ciclosporin increased by ●grapefruit juice (increased risk of toxicity)
- **Hormone Antagonists**: metabolism of ciclosporin inhibited by ●danazol (increased plasma concentration); plasma concentration of ciclosporin reduced by lanreotide and ●octreotide
- **Lipid-regulating Drugs**: increased risk of renal impairment when ciclosporin given with bezafibrate or fenofibrate; increased risk of myopathy when ciclosporin given with ●rosuvastatin (avoid concomitant use); plasma concentration of both drugs may increase when ciclosporin given with ●ezetimibe; increased risk of myopathy when ciclosporin given with ●statins
Mannitol: possible increased risk of nephrotoxicity when ciclosporin given with mannitol
- **Metoclopramide**: plasma concentration of ciclosporin increased by ●metoclopramide
Mifamurtide: avoidance of ciclosporin advised by manufacturer of mifamurtide
- **Modafinil**: plasma concentration of ciclosporin reduced by ●modafinil
Oestrogens: plasma concentration of ciclosporin possibly increased by oestrogens
- **Orlistat**: absorption of ciclosporin possibly reduced by ●orlistat
- **Potassium Salts**: increased risk of hyperkalaemia when ciclosporin given with ●potassium salts
- **Progestogens**: metabolism of ciclosporin inhibited by ●progestogens (increased plasma concentration)
Ranolazine: ciclosporin possibly increases plasma concentration of ranolazine
Sevelamer: plasma concentration of ciclosporin possibly reduced by sevelamer
Sirolimus: ciclosporin increases plasma concentration of sirolimus
Sitaxentan: ciclosporin increases plasma concentration of ●sitaxentan—avoid concomitant use
- **Sulfinpyrazone**: plasma concentration of ciclosporin reduced by ●sulfinpyrazone
- **Tacrolimus**: plasma concentration of ciclosporin increased by ●tacrolimus (increased risk of nephrotoxicity)—avoid concomitant use
- **Ulcer-healing Drugs**: plasma concentration of ciclosporin possibly increased by ●cimetidine; plasma concentration of ciclosporin possibly affected by omeprazole

Ciclosporin *(continued)*
Vitamins: plasma concentration of ciclosporin possibly affected by vitamin E

Cidofovir
Antivirals: combination of cidofovir with tenofovir may increase plasma concentration of either drug (or both)

Cilazapril *see* ACE Inhibitors

Cilostazol
- Anagrelide: avoidance of cilostazol advised by manufacturer of ●anagrelide
Analgesics: manufacturer of cilostazol recommends dose of concomitant aspirin should not exceed 80 mg daily
- Antibacterials: plasma concentration of cilostazol increased by ●erythromycin (also plasma concentration of erythromycin reduced)—avoid concomitant use
- Antifungals: plasma concentration of cilostazol possibly increased by ●ketoconazole—avoid concomitant use
- Antivirals: plasma concentration of cilostazol possibly increased by ●fosamprenavir, ●indinavir, ●lopinavir, ●nelfinavir, ●ritonavir and ●saquinavir—avoid concomitant use
- Calcium-channel Blockers: plasma concentration of cilostazol increased by ●diltiazem—avoid concomitant use
- Ulcer-healing Drugs: plasma concentration of cilostazol possibly increased by ●cimetidine and ●lansoprazole—avoid concomitant use; plasma concentration of cilostazol increased by ●omeprazole (risk of toxicity)—avoid concomitant use

Cimetidine *see* Histamine H₂-antagonists

Cinacalcet
Antifungals: metabolism of cinacalcet inhibited by ketoconazole (increased plasma concentration)
Tobacco: metabolism of cinacalcet increased by tobacco smoking (reduced plasma concentration)

Cinnarizine *see* Antihistamines

Ciprofibrate *see* Fibrates

Ciprofloxacin *see* Quinolones

Cisatracurium *see* Muscle Relaxants

Cisplatin *see* Platinum Compounds

Citalopram *see* Antidepressants, SSRI

Clarithromycin *see* Macrolides

Clemastine *see* Antihistamines

Clindamycin
- Muscle Relaxants: clindamycin enhances effects of ●non-depolarising muscle relaxants and ●suxamethonium
Oestrogens: antibacterials that do not induce liver enzymes possibly reduce contraceptive effect of oestrogens (risk probably small, see p. 486)
Parasympathomimetics: clindamycin antagonises effects of neostigmine and pyridostigmine
Vaccines: antibacterials inactivate oral typhoid vaccine–see p. 760

Clobazam *see* Anxiolytics and Hypnotics

Clomethiazole *see* Anxiolytics and Hypnotics

Clomipramine *see* Antidepressants, Tricyclic

Clonazepam *see* Anxiolytics and Hypnotics

Clonidine
ACE Inhibitors: enhanced hypotensive effect when clonidine given with ACE inhibitors; previous treatment with clonidine possibly delays antihypertensive effect of captopril
Adrenergic Neurone Blockers: enhanced hypotensive effect when clonidine given with adrenergic neurone blockers
Alcohol: enhanced hypotensive effect when clonidine given with alcohol
Aldesleukin: enhanced hypotensive effect when clonidine given with aldesleukin
Alpha-blockers: enhanced hypotensive effect when clonidine given with alpha-blockers

Clonidine *(continued)*
Anaesthetics, General: enhanced hypotensive effect when clonidine given with general anaesthetics
Analgesics: hypotensive effect of clonidine antagonised by NSAIDs
Angiotensin-II Receptor Antagonists: enhanced hypotensive effect when clonidine given with angiotensin-II receptor antagonists
- Antidepressants: enhanced hypotensive effect when clonidine given with MAOIs; hypotensive effect of clonidine antagonised by ●tricyclics, also increased risk of hypertension on clonidine withdrawal
Antipsychotics: enhanced hypotensive effect when clonidine given with phenothiazines
Anxiolytics and Hypnotics: enhanced hypotensive effect when clonidine given with anxiolytics and hypnotics
- Beta-blockers: increased risk of withdrawal hypertension when clonidine given with ●beta-blockers (withdraw beta-blockers several days before slowly withdrawing clonidine)
Calcium-channel Blockers: enhanced hypotensive effect when clonidine given with calcium-channel blockers
Corticosteroids: hypotensive effect of clonidine antagonised by corticosteroids
Diazoxide: enhanced hypotensive effect when clonidine given with diazoxide
Diuretics: enhanced hypotensive effect when clonidine given with diuretics
Dopaminergics: enhanced hypotensive effect when clonidine given with levodopa
Methyldopa: enhanced hypotensive effect when clonidine given with methyldopa
Moxisylyte: enhanced hypotensive effect when clonidine given with moxisylyte
Moxonidine: enhanced hypotensive effect when clonidine given with moxonidine
Muscle Relaxants: enhanced hypotensive effect when clonidine given with baclofen or tizanidine
Nitrates: enhanced hypotensive effect when clonidine given with nitrates
Oestrogens: hypotensive effect of clonidine antagonised by oestrogens
Prostaglandins: enhanced hypotensive effect when clonidine given with alprostadil
- Sympathomimetics: possible risk of hypertension when clonidine given with adrenaline (epinephrine) or noradrenaline (norepinephrine); serious adverse events reported with concomitant use of clonidine and ●methylphenidate (causality not established)
Vasodilator Antihypertensives: enhanced hypotensive effect when clonidine given with hydralazine, minoxidil or sodium nitroprusside

Clopamide *see* Diuretics

Clopidogrel
Analgesics: increased risk of bleeding when clopidogrel given with NSAIDs or aspirin
- Antibacterials: antiplatelet effect of clopidogrel possibly reduced by ●chloramphenicol, ●ciprofloxacin and ●erythromycin
- Anticoagulants: manufacturer of clopidogrel advises avoid concomitant use with ●warfarin; antiplatelet action of clopidogrel enhances anticoagulant effect of ●coumarins and ●phenindione; increased risk of bleeding when clopidogrel given with heparins
- Antidepressants: antiplatelet effect of clopidogrel possibly reduced by ●fluoxetine, ●fluvoxamine and ●moclobemide
- Antiepileptics: antiplatelet effect of clopidogrel possibly reduced by ●carbamazepine and ●oxcarbazepine
- Antifungals: antiplatelet effect of clopidogrel possibly reduced by ●fluconazole, ●itraconazole, ●ketoconazole and ●voriconazole
- Antivirals: antiplatelet effect of clopidogrel possibly reduced by ●etravirine

Appendix 1: Interactions

Clopidogrel *(continued)*

Dipyridamole: increased risk of bleeding when clopidogrel given with dipyridamole

Iloprost: increased risk of bleeding when clopidogrel given with iloprost

Prasugrel: possible increased risk of bleeding when clopidogrel given with prasugrel

• Ulcer-healing Drugs: antiplatelet effect of clopidogrel possibly reduced by ●cimetidine, lansoprazole, pantoprazole and rabeprazole; antiplatelet effect of clopidogrel reduced by ●esomeprazole and ●omeprazole

Clotrimazole *see* Antifungals, Imidazole

Clozapine *see* Antipsychotics

Co-amoxiclav *see* Penicillins

Co-beneldopa *see* Levodopa

Co-careldopa *see* Levodopa

Codeine *see* Opioid Analgesics

Co-fluampicil *see* Penicillins

Colchicine

• Antibacterials: increased risk of colchicine toxicity when given with ●clarithromycin or ●erythromycin

• Ciclosporin: possible increased risk of nephrotoxicity and myotoxicity when colchicine given with ●ciclosporin (increased plasma concentration of ciclosporin)

• Lipid-regulating Drugs: possible increased risk of myopathy when colchicine given with ●statins

Colesevelam

Note. Other drugs should be taken at least 1 hour before or 4 hours after colesevelam to reduce possible interference with absorption

Colestipol

Note. Other drugs should be taken at least 1 hour before or 4–6 hours after colestipol to reduce possible interference with absorption

Antibacterials: colestipol possibly reduces absorption of tetracycline

Bile Acids: colestipol possibly reduces absorption of bile acids

Cardiac Glycosides: colestipol possibly reduces absorption of cardiac glycosides

Diuretics: colestipol reduces absorption of thiazides and related diuretics (give at least 2 hours apart)

Thyroid Hormones: colestipol reduces absorption of thyroid hormones

Colestyramine

Note. Other drugs should be taken at least 1 hour before or 4–6 hours after colestyramine to reduce possible interference with absorption

Analgesics: colestyramine increases the excretion of meloxicam; colestyramine reduces absorption of paracetamol

Antibacterials: colestyramine possibly reduces absorption of tetracycline; colestyramine antagonises effects of *oral* vancomycin

• Anticoagulants: colestyramine may enhance or reduce anticoagulant effect of ●coumarins and ●phenindione

Antidiabetics: colestyramine possibly enhances hypoglycaemic effect of acarbose

Antiepileptics: colestyramine possibly reduces absorption of valproate

Bile Acids: colestyramine possibly reduces absorption of bile acids

Cardiac Glycosides: colestyramine possibly reduces absorption of cardiac glycosides

Diuretics: colestyramine reduces absorption of thiazides and related diuretics (give at least 2 hours apart)

Leflunomide: colestyramine significantly decreases effect of leflunomide (enhanced elimination)—avoid unless drug elimination desired

Mycophenolate: colestyramine reduces absorption of mycophenolate

Colestyramine *(continued)*

Raloxifene: colestyramine reduces absorption of raloxifene (manufacturer of raloxifene advises avoid concomitant administration)

Thyroid Hormones: colestyramine reduces absorption of thyroid hormones

Colistin *see* Polymyxins

Contraceptives, oral *see* Oestrogens and Progestogens

Corticosteroids

Note. Interactions do not generally apply to corticosteroids used for topical action (including inhalation) unless specified

ACE Inhibitors: corticosteroids antagonise hypotensive effect of ACE inhibitors

Adrenergic Neurone Blockers: corticosteroids antagonise hypotensive effect of adrenergic neurone blockers

• Aldesleukin: avoidance of corticosteroids advised by manufacturer of ●aldesleukin

Alpha-blockers: corticosteroids antagonise hypotensive effect of alpha-blockers

Analgesics: increased risk of gastro-intestinal bleeding and ulceration when corticosteroids given with NSAIDs; increased risk of gastro-intestinal bleeding and ulceration when corticosteroids given with aspirin, also corticosteroids reduce plasma concentration of salicylate

Angiotensin-II Receptor Antagonists: corticosteroids antagonise hypotensive effect of angiotensin-II receptor antagonists

Antacids: absorption of deflazacort reduced by antacids

• Antibacterials: plasma concentration of methylprednisolone possibly increased by clarithromycin; metabolism of corticosteroids possibly inhibited by erythromycin; metabolism of methylprednisolone inhibited by erythromycin; corticosteroids possibly reduce plasma concentration of isoniazid; metabolism of corticosteroids accelerated by ●rifamycins (reduced effect)

• Anticoagulants: corticosteroids may enhance or reduce anticoagulant effect of ●coumarins (high-dose corticosteroids enhance anticoagulant effect)

Antidiabetics: corticosteroids antagonise hypoglycaemic effect of antidiabetics

• Antiepileptics: metabolism of corticosteroids accelerated by ●carbamazepine, ●phenytoin and ●primidone (reduced effect)

• Antifungals: metabolism of corticosteroids possibly inhibited by itraconazole and ketoconazole; plasma concentration of active metabolite of ciclesonide increased by ketoconazole; plasma concentration of *inhaled* mometasone increased by ketoconazole; plasma concentration of *inhaled* and *oral* budesonide increased by ketoconazole; metabolism of methylprednisolone inhibited by ketoconazole; increased risk of hypokalaemia when corticosteroids given with ●amphotericin—avoid concomitant use unless corticosteroids needed to control reactions; plasma concentration of *inhaled* budesonide increased by itraconazole; metabolism of methylprednisolone possibly inhibited by itraconazole; dexamethasone possibly reduces plasma concentration of caspofungin—consider increasing dose of caspofungin

• Antivirals: dexamethasone possibly reduces plasma concentration of indinavir, lopinavir and saquinavir; plasma concentration of *inhaled* and *intranasal* fluticasone possibly increased by nelfinavir; plasma concentration of corticosteroids, dexamethasone and prednisolone possibly increased by ritonavir; plasma concentration of *inhaled* and *intranasal* budesonide and fluticasone increased by ●ritonavir

Aprepitant: metabolism of dexamethasone and methylprednisolone inhibited by aprepitant (reduce dose of dexamethasone and methylprednisolone)

Corticosteroids *(continued)*

- Barbiturates: metabolism of corticosteroids accelerated by ●barbiturates (reduced effect)

  Beta-blockers: corticosteroids antagonise hypotensive effect of beta-blockers

  Calcium Salts: corticosteroids reduce absorption of calcium salts

  Calcium-channel Blockers: corticosteroids antagonise hypotensive effect of calcium-channel blockers

  Cardiac Glycosides: increased risk of hypokalaemia when corticosteroids given with cardiac glycosides

- Ciclosporin: high-dose methylprednisolone increases plasma concentration of ●ciclosporin (risk of convulsions); plasma concentration of prednisolone increased by ciclosporin

  Clonidine: corticosteroids antagonise hypotensive effect of clonidine

  Diazoxide: corticosteroids antagonise hypotensive effect of diazoxide

  Diuretics: corticosteroids antagonise diuretic effect of diuretics; increased risk of hypokalaemia when corticosteroids given with acetazolamide, loop diuretics or thiazides and related diuretics

  Methyldopa: corticosteroids antagonise hypotensive effect of methyldopa

  Mifamurtide: avoidance of corticosteroids advised by manufacturer of mifamurtide

  Mifepristone: effect of corticosteroids (including *inhaled* corticosteroids) may be reduced for 3–4 days after mifepristone

  Moxonidine: corticosteroids antagonise hypotensive effect of moxonidine

  Muscle Relaxants: corticosteroids possibly antagonise effects of pancuronium and vecuronium

  Nitrates: corticosteroids antagonise hypotensive effect of nitrates

  Oestrogens: plasma concentration of corticosteroids increased by oral contraceptives containing oestrogens

  Sodium Benzoate: corticosteroids possibly reduce effects of sodium benzoate

  Sodium Phenylbutyrate: corticosteroids possibly reduce effects of sodium phenylbutyrate

  Somatropin: corticosteroids may inhibit growth-promoting effect of somatropin

  Sympathomimetics: metabolism of dexamethasone accelerated by ephedrine

  Sympathomimetics, Beta₂: increased risk of hypokalaemia when corticosteroids given with high doses of beta₂ sympathomimetics—see Hypokalaemia, p. 177

  Theophylline: increased risk of hypokalaemia when corticosteroids given with theophylline

- Vaccines: high doses of corticosteroids impair immune response to ●vaccines, avoid concomitant use with live vaccines (see p. 733)

  Vasodilator Antihypertensives: corticosteroids antagonise hypotensive effect of hydralazine, minoxidil and sodium nitroprusside

Cortisone *see* Corticosteroids

Co-trimoxazole *see* Trimethoprim and Sulfamethoxazole

Coumarins

Note. Change in patient's clinical condition, particularly associated with liver disease, intercurrent illness, or drug administration, necessitates more frequent testing. Major changes in diet (especially involving salads and vegetables) and in alcohol consumption may also affect anticoagulant control

- Alcohol: anticoagulant control with coumarins may be affected by major changes in consumption of ●alcohol

  Allopurinol: anticoagulant effect of coumarins possibly enhanced by allopurinol

- Anabolic Steroids: anticoagulant effect of coumarins enhanced by ●anabolic steroids

- Analgesics: anticoagulant effect of coumarins possibly enhanced by ●NSAIDs; anticoagulant effect of coumarins enhanced by ●azapropazone (avoid con-

Coumarins

- Analgesics *(continued)*

  comitant use); increased risk of haemorrhage when anticoagulants given with *intravenous* ●diclofenac (avoid concomitant use, including low-dose heparins); increased risk of haemorrhage when anticoagulants given with ●ketorolac (avoid concomitant use, including low-dose heparins); anticoagulant effect of coumarins enhanced by ●tramadol; increased risk of bleeding when coumarins given with ●aspirin (due to antiplatelet effect); anticoagulant effect of coumarins possibly enhanced by prolonged regular use of paracetamol

- Anti-arrhythmics: metabolism of coumarins inhibited by ●amiodarone (enhanced anticoagulant effect); anticoagulant effect of coumarins enhanced by ●propafenone

- Antibacterials: experience in anticoagulant clinics suggests that INR possibly altered when coumarins are given with ●neomycin (given for local action on gut); anticoagulant effect of coumarins possibly enhanced by ●azithromycin, ●aztreonam, ●cephalosporins, levofloxacin, ●tetracyclines, tigecycline and trimethoprim; anticoagulant effect of coumarins enhanced by ●chloramphenicol, ●ciprofloxacin, ●clarithromycin, ●erythromycin, ●metronidazole, ●nalidixic acid, ●norfloxacin, ●ofloxacin and ●sulphonamides; studies have failed to demonstrate an interaction with coumarins, but common experience in anticoagulant clinics is that INR can be altered by a course of broad-spectrum penicillins such as ampicillin; metabolism of coumarins accelerated by ●rifamycins (reduced anticoagulant effect)

- Antidepressants: anticoagulant effect of warfarin possibly enhanced by ●venlafaxine; anticoagulant effect of warfarin may be enhanced or reduced by trazodone; anticoagulant effect of coumarins possibly enhanced by ●SSRIs; anticoagulant effect of coumarins reduced by ●St John's wort (avoid concomitant use); anticoagulant effect of warfarin enhanced by mirtazapine; anticoagulant effect of coumarins may be enhanced or reduced by ●tricyclics

- Antidiabetics: anticoagulant effect of warfarin possibly enhanced by exenatide; coumarins possibly enhance hypoglycaemic effect of ●sulphonylureas, also possible changes to anticoagulant effect

- Antiepileptics: metabolism of coumarins accelerated by ●carbamazepine and ●primidone (reduced anticoagulant effect); plasma concentration of warfarin reduced by eslicarbazepine; metabolism of coumarins accelerated by ●phenytoin (possibility of reduced anticoagulant effect, but enhancement also reported); anticoagulant effect of coumarins possibly enhanced by valproate

- Antifungals: anticoagulant effect of coumarins enhanced by ●fluconazole, ●itraconazole, ●ketoconazole and ●voriconazole; anticoagulant effect of coumarins enhanced by ●miconazole (miconazole oral gel and possibly vaginal formulations absorbed); anticoagulant effect of coumarins reduced by ●griseofulvin

  Antimalarials: isolated reports that anticoagulant effect of warfarin may be enhanced by proguanil

- Antivirals: anticoagulant effect of warfarin may be enhanced or reduced by atazanavir, ●nevirapine and ●ritonavir; plasma concentration of warfarin possibly affected by efavirenz; anticoagulant effect of coumarins may be enhanced or reduced by fosamprenavir; anticoagulant effect of coumarins possibly enhanced by ●ritonavir; anticoagulant effect of warfarin possibly enhanced by saquinavir

  Anxiolytics and Hypnotics: anticoagulant effect of coumarins may transiently be enhanced by chloral and triclofos

Appendix 1: Interactions

Coumarins *(continued)*

Aprepitant: anticoagulant effect of warfarin possibly reduced by aprepitant

● Azathioprine: anticoagulant effect of coumarins possibly reduced by ●azathioprine

● Barbiturates: metabolism of coumarins accelerated by ●barbiturates (reduced anticoagulant effect)

Bosentan: monitoring anticoagulant effect of coumarins recommended by manufacturer of bosentan

● Clopidogrel: anticoagulant effect of coumarins enhanced due to antiplatelet action of ●clopidogrel; avoidance of warfarin advised by manufacturer of ●clopidogrel

● Corticosteroids: anticoagulant effect of coumarins may be enhanced or reduced by ●corticosteroids (high-dose corticosteroids enhance anticoagulant effect)

● Cranberry Juice: anticoagulant effect of coumarins possibly enhanced by ●cranberry juice—avoid concomitant use

● Cytotoxics: anticoagulant effect of coumarins possibly enhanced by ●etoposide, ●ifosfamide and ●sorafenib; anticoagulant effect of coumarins enhanced by ●fluorouracil; anticoagulant effect of warfarin possibly enhanced by ●gefitinib and gemcitabine; anticoagulant effect of coumarins possibly reduced by ●mercaptopurine and ●mitotane; increased risk of bleeding when coumarins given with ●erlotinib; replacement of warfarin with a heparin advised by manufacturer of ●imatinib (possibility of enhanced warfarin effect)

● Dipyridamole: anticoagulant effect of coumarins enhanced due to antiplatelet action of ●dipyridamole

● Disulfiram: anticoagulant effect of coumarins enhanced by ●disulfiram

● Dopaminergics: anticoagulant effect of warfarin enhanced by ●entacapone

● Enteral Foods: anticoagulant effect of coumarins antagonised by vitamin K (present in some ●enteral feeds)

● Glucosamine: anticoagulant effect of warfarin enhanced by ●glucosamine (avoid concomitant use)

● Hormone Antagonists: anticoagulant effect of coumarins possibly enhanced by bicalutamide and ●toremifene; metabolism of coumarins inhibited by ●danazol (enhanced anticoagulant effect); anticoagulant effect of coumarins enhanced by ●flutamide and ●tamoxifen

Iloprost: anticoagulant effect of coumarins possibly enhanced by iloprost

Lactulose: anticoagulant effect of coumarins possibly enhanced by lactulose

Leflunomide: anticoagulant effect of warfarin possibly enhanced by leflunomide

Leukotriene Receptor Antagonists: anticoagulant effect of warfarin enhanced by zafirlukast

● Levamisole: anticoagulant effect of warfarin possibly enhanced by ●levamisole

● Lipid-regulating Drugs: anticoagulant effect of coumarins may be enhanced or reduced by ●colestyramine; anticoagulant effect of warfarin may be transiently reduced by atorvastatin; anticoagulant effect of coumarins enhanced by ●fibrates, ●fluvastatin and simvastatin; anticoagulant effect of coumarins possibly enhanced by ezetimibe and ●rosuvastatin

Memantine: anticoagulant effect of warfarin possibly enhanced by memantine

● Oestrogens: anticoagulant effect of coumarins may be enhanced or reduced by ●oestrogens

Orlistat: monitoring anticoagulant effect of coumarins recommended by manufacturer of orlistat

Prasugrel: possible increased risk of bleeding when coumarins given with prasugrel

● Progestogens: anticoagulant effect of coumarins may be enhanced or reduced by ●progestogens

Coumarins *(continued)*

Raloxifene: anticoagulant effect of coumarins antagonised by raloxifene

● Retinoids: anticoagulant effect of coumarins possibly reduced by ●acitretin

Sibutramine: increased risk of bleeding when anticoagulants given with sibutramine

● Sitaxentan: anticoagulant effect of coumarins enhanced by ●sitaxentan

● Sulfinpyrazone: anticoagulant effect of coumarins enhanced by ●sulfinpyrazone

● Sympathomimetics: anticoagulant effect of coumarins possibly enhanced by ●methylphenidate

Terpene Mixture: anticoagulant effect of coumarins possibly reduced by Rowachol®

● Testolactone: anticoagulant effect of coumarins enhanced by ●testolactone

● Testosterone: anticoagulant effect of coumarins enhanced by ●testosterone

● Thyroid Hormones: anticoagulant effect of coumarins enhanced by ●thyroid hormones

Ubidecarenone: anticoagulant effect of warfarin may be enhanced or reduced by ubidecarenone

● Ulcer-healing Drugs: metabolism of coumarins inhibited by ●cimetidine (enhanced anticoagulant effect); anticoagulant effect of coumarins possibly enhanced by ●esomeprazole, ●omeprazole and pantoprazole; absorption of coumarins possibly reduced by ●sucralfate (reduced anticoagulant effect)

Vaccines: anticoagulant effect of warfarin enhanced by influenza vaccine

● Vitamins: anticoagulant effect of coumarins possibly enhanced by ●vitamin E; anticoagulant effect of coumarins antagonised by ●vitamin K

Cranberry Juice

● Anticoagulants: cranberry juice possibly enhances anticoagulant effect of ●coumarins—avoid concomitant use

Cyclizine *see* Antihistamines

Cyclopenthiazide *see* Diuretics

Cyclopentolate *see* Antimuscarinics

Cyclophosphamide

Antiepileptics: cytotoxics possibly reduce absorption of phenytoin

Antifungals: side-effects of cyclophosphamide possibly increased by itraconazole

● Antipsychotics: avoid concomitant use of cytotoxics with ●clozapine (increased risk of agranulocytosis)

Cardiac Glycosides: cytotoxics reduce absorption of digoxin tablets

● Cytotoxics: increased toxicity when high-dose cyclophosphamide given with ●pentostatin—avoid concomitant use

Muscle Relaxants: cyclophosphamide enhances effects of suxamethonium

Cycloserine

● Alcohol: increased risk of convulsions when cycloserine given with ●alcohol

Antibacterials: increased risk of CNS toxicity when cycloserine given with isoniazid

Oestrogens: antibacterials that do not induce liver enzymes possibly reduce contraceptive effect of oestrogens (risk probably small, see p. 486)

Vaccines: antibacterials inactivate oral typhoid vaccine–see p. 760

Cyproheptadine *see* Antihistamines

Cytarabine

Antiepileptics: cytotoxics possibly reduce absorption of phenytoin

Antifungals: cytarabine possibly reduces plasma concentration of flucytosine

● Antipsychotics: avoid concomitant use of cytotoxics with ●clozapine (increased risk of agranulocytosis)

Cardiac Glycosides: cytotoxics reduce absorption of digoxin tablets

Cytarabine *(continued)*

Cytotoxics: intracellular concentration of cytarabine increased by fludarabine

Cytotoxics *see* individual drugs

Dabigatran Etexilate

- Analgesics: possible increased risk of bleeding when dabigatran etexilate given with ●NSAIDs; increased risk of haemorrhage when anticoagulants given with *intravenous* ●diclofenac (avoid concomitant use, including low-dose heparins); increased risk of haemorrhage when anticoagulants given with ●ketorolac (avoid concomitant use, including low-dose heparins)
- Anti-arrhythmics: plasma concentration of dabigatran etexilate increased by ●amiodarone (reduce dose of dabigatran etexilate)

Sibutramine: increased risk of bleeding when anti-coagulants given with sibutramine

Dacarbazine

- Aldesleukin: avoidance of dacarbazine advised by manufacturer of ●aldesleukin

Antiepileptics: cytotoxics possibly reduce absorption of phenytoin

- Antipsychotics: avoid concomitant use of cytotoxics with ●clozapine (increased risk of agranulocytosis)

Cardiac Glycosides: cytotoxics reduce absorption of digoxin tablets

Dairy Products

Antibacterials: dairy products reduce absorption of ciprofloxacin and norfloxacin; dairy products reduce absorption of tetracyclines (except doxycycline and minocycline)

Dalteparin *see* Heparins

Danazol

- Anticoagulants: danazol inhibits metabolism of ●coumarins (enhanced anticoagulant effect)
- Antiepileptics: danazol inhibits metabolism of ●carbamazepine (increased risk of toxicity)
- Ciclosporin: danazol inhibits metabolism of ●ciclosporin (increased plasma concentration)
- Lipid-regulating Drugs: possible increased risk of myopathy when danazol given with ●simvastatin

Tacrolimus: danazol possibly increases plasma concentration of tacrolimus

Dantrolene *see* Muscle Relaxants

Dapsone

Antibacterials: plasma concentration of dapsone reduced by rifamycins; plasma concentration of both drugs may increase when dapsone given with trimethoprim

Antivirals: plasma concentration of dapsone possibly increased by fosamprenavir

Oestrogens: antibacterials that do not induce liver enzymes possibly reduce contraceptive effect of oestrogens (risk probably small, see p. 486)

Probenecid: excretion of dapsone reduced by pro-benecid (increased risk of side-effects)

Vaccines: antibacterials inactivate oral typhoid vaccine–see p. 760

Daptomycin

- Ciclosporin: increased risk of myopathy when dapto-mycin given with ●ciclosporin (preferably avoid concomitant use)
- Lipid-regulating Drugs: increased risk of myopathy when daptomycin given with ●fibrates or ●statins (preferably avoid concomitant use)

Oestrogens: antibacterials that do not induce liver enzymes possibly reduce contraceptive effect of oestrogens (risk probably small, see p. 486)

Vaccines: antibacterials inactivate oral typhoid vaccine–see p. 760

Darifenacin *see* Antimuscarinics

Darunavir

Anti-arrhythmics: darunavir possibly increases plasma concentration of lidocaine—avoid concomitant use

Darunavir *(continued)*

- Antibacterials: darunavir increases plasma concentration of ●rifabutin (reduce dose of rifabutin); plasma concentration of darunavir significantly reduced by ●rifampicin—avoid concomitant use

Anticoagulants: avoidance of darunavir advised by manufacturer of rivaroxaban

- Antidepressants: darunavir possibly reduces plasma concentration of paroxetine and sertraline; plasma concentration of darunavir reduced by ●St John's wort—avoid concomitant use

Antiepileptics: plasma concentration of darunavir possibly reduced by carbamazepine and phenytoin

Antifungals: plasma concentration of both drugs increased when darunavir given with ketoconazole

Antimalarials: caution with darunavir advised by manufacturer of artemether/lumefantrine

- Antivirals: plasma concentration of darunavir reduced by efavirenz and saquinavir; plasma concentration of both drugs increased when darunavir given with indinavir; plasma concentration of darunavir reduced by ●lopinavir, also plasma concentration of lopinavir increased (avoid concomitant use); daru-navir increases plasma concentration of ●maraviroc (consider reducing dose of maraviroc)

Barbiturates: plasma concentration of darunavir pos-sibly reduced by phenobarbital

- Cytotoxics: darunavir possibly increases plasma concentration of ●everolimus—manufacturer of ever-olimus advises avoid concomitant use
- Lipid-regulating Drugs: darunavir possibly increases plasma concentration of pravastatin; possible increased risk of myopathy when darunavir given with ●rosuvastatin—avoid concomitant use
- Ranolazine: darunavir possibly increases plasma con-centration of ●ranolazine—manufacturer of ranola-zine advises avoid concomitant use

Dasatinib

- Antibacterials: metabolism of dasatinib accelerated by ●rifampicin (reduced plasma concentration—avoid concomitant use)

Antiepileptics: cytotoxics possibly reduce absorption of phenytoin

Antifungals: plasma concentration of dasatinib possibly increased by ketoconazole

- Antipsychotics: avoid concomitant use of cytotoxics with ●clozapine (increased risk of agranulocytosis)

Cardiac Glycosides: cytotoxics reduce absorption of digoxin tablets

Lipid-regulating Drugs: dasatinib possibly increases plasma concentration of simvastatin

Ulcer-healing Drugs: plasma concentration of dasatinib possibly reduced by famotidine

Deferasirox

Antacids: absorption of deferasirox possibly reduced by antacids containing aluminium (manufacturer of deferasirox advises avoid concomitant use)

Antibacterials: plasma concentration of deferasirox reduced by rifampicin

Antidiabetics: deferasirox increases plasma concen-tration of repaglinide

Anxiolytics and Hypnotics: deferasirox possibly reduces plasma concentration of midazolam

Deflazacort *see* Corticosteroids

Demeclocycline *see* Tetracyclines

Desferrioxamine

Antipsychotics: avoidance of desferrioxamine advised by manufacturer of levomepromazine; manufacturer of desferrioxamine advises avoid concomitant use with prochlorperazine

Desflurane *see* Anaesthetics, General

Desloratadine *see* Antihistamines

Desmopressin

Analgesics: effects of desmopressin enhanced by indometacin

Desmopressin (continued)

Loperamide: plasma concentration of *oral* desmopressin increased by loperamide

Desogestrel see Progestogens

Dexamethasone see Corticosteroids

Dexamfetamine see Sympathomimetics

Dexibuprofen see NSAIDs

Dexketoprofen see NSAIDs

Dextromethorphan see Opioid Analgesics

Dextropropoxyphene see Opioid Analgesics

Diamorphine see Opioid Analgesics

Diazepam see Anxiolytics and Hypnotics

Diazoxide

ACE Inhibitors: enhanced hypotensive effect when diazoxide given with ACE inhibitors

Adrenergic Neurone Blockers: enhanced hypotensive effect when diazoxide given with adrenergic neurone blockers

Alcohol: enhanced hypotensive effect when diazoxide given with alcohol

Aldesleukin: enhanced hypotensive effect when diazoxide given with aldesleukin

Alpha-blockers: enhanced hypotensive effect when diazoxide given with alpha-blockers

Anaesthetics, General: enhanced hypotensive effect when diazoxide given with general anaesthetics

Analgesics: hypotensive effect of diazoxide antagonised by NSAIDs

Angiotensin-II Receptor Antagonists: enhanced hypotensive effect when diazoxide given with angiotensin-II receptor antagonists

Antidepressants: enhanced hypotensive effect when diazoxide given with MAOIs or tricyclic-related antidepressants

Antidiabetics: diazoxide antagonises hypoglycaemic effect of antidiabetics

Antiepileptics: diazoxide reduces plasma concentration of phenytoin, also effect of diazoxide may be reduced

Antipsychotics: enhanced hypotensive effect when diazoxide given with phenothiazines

Anxiolytics and Hypnotics: enhanced hypotensive effect when diazoxide given with anxiolytics and hypnotics

Beta-blockers: enhanced hypotensive effect when diazoxide given with beta-blockers

Calcium-channel Blockers: enhanced hypotensive effect when diazoxide given with calcium-channel blockers

Clonidine: enhanced hypotensive effect when diazoxide given with clonidine

Corticosteroids: hypotensive effect of diazoxide antagonised by corticosteroids

Diuretics: enhanced hypotensive and hyperglycaemic effects when diazoxide given with diuretics

Dopaminergics: enhanced hypotensive effect when diazoxide given with levodopa

Methyldopa: enhanced hypotensive effect when diazoxide given with methyldopa

Moxisylyte: enhanced hypotensive effect when diazoxide given with moxisylyte

Moxonidine: enhanced hypotensive effect when diazoxide given with moxonidine

Muscle Relaxants: enhanced hypotensive effect when diazoxide given with baclofen or tizanidine

Nitrates: enhanced hypotensive effect when diazoxide given with nitrates

Oestrogens: hypotensive effect of diazoxide antagonised by oestrogens

Prostaglandins: enhanced hypotensive effect when diazoxide given with alprostadil

Vasodilator Antihypertensives: enhanced hypotensive effect when diazoxide given with hydralazine, minoxidil or sodium nitroprusside

Diclofenac see NSAIDs

Dicycloverine see Antimuscarinics

Didanosine

Note. Antacids in tablet formulation may affect absorption of other drugs

• Allopurinol: plasma concentration of didanosine increased by ●allopurinol (risk of toxicity)—avoid concomitant use

Analgesics: plasma concentration of didanosine possibly reduced by methadone

• Antivirals: plasma concentration of didanosine possibly increased by ganciclovir; increased risk of side-effects when didanosine given with ●ribavirin—avoid concomitant use; increased risk of side-effects when didanosine given with ●stavudine; plasma concentration of didanosine increased by ●tenofovir (increased risk of toxicity)—avoid concomitant use; plasma concentration of didanosine reduced by ●tipranavir

• Cytotoxics: increased risk of toxicity when didanosine given with ●hydroxycarbamide—avoid concomitant use

Dienogest see Progestogens

Digitoxin see Cardiac Glycosides

Digoxin see Cardiac Glycosides

Dihydrocodeine see Opioid Analgesics

Diltiazem see Calcium-channel Blockers

Dimercaprol

• Iron: avoid concomitant use of dimercaprol with ●iron

Dimethyl sulfoxide

• Analgesics: avoid concomitant use of dimethyl sulfoxide with ●sulindac

Dinoprostone see Prostaglandins

Diphenoxylate see Opioid Analgesics

Dipipanone see Opioid Analgesics

Dipivefrine see Sympathomimetics

Dipyridamole

Antacids: absorption of dipyridamole possibly reduced by antacids

• Anti-arrhythmics: dipyridamole enhances and extends the effects of ●adenosine (important risk of toxicity)

• Anticoagulants: antiplatelet action of dipyridamole enhances anticoagulant effect of ●coumarins and ●phenindione; dipyridamole enhances anticoagulant effect of heparins

Clopidogrel: increased risk of bleeding when dipyridamole given with clopidogrel

Cytotoxics: dipyridamole possibly reduces effects of fludarabine

Disodium Etidronate see Bisphosphonates

Disodium Pamidronate see Bisphosphonates

Disopyramide

Anaesthetics, Local: increased myocardial depression when anti-arrhythmics given with bupivacaine, levobupivacaine, prilocaine or ropivacaine

• Anti-arrhythmics: increased myocardial depression when anti-arrhythmics given with other ●anti-arrhythmics; increased risk of ventricular arrhythmias when disopyramide given with ●amiodarone—avoid concomitant use

• Antibacterials: plasma concentration of disopyramide possibly increased by ●clarithromycin (increased risk of toxicity); plasma concentration of disopyramide increased by ●erythromycin (increased risk of toxicity); increased risk of ventricular arrhythmias when disopyramide given with ●moxifloxacin or ●quinupristin/dalfopristin—avoid concomitant use; metabolism of disopyramide accelerated by ●rifamycins (reduced plasma concentration)

• Antidepressants: increased risk of ventricular arrhythmias when disopyramide given with ●tricyclics

Antidiabetics: disopyramide possibly enhances hypoglycaemic effect of gliclazide, insulin and metformin

Antiepileptics: plasma concentration of disopyramide reduced by phenytoin; metabolism of disopyramide accelerated by primidone (reduced plasma concentration)

Disopyramide *(continued)*
- Antifungals: increased risk of ventricular arrhythmias when disopyramide given with ●ketoconazole—avoid concomitant use; avoidance of disopyramide advised by manufacturer of ●itraconazole
- Antihistamines: increased risk of ventricular arrhythmias when disopyramide given with ●mizolastine—avoid concomitant use
- Antimalarials: avoidance of disopyramide advised by manufacturer of ●artemether/lumefantrine (risk of ventricular arrhythmias)
- Antimuscarinics: increased risk of antimuscarinic side-effects when disopyramide given with antimuscarinics; increased risk of ventricular arrhythmias when disopyramide given with ●tolterodine
- Antipsychotics: increased risk of ventricular arrhythmias when anti-arrhythmics that prolong the QT interval given with ●antipsychotics that prolong the QT interval; increased risk of ventricular arrhythmias when disopyramide given with ●amisulpride, ●droperidol, ●pimozide, ●sertindole or ●zuclopenthixol—avoid concomitant use; possible increased risk of ventricular arrhythmias when disopyramide given with ●haloperidol—avoid concomitant use; increased risk of ventricular arrhythmias when disopyramide given with ●phenothiazines or ●sulpiride
- Antivirals: plasma concentration of disopyramide possibly increased by ●ritonavir (increased risk of toxicity)
- Atomoxetine: increased risk of ventricular arrhythmias when disopyramide given with ●atomoxetine
  Barbiturates: metabolism of disopyramide accelerated by barbiturates (reduced plasma concentration)
- Beta-blockers: increased myocardial depression when anti-arrhythmics given with ●beta-blockers; increased risk of ventricular arrhythmias when disopyramide given with ●sotalol—avoid concomitant use
- Calcium-channel Blockers: increased risk of myocardial depression and asystole when disopyramide given with ●verapamil
- Cytotoxics: increased risk of ventricular arrhythmias when disopyramide given with ●arsenic trioxide
- Diuretics: increased cardiac toxicity with disopyramide if hypokalaemia occurs with ●acetazolamide, ●loop diuretics or ●thiazides and related diuretics
- Ivabradine: increased risk of ventricular arrhythmias when disopyramide given with ●ivabradine
  Nitrates: disopyramide reduces effects of sublingual tablets of nitrates (failure to dissolve under tongue owing to dry mouth)
- Ranolazine: avoidance of disopyramide advised by manufacturer of ●ranolazine

Distigmine *see Parasympathomimetics*

Disulfiram
  Alcohol: disulfiram reaction when disulfiram given with alcohol (see BNF section 4.10)
  Antibacterials: psychotic reaction reported when disulfiram given with metronidazole; CNS effects of disulfiram possibly increased by isoniazid
- Anticoagulants: disulfiram enhances anticoagulant effect of ●coumarins
  Antidepressants: increased disulfiram reaction with alcohol reported when concomitant amitriptyline; disulfiram inhibits metabolism of tricyclics (increased plasma concentration)
- Antiepileptics: disulfiram inhibits metabolism of ●phenytoin (increased risk of toxicity)
  Anxiolytics and Hypnotics: disulfiram increases risk of temazepam toxicity; disulfiram inhibits metabolism of benzodiazepines (increased sedative effects)
- Paraldehyde: risk of toxicity when disulfiram given with ●paraldehyde
  Theophylline: disulfiram inhibits metabolism of theophylline (increased risk of toxicity)

Diuretics
  Note. Since systemic absorption may follow topical application of brinzolamide to the eye, the possibility of interactions should be borne in mind
  Note. Since systemic absorption may follow topical application of dorzolamide to the eye, the possibility of interactions should be borne in mind
- ACE Inhibitors: enhanced hypotensive effect when diuretics given with ●ACE inhibitors; increased risk of severe hyperkalaemia when potassium-sparing diuretics and aldosterone antagonists given with ●ACE inhibitors (monitor potassium concentration with low-dose spironolactone in heart failure)
  Adrenergic Neurone Blockers: enhanced hypotensive effect when diuretics given with adrenergic neurone blockers
  Alcohol: enhanced hypotensive effect when diuretics given with alcohol
  Aldesleukin: enhanced hypotensive effect when diuretics given with aldesleukin
  Aliskiren: plasma concentration of furosemide reduced by aliskiren; increased risk of hyperkalaemia when potassium-sparing diuretics and aldosterone antagonists given with aliskiren
  Allopurinol: increased risk of hypersensitivity when thiazides and related diuretics given with allopurinol especially in renal impairment
- Alpha-blockers: enhanced hypotensive effect when diuretics given with ●alpha-blockers, also increased risk of first-dose hypotension with post-synaptic alpha-blockers such as prazosin
  Anaesthetics, General: enhanced hypotensive effect when diuretics given with general anaesthetics
- Analgesics: Diuretic effect of potassium canrenoate possibly antagonised by NSAIDs; possibly increased risk of hyperkalaemia when potassium-sparing diuretics and aldosterone antagonists given with NSAIDs; diuretics increase risk of nephrotoxicity of NSAIDs, also antagonism of diuretic effect; effects of diuretics antagonised by indometacin and ketorolac; increased risk of hyperkalaemia when potassium-sparing diuretics and aldosterone antagonists given with indometacin; occasional reports of reduced renal function when triamterene given with ●indometacin—avoid concomitant use; diuretic effect of spironolactone antagonised by aspirin; increased risk of toxicity when carbonic anhydrase inhibitors given with high-dose aspirin
- Angiotensin-II Receptor Antagonists: enhanced hypotensive effect when diuretics given with ●angiotensin-II receptor antagonists; increased risk of hyperkalaemia when potassium-sparing diuretics and aldosterone antagonists given with ●angiotensin-II receptor antagonists
- Anti-arrhythmics: hypokalaemia caused by acetazolamide, loop diuretics or thiazides and related diuretics increases cardiac toxicity with amiodarone; plasma concentration of eplerenone increased by amiodarone (reduce dose of eplerenone); hypokalaemia caused by acetazolamide, loop diuretics or thiazides and related diuretics increases cardiac toxicity with ●disopyramide; hypokalaemia caused by acetazolamide, loop diuretics or thiazides and related diuretics increases cardiac toxicity with ●flecainide; hypokalaemia caused by acetazolamide, loop diuretics or thiazides and related diuretics increases cardiac toxicity with ●lidocaine
- Antibacterials: plasma concentration of eplerenone increased by ●clarithromycin and ●telithromycin—avoid concomitant use; plasma concentration of eplerenone increased by erythromycin (reduce dose of eplerenone); plasma concentration of eplerenone reduced by ●rifampicin—avoid concomitant use; avoidance of diuretics advised by manufacturer of lymecycline; increased risk of ototoxicity when loop diuretics given with ●aminoglycosides, ●polymyxins or ●vancomycin; acetazolamide antag-

Diuretics

- Antibacterials (continued)
  onises effects of •methenamine; increased risk of hyperkalaemia when eplerenone given with trimethoprim

- Antidepressants: possible increased risk of hypokalaemia when loop diuretics or thiazides and related diuretics given with reboxetine; enhanced hypotensive effect when diuretics given with MAOIs; plasma concentration of eplerenone reduced by •St John's wort—avoid concomitant use; increased risk of postural hypotension when diuretics given with tricyclics

  Antidiabetics: loop diuretics and thiazides and related diuretics antagonise hypoglycaemic effect of antidiabetics

- Antiepileptics: increased risk of hyponatraemia when diuretics given with carbamazepine; acetazolamide increases plasma concentration of carbamazepine; plasma concentration of eplerenone reduced by •carbamazepine and •phenytoin—avoid concomitant use; increased risk of osteomalacia when carbonic anhydrase inhibitors given with phenytoin or primidone; effects of furosemide antagonised by phenytoin; acetazolamide possibly reduces plasma concentration of primidone

- Antifungals: plasma concentration of eplerenone increased by •itraconazole and •ketoconazole—avoid concomitant use; increased risk of hypokalaemia when loop diuretics or thiazides and related diuretics given with amphotericin; hydrochlorothiazide increases plasma concentration of fluconazole; plasma concentration of eplerenone increased by fluconazole (reduce dose of eplerenone)

- Antipsychotics: hypokalaemia caused by diuretics increases risk of ventricular arrhythmias with •amisulpride or •sertindole; enhanced hypotensive effect when diuretics given with phenothiazines; hypokalaemia caused by diuretics increases risk of ventricular arrhythmias with •pimozide (avoid concomitant use)

- Antivirals: plasma concentration of eplerenone increased by •nelfinavir and •ritonavir—avoid concomitant use; plasma concentration of eplerenone increased by saquinavir (reduce dose of eplerenone)

  Anxiolytics and Hypnotics: enhanced hypotensive effect when diuretics given with anxiolytics and hypnotics; administration of parenteral furosemide with chloral or triclofos may displace thyroid hormone from binding sites

- Atomoxetine: hypokalaemia caused by diuretics increases risk of ventricular arrhythmias with •atomoxetine

- Barbiturates: plasma concentration of eplerenone reduced by •phenobarbital—avoid concomitant use; increased risk of osteomalacia when carbonic anhydrase inhibitors given with phenobarbital

- Beta-blockers: enhanced hypotensive effect when diuretics given with beta-blockers; hypokalaemia caused by loop diuretics or thiazides and related diuretics increases risk of ventricular arrhythmias with •sotalol

  Calcium Salts: increased risk of hypercalcaemia when thiazides and related diuretics given with calcium salts

  Calcium-channel Blockers: enhanced hypotensive effect when diuretics given with calcium-channel blockers; plasma concentration of eplerenone increased by diltiazem and verapamil (reduce dose of eplerenone)

- Cardiac Glycosides: hypokalaemia caused by acetazolamide, loop diuretics or thiazides and related diuretics increases cardiac toxicity with •cardiac glycosides; spironolactone possibly affects plasma concentration of digitoxin; potassium cannrenoate possibly increases plasma concentration of digoxin;

Diuretics

- Cardiac Glycosides (continued)
  spironolactone increases plasma concentration of •digoxin

- Ciclosporin: increased risk of nephrotoxicity and possibly hypermagnesaemia when thiazides and related diuretics given with ciclosporin; increased risk of hyperkalaemia when potassium-sparing diuretics and aldosterone antagonists given with •ciclosporin

  Clonidine: enhanced hypotensive effect when diuretics given with clonidine

  Corticosteroids: diuretic effect of diuretics antagonised by corticosteroids; increased risk of hypokalaemia when acetazolamide, loop diuretics or thiazides and related diuretics given with corticosteroids

- Cytotoxics: hypokalaemia caused by acetazolamide, loop diuretics or thiazides and related diuretics increases risk of ventricular arrhythmias with •arsenic trioxide; avoidance of spironolactone advised by manufacturer of mitotane (antagonism of effect); increased risk of nephrotoxicity and ototoxicity when diuretics given with platinum compounds

  Diazoxide: enhanced hypotensive and hyperglycaemic effects when diuretics given with diazoxide

  Diuretics: increased risk of hypokalaemia when loop diuretics or thiazides and related diuretics given with acetazolamide; profound diuresis possible when metolazone given with furosemide; increased risk of hypokalaemia when thiazides and related diuretics given with loop diuretics

  Dopaminergics: enhanced hypotensive effect when diuretics given with levodopa

  Hormone Antagonists: increased risk of hypercalcaemia when thiazides and related diuretics given with toremifene; increased risk of hyperkalaemia when potassium-sparing diuretics and aldosterone antagonists given with trilostane

  Lipid-regulating Drugs: absorption of thiazides and related diuretics reduced by colestipol and colestyramine (give at least 2 hours apart)

- Lithium: loop diuretics and thiazides and related diuretics reduce excretion of •lithium (increased plasma concentration and risk of toxicity)—loop diuretics safer than thiazides; potassium-sparing diuretics and aldosterone antagonists reduce excretion of •lithium (increased plasma concentration and risk of toxicity); acetazolamide increases the excretion of •lithium

  Methyldopa: enhanced hypotensive effect when diuretics given with methyldopa

  Moxisylyte: enhanced hypotensive effect when diuretics given with moxisylyte

  Moxonidine: enhanced hypotensive effect when diuretics given with moxonidine

  Muscle Relaxants: enhanced hypotensive effect when diuretics given with baclofen or tizanidine

  Nitrates: enhanced hypotensive effect when diuretics given with nitrates

  Oestrogens: diuretic effect of diuretics antagonised by oestrogens

- Potassium Salts: increased risk of hyperkalaemia when potassium-sparing diuretics and aldosterone antagonists given with •potassium salts

  Progestogens: risk of hyperkalaemia when potassium-sparing diuretics and aldosterone antagonists given with drospirenone (monitor serum potassium during first cycle)

  Prostaglandins: enhanced hypotensive effect when diuretics given with alprostadil

  Sympathomimetics, Beta₂: increased risk of hypokalaemia when acetazolamide, loop diuretics or thiazides and related diuretics given with high doses of beta₂ sympathomimetics—see Hypokalaemia, p. 177

Diuretics *(continued)*

- Tacrolimus: increased risk of hyperkalaemia when potassium-sparing diuretics and aldosterone antagonists given with ●tacrolimus

  Theophylline: increased risk of hypokalaemia when acetazolamide, loop diuretics or thiazides and related diuretics given with theophylline

  Vasodilator Antihypertensives: enhanced hypotensive effect when diuretics given with hydralazine, minoxidil or sodium nitroprusside

  Vitamins: increased risk of hypercalcaemia when thiazides and related diuretics given with vitamin D

Diuretics, Loop *see* Diuretics

Diuretics, Potassium-sparing and Aldosterone Antagonists *see* Diuretics

Diuretics, Thiazide and related *see* Diuretics

Dobutamine *see* Sympathomimetics

Docetaxel

  Antibacterials: *in vitro* studies suggest a possible interaction between docetaxel and erythromycin (consult docetaxel product literature)

  Antiepileptics: cytotoxics possibly reduce absorption of phenytoin

  Antifungals: *in vitro* studies suggest a possible interaction between docetaxel and ketoconazole (consult docetaxel product literature)

- Antipsychotics: avoid concomitant use of cytotoxics with ●clozapine (increased risk of agranulocytosis)

  Cardiac Glycosides: cytotoxics reduce absorption of digoxin tablets

  Ciclosporin: *in vitro* studies suggest a possible interaction between docetaxel and ciclosporin (consult docetaxel product literature)

  Cytotoxics: plasma concentration of docetaxel increased by sorafenib

Domperidone

  Analgesics: effects of domperidone on gastro-intestinal activity antagonised by opioid analgesics

- Antifungals: risk of arrhythmias with domperidone possibly increased by ●ketoconazole

  Antimuscarinics: effects of domperidone on gastro-intestinal activity antagonised by antimuscarinics

  Dopaminergics: domperidone possibly antagonises hypoprolactinaemic effects of bromocriptine and cabergoline

Donepezil *see* Parasympathomimetics

Dopamine *see* Sympathomimetics

Dopaminergics *see* Amantadine, Apomorphine, Bromocriptine, Cabergoline, Entacapone, Levodopa, Pergolide, Pramipexole, Quinagolide, Rasagiline, Ropinirole, Rotigotine, Selegiline, and Tolcapone

Dopexamine *see* Sympathomimetics

Doripenem

- Antiepileptics: carbapenems reduce plasma concentration of ●valproate (possible therapeutic failure of valproate)

  Oestrogens: antibacterials that do not induce liver enzymes possibly reduce contraceptive effect of oestrogens (risk probably small, see p. 486)

  Probenecid: excretion of doripenem reduced by probenecid (manufacturers of doripenem advise avoid concomitant use)

  Vaccines: antibacterials inactivate oral typhoid vaccine—see p. 760

Dorzolamide *see* Diuretics

Dosulepin *see* Antidepressants, Tricyclic

Doxapram

  Antidepressants: effects of doxapram enhanced by MAOIs

  Sympathomimetics: increased risk of hypertension when doxapram given with sympathomimetics

  Theophylline: increased CNS stimulation when doxapram given with theophylline

Doxazosin *see* Alpha-blockers

Doxepin *see* Antidepressants, Tricyclic

Doxorubicin

  Antiepileptics: cytotoxics possibly reduce absorption of phenytoin

- Antipsychotics: avoid concomitant use of cytotoxics with ●clozapine (increased risk of agranulocytosis)

  Antivirals: doxorubicin possibly inhibits effects of stavudine

  Cardiac Glycosides: cytotoxics reduce absorption of digoxin tablets

- Ciclosporin: increased risk of neurotoxicity when doxorubicin given with ●ciclosporin

  Cytotoxics: plasma concentration of doxorubicin possibly increased by sorafenib

Doxycycline *see* Tetracyclines

Droperidol *see* Antipsychotics

Drospirenone *see* Progestogens

Drotrecogin Alfa

- Anticoagulants: manufacturer of drotrecogin alfa advises avoid concomitant use with high doses of ●heparins—consult product literature

Duloxetine

  Analgesics: possible increased serotonergic effects when duloxetine given with pethidine or tramadol

- Antibacterials: metabolism of duloxetine inhibited by ●ciprofloxacin—avoid concomitant use

- Antidepressants: metabolism of duloxetine inhibited by ●fluvoxamine—avoid concomitant use; possible increased serotonergic effects when duloxetine given with SSRIs, St John's wort, amitriptyline, clomipramine, ●moclobemide, tryptophan or venlafaxine; duloxetine should not be started until 2 weeks after stopping ●MAOIs, also MAOIs should not be started until at least 5 days after stopping duloxetine; after stopping SSRI-related antidepressants do not start ●moclobemide for at least 1 week

- Antimalarials: avoidance of antidepressants advised by manufacturer of ●artemether/lumefantrine

  Atomoxetine: possible increased risk of convulsions when antidepressants given with atomoxetine

- Hormone Antagonists: duloxetine possibly inhibits metabolism of ●tamoxifen to active metabolite (avoid concomitant use)

  5HT$_1$ Agonists: possible increased serotonergic effects when duloxetine given with 5HT$_1$ agonists

- Sibutramine: increased risk of CNS toxicity when SSRI-related antidepressants given with ●sibutramine (manufacturer of sibutramine advises avoid concomitant use)

Dutasteride

  Calcium-channel Blockers: plasma concentration of dutasteride increased by diltiazem and verapamil

Dydrogesterone *see* Progestogens

Edrophonium *see* Parasympathomimetics

Efavirenz

  Analgesics: efavirenz reduces plasma concentration of methadone

  Antibacterials: increased risk of rash when efavirenz given with clarithromycin; efavirenz reduces plasma concentration of rifabutin—increase dose of rifabutin; plasma concentration of efavirenz reduced by rifampicin—increase dose of efavirenz

- Anticoagulants: efavirenz possibly affects plasma concentration of ●warfarin

- Antidepressants: plasma concentration of efavirenz reduced by ●St John's wort—avoid concomitant use

  Antiepileptics: plasma concentration of both drugs reduced when efavirenz given with carbamazepine

  Antifungals: efavirenz reduces plasma concentration of itraconazole and ●posaconazole; efavirenz reduces plasma concentration of ●voriconazole, also plasma concentration of efavirenz increased (increase voriconazole dose and reduce efavirenz dose); efavirenz possibly reduces plasma concentration of caspofungin—consider increasing dose of caspofungin

- Antipsychotics: efavirenz possibly reduces plasma concentration of ●aripiprazole—increase dose of

Efavirenz

- Antipsychotics *(continued)*
  aripiprazole; efavirenz possibly increases plasma concentration of ●pimozide (increased risk of ventricular arrhythmias—avoid concomitant use)
- Antivirals: avoidance of efavirenz advised by manufacturer of ●atazanavir (plasma concentration of atazanavir reduced); efavirenz reduces plasma concentration of darunavir, fosamprenavir and indinavir; efavirenz possibly reduces plasma concentration of ●etravirine—avoid concomitant use; efavirenz reduces plasma concentration of ●lopinavir—consider increasing dose of lopinavir; efavirenz possibly reduces plasma concentration of ●maraviroc—consider increasing dose of maraviroc; plasma concentration of efavirenz reduced by nevirapine; toxicity of efavirenz increased by ritonavir, monitor liver function tests; efavirenz significantly reduces plasma concentration of saquinavir
- Anxiolytics and Hypnotics: increased risk of prolonged sedation when efavirenz given with ●midazolam—avoid concomitant use
  Calcium-channel Blockers: efavirenz reduces plasma concentration of diltiazem
- Ciclosporin: efavirenz possibly reduces plasma concentration of ●ciclosporin
- Ergot Alkaloids: increased risk of ergotism when efavirenz given with ●ergot alkaloids—avoid concomitant use
  Grapefruit Juice: plasma concentration of efavirenz possibly increased by grapefruit juice
  Lipid-regulating Drugs: efavirenz reduces plasma concentration of atorvastatin, pravastatin and simvastatin
  Oestrogens: efavirenz possibly reduces contraceptive effect of oestrogens
- Progestogens: efavirenz possibly reduces contraceptive effect of ●progestogens
- Tacrolimus: efavirenz possibly affects plasma concentration of ●tacrolimus

Eletriptan *see* 5HT$_1$ Agonists

Emtricitabine

Antivirals: manufacturer of emtricitabine advises avoid concomitant use with lamivudine

Enalapril *see* ACE Inhibitors

Enoxaparin *see* Heparins

Enoximone *see* Phosphodiesterase Inhibitors

Entacapone

- Anticoagulants: entacapone enhances anticoagulant effect of ●warfarin
- Antidepressants: manufacturer of entacapone advises caution with moclobemide, paroxetine, tricyclics and venlafaxine; avoid concomitant use of entacapone with non-selective ●MAOIs
  Dopaminergics: entacapone possibly enhances effects of apomorphine; entacapone possibly reduces plasma concentration of rasagiline; manufacturer of entacapone advises max. dose of 10 mg selegiline if used concomitantly
  Iron: absorption of entacapone reduced by *oral* iron
  Memantine: effects of dopaminergics possibly enhanced by memantine
  Methyldopa: entacapone possibly enhances effects of methyldopa; antiparkinsonian effect of dopaminergics antagonised by methyldopa
  Sympathomimetics: entacapone possibly enhances effects of adrenaline (epinephrine), dobutamine, dopamine and noradrenaline (norepinephrine)

Enteral Foods

- Anticoagulants: the presence of vitamin K in some enteral feeds can antagonise the anticoagulant effect of ●coumarins and ●phenindione
  Antiepileptics: enteral feeds possibly reduce absorption of phenytoin

Ephedrine *see* Sympathomimetics

Epinephrine (adrenaline) *see* Sympathomimetics

Epirubicin

Antiepileptics: cytotoxics possibly reduce absorption of phenytoin
- Antipsychotics: avoid concomitant use of cytotoxics with ●clozapine (increased risk of agranulocytosis)
  Cardiac Glycosides: cytotoxics reduce absorption of digoxin tablets
- Ciclosporin: plasma concentration of epirubicin increased by ●ciclosporin
- Ulcer-healing Drugs: plasma concentration of epirubicin increased by ●cimetidine

Eplerenone *see* Diuretics

Eprosartan *see* Angiotensin-II Receptor Antagonists

Eptifibatide

Iloprost: increased risk of bleeding when eptifibatide given with iloprost

Ergometrine *see* Ergot Alkaloids

Ergot Alkaloids

Anaesthetics, General: effects of ergometrine on the parturient uterus reduced by halothane
- Antibacterials: increased risk of ergotism when ergotamine and methysergide given with ●macrolides or ●telithromycin—avoid concomitant use; avoidance of ergotamine and methysergide advised by manufacturer of ●quinupristin/dalfopristin; increased risk of ergotism when ergotamine and methysergide given with tetracyclines
  Antidepressants: possible risk of hypertension when ergotamine and methysergide given with reboxetine
- Antifungals: increased risk of ergotism when ergotamine and methysergide given with ●imidazoles or ●triazoles—avoid concomitant use
- Antivirals: plasma concentration of ergot alkaloids possibly increased by ●atazanavir—avoid concomitant use; increased risk of ergotism when ergot alkaloids given with ●efavirenz—avoid concomitant use; increased risk of ergotism when ergotamine and methysergide given with ●fosamprenavir, ●indinavir, ●nelfinavir, ●ritonavir or ●saquinavir—avoid concomitant use
  Beta-blockers: increased peripheral vasoconstriction when ergotamine and methysergide given with beta-blockers
- 5HT$_1$ Agonists: increased risk of vasospasm when ergotamine and methysergide given with ●almotriptan, ●rizatriptan, ●sumatriptan or ●zolmitriptan (avoid ergotamine and methysergide for 6 hours after almotriptan, rizatriptan, sumatriptan or zolmitriptan, avoid almotriptan, rizatriptan, sumatriptan or zolmitriptan for 24 hours after ergotamine and methysergide); increased risk of vasospasm when ergotamine and methysergide given with ●eletriptan or ●frovatriptan (avoid ergotamine and methysergide for 24 hours after eletriptan or frovatriptan, avoid eletriptan or frovatriptan for 24 hours after ergotamine and methysergide); avoid concomitant use of ergotamine and methysergide with ●naratriptan
  Sympathomimetics: increased risk of ergotism when ergotamine and methysergide given with sympathomimetics
- Ulcer-healing Drugs: increased risk of ergotism when ergotamine and methysergide given with ●cimetidine—avoid concomitant use

Ergotamine and Methysergide *see* Ergot Alkaloids

Erlotinib

- Analgesics: increased risk of bleeding when erlotinib given with ●NSAIDs
  Antibacterials: plasma concentration of erlotinib increased by ciprofloxacin; metabolism of erlotinib accelerated by rifampicin (reduced plasma concentration)
- Anticoagulants: increased risk of bleeding when erlotinib given with ●coumarins
  Antiepileptics: cytotoxics possibly reduce absorption of phenytoin

Erlotinib (continued)

Antifungals: metabolism of erlotinib inhibited by keto-conazole (increased plasma concentration)

● Antipsychotics: avoid concomitant use of cytotoxics with ●clozapine (increased risk of agranulocytosis)

Cardiac Glycosides: cytotoxics reduce absorption of digoxin tablets

Cytotoxics: plasma concentration of erlotinib possibly increased by capecitabine

Tobacco: plasma concentration of erlotinib reduced by tobacco smoking

Ertapenem

● Antiepileptics: carbapenems reduce plasma concentration of ●valproate (possible therapeutic failure of valproate)

Oestrogens: antibacterials that do not induce liver enzymes possibly reduce contraceptive effect of oestrogens (risk probably small, see p. 486)

Vaccines: antibacterials inactivate oral typhoid vaccine–see p. 760

Erythromycin see Macrolides

Escitalopram see Antidepressants, SSRI

Eslicarbazepine

Anticoagulants: eslicarbazepine reduces plasma concentration of warfarin

● Antidepressants: anticonvulsant effect of antiepileptics possibly antagonised by MAOIs and ●tricyclic-related antidepressants (convulsive threshold lowered); anticonvulsant effect of antiepileptics antagonised by ●SSRIs and ●tricyclics (convulsive threshold lowered); avoid concomitant use of anti-epileptics with ●St John's wort

Antiepileptics: plasma concentration of both drugs reduced when eslicarbazepine given with carbamazepine; manufacturer of eslicarbazepine advises avoid concomitant use with oxcarbazepine; plasma concentration of eslicarbazepine reduced by phenytoin, also plasma concentration of phenytoin increased

● Antimalarials: possible increased risk of convulsions when antiepileptics given with chloroquine and hydroxychloroquine; anticonvulsant effect of anti-epileptics antagonised by ●mefloquine

● Oestrogens: eslicarbazepine accelerates metabolism of ●oestrogens (reduced contraceptive effect—see p. 486)

● Orlistat: possible increased risk of convulsions when antiepileptics given with ●orlistat

● Progestogens: eslicarbazepine accelerates metabolism of ●progestogens (reduced contraceptive effect—see p. 486)

Esmolol see Beta-blockers

Esomeprazole see Proton Pump Inhibitors

Estradiol see Oestrogens

Estramustine

Antiepileptics: cytotoxics possibly reduce absorption of phenytoin

● Antipsychotics: avoid concomitant use of cytotoxics with ●clozapine (increased risk of agranulocytosis)

● Bisphosphonates: plasma concentration of estra-mustine increased by ●sodium clodronate

Cardiac Glycosides: cytotoxics reduce absorption of digoxin tablets

Estriol see Oestrogens

Estrone see Oestrogens

Estropipate see Oestrogens

Etanercept

● Abatacept: avoid concomitant use of etanercept with ●abatacept

● Anakinra: avoid concomitant use of etanercept with ●anakinra

● Vaccines: avoid concomitant use of etanercept with live ●vaccines (see p. 733)

Ethinylestradiol see Oestrogens

Ethosuximide

● Antibacterials: metabolism of ethosuximide inhibited by ●isoniazid (increased plasma concentration and risk of toxicity)

● Antidepressants: anticonvulsant effect of antiepileptics possibly antagonised by MAOIs and ●tricyclic-related antidepressants (convulsive threshold lowered); anticonvulsant effect of antiepileptics antagonised by ●SSRIs and ●tricyclics (convulsive threshold lowered); avoid concomitant use of anti-epileptics with ●St John's wort

● Antiepileptics: plasma concentration of ethosuximide possibly reduced by carbamazepine and primidone; plasma concentration of ethosuximide possibly reduced by ●phenytoin, also plasma concentration of phenytoin possibly increased; plasma concentration of ethosuximide possibly increased by valproate

● Antimalarials: possible increased risk of convulsions when antiepileptics given with chloroquine and hydroxychloroquine; anticonvulsant effect of anti-epileptics antagonised by ●mefloquine

● Antipsychotics: anticonvulsant effect of ethosuximide antagonised by ●antipsychotics (convulsive threshold lowered)

Barbiturates: plasma concentration of ethosuximide possibly reduced by phenobarbital

● Orlistat: possible increased risk of convulsions when antiepileptics given with ●orlistat

Etodolac see NSAIDs

Etomidate see Anaesthetics, General

Etonogestrel see Progestogens

Etoposide

● Anticoagulants: etoposide possibly enhances antic-oagulant effect of ●coumarins

Antiepileptics: plasma concentration of etoposide possibly reduced by phenytoin; cytotoxics possibly reduce absorption of phenytoin

● Antipsychotics: avoid concomitant use of cytotoxics with ●clozapine (increased risk of agranulocytosis)

Barbiturates: plasma concentration of etoposide possibly reduced by phenobarbital

Cardiac Glycosides: cytotoxics reduce absorption of digoxin tablets

Ciclosporin: plasma concentration of etoposide possibly increased by ciclosporin (increased risk of toxicity)

Etoricoxib see NSAIDs

Etravirine

● Antibacterials: plasma concentration of etravirine increased by ●clarithromycin, also plasma concentration of clarithromycin reduced; plasma concentration of both drugs reduced when etravirine given with ●rifabutin; manufacturer of etravirine advises avoid concomitant use with rifampicin

Antidepressants: manufacturer of etravirine advises avoid concomitant use with St John's wort

Antiepileptics: manufacturer of etravirine advises avoid concomitant use with carbamazepine and phenytoin

● Antivirals: plasma concentration of etravirine possibly reduced by ●efavirenz and ●nevirapine—avoid concomitant use; etravirine increases plasma concentration of ●fosamprenavir (consider reducing dose of fosamprenavir); etravirine possibly reduces plasma concentration of ●indinavir—avoid concomitant use; etravirine possibly reduces plasma concentration of maraviroc; etravirine possibly increases plasma concentration of nelfinavir—avoid concomitant use; plasma concentration of etravirine reduced by ●tipranavir, also plasma concentration of tipranavir increased (avoid concomitant use)

Barbiturates: manufacturer of etravirine advises avoid concomitant use with phenobarbital

Cardiac Glycosides: etravirine increases plasma concentration of digoxin

Clopidogrel: etravirine possibly reduces antiplatelet effect of ●clopidogrel

Etravirine *(continued)*

Lipid-regulating Drugs: etravirine possibly reduces plasma concentration of atorvastatin

Sildenafil: etravirine reduces plasma concentration of sildenafil

Etynodiol *see* Progestogens

Everolimus

● Antibacterials: plasma concentration of everolimus possibly increased by ●clarithromycin and ●telithromycin—manufacturer of everolimus advises avoid concomitant use; plasma concentration of everolimus increased by ●erythromycin; plasma concentration of everolimus reduced by ●rifampicin

Antidepressants: plasma concentration of everolimus possibly reduced by St John's wort—manufacturer of everolimus advises avoid concomitant use

Antiepileptics: cytotoxics possibly reduce absorption of phenytoin

● Antifungals: plasma concentration of everolimus increased by ●ketoconazole—avoid concomitant use; plasma concentration of everolimus possibly increased by ●itraconazole, ●posaconazole and ●voriconazole—manufacturer of everolimus advises avoid concomitant use

● Antipsychotics: avoid concomitant use of cytotoxics with ●clozapine (increased risk of agranulocytosis)

● Antivirals: plasma concentration of everolimus possibly increased by ●atazanavir, ●darunavir, ●indinavir, ●nelfinavir, ●ritonavir and ●saquinavir—manufacturer of everolimus advises avoid concomitant use

● Calcium-channel Blockers: plasma concentration of both drugs may increase when everolimus given with ●verapamil

Cardiac Glycosides: cytotoxics reduce absorption of digoxin tablets

● Ciclosporin: plasma concentration of everolimus increased by ●ciclosporin

Grapefruit Juice: manufacturer of everolimus advises avoid concomitant use with grapefruit juice

Exemestane

Antibacterials: plasma concentration of exemestane possibly reduced by rifampicin

Ezetimibe

Anticoagulants: ezetimibe possibly enhances anticoagulant effect of coumarins

● Ciclosporin: plasma concentration of both drugs may increase when ezetimibe given with ●ciclosporin

Lipid-regulating Drugs: increased risk of cholelithiasis and gallbladder disease when ezetimibe given with fibrates—discontinue if suspected

Famciclovir

Probenecid: excretion of famciclovir possibly reduced by probenecid (increased plasma concentration)

Famotidine *see* Histamine H$_2$-antagonists

Felodipine *see* Calcium-channel Blockers

Fenbufen *see* NSAIDs

Fenofibrate *see* Fibrates

Fenoprofen *see* NSAIDs

Fenoterol *see* Sympathomimetics, Beta$_2$

Fentanyl *see* Opioid Analgesics

Ferrous Salts *see* Iron

Fesoterodine *see* Antimuscarinics

Fexofenadine *see* Antihistamines

Fibrates

● Antibacterials: increased risk of myopathy when fibrates given with ●daptomycin (preferably avoid concomitant use)

● Anticoagulants: fibrates enhance anticoagulant effect of ●coumarins and ●phenindione

● Antidiabetics: gemfibrozil increases plasma concentration of ●rosiglitazone (consider reducing dose of rosiglitazone); fibrates may improve glucose tolerance and have an additive effect with insulin or sulphonylureas; gemfibrozil possibly enhances hypoglycaemic effect of nateglinide; increased risk of

Fibrates

● Antidiabetics *(continued)*

severe hypoglycaemia when gemfibrozil given with ●repaglinide—avoid concomitant use

Ciclosporin: increased risk of renal impairment when bezafibrate or fenofibrate given with ciclosporin

● Cytotoxics: gemfibrozil increases plasma concentration of ●bexarotene—avoid concomitant use

● Lipid-regulating Drugs: increased risk of cholelithiasis and gallbladder disease when fibrates given with ezetimibe—discontinue if suspected; increased risk of myopathy when fibrates given with ●statins; increased risk of myopathy when gemfibrozil given with ●statins (preferably avoid concomitant use)

Filgrastim

Note. Pegfilgrastim interactions as for filgrastim

Cytotoxics: neutropenia possibly exacerbated when filgrastim given with fluorouracil

Flavoxate *see* Antimuscarinics

Flecainide

Anaesthetics, Local: increased myocardial depression when anti-arrhythmics given with bupivacaine, levobupivacaine, prilocaine or ropivacaine

● Anti-arrhythmics: increased myocardial depression when anti-arrhythmics given with other ●anti-arrhythmics; plasma concentration of flecainide increased by ●amiodarone (halve dose of flecainide)

● Antidepressants: plasma concentration of flecainide increased by fluoxetine; increased risk of ventricular arrhythmias when flecainide given with ●tricyclics

● Antihistamines: increased risk of ventricular arrhythmias when flecainide given with ●mizolastine—avoid concomitant use

● Antimalarials: avoidance of flecainide advised by manufacturer of ●artemether/lumefantrine (risk of ventricular arrhythmias); plasma concentration of flecainide increased by ●quinine

● Antimuscarinics: increased risk of ventricular arrhythmias when flecainide given with ●tolterodine

● Antipsychotics: increased risk of ventricular arrhythmias when anti-arrhythmics that prolong the QT interval given with ●antipsychotics that prolong the QT interval; increased risk of arrhythmias when flecainide given with ●clozapine

● Antivirals: plasma concentration of flecainide possibly increased by ●fosamprenavir, ●indinavir, ●lopinavir and ●ritonavir (increased risk of ventricular arrhythmias—avoid concomitant use)

● Beta-blockers: increased risk of myocardial depression and bradycardia when flecainide given with ●beta-blockers; increased myocardial depression when anti-arrhythmics given with ●beta-blockers

● Calcium-channel Blockers: increased risk of myocardial depression and asystole when flecainide given with ●verapamil

● Diuretics: increased cardiac toxicity with flecainide if hypokalaemia occurs with ●acetazolamide, ●loop diuretics or ●thiazides and related diuretics

Ulcer-healing Drugs: metabolism of flecainide inhibited by cimetidine (increased plasma concentration)

Flucloxacillin *see* Penicillins

Fluconazole *see* Antifungals, Triazole

Flucytosine

Antifungals: renal excretion of flucytosine decreased and cellular uptake increased by amphotericin (toxicity possibly increased)

Cytotoxics: plasma concentration of flucytosine possibly reduced by cytarabine

Fludarabine

Antiepileptics: cytotoxics possibly reduce absorption of phenytoin

● Antipsychotics: avoid concomitant use of cytotoxics with ●clozapine (increased risk of agranulocytosis)

Cardiac Glycosides: cytotoxics reduce absorption of digoxin tablets

Fludarabine *(continued)*
- Cytotoxics: fludarabine increases intracellular concentration of cytarabine; increased pulmonary toxicity when fludarabine given with ●pentostatin (unacceptably high incidence of fatalities)

  Dipyridamole: effects of fludarabine possibly reduced by dipyridamole

Fludrocortisone *see* Corticosteroids

Flunisolide *see* Corticosteroids

Fluorides

  Calcium Salts: absorption of fluorides reduced by calcium salts

Fluorouracil

  Note. Capecitabine is a prodrug of fluorouracil

  Note. Tegafur is a prodrug of fluorouracil
- Allopurinol: manufacturer of capecitabine advises avoid concomitant use with ●allopurinol

  Antibacterials: metabolism of fluorouracil inhibited by metronidazole (increased toxicity)
- Anticoagulants: fluorouracil enhances anticoagulant effect of ●coumarins

  Antiepileptics: fluorouracil possibly inhibits metabolism of phenytoin (increased risk of toxicity); cytotoxics possibly reduce absorption of phenytoin
- Antipsychotics: avoid concomitant use of cytotoxics with ●clozapine (increased risk of agranulocytosis)

  Cardiac Glycosides: cytotoxics reduce absorption of digoxin tablets

  Cytotoxics: capecitabine possibly increases plasma concentration of erlotinib

  Filgrastim: neutropenia possibly exacerbated when fluorouracil given with filgrastim
- Temoporfin: increased skin photosensitivity when *topical* fluorouracil used with ●temoporfin

  Ulcer-healing Drugs: metabolism of fluorouracil inhibited by cimetidine (increased plasma concentration)

Fluoxetine *see* Antidepressants, SSRI

Flupentixol *see* Antipsychotics

Fluphenazine *see* Antipsychotics

Flurazepam *see* Anxiolytics and Hypnotics

Flurbiprofen *see* NSAIDs

Flutamide
- Anticoagulants: flutamide enhances anticoagulant effect of ●coumarins

Fluticasone *see* Corticosteroids

Fluvastatin *see* Statins

Fluvoxamine *see* Antidepressants, SSRI

Folates

  Aminosalicylates: absorption of folic acid possibly reduced by sulfasalazine

  Antiepileptics: folates possibly reduce plasma concentration of phenytoin and primidone

  Barbiturates: folates possibly reduce plasma concentration of phenobarbital
- Cytotoxics: avoidance of folates advised by manufacturer of ●raltitrexed

Folic Acid *see* Folates

Folinic Acid *see* Folates

Formoterol *see* Sympathomimetics, Beta$_2$

Fosamprenavir

  Note. Fosamprenavir is a prodrug of amprenavir

  Analgesics: fosamprenavir reduces plasma concentration of methadone

  Antacids: absorption of fosamprenavir possibly reduced by antacids
- Anti-arrhythmics: fosamprenavir possibly increases plasma concentration of ●amiodarone, ●flecainide and ●propafenone (increased risk of ventricular arrhythmias—avoid concomitant use); fosamprenavir possibly increases plasma concentration of ●lidocaine—avoid concomitant use
- Antibacterials: plasma concentration of both drugs increased when fosamprenavir given with erythromycin; fosamprenavir increases plasma concentration of ●rifabutin (reduce dose of rifabutin); plasma concentration of fosamprenavir significantly reduced

Fosamprenavir
- Antibacterials *(continued)*

  by ●rifampicin—avoid concomitant use; fosamprenavir possibly increases plasma concentration of dapsone; avoidance of concomitant fosamprenavir in severe renal and hepatic impairment advised by manufacturer of ●telithromycin

  Anticoagulants: fosamprenavir may enhance or reduce anticoagulant effect of coumarins; avoidance of fosamprenavir advised by manufacturer of rivaroxaban
- Antidepressants: plasma concentration of fosamprenavir reduced by ●St John's wort—avoid concomitant use; fosamprenavir possibly increases side-effects of tricyclics

  Antiepileptics: plasma concentration of fosamprenavir possibly reduced by carbamazepine and phenytoin

  Antifungals: fosamprenavir increases plasma concentration of ketoconazole; fosamprenavir possibly increases plasma concentration of itraconazole

  Antihistamines: fosamprenavir possibly increases plasma concentration of loratadine

  Antimalarials: caution with fosamprenavir advised by manufacturer of artemether/lumefantrine

  Antimuscarinics: avoidance of fosamprenavir advised by manufacturer of darifenacin and tolterodine
- Antipsychotics: fosamprenavir possibly inhibits metabolism of ●aripiprazole (reduce dose of aripiprazole); fosamprenavir possibly increases plasma concentration of clozapine; fosamprenavir increases plasma concentration of ●pimozide and ●sertindole (increased risk of ventricular arrhythmias—avoid concomitant use)
- Antivirals: plasma concentration of fosamprenavir reduced by efavirenz and ●tipranavir; plasma concentration of fosamprenavir increased by ●etravirine (consider reducing dose of fosamprenavir); plasma concentration of fosamprenavir reduced by lopinavir, effect on lopinavir plasma concentration not predictable—avoid concomitant use; plasma concentration of fosamprenavir possibly reduced by nevirapine
- Anxiolytics and Hypnotics: increased risk of prolonged sedation and respiratory depression when fosamprenavir given with ●alprazolam, clonazepam, ●diazepam, ●flurazepam or ●midazolam

  Barbiturates: plasma concentration of fosamprenavir possibly reduced by phenobarbital
- Cilostazol: fosamprenavir possibly increases plasma concentration of ●cilostazol—avoid concomitant use
- Ergot Alkaloids: increased risk of ergotism when fosamprenavir given with ●ergotamine and methysergide—avoid concomitant use
- Lipid-regulating Drugs: possible increased risk of myopathy when fosamprenavir given with atorvastatin; possible increased risk of myopathy when fosamprenavir given with ●rosuvastatin or ●simvastatin—avoid concomitant use

  Oestrogens: fosamprenavir increases plasma concentration of oestrogens, also plasma concentration of fosamprenavir reduced—alternative contraception recommended

  Progestogens: fosamprenavir increases plasma concentration of progestogens, also plasma concentration of fosamprenavir reduced—alternative contraception recommended
- Ranolazine: fosamprenavir possibly increases plasma concentration of ●ranolazine—manufacturer of ranolazine advises avoid concomitant use

  Sildenafil: fosamprenavir possibly increases plasma concentration of sildenafil—reduce initial dose of sildenafil

  Tadalafil: fosamprenavir possibly increases plasma concentration of tadalafil

  Ulcer-healing Drugs: fosamprenavir possibly increases plasma concentration of cimetidine

Fosamprenavir *(continued)*

Vardenafil: fosamprenavir possibly increases plasma concentration of vardenafil

Fosaprepitant *see* Aprepitant

Foscarnet

Antivirals: avoidance of foscarnet advised by manufacturer of lamivudine

- Pentamidine Isetionate: increased risk of hypocalcaemia when foscarnet given with *parenteral* ●pentamidine isetionate

Fosinopril *see* ACE Inhibitors

Fosphenytoin *see* Phenytoin

Framycetin *see* Aminoglycosides

Frovatriptan *see* 5HT$_1$ Agonists

Furosemide *see* Diuretics

Fusidic Acid

- Antivirals: plasma concentration of both drugs increased when fusidic acid given with ●ritonavir—avoid concomitant use
- Lipid-regulating Drugs: possible increased risk of myopathy when fusidic acid given with atorvastatin; increased risk of myopathy when fusidic acid given with ●simvastatin

Oestrogens: antibacterials that do not induce liver enzymes possibly reduce contraceptive effect of oestrogens (risk probably small, see p. 486)

Sugammadex: fusidic acid possibly reduces response to sugammadex

Vaccines: antibacterials inactivate oral typhoid vaccine–see p. 760

Gabapentin

Analgesics: bioavailability of gabapentin increased by morphine

Antacids: absorption of gabapentin reduced by antacids

- Antidepressants: anticonvulsant effect of antiepileptics possibly antagonised by MAOIs and ●tricyclic-related antidepressants (convulsive threshold lowered); anticonvulsant effect of antiepileptics antagonised by ●SSRIs and ●tricyclics (convulsive threshold lowered); avoid concomitant use of antiepileptics with ●St John's wort
- Antimalarials: possible increased risk of convulsions when antiepileptics given with chloroquine and hydroxychloroquine; anticonvulsant effect of antiepileptics antagonised by ●mefloquine
- Orlistat: possible increased risk of convulsions when antiepileptics given with ●orlistat

Galantamine *see* Parasympathomimetics

Ganciclovir

Note. Increased risk of myelosuppression with other myelosuppressive drugs—consult product literature

Note. Valganciclovir interactions as for ganciclovir

- Antibacterials: increased risk of convulsions when ganciclovir given with ●imipenem with cilastatin
- Antivirals: ganciclovir possibly increases plasma concentration of didanosine; avoidance of *intravenous* ganciclovir advised by manufacturer of lamivudine; profound myelosuppression when ganciclovir given with ●zidovudine (if possible avoid concomitant administration, particularly during initial ganciclovir therapy)

Mycophenolate: plasma concentration of ganciclovir possibly increased by mycophenolate, also plasma concentration of inactive metabolite of mycophenolate possibly increased

Probenecid: excretion of ganciclovir reduced by probenecid (increased plasma concentration and risk of toxicity)

Tacrolimus: possible increased risk of nephrotoxicity when ganciclovir given with tacrolimus

Gefitinib

- Antibacterials: plasma concentration of gefitinib reduced by ●rifampicin—avoid concomitant use
- Anticoagulants: gefitinib possibly enhances anticoagulant effect of ●warfarin

Gefitinib *(continued)*

Antidepressants: manufacturer of gefitinib advises avoid concomitant use with St John's wort

Antiepileptics: manufacturer of gefitinib advises avoid concomitant use with carbamazepine and phenytoin; cytotoxics possibly reduce absorption of phenytoin

Antifungals: plasma concentration of gefitinib increased by itraconazole

- Antipsychotics: avoid concomitant use of cytotoxics with ●clozapine (increased risk of agranulocytosis)

Barbiturates: manufacturer of gefitinib advises avoid concomitant use with barbiturates

Cardiac Glycosides: cytotoxics reduce absorption of digoxin tablets

Ulcer-healing Drugs: plasma concentration of gefitinib possibly reduced by ranitidine

Gemcitabine

Anticoagulants: gemcitabine possibly enhances anticoagulant effect of warfarin

Antiepileptics: cytotoxics possibly reduce absorption of phenytoin

- Antipsychotics: avoid concomitant use of cytotoxics with ●clozapine (increased risk of agranulocytosis)

Cardiac Glycosides: cytotoxics reduce absorption of digoxin tablets

Gemeprost *see* Prostaglandins

Gemfibrozil *see* Fibrates

Gentamicin *see* Aminoglycosides

Gestodene *see* Progestogens

Glibenclamide *see* Antidiabetics

Gliclazide *see* Antidiabetics

Glimepiride *see* Antidiabetics

Glipizide *see* Antidiabetics

Glucosamine

- Anticoagulants: glucosamine enhances anticoagulant effect of ●warfarin (avoid concomitant use)

Glyceryl Trinitrate *see* Nitrates

Glycopyrronium *see* Antimuscarinics

Gold

Penicillamine: avoidance of gold advised by manufacturer of penicillamine (increased risk of toxicity)

Grapefruit Juice

Anti-arrhythmics: grapefruit juice increases plasma concentration of amiodarone

- Antihistamines: grapefruit juice increases plasma concentration of ●rupatadine—avoid concomitant use

Antimalarials: grapefruit juice possibly increases plasma concentration of artemether/lumefantrine

Antivirals: grapefruit juice possibly increases plasma concentration of efavirenz

Anxiolytics and Hypnotics: grapefruit juice increases plasma concentration of buspirone

Calcium-channel Blockers: grapefruit juice increases plasma concentration of felodipine, isradipine, lacidipine, lercanidipine, nicardipine, nifedipine, nimodipine and verapamil

- Ciclosporin: grapefruit juice increases plasma concentration of ●ciclosporin (increased risk of toxicity)
- Cytotoxics: avoidance of grapefruit juice advised by manufacturer of everolimus, ●lapatinib and ●nilotinib

Ivabradine: grapefruit juice increases plasma concentration of ivabradine

- Lipid-regulating Drugs: grapefruit juice possibly increases plasma concentration of atorvastatin; grapefruit juice increases plasma concentration of ●simvastatin—avoid concomitant use
- Ranolazine: grapefruit juice possibly increases plasma concentration of ●ranolazine—manufacturer of ranolazine advises avoid concomitant use

Sildenafil: grapefruit juice possibly increases plasma concentration of sildenafil

- Sirolimus: grapefruit juice increases plasma concentration of ●sirolimus—avoid concomitant use
- Tacrolimus: grapefruit juice increases plasma concentration of ●tacrolimus

Grapefruit Juice *(continued)*

Tadalafil: grapefruit juice possibly increases plasma concentration of tadalafil

• Tolvaptan: grapefruit juice increases plasma concentration of •tolvaptan—avoid concomitant use

• Vardenafil: grapefruit juice possibly increases plasma concentration of •vardenafil—avoid concomitant use

Griseofulvin

Alcohol: griseofulvin possibly enhances effects of alcohol

• Anticoagulants: griseofulvin reduces anticoagulant effect of •coumarins

Antiepileptics: absorption of griseofulvin reduced by primidone (reduced effect)

Barbiturates: absorption of griseofulvin reduced by phenobarbital (reduced effect)

Ciclosporin: griseofulvin possibly reduces plasma concentration of ciclosporin

• Oestrogens: griseofulvin accelerates metabolism of •oestrogens (reduced contraceptive effect—see p. 486)

• Progestogens: griseofulvin accelerates metabolism of •progestogens (reduced contraceptive effect—see p. 486)

Guanethidine *see* Adrenergic Neurone Blockers

Haloperidol *see* Antipsychotics

Halothane *see* Anaesthetics, General

Heparin *see* Heparins

Heparins

ACE Inhibitors: increased risk of hyperkalaemia when heparins given with ACE inhibitors

Aliskiren: increased risk of hyperkalaemia when heparins given with aliskiren

• Analgesics: possible increased risk of bleeding when heparins given with NSAIDs; increased risk of haemorrhage when anticoagulants given with *intravenous* •diclofenac (avoid concomitant use, including low-dose heparins); increased risk of haemorrhage when anticoagulants given with •ketorolac (avoid concomitant use, including low-dose heparins); anticoagulant effect of heparins enhanced by •aspirin

Angiotensin-II Receptor Antagonists: increased risk of hyperkalaemia when heparins given with angiotensin-II receptor antagonists

Clopidogrel: increased risk of bleeding when heparins given with clopidogrel

Dipyridamole: anticoagulant effect of heparins enhanced by dipyridamole

• Drotrecogin Alfa: avoidance of concomitant use of high doses of heparins with drotrecogin alfa advised by manufacturer of •drotrecogin alfa—consult product literature

Iloprost: anticoagulant effect of heparins possibly enhanced by iloprost

• Nitrates: anticoagulant effect of heparins reduced by *infusion* of •glyceryl trinitrate

Sibutramine: increased risk of bleeding when anticoagulants given with sibutramine

Histamine H$_2$-antagonists

• Alpha-blockers: cimetidine and ranitidine antagonise effects of •tolazoline

Analgesics: cimetidine possibly increases plasma concentration of azapropazone; cimetidine inhibits metabolism of opioid analgesics (increased plasma concentration)

• Anti-arrhythmics: cimetidine increases plasma concentration of amiodarone and •propafenone; cimetidine inhibits metabolism of flecainide (increased plasma concentration); cimetidine increases plasma concentration of •lidocaine (increased risk of toxicity)

Antibacterials: histamine H$_2$-antagonists reduce absorption of cefpodoxime; cimetidine increases plasma concentration of erythromycin (increased

Histamine H$_2$-antagonists

Antibacterials *(continued)*

risk of toxicity, including deafness); cimetidine inhibits metabolism of metronidazole (increased plasma concentration); metabolism of cimetidine accelerated by rifampicin (reduced plasma concentration)

• Anticoagulants: cimetidine inhibits metabolism of •coumarins (enhanced anticoagulant effect)

Antidepressants: cimetidine increases plasma concentration of citalopram, escitalopram, mirtazapine and sertraline; cimetidine inhibits metabolism of amitriptyline, doxepin, imipramine and nortriptyline (increased plasma concentration); cimetidine increases plasma concentration of moclobemide (halve dose of moclobemide); cimetidine possibly increases plasma concentration of tricyclics

Antidiabetics: cimetidine reduces excretion of metformin (increased plasma concentration); cimetidine enhances hypoglycaemic effect of sulphonylureas

• Antiepileptics: cimetidine inhibits metabolism of •carbamazepine, •phenytoin and •valproate (increased plasma concentration)

• Antifungals: histamine H$_2$-antagonists reduce absorption of itraconazole and ketoconazole; cimetidine reduces plasma concentration of •posaconazole; cimetidine increases plasma concentration of terbinafine

Antihistamines: manufacturer of loratadine advises cimetidine possibly increases plasma concentration of loratadine

• Antimalarials: avoidance of cimetidine advised by manufacturer of •artemether/lumefantrine; cimetidine inhibits metabolism of chloroquine and hydroxychloroquine and quinine (increased plasma concentration)

• Antipsychotics: cimetidine possibly enhances effects of antipsychotics, chlorpromazine and clozapine; increased risk of ventricular arrhythmias when cimetidine given with •sertindole—avoid concomitant use

Antivirals: histamine H$_2$-antagonists possibly reduce plasma concentration of atazanavir; plasma concentration of cimetidine possibly increased by fosamprenavir; histamine H$_2$-antagonists possibly increase plasma concentration of raltegravir—manufacturer of raltegravir advises avoid concomitant use; cimetidine possibly increases plasma concentration of saquinavir

Anxiolytics and Hypnotics: cimetidine inhibits metabolism of benzodiazepines, clomethiazole and zaleplon (increased plasma concentration); cimetidine increases plasma concentration of melatonin

Beta-blockers: cimetidine increases plasma concentration of labetalol, metoprolol and propranolol

Calcium-channel Blockers: cimetidine possibly inhibits metabolism of calcium-channel blockers (increased plasma concentration); cimetidine increases plasma concentration of isradipine (halve dose of isradipine)

• Ciclosporin: cimetidine possibly increases plasma concentration of •ciclosporin

• Cilostazol: cimetidine possibly increases plasma concentration of •cilostazol—avoid concomitant use

• Clopidogrel: cimetidine possibly reduces antiplatelet effect of •clopidogrel

• Cytotoxics: cimetidine possibly enhances myelosuppressive effects of carmustine and lomustine; cimetidine increases plasma concentration of •epirubicin; cimetidine inhibits metabolism of fluorouracil (increased plasma concentration); famotidine possibly reduces plasma concentration of dasatinib; ranitidine possibly reduces plasma concentration of gefitinib; histamine H$_2$-antagonists possibly reduce absorption of lapatinib

Dopaminergics: cimetidine reduces excretion of pramipexole (increased plasma concentration)

Histamine H₂-antagonists *(continued)*

- Ergot Alkaloids: increased risk of ergotism when cimetidine given with ●ergotamine and methysergide—avoid concomitant use

  Hormone Antagonists: absorption of cimetidine possibly delayed by octreotide

  5HT₁ Agonists: cimetidine inhibits metabolism of zolmitriptan (reduce dose of zolmitriptan)

  Mebendazole: cimetidine possibly inhibits metabolism of mebendazole (increased plasma concentration)

  Sildenafil: cimetidine increases plasma concentration of sildenafil (reduce initial dose of sildenafil)

- Theophylline: cimetidine inhibits metabolism of ●theophylline (increased plasma concentration)

  Thyroid Hormones: cimetidine reduces absorption of levothyroxine

- Ulipristal: avoidance of histamine H₂-antagonists advised by manufacturer of ●ulipristal (plasma concentration of ulipristal possibly reduced)

Homatropine *see* Antimuscarinics

Hormone Antagonists *see* Bicalutamide, Danazol, Dutasteride, Exemestane, Flutamide, Lanreotide, Octreotide, Tamoxifen, Toremifene, and Trilostane

5HT₁ Agonists

- Antibacterials: plasma concentration of eletriptan increased by ●clarithromycin and ●erythromycin (risk of toxicity)—avoid concomitant use; metabolism of zolmitriptan possibly inhibited by quinolones (reduce dose of zolmitriptan)

- Antidepressants: increased risk of CNS toxicity when sumatriptan given with ●citalopram, ●escitalopram, ●fluoxetine, ●fluvoxamine or ●paroxetine; metabolism of frovatriptan inhibited by fluvoxamine; metabolism of zolmitriptan possibly inhibited by fluvoxamine (reduce dose of zolmitriptan); CNS toxicity reported when sumatriptan given with sertraline; possible increased serotonergic effects when 5HT₁ agonists given with duloxetine; risk of CNS toxicity when rizatriptan or sumatriptan given with ●MAOIs (avoid rizatriptan or sumatriptan for 2 weeks after MAOIs); increased risk of CNS toxicity when zolmitriptan given with ●MAOIs; risk of CNS toxicity when rizatriptan or sumatriptan given with ●moclobemide (avoid rizatriptan or sumatriptan for 2 weeks after moclobemide); risk of CNS toxicity when zolmitriptan given with ●moclobemide (reduce dose of zolmitriptan); increased serotonergic effects when 5HT₁ agonists given with ●St John's wort—avoid concomitant use

- Antifungals: plasma concentration of eletriptan increased by ●itraconazole and ●ketoconazole (risk of toxicity)—avoid concomitant use; plasma concentration of almotriptan increased by ketoconazole (increased risk of toxicity)

- Antivirals: plasma concentration of eletriptan increased by ●indinavir, ●nelfinavir and ●ritonavir (risk of toxicity)—avoid concomitant use

  Beta-blockers: plasma concentration of rizatriptan increased by propranolol (manufacturer of rizatriptan advises halve dose and avoid within 2 hours of propranolol)

- Ergot Alkaloids: increased risk of vasospasm when almotriptan, rizatriptan, sumatriptan or zolmitriptan given with ●ergotamine and methysergide (avoid ergotamine and methysergide for 6 hours after almotriptan, rizatriptan, sumatriptan or zolmitriptan, avoid almotriptan, rizatriptan, sumatriptan or zolmitriptan for 24 hours after ergotamine and methysergide); avoid concomitant use of naratriptan with ●ergotamine and methysergide; increased risk of vasospasm when eletriptan or frovatriptan given with ●ergotamine and methysergide (avoid ergotamine and methysergide for 24 hours after eletriptan or frovatriptan, avoid eletriptan or frovatriptan for 24 hours after ergotamine and methysergide)

5HT₁ Agonists *(continued)*

Ulcer-healing Drugs: metabolism of zolmitriptan inhibited by cimetidine (reduce dose of zolmitriptan)

5HT₃ Antagonists

Analgesics: ondansetron possibly antagonises effects of tramadol

Antibacterials: metabolism of ondansetron accelerated by rifampicin (reduced effect)

Antiepileptics: metabolism of ondansetron accelerated by carbamazepine and phenytoin (reduced effect)

Hydralazine *see* Vasodilator Antihypertensives

Hydrochlorothiazide *see* Diuretics

Hydrocortisone *see* Corticosteroids

Hydroflumethiazide *see* Diuretics

Hydromorphone *see* Opioid Analgesics

Hydrotalcite *see* Antacids

Hydroxocobalamin

Antibacterials: response to hydroxocobalamin reduced by chloramphenicol

Hydroxycarbamide

Antiepileptics: cytotoxics possibly reduce absorption of phenytoin

- Antipsychotics: avoid concomitant use of cytotoxics with ●clozapine (increased risk of agranulocytosis)

- Antivirals: increased risk of toxicity when hydroxycarbamide given with ●didanosine and ●stavudine—avoid concomitant use

  Cardiac Glycosides: cytotoxics reduce absorption of digoxin tablets

Hydroxychloroquine *see* Chloroquine and Hydroxychloroquine

Hydroxyzine *see* Antihistamines

Hyoscine *see* Antimuscarinics

Ibandronic Acid *see* Bisphosphonates

Ibuprofen *see* NSAIDs

Idarubicin

Antiepileptics: cytotoxics possibly reduce absorption of phenytoin

- Antipsychotics: avoid concomitant use of cytotoxics with ●clozapine (increased risk of agranulocytosis)

  Cardiac Glycosides: cytotoxics reduce absorption of digoxin tablets

- Ciclosporin: plasma concentration of idarubicin increased by ●ciclosporin

Ifosfamide

- Anticoagulants: ifosfamide possibly enhances anticoagulant effect of ●coumarins

  Antiepileptics: cytotoxics possibly reduce absorption of phenytoin

- Antipsychotics: avoid concomitant use of cytotoxics with ●clozapine (increased risk of agranulocytosis)

  Cardiac Glycosides: cytotoxics reduce absorption of digoxin tablets

Iloprost

Analgesics: increased risk of bleeding when iloprost given with NSAIDs or aspirin

Anticoagulants: iloprost possibly enhances anticoagulant effect of coumarins and heparins; increased risk of bleeding when iloprost given with phenindione

Clopidogrel: increased risk of bleeding when iloprost given with clopidogrel

Eptifibatide: increased risk of bleeding when iloprost given with eptifibatide

Tirofiban: increased risk of bleeding when iloprost given with tirofiban

Imatinib

- Antibacterials: plasma concentration of imatinib reduced by ●rifampicin—avoid concomitant use

  Anticoagulants: manufacturer of imatinib advises replacement of warfarin with a heparin (possibility of enhanced warfarin effect)

- Antidepressants: plasma concentration of imatinib reduced by ●St John's wort—avoid concomitant use

- Antiepileptics: plasma concentration of imatinib reduced by ●carbamazepine, ●oxcarbazepine and

Imatinib
- Antiepileptics *(continued)*
  - ●phenytoin—avoid concomitant use; cytotoxics possibly reduce absorption of phenytoin
  - Antifungals: plasma concentration of imatinib increased by ketoconazole
- Antipsychotics: avoid concomitant use of cytotoxics with ●clozapine (increased risk of agranulocytosis)
  - Cardiac Glycosides: cytotoxics reduce absorption of digoxin tablets
  - Ciclosporin: imatinib possibly increases plasma concentration of ciclosporin
  - Lipid-regulating Drugs: imatinib increases plasma concentration of simvastatin
  - Thyroid Hormones: imatinib possibly reduces plasma concentration of levothyroxine

Imidapril *see* ACE Inhibitors

Imipenem with Cilastatin
- Antiepileptics: carbapenems reduce plasma concentration of ●valproate (possible therapeutic failure of valproate)
- Antivirals: increased risk of convulsions when imipenem with cilastatin given with ●ganciclovir
  - Oestrogens: antibacterials that do not induce liver enzymes possibly reduce contraceptive effect of oestrogens (risk probably small, see p. 486)
  - Vaccines: antibacterials inactivate oral typhoid vaccine–see p. 760

Imipramine *see* Antidepressants, Tricyclic

Immunoglobulins
  Note. For advice on immunoglobulins and live virus vaccines, see under Normal Immunoglobulin, p. 763

Indapamide *see* Diuretics

Indinavir
  Aldesleukin: plasma concentration of indinavir possibly increased by aldesleukin
- Anti-arrhythmics: indinavir possibly increases plasma concentration of ●amiodarone—avoid concomitant use; indinavir possibly increases plasma concentration of ●flecainide (increased risk of ventricular arrhythmias—avoid concomitant use)
- Antibacterials: indinavir increases plasma concentration of ●rifabutin—avoid concomitant use; metabolism of indinavir accelerated by ●rifampicin (reduced plasma concentration—avoid concomitant use); avoidance of concomitant indinavir in severe renal and hepatic impairment advised by manufacturer of ●telithromycin
  Anticoagulants: avoidance of indinavir advised by manufacturer of rivaroxaban
- Antidepressants: plasma concentration of indinavir reduced by ●St John's wort—avoid concomitant use
- Antiepileptics: plasma concentration of indinavir possibly reduced by ●carbamazepine and ●phenytoin, also plasma concentration of carbamazepine and phenytoin possibly increased; plasma concentration of indinavir possibly reduced by ●primidone
- Antifungals: plasma concentration of indinavir increased by ●itraconazole and ●ketoconazole (consider reducing dose of indinavir)
  Antimalarials: caution with indinavir advised by manufacturer of artemether/lumefantrine
  Antimuscarinics: avoidance of indinavir advised by manufacturer of darifenacin and tolterodine; manufacturer of fesoterodine advises dose reduction when indinavir given with fesoterodine—consult fesoterodine product literature
- Antipsychotics: indinavir possibly inhibits metabolism of ●aripiprazole (reduce dose of aripiprazole); indinavir possibly increases plasma concentration of ●pimozide (increased risk of ventricular arrhythmias—avoid concomitant use); indinavir increases plasma concentration of ●sertindole (increased risk of ventricular arrhythmias—avoid concomitant use)
- Antivirals: avoid concomitant use of indinavir with ●atazanavir; plasma concentration of both drugs

Indinavir
- Antivirals *(continued)*
  increased when indinavir given with darunavir; plasma concentration of indinavir reduced by efavirenz and nevirapine; plasma concentration of indinavir possibly reduced by ●etravirine—avoid concomitant use; indinavir increases plasma concentration of ●maraviroc (consider reducing dose of maraviroc); combination of indinavir with nelfinavir may increase plasma concentration of either drug (or both); plasma concentration of indinavir increased by ritonavir; indinavir increases plasma concentration of saquinavir
- Anxiolytics and Hypnotics: increased risk of prolonged sedation when indinavir given with ●alprazolam—avoid concomitant use; indinavir possibly increases plasma concentration of ●midazolam (risk of prolonged sedation—avoid concomitant use of *oral* midazolam)
  Atovaquone: plasma concentration of indinavir possibly reduced by atovaquone
- Barbiturates: plasma concentration of indinavir possibly reduced by ●barbiturates; plasma concentration of indinavir possibly reduced by ●phenobarbital, also plasma concentration of phenobarbital possibly increased
- Ciclosporin: indinavir increases plasma concentration of ●ciclosporin
- Cilostazol: indinavir possibly increases plasma concentration of ●cilostazol—avoid concomitant use
  Corticosteroids: plasma concentration of indinavir possibly reduced by dexamethasone
- Cytotoxics: indinavir possibly increases plasma concentration of ●everolimus—manufacturer of everolimus advises avoid concomitant use
- Ergot Alkaloids: increased risk of ergotism when indinavir given with ●ergotamine and methysergide—avoid concomitant use
- 5HT$_1$ Agonists: indinavir increases plasma concentration of ●eletriptan (risk of toxicity)—avoid concomitant use
- Lipid-regulating Drugs: possible increased risk of myopathy when indinavir given with atorvastatin; possible increased risk of myopathy when indinavir given with ●rosuvastatin—avoid concomitant use; increased risk of myopathy when indinavir given with ●simvastatin (avoid concomitant use)
- Ranolazine: indinavir possibly increases plasma concentration of ●ranolazine—manufacturer of ranolazine advises avoid concomitant use
- Sildenafil: indinavir increases plasma concentration of ●sildenafil—reduce initial dose of sildenafil
  Tadalafil: indinavir possibly increases plasma concentration of tadalafil
- Vardenafil: indinavir increases plasma concentration of ●vardenafil—avoid concomitant use

Indometacin *see* NSAIDs

Indoramin *see* Alpha-blockers

Infliximab
- Abatacept: avoid concomitant use of infliximab with ●abatacept
- Anakinra: avoid concomitant use of infliximab with ●anakinra
- Vaccines: avoid concomitant use of infliximab with live ●vaccines (see p. 733)

Influenza Vaccine *see* Vaccines

Insulin *see* Antidiabetics

Interferon Alfa *see* Interferons

Interferon Gamma *see* Interferons

Interferons
  Note. Peginterferon alfa interactions as for interferon alfa
- Antivirals: increased risk of peripheral neuropathy when interferon alfa given with ●telbivudine
  Theophylline: interferon alfa inhibits metabolism of theophylline (increased plasma concentration)

Interferons *(continued)*

Vaccines: manufacturer of interferon gamma advises avoid concomitant use with vaccines

Ipratropium *see* Antimuscarinics

Irbesartan *see* Angiotensin-II Receptor Antagonists

Irinotecan

- Antidepressants: metabolism of irinotecan accelerated by ●St John's wort (reduced plasma concentration—avoid concomitant use)

  Antiepileptics: plasma concentration of irinotecan and its active metabolite reduced by carbamazepine and phenytoin; cytotoxics possibly reduce absorption of phenytoin

- Antifungals: plasma concentration of irinotecan reduced by ●ketoconazole (but concentration of active metabolite of irinotecan increased)—avoid concomitant use

- Antipsychotics: avoid concomitant use of cytotoxics with ●clozapine (increased risk of agranulocytosis)

- Antivirals: metabolism of irinotecan possibly inhibited by ●atazanavir (increased risk of toxicity)

  Barbiturates: plasma concentration of irinotecan and its active metabolite reduced by phenobarbital

  Cardiac Glycosides: cytotoxics reduce absorption of digoxin tablets

  Cytotoxics: plasma concentration of irinotecan possibly increased by sorafenib

Iron

Antacids: absorption of *oral* iron reduced by oral magnesium salts (as magnesium trisilicate)

Antibacterials: *oral* iron reduces absorption of ciprofloxacin, levofloxacin, moxifloxacin, norfloxacin and ofloxacin; *oral* iron reduces absorption of tetracyclines, also absorption of *oral* iron reduced by tetracyclines

Bisphosphonates: *oral* iron reduces absorption of bisphosphonates

Calcium Salts: absorption of *oral* iron reduced by calcium salts

- Dimercaprol: avoid concomitant use of iron with ●dimercaprol

  Dopaminergics: *oral* iron reduces absorption of entacapone; *oral* iron possibly reduces absorption of levodopa

  Methyldopa: *oral* iron antagonises hypotensive effect of methyldopa

  Mycophenolate: *oral* iron reduces absorption of mycophenolate

  Penicillamine: *oral* iron reduces absorption of penicillamine

  Thyroid Hormones: *oral* iron reduces absorption of levothyroxine (give at least 2 hours apart)

  Trientine: absorption of *oral* iron reduced by trientine

  Zinc: *oral* iron reduces absorption of zinc, also absorption of *oral* iron reduced by zinc

Isocarboxazid *see* MAOIs

Isoflurane *see* Anaesthetics, General

Isometheptene *see* Sympathomimetics

Isoniazid

Antacids: absorption of isoniazid reduced by antacids

Antibacterials: increased risk of CNS toxicity when isoniazid given with cycloserine

- Antiepileptics: isoniazid increases plasma concentration of ●carbamazepine (also possibly increased isoniazid hepatotoxicity); isoniazid inhibits metabolism of ●ethosuximide (increased plasma concentration and risk of toxicity); isoniazid inhibits metabolism of ●phenytoin (increased plasma concentration)

  Antifungals: isoniazid possibly reduces plasma concentration of ketoconazole

  Anxiolytics and Hypnotics: isoniazid inhibits the metabolism of diazepam

  Corticosteroids: plasma concentration of isoniazid possibly reduced by corticosteroids

Isoniazid *(continued)*

Disulfiram: isoniazid possibly increases CNS effects of disulfiram

Dopaminergics: isoniazid possibly reduces effects of levodopa

Oestrogens: antibacterials that do not induce liver enzymes possibly reduce contraceptive effect of oestrogens (risk probably small, see p. 486)

Theophylline: isoniazid possibly increases plasma concentration of theophylline

Vaccines: antibacterials inactivate oral typhoid vaccine–see p. 760

Isosorbide Dinitrate *see* Nitrates

Isosorbide Mononitrate *see* Nitrates

Isotretinoin *see* Retinoids

Isradipine *see* Calcium-channel Blockers

Itraconazole *see* Antifungals, Triazole

Ivabradine

- Anti-arrhythmics: increased risk of ventricular arrhythmias when ivabradine given with ●amiodarone or ●disopyramide

- Antibacterials: plasma concentration of ivabradine possibly increased by ●clarithromycin and ●telithromycin—avoid concomitant use; increased risk of ventricular arrhythmias when ivabradine given with ●erythromycin—avoid concomitant use

  Antidepressants: plasma concentration of ivabradine reduced by St John's wort—avoid concomitant use

- Antifungals: plasma concentration of ivabradine increased by ●ketoconazole—avoid concomitant use; plasma concentration of ivabradine increased by fluconazole—reduce initial dose of ivabradine; plasma concentration of ivabradine possibly increased by ●itraconazole—avoid concomitant use

- Antimalarials: increased risk of ventricular arrhythmias when ivabradine given with ●mefloquine

- Antipsychotics: increased risk of ventricular arrhythmias when ivabradine given with ●pimozide or ●sertindole

- Antivirals: plasma concentration of ivabradine possibly increased by ●nelfinavir and ●ritonavir—avoid concomitant use

- Beta-blockers: increased risk of ventricular arrhythmias when ivabradine given with ●sotalol

- Calcium-channel Blockers: plasma concentration of ivabradine increased by ●diltiazem and ●verapamil—avoid concomitant use

  Grapefruit Juice: plasma concentration of ivabradine increased by grapefruit juice

- Pentamidine Isetionate: increased risk of ventricular arrhythmias when ivabradine given with ●pentamidine isetionate

Kaolin

Analgesics: kaolin possibly reduces absorption of aspirin

Antibacterials: kaolin possibly reduces absorption of tetracyclines

Antimalarials: kaolin reduces absorption of chloroquine and hydroxychloroquine

Antipsychotics: kaolin possibly reduces absorption of phenothiazines

Ketamine *see* Anaesthetics, General

Ketoconazole *see* Antifungals, Imidazole

Ketoprofen *see* NSAIDs

Ketorolac *see* NSAIDs

Ketotifen *see* Antihistamines

Labetalol *see* Beta-blockers

Lacidipine *see* Calcium-channel Blockers

Lacosamide

- Antidepressants: anticonvulsant effect of antiepileptics possibly antagonised by MAOIs and ●tricyclic-related antidepressants (convulsive threshold lowered); anticonvulsant effect of antiepileptics antagonised by ●SSRIs and ●tricyclics (convulsive threshold lowered); avoid concomitant use of antiepileptics with ●St John's wort

Lacosamide *(continued)*
- Antimalarials: possible increased risk of convulsions when antiepileptics given with chloroquine and hydroxychloroquine; anticonvulsant effect of antiepileptics antagonised by ●mefloquine
- Orlistat: possible increased risk of convulsions when antiepileptics given with ●orlistat

Lactulose
  Anticoagulants: lactulose possibly enhances anticoagulant effect of coumarins

Lamivudine
  Antibacterials: plasma concentration of lamivudine increased by trimethoprim (as co-trimoxazole)—avoid concomitant use of high-dose co-trimoxazole
  Antivirals: avoidance of lamivudine advised by manufacturer of emtricitabine; manufacturer of lamivudine advises avoid concomitant use with foscarnet; manufacturer of lamivudine advises avoid concomitant use of *intravenous* ganciclovir

Lamotrigine
- Antibacterials: plasma concentration of lamotrigine reduced by ●rifampicin
- Antidepressants: anticonvulsant effect of antiepileptics possibly antagonised by MAOIs and ●tricyclic-related antidepressants (convulsive threshold lowered); anticonvulsant effect of antiepileptics antagonised by ●SSRIs and ●tricyclics (convulsive threshold lowered); avoid concomitant use of antiepileptics with ●St John's wort
  Antiepileptics: plasma concentration of lamotrigine often reduced by carbamazepine, also plasma concentration of an active metabolite of carbamazepine sometimes raised (but evidence is conflicting); plasma concentration of lamotrigine reduced by phenytoin and primidone; plasma concentration of lamotrigine increased by valproate
- Antimalarials: possible increased risk of convulsions when antiepileptics given with chloroquine and hydroxychloroquine; anticonvulsant effect of antiepileptics antagonised by ●mefloquine
  Antivirals: plasma concentration of lamotrigine possibly reduced by ritonavir
  Barbiturates: plasma concentration of lamotrigine reduced by phenobarbital
- Oestrogens: plasma concentration of lamotrigine possibly reduced by ●oestrogens—consider increasing dose of lamotrigine
- Orlistat: possible increased risk of convulsions when antiepileptics given with ●orlistat
- Progestogens: plasma concentration of lamotrigine possibly reduced by ●progestogens—consider increasing dose of lamotrigine

Lanreotide
  Antidiabetics: lanreotide possibly reduces requirements for insulin, metformin, repaglinide and sulphonylureas
  Ciclosporin: lanreotide reduces plasma concentration of ciclosporin

Lansoprazole *see* Proton Pump Inhibitors

Lanthanum
  Antifungals: lanthanum possibly reduces absorption of ketoconazole (give at least 2 hours apart)
  Antimalarials: lanthanum possibly reduces absorption of chloroquine and hydroxychloroquine (give at least 2 hours apart)

Lapatinib
- Antibacterials: manufacturer of lapatinib advises avoid concomitant use with ●rifabutin, ●rifampicin and ●telithromycin
- Antidepressants: manufacturer of lapatinib advises avoid concomitant use with ●St John's wort
- Antidiabetics: manufacturer of lapatinib advises avoid concomitant use with ●repaglinide
- Antiepileptics: plasma concentration of lapatinib reduced by ●carbamazepine—avoid concomitant use; cytotoxics possibly reduce absorption of

Lapatinib
- Antiepileptics *(continued)*
  phenytoin; manufacturer of lapatinib advises avoid concomitant use with ●phenytoin
- Antifungals: plasma concentration of lapatinib increased by ●ketoconazole—avoid concomitant use; manufacturer of lapatinib advises avoid concomitant use with ●itraconazole, ●posaconazole and ●voriconazole
- Antipsychotics: avoid concomitant use of cytotoxics with ●clozapine (increased risk of agranulocytosis); manufacturer of lapatinib advises avoid concomitant use with ●pimozide
- Antivirals: manufacturer of lapatinib advises avoid concomitant use with ●ritonavir and ●saquinavir
  Cardiac Glycosides: cytotoxics reduce absorption of digoxin tablets
- Grapefruit Juice: manufacturer of lapatinib advises avoid concomitant use with ●grapefruit juice
  Ulcer-healing Drugs: absorption of lapatinib possibly reduced by histamine H_2-antagonists and proton pump inhibitors

Laronidase
  Antimalarials: effects of laronidase possibly inhibited by chloroquine and hydroxychloroquine (manufacturer of laronidase advises avoid concomitant use)

Leflunomide
  Note. Increased risk of toxicity with other haematotoxic and hepatotoxic drugs
  Antibacterials: plasma concentration of active metabolite of leflunomide possibly increased by rifampicin
  Anticoagulants: leflunomide possibly enhances anticoagulant effect of warfarin
  Antidiabetics: leflunomide possibly enhances hypoglycaemic effect of tolbutamide
  Antiepileptics: leflunomide possibly increases plasma concentration of phenytoin
- Cytotoxics: risk of toxicity when leflunomide given with ●methotrexate
  Lipid-regulating Drugs: the effect of leflunomide is significantly decreased by colestyramine (enhanced elimination)—avoid unless drug elimination desired
- Vaccines: avoid concomitant use of leflunomide with live ●vaccines (see p. 733)

Lenalidomide
  Cardiac Glycosides: lenalidomide possibly increases plasma concentration of digoxin

Lercanidipine *see* Calcium-channel Blockers

Leukotriene Receptor Antagonists
  Analgesics: plasma concentration of zafirlukast increased by aspirin
  Antibacterials: plasma concentration of zafirlukast reduced by erythromycin
  Anticoagulants: zafirlukast enhances anticoagulant effect of warfarin
  Antiepileptics: plasma concentration of montelukast reduced by primidone
  Barbiturates: plasma concentration of montelukast reduced by phenobarbital
  Theophylline: zafirlukast possibly increases plasma concentration of theophylline, also plasma concentration of zafirlukast reduced

Levamisole
  Alcohol: possibility of disulfiram-like reaction when levamisole given with alcohol
- Anticoagulants: levamisole possibly enhances anticoagulant effect of ●warfarin
  Antiepileptics: levamisole possibly increases plasma concentration of phenytoin

Levetiracetam
- Antidepressants: anticonvulsant effect of antiepileptics possibly antagonised by MAOIs and ●tricyclic-related antidepressants (convulsive threshold lowered); anticonvulsant effect of antiepileptics antagonised by ●SSRIs and ●tricyclics (convulsive

Levetiracetam
- Antidepressants *(continued)*
  threshold lowered); avoid concomitant use of anti-epileptics with ●St John's wort
  Antiepileptics: levetiracetam possibly increases risk of carbamazepine toxicity
- Antimalarials: possible increased risk of convulsions when antiepileptics given with chloroquine and hydroxychloroquine; anticonvulsant effect of anti-epileptics antagonised by ●mefloquine
- Orlistat: possible increased risk of convulsions when antiepileptics given with ●orlistat

Levobunolol *see* Beta-blockers

Levobupivacaine
  Anti-arrhythmics: increased myocardial depression when levobupivacaine given with anti-arrhythmics

Levocetirizine *see* Antihistamines

Levodopa
  ACE Inhibitors: enhanced hypotensive effect when levodopa given with ACE inhibitors
  Adrenergic Neurone Blockers: enhanced hypotensive effect when levodopa given with adrenergic neurone blockers
  Alpha-blockers: enhanced hypotensive effect when levodopa given with alpha-blockers
- Anaesthetics, General: increased risk of arrhythmias when levodopa given with ●volatile liquid general anaesthetics
  Angiotensin-II Receptor Antagonists: enhanced hypotensive effect when levodopa given with angiotensin-II receptor antagonists
  Antibacterials: effects of levodopa possibly reduced by isoniazid
- Antidepressants: risk of hypertensive crisis when levodopa given with ●MAOIs, avoid levodopa for at least 2 weeks after stopping MAOIs; increased risk of side-effects when levodopa given with moclobemide
  Antiepileptics: effects of levodopa possibly reduced by phenytoin
  Antimuscarinics: absorption of levodopa possibly reduced by antimuscarinics
  Antipsychotics: effects of levodopa antagonised by antipsychotics; avoidance of levodopa advised by manufacturer of amisulpride (antagonism of effect)
  Anxiolytics and Hypnotics: effects of levodopa possibly antagonised by benzodiazepines
  Beta-blockers: enhanced hypotensive effect when levodopa given with beta-blockers
  Bupropion: increased risk of side-effects when levodopa given with bupropion
  Calcium-channel Blockers: enhanced hypotensive effect when levodopa given with calcium-channel blockers
  Clonidine: enhanced hypotensive effect when levodopa given with clonidine
  Diazoxide: enhanced hypotensive effect when levodopa given with diazoxide
  Diuretics: enhanced hypotensive effect when levodopa given with diuretics
  Dopaminergics: enhanced effects and increased toxicity of levodopa when given with selegiline (reduce dose of levodopa)
  Iron: absorption of levodopa possibly reduced by *oral* iron
  Memantine: effects of dopaminergics possibly enhanced by memantine
  Methyldopa: enhanced hypotensive effect when levodopa given with methyldopa; antiparkinsonian effect of dopaminergics antagonised by methyldopa
  Moxonidine: enhanced hypotensive effect when levodopa given with moxonidine
  Muscle Relaxants: possible agitation, confusion and hallucinations when levodopa given with baclofen
  Nitrates: enhanced hypotensive effect when levodopa given with nitrates

Levodopa *(continued)*
  Vasodilator Antihypertensives: enhanced hypotensive effect when levodopa given with hydralazine, minoxidil or sodium nitroprusside
  Vitamins: effects of levodopa reduced by pyridoxine when given without dopa-decarboxylase inhibitor

Levofloxacin *see* Quinolones

Levomepromazine *see* Antipsychotics

Levonorgestrel *see* Progestogens

Levothyroxine *see* Thyroid Hormones

Lidocaine
  Note. Interactions less likely when lidocaine used topically
  Anaesthetics, Local: increased myocardial depression when anti-arrhythmics given with bupivacaine, levobupivacaine, prilocaine or ropivacaine
- Anti-arrhythmics: increased myocardial depression when anti-arrhythmics given with other ●anti-arrhythmics
- Antibacterials: increased risk of ventricular arrhythmias when lidocaine given with ●quinupristin/dalfopristin—avoid concomitant use
- Antipsychotics: increased risk of ventricular arrhythmias when anti-arrhythmics that prolong the QT interval given with ●antipsychotics that prolong the QT interval
- Antivirals: plasma concentration of lidocaine possibly increased by ●atazanavir and lopinavir; plasma concentration of lidocaine possibly increased by darunavir and ●fosamprenavir—avoid concomitant use
- Beta-blockers: increased myocardial depression when anti-arrhythmics given with ●beta-blockers; increased risk of lidocaine toxicity when given with ●propranolol
- Diuretics: action of lidocaine antagonised by hypokalaemia caused by ●acetazolamide, ●loop diuretics or ●thiazides and related diuretics
  Muscle Relaxants: neuromuscular blockade enhanced and prolonged when lidocaine given with suxamethonium
- Ulcer-healing Drugs: plasma concentration of lidocaine increased by ●cimetidine (increased risk of toxicity)

Linezolid
  Note. Linezolid is a reversible, non-selective MAO inhibitor—see interactions of MAOIs
  Antibacterials: plasma concentration of linezolid reduced by rifampicin (possible therapeutic failure of linezolid)
  Oestrogens: antibacterials that do not induce liver enzymes possibly reduce contraceptive effect of oestrogens (risk probably small, see p. 486)
  Vaccines: antibacterials inactivate oral typhoid vaccine—see p. 760

Liothyronine *see* Thyroid Hormones

Lipid-regulating Drugs *see* Colestipol, Colestyramine, Ezetimibe, Fibrates, Nicotinic Acid, and Statins

Liraglutide *see* Antidiabetics

Lisinopril *see* ACE Inhibitors

Lithium
- ACE Inhibitors: excretion of lithium reduced by ●ACE inhibitors (increased plasma concentration)
- Analgesics: excretion of lithium reduced by ●NSAIDs (increased risk of toxicity); excretion of lithium reduced by ●ketorolac (increased risk of toxicity)—avoid concomitant use
- Angiotensin-II Receptor Antagonists: excretion of lithium reduced by ●angiotensin-II receptor antagonists (increased plasma concentration)
  Antacids: excretion of lithium increased by sodium bicarbonate (reduced plasma concentration)
- Anti-arrhythmics: avoidance of lithium advised by manufacturer of ●amiodarone (risk of ventricular arrhythmias)
  Antibacterials: increased risk of lithium toxicity when given with metronidazole

Lithium *(continued)*

- Antidepressants: possible increased serotonergic effects when lithium given with venlafaxine; increased risk of CNS effects when lithium given with ●SSRIs (lithium toxicity reported); risk of toxicity when lithium given with tricyclics

  Antiepileptics: neurotoxicity may occur when lithium given with carbamazepine or phenytoin without increased plasma concentration of lithium; plasma concentration of lithium possibly affected by topiramate

- Antipsychotics: increased risk of extrapyramidal side-effects and possibly neurotoxicity when lithium given with clozapine, flupentixol, haloperidol, phenothiazines or zuclopenthixol; increased risk of ventricular arrhythmias when lithium given with ●sertindole—avoid concomitant use; increased risk of extrapyramidal side-effects when lithium given with sulpiride

  Calcium-channel Blockers: neurotoxicity may occur when lithium given with diltiazem or verapamil without increased plasma concentration of lithium

- Cytotoxics: increased risk of ventricular arrhythmias when lithium given with ●arsenic trioxide

- Diuretics: excretion of lithium increased by ●acetazolamide; excretion of lithium reduced by ●loop diuretics and ●thiazides and related diuretics (increased plasma concentration and risk of toxicity)—loop diuretics safer than thiazides; excretion of lithium reduced by ●potassium-sparing diuretics and aldosterone antagonists (increased plasma concentration and risk of toxicity)

- Methyldopa: neurotoxicity may occur when lithium given with ●methyldopa without increased plasma concentration of lithium

  Muscle Relaxants: lithium enhances effects of muscle relaxants; hyperkinesis caused by lithium possibly aggravated by baclofen

  Parasympathomimetics: lithium antagonises effects of neostigmine and pyridostigmine

  Theophylline: excretion of lithium increased by theophylline (reduced plasma concentration)

Lofepramine *see* Antidepressants, Tricyclic

Lofexidine

  Alcohol: increased sedative effect when lofexidine given with alcohol

  Anxiolytics and Hypnotics: increased sedative effect when lofexidine given with anxiolytics and hypnotics

  Barbiturates: increased sedative effect when lofexidine given with barbiturates

Lomustine

  Antiepileptics: cytotoxics possibly reduce absorption of phenytoin

- Antipsychotics: avoid concomitant use of cytotoxics with ●clozapine (increased risk of agranulocytosis)

  Cardiac Glycosides: cytotoxics reduce absorption of digoxin tablets

  Ulcer-healing Drugs: myelosuppressive effects of lomustine possibly enhanced by cimetidine

Loperamide

  Desmopressin: loperamide increases plasma concentration of *oral* desmopressin

Lopinavir

  Note. In combination with ritonavir as *Kaletra*® (ritonavir is present to inhibit lopinavir metabolism and increase plasma-lopinavir concentration)—see also Ritonavir

- Anti-arrhythmics: lopinavir possibly increases plasma concentration of ●flecainide (increased risk of ventricular arrhythmias—avoid concomitant use); lopinavir possibly increases plasma concentration of lidocaine

- Antibacterials: plasma concentration of lopinavir reduced by ●rifampicin—avoid concomitant use; avoidance of concomitant lopinavir in severe renal and hepatic impairment advised by manufacturer of ●telithromycin

Lopinavir *(continued)*

  Anticoagulants: avoidance of lopinavir advised by manufacturer of rivaroxaban

- Antidepressants: plasma concentration of lopinavir reduced by ●St John's wort—avoid concomitant use

- Antiepileptics: plasma concentration of lopinavir possibly reduced by carbamazepine, phenytoin and ●primidone

  Antihistamines: lopinavir possibly increases plasma concentration of chlorphenamine

  Antimalarials: caution with lopinavir advised by manufacturer of artemether/lumefantrine

  Antimuscarinics: avoidance of lopinavir advised by manufacturer of darifenacin and tolterodine

- Antipsychotics: lopinavir possibly inhibits metabolism of ●aripiprazole (reduce dose of aripiprazole); lopinavir increases plasma concentration of ●sertindole (increased risk of ventricular arrhythmias—avoid concomitant use)

- Antivirals: lopinavir reduces plasma concentration of ●darunavir, also plasma concentration of lopinavir increased (avoid concomitant use); plasma concentration of lopinavir reduced by ●efavirenz—consider increasing dose of lopinavir; lopinavir reduces plasma concentration of fosamprenavir, effect on lopinavir plasma concentration not predictable—avoid concomitant use; lopinavir increases plasma concentration of ●maraviroc (consider reducing dose of maraviroc); plasma concentration of lopinavir reduced by nelfinavir, also plasma concentration of active metabolite of nelfinavir increased; plasma concentration of lopinavir possibly reduced by ●nevirapine—consider increasing dose of lopinavir; lopinavir increases plasma concentration of tenofovir; plasma concentration of lopinavir reduced by ●tipranavir

- Barbiturates: plasma concentration of lopinavir possibly reduced by ●phenobarbital

- Cilostazol: lopinavir possibly increases plasma concentration of ●cilostazol—avoid concomitant use

  Corticosteroids: plasma concentration of lopinavir possibly reduced by dexamethasone

- Lipid-regulating Drugs: possible increased risk of myopathy when lopinavir given with atorvastatin; possible increased risk of myopathy when lopinavir given with ●rosuvastatin or ●simvastatin—avoid concomitant use

- Ranolazine: lopinavir possibly increases plasma concentration of ●ranolazine—manufacturer of ranolazine advises avoid concomitant use

  Sirolimus: lopinavir possibly increases plasma concentration of sirolimus

Loprazolam *see* Anxiolytics and Hypnotics

Loratadine *see* Antihistamines

Lorazepam *see* Anxiolytics and Hypnotics

Lormetazepam *see* Anxiolytics and Hypnotics

Losartan *see* Angiotensin-II Receptor Antagonists

Lumefantrine *see* Artemether with Lumefantrine

Lymecycline *see* Tetracyclines

Macrolides

  Note. See also Telithromycin

  Note. Interactions do not apply to small amounts of erythromycin used topically

  Analgesics: erythromycin increases plasma concentration of alfentanil

  Antacids: absorption of azithromycin reduced by antacids

- Anti-arrhythmics: increased risk of ventricular arrhythmias when *parenteral* erythromycin given with ●amiodarone—avoid concomitant use; clarithromycin possibly increases plasma concentration of ●disopyramide (increased risk of toxicity); erythromycin increases plasma concentration of ●disopyramide (increased risk of toxicity)

- Antibacterials: increased risk of ventricular arrhythmias when *parenteral* erythromycin given with

Appendix 1: Interactions

Macrolides

- Antibacterials *(continued)*
    - moxifloxacin—avoid concomitant use; macrolides possibly increase plasma concentration of ●rifabutin (increased risk of uveitis—reduce rifabutin dose); clarithromycin increases plasma concentration of ●rifabutin (increased risk of uveitis—reduce rifabutin dose); plasma concentration of clarithromycin reduced by rifamycins
- Anticoagulants: clarithromycin and erythromycin enhance anticoagulant effect of ●coumarins; azithromycin possibly enhances anticoagulant effect of ●coumarins
- Antidepressants: avoidance of macrolides advised by manufacturer of ●reboxetine

    Antidiabetics: clarithromycin enhances effects of repaglinide
- Antiepileptics: clarithromycin and erythromycin increase plasma concentration of ●carbamazepine; clarithromycin inhibits metabolism of phenytoin (increased plasma concentration); erythromycin possibly inhibits metabolism of valproate (increased plasma concentration)

    Antifungals: clarithromycin increases plasma concentration of itraconazole
- Antihistamines: manufacturer of loratadine advises erythromycin possibly increases plasma concentration of loratadine; macrolides possibly inhibit metabolism of ●mizolastine (avoid concomitant use); erythromycin inhibits metabolism of ●mizolastine—avoid concomitant use; erythromycin increases plasma concentration of rupatadine
- Antimalarials: avoidance of macrolides advised by manufacturer of ●artemether/lumefantrine

    Antimuscarinics: erythromycin possibly increases plasma concentration of darifenacin; manufacturer of fesoterodine advises dose reduction when clarithromycin given with fesoterodine—consult fesoterodine product literature; avoidance of clarithromycin and erythromycin advised by manufacturer of tolterodine
- Antipsychotics: avoidance of macrolides advised by manufacturer of ●droperidol (risk of ventricular arrhythmias); increased risk of ventricular arrhythmias when *parenteral* erythromycin given with ●amisulpride or ●zuclopenthixol—avoid concomitant use; erythromycin possibly increases plasma concentration of ●clozapine (possible increased risk of convulsions); possible increased risk of ventricular arrhythmias when erythromycin given with ●pimozide—avoid concomitant use; increased risk of ventricular arrhythmias when clarithromycin given with ●pimozide—avoid concomitant use; macrolides possibly increase plasma concentration of quetiapine (reduce dose of quetiapine); increased risk of ventricular arrhythmias when erythromycin given with ●sertindole—avoid concomitant use; possible increased risk of ventricular arrhythmias when macrolides given with ●sertindole—avoid concomitant use; increased risk of ventricular arrhythmias when *parenteral* erythromycin given with ●sulpiride
- Antivirals: plasma concentration of both drugs increased when clarithromycin given with atazanavir; increased risk of rash when clarithromycin given with efavirenz; clarithromycin increases plasma concentration of ●etravirine, also plasma concentration of clarithromycin reduced; plasma concentration of both drugs increased when erythromycin given with fosamprenavir; clarithromycin possibly increases plasma concentration of ●maraviroc (consider reducing dose of maraviroc); plasma concentration of clarithromycin increased by ●ritonavir (reduce dose of clarithromycin in renal impairment); plasma concentration of azithromycin and erythromycin possibly increased by ritonavir; plasma concentration of clarithromycin increased by ●tipranavir (reduce dose of clarithromycin in renal impairment),

Macrolides

- Antivirals *(continued)*
    also clarithromycin increases plasma concentration of tipranavir; clarithromycin tablets reduce absorption of zidovudine (give at least 2 hours apart)
- Anxiolytics and Hypnotics: clarithromycin and erythromycin inhibit metabolism of ●midazolam (increased plasma concentration with increased sedation); erythromycin increases plasma concentration of buspirone (reduce dose of buspirone); erythromycin inhibits the metabolism of zopiclone

    Aprepitant: clarithromycin possibly increases plasma concentration of aprepitant
- Atomoxetine: increased risk of ventricular arrhythmias when *parenteral* erythromycin given with ●atomoxetine
- Calcium-channel Blockers: erythromycin possibly inhibits metabolism of felodipine (increased plasma concentration); avoidance of erythromycin advised by manufacturer of lercanidipine; clarithromycin and erythromycin possibly inhibit metabolism of ●verapamil (increased risk of toxicity)

    Cardiac Glycosides: macrolides increase plasma concentration of digoxin (increased risk of toxicity)
- Ciclosporin: macrolides possibly inhibit metabolism of ●ciclosporin (increased plasma concentration); clarithromycin and erythromycin inhibit metabolism of ●ciclosporin (increased plasma concentration)
- Cilostazol: erythromycin increases plasma concentration of ●cilostazol (also plasma concentration of erythromycin reduced)—avoid concomitant use
- Clopidogrel: erythromycin possibly reduces antiplatelet effect of ●clopidogrel
- Colchicine: clarithromycin or erythromycin increase risk of ●colchicine toxicity

    Corticosteroids: erythromycin possibly inhibits metabolism of corticosteroids; erythromycin inhibits the metabolism of methylprednisolone; clarithromycin possibly increases plasma concentration of methylprednisolone
- Cytotoxics: clarithromycin possibly increases plasma concentration of ●everolimus—manufacturer of everolimus advises avoid concomitant use; erythromycin increases plasma concentration of ●everolimus; avoidance of clarithromycin advised by manufacturer of ●nilotinib; *in vitro* studies suggest a possible interaction between erythromycin and docetaxel (consult docetaxel product literature); increased risk of ventricular arrhythmias when erythromycin given with ●arsenic trioxide; erythromycin increases toxicity of ●vinblastine—avoid concomitant use; possible increased risk of neutropenia when clarithromycin given with ●vinorelbine
- Diuretics: clarithromycin increases plasma concentration of ●eplerenone—avoid concomitant use; erythromycin increases plasma concentration of eplerenone (reduce dose of eplerenone)

    Dopaminergics: erythromycin increases plasma concentration of bromocriptine and cabergoline (increased risk of toxicity); macrolides possibly increase plasma concentration of bromocriptine and cabergoline (increased risk of toxicity)
- Ergot Alkaloids: increased risk of ergotism when macrolides given with ●ergotamine and methysergide—avoid concomitant use
- 5HT₁ Agonists: clarithromycin and erythromycin increase plasma concentration of ●eletriptan (risk of toxicity)—avoid concomitant use
- Ivabradine: clarithromycin possibly increases plasma concentration of ●ivabradine—avoid concomitant use; increased risk of ventricular arrhythmias when erythromycin given with ●ivabradine—avoid concomitant use

    Leukotriene Receptor Antagonists: erythromycin reduces plasma concentration of zafirlukast

Macrolides (continued)
- Lipid-regulating Drugs: clarithromycin increases plasma concentration of ●atorvastatin and prava-statin; possible increased risk of myopathy when erythromycin given with atorvastatin; erythromycin increases plasma concentration of pravastatin; erythromycin reduces plasma concentration of rosuvastatin; increased risk of myopathy when clarithromycin or erythromycin given with ●simvastatin (avoid concomitant use)

Oestrogens: antibacterials that do not induce liver enzymes possibly reduce contraceptive effect of oestrogens (risk probably small, see p. 486)

Parasympathomimetics: erythromycin increases plasma concentration of galantamine

- Pentamidine Isetionate: increased risk of ventricular arrhythmias when *parenteral* erythromycin given with ●pentamidine isetionate

- Ranolazine: clarithromycin possibly increases plasma concentration of ●ranolazine—manufacturer of ranolazine advises avoid concomitant use

Sildenafil: clarithromycin possibly increases plasma concentration of sildenafil—reduce initial dose of sildenafil; erythromycin increases plasma concentration of sildenafil—reduce initial dose of sildenafil

Sirolimus: clarithromycin increases plasma concentration of ●sirolimus—avoid concomitant use; plasma concentration of both drugs increased when erythromycin given with ●sirolimus

- Tacrolimus: clarithromycin and erythromycin increase plasma concentration of ●tacrolimus

Tadalafil: clarithromycin and erythromycin possibly increase plasma concentration of tadalafil

- Theophylline: azithromycin possibly increases plasma concentration of theophylline; clarithromycin inhibits metabolism of ●theophylline (increased plasma concentration); erythromycin inhibits metabolism of ●theophylline (increased plasma concentration), if erythromycin given *by mouth*, also decreased plasma-erythromycin concentration

Ulcer-healing Drugs: plasma concentration of erythromycin increased by cimetidine (increased risk of toxicity, including deafness); plasma concentration of both drugs increased when clarithromycin given with omeprazole

Vaccines: antibacterials inactivate oral typhoid vaccine–see p. 760

Vardenafil: erythromycin increases plasma concentration of vardenafil (reduce dose of vardenafil)

Magnesium (parenteral)
- Calcium-channel Blockers: profound hypotension reported with concomitant use of parenteral magnesium and ●nifedipine in pre-eclampsia

Muscle Relaxants: parenteral magnesium enhances effects of non-depolarising muscle relaxants and suxamethonium

Magnesium Salts (oral) *see* Antacids

Mannitol

Ciclosporin: possible increased risk of nephrotoxicity when mannitol given with ciclosporin

MAOIs

Note. For interactions of reversible MAO-A inhibitors (RIMAs) see Moclobemide, and for interactions of MAO-B inhibitors see Rasagiline and Selegiline; the antibacterial Linezolid is a reversible, non-selective MAO inhibitor

ACE Inhibitors: MAOIs possibly enhance hypotensive effect of ACE inhibitors

Adrenergic Neurone Blockers: enhanced hypotensive effect when MAOIs given with adrenergic neurone blockers

- Alcohol: MAOIs interact with tyramine found in some beverages containing ●alcohol and some dealcoho-lised beverages (hypertensive crisis)—if no tyramine, enhanced hypotensive effect

Alpha₂-adrenoceptor Stimulants: avoidance of MAOIs advised by manufacturer of apraclonidine and bri-monidine

MAOIs (continued)
- Alpha-blockers: avoidance of MAOIs advised by manufacturer of ●indoramin; enhanced hypotensive effect when MAOIs given with alpha-blockers

- Anaesthetics, General: Because of hazardous interactions between MAOIs and ●general anaesthetics, MAOIs should normally be stopped 2 weeks before surgery

- Analgesics: CNS excitation or depression (hypertension or hypotension) when MAOIs given with ●pethidine—avoid concomitant use and for 2 weeks after stopping MAOIs; avoidance of MAOIs advised by manufacturer of ●nefopam; possible CNS excitation or depression (hypertension or hypotension) when MAOIs given with ●opioid analgesics—avoid concomitant use and for 2 weeks after stopping MAOIs

Angiotensin-II Receptor Antagonists: MAOIs possibly enhance hypotensive effect of angiotensin-II receptor antagonists

- Antidepressants: increased risk of hypertension and CNS excitation when MAOIs given with ●reboxetine (MAOIs should not be started until 1 week after stopping reboxetine, avoid reboxetine for 2 weeks after stopping MAOIs); after stopping MAOIs do not start ●citalopram, ●escitalopram, ●fluvoxamine, ●paroxetine or ●sertraline for 2 weeks, also MAOIs should not be started until at least 1 week after stopping citalopram, escitalopram, fluvoxamine, paroxetine or sertraline; after stopping MAOIs do not start ●fluoxetine for 2 weeks, also MAOIs should not be started until at least 5 weeks after stopping fluoxetine; after stopping MAOIs do not start ●duloxetine for 2 weeks, also MAOIs should not be started until at least 5 days after stopping duloxetine; enhanced CNS effects and toxicity when MAOIs given with ●venlafaxine (venlafaxine should not be started until 2 weeks after stopping MAOIs, avoid MAOIs for 1 week after stopping venlafaxine); increased risk of hypertension and CNS excitation when MAOIs given with other ●MAOIs (avoid for at least 2 weeks after stopping previous MAOIs and then start at a reduced dose); after stopping MAOIs do not start ●moclobemide for at least 1 week; MAOIs increase CNS effects of ●SSRIs (risk of serious toxicity); after stopping MAOIs do not start ●mirtazapine for 2 weeks, also MAOIs should not be started until at least 2 weeks after stopping mirtazapine; after stopping MAOIs do not start ●tricyclic-related antidepressants for 2 weeks, also MAOIs should not be started until at least 1–2 weeks after stopping tricyclic-related antidepressants; increased risk of hypertension and CNS excitation when MAOIs given with ●tricyclics, tricyclics should not be started until 2 weeks after stopping MAOIs (3 weeks if starting clomipramine or imipramine), also MAOIs should not be started for at least 1–2 weeks after stopping tricyclics (3 weeks in the case of clomipramine or imipramine); CNS excitation and confusion when MAOIs given with ●tryptophan (reduce dose of tryptophan)

Antidiabetics: MAOIs possibly enhance hypoglycaemic effect of antidiabetics; MAOIs enhance hypoglycaemic effect of insulin, metformin and sulphonylureas

- Antiepileptics: MAOIs possibly antagonise anticonvulsant effect of antiepileptics (convulsive threshold lowered); avoidance for 2 weeks after stopping MAOIs advised by manufacturer of ●carbamazepine, also antagonism of anticonvulsant effect

Antihistamines: increased antimuscarinic and sedative effects when MAOIs given with antihistamines

- Antimalarials: avoidance of antidepressants advised by manufacturer of ●artemether/lumefantrine

Antimuscarinics: increased risk of antimuscarinic side-effects when MAOIs given with antimuscarinics

MAOIs *(continued)*

- Antipsychotics: CNS effects of MAOIs possibly increased by ●clozapine

  Anxiolytics and Hypnotics: avoidance of MAOIs advised by manufacturer of buspirone

- Atomoxetine: after stopping MAOIs do not start ●atomoxetine for 2 weeks, also MAOIs should not be started until at least 2 weeks after stopping atomoxetine; possible increased risk of convulsions when antidepressants given with atomoxetine

  Barbiturates: MAOIs possibly antagonise anticonvulsant effect of barbiturates (convulsive threshold lowered)

  Beta-blockers: enhanced hypotensive effect when MAOIs given with beta-blockers

- Bupropion: avoidance of bupropion for 2 weeks after stopping MAOIs advised by manufacturer of ●bupropion

  Calcium-channel Blockers: enhanced hypotensive effect when MAOIs given with calcium-channel blockers

  Clonidine: enhanced hypotensive effect when MAOIs given with clonidine

  Diazoxide: enhanced hypotensive effect when MAOIs given with diazoxide

  Diuretics: enhanced hypotensive effect when MAOIs given with diuretics

- Dopaminergics: avoid concomitant use of non-selective MAOIs with ●entacapone; risk of hypertensive crisis when MAOIs given with ●levodopa, avoid levodopa for at least 2 weeks after stopping MAOIs; risk of hypertensive crisis when MAOIs given with ●rasagiline, avoid MAOIs for at least 2 weeks after stopping rasagiline; enhanced hypotensive effect when MAOIs given with selegiline; avoid concomitant use of MAOIs with tolcapone

  Doxapram: MAOIs enhance effects of doxapram

- $5HT_1$ Agonists: risk of CNS toxicity when MAOIs given with ●rizatriptan or ●sumatriptan (avoid rizatriptan or sumatriptan for 2 weeks after MAOIs); increased risk of CNS toxicity when MAOIs given with ●zolmitriptan

- Methyldopa: avoidance of MAOIs advised by manufacturer of ●methyldopa

  Moxonidine: enhanced hypotensive effect when MAOIs given with moxonidine

  Muscle Relaxants: phenelzine enhances effects of suxamethonium

  Nicorandil: enhanced hypotensive effect when MAOIs given with nicorandil

  Nitrates: enhanced hypotensive effect when MAOIs given with nitrates

- Sibutramine: increased CNS toxicity when MAOIs given with ●sibutramine (manufacturer of sibutramine advises avoid concomitant use), also avoid sibutramine for 2 weeks after stopping MAOIs

- Sympathomimetics: risk of hypertensive crisis when MAOIs given with ●sympathomimetics; risk of hypertensive crisis when MAOIs given with ●methylphenidate, some manufacturers advise avoid methylphenidate for at least 2 weeks after stopping MAOIs

- Tetrabenazine: risk of CNS excitation and hypertension when MAOIs given with ●tetrabenazine

  Vasodilator Antihypertensives: enhanced hypotensive effect when MAOIs given with hydralazine, minoxidil or sodium nitroprusside

MAOIs, reversible *see* Moclobemide

Maraviroc

- Antibacterials: plasma concentration of maraviroc possibly increased by ●clarithromycin and ●telithromycin (consider reducing dose of maraviroc); plasma concentration of maraviroc reduced by ●rifampicin—consider increasing dose of maraviroc

Maraviroc *(continued)*

- Antidepressants: plasma concentration of maraviroc possibly reduced by ●St John's wort—avoid concomitant use

- Antifungals: plasma concentration of maraviroc increased by ●ketoconazole (consider reducing dose of maraviroc)

- Antivirals: plasma concentration of maraviroc increased by ●atazanavir, ●darunavir, ●indinavir, ●lopinavir and ●saquinavir (consider reducing dose of maraviroc); plasma concentration of maraviroc possibly reduced by ●efavirenz—consider increasing dose of maraviroc; plasma concentration of maraviroc possibly reduced by etravirine; plasma concentration of maraviroc possibly increased by ●nelfinavir (consider reducing dose of maraviroc); plasma concentration of maraviroc increased by ritonavir

Mebendazole

  Ulcer-healing Drugs: metabolism of mebendazole possibly inhibited by cimetidine (increased plasma concentration)

Medroxyprogesterone *see* Progestogens

Mefenamic Acid *see* NSAIDs

Mefloquine

- Anti-arrhythmics: increased risk of ventricular arrhythmias when mefloquine given with ●amiodarone—avoid concomitant use

- Antibacterials: increased risk of ventricular arrhythmias when mefloquine given with ●moxifloxacin—avoid concomitant use; plasma concentration of mefloquine reduced by ●rifampicin—avoid concomitant use

- Antiepileptics: mefloquine antagonises anticonvulsant effect of ●antiepileptics

  Antifungals: plasma concentration of mefloquine increased by ketoconazole

- Antimalarials: avoidance of antimalarials advised by manufacturer of ●artemether/lumefantrine; increased risk of convulsions when mefloquine given with ●chloroquine and hydroxychloroquine; increased risk of convulsions when mefloquine given with ●quinine (but should not prevent the use of *intravenous* quinine in severe cases)

- Antipsychotics: possible increased risk of ventricular arrhythmias when mefloquine given with ●haloperidol—avoid concomitant use; increased risk of ventricular arrhythmias when mefloquine given with ●pimozide—avoid concomitant use

- Atomoxetine: increased risk of ventricular arrhythmias when mefloquine given with ●atomoxetine

  Beta-blockers: increased risk of bradycardia when mefloquine given with beta-blockers

  Calcium-channel Blockers: possible increased risk of bradycardia when mefloquine given with calcium-channel blockers

  Cardiac Glycosides: possible increased risk of bradycardia when mefloquine given with digoxin

- Ivabradine: increased risk of ventricular arrhythmias when mefloquine given with ●ivabradine

  Vaccines: antimalarials inactivate oral typhoid vaccine—see p. 760

Megestrol *see* Progestogens

Melatonin *see* Anxiolytics and Hypnotics

Meloxicam *see* NSAIDs

Melphalan

  Antibacterials: increased risk of melphalan toxicity when given with nalidixic acid

  Antiepileptics: cytotoxics possibly reduce absorption of phenytoin

- Antipsychotics: avoid concomitant use of cytotoxics with ●clozapine (increased risk of agranulocytosis)

  Cardiac Glycosides: cytotoxics reduce absorption of digoxin tablets

- Ciclosporin: increased risk of nephrotoxicity when melphalan given with ●ciclosporin

Memantine

- Anaesthetics, General: increased risk of CNS toxicity when memantine given with ●ketamine (manufacturer of memantine advises avoid concomitant use)
- Analgesics: increased risk of CNS toxicity when memantine given with ●dextromethorphan (manufacturer of memantine advises avoid concomitant use)

  Anticoagulants: memantine possibly enhances anticoagulant effect of warfarin

  Antiepileptics: memantine possibly reduces effects of primidone

  Antimuscarinics: memantine possibly enhances effects of antimuscarinics

  Antipsychotics: memantine possibly reduces effects of antipsychotics

  Barbiturates: memantine possibly reduces effects of barbiturates
- Dopaminergics: memantine possibly enhances effects of dopaminergics and selegiline; increased risk of CNS toxicity when memantine given with ●amantadine (manufacturer of memantine advises avoid concomitant use)

  Muscle Relaxants: memantine possibly modifies effects of baclofen and dantrolene

Mepacrine

Antimalarials: mepacrine increases plasma concentration of primaquine (increased risk of toxicity)

Meprobamate *see* Anxiolytics and Hypnotics

Meptazinol *see* Opioid Analgesics

Mercaptopurine

- Allopurinol: enhanced effects and increased toxicity of mercaptopurine when given with ●allopurinol (reduce dose of mercaptopurine to one quarter of usual dose)

  Aminosalicylates: possible increased risk of leucopenia when mercaptopurine given with aminosalicylates
- Antibacterials: increased risk of haematological toxicity when mercaptopurine given with ●sulfamethoxazole (as co-trimoxazole); increased risk of haematological toxicity when mercaptopurine given with ●trimethoprim (also with co-trimoxazole)
- Anticoagulants: mercaptopurine possibly reduces anticoagulant effect of ●coumarins

  Antiepileptics: cytotoxics possibly reduce absorption of phenytoin
- Antipsychotics: avoid concomitant use of cytotoxics with ●clozapine (increased risk of agranulocytosis)

  Cardiac Glycosides: cytotoxics reduce absorption of digoxin tablets

Meropenem

- Antiepileptics: carbapenems reduce plasma concentration of ●valproate (possible therapeutic failure of valproate)

  Oestrogens: antibacterials that do not induce liver enzymes possibly reduce contraceptive effect of oestrogens (risk probably small, see p. 486)

  Probenecid: excretion of meropenem reduced by probenecid (manufacturers of meropenem advise avoid concomitant use)

  Vaccines: antibacterials inactivate oral typhoid vaccine–see p. 760

Mesalazine *see* Aminosalicylates

Mestranol *see* Oestrogens

Metaraminol *see* Sympathomimetics

Metformin *see* Antidiabetics

Methadone *see* Opioid Analgesics

Methenamine

- Antibacterials: increased risk of crystalluria when methenamine given with ●sulphonamides
- Diuretics: effects of methenamine antagonised by ●acetazolamide

  Oestrogens: antibacterials that do not induce liver enzymes possibly reduce contraceptive effect of oestrogens (risk probably small, see p. 486)

Methenamine *(continued)*

Potassium Salts: avoid concomitant use of methenamine with potassium citrate

Vaccines: antibacterials inactivate oral typhoid vaccine–see p. 760

Methocarbamol *see* Muscle Relaxants

Methotrexate

- Anaesthetics, General: antifolate effect of methotrexate increased by ●nitrous oxide—avoid concomitant use
- Analgesics: excretion of methotrexate probably reduced by ●NSAIDs (increased risk of toxicity); excretion of methotrexate reduced by ●azapropazone (avoid concomitant use); excretion of methotrexate reduced by ●aspirin, ●diclofenac, ●ibuprofen, ●indometacin, ●ketoprofen, ●meloxicam and ●naproxen (increased risk of toxicity)
- Antibacterials: absorption of methotrexate possibly reduced by neomycin; excretion of methotrexate possibly reduced by ciprofloxacin (increased risk of toxicity); increased risk of haematological toxicity when methotrexate given with ●sulfamethoxazole (as co-trimoxazole); increased risk of methotrexate toxicity when given with doxycycline, sulphonamides or tetracycline; excretion of methotrexate reduced by penicillins (increased risk of toxicity); increased risk of haematological toxicity when methotrexate given with ●trimethoprim (also with co-trimoxazole)

  Antiepileptics: antifolate effect of methotrexate increased by phenytoin; cytotoxics possibly reduce absorption of phenytoin
- Antimalarials: antifolate effect of methotrexate increased by ●pyrimethamine
- Antipsychotics: avoid concomitant use of cytotoxics with ●clozapine (increased risk of agranulocytosis)

  Cardiac Glycosides: cytotoxics reduce absorption of digoxin tablets
- Ciclosporin: risk of toxicity when methotrexate given with ●ciclosporin
- Cytotoxics: increased pulmonary toxicity when methotrexate given with ●cisplatin
- Leflunomide: risk of toxicity when methotrexate given with ●leflunomide
- Probenecid: excretion of methotrexate reduced by ●probenecid (increased risk of toxicity)
- Retinoids: plasma concentration of methotrexate increased by ●acitretin (also increased risk of hepatotoxicity)—avoid concomitant use

  Theophylline: methotrexate possibly increases plasma concentration of theophylline

  Ulcer-healing Drugs: excretion of methotrexate possibly reduced by omeprazole (increased risk of toxicity)

Methoxamine *see* Sympathomimetics

Methyldopa

ACE Inhibitors: enhanced hypotensive effect when methyldopa given with ACE inhibitors

Adrenergic Neurone Blockers: enhanced hypotensive effect when methyldopa given with adrenergic neurone blockers

Alcohol: enhanced hypotensive effect when methyldopa given with alcohol

Aldesleukin: enhanced hypotensive effect when methyldopa given with aldesleukin

Alpha-blockers: enhanced hypotensive effect when methyldopa given with alpha-blockers

Anaesthetics, General: enhanced hypotensive effect when methyldopa given with general anaesthetics

Analgesics: hypotensive effect of methyldopa antagonised by NSAIDs

Angiotensin-II Receptor Antagonists: enhanced hypotensive effect when methyldopa given with angiotensin-II receptor antagonists
- Antidepressants: manufacturer of methyldopa advises avoid concomitant use with ●MAOIs

Methyldopa (continued)

Antipsychotics: enhanced hypotensive effect when methyldopa given with antipsychotics (also increased risk of extrapyramidal effects)

Anxiolytics and Hypnotics: enhanced hypotensive effect when methyldopa given with anxiolytics and hypnotics

Beta-blockers: enhanced hypotensive effect when methyldopa given with beta-blockers

Calcium-channel Blockers: enhanced hypotensive effect when methyldopa given with calcium-channel blockers

Clonidine: enhanced hypotensive effect when methyldopa given with clonidine

Corticosteroids: hypotensive effect of methyldopa antagonised by corticosteroids

Diazoxide: enhanced hypotensive effect when methyldopa given with diazoxide

Diuretics: enhanced hypotensive effect when methyldopa given with diuretics

Dopaminergics: methyldopa antagonises antiparkinsonian effect of dopaminergics; increased risk of extrapyramidal side-effects when methyldopa given with amantadine; effects of methyldopa possibly enhanced by entacapone; enhanced hypotensive effect when methyldopa given with levodopa

Iron: hypotensive effect of methyldopa antagonised by *oral* iron

- Lithium: neurotoxicity may occur when methyldopa given with ●lithium without increased plasma concentration of lithium

Moxisylyte: enhanced hypotensive effect when methyldopa given with moxisylyte

Moxonidine: enhanced hypotensive effect when methyldopa given with moxonidine

Muscle Relaxants: enhanced hypotensive effect when methyldopa given with baclofen or tizanidine

Nitrates: enhanced hypotensive effect when methyldopa given with nitrates

Oestrogens: hypotensive effect of methyldopa antagonised by oestrogens

Prostaglandins: enhanced hypotensive effect when methyldopa given with alprostadil

- Sympathomimetics, Beta$_2$: acute hypotension reported when methyldopa given with *infusion* of ●salbutamol

Vasodilator Antihypertensives: enhanced hypotensive effect when methyldopa given with hydralazine, minoxidil or sodium nitroprusside

Methylphenidate *see* Sympathomimetics
Methylprednisolone *see* Corticosteroids
Methysergide *see* Ergot Alkaloids
Metipranolol *see* Beta-blockers
Metoclopramide

Analgesics: metoclopramide increases rate of absorption of aspirin (enhanced effect); effects of metoclopramide on gastro-intestinal activity antagonised by opioid analgesics; metoclopramide increases rate of absorption of paracetamol

Antimuscarinics: effects of metoclopramide on gastrointestinal activity antagonised by antimuscarinics

Antipsychotics: increased risk of extrapyramidal side-effects when metoclopramide given with antipsychotics

Atovaquone: metoclopramide reduces plasma concentration of atovaquone

- Ciclosporin: metoclopramide increases plasma concentration of ●ciclosporin

Dopaminergics: metoclopramide antagonises hypoprolactinaemic effects of bromocriptine and cabergoline; metoclopramide antagonises antiparkinsonian effect of pergolide; avoidance of metoclopramide advised by manufacturer of ropinirole and rotigotine (antagonism of effect)

Muscle Relaxants: metoclopramide enhances effects of suxamethonium

Metoclopramide (continued)

Tetrabenazine: increased risk of extrapyramidal side-effects when metoclopramide given with tetrabenazine

Metolazone *see* Diuretics
Metoprolol *see* Beta-blockers
Metronidazole

Note. Interactions do not apply to topical metronidazole preparations

Alcohol: disulfiram-like reaction when metronidazole given with alcohol

- Anticoagulants: metronidazole enhances anticoagulant effect of ●coumarins
- Antiepileptics: metronidazole inhibits metabolism of ●phenytoin (increased plasma concentration); metabolism of metronidazole accelerated by primidone (reduced plasma concentration)

Barbiturates: metabolism of metronidazole accelerated by barbiturates (reduced plasma concentration)

- Cytotoxics: metronidazole increases plasma concentration of ●busulfan (increased risk of toxicity); metronidazole inhibits metabolism of fluorouracil (increased toxicity)

Disulfiram: psychotic reaction reported when metronidazole given with disulfiram

Lithium: metronidazole increases risk of lithium toxicity

Mycophenolate: metronidazole possibly reduces bioavailability of mycophenolate

Oestrogens: antibacterials that do not induce liver enzymes possibly reduce contraceptive effect of oestrogens (risk probably small, see p. 486)

Ulcer-healing Drugs: metabolism of metronidazole inhibited by cimetidine (increased plasma concentration)

Vaccines: antibacterials inactivate oral typhoid vaccine–see p. 760

Mianserin *see* Antidepressants, Tricyclic (related)
Micafungin

Antifungals: micafungin increases plasma concentration of itraconazole (consider reducing dose of itraconazole)

Calcium-channel Blockers: micafungin increases plasma concentration of nifedipine

Ciclosporin: micafungin possibly increases plasma concentration of ciclosporin

Sirolimus: micafungin increases plasma concentration of sirolimus

Miconazole *see* Antifungals, Imidazole
Midazolam *see* Anxiolytics and Hypnotics
Mifamurtide

Analgesics: manufacturer of mifamurtide advises avoid concomitant use with high doses of NSAIDs

Ciclosporin: manufacturer of mifamurtide advises avoid concomitant use with ciclosporin

Corticosteroids: manufacturer of mifamurtide advises avoid concomitant use with corticosteroids

Tacrolimus: manufacturer of mifamurtide advises avoid concomitant use with tacrolimus

Mifepristone

Corticosteroids: mifepristone may reduce effect of corticosteroids (including *inhaled* corticosteroids) for 3–4 days

Milrinone *see* Phosphodiesterase Inhibitors
Minocycline *see* Tetracyclines
Minoxidil *see* Vasodilator Antihypertensives
Mirtazapine

- Alcohol: increased sedative effect when mirtazapine given with ●alcohol

Analgesics: possible increased serotonergic effects when mirtazapine given with tramadol

Anticoagulants: mirtazapine enhances anticoagulant effect of warfarin

- Antidepressants: possible increased serotonergic effects when mirtazapine given with fluoxetine, fluvoxamine or venlafaxine; mirtazapine should not

Mirtazapine
- Antidepressants *(continued)*
  be started until 2 weeks after stopping ●MAOIs, also MAOIs should not be started until at least 2 weeks after stopping mirtazapine; after stopping mirtazapine do not start ●moclobemide for at least 1 week

  Antiepileptics: plasma concentration of mirtazapine reduced by carbamazepine and phenytoin

  Antifungals: plasma concentration of mirtazapine increased by ketoconazole
- Antimalarials: avoidance of antidepressants advised by manufacturer of ●artemether/lumefantrine

  Anxiolytics and Hypnotics: increased sedative effect when mirtazapine given with anxiolytics and hypnotics

  Atomoxetine: possible increased risk of convulsions when antidepressants given with atomoxetine
- Sibutramine: increased risk of CNS toxicity when mirtazapine given with ●sibutramine (manufacturer of sibutramine advises avoid concomitant use)

  Ulcer-healing Drugs: plasma concentration of mirtazapine increased by cimetidine

Mitomycin
  Antiepileptics: cytotoxics possibly reduce absorption of phenytoin
- Antipsychotics: avoid concomitant use of cytotoxics with ●clozapine (increased risk of agranulocytosis)

  Cardiac Glycosides: cytotoxics reduce absorption of digoxin tablets

Mitotane
- Anticoagulants: mitotane possibly reduces anticoagulant effect of ●coumarins

  Antiepileptics: cytotoxics possibly reduce absorption of phenytoin
- Antipsychotics: avoid concomitant use of cytotoxics with ●clozapine (increased risk of agranulocytosis)

  Cardiac Glycosides: cytotoxics reduce absorption of digoxin tablets

  Diuretics: manufacturer of mitotane advises avoid concomitant use of spironolactone (antagonism of effect)

Mitoxantrone
  Antiepileptics: cytotoxics possibly reduce absorption of phenytoin
- Antipsychotics: avoid concomitant use of cytotoxics with ●clozapine (increased risk of agranulocytosis)

  Cardiac Glycosides: cytotoxics reduce absorption of digoxin tablets

  Ciclosporin: excretion of mitoxantrone reduced by ciclosporin (increased plasma concentration)

Mivacurium *see* Muscle Relaxants

Mizolastine *see* Antihistamines

Moclobemide
- Analgesics: possible CNS excitation or depression (hypertension or hypotension) when moclobemide given with ●dextromethorphan or ●pethidine—avoid concomitant use; possible CNS excitation or depression (hypertension or hypotension) when moclobemide given with ●opioid analgesics
- Antidepressants: moclobemide should not be started for at least 1 week after stopping ●MAOIs, ●SSRI-related antidepressants, ●citalopram, ●fluvoxamine, ●mirtazapine, ●paroxetine, ●sertraline, ●tricyclic-related antidepressants or ●tricyclics; increased risk of CNS toxicity when moclobemide given with ●escitalopram, preferably avoid concomitant use; moclobemide should not be started until 5 weeks after stopping ●fluoxetine; possible increased serotonergic effects when moclobemide given with ●duloxetine
- Antimalarials: avoidance of antidepressants advised by manufacturer of ●artemether/lumefantrine

  Atomoxetine: possible increased risk of convulsions when antidepressants given with atomoxetine
- Bupropion: avoidance of moclobemide advised by manufacturer of ●bupropion

Moclobemide *(continued)*
- Clopidogrel: moclobemide possibly reduces antiplatelet effect of ●clopidogrel
- Dopaminergics: caution with moclobemide advised by manufacturer of entacapone; increased risk of side-effects when moclobemide given with levodopa; avoid concomitant use of moclobemide with ●selegiline
- 5HT₁ Agonists: risk of CNS toxicity when moclobemide given with ●rizatriptan or ●sumatriptan (avoid rizatriptan or sumatriptan for 2 weeks after moclobemide); risk of CNS toxicity when moclobemide given with ●zolmitriptan (reduce dose of zolmitriptan)
- Sibutramine: increased CNS toxicity when moclobemide given with ●sibutramine (manufacturer of sibutramine advises avoid concomitant use, also avoid sibutramine for 2 weeks after stopping moclobemide)
- Sympathomimetics: risk of hypertensive crisis when moclobemide given with ●sympathomimetics

  Ulcer-healing Drugs: plasma concentration of moclobemide increased by cimetidine (halve dose of moclobemide)

Modafinil
  Antiepileptics: modafinil possibly increases plasma concentration of phenytoin
- Ciclosporin: modafinil reduces plasma concentration of ●ciclosporin
- Oestrogens: modafinil accelerates metabolism of ●oestrogens (reduced contraceptive effect—see p. 486)

Moexipril *see* ACE Inhibitors

Mometasone *see* Corticosteroids

Monobactams *see* Aztreonam

Montelukast *see* Leukotriene Receptor Antagonists

Morphine *see* Opioid Analgesics

Moxifloxacin *see* Quinolones

Moxisylyte
  ACE Inhibitors: enhanced hypotensive effect when moxisylyte given with ACE inhibitors

  Adrenergic Neurone Blockers: enhanced hypotensive effect when moxisylyte given with adrenergic neurone blockers
- Alpha-blockers: possible severe postural hypotension when moxisylyte given with ●alpha-blockers

  Angiotensin-II Receptor Antagonists: enhanced hypotensive effect when moxisylyte given with angiotensin-II receptor antagonists
- Beta-blockers: possible severe postural hypotension when moxisylyte given with ●beta-blockers

  Calcium-channel Blockers: enhanced hypotensive effect when moxisylyte given with calcium-channel blockers

  Clonidine: enhanced hypotensive effect when moxisylyte given with clonidine

  Diazoxide: enhanced hypotensive effect when moxisylyte given with diazoxide

  Diuretics: enhanced hypotensive effect when moxisylyte given with diuretics

  Methyldopa: enhanced hypotensive effect when moxisylyte given with methyldopa

  Moxonidine: enhanced hypotensive effect when moxisylyte given with moxonidine

  Nitrates: enhanced hypotensive effect when moxisylyte given with nitrates

  Vasodilator Antihypertensives: enhanced hypotensive effect when moxisylyte given with hydralazine, minoxidil or sodium nitroprusside

Moxonidine
  ACE Inhibitors: enhanced hypotensive effect when moxonidine given with ACE inhibitors

  Adrenergic Neurone Blockers: enhanced hypotensive effect when moxonidine given with adrenergic neurone blockers

Moxonidine (continued)

Alcohol: enhanced hypotensive effect when moxonidine given with alcohol

Aldesleukin: enhanced hypotensive effect when moxonidine given with aldesleukin

Alpha-blockers: enhanced hypotensive effect when moxonidine given with alpha-blockers

Anaesthetics, General: enhanced hypotensive effect when moxonidine given with general anaesthetics

Analgesics: hypotensive effect of moxonidine antagonised by NSAIDs

Angiotensin-II Receptor Antagonists: enhanced hypotensive effect when moxonidine given with angiotensin-II receptor antagonists

Antidepressants: enhanced hypotensive effect when moxonidine given with MAOIs

Antipsychotics: enhanced hypotensive effect when moxonidine given with phenothiazines

Anxiolytics and Hypnotics: enhanced hypotensive effect when moxonidine given with anxiolytics and hypnotics; sedative effects possibly increased when moxonidine given with benzodiazepines

Beta-blockers: enhanced hypotensive effect when moxonidine given with beta-blockers

Calcium-channel Blockers: enhanced hypotensive effect when moxonidine given with calcium-channel blockers

Clonidine: enhanced hypotensive effect when moxonidine given with clonidine

Corticosteroids: hypotensive effect of moxonidine antagonised by corticosteroids

Diazoxide: enhanced hypotensive effect when moxonidine given with diazoxide

Diuretics: enhanced hypotensive effect when moxonidine given with diuretics

Dopaminergics: enhanced hypotensive effect when moxonidine given with levodopa

Methyldopa: enhanced hypotensive effect when moxonidine given with methyldopa

Moxisylyte: enhanced hypotensive effect when moxonidine given with moxisylyte

Muscle Relaxants: enhanced hypotensive effect when moxonidine given with baclofen or tizanidine

Nitrates: enhanced hypotensive effect when moxonidine given with nitrates

Oestrogens: hypotensive effect of moxonidine antagonised by oestrogens

Prostaglandins: enhanced hypotensive effect when moxonidine given with alprostadil

Vasodilator Antihypertensives: enhanced hypotensive effect when moxonidine given with hydralazine, minoxidil or sodium nitroprusside

Muscle Relaxants

ACE Inhibitors: enhanced hypotensive effect when baclofen or tizanidine given with ACE inhibitors

Adrenergic Neurone Blockers: enhanced hypotensive effect when baclofen or tizanidine given with adrenergic neurone blockers

Alcohol: increased sedative effect when baclofen, methocarbamol or tizanidine given with alcohol

Alpha-blockers: enhanced hypotensive effect when baclofen or tizanidine given with alpha-blockers

● Anaesthetics, General: effects of atracurium enhanced by ketamine; increased risk of myocardial depression and bradycardia when suxamethonium given with ●propofol; effects of non-depolarising muscle relaxants and suxamethonium enhanced by volatile liquid general anaesthetics

Analgesics: excretion of baclofen possibly reduced by NSAIDs (increased risk of toxicity); excretion of baclofen reduced by ibuprofen (increased risk of toxicity); increased sedative effect when baclofen given with fentanyl or morphine

Angiotensin-II Receptor Antagonists: enhanced hypotensive effect when baclofen or tizanidine given with angiotensin-II receptor antagonists

Muscle Relaxants (continued)

Anti-arrhythmics: neuromuscular blockade enhanced and prolonged when suxamethonium given with lidocaine

● Antibacterials: effects of non-depolarising muscle relaxants and suxamethonium enhanced by piperacillin; plasma concentration of tizanidine increased by ●ciprofloxacin (increased risk of toxicity)—avoid concomitant use; plasma concentration of tizanidine possibly increased by norfloxacin (increased risk of toxicity); effects of non-depolarising muscle relaxants and suxamethonium enhanced by ●aminoglycosides; effects of non-depolarising muscle relaxants and suxamethonium enhanced by ●clindamycin; effects of non-depolarising muscle relaxants and suxamethonium enhanced by ●polymyxins; effects of suxamethonium enhanced by ●vancomycin

● Antidepressants: plasma concentration of tizanidine increased by ●fluvoxamine (increased risk of toxicity)—avoid concomitant use; effects of suxamethonium enhanced by phenelzine; muscle relaxant effect of baclofen enhanced by tricyclics

Antiepileptics: muscle relaxant effect of non-depolarising muscle relaxants antagonised by carbamazepine and phenytoin (accelerated recovery from neuromuscular blockade)

Antimalarials: effects of suxamethonium possibly enhanced by quinine

Antipsychotics: effects of suxamethonium possibly enhanced by promazine

Anxiolytics and Hypnotics: increased sedative effect when baclofen or tizanidine given with anxiolytics and hypnotics

Beta-blockers: enhanced hypotensive effect when baclofen given with beta-blockers; possible enhanced hypotensive effect and bradycardia when tizanidine given with beta-blockers; effects of muscle relaxants enhanced by propranolol

Calcium-channel Blockers: enhanced hypotensive effect when baclofen or tizanidine given with calcium-channel blockers; effects of non-depolarising muscle relaxants possibly enhanced by calcium-channel blockers; risk of arrhythmias when *intravenous* dantrolene given with diltiazem; effects of non-depolarising muscle relaxants and suxamethonium enhanced by verapamil; hypotension, myocardial depression, and hyperkalaemia when *intravenous* dantrolene given with verapamil

Cardiac Glycosides: possible increased risk of bradycardia when tizanidine given with cardiac glycosides; risk of ventricular arrhythmias when suxamethonium given with cardiac glycosides

Clonidine: enhanced hypotensive effect when baclofen or tizanidine given with clonidine

Corticosteroids: effects of pancuronium and vecuronium possibly antagonised by corticosteroids

Cytotoxics: effects of suxamethonium enhanced by cyclophosphamide and thiotepa

Diazoxide: enhanced hypotensive effect when baclofen or tizanidine given with diazoxide

Diuretics: enhanced hypotensive effect when baclofen or tizanidine given with diuretics

Dopaminergics: possible agitation, confusion and hallucinations when baclofen given with levodopa

Lithium: effects of muscle relaxants enhanced by lithium; baclofen possibly aggravates hyperkinesis caused by lithium

Magnesium (parenteral): effects of non-depolarising muscle relaxants and suxamethonium enhanced by parenteral magnesium

Memantine: effects of baclofen and dantrolene possibly modified by memantine

Methyldopa: enhanced hypotensive effect when baclofen or tizanidine given with methyldopa

Muscle Relaxants *(continued)*

Metoclopramide: effects of suxamethonium enhanced by metoclopramide

Moxonidine: enhanced hypotensive effect when baclofen or tizanidine given with moxonidine

Nitrates: enhanced hypotensive effect when baclofen or tizanidine given with nitrates

Oestrogens: plasma concentration of tizanidine possibly increased by oestrogens (increased risk of toxicity)

Parasympathomimetics: effects of non-depolarising muscle relaxants possibly antagonised by donepezil; effects of suxamethonium possibly enhanced by donepezil; effects of non-depolarising muscle relaxants antagonised by edrophonium, neostigmine, pyridostigmine and rivastigmine; effects of suxamethonium enhanced by edrophonium, galantamine, neostigmine, pyridostigmine and rivastigmine

Progestogens: plasma concentration of tizanidine possibly increased by progestogens (increased risk of toxicity)

Sympathomimetics, Beta$_2$: effects of suxamethonium enhanced by bambuterol

Vasodilator Antihypertensives: enhanced hypotensive effect when baclofen or tizanidine given with hydralazine; enhanced hypotensive effect when baclofen or tizanidine given with minoxidil; enhanced hypotensive effect when baclofen or tizanidine given with sodium nitroprusside

Muscle Relaxants, depolarising *see* Muscle Relaxants
Muscle Relaxants, non-depolarising *see* Muscle Relaxants
Mycophenolate

Antacids: absorption of mycophenolate reduced by antacids

• Antibacterials: bioavailability of mycophenolate possibly reduced by metronidazole and norfloxacin; plasma concentration of active metabolite of mycophenolate reduced by ●rifampicin

Antivirals: mycophenolate increases plasma concentration of aciclovir, also plasma concentration of inactive metabolite of mycophenolate increased; mycophenolate possibly increases plasma concentration of ganciclovir, also plasma concentration of inactive metabolite of mycophenolate possibly increased

Iron: absorption of mycophenolate reduced by *oral* iron

Lipid-regulating Drugs: absorption of mycophenolate reduced by colestyramine

Sevelamer: plasma concentration of mycophenolate possibly reduced by sevelamer

Mycophenolate Mofetil *see* Mycophenolate
Mycophenolate Sodium *see* Mycophenolate
Mycophenolic Acid *see* Mycophenolate
Nabilone

Alcohol: increased sedative effect when nabilone given with alcohol

Anxiolytics and Hypnotics: increased sedative effect when nabilone given with anxiolytics and hypnotics

Nabumetone *see* NSAIDs
Nadolol *see* Beta-blockers
Nalidixic Acid *see* Quinolones
Nandrolone *see* Anabolic Steroids
Naproxen *see* NSAIDs
Naratriptan *see* 5HT$_1$ Agonists
Nateglinide *see* Antidiabetics
Nebivolol *see* Beta-blockers
Nefopam

• Antidepressants: manufacturer of nefopam advises avoid concomitant use with ●MAOIs; side-effects possibly increased when nefopam given with tricyclics

Antimuscarinics: increased risk of antimuscarinic side-effects when nefopam given with antimuscarinics

Nelfinavir

Analgesics: nelfinavir reduces plasma concentration of methadone

Nelfinavir *(continued)*

• Anti-arrhythmics: increased risk of ventricular arrhythmias when nelfinavir given with ●amiodarone—avoid concomitant use

• Antibacterials: nelfinavir increases plasma concentration of ●rifabutin (halve dose of rifabutin); plasma concentration of nelfinavir significantly reduced by ●rifampicin—avoid concomitant use; avoidance of concomitant nelfinavir in severe renal and hepatic impairment advised by manufacturer of ●telithromycin

Anticoagulants: avoidance of nelfinavir advised by manufacturer of rivaroxaban

• Antidepressants: plasma concentration of nelfinavir reduced by ●St John's wort—avoid concomitant use

• Antiepileptics: plasma concentration of nelfinavir possibly reduced by carbamazepine and ●primidone; nelfinavir reduces plasma concentration of phenytoin

Antimalarials: caution with nelfinavir advised by manufacturer of artemether/lumefantrine

Antimuscarinics: avoidance of nelfinavir advised by manufacturer of darifenacin and tolterodine; manufacturer of fesoterodine advises dose reduction when nelfinavir given with fesoterodine—consult fesoterodine product literature; nelfinavir increases plasma concentration of solifenacin

• Antipsychotics: nelfinavir possibly inhibits metabolism of ●aripiprazole (reduce dose of aripiprazole); nelfinavir possibly increases plasma concentration of ●pimozide (increased risk of ventricular arrhythmias—avoid concomitant use); nelfinavir increases plasma concentration of ●sertindole (increased risk of ventricular arrhythmias—avoid concomitant use)

• Antivirals: plasma concentration of nelfinavir possibly increased by etravirine—avoid concomitant use; combination of nelfinavir with indinavir, ritonavir or saquinavir may increase plasma concentration of either drug (or both); nelfinavir reduces plasma concentration of lopinavir, also plasma concentration of active metabolite of nelfinavir increased; nelfinavir possibly increases plasma concentration of ●maraviroc (consider reducing dose of maraviroc)

• Anxiolytics and Hypnotics: nelfinavir possibly increases plasma concentration of ●midazolam (risk of prolonged sedation—avoid concomitant use of *oral* midazolam)

• Barbiturates: plasma concentration of nelfinavir possibly reduced by ●barbiturates

• Ciclosporin: nelfinavir possibly increases plasma concentration of ●ciclosporin

• Cilostazol: nelfinavir possibly increases plasma concentration of ●cilostazol—avoid concomitant use

Corticosteroids: nelfinavir possibly increases plasma concentration of *inhaled* and *intranasal* fluticasone

• Cytotoxics: nelfinavir possibly increases plasma concentration of ●everolimus—manufacturer of everolimus advises avoid concomitant use; nelfinavir increases plasma concentration of paclitaxel

• Diuretics: nelfinavir increases plasma concentration of ●eplerenone—avoid concomitant use

• Ergot Alkaloids: increased risk of ergotism when nelfinavir given with ●ergotamine and methysergide—avoid concomitant use

• 5HT$_1$ Agonists: nelfinavir increases plasma concentration of ●eletriptan (risk of toxicity)—avoid concomitant use

• Ivabradine: nelfinavir possibly increases plasma concentration of ●ivabradine—avoid concomitant use

• Lipid-regulating Drugs: possible increased risk of myopathy when nelfinavir given with atorvastatin; possible increased risk of myopathy when nelfinavir given with ●rosuvastatin—manufacturer of rosuvastatin advises avoid concomitant use; increased risk of myopathy when nelfinavir given with ●simvastatin (avoid concomitant use)

Nelfinavir *(continued)*
- Oestrogens: nelfinavir accelerates metabolism of
  ●oestrogens (reduced contraceptive effect—see
  p. 486)

  Progestogens: nelfinavir possibly reduces contraceptive effect of progestogens
- Ranolazine: nelfinavir possibly increases plasma concentration of ●ranolazine—manufacturer of ranolazine advises avoid concomitant use

  Sildenafil: nelfinavir possibly increases plasma concentration of sildenafil—reduce initial dose of
  sildenafil
- Tacrolimus: nelfinavir possibly increases plasma concentration of ●tacrolimus
- Ulcer-healing Drugs: plasma concentration of nelfinavir reduced by ●omeprazole—avoid concomitant use

Neomycin *see* Aminoglycosides
Neostigmine *see* Parasympathomimetics
Nevirapine
  Analgesics: nevirapine possibly reduces plasma concentration of methadone
- Antibacterials: nevirapine possibly increases plasma concentration of rifabutin; plasma concentration of
  nevirapine reduced by ●rifampicin—avoid concomitant use
- Anticoagulants: nevirapine may enhance or reduce anticoagulant effect of ●warfarin
- Antidepressants: plasma concentration of nevirapine reduced by ●St John's wort—avoid concomitant use
- Antifungals: nevirapine reduces plasma concentration of ●ketoconazole—avoid concomitant use; plasma concentration of nevirapine increased by ●fluconazole; nevirapine possibly reduces plasma concentration of caspofungin and itraconazole—consider increasing dose of caspofungin and itraconazole
- Antipsychotics: nevirapine possibly reduces plasma concentration of ●aripiprazole—increase dose of aripiprazole
- Antivirals: nevirapine possibly reduces plasma concentration of ●atazanavir and ●etravirine—avoid concomitant use; nevirapine reduces plasma concentration of efavirenz and indinavir; nevirapine possibly reduces plasma concentration of fosamprenavir; nevirapine possibly reduces plasma concentration of ●lopinavir—consider increasing dose of lopinavir
- Oestrogens: nevirapine accelerates metabolism of ●oestrogens (reduced contraceptive effect—see p. 486)
- Progestogens: nevirapine accelerates metabolism of ●progestogens (reduced contraceptive effect—see p. 486)

Nicardipine *see* Calcium-channel Blockers
Nicorandil
  Alcohol: hypotensive effect of nicorandil possibly enhanced by alcohol
  Antidepressants: enhanced hypotensive effect when nicorandil given with MAOIs; hypotensive effect of nicorandil possibly enhanced by tricyclics
- Sildenafil: hypotensive effect of nicorandil significantly enhanced by ●sildenafil (avoid concomitant use)
- Tadalafil: hypotensive effect of nicorandil significantly enhanced by ●tadalafil (avoid concomitant use)
- Vardenafil: possible increased hypotensive effect when nicorandil given with ●vardenafil—avoid concomitant use
  Vasodilator Antihypertensives: possible enhanced hypotensive effect when nicorandil given with hydralazine, minoxidil or sodium nitroprusside

Nicotine
  Anti-arrhythmics: nicotine possibly enhances effects of adenosine

Nicotinic Acid
  Note. Interactions apply to lipid-regulating doses of nicotinic acid
- Lipid-regulating Drugs: increased risk of myopathy when nicotinic acid given with ●statins (applies to lipid regulating doses of nicotinic acid)

Nifedipine *see* Calcium-channel Blockers
Nilotinib
- Antibacterials: manufacturer of nilotinib advises avoid concomitant use with ●clarithromycin and ●telithromycin; plasma concentration of nilotinib reduced by ●rifampicin—avoid concomitant use
  Antiepileptics: cytotoxics possibly reduce absorption of phenytoin
- Antifungals: plasma concentration of nilotinib increased by ●ketoconazole—avoid concomitant use; manufacturer of nilotinib advises avoid concomitant use with ●itraconazole and ●voriconazole
- Antipsychotics: avoid concomitant use of cytotoxics with ●clozapine (increased risk of agranulocytosis)
- Antivirals: manufacturer of nilotinib advises avoid concomitant use with ●ritonavir
  Anxiolytics and Hypnotics: nilotinib increases plasma concentration of midazolam
  Cardiac Glycosides: cytotoxics reduce absorption of digoxin tablets
- Grapefruit Juice: manufacturer of nilotinib advises avoid concomitant use with ●grapefruit juice

Nimodipine *see* Calcium-channel Blockers
Nitrates
  ACE Inhibitors: enhanced hypotensive effect when nitrates given with ACE inhibitors
  Adrenergic Neurone Blockers: enhanced hypotensive effect when nitrates given with adrenergic neurone blockers
  Alcohol: enhanced hypotensive effect when nitrates given with alcohol
  Aldesleukin: enhanced hypotensive effect when nitrates given with aldesleukin
  Alpha-blockers: enhanced hypotensive effect when nitrates given with alpha-blockers
  Anaesthetics, General: enhanced hypotensive effect when nitrates given with general anaesthetics
  Analgesics: hypotensive effect of nitrates antagonised by NSAIDs
  Angiotensin-II Receptor Antagonists: enhanced hypotensive effect when nitrates given with angiotensin-II receptor antagonists
  Anti-arrhythmics: effects of sublingual tablets of nitrates reduced by disopyramide (failure to dissolve under tongue owing to dry mouth)
- Anticoagulants: *infusion* of glyceryl trinitrate reduces anticoagulant effect of ●heparins
  Antidepressants: enhanced hypotensive effect when nitrates given with MAOIs; effects of sublingual tablets of nitrates possibly reduced by tricyclic-related antidepressants (failure to dissolve under tongue owing to dry mouth); effects of sublingual tablets of nitrates reduced by tricyclics (failure to dissolve under tongue owing to dry mouth)
  Antimuscarinics: effects of sublingual tablets of nitrates possibly reduced by antimuscarinics (failure to dissolve under tongue owing to dry mouth)
  Antipsychotics: enhanced hypotensive effect when nitrates given with phenothiazines
  Anxiolytics and Hypnotics: enhanced hypotensive effect when nitrates given with anxiolytics and hypnotics
  Beta-blockers: enhanced hypotensive effect when nitrates given with beta-blockers
  Calcium-channel Blockers: enhanced hypotensive effect when nitrates given with calcium-channel blockers
  Clonidine: enhanced hypotensive effect when nitrates given with clonidine

Nitrates *(continued)*

Corticosteroids: hypotensive effect of nitrates antagonised by corticosteroids

Diazoxide: enhanced hypotensive effect when nitrates given with diazoxide

Diuretics: enhanced hypotensive effect when nitrates given with diuretics

Dopaminergics: enhanced hypotensive effect when nitrates given with levodopa

Methyldopa: enhanced hypotensive effect when nitrates given with methyldopa

Moxisylyte: enhanced hypotensive effect when nitrates given with moxisylyte

Moxonidine: enhanced hypotensive effect when nitrates given with moxonidine

Muscle Relaxants: enhanced hypotensive effect when nitrates given with baclofen or tizanidine

Oestrogens: hypotensive effect of nitrates antagonised by oestrogens

Prostaglandins: enhanced hypotensive effect when nitrates given with alprostadil

- Sildenafil: hypotensive effect of nitrates significantly enhanced by ●sildenafil (avoid concomitant use)
- Tadalafil: hypotensive effect of nitrates significantly enhanced by ●tadalafil (avoid concomitant use)
- Vardenafil: possible increased hypotensive effect when nitrates given with ●vardenafil—avoid concomitant use

Vasodilator Antihypertensives: enhanced hypotensive effect when nitrates given with hydralazine, minoxidil or sodium nitroprusside

Nitrazepam *see* Anxiolytics and Hypnotics

Nitrofurantoin

Antacids: absorption of nitrofurantoin reduced by oral magnesium salts (as magnesium trisilicate)

Oestrogens: antibacterials that do not induce liver enzymes possibly reduce contraceptive effect of oestrogens (risk probably small, see p. 486)

Probenecid: excretion of nitrofurantoin reduced by probenecid (increased risk of side-effects)

Sulfinpyrazone: excretion of nitrofurantoin reduced by sulfinpyrazone (increased risk of toxicity)

Vaccines: antibacterials inactivate oral typhoid vaccine–see p. 760

Nitroimidazoles *see* Metronidazole and Tinidazole

Nitrous Oxide *see* Anaesthetics, General

Nizatidine *see* Histamine H_2-antagonists

Noradrenaline (norepinephrine) *see* Sympathomimetics

Norelgestromin *see* Progestogens

Norepinephrine (noradrenaline) *see* Sympathomimetics

Norethisterone *see* Progestogens

Norfloxacin *see* Quinolones

Norgestimate *see* Progestogens

Norgestrel *see* Progestogens

Nortriptyline *see* Antidepressants, Tricyclic

NSAIDs

Note. See also Aspirin. Interactions do not generally apply to topical NSAIDs

ACE Inhibitors: increased risk of renal impairment when NSAIDs given with ACE inhibitors, also hypotensive effect antagonised

Adrenergic Neurone Blockers: NSAIDs antagonise hypotensive effect of adrenergic neurone blockers

Alpha-blockers: NSAIDs antagonise hypotensive effect of alpha-blockers

Analgesics: avoid concomitant use of NSAIDs with ●NSAIDs or ●aspirin (increased side-effects); avoid concomitant use of NSAIDs with ●ketorolac (increased side-effects and haemorrhage); ibuprofen possibly reduces antiplatelet effect of aspirin

Angiotensin-II Receptor Antagonists: increased risk of renal impairment when NSAIDs given with angiotensin-II receptor antagonists, also hypotensive effect antagonised

- Antibacterials: indometacin possibly increases plasma concentration of amikacin and gentamicin in neo-

NSAIDs

- Antibacterials *(continued)*
nates; plasma concentration of etoricoxib reduced by rifampicin; possible increased risk of convulsions when NSAIDs given with ●quinolones
- Anticoagulants: increased risk of haemorrhage when *intravenous* diclofenac given with ●anticoagulants (avoid concomitant use, including low-dose heparins); increased risk of haemorrhage when ketorolac given with ●anticoagulants (avoid concomitant use, including low-dose heparins); azapropazone enhances anticoagulant effect of ●coumarins (avoid concomitant use); NSAIDs possibly enhance anticoagulant effect of ●coumarins and ●phenindione; possible increased risk of bleeding when NSAIDs given with ●dabigatran etexilate or heparins
- Antidepressants: increased risk of bleeding when NSAIDs given with ●SSRIs or ●venlafaxine
- Antidiabetics: azapropazone enhances effects of ●tolbutamide (avoid concomitant use); NSAIDs possibly enhance effects of ●sulphonylureas
- Antiepileptics: azapropazone significantly increases plasma concentration of ●phenytoin—avoid concomitant use; NSAIDs possibly enhance effects of ●phenytoin

Antifungals: plasma concentration of parecoxib increased by fluconazole (reduce dose of parecoxib); plasma concentration of celecoxib increased by fluconazole (halve dose of celecoxib); plasma concentration of diclofenac and ibuprofen increased by voriconazole

- Antipsychotics: possible severe drowsiness when indometacin given with haloperidol; avoid concomitant use of azapropazone with ●clozapine (increased risk of agranulocytosis)
- Antivirals: plasma concentration of NSAIDs possibly increased by ritonavir; plasma concentration of piroxicam increased by ●ritonavir (risk of toxicity)—avoid concomitant use; increased risk of haematological toxicity when NSAIDs given with zidovudine

Beta-blockers: NSAIDs antagonise hypotensive effect of beta-blockers

Bisphosphonates: indometacin increases bioavailability of tiludronic acid

Calcium-channel Blockers: NSAIDs antagonise hypotensive effect of calcium-channel blockers

Cardiac Glycosides: NSAIDs possibly increase plasma concentration of cardiac glycosides, also possible exacerbation of heart failure and reduction of renal function

- Ciclosporin: increased risk of nephrotoxicity when NSAIDs given with ●ciclosporin; plasma concentration of diclofenac increased by ●ciclosporin (halve dose of diclofenac)

Clonidine: NSAIDs antagonise hypotensive effect of clonidine

Clopidogrel: increased risk of bleeding when NSAIDs given with clopidogrel

Corticosteroids: increased risk of gastro-intestinal bleeding and ulceration when NSAIDs given with corticosteroids

- Cytotoxics: NSAIDs probably reduce excretion of ●methotrexate (increased risk of toxicity); azapropazone reduces excretion of ●methotrexate (avoid concomitant use); diclofenac, ibuprofen, indometacin, ketoprofen, meloxicam and naproxen reduce excretion of ●methotrexate (increased risk of toxicity); increased risk of bleeding when NSAIDs given with ●erlotinib

Desmopressin: indometacin enhances effects of desmopressin

Diazoxide: NSAIDs antagonise hypotensive effect of diazoxide

- Dimethyl sulfoxide: avoid concomitant use of sulindac with ●dimethyl sulfoxide

NSAIDs *(continued)*

- Diuretics: risk of nephrotoxicity of NSAIDs increased by diuretics, also antagonism of diuretic effect; indometacin and ketorolac antagonise effects of diuretics; NSAIDs possibly antagonise diuretic effect of potassium canrenoate; occasional reports of reduced renal function when indometacin given with ●triamterene—avoid concomitant use; increased risk of hyperkalaemia when indometacin given with potassium-sparing diuretics and aldosterone antagonists; possibly increased risk of hyperkalaemia when NSAIDs given with potassium-sparing diuretics and aldosterone antagonists

  Iloprost: increased risk of bleeding when NSAIDs given with iloprost

  Lipid-regulating Drugs: excretion of meloxicam increased by colestyramine

- Lithium: NSAIDs reduce excretion of ●lithium (increased risk of toxicity); ketorolac reduces excretion of ●lithium (increased risk of toxicity)—avoid concomitant use

  Methyldopa: NSAIDs antagonise hypotensive effect of methyldopa

  Mifamurtide: avoidance of high doses of NSAIDs advised by manufacturer of mifamurtide

  Moxonidine: NSAIDs antagonise hypotensive effect of moxonidine

  Muscle Relaxants: NSAIDs possibly reduce excretion of baclofen (increased risk of toxicity); ibuprofen reduces excretion of baclofen (increased risk of toxicity)

  Nitrates: NSAIDs antagonise hypotensive effect of nitrates

  Oestrogens: etoricoxib increases plasma concentration of ethinylestradiol

  Penicillamine: possible increased risk of nephrotoxicity when NSAIDs given with penicillamine

- Pentoxifylline: possible increased risk of bleeding when NSAIDs given with pentoxifylline; increased risk of bleeding when ketorolac given with ●pentoxifylline (avoid concomitant use)

  Prasugrel: possible increased risk of bleeding when NSAIDs given with prasugrel

- Probenecid: excretion of dexketoprofen, indometacin, ketoprofen and naproxen reduced by ●probenecid (increased plasma concentration); excretion of ketorolac reduced by ●probenecid (increased plasma concentration)—avoid concomitant use

  Sibutramine: increased risk of bleeding when NSAIDs given with sibutramine

- Tacrolimus: possible increased risk of nephrotoxicity when NSAIDs given with tacrolimus; increased risk of nephrotoxicity when ibuprofen given with ●tacrolimus

  Ulcer-healing Drugs: plasma concentration of azapropazone possibly increased by cimetidine

  Vasodilator Antihypertensives: NSAIDs antagonise hypotensive effect of hydralazine, minoxidil and sodium nitroprusside

Octreotide

  Antidiabetics: octreotide possibly reduces requirements for insulin, metformin, repaglinide and sulphonylureas

- Ciclosporin: octreotide reduces plasma concentration of ●ciclosporin

  Dopaminergics: octreotide increases plasma concentration of bromocriptine

  Ulcer-healing Drugs: octreotide possibly delays absorption of cimetidine

Oestrogens

  Note. Interactions of combined oral contraceptives may also apply to combined contraceptive patches and vaginal rings

  ACE Inhibitors: oestrogens antagonise hypotensive effect of ACE inhibitors

Oestrogens *(continued)*

  Adrenergic Neurone Blockers: oestrogens antagonise hypotensive effect of adrenergic neurone blockers

  Alpha-blockers: oestrogens antagonise hypotensive effect of alpha-blockers

  Analgesics: plasma concentration of ethinylestradiol increased by etoricoxib

  Angiotensin-II Receptor Antagonists: oestrogens antagonise hypotensive effect of angiotensin-II receptor antagonists

- Antibacterials: contraceptive effect of oestrogens possibly reduced by antibacterials that do not induce liver enzymes (risk probably small, see p. 486); metabolism of oestrogens accelerated by ●rifamycins (reduced contraceptive effect—see p. 486)

- Anticoagulants: oestrogens may enhance or reduce anticoagulant effect of ●coumarins; oestrogens antagonise anticoagulant effect of ●phenindione

- Antidepressants: contraceptive effect of oestrogens reduced by ●St John's wort (avoid concomitant use); oestrogens antagonise antidepressant effect of tricyclics (but side-effects of tricyclics possibly increased due to increased plasma concentration)

  Antidiabetics: oestrogens antagonise hypoglycaemic effect of antidiabetics

- Antiepileptics: metabolism of oestrogens accelerated by ●carbamazepine, ●eslicarbazepine, ●oxcarbazepine, ●phenytoin, ●primidone, ●rufinamide and ●topiramate (reduced contraceptive effect—see p. 486); oestrogens possibly reduce plasma concentration of ●lamotrigine—consider increasing dose of lamotrigine

- Antifungals: anecdotal reports of contraceptive failure when oestrogens given with fluconazole, imidazoles, itraconazole or ketoconazole; metabolism of oestrogens accelerated by ●griseofulvin (reduced contraceptive effect—see p. 486); occasional reports of breakthrough bleeding when oestrogens (used for contraception) given with terbinafine

- Antivirals: plasma concentration of ethinylestradiol increased by atazanavir; contraceptive effect of oestrogens possibly reduced by efavirenz; plasma concentration of oestrogens increased by fosamprenavir, also plasma concentration of fosamprenavir reduced—alternative contraception recommended; metabolism of oestrogens accelerated by ●nelfinavir, ●nevirapine and ●ritonavir (reduced contraceptive effect—see p. 486)

  Anxiolytics and Hypnotics: oestrogens increase plasma concentration of melatonin

- Aprepitant: possible contraceptive failure of hormonal contraceptives containing oestrogens when given with ●aprepitant (alternative contraception recommended)

- Barbiturates: metabolism of oestrogens accelerated by ●barbiturates (reduced contraceptive effect—see p. 486)

  Beta-blockers: oestrogens antagonise hypotensive effect of beta-blockers

  Bile Acids: elimination of cholesterol in bile increased when oestrogens given with bile acids

- Bosentan: possible contraceptive failure of hormonal contraceptives containing oestrogens when given with ●bosentan (alternative contraception recommended)

  Calcium-channel Blockers: oestrogens antagonise hypotensive effect of calcium-channel blockers

  Ciclosporin: oestrogens possibly increase plasma concentration of ciclosporin

  Clonidine: oestrogens antagonise hypotensive effect of clonidine

  Corticosteroids: oral contraceptives containing oestrogens increase plasma concentration of corticosteroids

  Diazoxide: oestrogens antagonise hypotensive effect of diazoxide

Oestrogens (continued)

Diuretics: oestrogens antagonise diuretic effect of diuretics

Dopaminergics: oestrogens increase plasma concentration of ropinirole; oestrogens increase plasma concentration of selegiline (increased risk of toxicity)

Lipid-regulating Drugs: plasma concentration of ethinylestradiol increased by atorvastatin and rosuvastatin

Methyldopa: oestrogens antagonise hypotensive effect of methyldopa

• Modafinil: metabolism of oestrogens accelerated by ●modafinil (reduced contraceptive effect—see p. 486)

Moxonidine: oestrogens antagonise hypotensive effect of moxonidine

Muscle Relaxants: oestrogens possibly increase plasma concentration of tizanidine (increased risk of toxicity)

Nitrates: oestrogens antagonise hypotensive effect of nitrates

Sitaxentan: plasma concentration of oestrogens increased by sitaxentan

Somatropin: oestrogens (when used as oral replacement therapy) may increase dose requirements of somatropin

Sugammadex: plasma concentration of oestrogens possibly reduced by sugammadex

Tacrolimus: metabolism of oestrogens possibly inhibited by tacrolimus; ethinylestradiol possibly increases plasma concentration of tacrolimus

Theophylline: oestrogens reduce excretion of theophylline (increased plasma concentration)

Thyroid Hormones: oestrogens may increase requirements for thyroid hormones in hypothyroidism

Vasodilator Antihypertensives: oestrogens antagonise hypotensive effect of hydralazine, minoxidil and sodium nitroprusside

Oestrogens, conjugated see Oestrogens

Ofloxacin see Quinolones

Olanzapine see Antipsychotics

Olmesartan see Angiotensin-II Receptor Antagonists

Olsalazine see Aminosalicylates

Omeprazole see Proton Pump Inhibitors

Ondansetron see 5HT$_3$ Antagonists

Opioid Analgesics

Alcohol: enhanced hypotensive and sedative effects when opioid analgesics given with alcohol

Anaesthetics, General: opioid analgesics possibly enhance effects of intravenous general anaesthetics and volatile liquid general anaesthetics

Antibacterials: plasma concentration of alfentanil increased by erythromycin; avoidance of premedication with opioid analgesics advised by manufacturer of ciprofloxacin (reduced plasma concentration of ciprofloxacin) when ciprofloxacin used for surgical prophylaxis; metabolism of alfentanil, codeine, fentanyl, methadone and morphine accelerated by rifampicin (reduced effect); metabolism of oxycodone possibly accelerated by rifampicin

• Anticoagulants: tramadol enhances anticoagulant effect of ●coumarins

• Antidepressants: plasma concentration of methadone possibly increased by fluoxetine, fluvoxamine, paroxetine and sertraline; possible increased serotonergic effects when pethidine or tramadol given with duloxetine; possible increased serotonergic effects when tramadol given with mirtazapine or venlafaxine; possible CNS excitation or depression (hypertension or hypotension) when opioid analgesics given with ●MAOIs—avoid concomitant use and for 2 weeks after stopping MAOIs; CNS excitation or depression (hypertension or hypotension) when pethidine given with ●MAOIs—avoid concomitant use and for 2 weeks after stopping MAOIs; possible CNS excitation or depression (hypertension or hypotension) when opioid anal-

Opioid Analgesics

• Antidepressants (continued)

gesics given with ●moclobemide; possible CNS excitation or depression (hypertension or hypotension) when dextromethorphan or pethidine given with ●moclobemide—avoid concomitant use; increased risk of CNS toxicity when tramadol given with ●SSRIs or ●tricyclics; plasma concentration of methadone possibly reduced by St John's wort; sedative effects possibly increased when opioid analgesics given with tricyclics

• Antiepileptics: plasma concentration of methadone reduced by carbamazepine; dextropropoxyphene enhances effects of ●carbamazepine; effects of tramadol reduced by carbamazepine; morphine increases bioavailability of gabapentin; metabolism of methadone accelerated by phenytoin (reduced effect and risk of withdrawal effects); plasma concentration of methadone possibly reduced by primidone

• Antifungals: metabolism of buprenorphine inhibited by ●ketoconazole (reduce dose of buprenorphine); metabolism of alfentanil inhibited by fluconazole (risk of prolonged or delayed respiratory depression); plasma concentration of fentanyl possibly increased by fluconazole and itraconazole; metabolism of alfentanil possibly inhibited by itraconazole; plasma concentration of alfentanil and methadone increased by ●voriconazole (consider reducing dose of alfentanil and methadone)

• Antihistamines: sedative effects possibly increased when opioid analgesics given with ●sedating antihistamines

• Antipsychotics: enhanced hypotensive and sedative effects when opioid analgesics given with antipsychotics; increased risk of ventricular arrhythmias when methadone given with ●antipsychotics that prolong the QT interval; increased risk of convulsions when tramadol given with antipsychotics; increased risk of ventricular arrhythmias when methadone given with ●amisulpride—avoid concomitant use

• Antivirals: plasma concentration of methadone possibly reduced by abacavir and nevirapine; methadone possibly reduces plasma concentration of didanosine; plasma concentration of methadone reduced by efavirenz, fosamprenavir, nelfinavir and ritonavir; plasma concentration of alfentanil and fentanyl increased by ●ritonavir; plasma concentration of dextropropoxyphene increased by ●ritonavir (risk of toxicity)—avoid concomitant use; plasma concentration of buprenorphine possibly increased by ritonavir; plasma concentration of pethidine reduced by ●ritonavir, but plasma concentration of toxic pethidine metabolite increased (avoid concomitant use); plasma concentration of morphine possibly reduced by ritonavir; buprenorphine possibly reduces plasma concentration of tipranavir; methadone possibly increases plasma concentration of zidovudine

Anxiolytics and Hypnotics: increased sedative effect when opioid analgesics given with anxiolytics and hypnotics

• Atomoxetine: increased risk of ventricular arrhythmias when methadone given with ●atomoxetine; possible increased risk of convulsions when tramadol given with atomoxetine

Barbiturates: CNS effects of opioid analgesics possibly increased by barbiturates; plasma concentration of methadone reduced by phenobarbital

Beta-blockers: morphine possibly increases plasma concentration of esmolol

Calcium-channel Blockers: metabolism of alfentanil inhibited by diltiazem (risk of prolonged or delayed respiratory depression)

Opioid Analgesics *(continued)*

Domperidone: opioid analgesics antagonise effects of domperidone on gastro-intestinal activity

• Dopaminergics: risk of CNS toxicity when pethidine given with ●rasagiline (avoid pethidine for 2 weeks after rasagiline); avoid concomitant use of dextromethorphan with ●rasagiline; caution with tramadol advised by manufacturer of selegiline; hyperpyrexia and CNS toxicity reported when pethidine given with ●selegiline (avoid concomitant use)

5HT₃ Antagonists: effects of tramadol possibly antagonised by ondansetron

• Memantine: increased risk of CNS toxicity when dextromethorphan given with ●memantine (manufacturer of memantine advises avoid concomitant use)

Metoclopramide: opioid analgesics antagonise effects of metoclopramide on gastro-intestinal activity

Muscle Relaxants: increased sedative effect when fentanyl or morphine given with baclofen

• Sodium Oxybate: opioid analgesics enhance effects of ●sodium oxybate (avoid concomitant use)

Ulcer-healing Drugs: metabolism of opioid analgesics inhibited by cimetidine (increased plasma concentration)

Orciprenaline *see* Sympathomimetics

Orlistat

Anti-arrhythmics: orlistat possibly reduces plasma concentration of amiodarone

Anticoagulants: manufacturer of orlistat recommends monitoring anticoagulant effect of coumarins

Antidiabetics: manufacturer of orlistat advises avoid concomitant use with acarbose

• Antiepileptics: possible increased risk of convulsions when orlistat given with ●antiepileptics

• Ciclosporin: orlistat possibly reduces absorption of ●ciclosporin

Thyroid Hormones: possible increased risk of hypothyroidism when orlistat given with levothyroxine

Orphenadrine *see* Antimuscarinics

Oxaliplatin *see* Platinum Compounds

Oxandrolone *see* Anabolic Steroids

Oxazepam *see* Anxiolytics and Hypnotics

Oxcarbazepine

• Antidepressants: anticonvulsant effect of antiepileptics possibly antagonised by MAOIs and ●tricyclic-related antidepressants (convulsive threshold lowered); anticonvulsant effect of antiepileptics antagonised by ●SSRIs and ●tricyclics (convulsive threshold lowered); avoid concomitant use of antiepileptics with ●St John's wort

Antiepileptics: oxcarbazepine sometimes reduces plasma concentration of carbamazepine (but concentration of an active metabolite of carbamazepine may be increased), also plasma concentration of an active metabolite of oxcarbazepine often reduced; avoidance of oxcarbazepine advised by manufacturer of eslicarbazepine; oxcarbazepine increases plasma concentration of phenytoin, also plasma concentration of an active metabolite of oxcarbazepine reduced; plasma concentration of an active metabolite of oxcarbazepine sometimes reduced by valproate

Antimalarials: possible increased risk of convulsions when antiepileptics given with chloroquine and hydroxychloroquine; anticonvulsant effect of antiepileptics antagonised by ●mefloquine

• Antipsychotics: anticonvulsant effect of oxcarbazepine antagonised by ●antipsychotics (convulsive threshold lowered)

Barbiturates: oxcarbazepine increases plasma concentration of phenobarbital, also plasma concentration of an active metabolite of oxcarbazepine reduced

Ciclosporin: oxcarbazepine possibly reduces plasma concentration of ciclosporin

Oxcarbazepine *(continued)*

• Clopidogrel: oxcarbazepine possibly reduces antiplatelet effect of ●clopidogrel

• Cytotoxics: oxcarbazepine reduces plasma concentration of ●imatinib—avoid concomitant use

• Oestrogens: oxcarbazepine accelerates metabolism of ●oestrogens (reduced contraceptive effect—see p. 486)

• Orlistat: possible increased risk of convulsions when antiepileptics given with ●orlistat

• Progestogens: oxcarbazepine accelerates metabolism of ●progestogens (reduced contraceptive effect—see p. 486)

Oxprenolol *see* Beta-blockers

Oxybutynin *see* Antimuscarinics

Oxycodone *see* Opioid Analgesics

Oxymetazoline *see* Sympathomimetics

Oxytetracycline *see* Tetracyclines

Oxytocin

Anaesthetics, General: oxytocic effect possibly reduced, also enhanced hypotensive effect and risk of arrhythmias when oxytocin given with volatile liquid general anaesthetics

Prostaglandins: uterotonic effect of oxytocin potentiated by prostaglandins

Sympathomimetics: risk of hypertension when oxytocin given with vasoconstrictor sympathomimetics (due to enhanced vasopressor effect)

Paclitaxel

Antidiabetics: paclitaxel possibly inhibits metabolism of rosiglitazone

Antiepileptics: cytotoxics possibly reduce absorption of phenytoin

• Antipsychotics: avoid concomitant use of cytotoxics with ●clozapine (increased risk of agranulocytosis)

Antivirals: plasma concentration of paclitaxel increased by nelfinavir and ritonavir

Cardiac Glycosides: cytotoxics reduce absorption of digoxin tablets

Paliperidone *see* Antipsychotics

Pancreatin

Antidiabetics: pancreatin antagonises hypoglycaemic effect of acarbose

Pancuronium *see* Muscle Relaxants

Pantoprazole *see* Proton Pump Inhibitors

Papaveretum *see* Opioid Analgesics

Paracetamol

Anticoagulants: prolonged regular use of paracetamol possibly enhances anticoagulant effect of coumarins

Antiepileptics: metabolism of paracetamol possibly accelerated by carbamazepine

Cytotoxics: paracetamol possibly inhibits metabolism of *intravenous* busulfan (manufacturer of *intravenous* busulfan advises caution within 72 hours of paracetamol)

Lipid-regulating Drugs: absorption of paracetamol reduced by colestyramine

Metoclopramide: rate of absorption of paracetamol increased by metoclopramide

Paraldehyde

• Alcohol: increased sedative effect when paraldehyde given with ●alcohol

• Disulfiram: risk of toxicity when paraldehyde given with ●disulfiram

Parasympathomimetics

Anti-arrhythmics: effects of neostigmine and pyridostigmine possibly antagonised by propafenone

• Antibacterials: plasma concentration of galantamine increased by erythromycin; effects of neostigmine and pyridostigmine antagonised by ●aminoglycosides; effects of neostigmine and pyridostigmine antagonised by clindamycin; effects of neostigmine and pyridostigmine antagonised by ●polymyxins

Antidepressants: plasma concentration of galantamine increased by paroxetine

Parasympathomimetics *(continued)*

Antifungals: plasma concentration of galantamine increased by ketoconazole

Antimalarials: effects of neostigmine and pyridostigmine may be diminished because of potential for chloroquine and hydroxychloroquine to increase symptoms of myasthenia gravis

Antimuscarinics: effects of parasympathomimetics antagonised by antimuscarinics

Beta-blockers: increased risk of arrhythmias when pilocarpine given with beta-blockers; effects of neostigmine and pyridostigmine antagonised by propranolol

Lithium: effects of neostigmine and pyridostigmine antagonised by lithium

Muscle Relaxants: donepezil possibly enhances effects of suxamethonium; edrophonium, galantamine, neostigmine, pyridostigmine and rivastigmine enhance effects of suxamethonium; donepezil possibly antagonises effects of non-depolarising muscle relaxants; edrophonium, neostigmine, pyridostigmine and rivastigmine antagonise effects of non-depolarising muscle relaxants

Parecoxib *see* NSAIDs

Paricalcitol *see* Vitamins

Paroxetine *see* Antidepressants, SSRI

Pegfilgrastim *see* Filgrastim

Peginterferon Alfa *see* Interferons

Pemetrexed

Antiepileptics: cytotoxics possibly reduce absorption of phenytoin

● Antimalarials: antifolate effect of pemetrexed increased by ●pyrimethamine

● Antipsychotics: avoid concomitant use of cytotoxics with ●clozapine (increased risk of agranulocytosis)

Cardiac Glycosides: cytotoxics reduce absorption of digoxin tablets

Penicillamine

Analgesics: possible increased risk of nephrotoxicity when penicillamine given with NSAIDs

Antacids: absorption of penicillamine reduced by antacids

● Antipsychotics: avoid concomitant use of penicillamine with ●clozapine (increased risk of agranulocytosis)

Cardiac Glycosides: penicillamine possibly reduces plasma concentration of digoxin

Gold: manufacturer of penicillamine advises avoid concomitant use with gold (increased risk of toxicity)

Iron: absorption of penicillamine reduced by *oral* iron

Zinc: penicillamine reduces absorption of zinc, also absorption of penicillamine reduced by zinc

Penicillins

Allopurinol: increased risk of rash when amoxicillin or ampicillin given with allopurinol

Antibacterials: absorption of phenoxymethylpenicillin reduced by neomycin; effects of penicillins possibly antagonised by tetracyclines

Anticoagulants: common experience in anticoagulant clinics is that INR can be altered by a course of broad-spectrum penicillins such as ampicillin, although studies have failed to demonstrate an interaction with coumarins or phenindione

Cytotoxics: penicillins reduce excretion of methotrexate (increased risk of toxicity)

Muscle Relaxants: piperacillin enhances effects of non-depolarising muscle relaxants and suxamethonium

Oestrogens: antibacterials that do not induce liver enzymes possibly reduce contraceptive effect of oestrogens (risk probably small, see p. 486)

Probenecid: excretion of penicillins reduced by probenecid (increased plasma concentration)

Sulfinpyrazone: excretion of penicillins reduced by sulfinpyrazone

Penicillins *(continued)*

Vaccines: antibacterials inactivate oral typhoid vaccine–see p. 760

Pentamidine Isetionate

● Anti-arrhythmics: increased risk of ventricular arrhythmias when pentamidine isetionate given with ●amiodarone—avoid concomitant use

● Antibacterials: increased risk of ventricular arrhythmias when pentamidine isetionate given with *parenteral* ●erythromycin; increased risk of ventricular arrhythmias when pentamidine isetionate given with ●moxifloxacin—avoid concomitant use

● Antidepressants: increased risk of ventricular arrhythmias when pentamidine isetionate given with ●tricyclics

Antifungals: possible increased risk of nephrotoxicity when pentamidine isetionate given with amphotericin

● Antipsychotics: increased risk of ventricular arrhythmias when pentamidine isetionate given with ●amisulpride or ●droperidol—avoid concomitant use; increased risk of ventricular arrhythmias when pentamidine isetionate given with ●phenothiazines

● Antivirals: increased risk of hypocalcaemia when *parenteral* pentamidine isetionate given with ●foscarnet

● Ivabradine: increased risk of ventricular arrhythmias when pentamidine isetionate given with ●ivabradine

Pentazocine *see* Opioid Analgesics

Pentostatin

Antiepileptics: cytotoxics possibly reduce absorption of phenytoin

● Antipsychotics: avoid concomitant use of cytotoxics with ●clozapine (increased risk of agranulocytosis)

Cardiac Glycosides: cytotoxics reduce absorption of digoxin tablets

● Cytotoxics: increased toxicity when pentostatin given with high-dose ●cyclophosphamide—avoid concomitant use; increased pulmonary toxicity when pentostatin given with ●fludarabine (unacceptably high incidence of fatalities)

Pentoxifylline

● Analgesics: possible increased risk of bleeding when pentoxifylline given with NSAIDs; increased risk of bleeding when pentoxifylline given with ●ketorolac (avoid concomitant use)

Theophylline: pentoxifylline increases plasma concentration of theophylline

Pergolide

Antipsychotics: effects of pergolide antagonised by antipsychotics

Memantine: effects of dopaminergics possibly enhanced by memantine

Methyldopa: antiparkinsonian effect of dopaminergics antagonised by methyldopa

Metoclopramide: antiparkinsonian effect of pergolide antagonised by metoclopramide

Pericyazine *see* Antipsychotics

Perindopril *see* ACE Inhibitors

Perphenazine *see* Antipsychotics

Pethidine *see* Opioid Analgesics

Phenazocine *see* Opioid Analgesics

Phenelzine *see* MAOIs

Phenindione

Note. Change in patient's clinical condition particularly associated with liver disease, intercurrent illness, or drug administration, necessitates more frequent testing. Major changes in diet (especially involving salads and vegetables) and in alcohol consumption may also affect anticoagulant control

● Alcohol: anticoagulant control with phenindione may be affected by major changes in consumption of ●alcohol

● Anabolic Steroids: anticoagulant effect of phenindione enhanced by ●anabolic steroids

Phenindione *(continued)*
- Analgesics: anticoagulant effect of phenindione possibly enhanced by ●NSAIDs; increased risk of haemorrhage when anticoagulants given with *intravenous* ●diclofenac (avoid concomitant use, including low-dose heparins); increased risk of haemorrhage when anticoagulants given with ●ketorolac (avoid concomitant use, including low-dose heparins); increased risk of bleeding when phenindione given with ●aspirin (due to antiplatelet effect)
- Anti-arrhythmics: metabolism of phenindione inhibited by ●amiodarone (enhanced anticoagulant effect)
- Antibacterials: experience in anticoagulant clinics suggests that INR possibly altered when phenindione is given with ●neomycin (given for local action on gut); anticoagulant effect of phenindione possibly enhanced by levofloxacin and ●tetracyclines; studies have failed to demonstrate an interaction with phenindione, but common experience in anticoagulant clinics is that INR can be altered by a course of broad-spectrum penicillins such as ampicillin
- Antivirals: anticoagulant effect of phenindione possibly enhanced by ●ritonavir
- Clopidogrel: anticoagulant effect of phenindione enhanced due to antiplatelet action of ●clopidogrel
- Dipyridamole: anticoagulant effect of phenindione enhanced due to antiplatelet action of ●dipyridamole
- Enteral Foods: anticoagulant effect of phenindione antagonised by vitamin K (present in some ●enteral feeds)
  Iloprost: increased risk of bleeding when phenindione given with iloprost
- Lipid-regulating Drugs: anticoagulant effect of phenindione may be enhanced or reduced by ●colestyramine; anticoagulant effect of phenindione possibly enhanced by ●rosuvastatin; anticoagulant effect of phenindione enhanced by ●fibrates
- Oestrogens: anticoagulant effect of phenindione antagonised by ●oestrogens
  Prasugrel: possible increased risk of bleeding when phenindione given with prasugrel
- Progestogens: anticoagulant effect of phenindione antagonised by ●progestogens
  Sibutramine: increased risk of bleeding when anticoagulants given with sibutramine
- Testolactone: anticoagulant effect of phenindione enhanced by ●testolactone
- Testosterone: anticoagulant effect of phenindione enhanced by ●testosterone
- Thyroid Hormones: anticoagulant effect of phenindione enhanced by ●thyroid hormones
- Vitamins: anticoagulant effect of phenindione antagonised by ●vitamin K

Phenobarbital *see* Barbiturates
Phenothiazines *see* Antipsychotics
Phenoxybenzamine *see* Alpha-blockers
Phenoxymethylpenicillin *see* Penicillins
Phentolamine *see* Alpha-blockers
Phenylephrine *see* Sympathomimetics
Phenytoin
  Note. Fosphenytoin interactions as for phenytoin
- Analgesics: effects of phenytoin possibly enhanced by ●NSAIDs; plasma concentration of phenytoin significantly increased by ●azapropazone—avoid concomitant use; phenytoin accelerates metabolism of methadone (reduced effect and risk of withdrawal effects); effects of phenytoin enhanced by aspirin
  Antacids: absorption of phenytoin reduced by antacids
- Anti-arrhythmics: metabolism of phenytoin inhibited by ●amiodarone (increased plasma concentration); phenytoin reduces plasma concentration of disopyramide
- Antibacterials: metabolism of phenytoin inhibited by clarithromycin, ●isoniazid and ●metronidazole (increased plasma concentration); plasma concentration of phenytoin increased or decreased by ciprofloxacin; phenytoin accelerates metabolism of

Phenytoin
- Antibacterials *(continued)*
  doxycycline (reduced plasma concentration); plasma concentration of phenytoin increased by ●chloramphenicol (increased risk of toxicity); metabolism of phenytoin accelerated by ●rifamycins (reduced plasma concentration); plasma concentration of phenytoin possibly increased by sulphonamides; phenytoin reduces plasma concentration of ●telithromycin (avoid during and for 2 weeks after phenytoin); plasma concentration of phenytoin increased by ●trimethoprim (also increased antifolate effect)
- Anticoagulants: phenytoin accelerates metabolism of ●coumarins (possibility of reduced anticoagulant effect, but enhancement also reported)
- Antidepressants: plasma concentration of phenytoin increased by ●fluoxetine and ●fluvoxamine; phenytoin reduces plasma concentration of ●mianserin, mirtazapine and paroxetine; anticonvulsant effect of antiepileptics possibly antagonised by MAOIs and ●tricyclic-related antidepressants (convulsive threshold lowered); anticonvulsant effect of antiepileptics antagonised by ●SSRIs and ●tricyclics (convulsive threshold lowered); avoid concomitant use of antiepileptics with ●St John's wort; phenytoin possibly reduces plasma concentration of ●tricyclics
  Antidiabetics: plasma concentration of phenytoin transiently increased by tolbutamide (possibility of toxicity)
- Antiepileptics: plasma concentration of both drugs often reduced when phenytoin given with carbamazepine, also plasma concentration of phenytoin may be increased; phenytoin reduces plasma concentration of eslicarbazepine, also plasma concentration of phenytoin increased; plasma concentration of phenytoin possibly increased by ●ethosuximide, also plasma concentration of ethosuximide possibly reduced; phenytoin reduces plasma concentration of lamotrigine, tiagabine and zonisamide; plasma concentration of phenytoin increased by oxcarbazepine, also plasma concentration of an active metabolite of oxcarbazepine reduced; phenytoin possibly reduces plasma concentration of primidone (but concentration of an active metabolite increased), plasma concentration of phenytoin often reduced but may be increased; plasma concentration of phenytoin possibly increased by rufinamide; plasma concentration of phenytoin increased by ●stiripentol; plasma concentration of phenytoin increased by ●topiramate (also plasma concentration of topiramate reduced); plasma concentration of phenytoin increased or possibly reduced when given with valproate, also plasma concentration of valproate reduced; plasma concentration of phenytoin reduced by vigabatrin
- Antifungals: phenytoin reduces plasma concentration of ●ketoconazole and ●posaconazole; anticonvulsant effect of phenytoin enhanced by ●miconazole (plasma concentration of phenytoin increased); plasma concentration of phenytoin increased by ●fluconazole (consider reducing dose of phenytoin); phenytoin reduces plasma concentration of ●itraconazole—avoid concomitant use; plasma concentration of phenytoin increased by ●voriconazole, also phenytoin reduces plasma concentration of voriconazole (increase dose of voriconazole and also monitor for phenytoin toxicity); phenytoin possibly reduces plasma concentration of caspofungin—consider increasing dose of caspofungin
- Antimalarials: possible increased risk of convulsions when antiepileptics given with chloroquine and hydroxychloroquine; anticonvulsant effect of antiepileptics antagonised by ●mefloquine; anticonvulsant effect of phenytoin antagonised by ●pyrimethamine, also increased antifolate effect

Phenytoin *(continued)*

- Antipsychotics: anticonvulsant effect of phenytoin antagonised by ●antipsychotics (convulsive threshold lowered); phenytoin possibly reduces plasma concentration of ●aripiprazole—increase dose of aripiprazole; phenytoin accelerates metabolism of clozapine, quetiapine and sertindole (reduced plasma concentration)

- Antivirals: phenytoin possibly reduces plasma concentration of abacavir, darunavir, fosamprenavir, lopinavir and saquinavir; avoidance of phenytoin advised by manufacturer of etravirine; phenytoin possibly reduces plasma concentration of ●indinavir, also plasma concentration of phenytoin possibly increased; plasma concentration of phenytoin reduced by nelfinavir; phenytoin possibly reduces plasma concentration of ritonavir, also plasma concentration of phenytoin possibly affected; plasma concentration of phenytoin increased or decreased by zidovudine

  Anxiolytics and Hypnotics: phenytoin often reduces plasma concentration of clonazepam; plasma concentration of phenytoin increased or decreased by diazepam; plasma concentration of phenytoin possibly increased or decreased by benzodiazepines

  Aprepitant: phenytoin possibly reduces plasma concentration of aprepitant

  Barbiturates: phenytoin often increases plasma concentration of phenobarbital, plasma concentration of phenytoin often reduced but may be increased

  Bupropion: phenytoin reduces plasma concentration of bupropion

- Calcium-channel Blockers: phenytoin reduces effects of felodipine, isradipine and verapamil; phenytoin probably reduces effects of dihydropyridines, nicardipine and ●nifedipine; plasma concentration of phenytoin increased by ●diltiazem but also effect of diltiazem reduced

  Cardiac Glycosides: phenytoin accelerates metabolism of digitoxin (reduced effect); phenytoin possibly reduces plasma concentration of digoxin

- Ciclosporin: phenytoin accelerates metabolism of ●ciclosporin (reduced plasma concentration)

- Corticosteroids: phenytoin accelerates metabolism of ●corticosteroids (reduced effect)

- Cytotoxics: phenytoin possibly reduces plasma concentration of busulfan and etoposide; metabolism of phenytoin possibly inhibited by fluorouracil (increased risk of toxicity); phenytoin increases antifolate effect of methotrexate; absorption of phenytoin possibly reduced by cytotoxics; avoidance of phenytoin advised by manufacturer of gefitinib and ●lapatinib; phenytoin reduces plasma concentration of ●imatinib—avoid concomitant use; phenytoin reduces plasma concentration of irinotecan and its active metabolite

  Diazoxide: plasma concentration of phenytoin reduced by diazoxide, also effect of diazoxide may be reduced

- Disulfiram: metabolism of phenytoin inhibited by ●disulfiram (increased risk of toxicity)

- Diuretics: phenytoin antagonises effects of furosemide; phenytoin reduces plasma concentration of ●eplerenone—avoid concomitant use; increased risk of osteomalacia when phenytoin given with carbonic anhydrase inhibitors

  Dopaminergics: phenytoin possibly reduces effects of levodopa

  Enteral Foods: absorption of phenytoin possibly reduced by enteral feeds

  Folates: plasma concentration of phenytoin possibly reduced by folates

  Hormone Antagonists: phenytoin possibly accelerates metabolism of toremifene

  5HT$_3$ Antagonists: phenytoin accelerates metabolism of ondansetron (reduced effect)

Phenytoin *(continued)*

  Leflunomide: plasma concentration of phenytoin possibly increased by leflunomide

  Levamisole: plasma concentration of phenytoin possibly increased by levamisole

  Lipid-regulating Drugs: combination of phenytoin with fluvastatin may increase plasma concentration of either drug (or both)

  Lithium: neurotoxicity may occur when phenytoin given with lithium without increased plasma concentration of lithium

  Modafinil: plasma concentration of phenytoin possibly increased by modafinil

  Muscle Relaxants: phenytoin antagonises muscle relaxant effect of non-depolarising muscle relaxants (accelerated recovery from neuromuscular blockade)

- Oestrogens: phenytoin accelerates metabolism of ●oestrogens (reduced contraceptive effect—see p. 486)

- Orlistat: possible increased risk of convulsions when antiepileptics given with ●orlistat

- Progestogens: phenytoin accelerates metabolism of ●progestogens (reduced contraceptive effect—see p. 486)

- Sulfinpyrazone: plasma concentration of phenytoin increased by ●sulfinpyrazone

  Sympathomimetics: plasma concentration of phenytoin increased by methylphenidate

  Tacrolimus: phenytoin reduces plasma concentration of tacrolimus, also plasma concentration of phenytoin possibly increased

- Theophylline: plasma concentration of both drugs reduced when phenytoin given with ●theophylline

  Thyroid Hormones: phenytoin accelerates metabolism of thyroid hormones (may increase requirements in hypothyroidism), also plasma concentration of phenytoin possibly increased

  Tibolone: phenytoin accelerates metabolism of tibolone

- Ulcer-healing Drugs: metabolism of phenytoin inhibited by ●cimetidine (increased plasma concentration); effects of phenytoin enhanced by ●esomeprazole; effects of phenytoin possibly enhanced by omeprazole; absorption of phenytoin reduced by ●sucralfate

- Ulipristal: avoidance of phenytoin advised by manufacturer of ●ulipristal (contraceptive effect of ulipristal possibly reduced)

  Vaccines: effects of phenytoin enhanced by influenza vaccine

  Vitamins: phenytoin possibly increases requirements for vitamin D

Phosphodiesterase Inhibitors

- Anagrelide: avoidance of enoximone and milrinone advised by manufacturer of ●anagrelide

Physostigmine *see* Parasympathomimetics

Pilocarpine *see* Parasympathomimetics

Pimozide *see* Antipsychotics

Pindolol *see* Beta-blockers

Pioglitazone *see* Antidiabetics

Piperacillin *see* Penicillins

Pipotiazine *see* Antipsychotics

Piroxicam *see* NSAIDs

Pivmecillinam *see* Penicillins

Pizotifen

  Adrenergic Neurone Blockers: pizotifen antagonises hypotensive effect of adrenergic neurone blockers

Platinum Compounds

- Aldesleukin: avoidance of cisplatin advised by manufacturer of ●aldesleukin

- Antibacterials: increased risk of nephrotoxicity and possibly of ototoxicity when platinum compounds given with ●aminoglycosides or ●polymyxins; increased risk of nephrotoxicity and ototoxicity when platinum compounds given with capreomycin;

Platinum Compounds

- Antibacterials *(continued)*
  increased risk of nephrotoxicity and possibly of ototoxicity when cisplatin given with vancomycin

  Antiepileptics: cytotoxics possibly reduce absorption of phenytoin
- Antipsychotics: avoid concomitant use of cytotoxics with •clozapine (increased risk of agranulocytosis)

  Cardiac Glycosides: cytotoxics reduce absorption of digoxin tablets
- Cytotoxics: increased pulmonary toxicity when cisplatin given with •bleomycin and •methotrexate

  Diuretics: increased risk of nephrotoxicity and ototoxicity when platinum compounds given with diuretics

Polymyxin B *see* Polymyxins

Polymyxins

  Antibacterials: increased risk of nephrotoxicity when colistin or polymyxins given with aminoglycosides; increased risk of nephrotoxicity when colistin or polymyxins given with capreomycin; increased risk of nephrotoxicity and ototoxicity when colistin given with teicoplanin or vancomycin; increased risk of nephrotoxicity when polymyxins given with vancomycin

  Antifungals: increased risk of nephrotoxicity when polymyxins given with amphotericin
- Ciclosporin: increased risk of nephrotoxicity when polymyxins given with •ciclosporin
- Cytotoxics: increased risk of nephrotoxicity and possibly of ototoxicity when polymyxins given with •platinum compounds
- Diuretics: increased risk of ototoxicity when polymyxins given with •loop diuretics
- Muscle Relaxants: polymyxins enhance effects of •non-depolarising muscle relaxants and •suxamethonium

  Oestrogens: antibacterials that do not induce liver enzymes possibly reduce contraceptive effect of oestrogens (risk probably small, see p. 486)
- Parasympathomimetics: polymyxins antagonise effects of •neostigmine and •pyridostigmine

  Vaccines: antibacterials inactivate oral typhoid vaccine—see p. 760

Polystyrene Sulphonate Resins

  Thyroid Hormones: polystyrene sulphonate resins reduce absorption of levothyroxine

Posaconazole *see* Antifungals, Triazole

Potassium Canrenoate *see* Diuretics

Potassium Aminobenzoate

  Antibacterials: potassium aminobenzoate inhibits effects of sulphonamides

Potassium Bicarbonate *see* Potassium Salts

Potassium Chloride *see* Potassium Salts

Potassium Citrate *see* Potassium Salts

Potassium Salts

  Note. Includes salt substitutes
- ACE Inhibitors: increased risk of severe hyperkalaemia when potassium salts given with •ACE inhibitors

  Aliskiren: increased risk of hyperkalaemia when potassium salts given with aliskiren
- Angiotensin-II Receptor Antagonists: increased risk of hyperkalaemia when potassium salts given with •angiotensin-II receptor antagonists

  Antibacterials: avoid concomitant use of potassium citrate with methenamine
- Ciclosporin: increased risk of hyperkalaemia when potassium salts given with •ciclosporin
- Diuretics: increased risk of hyperkalaemia when potassium salts given with •potassium-sparing diuretics and aldosterone antagonists
- Tacrolimus: increased risk of hyperkalaemia when potassium salts given with •tacrolimus

Pramipexole

  Antipsychotics: manufacturer of pramipexole advises avoid concomitant use of antipsychotics (antagonism of effect)

  Memantine: effects of dopaminergics possibly enhanced by memantine

  Methyldopa: antiparkinsonian effect of dopaminergics antagonised by methyldopa

  Ulcer-healing Drugs: excretion of pramipexole reduced by cimetidine (increased plasma concentration)

Prasugrel

  Analgesics: possible increased risk of bleeding when prasugrel given with NSAIDs

  Anticoagulants: possible increased risk of bleeding when prasugrel given with coumarins or phenindione

  Clopidogrel: possible increased risk of bleeding when prasugrel given with clopidogrel

Pravastatin *see* Statins

Prazosin *see* Alpha-blockers

Prednisolone *see* Corticosteroids

Prilocaine

  Anti-arrhythmics: increased myocardial depression when prilocaine given with anti-arrhythmics

  Antibacterials: increased risk of methaemoglobinaemia when prilocaine given with sulphonamides

Primaquine

- Antimalarials: avoidance of antimalarials advised by manufacturer of •artemether/lumefantrine

  Mepacrine: plasma concentration of primaquine increased by mepacrine (increased risk of toxicity)

  Vaccines: antimalarials inactivate oral typhoid vaccine—see p. 760

Primidone

  Alcohol: increased sedative effect when primidone given with alcohol

  Analgesics: primidone possibly reduces plasma concentration of methadone

  Anti-arrhythmics: primidone accelerates metabolism of disopyramide (reduced plasma concentration)
- Antibacterials: primidone accelerates metabolism of •chloramphenicol, doxycycline and metronidazole (reduced plasma concentration); primidone reduces plasma concentration of •telithromycin (avoid during and for 2 weeks after primidone)
- Anticoagulants: primidone accelerates metabolism of •coumarins (reduced anticoagulant effect)
- Antidepressants: primidone reduces plasma concentration of paroxetine; primidone accelerates metabolism of •mianserin (reduced plasma concentration); anticonvulsant effect of antiepileptics possibly antagonised by MAOIs and •tricyclic-related antidepressants (convulsive threshold lowered); anticonvulsant effect of antiepileptics antagonised by •SSRIs and •tricyclics (convulsive threshold lowered); avoid concomitant use of antiepileptics with •St John's wort; anticonvulsant effect of primidone antagonised by •tricyclics (convulsive threshold lowered), also metabolism of tricyclics possibly accelerated (reduced plasma concentration)
- Antiepileptics: primidone often reduces plasma concentration of carbamazepine, also plasma concentration of primidone sometimes reduced (but concentration of an active metabolite of primidone often increased); primidone possibly reduces plasma concentration of ethosuximide; primidone reduces plasma concentration of lamotrigine and tiagabine; plasma concentration of primidone possibly reduced by phenytoin (but concentration of an active metabolite increased), plasma concentration of phenytoin often reduced but may be increased; plasma concentration of primidone possibly increased by •valproate (plasma concentration of active metabolite of primidone increased), also plasma concentration of valproate reduced; plasma

Primidone

- Antiepileptics *(continued)*
  concentration of primidone possibly reduced by vigabatrin
- Antifungals: primidone possibly reduces plasma concentration of ●posaconazole; primidone possibly reduces plasma concentration of ●voriconazole—avoid concomitant use; primidone reduces absorption of griseofulvin (reduced effect)
- Antimalarials: possible increased risk of convulsions when antiepileptics given with chloroquine and hydroxychloroquine; anticonvulsant effect of antiepileptics antagonised by ●mefloquine
- Antipsychotics: anticonvulsant effect of primidone antagonised by ●antipsychotics (convulsive threshold lowered); primidone accelerates metabolism of haloperidol (reduced plasma concentration); primidone possibly reduces plasma concentration of ●aripiprazole—increase dose of aripiprazole
- Antivirals: primidone possibly reduces plasma concentration of ●indinavir, ●lopinavir, ●nelfinavir and ●saquinavir
  Anxiolytics and Hypnotics: primidone often reduces plasma concentration of clonazepam
  Barbiturates: increased sedative effect when primidone given with barbiturates
- Calcium-channel Blockers: primidone reduces effects of ●felodipine and ●isradipine; primidone probably reduces effects of ●dihydropyridines, ●diltiazem and ●verapamil
  Cardiac Glycosides: primidone accelerates metabolism of digitoxin (reduced effect)
- Ciclosporin: primidone accelerates metabolism of ●ciclosporin (reduced effect)
- Corticosteroids: primidone accelerates metabolism of ●corticosteroids (reduced effect)
  Diuretics: plasma concentration of primidone possibly reduced by acetazolamide; increased risk of osteomalacia when primidone given with carbonic anhydrase inhibitors
  Folates: plasma concentration of primidone possibly reduced by folates
  Hormone Antagonists: primidone accelerates metabolism of toremifene (reduced plasma concentration)
  Leukotriene Receptor Antagonists: primidone reduces plasma concentration of montelukast
  Memantine: effects of primidone possibly reduced by memantine
- Oestrogens: primidone accelerates metabolism of ●oestrogens (reduced contraceptive effect—see p. 486)
- Orlistat: possible increased risk of convulsions when antiepileptics given with ●orlistat
- Progestogens: primidone accelerates metabolism of ●progestogens (reduced contraceptive effect—see p. 486)
  Sympathomimetics: plasma concentration of primidone possibly increased by methylphenidate
  Theophylline: primidone accelerates metabolism of theophylline (reduced effect)
  Thyroid Hormones: primidone accelerates metabolism of thyroid hormones (may increase requirements for thyroid hormones in hypothyroidism)
  Tibolone: primidone accelerates metabolism of tibolone (reduced plasma concentration)
  Vitamins: primidone possibly increases requirements for vitamin D

Probenecid

  ACE Inhibitors: probenecid reduces excretion of captopril
  Anaesthetics, General: probenecid possibly enhances effects of thiopental
- Analgesics: probenecid reduces excretion of ●dexketoprofen, ●indometacin, ●ketoprofen and ●naproxen (increased plasma concentration); probenecid reduces excretion of ●ketorolac (increased

Probenecid

- Analgesics *(continued)*
  plasma concentration)—avoid concomitant use; effects of probenecid antagonised by aspirin
  Antibacterials: probenecid reduces excretion of doripenem and meropenem (manufacturers of doripenem and meropenem advise avoid concomitant use); probenecid reduces excretion of cephalosporins, ciprofloxacin, nalidixic acid, norfloxacin and penicillins (increased plasma concentration); probenecid reduces excretion of dapsone and nitrofurantoin (increased risk of side-effects); effects of probenecid antagonised by pyrazinamide
- Antivirals: probenecid reduces excretion of aciclovir (increased plasma concentration); probenecid possibly reduces excretion of famciclovir (increased plasma concentration); probenecid reduces excretion of ganciclovir and ●zidovudine (increased plasma concentration and risk of toxicity)
  Anxiolytics and Hypnotics: probenecid reduces excretion of lorazepam (increased plasma concentration); probenecid possibly reduces excretion of nitrazepam (increased plasma concentration)
- Cytotoxics: probenecid reduces excretion of ●methotrexate (increased risk of toxicity)
  Sodium Benzoate: probenecid possibly reduces excretion of conjugate formed by sodium benzoate
  Sodium Phenylbutyrate: probenecid possibly reduces excretion of conjugate formed by sodium phenylbutyrate

Procarbazine

  Alcohol: disulfiram-like reaction when procarbazine given with alcohol
  Antiepileptics: cytotoxics possibly reduce absorption of phenytoin
- Antipsychotics: avoid concomitant use of cytotoxics with ●clozapine (increased risk of agranulocytosis)
  Cardiac Glycosides: cytotoxics reduce absorption of digoxin tablets

Prochlorperazine *see* Antipsychotics

Procyclidine *see* Antimuscarinics

Progesterone *see* Progestogens

Progestogens

  Note. Interactions of combined oral contraceptives may also apply to combined contraceptive patches and vaginal rings
- Antibacterials: metabolism of progestogens accelerated by ●rifamycins (reduced contraceptive effect—see p. 486)
- Anticoagulants: progestogens may enhance or reduce anticoagulant effect of ●coumarins; progestogens antagonise anticoagulant effect of ●phenindione
- Antidepressants: contraceptive effect of progestogens reduced by ●St John's wort (avoid concomitant use)
  Antidiabetics: progestogens antagonise hypoglycaemic effect of antidiabetics
- Antiepileptics: metabolism of progestogens accelerated by ●carbamazepine, ●eslicarbazepine, ●oxcarbazepine, ●phenytoin, ●primidone, ●rufinamide and ●topiramate (reduced contraceptive effect—see p. 486); progestogens possibly reduce plasma concentration of ●lamotrigine—consider increasing dose of lamotrigine
- Antifungals: metabolism of progestogens accelerated by ●griseofulvin (reduced contraceptive effect—see p. 486); occasional reports of breakthrough bleeding when progestogens (used for contraception) given with terbinafine
- Antivirals: contraceptive effect of progestogens possibly reduced by ●efavirenz and nelfinavir; plasma concentration of progestogens increased by fosamprenavir, also plasma concentration of fosamprenavir reduced—alternative contraception recommended; metabolism of progestogens accelerated by ●nevirapine (reduced contraceptive effect—see p. 486)

Progestogens *(continued)*

- Aprepitant: possible contraceptive failure of hormonal contraceptives containing progestogens when given with ●aprepitant (alternative contraception recommended)
- Barbiturates: metabolism of progestogens accelerated by ●barbiturates (reduced contraceptive effect—see p. 486)
- Bosentan: possible contraceptive failure of hormonal contraceptives containing progestogens when given with ●bosentan (alternative contraception recommended)
- Ciclosporin: progestogens inhibit metabolism of ●ciclosporin (increased plasma concentration)

  Diuretics: risk of hyperkalaemia when drospirenone given with potassium-sparing diuretics and aldosterone antagonists (monitor serum potassium during first cycle)

  Dopaminergics: progestogens increase plasma concentration of selegiline (increased risk of toxicity)

  Lipid-regulating Drugs: plasma concentration of norethisterone increased by atorvastatin; plasma concentration of norgestrel increased by rosuvastatin

  Muscle Relaxants: progestogens possibly increase plasma concentration of tizanidine (increased risk of toxicity)

  Sitaxentan: plasma concentration of progestogens increased by sitaxentan

  Sugammadex: plasma concentration of progestogens possibly reduced by sugammadex

  Tacrolimus: metabolism of progestogens possibly inhibited by tacrolimus
- Ulipristal: contraceptive effect of progestogens possibly reduced by ●ulipristal

Proguanil

  Antacids: absorption of proguanil reduced by oral magnesium salts (as magnesium trisilicate)

  Anticoagulants: isolated reports that proguanil may enhance anticoagulant effect of warfarin
- Antimalarials: avoidance of antimalarials advised by manufacturer of ●artemether/lumefantrine; increased antifolate effect when proguanil given with pyrimethamine

  Vaccines: antimalarials inactivate oral typhoid vaccine–see p. 760

Promazine *see* Antipsychotics

Promethazine *see* Antihistamines

Propafenone

  Anaesthetics, Local: increased myocardial depression when anti-arrhythmics given with bupivacaine, levobupivacaine, prilocaine or ropivacaine
- Anti-arrhythmics: increased myocardial depression when anti-arrhythmics given with other ●anti-arrhythmics
- Antibacterials: metabolism of propafenone accelerated by ●rifampicin (reduced effect)
- Anticoagulants: propafenone enhances anticoagulant effect of ●coumarins
- Antidepressants: metabolism of propafenone possibly inhibited by paroxetine (increased risk of toxicity); increased risk of arrhythmias when propafenone given with ●tricyclics
- Antihistamines: increased risk of ventricular arrhythmias when propafenone given with ●mizolastine—avoid concomitant use
- Antipsychotics: increased risk of ventricular arrhythmias when anti-arrhythmics that prolong the QT interval given with ●antipsychotics that prolong the QT interval
- Antivirals: plasma concentration of propafenone possibly increased by ●fosamprenavir (increased risk of ventricular arrhythmias—avoid concomitant use); plasma concentration of propafenone increased by ●ritonavir (increased risk of ventricular arrhythmias—avoid concomitant use)

Propafenone *(continued)*

- Beta-blockers: increased myocardial depression when anti-arrhythmics given with ●beta-blockers; propafenone increases plasma concentration of metoprolol and propranolol
- Cardiac Glycosides: propafenone increases plasma concentration of ●digoxin (halve dose of digoxin)

  Ciclosporin: propafenone possibly increases plasma concentration of ciclosporin

  Parasympathomimetics: propafenone possibly antagonises effects of neostigmine and pyridostigmine

  Theophylline: propafenone increases plasma concentration of theophylline
- Ulcer-healing Drugs: plasma concentration of propafenone increased by ●cimetidine

Propantheline *see* Antimuscarinics

Propiverine *see* Antimuscarinics

Propofol *see* Anaesthetics, General

Propranolol *see* Beta-blockers

Prostaglandins

  ACE Inhibitors: enhanced hypotensive effect when alprostadil given with ACE inhibitors

  Adrenergic Neurone Blockers: enhanced hypotensive effect when alprostadil given with adrenergic neurone blockers

  Alpha-blockers: enhanced hypotensive effect when alprostadil given with alpha-blockers

  Angiotensin-II Receptor Antagonists: enhanced hypotensive effect when alprostadil given with angiotensin-II receptor antagonists

  Beta-blockers: enhanced hypotensive effect when alprostadil given with beta-blockers

  Calcium-channel Blockers: enhanced hypotensive effect when alprostadil given with calcium-channel blockers

  Clonidine: enhanced hypotensive effect when alprostadil given with clonidine

  Diazoxide: enhanced hypotensive effect when alprostadil given with diazoxide

  Diuretics: enhanced hypotensive effect when alprostadil given with diuretics

  Methyldopa: enhanced hypotensive effect when alprostadil given with methyldopa

  Moxonidine: enhanced hypotensive effect when alprostadil given with moxonidine

  Nitrates: enhanced hypotensive effect when alprostadil given with nitrates

  Oxytocin: prostaglandins potentiate uterotonic effect of oxytocin

  Vasodilator Antihypertensives: enhanced hypotensive effect when alprostadil given with hydralazine, minoxidil or sodium nitroprusside

Protein Kinase Inhibitors *see* Dasatinib, Erlotinib, Everolimus, Gefitinib, Imatinib, Lapatinib, Nilotinib, Sorafenib, Sunitinib, and Temsirolimus

Proton Pump Inhibitors

  Antacids: absorption of lansoprazole possibly reduced by antacids

  Antibacterials: plasma concentration of both drugs increased when omeprazole given with clarithromycin
- Anticoagulants: esomeprazole, omeprazole and pantoprazole possibly enhance anticoagulant effect of ●coumarins

  Antidepressants: omeprazole increases plasma concentration of escitalopram; plasma concentration of lansoprazole possibly increased by fluvoxamine; plasma concentration of omeprazole possibly reduced by St John's wort
- Antiepileptics: omeprazole possibly enhances effects of phenytoin; esomeprazole enhances effects of ●phenytoin

  Antifungals: proton pump inhibitors reduce absorption of itraconazole and ketoconazole; plasma concentration of esomeprazole possibly increased by voriconazole; plasma concentration of omeprazole

Proton Pump Inhibitors

Antifungals *(continued)*
increased by voriconazole (consider reducing dose of omeprazole)

Antipsychotics: omeprazole possibly reduces plasma concentration of clozapine

- Antivirals: proton pump inhibitors reduce plasma concentration of ●atazanavir; omeprazole reduces plasma concentration of ●nelfinavir—avoid concomitant use; omeprazole increases plasma concentration of ●raltegravir—avoid concomitant use; proton pump inhibitors possibly increase plasma concentration of raltegravir—manufacturer of raltegravir advises avoid concomitant use; omeprazole increases plasma concentration of saquinavir; plasma concentration of esomeprazole and omeprazole reduced by ●tipranavir

Anxiolytics and Hypnotics: esomeprazole and omeprazole possibly inhibit metabolism of diazepam (increased plasma concentration)

Cardiac Glycosides: proton pump inhibitors possibly slightly increase plasma concentration of digoxin

Ciclosporin: omeprazole possibly affects plasma concentration of ciclosporin

- Cilostazol: omeprazole increases plasma concentration of ●cilostazol (risk of toxicity)—avoid concomitant use; lansoprazole possibly increases plasma concentration of ●cilostazol—avoid concomitant use

- Clopidogrel: esomeprazole and omeprazole reduce antiplatelet effect of ●clopidogrel; lansoprazole, pantoprazole and rabeprazole possibly reduce antiplatelet effect of clopidogrel

Cytotoxics: omeprazole possibly reduces excretion of methotrexate (increased risk of toxicity); proton pump inhibitors possibly reduce absorption of lapatinib

Tacrolimus: omeprazole possibly increases plasma concentration of tacrolimus

Ulcer-healing Drugs: absorption of lansoprazole possibly reduced by sucralfate

- Ulipristal: avoidance of proton pump inhibitors advised by manufacturer of ●ulipristal (plasma concentration of ulipristal possibly reduced)

Pseudoephedrine *see* Sympathomimetics

Pyrazinamide

Oestrogens: antibacterials that do not induce liver enzymes possibly reduce contraceptive effect of oestrogens (risk probably small, see p. 486)

Probenecid: pyrazinamide antagonises effects of probenecid

Sulfinpyrazone: pyrazinamide antagonises effects of sulfinpyrazone

Vaccines: antibacterials inactivate oral typhoid vaccine–see p. 760

Pyridostigmine *see* Parasympathomimetics

Pyridoxine *see* Vitamins

Pyrimethamine

- Antibacterials: increased antifolate effect when pyrimethamine given with ●sulphonamides or ●trimethoprim

- Antiepileptics: pyrimethamine antagonises anticonvulsant effect of ●phenytoin, also increased antifolate effect

- Antimalarials: avoidance of antimalarials advised by manufacturer of ●artemether/lumefantrine; increased antifolate effect when pyrimethamine given with proguanil

Antivirals: increased antifolate effect when pyrimethamine given with zidovudine

- Cytotoxics: pyrimethamine increases antifolate effect of ●methotrexate and ●pemetrexed

Vaccines: antimalarials inactivate oral typhoid vaccine–see p. 760

Quetiapine *see* Antipsychotics

Quinagolide

Memantine: effects of dopaminergics possibly enhanced by memantine

Quinagolide *(continued)*

Methyldopa: antiparkinsonian effect of dopaminergics antagonised by methyldopa

Quinapril *see* ACE Inhibitors

Quinine

- Anti-arrhythmics: increased risk of ventricular arrhythmias when quinine given with ●amiodarone—avoid concomitant use; quinine increases plasma concentration of ●flecainide

- Antibacterials: increased risk of ventricular arrhythmias when quinine given with ●moxifloxacin—avoid concomitant use; plasma concentration of quinine reduced by ●rifampicin

- Antimalarials: increased risk of ventricular arrhythmias when quinine given with ●artemether/lumefantrine; avoidance of antimalarials advised by manufacturer of ●artemether/lumefantrine; increased risk of convulsions when quinine given with ●mefloquine (but should not prevent the use of *intravenous* quinine in severe cases)

- Antipsychotics: increased risk of ventricular arrhythmias when quinine given with ●droperidol or ●pimozide—avoid concomitant use; possible increased risk of ventricular arrhythmias when quinine given with ●haloperidol—avoid concomitant use

- Cardiac Glycosides: quinine increases plasma concentration of ●digoxin

Muscle Relaxants: quinine possibly enhances effects of suxamethonium

Ulcer-healing Drugs: metabolism of quinine inhibited by cimetidine (increased plasma concentration)

Vaccines: antimalarials inactivate oral typhoid vaccine–see p. 760

Quinolones

- Analgesics: possible increased risk of convulsions when quinolones given with ●NSAIDs; manufacturer of ciprofloxacin advises avoid premedication with opioid analgesics (reduced plasma concentration of ciprofloxacin) when ciprofloxacin used for surgical prophylaxis

Antacids: absorption of ciprofloxacin, levofloxacin, moxifloxacin, norfloxacin and ofloxacin reduced by antacids

- Anti-arrhythmics: increased risk of ventricular arrhythmias when levofloxacin or moxifloxacin given with ●amiodarone—avoid concomitant use; increased risk of ventricular arrhythmias when moxifloxacin given with ●disopyramide—avoid concomitant use

- Antibacterials: increased risk of ventricular arrhythmias when moxifloxacin given with *parenteral* ●erythromycin—avoid concomitant use

- Anticoagulants: levofloxacin possibly enhances anticoagulant effect of coumarins and phenindione; ciprofloxacin, nalidixic acid, norfloxacin and ofloxacin enhance anticoagulant effect of ●coumarins

- Antidepressants: ciprofloxacin inhibits metabolism of ●duloxetine—avoid concomitant use; avoidance of ciprofloxacin advised by manufacturer of ●agomelatine; increased risk of ventricular arrhythmias when moxifloxacin given with ●tricyclics—avoid concomitant use

Antidiabetics: ciprofloxacin and norfloxacin possibly enhance effects of glibenclamide

Antiepileptics: ciprofloxacin increases or decreases plasma concentration of phenytoin

- Antihistamines: increased risk of ventricular arrhythmias when moxifloxacin given with ●mizolastine—avoid concomitant use

- Antimalarials: avoidance of quinolones advised by manufacturer of ●artemether/lumefantrine; increased risk of ventricular arrhythmias when moxifloxacin given with ●chloroquine and hydroxychloroquine, ●mefloquine or ●quinine—avoid concomitant use

Quinolones *(continued)*

- Antipsychotics: increased risk of ventricular arrhythmias when moxifloxacin given with ●benperidol—manufacturer of benperidol advises avoid concomitant use; increased risk of ventricular arrhythmias when moxifloxacin given with ●droperidol, ●haloperidol, ●phenothiazines, ●pimozide, ●sertindole or ●zuclopenthixol—avoid concomitant use; ciprofloxacin increases plasma concentration of clozapine; ciprofloxacin possibly increases plasma concentration of olanzapine
- Atomoxetine: increased risk of ventricular arrhythmias when moxifloxacin given with ●atomoxetine
- Beta-blockers: increased risk of ventricular arrhythmias when moxifloxacin given with ●sotalol—avoid concomitant use

  Calcium Salts: absorption of ciprofloxacin reduced by calcium salts
- Ciclosporin: increased risk of nephrotoxicity when quinolones given with ●ciclosporin
- Clopidogrel: ciprofloxacin possibly reduces antiplatelet effect of ●clopidogrel
- Cytotoxics: nalidixic acid increases risk of melphalan toxicity; ciprofloxacin possibly reduces excretion of methotrexate (increased risk of toxicity); ciprofloxacin increases plasma concentration of erlotinib; increased risk of ventricular arrhythmias when levofloxacin or moxifloxacin given with ●arsenic trioxide

  Dairy Products: absorption of ciprofloxacin and norfloxacin reduced by dairy products

  Dopaminergics: ciprofloxacin inhibits metabolism of ropinirole (increased plasma concentration)

  $5HT_1$ Agonists: quinolones possibly inhibit metabolism of zolmitriptan (reduce dose of zolmitriptan)

  Iron: absorption of ciprofloxacin, levofloxacin, moxifloxacin, norfloxacin and ofloxacin reduced by *oral* iron
- Muscle Relaxants: norfloxacin possibly increases plasma concentration of tizanidine (increased risk of toxicity); ciprofloxacin increases plasma concentration of ●tizanidine (increased risk of toxicity)—avoid concomitant use

  Mycophenolate: norfloxacin possibly reduces bioavailability of mycophenolate

  Oestrogens: antibacterials that do not induce liver enzymes possibly reduce contraceptive effect of oestrogens (risk probably small, see p. 486)
- Pentamidine Isetionate: increased risk of ventricular arrhythmias when moxifloxacin given with ●pentamidine isetionate—avoid concomitant use

  Probenecid: excretion of ciprofloxacin, nalidixic acid and norfloxacin reduced by probenecid (increased plasma concentration)

  Sevelamer: bioavailability of ciprofloxacin reduced by sevelamer

  Strontium Ranelate: absorption of quinolones reduced by strontium ranelate (manufacturer of strontium ranelate advises avoid concomitant use)
- Theophylline: possible increased risk of convulsions when quinolones given with ●theophylline; ciprofloxacin and norfloxacin increase plasma concentration of ●theophylline

  Ulcer-healing Drugs: absorption of ciprofloxacin, levofloxacin, moxifloxacin, norfloxacin and ofloxacin reduced by sucralfate

  Vaccines: antibacterials inactivate oral typhoid vaccine–see p. 760

  Zinc: absorption of ciprofloxacin, levofloxacin, moxifloxacin, norfloxacin and ofloxacin reduced by zinc

Quinupristin with Dalfopristin

- Anti-arrhythmics: increased risk of ventricular arrhythmias when quinupristin/dalfopristin given with ●disopyramide or ●lidocaine—avoid concomitant use

Quinupristin with Dalfopristin *(continued)*

  Antibacterials: manufacturer of quinupristin/dalfopristin recommends monitoring liver function when given with rifampicin

  Antivirals: quinupristin/dalfopristin possibly increases plasma concentration of saquinavir
- Anxiolytics and Hypnotics: quinupristin/dalfopristin inhibits metabolism of ●midazolam (increased plasma concentration with increased sedation); quinupristin/dalfopristin inhibits the metabolism of zopiclone
- Calcium-channel Blockers: quinupristin/dalfopristin increases plasma concentration of ●nifedipine
- Ciclosporin: quinupristin/dalfopristin increases plasma concentration of ●ciclosporin
- Ergot Alkaloids: manufacturer of quinupristin/dalfopristin advises avoid concomitant use with ●ergotamine and methysergide

  Oestrogens: antibacterials that do not induce liver enzymes possibly reduce contraceptive effect of oestrogens (risk probably small, see p. 486)
- Tacrolimus: quinupristin/dalfopristin increases plasma concentration of ●tacrolimus

  Vaccines: antibacterials inactivate oral typhoid vaccine–see p. 760

Rabeprazole *see* Proton Pump Inhibitors

Raloxifene

  Anticoagulants: raloxifene antagonises anticoagulant effect of coumarins

  Lipid-regulating Drugs: absorption of raloxifene reduced by colestyramine (manufacturer of raloxifene advises avoid concomitant administration)

Raltegravir

- Antibacterials: plasma concentration of raltegravir reduced by ●rifampicin—consider increasing dose of raltegravir
- Ulcer-healing Drugs: plasma concentration of raltegravir increased by ●omeprazole—avoid concomitant use; plasma concentration of raltegravir possibly increased by histamine H_2-antagonists and proton pump inhibitors—manufacturer of raltegravir advises avoid concomitant use

Raltitrexed

  Antiepileptics: cytotoxics possibly reduce absorption of phenytoin
- Antipsychotics: avoid concomitant use of cytotoxics with ●clozapine (increased risk of agranulocytosis)

  Cardiac Glycosides: cytotoxics reduce absorption of digoxin tablets
- Folates: manufacturer of raltitrexed advises avoid concomitant use with ●folates

Ramipril *see* ACE Inhibitors

Ranitidine *see* Histamine H_2-antagonists

Ranolazine

- Anti-arrhythmics: manufacturer of ranolazine advises avoid concomitant use with ●disopyramide
- Antibacterials: plasma concentration of ranolazine possibly increased by ●clarithromycin and ●telithromycin—manufacturer of ranolazine advises avoid concomitant use; plasma concentration of ranolazine reduced by ●rifampicin—manufacturer of ranolazine advises avoid concomitant use

  Antidepressants: plasma concentration of ranolazine increased by paroxetine
- Antifungals: plasma concentration of ranolazine increased by ●ketoconazole—avoid concomitant use; plasma concentration of ranolazine possibly increased by ●itraconazole, ●posaconazole and ●voriconazole—manufacturer of ranolazine advises avoid concomitant use
- Antivirals: plasma concentration of ranolazine possibly increased by ●atazanavir, ●darunavir, ●fosamprenavir, ●indinavir, ●lopinavir, ●nelfinavir,

Ranolazine

- Antivirals (continued)
  - ●ritonavir, ●saquinavir and ●tipranavir—manufacturer of ranolazine advises avoid concomitant use
- Beta-blockers: manufacturer of ranolazine advises avoid concomitant use with ●sotalol

  Calcium-channel Blockers: plasma concentration of ranolazine increased by diltiazem and verapamil (consider reducing dose of ranolazine)

  Cardiac Glycosides: ranolazine increases plasma concentration of digoxin

  Ciclosporin: plasma concentration of ranolazine possibly increased by ciclosporin
- Grapefruit Juice: plasma concentration of ranolazine possibly increased by ●grapefruit juice—manufacturer of ranolazine advises avoid concomitant use

  Lipid-regulating Drugs: ranolazine increases plasma concentration of simvastatin (consider reducing dose of simvastatin)

Rasagiline

Note. Rasagiline is a MAO-B inhibitor
- Analgesics: avoid concomitant use of rasagiline with ●dextromethorphan; risk of CNS toxicity when rasagiline given with ●pethidine (avoid pethidine for 2 weeks after rasagiline)
- Antidepressants: after stopping rasagiline do not start ●fluoxetine for 2 weeks, also rasagiline should not be started until at least 5 weeks after stopping fluoxetine; after stopping rasagiline do not start ●fluvoxamine for 2 weeks; risk of hypertensive crisis when rasagiline given with ●MAOIs, avoid MAOIs for at least 2 weeks after stopping rasagiline; increased risk of CNS toxicity when rasagiline given with ●SSRIs or ●tricyclics

  Dopaminergics: plasma concentration of rasagiline possibly reduced by entacapone

  Memantine: effects of dopaminergics possibly enhanced by memantine

  Methyldopa: antiparkinsonian effect of dopaminergics antagonised by methyldopa
- Sympathomimetics: avoid concomitant use of rasagiline with ●sympathomimetics

Reboxetine

- Antibacterials: manufacturer of reboxetine advises avoid concomitant use with ●macrolides
- Antidepressants: manufacturer of reboxetine advises avoid concomitant use with ●fluvoxamine; increased risk of hypertension and CNS excitation when reboxetine given with ●MAOIs (MAOIs should not be started until 1 week after stopping reboxetine, avoid reboxetine for 2 weeks after stopping MAOIs)
- Antifungals: manufacturer of reboxetine advises avoid concomitant use with ●imidazoles and ●triazoles
- Antimalarials: avoidance of antidepressants advised by manufacturer of ●artemether/lumefantrine

  Atomoxetine: possible increased risk of convulsions when antidepressants given with atomoxetine

  Diuretics: possible increased risk of hypokalaemia when reboxetine given with loop diuretics or thiazides and related diuretics

  Ergot Alkaloids: possible risk of hypertension when reboxetine given with ergotamine and methysergide
- Sibutramine: increased risk of CNS toxicity when noradrenaline re-uptake inhibitors given with ●sibutramine (manufacturer of sibutramine advises avoid concomitant use)

Remifentanil see Opioid Analgesics

Repaglinide see Antidiabetics

Retinoids

- Alcohol: etretinate formed from acitretin in presence of ●alcohol (increased risk of teratogenicity in women of child-bearing potential)
- Antibacterials: possible increased risk of benign intracranial hypertension when retinoids given with ●tetracyclines (avoid concomitant use)

Retinoids (continued)

- Anticoagulants: acitretin possibly reduces anticoagulant effect of ●coumarins

  Antiepileptics: isotretinoin possibly reduces plasma concentration of carbamazepine

  Antifungals: plasma concentration of alitretinoin increased by ketoconazole
- Cytotoxics: acitretin increases plasma concentration of ●methotrexate (also increased risk of hepatotoxicity)—avoid concomitant use

  Lipid-regulating Drugs: alitretinoin reduces plasma concentration of simvastatin

  Vitamins: risk of hypervitaminosis A when retinoids given with vitamin A

Ribavirin

- Antivirals: increased risk of side-effects when ribavirin given with ●didanosine—avoid concomitant use; ribavirin possibly inhibits effects of ●stavudine; increased risk of anaemia when ribavirin given with ●zidovudine—avoid concomitant use

Rifabutin see Rifamycins

Rifampicin see Rifamycins

Rifamycins

  ACE Inhibitors: rifampicin reduces plasma concentration of active metabolite of imidapril (reduced antihypertensive effect)

  Analgesics: rifampicin reduces plasma concentration of etoricoxib; rifampicin accelerates metabolism of alfentanil, codeine, fentanyl, methadone and morphine (reduced effect); rifampicin possibly accelerates metabolism of oxycodone

  Angiotensin-II Receptor Antagonists: rifampicin reduces plasma concentration of losartan and its active metabolite

  Antacids: absorption of rifampicin reduced by antacids
- Anti-arrhythmics: rifampicins accelerate metabolism of ●disopyramide (reduced plasma concentration); rifampicin accelerates metabolism of ●propafenone (reduced effect)
- Antibacterials: rifampicins reduce plasma concentration of clarithromycin and dapsone; plasma concentration of rifabutin increased by ●clarithromycin (increased risk of uveitis—reduce rifabutin dose); rifampicin reduces plasma concentration of doxycycline—consider increasing dose of doxycycline; rifampicin accelerates metabolism of chloramphenicol (reduced plasma concentration); rifampicin reduces plasma concentration of linezolid (possible therapeutic failure of linezolid); plasma concentration of rifabutin possibly increased by ●macrolides (increased risk of uveitis—reduce rifabutin dose); monitoring of liver function with rifampicin recommended by manufacturer of quinupristin/dalfopristin; rifampicin reduces plasma concentration of ●telithromycin (avoid during and for 2 weeks after rifampicin); rifampicin possibly reduces plasma concentration of trimethoprim
- Anticoagulants: rifamycins accelerate metabolism of ●coumarins (reduced anticoagulant effect); rifampicin reduces plasma concentration of rivaroxaban
- Antidiabetics: rifamycins accelerate metabolism of ●tolbutamide (reduced effect); rifampicin reduces plasma concentration of ●rosiglitazone—consider increasing dose of rosiglitazone; rifampicin reduces plasma concentration of nateglinide; rifampicin possibly antagonises hypoglycaemic effect of repaglinide; rifampicins possibly accelerate metabolism of ●sulphonylureas (reduced effect)
- Antiepileptics: rifabutin reduces plasma concentration of ●carbamazepine; rifampicin reduces plasma concentration of ●lamotrigine; rifamycins accelerate metabolism of ●phenytoin (reduced plasma concentration)
- Antifungals: rifampicin accelerates metabolism of ●ketoconazole (reduced plasma concentration), also

Rifamycins

- Antifungals *(continued)*

    plasma concentration of rifampicin may be reduced by ketoconazole; plasma concentration of rifabutin increased by ●fluconazole (increased risk of uveitis—reduce rifabutin dose); rifampicin accelerates metabolism of ●fluconazole and ●itraconazole (reduced plasma concentration); rifabutin reduces plasma concentration of ●itraconazole—avoid concomitant use; plasma concentration of rifabutin increased by ●posaconazole (also plasma concentration of posaconazole reduced); rifampicin reduces plasma concentration of ●posaconazole and ●terbinafine; plasma concentration of rifabutin increased by ●voriconazole, also rifabutin reduces plasma concentration of voriconazole (increase dose of voriconazole and also monitor for rifabutin toxicity); rifampicin reduces plasma concentration of ●voriconazole—avoid concomitant use; rifampicin initially increases and then reduces plasma concentration of caspofungin (consider increasing dose of caspofungin); plasma concentration of rifabutin possibly increased by ●triazoles (increased risk of uveitis—reduce rifabutin dose)

- Antimalarials: rifampicin reduces plasma concentration of ●mefloquine—avoid concomitant use; rifampicin reduces plasma concentration of ●quinine

    Antimuscarinics: rifampicin reduces plasma concentration of active metabolite of fesoterodine

- Antipsychotics: rifampicin accelerates metabolism of ●haloperidol (reduced plasma concentration); rifabutin and rifampicin possibly reduce plasma concentration of ●aripiprazole—increase dose of aripiprazole; rifampicin possibly reduces plasma concentration of clozapine

- Antivirals: rifampicin possibly reduces plasma concentration of abacavir and ritonavir; plasma concentration of rifabutin increased by ●atazanavir, ●darunavir, ●fosamprenavir and ●tipranavir (reduce dose of rifabutin); rifampicin reduces plasma concentration of ●atazanavir, ●lopinavir and ●nevirapine—avoid concomitant use; rifampicin significantly reduces plasma concentration of ●darunavir, ●fosamprenavir and ●nelfinavir—avoid concomitant use; rifampicin reduces plasma concentration of efavirenz—increase dose of efavirenz; plasma concentration of rifabutin reduced by efavirenz—increase dose of rifabutin; avoidance of rifampicin advised by manufacturer of etravirine and zidovudine; plasma concentration of both drugs reduced when rifabutin given with ●etravirine; plasma concentration of rifabutin increased by ●indinavir—avoid concomitant use; rifampicin accelerates metabolism of ●indinavir (reduced plasma concentration—avoid concomitant use); rifampicin reduces plasma concentration of ●maraviroc and ●raltegravir—consider increasing dose of maraviroc and raltegravir; plasma concentration of rifabutin increased by ●nelfinavir (halve dose of rifabutin); plasma concentration of rifabutin possibly increased by nevirapine; plasma concentration of rifabutin increased by ●ritonavir (increased risk of toxicity); rifampicin significantly reduces plasma concentration of ●saquinavir, also risk of hepatotoxicity—avoid concomitant use; rifabutin reduces plasma concentration of ●saquinavir; rifampicin possibly reduces plasma concentration of ●tipranavir—avoid concomitant use

    Anxiolytics and Hypnotics: rifampicin accelerates metabolism of diazepam (reduced plasma concentration); rifampicin possibly accelerates metabolism of benzodiazepines (reduced plasma concentration); rifampicin possibly accelerates metabolism of buspirone and zaleplon; rifampicin accelerates metabolism of zolpidem (reduced plasma concen-

Rifamycins

    Anxiolytics and Hypnotics *(continued)*
    tration and reduced effect); rifampicin significantly reduces plasma concentration of zopiclone

    Aprepitant: rifampicin reduces plasma concentration of aprepitant

- Atovaquone: rifabutin and rifampicin reduce plasma concentration of ●atovaquone (possible therapeutic failure of atovaquone)

    Barbiturates: plasma concentration of rifampicin possibly reduced by phenobarbital

    Beta-blockers: rifampicin accelerates metabolism of bisoprolol and propranolol (plasma concentration significantly reduced); rifampicin reduces plasma concentration of carvedilol, celiprolol and metoprolol

- Bosentan: rifampicin reduces plasma concentration of ●bosentan—avoid concomitant use

- Calcium-channel Blockers: rifampicin possibly accelerates metabolism of ●isradipine and ●nicardipine (possible significantly reduced plasma concentration); rifampicin accelerates metabolism of ●diltiazem, ●nifedipine, ●nimodipine and ●verapamil (plasma concentration significantly reduced)

    Cardiac Glycosides: rifamycins accelerate metabolism of digitoxin (reduced effect); rifampicin possibly reduces plasma concentration of digoxin

- Ciclosporin: rifampicin accelerates metabolism of ●ciclosporin (reduced plasma concentration)

- Corticosteroids: rifamycins accelerate metabolism of ●corticosteroids (reduced effect)

- Cytotoxics: rifampicin accelerates metabolism of ●dasatinib (reduced plasma concentration—avoid concomitant use); rifampicin accelerates metabolism of erlotinib and sunitinib (reduced plasma concentration); rifampicin reduces plasma concentration of ●everolimus and sorafenib; rifampicin reduces plasma concentration of ●gefitinib, ●imatinib and ●nilotinib—avoid concomitant use; avoidance of rifabutin and rifampicin advised by manufacturer of ●lapatinib; rifampicin reduces plasma concentration of active metabolite of ●temsirolimus—avoid concomitant use

    Deferasirox: rifampicin reduces plasma concentration of deferasirox

- Diuretics: rifampicin reduces plasma concentration of ●eplerenone—avoid concomitant use

    Hormone Antagonists: rifampicin possibly reduces plasma concentration of exemestane; rifampicin accelerates metabolism of tamoxifen (reduced plasma concentration)

    5HT$_3$ Antagonists: rifampicin accelerates metabolism of ondansetron (reduced effect)

    Leflunomide: rifampicin possibly increases plasma concentration of active metabolite of leflunomide

    Lipid-regulating Drugs: rifampicin possibly reduces plasma concentration of atorvastatin and simvastatin; rifampicin accelerates metabolism of fluvastatin (reduced effect)

- Mycophenolate: rifampicin reduces plasma concentration of active metabolite of ●mycophenolate

- Oestrogens: rifamycins accelerate metabolism of ●oestrogens (reduced contraceptive effect—see p. 486); antibacterials that do not induce liver enzymes possibly reduce contraceptive effect of oestrogens (risk probably small, see p. 486)

- Progestogens: rifamycins accelerate metabolism of ●progestogens (reduced contraceptive effect—see p. 486)

- Ranolazine: rifampicin reduces plasma concentration of ●ranolazine—manufacturer of ranolazine advises avoid concomitant use

- Sirolimus: rifabutin and rifampicin reduce plasma concentration of ●sirolimus—avoid concomitant use

Rifamycins *(continued)*

- Tacrolimus: rifabutin possibly reduces plasma concentration of tacrolimus; rifampicin reduces plasma concentration of ●tacrolimus

  Tadalafil: rifampicin reduces plasma concentration of tadalafil

  Theophylline: rifampicin accelerates metabolism of theophylline (reduced plasma concentration)

  Thyroid Hormones: rifampicin accelerates metabolism of levothyroxine (may increase requirements for levothyroxine in hypothyroidism)

  Tibolone: rifampicin accelerates metabolism of tibolone (reduced plasma concentration)

  Tolvaptan: rifampicin reduces plasma concentration of tolvaptan

  Ulcer-healing Drugs: rifampicin accelerates metabolism of cimetidine (reduced plasma concentration)

- Ulipristal: avoidance of rifampicin advised by manufacturer of ●ulipristal (contraceptive effect of ulipristal possibly reduced)

  Vaccines: antibacterials inactivate oral typhoid vaccine–see p. 760

Risedronate Sodium *see* Bisphosphonates

Risperidone *see* Antipsychotics

Ritodrine *see* Sympathomimetics, Beta$_2$

Ritonavir

- Alpha-blockers: ritonavir possibly increases plasma concentration of ●alfuzosin—avoid concomitant use

- Analgesics: ritonavir possibly increases plasma concentration of NSAIDs and buprenorphine; ritonavir increases plasma concentration of ●dextropropoxyphene and ●piroxicam (risk of toxicity)—avoid concomitant use; ritonavir increases plasma concentration of ●alfentanil and ●fentanyl; ritonavir reduces plasma concentration of methadone; ritonavir possibly reduces plasma concentration of morphine; ritonavir reduces plasma concentration of ●pethidine, but increases plasma concentration of toxic metabolite of pethidine (avoid concomitant use)

- Anti-arrhythmics: ritonavir increases plasma concentration of ●amiodarone and ●propafenone (increased risk of ventricular arrhythmias—avoid concomitant use); ritonavir possibly increases plasma concentration of ●disopyramide (increased risk of toxicity); ritonavir possibly increases plasma concentration of ●flecainide (increased risk of ventricular arrhythmias—avoid concomitant use)

- Antibacterials: ritonavir possibly increases plasma concentration of azithromycin and erythromycin; ritonavir increases plasma concentration of ●clarithromycin (reduce dose of clarithromycin in renal impairment); ritonavir increases plasma concentration of ●rifabutin (increased risk of toxicity); plasma concentration of ritonavir possibly reduced by rifampicin; plasma concentration of both drugs increased when ritonavir given with ●fusidic acid—avoid concomitant use; avoidance of concomitant ritonavir in severe renal and hepatic impairment advised by manufacturer of ●telithromycin

- Anticoagulants: ritonavir may enhance or reduce anticoagulant effect of ●warfarin; ritonavir possibly enhances anticoagulant effect of ●coumarins and ●phenindione; ritonavir increases plasma concentration of ●rivaroxaban—manufacturer of rivaroxaban advises avoid concomitant use

- Antidepressants: ritonavir possibly reduces plasma concentration of paroxetine; side-effects possibly increased when ritonavir given with trazodone; ritonavir possibly increases plasma concentration of ●SSRIs and ●tricyclics; plasma concentration of ritonavir reduced by ●St John's wort—avoid concomitant use

  Antidiabetics: ritonavir possibly increases plasma concentration of tolbutamide

Ritonavir *(continued)*

- Antiepileptics: ritonavir possibly increases plasma concentration of ●carbamazepine; ritonavir possibly reduces plasma concentration of lamotrigine; plasma concentration of ritonavir possibly reduced by phenytoin, also plasma concentration of phenytoin possibly affected

- Antifungals: combination of ritonavir with ●itraconazole or ●ketoconazole may increase plasma concentration of either drug (or both); plasma concentration of ritonavir increased by fluconazole; ritonavir reduces plasma concentration of ●voriconazole—avoid concomitant use

  Antihistamines: ritonavir possibly increases plasma concentration of non-sedating antihistamines

  Antimalarials: caution with ritonavir advised by manufacturer of artemether/lumefantrine

  Antimuscarinics: avoidance of ritonavir advised by manufacturer of darifenacin and tolterodine; manufacturer of fesoterodine advises dose reduction when ritonavir given with fesoterodine—consult fesoterodine product literature; ritonavir increases plasma concentration of solifenacin

- Antipsychotics: ritonavir possibly increases plasma concentration of ●antipsychotics; ritonavir possibly inhibits metabolism of ●aripiprazole (reduce dose of aripiprazole); ritonavir increases plasma concentration of ●clozapine (increased risk of toxicity)—avoid concomitant use; ritonavir reduces plasma concentration of olanzapine—consider increasing dose of olanzapine; ritonavir increases plasma concentration of ●pimozide and ●sertindole (increased risk of ventricular arrhythmias—avoid concomitant use)

- Antivirals: ritonavir increases toxicity of efavirenz, monitor liver function tests; ritonavir increases plasma concentration of indinavir, maraviroc and ●saquinavir; combination of ritonavir with nelfinavir may increase plasma concentration of either drug (or both)

- Anxiolytics and Hypnotics: ritonavir possibly increases plasma concentration of ●anxiolytics and hypnotics; ritonavir possibly increases plasma concentration of ●alprazolam, ●diazepam, ●flurazepam and ●zolpidem (risk of extreme sedation and respiratory depression—avoid concomitant use); ritonavir possibly increases plasma concentration of ●midazolam (risk of prolonged sedation—avoid concomitant use of *oral* midazolam); ritonavir increases plasma concentration of buspirone (increased risk of toxicity)

  Aprepitant: ritonavir possibly increases plasma concentration of aprepitant

  Bosentan: ritonavir possibly increases plasma concentration of bosentan

  Bupropion: ritonavir reduces plasma concentration of bupropion

- Calcium-channel Blockers: ritonavir possibly increases plasma concentration of ●calcium-channel blockers; avoidance of ritonavir advised by manufacturer of lercanidipine

  Cardiac Glycosides: ritonavir possibly increases plasma concentration of digoxin

- Ciclosporin: ritonavir possibly increases plasma concentration of ●ciclosporin

- Cilostazol: ritonavir possibly increases plasma concentration of ●cilostazol—avoid concomitant use

- Corticosteroids: ritonavir possibly increases plasma concentration of corticosteroids, dexamethasone and prednisolone; ritonavir increases plasma concentration of *inhaled* and *intranasal* budesonide and ●fluticasone

- Cytotoxics: ritonavir possibly increases plasma concentration of ●everolimus—manufacturer of everolimus advises avoid concomitant use; avoidance of ritonavir advised by manufacturer of ●lapatinib and ●nilotinib; ritonavir increases plasma concentration

Appendix 1: Interactions

Ritonavir
- Cytotoxics *(continued)*
  of paclitaxel; ritonavir possibly increases plasma concentration of vinblastine
- Diuretics: ritonavir increases plasma concentration of ●eplerenone—avoid concomitant use
- Ergot Alkaloids: increased risk of ergotism when ritonavir given with ●ergotamine and methysergide—avoid concomitant use
- 5HT$_1$ Agonists: ritonavir increases plasma concentration of ●eletriptan (risk of toxicity)—avoid concomitant use
- Ivabradine: ritonavir possibly increases plasma concentration of ●ivabradine—avoid concomitant use
- Lipid-regulating Drugs: possible increased risk of myopathy when ritonavir given with atorvastatin; possible increased risk of myopathy when ritonavir given with ●rosuvastatin—avoid concomitant use; increased risk of myopathy when ritonavir given with ●simvastatin (avoid concomitant use)
- Oestrogens: ritonavir accelerates metabolism of ●oestrogens (reduced contraceptive effect—see p. 486)
- Ranolazine: ritonavir possibly increases plasma concentration of ●ranolazine—manufacturer of ranolazine advises avoid concomitant use
- Sildenafil: ritonavir significantly increases plasma concentration of ●sildenafil—avoid concomitant use
  Sympathomimetics: ritonavir possibly increases plasma concentration of dexamfetamine
- Tacrolimus: ritonavir possibly increases plasma concentration of ●tacrolimus
  Tadalafil: ritonavir increases plasma concentration of tadalafil
- Theophylline: ritonavir accelerates metabolism of ●theophylline (reduced plasma concentration)
- Ulipristal: avoidance of ritonavir advised by manufacturer of ●ulipristal (contraceptive effect of ulipristal possibly reduced)
- Vardenafil: ritonavir increases plasma concentration of ●vardenafil—avoid concomitant use

Rivaroxaban
- Analgesics: increased risk of haemorrhage when anticoagulants given with *intravenous* ●diclofenac (avoid concomitant use, including low-dose heparins); increased risk of haemorrhage when anticoagulants given with ●ketorolac (avoid concomitant use, including low-dose heparins)
  Antibacterials: plasma concentration of rivaroxaban reduced by rifampicin
- Antifungals: plasma concentration of rivaroxaban increased by ●ketoconazole—avoid concomitant use; manufacturer of rivaroxaban advises avoid concomitant use with itraconazole, posaconazole and voriconazole
- Antivirals: manufacturer of rivaroxaban advises avoid concomitant use with atazanavir, darunavir, fosamprenavir, indinavir, lopinavir, nelfinavir, saquinavir and tipranavir; plasma concentration of rivaroxaban increased by ●ritonavir—manufacturer of rivaroxaban advises avoid concomitant use
  Sibutramine: increased risk of bleeding when anticoagulants given with sibutramine

Rivastigmine *see* Parasympathomimetics
Rizatriptan *see* 5HT$_1$ Agonists
Rocuronium *see* Muscle Relaxants
Ropinirole
  Antibacterials: metabolism of ropinirole inhibited by ciprofloxacin (increased plasma concentration)
  Antipsychotics: manufacturer of ropinirole advises avoid concomitant use of antipsychotics (antagonism of effect)
  Memantine: effects of dopaminergics possibly enhanced by memantine
  Methyldopa: antiparkinsonian effect of dopaminergics antagonised by methyldopa

Ropinirole *(continued)*
  Metoclopramide: manufacturer of ropinirole advises avoid concomitant use of metoclopramide (antagonism of effect)
  Oestrogens: plasma concentration of ropinirole increased by oestrogens
Ropivacaine
  Anti-arrhythmics: increased myocardial depression when ropivacaine given with anti-arrhythmics
  Antidepressants: metabolism of ropivacaine inhibited by fluvoxamine—avoid prolonged administration of ropivacaine
Rosiglitazone *see* Antidiabetics
Rosuvastatin *see* Statins
Rotigotine
  Antipsychotics: manufacturer of rotigotine advises avoid concomitant use of antipsychotics (antagonism of effect)
  Memantine: effects of dopaminergics possibly enhanced by memantine
  Methyldopa: antiparkinsonian effect of dopaminergics antagonised by methyldopa
  Metoclopramide: manufacturer of rotigotine advises avoid concomitant use of metoclopramide (antagonism of effect)
Rowachol®
  Anticoagulants: Rowachol® possibly reduces anticoagulant effect of coumarins
Rufinamide
- Antidepressants: anticonvulsant effect of antiepileptics possibly antagonised by MAOIs and ●tricyclic-related antidepressants (convulsive threshold lowered); anticonvulsant effect of antiepileptics antagonised by ●SSRIs and ●tricyclics (convulsive threshold lowered); avoid concomitant use of antiepileptics with ●St John's wort
  Antiepileptics: rufinamide possibly increases plasma concentration of phenytoin; plasma concentration of rufinamide possibly increased by valproate (reduce dose of rufinamide)
- Antimalarials: possible increased risk of convulsions when antiepileptics given with chloroquine and hydroxychloroquine; anticonvulsant effect of antiepileptics antagonised by ●mefloquine
- Oestrogens: rufinamide accelerates metabolism of ●oestrogens (reduced contraceptive effect—see p. 486)
- Orlistat: possible increased risk of convulsions when antiepileptics given with ●orlistat
- Progestogens: rufinamide accelerates metabolism of ●progestogens (reduced contraceptive effect—see p. 486)
Rupatadine *see* Antihistamines
St John's Wort
  Analgesics: St John's wort possibly reduces plasma concentration of methadone
- Antibacterials: St John's wort reduces plasma concentration of ●telithromycin (avoid during and for 2 weeks after St John's wort)
- Anticoagulants: St John's wort reduces anticoagulant effect of ●coumarins (avoid concomitant use)
- Antidepressants: possible increased serotonergic effects when St John's wort given with duloxetine or venlafaxine; St John's wort reduces plasma concentration of amitriptyline; increased serotonergic effects when St John's wort given with ●SSRIs—avoid concomitant use
- Antiepileptics: avoid concomitant use of St John's wort with ●antiepileptics
- Antifungals: St John's wort reduces plasma concentration of ●voriconazole—avoid concomitant use
- Antimalarials: avoidance of antidepressants advised by manufacturer of ●artemether/lumefantrine
- Antipsychotics: St John's wort possibly reduces plasma concentration of ●aripiprazole—increase dose of aripiprazole

St John's Wort *(continued)*

- Antivirals: St John's wort reduces plasma concentration of ●atazanavir, ●darunavir, ●efavirenz, ●fosamprenavir, ●indinavir, ●lopinavir, ●nelfinavir, ●nevirapine, ●ritonavir and ●saquinavir—avoid concomitant use; avoidance of St John's wort advised by manufacturer of etravirine; St John's wort possibly reduces plasma concentration of ●maraviroc and ●tipranavir—avoid concomitant use

  Anxiolytics and Hypnotics: St John's wort possibly reduces plasma concentration of *oral* midazolam

- Aprepitant: avoidance of St John's wort advised by manufacturer of ●aprepitant

  Atomoxetine: possible increased risk of convulsions when antidepressants given with atomoxetine

- Barbiturates: avoid concomitant use of St John's wort with ●phenobarbital
- Calcium-channel Blockers: St John's wort possibly reduces plasma concentration of amlodipine; St John's wort reduces plasma concentration of nifedipine; St John's wort significantly reduces plasma concentration of ●verapamil
- Cardiac Glycosides: St John's wort reduces plasma concentration of ●digoxin—avoid concomitant use
- Ciclosporin: St John's wort reduces plasma concentration of ●ciclosporin—avoid concomitant use
- Cytotoxics: St John's wort possibly reduces plasma concentration of everolimus—manufacturer of everolimus advises avoid concomitant use; avoidance of St John's wort advised by manufacturer of gefitinib and ●lapatinib; St John's wort reduces plasma concentration of ●imatinib—avoid concomitant use; St John's wort accelerates metabolism of ●irinotecan (reduced plasma concentration—avoid concomitant use)
- Diuretics: St John's wort reduces plasma concentration of ●eplerenone—avoid concomitant use
- 5HT$_1$ Agonists: increased serotonergic effects when St John's wort given with ●5HT$_1$ agonists—avoid concomitant use

  Ivabradine: St John's wort reduces plasma concentration of ivabradine—avoid concomitant use

  Lipid-regulating Drugs: St John's wort reduces plasma concentration of simvastatin

- Oestrogens: St John's wort reduces contraceptive effect of ●oestrogens (avoid concomitant use)
- Progestogens: St John's wort reduces contraceptive effect of ●progestogens (avoid concomitant use)
- Tacrolimus: St John's wort reduces plasma concentration of ●tacrolimus—avoid concomitant use
- Theophylline: St John's wort reduces plasma concentration of ●theophylline—avoid concomitant use

  Ulcer-healing Drugs: St John's wort possibly reduces plasma concentration of omeprazole

- Ulipristal: avoidance of St John's wort advised by manufacturer of ●ulipristal (contraceptive effect of ulipristal possibly reduced)

Salbutamol *see* Sympathomimetics, Beta$_2$
Salmeterol *see* Sympathomimetics, Beta$_2$
Saquinavir

- Antibacterials: plasma concentration of saquinavir reduced by ●rifabutin; plasma concentration of saquinavir significantly reduced by ●rifampicin, also risk of hepatotoxicity—avoid concomitant use; plasma concentration of saquinavir possibly increased by quinupristin/dalfopristin; avoidance of concomitant saquinavir in severe renal and hepatic impairment advised by manufacturer of ●telithromycin

  Anticoagulants: saquinavir possibly enhances anticoagulant effect of warfarin; avoidance of saquinavir advised by manufacturer of rivaroxaban

- Antidepressants: plasma concentration of saquinavir reduced by ●St John's wort—avoid concomitant use

Saquinavir *(continued)*

- Antiepileptics: plasma concentration of saquinavir possibly reduced by carbamazepine, phenytoin and ●primidone

  Antifungals: plasma concentration of saquinavir increased by ketoconazole; plasma concentration of saquinavir possibly increased by imidazoles and triazoles

  Antimalarials: caution with saquinavir advised by manufacturer of artemether/lumefantrine

  Antimuscarinics: avoidance of saquinavir advised by manufacturer of darifenacin and tolterodine; manufacturer of fesoterodine advises dose reduction when saquinavir given with fesoterodine—consult fesoterodine product literature

- Antipsychotics: saquinavir possibly inhibits metabolism of ●aripiprazole (reduce dose of aripiprazole); saquinavir possibly increases plasma concentration of ●pimozide (increased risk of ventricular arrhythmias—avoid concomitant use); saquinavir increases plasma concentration of ●sertindole (increased risk of ventricular arrhythmias—avoid concomitant use)
- Antivirals: plasma concentration of saquinavir increased by atazanavir, indinavir and ●ritonavir; saquinavir reduces plasma concentration of darunavir; plasma concentration of saquinavir significantly reduced by efavirenz; saquinavir increases plasma concentration of ●maraviroc (consider reducing dose of maraviroc); combination of saquinavir with nelfinavir may increase plasma concentration of either drug (or both); plasma concentration of saquinavir reduced by ●tipranavir
- Anxiolytics and Hypnotics: saquinavir increases plasma concentration of ●midazolam (risk of prolonged sedation—avoid concomitant use of *oral* midazolam)
- Barbiturates: plasma concentration of saquinavir possibly reduced by ●barbiturates
- Ciclosporin: plasma concentration of both drugs increased when saquinavir given with ●ciclosporin
- Cilostazol: saquinavir possibly increases plasma concentration of ●cilostazol—avoid concomitant use

  Corticosteroids: plasma concentration of saquinavir possibly reduced by dexamethasone

- Cytotoxics: saquinavir possibly increases plasma concentration of ●everolimus—manufacturer of everolimus advises avoid concomitant use; avoidance of saquinavir advised by manufacturer of ●lapatinib

  Diuretics: saquinavir increases plasma concentration of eplerenone (reduce dose of eplerenone)

- Ergot Alkaloids: increased risk of ergotism when saquinavir given with ●ergotamine and methysergide—avoid concomitant use
- Lipid-regulating Drugs: possible increased risk of myopathy when saquinavir given with atorvastatin; possible increased risk of myopathy when saquinavir given with ●rosuvastatin—avoid concomitant use; increased risk of myopathy when saquinavir given with ●simvastatin (avoid concomitant use)
- Ranolazine: saquinavir possibly increases plasma concentration of ●ranolazine—manufacturer of ranolazine advises avoid concomitant use

  Sildenafil: saquinavir possibly increases plasma concentration of sildenafil—reduce initial dose of sildenafil

- Tacrolimus: saquinavir increases plasma concentration of ●tacrolimus (consider reducing dose of tacrolimus)

  Tadalafil: saquinavir possibly increases plasma concentration of tadalafil—reduce initial dose of tadalafil

  Ulcer-healing Drugs: plasma concentration of saquinavir possibly increased by cimetidine; plasma concentration of saquinavir increased by omeprazole

  Vardenafil: saquinavir possibly increases plasma concentration of vardenafil—reduce initial dose of vardenafil

Saxagliptin see Antidiabetics
Secobarbital see Barbiturates
Selegiline
Note. Selegiline is a MAO-B inhibitor
- Analgesics: hyperpyrexia and CNS toxicity reported when selegiline given with ●pethidine (avoid concomitant use); manufacturer of selegiline advises caution with tramadol
- Antidepressants: theoretical risk of serotonin syndrome if selegiline given with citalopram (especially if dose of selegiline exceeds 10 mg daily); caution with selegiline advised by manufacturer of escitalopram; increased risk of hypertension and CNS excitation when selegiline given with ●fluoxetine (selegiline should not be started until 5 weeks after stopping fluoxetine, avoid fluoxetine for 2 weeks after stopping selegiline); increased risk of hypertension and CNS excitation when selegiline given with ●fluvoxamine, ●sertraline or ●venlafaxine (selegiline should not be started until 1 week after stopping fluvoxamine, sertraline or venlafaxine, avoid fluvoxamine, sertraline or venlafaxine for 2 weeks after stopping selegiline); increased risk of hypertension and CNS excitation when selegiline given with ●paroxetine (selegiline should not be started until 2 weeks after stopping paroxetine, avoid paroxetine for 2 weeks after stopping selegiline); enhanced hypotensive effect when selegiline given with MAOIs; avoid concomitant use of selegiline with ●moclobemide; CNS toxicity reported when selegiline given with ●tricyclics
  Dopaminergics: max. dose of 10 mg selegiline advised by manufacturer of entacapone if used concomitantly; selegiline enhances effects and increases toxicity of levodopa (reduce dose of levodopa)
  Memantine: effects of dopaminergics and selegiline possibly enhanced by memantine
  Methyldopa: antiparkinsonian effect of dopaminergics antagonised by methyldopa
  Oestrogens: plasma concentration of selegiline increased by oestrogens (increased risk of toxicity)
  Progestogens: plasma concentration of selegiline increased by progestogens (increased risk of toxicity)
- Sympathomimetics: risk of hypertensive crisis when selegiline given with ●dopamine
Selenium
  Vitamins: absorption of selenium possibly reduced by ascorbic acid (give at least 4 hours apart)
Sertindole see Antipsychotics
Sertraline see Antidepressants, SSRI
Sevelamer
  Antibacterials: sevelamer reduces bioavailability of ciprofloxacin
  Ciclosporin: sevelamer possibly reduces plasma concentration of ciclosporin
  Mycophenolate: sevelamer possibly reduces plasma concentration of mycophenolate
  Tacrolimus: sevelamer possibly reduces plasma concentration of tacrolimus
  Thyroid Hormones: sevelamer possibly reduces absorption of levothyroxine
Sevoflurane see Anaesthetics, General
Sibutramine
  Analgesics: increased risk of bleeding when sibutramine given with NSAIDs or aspirin
  Anticoagulants: increased risk of bleeding when sibutramine given with anticoagulants
- Antidepressants: increased CNS toxicity when sibutramine given with ●MAOIs or ●moclobemide (manufacturer of sibutramine advises avoid concomitant use), also avoid sibutramine for 2 weeks after stopping MAOIs or moclobemide; increased risk of CNS toxicity when sibutramine given with ●SSRI-related antidepressants, ●SSRIs, ●mirtazapine, ●noradrenaline re-uptake inhibitors, ●tricyclic-

Sibutramine
- Antidepressants (continued)
  related antidepressants, ●tricyclics or ●tryptophan (manufacturer of sibutramine advises avoid concomitant use)
- Antipsychotics: increased risk of CNS toxicity when sibutramine given with ●antipsychotics (manufacturer of sibutramine advises avoid concomitant use)
Sildenafil
- Alpha-blockers: enhanced hypotensive effect when sildenafil given with ●alpha-blockers (avoid alpha-blockers for 4 hours after sildenafil)—see also
  Antibacterials: plasma concentration of sildenafil possibly increased by clarithromycin and telithromycin—reduce initial dose of sildenafil; plasma concentration of sildenafil increased by erythromycin—reduce initial dose of sildenafil
  Antifungals: plasma concentration of sildenafil increased by itraconazole and ketoconazole—reduce initial dose of sildenafil
- Antivirals: side-effects of sildenafil possibly increased by ●atazanavir; plasma concentration of sildenafil reduced by etravirine; plasma concentration of sildenafil possibly increased by fosamprenavir, nelfinavir and saquinavir—reduce initial dose of sildenafil; plasma concentration of sildenafil increased by ●indinavir—reduce initial dose of sildenafil; plasma concentration of sildenafil significantly increased by ●ritonavir—avoid concomitant use
  Bosentan: plasma concentration of sildenafil reduced by bosentan
  Calcium-channel Blockers: enhanced hypotensive effect when sildenafil given with amlodipine
  Grapefruit Juice: plasma concentration of sildenafil possibly increased by grapefruit juice
- Nicorandil: sildenafil significantly enhances hypotensive effect of ●nicorandil (avoid concomitant use)
- Nitrates: sildenafil significantly enhances hypotensive effect of ●nitrates (avoid concomitant use)
  Ulcer-healing Drugs: plasma concentration of sildenafil increased by cimetidine (reduce initial dose of sildenafil)
Simvastatin see Statins
Sirolimus
- Antibacterials: plasma concentration of sirolimus increased by ●clarithromycin and ●telithromycin—avoid concomitant use; plasma concentration of both drugs increased when sirolimus given with ●erythromycin; plasma concentration of sirolimus reduced by ●rifabutin and ●rifampicin—avoid concomitant use
- Antifungals: plasma concentration of sirolimus increased by ●itraconazole, ●ketoconazole and ●voriconazole—avoid concomitant use; plasma concentration of sirolimus increased by micafungin and ●miconazole; plasma concentration of sirolimus possibly increased by posaconazole
- Antivirals: plasma concentration of sirolimus possibly increased by ●atazanavir and lopinavir
- Calcium-channel Blockers: plasma concentration of sirolimus increased by ●diltiazem; plasma concentration of both drugs increased when sirolimus given with ●verapamil
  Ciclosporin: plasma concentration of sirolimus increased by ciclosporin
- Grapefruit Juice: plasma concentration of sirolimus increased by ●grapefruit juice—avoid concomitant use
Sitagliptin see Antidiabetics
Sitaxentan
- Anticoagulants: sitaxentan enhances anticoagulant effect of ●coumarins
- Ciclosporin: plasma concentration of sitaxentan increased by ●ciclosporin—avoid concomitant use

Sitaxentan *(continued)*

　　Oestrogens: sitaxentan increases plasma concentration of oestrogens

　　Progestogens: sitaxentan increases plasma concentration of progestogens

Sodium Aurothiomalate *see* Gold

Sodium Benzoate

　　Antiepileptics: effects of sodium benzoate possibly reduced by valproate

　　Antipsychotics: effects of sodium benzoate possibly reduced by haloperidol

　　Corticosteroids: effects of sodium benzoate possibly reduced by corticosteroids

　　Probenecid: excretion of conjugate formed by sodium benzoate possibly reduced by probenecid

Sodium Bicarbonate *see* Antacids

Sodium Clodronate *see* Bisphosphonates

Sodium Nitroprusside *see* Vasodilator Antihypertensives

Sodium Oxybate

- Analgesics: effects of sodium oxybate enhanced by ●opioid analgesics (avoid concomitant use)

　　Antidepressants: increased risk of side-effects when sodium oxybate given with tricyclics

　　Antipsychotics: effects of sodium oxybate possibly enhanced by antipsychotics

- Anxiolytics and Hypnotics: effects of sodium oxybate enhanced by ●benzodiazepines (avoid concomitant use)

- Barbiturates: effects of sodium oxybate enhanced by ●barbiturates (avoid concomitant use)

Sodium Phenylbutyrate

　　Antiepileptics: effects of sodium phenylbutyrate possibly reduced by valproate

　　Antipsychotics: effects of sodium phenylbutyrate possibly reduced by haloperidol

　　Corticosteroids: effects of sodium phenylbutyrate possibly reduced by corticosteroids

　　Probenecid: excretion of conjugate formed by sodium phenylbutyrate possibly reduced by probenecid

Sodium Valproate *see* Valproate

Solifenacin *see* Antimuscarinics

Somatropin

　　Corticosteroids: growth-promoting effect of somatropin may be inhibited by corticosteroids

　　Oestrogens: increased doses of somatropin may be needed when given with oestrogens (when used as oral replacement therapy)

Sorafenib

　　Antibacterials: bioavailability of sorafenib reduced by neomycin; plasma concentration of sorafenib reduced by rifampicin

- Anticoagulants: sorafenib possibly enhances anticoagulant effect of ●coumarins

　　Antiepileptics: cytotoxics possibly reduce absorption of phenytoin

- Antipsychotics: avoid concomitant use of cytotoxics with ●clozapine (increased risk of agranulocytosis)

　　Cardiac Glycosides: cytotoxics reduce absorption of digoxin tablets

　　Cytotoxics: sorafenib possibly increases plasma concentration of doxorubicin and irinotecan; sorafenib increases plasma concentration of docetaxel

Sotalol *see* Beta-blockers

Spironolactone *see* Diuretics

Statins

　　Antacids: absorption of rosuvastatin reduced by antacids

- Anti-arrhythmics: increased risk of myopathy when simvastatin given with ●amiodarone

- Antibacterials: plasma concentration of atorvastatin and pravastatin increased by ●clarithromycin; increased risk of myopathy when simvastatin given with ●clarithromycin, ●erythromycin or ●telithromycin (avoid concomitant use); plasma concentration of rosuvastatin reduced by erythromycin; possible increased risk of myopathy when atorvastatin given with erythromycin or

Statins

- Antibacterials *(continued)*

　　fusidic acid; plasma concentration of pravastatin increased by erythromycin; plasma concentration of atorvastatin and simvastatin possibly reduced by rifampicin; metabolism of fluvastatin accelerated by rifampicin (reduced effect); increased risk of myopathy when statins given with ●daptomycin (preferably avoid concomitant use); increased risk of myopathy when simvastatin given with ●fusidic acid; possible increased risk of myopathy when pravastatin given with telithromycin; increased risk of myopathy when atorvastatin given with ●telithromycin (avoid concomitant use)

- Anticoagulants: atorvastatin may transiently reduce anticoagulant effect of warfarin; fluvastatin and simvastatin enhance anticoagulant effect of ●coumarins; rosuvastatin possibly enhances anticoagulant effect of ●coumarins and ●phenindione

　　Antidepressants: plasma concentration of simvastatin reduced by St John's wort

　　Antidiabetics: fluvastatin possibly increases plasma concentration of glibenclamide

- Antiepileptics: plasma concentration of simvastatin reduced by ●carbamazepine—consider increasing dose of simvastatin; combination of fluvastatin with phenytoin may increase plasma concentration of either drug (or both)

- Antifungals: increased risk of myopathy when simvastatin given with ●itraconazole, ●ketoconazole or ●posaconazole (avoid concomitant use); possible increased risk of myopathy when simvastatin given with ●miconazole—avoid concomitant use; plasma concentration of fluvastatin increased by fluconazole; increased risk of myopathy when atorvastatin given with ●itraconazole or ●posaconazole (avoid concomitant use); possible increased risk of myopathy when atorvastatin or simvastatin given with imidazoles; possible increased risk of myopathy when atorvastatin or simvastatin given with triazoles

- Antivirals: increased risk of myopathy when simvastatin given with ●atazanavir, ●indinavir, ●nelfinavir, ●ritonavir or ●saquinavir (avoid concomitant use); possible increased risk of myopathy when atorvastatin given with atazanavir, fosamprenavir, indinavir, lopinavir, nelfinavir, ritonavir or saquinavir; possible increased risk of myopathy when rosuvastatin given with ●atazanavir, ●darunavir, ●fosamprenavir, ●indinavir, ●lopinavir, ●ritonavir or ●saquinavir—avoid concomitant use; plasma concentration of pravastatin possibly increased by darunavir; plasma concentration of atorvastatin, pravastatin and simvastatin reduced by efavirenz; plasma concentration of atorvastatin possibly reduced by etravirine; possible increased risk of myopathy when simvastatin given with ●fosamprenavir or ●lopinavir—avoid concomitant use; possible increased risk of myopathy when rosuvastatin given with ●nelfinavir—manufacturer of rosuvastatin advises avoid concomitant use; plasma concentration of simvastatin possibly increased by ●tipranavir—avoid concomitant use; plasma concentration of atorvastatin possibly increased by ●tipranavir (consider reducing dose of atorvastatin); plasma concentration of rosuvastatin possibly increased by ●tipranavir—manufacturer of rosuvastatin advises avoid concomitant use

　　Bosentan: plasma concentration of simvastatin reduced by bosentan

- Calcium-channel Blockers: plasma concentration of atorvastatin increased by diltiazem; possible increased risk of myopathy when simvastatin given with diltiazem; increased risk of myopathy when simvastatin given with ●verapamil

　　Cardiac Glycosides: atorvastatin possibly increases plasma concentration of digoxin

Statins *(continued)*

- Ciclosporin: increased risk of myopathy when statins given with ●ciclosporin; increased risk of myopathy when rosuvastatin given with ●ciclosporin (avoid concomitant use)
- Colchicine: possible increased risk of myopathy when statins given with ●colchicine

  Cytotoxics: plasma concentration of simvastatin possibly increased by dasatinib; plasma concentration of simvastatin increased by imatinib
- Grapefruit Juice: plasma concentration of atorvastatin possibly increased by grapefruit juice; plasma concentration of simvastatin increased by ●grapefruit juice—avoid concomitant use
- Hormone Antagonists: possible increased risk of myopathy when simvastatin given with ●danazol
- Lipid-regulating Drugs: increased risk of myopathy when statins given with ●gemfibrozil (preferably avoid concomitant use); increased risk of myopathy when statins given with ●fibrates; increased risk of myopathy when statins given with ●nicotinic acid (applies to lipid regulating doses of nicotinic acid)

  Oestrogens: atorvastatin and rosuvastatin increase plasma concentration of ethinylestradiol

  Progestogens: atorvastatin increases plasma concentration of norethisterone; rosuvastatin increases plasma concentration of norgestrel

  Ranolazine: plasma concentration of simvastatin increased by ranolazine (consider reducing dose of simvastatin)

  Retinoids: plasma concentration of simvastatin reduced by alitretinoin

Stavudine

- Antivirals: increased risk of side-effects when stavudine given with ●didanosine; effects of stavudine possibly inhibited by ●ribavirin; effects of stavudine possibly inhibited by ●zidovudine (manufacturers advise avoid concomitant use)
- Cytotoxics: effects of stavudine possibly inhibited by doxorubicin; increased risk of toxicity when stavudine given with ●hydroxycarbamide—avoid concomitant use

Stiripentol

- Antidepressants: anticonvulsant effect of antiepileptics possibly antagonised by MAOIs and ●tricyclic-related antidepressants (convulsive threshold lowered); anticonvulsant effect of antiepileptics antagonised by ●SSRIs and ●tricyclics (convulsive threshold lowered); avoid concomitant use of antiepileptics with ●St John's wort
- Antiepileptics: stiripentol increases plasma concentration of ●carbamazepine and ●phenytoin
- Antimalarials: possible increased risk of convulsions when antiepileptics given with chloroquine and hydroxychloroquine; anticonvulsant effect of antiepileptics antagonised by ●mefloquine

  Anxiolytics and Hypnotics: stiripentol increases plasma concentration of clobazam
- Barbiturates: stiripentol increases plasma concentration of ●phenobarbital
- Orlistat: possible increased risk of convulsions when antiepileptics given with ●orlistat

Streptomycin *see* Aminoglycosides

Strontium Ranelate

  Antibacterials: strontium ranelate reduces absorption of quinolones and tetracyclines (manufacturer of strontium ranelate advises avoid concomitant use)

Sucralfate

  Antibacterials: sucralfate reduces absorption of ciprofloxacin, levofloxacin, moxifloxacin, norfloxacin, ofloxacin and tetracyclines
- Anticoagulants: sucralfate possibly reduces absorption of ●coumarins (reduced anticoagulant effect)
- Antiepileptics: sucralfate reduces absorption of ●phenytoin

Sucralfate *(continued)*

  Antifungals: sucralfate reduces absorption of ketoconazole

  Antipsychotics: sucralfate reduces absorption of sulpiride

  Cardiac Glycosides: sucralfate possibly reduces absorption of cardiac glycosides

  Theophylline: sucralfate possibly reduces absorption of theophylline (give at least 2 hours apart)

  Thyroid Hormones: sucralfate reduces absorption of levothyroxine

  Ulcer-healing Drugs: sucralfate possibly reduces absorption of lansoprazole

Sugammadex

  Antibacterials: response to sugammadex possibly reduced by flucloxacillin and fusidic acid

  Hormone Antagonists: response to sugammadex possibly reduced by toremifene

  Oestrogens: sugammadex possibly reduces plasma concentration of oestrogens

  Progestogens: sugammadex possibly reduces plasma concentration of progestogens

Sulfadiazine *see* Sulphonamides

Sulfadoxine *see* Sulphonamides

Sulfamethoxazole *see* Sulphonamides

Sulfasalazine *see* Aminosalicylates

Sulfinpyrazone

  Analgesics: effects of sulfinpyrazone antagonised by aspirin

  Antibacterials: sulfinpyrazone reduces excretion of nitrofurantoin (increased risk of toxicity); sulfinpyrazone reduces excretion of penicillins; effects of sulfinpyrazone antagonised by pyrazinamide
- Anticoagulants: sulfinpyrazone enhances anticoagulant effect of ●coumarins
- Antidiabetics: sulfinpyrazone enhances effects of ●sulphonylureas
- Antiepileptics: sulfinpyrazone increases plasma concentration of ●phenytoin
- Ciclosporin: sulfinpyrazone reduces plasma concentration of ●ciclosporin

  Theophylline: sulfinpyrazone reduces plasma concentration of theophylline

Sulindac *see* NSAIDs

Sulphonamides

  Anaesthetics, General: sulphonamides enhance effects of thiopental

  Anaesthetics, Local: increased risk of methaemoglobinaemia when sulphonamides given with prilocaine
- Anti-arrhythmics: increased risk of ventricular arrhythmias when sulfamethoxazole (as co-trimoxazole) given with ●amiodarone—avoid concomitant use of co-trimoxazole
- Antibacterials: increased risk of crystalluria when sulphonamides given with ●methenamine
- Anticoagulants: sulphonamides enhance anticoagulant effect of ●coumarins

  Antidiabetics: sulphonamides rarely enhance the effects of sulphonylureas

  Antiepileptics: sulphonamides possibly increase plasma concentration of phenytoin
- Antimalarials: increased antifolate effect when sulphonamides given with ●pyrimethamine
- Antipsychotics: avoid concomitant use of sulphonamides with ●clozapine (increased risk of agranulocytosis)
- Azathioprine: increased risk of haematological toxicity when sulfamethoxazole (as co-trimoxazole) given with ●azathioprine
- Ciclosporin: increased risk of nephrotoxicity when sulphonamides given with ●ciclosporin; sulfadiazine possibly reduces plasma concentration of ●ciclosporin
- Cytotoxics: increased risk of haematological toxicity when sulfamethoxazole (as co-trimoxazole) given

Sulphonamides
- Cytotoxics *(continued)*
  with ●mercaptopurine or ●methotrexate; sulphonamides increase risk of methotrexate toxicity

  Oestrogens: antibacterials that do not induce liver enzymes possibly reduce contraceptive effect of oestrogens (risk probably small, see p. 486)

  Potassium Aminobenzoate: effects of sulphonamides inhibited by potassium aminobenzoate

  Vaccines: antibacterials inactivate oral typhoid vaccine–see p. 760

Sulphonylureas *see* Antidiabetics

Sulpiride *see* Antipsychotics

Sumatriptan *see* 5HT₁ Agonists

Sunitinib
Antibacterials: metabolism of sunitinib accelerated by rifampicin (reduced plasma concentration)

Antiepileptics: cytotoxics possibly reduce absorption of phenytoin

Antifungals: metabolism of sunitinib inhibited by ketoconazole (increased plasma concentration)
- Antipsychotics: avoid concomitant use of cytotoxics with ●clozapine (increased risk of agranulocytosis)

Cardiac Glycosides: cytotoxics reduce absorption of digoxin tablets

Suxamethonium *see* Muscle Relaxants

Sympathomimetics
- Adrenergic Neurone Blockers: ephedrine, isometheptene, metaraminol, methylphenidate, noradrenaline (norepinephrine), oxymetazoline, phenylephrine, pseudoephedrine and xylometazoline antagonise hypotensive effect of ●adrenergic neurone blockers; dexamfetamine antagonises hypotensive effect of ●guanethidine

  Alcohol: effects of methylphenidate possibly enhanced by alcohol
- Alpha-blockers: avoid concomitant use of adrenaline (epinephrine) or dopamine with ●tolazoline
- Anaesthetics, General: increased risk of hypertension when methylphenidate given with ●volatile liquid general anaesthetics; increased risk of arrhythmias when adrenaline (epinephrine) given with ●volatile liquid general anaesthetics
- Anticoagulants: methylphenidate possibly enhances anticoagulant effect of ●coumarins
- Antidepressants: risk of hypertensive crisis when methylphenidate given with ●MAOIs, some manufacturers advise avoid methylphenidate for at least 2 weeks after stopping MAOIs; risk of hypertensive crisis when sympathomimetics given with ●MAOIs or ●moclobemide; methylphenidate possibly inhibits metabolism of SSRIs and tricyclics; increased risk of hypertension and arrhythmias when noradrenaline (norepinephrine) given with ●tricyclics; increased risk of hypertension and arrhythmias when adrenaline (epinephrine) given with ●tricyclics (but local anaesthetics with adrenaline appear to be safe)

  Antiepileptics: methylphenidate increases plasma concentration of phenytoin; methylphenidate possibly increases plasma concentration of primidone

  Antipsychotics: hypertensive effect of sympathomimetics antagonised by antipsychotics; dexamfetamine possibly antagonises antipsychotic effects of chlorpromazine; methylphenidate possibly increases side-effects of risperidone

  Antivirals: plasma concentration of dexamfetamine possibly increased by ritonavir

  Barbiturates: methylphenidate possibly increases plasma concentration of phenobarbital
- Beta-blockers: increased risk of severe hypertension and bradycardia when adrenaline (epinephrine) given with non-cardioselective ●beta-blockers, also response to adrenaline (epinephrine) may be reduced; increased risk of severe hypertension and bradycardia when dobutamine given with non-

Sympathomimetics
- Beta-blockers *(continued)*
  cardioselective ●beta-blockers; possible increased risk of severe hypertension and bradycardia when noradrenaline (norepinephrine) given with non-cardioselective ●beta-blockers
- Clonidine: possible risk of hypertension when adrenaline (epinephrine) or noradrenaline (norepinephrine) given with clonidine; serious adverse events reported with concomitant use of methylphenidate and ●clonidine (causality not established)

  Corticosteroids: ephedrine accelerates metabolism of dexamethasone
- Dopaminergics: risk of toxicity when isometheptene given with ●bromocriptine; effects of adrenaline (epinephrine), dobutamine, dopamine and noradrenaline (norepinephrine) possibly enhanced by entacapone; avoid concomitant use of sympathomimetics with ●rasagiline; risk of hypertensive crisis when dopamine given with ●selegiline

  Doxapram: increased risk of hypertension when sympathomimetics given with doxapram

  Ergot Alkaloids: increased risk of ergotism when sympathomimetics given with ergotamine and methysergide

  Oxytocin: risk of hypertension when vasoconstrictor sympathomimetics given with oxytocin (due to enhanced vasopressor effect)
- Sympathomimetics: effects of adrenaline (epinephrine) possibly enhanced by ●dopexamine; dopexamine possibly enhances effects of ●noradrenaline (norepinephrine)

  Theophylline: avoidance of ephedrine in children advised by manufacturer of theophylline

Sympathomimetics, Beta₂
Atomoxetine: Increased risk of cardiovascular side-effects when *parenteral* salbutamol given with atomoxetine

Cardiac Glycosides: salbutamol possibly reduces plasma concentration of digoxin

Corticosteroids: increased risk of hypokalaemia when high doses of beta₂ sympathomimetics given with corticosteroids—see Hypokalaemia, p. 177

Diuretics: increased risk of hypokalaemia when high doses of beta₂ sympathomimetics given with acetazolamide, loop diuretics or thiazides and related diuretics—see Hypokalaemia, p. 177
- Methyldopa: acute hypotension reported when *infusion* of salbutamol given with ●methyldopa

  Muscle Relaxants: bambuterol enhances effects of suxamethonium

  Theophylline: increased risk of hypokalaemia when high doses of beta₂ sympathomimetics given with theophylline—see Hypokalaemia, p. 177

Tacrolimus
Note. Interactions do not generally apply to tacrolimus used topically; risk of facial flushing and skin irritation with alcohol consumption (p. 700) does not apply to tacrolimus taken systemically
- Analgesics: possible increased risk of nephrotoxicity when tacrolimus given with NSAIDs; increased risk of nephrotoxicity when tacrolimus given with ●ibuprofen

  Angiotensin-II Receptor Antagonists: increased risk of hyperkalaemia when tacrolimus given with angiotensin-II receptor antagonists
- Antibacterials: plasma concentration of tacrolimus increased by ●clarithromycin, ●erythromycin and ●quinupristin/dalfopristin; plasma concentration of tacrolimus possibly reduced by rifabutin; plasma concentration of tacrolimus reduced by ●rifampicin; increased risk of nephrotoxicity when tacrolimus given with ●aminoglycosides; plasma concentration of tacrolimus possibly increased by ●chloramphenicol and ●telithromycin;

Tacrolimus

- Antibacterials *(continued)*
  possible increased risk of nephrotoxicity when tacrolimus given with vancomycin
- Antidepressants: plasma concentration of tacrolimus reduced by ●St John's wort—avoid concomitant use
  Antiepileptics: plasma concentration of tacrolimus reduced by phenytoin, also plasma concentration of phenytoin possibly increased
- Antifungals: plasma concentration of tacrolimus increased by ●fluconazole, ●itraconazole, ●ketoconazole and ●voriconazole; increased risk of nephrotoxicity when tacrolimus given with ●amphotericin; plasma concentration of tacrolimus increased by ●posaconazole (reduce dose of tacrolimus); plasma concentration of tacrolimus reduced by ●caspofungin; plasma concentration of tacrolimus possibly increased by ●imidazoles and ●triazoles
- Antipsychotics: avoidance of tacrolimus advised by manufacturer of ●droperidol (risk of ventricular arrhythmias)
- Antivirals: possible increased risk of nephrotoxicity when tacrolimus given with aciclovir or ganciclovir; plasma concentration of tacrolimus possibly increased by ●atazanavir, ●nelfinavir and ●ritonavir; plasma concentration of tacrolimus possibly affected by efavirenz; plasma concentration of tacrolimus increased by ●saquinavir (consider reducing dose of tacrolimus)
- Barbiturates: plasma concentration of tacrolimus reduced by ●phenobarbital
- Calcium-channel Blockers: plasma concentration of tacrolimus possibly increased by felodipine, nicardipine and verapamil; plasma concentration of tacrolimus increased by ●diltiazem and ●nifedipine
- Ciclosporin: tacrolimus increases plasma concentration of ●ciclosporin (increased risk of nephrotoxicity)—avoid concomitant use
- Diuretics: increased risk of hyperkalaemia when tacrolimus given with ●potassium-sparing diuretics and aldosterone antagonists
- Grapefruit Juice: plasma concentration of tacrolimus increased by ●grapefruit juice
  Hormone Antagonists: plasma concentration of tacrolimus possibly increased by danazol
  Mifamurtide: avoidance of tacrolimus advised by manufacturer of mifamurtide
  Oestrogens: tacrolimus possibly inhibits metabolism of oestrogens; plasma concentration of tacrolimus possibly increased by ethinylestradiol
- Potassium Salts: increased risk of hyperkalaemia when tacrolimus given with ●potassium salts
  Progestogens: tacrolimus possibly inhibits metabolism of progestogens
  Sevelamer: plasma concentration of tacrolimus possibly reduced by sevelamer
  Ulcer-healing Drugs: plasma concentration of tacrolimus possibly increased by omeprazole

Tadalafil

- Alpha-blockers: enhanced hypotensive effect when tadalafil given with ●doxazosin—manufacturer of tadalafil advises avoid concomitant use; enhanced hypotensive effect when tadalafil given with ●alpha-blockers—see also
  Antibacterials: plasma concentration of tadalafil possibly increased by clarithromycin and erythromycin; plasma concentration of tadalafil reduced by rifampicin
  Antifungals: plasma concentration of tadalafil increased by ketoconazole; plasma concentration of tadalafil possibly increased by itraconazole
  Antivirals: plasma concentration of tadalafil possibly increased by fosamprenavir and indinavir; plasma concentration of tadalafil increased by ritonavir; plasma concentration of tadalafil possibly increased by saquinavir—reduce initial dose of tadalafil

Tadalafil *(continued)*

  Grapefruit Juice: plasma concentration of tadalafil possibly increased by grapefruit juice
- Nicorandil: tadalafil significantly enhances hypotensive effect of ●nicorandil (avoid concomitant use)
- Nitrates: tadalafil significantly enhances hypotensive effect of ●nitrates (avoid concomitant use)

Tamoxifen

  Antibacterials: metabolism of tamoxifen accelerated by rifampicin (reduced plasma concentration)
- Anticoagulants: tamoxifen enhances anticoagulant effect of ●coumarins
- Antidepressants: metabolism of tamoxifen to active metabolite possibly inhibited by ●duloxetine, ●fluoxetine and ●paroxetine (avoid concomitant use)
- Antipsychotics: avoidance of tamoxifen advised by manufacturer of ●droperidol (risk of ventricular arrhythmias)
- Bupropion: metabolism of tamoxifen to active metabolite possibly inhibited by ●bupropion (avoid concomitant use)

Tamsulosin *see Alpha-blockers*

Taxanes *see Docetaxel and Paclitaxel*

Tegafur with uracil *see Fluorouracil*

Teicoplanin

  Antibacterials: increased risk of nephrotoxicity and ototoxicity when teicoplanin given with colistin
  Oestrogens: antibacterials that do not induce liver enzymes possibly reduce contraceptive effect of oestrogens (risk probably small, see p. 486)
  Vaccines: antibacterials inactivate oral typhoid vaccine—see p. 760

Telbivudine

- Interferons: increased risk of peripheral neuropathy when telbivudine given with ●interferon alfa

Telithromycin

- Antibacterials: plasma concentration of telithromycin reduced by ●rifampicin (avoid during and for 2 weeks after rifampicin)
- Antidepressants: plasma concentration of telithromycin reduced by ●St John's wort (avoid during and for 2 weeks after St John's wort)
- Antiepileptics: plasma concentration of telithromycin reduced by ●carbamazepine, ●phenytoin and ●primidone (avoid during and for 2 weeks after carbamazepine, phenytoin and primidone)
- Antifungals: manufacturer of telithromycin advises avoid concomitant use with ●ketoconazole in severe renal and hepatic impairment
  Antimuscarinics: manufacturer of fesoterodine advises dose reduction when telithromycin given with fesoterodine—consult fesoterodine product literature
- Antipsychotics: increased risk of ventricular arrhythmias when telithromycin given with ●pimozide—avoid concomitant use
- Antivirals: manufacturer of telithromycin advises avoid concomitant use with ●atazanavir, ●fosamprenavir, ●indinavir, ●lopinavir, ●nelfinavir, ●ritonavir, ●saquinavir and ●tipranavir in severe renal and hepatic impairment; telithromycin possibly increases plasma concentration of ●maraviroc (consider reducing dose of maraviroc)
- Anxiolytics and Hypnotics: telithromycin inhibits metabolism of ●midazolam (increased plasma concentration with increased sedation)
  Aprepitant: telithromycin possibly increases plasma concentration of aprepitant
- Barbiturates: plasma concentration of telithromycin reduced by ●phenobarbital (avoid during and for 2 weeks after phenobarbital)
  Cardiac Glycosides: telithromycin possibly increases plasma concentration of digoxin
- Ciclosporin: telithromycin possibly increases plasma concentration of ●ciclosporin

Telithromycin *(continued)*

- Cytotoxics: telithromycin possibly increases plasma concentration of ●everolimus—manufacturer of everolimus advises avoid concomitant use; avoidance of telithromycin advised by manufacturer of ●lapatinib and ●nilotinib
- Diuretics: telithromycin increases plasma concentration of ●eplerenone—avoid concomitant use
- Ergot Alkaloids: increased risk of ergotism when telithromycin given with ●ergotamine and methysergide—avoid concomitant use
- Ivabradine: telithromycin possibly increases plasma concentration of ●ivabradine—avoid concomitant use
- Lipid-regulating Drugs: increased risk of myopathy when telithromycin given with ●atorvastatin or ●simvastatin (avoid concomitant use); possible increased risk of myopathy when telithromycin given with pravastatin

  Oestrogens: antibacterials that do not induce liver enzymes possibly reduce contraceptive effect of oestrogens (risk probably small, see p. 486)
- Ranolazine: telithromycin possibly increases plasma concentration of ●ranolazine—manufacturer of ranolazine advises avoid concomitant use

  Sildenafil: telithromycin possibly increases plasma concentration of sildenafil—reduce initial dose of sildenafil
- Sirolimus: telithromycin increases plasma concentration of ●sirolimus—avoid concomitant use
- Tacrolimus: telithromycin possibly increases plasma concentration of ●tacrolimus

  Vaccines: antibacterials inactivate oral typhoid vaccine—see p. 760

Telmisartan *see* Angiotensin-II Receptor Antagonists

Temazepam *see* Anxiolytics and Hypnotics

Temocillin *see* Penicillins

Temoporfin

- Cytotoxics: increased skin photosensitivity when temoporfin given with *topical* ●fluorouracil

Temozolomide

  Antiepileptics: cytotoxics possibly reduce absorption of phenytoin; plasma concentration of temozolomide increased by valproate
- Antipsychotics: avoid concomitant use of cytotoxics with ●clozapine (increased risk of agranulocytosis)

  Cardiac Glycosides: cytotoxics reduce absorption of digoxin tablets

Temsirolimus

  Note. The main active metabolite of temsirolimus is sirolimus—*see also* interactions of sirolimus and consult product literature
- Antibacterials: plasma concentration of active metabolite of temsirolimus reduced by ●rifampicin—avoid concomitant use

  Antiepileptics: cytotoxics possibly reduce absorption of phenytoin
- Antifungals: plasma concentration of active metabolite of temsirolimus increased by ●ketoconazole—avoid concomitant use
- Antipsychotics: avoid concomitant use of cytotoxics with ●clozapine (increased risk of agranulocytosis)

  Cardiac Glycosides: cytotoxics reduce absorption of digoxin tablets

Tenofovir

- Antivirals: manufacturer of tenofovir advises avoid concomitant use with adefovir; tenofovir reduces plasma concentration of atazanavir, also plasma concentration of tenofovir possibly increased; combination of tenofovir with cidofovir may increase plasma concentration of either drug (or both); tenofovir increases plasma concentration of ●didanosine (increased risk of toxicity)—avoid concomitant use; plasma concentration of tenofovir increased by lopinavir

Tenoxicam *see* NSAIDs

Terazosin *see* Alpha-blockers

Terbinafine

- Antibacterials: plasma concentration of terbinafine reduced by ●rifampicin

  Antidepressants: terbinafine possibly increases plasma concentration of imipramine and nortriptyline

  Ciclosporin: terbinafine possibly reduces plasma concentration of ciclosporin

  Oestrogens: occasional reports of breakthrough bleeding when terbinafine given with oestrogens (when used for contraception)

  Progestogens: occasional reports of breakthrough bleeding when terbinafine given with progestogens (when used for contraception)

  Ulcer-healing Drugs: plasma concentration of terbinafine increased by cimetidine

Terbutaline *see* Sympathomimetics, Beta₂

Terpene Mixture *see* Rowachol®

Testolactone

- Anticoagulants: testolactone enhances anticoagulant effect of ●coumarins and ●phenindione

Testosterone

- Anticoagulants: testosterone enhances anticoagulant effect of ●coumarins and ●phenindione

  Antidiabetics: testosterone possibly enhances hypoglycaemic effect of antidiabetics

Tetrabenazine

- Antidepressants: risk of CNS excitation and hypertension when tetrabenazine given with ●MAOIs

  Antipsychotics: increased risk of extrapyramidal side-effects when tetrabenazine given with antipsychotics

  Dopaminergics: increased risk of extrapyramidal side-effects when tetrabenazine given with amantadine

  Metoclopramide: increased risk of extrapyramidal side-effects when tetrabenazine given with metoclopramide

Tetracosactide *see* Corticosteroids

Tetracycline *see* Tetracyclines

Tetracyclines

  ACE Inhibitors: absorption of tetracyclines reduced by quinapril tablets (quinapril tablets contain magnesium carbonate)

  Adsorbents: absorption of tetracyclines possibly reduced by kaolin

  Antacids: absorption of tetracyclines reduced by antacids

  Antibacterials: plasma concentration of doxycycline reduced by rifampicin—consider increasing dose of doxycycline; tetracyclines possibly antagonise effects of penicillins
- Anticoagulants: tetracyclines possibly enhance anticoagulant effect of ●coumarins and ●phenindione

  Antidiabetics: tetracyclines possibly enhance hypoglycaemic effect of sulphonylureas

  Antiepileptics: metabolism of doxycycline accelerated by carbamazepine (reduced effect); metabolism of doxycycline accelerated by phenytoin and primidone (reduced plasma concentration)

  Atovaquone: tetracycline reduces plasma concentration of atovaquone

  Barbiturates: metabolism of doxycycline accelerated by barbiturates (reduced plasma concentration)

  Calcium Salts: absorption of tetracycline reduced by calcium salts
- Ciclosporin: doxycycline possibly increases plasma concentration of ●ciclosporin

  Cytotoxics: doxycycline or tetracycline increase risk of methotrexate toxicity

  Dairy Products: absorption of tetracyclines (except doxycycline and minocycline) reduced by dairy products

  Diuretics: manufacturer of lymecycline advises avoid concomitant use with diuretics

  Ergot Alkaloids: increased risk of ergotism when tetracyclines given with ergotamine and methysergide

Tetracyclines *(continued)*

Iron: absorption of tetracyclines reduced by *oral* iron, also absorption of *oral* iron reduced by tetracyclines

Lipid-regulating Drugs: absorption of tetracycline possibly reduced by colestipol and colestyramine

Oestrogens: antibacterials that do not induce liver enzymes possibly reduce contraceptive effect of oestrogens (risk probably small, see p. 486)

• Retinoids: possible increased risk of benign intracranial hypertension when tetracyclines given with ●retinoids (avoid concomitant use)

Strontium Ranelate: absorption of tetracyclines reduced by strontium ranelate (manufacturer of strontium ranelate advises avoid concomitant use)

Ulcer-healing Drugs: absorption of tetracyclines reduced by sucralfate and tripotassium dicitratobismuthate

Vaccines: antibacterials inactivate oral typhoid vaccine–see p. 760

Zinc: absorption of tetracyclines reduced by zinc, also absorption of zinc reduced by tetracyclines

Theophylline

Allopurinol: plasma concentration of theophylline possibly increased by allopurinol

Anaesthetics, General: increased risk of convulsions when theophylline given with ketamine; increased risk of arrhythmias when theophylline given with halothane

Anti-arrhythmics: theophylline antagonises anti-arrhythmic effect of adenosine; plasma concentration of theophylline increased by propafenone

• Antibacterials: plasma concentration of theophylline possibly increased by azithromycin and isoniazid; metabolism of theophylline inhibited by ●clarithromycin (increased plasma concentration); metabolism of theophylline inhibited by ●erythromycin (increased plasma concentration), if erythromycin given *by mouth*, also decreased plasma-erythromycin concentration; plasma concentration of theophylline increased by ●ciprofloxacin and ●norfloxacin; metabolism of theophylline accelerated by rifampicin (reduced plasma concentration); possible increased risk of convulsions when theophylline given with ●quinolones

• Antidepressants: plasma concentration of theophylline increased by ●fluvoxamine (concomitant use should usually be avoided, but where not possible halve theophylline dose and monitor plasma-theophylline concentration); plasma concentration of theophylline reduced by ●St John's wort—avoid concomitant use

• Antiepileptics: metabolism of theophylline accelerated by carbamazepine and primidone (reduced effect); plasma concentration of both drugs reduced when theophylline given with ●phenytoin

• Antifungals: plasma concentration of theophylline possibly increased by ●fluconazole and ●ketoconazole

• Antivirals: plasma concentration of theophylline possibly increased by aciclovir; metabolism of theophylline accelerated by ●ritonavir (reduced plasma concentration)

Anxiolytics and Hypnotics: theophylline possibly reduces effects of benzodiazepines

Barbiturates: metabolism of theophylline accelerated by barbiturates (reduced effect)

• Calcium-channel Blockers: plasma concentration of theophylline possibly increased by ●calcium-channel blockers (enhanced effect); plasma concentration of theophylline increased by diltiazem; plasma concentration of theophylline increased by ●verapamil (enhanced effect)

Corticosteroids: increased risk of hypokalaemia when theophylline given with corticosteroids

Cytotoxics: plasma concentration of theophylline possibly increased by methotrexate

Theophylline *(continued)*

Disulfiram: metabolism of theophylline inhibited by disulfiram (increased risk of toxicity)

Diuretics: increased risk of hypokalaemia when theophylline given with acetazolamide, loop diuretics or thiazides and related diuretics

Doxapram: increased CNS stimulation when theophylline given with doxapram

Interferons: metabolism of theophylline inhibited by interferon alfa (increased plasma concentration)

Leukotriene Receptor Antagonists: plasma concentration of theophylline possibly increased by zafirlukast, also plasma concentration of zafirlukast reduced

Lithium: theophylline increases excretion of lithium (reduced plasma concentration)

Oestrogens: excretion of theophylline reduced by oestrogens (increased plasma concentration)

Pentoxifylline: plasma concentration of theophylline increased by pentoxifylline

Sulfinpyrazone: plasma concentration of theophylline reduced by sulfinpyrazone

Sympathomimetics: manufacturer of theophylline advises avoid concomitant use with ephedrine in children

Sympathomimetics, Beta$_2$: increased risk of hypokalaemia when theophylline given with high doses of beta$_2$ sympathomimetics—see Hypokalaemia, p. 177

Tobacco: metabolism of theophylline increased by tobacco smoking (reduced plasma concentration)

• Ulcer-healing Drugs: metabolism of theophylline inhibited by ●cimetidine (increased plasma concentration); absorption of theophylline possibly reduced by sucralfate (give at least 2 hours apart)

Vaccines: plasma concentration of theophylline possibly increased by influenza vaccine

Thiazolidinediones *see* Antidiabetics

Thiopental *see* Anaesthetics, General

Thiotepa

Antiepileptics: cytotoxics possibly reduce absorption of phenytoin

• Antipsychotics: avoid concomitant use of cytotoxics with ●clozapine (increased risk of agranulocytosis)

Cardiac Glycosides: cytotoxics reduce absorption of digoxin tablets

Muscle Relaxants: thiotepa enhances effects of suxamethonium

Thioxanthenes *see* Antipsychotics

Thyroid Hormones

Antacids: absorption of levothyroxine possibly reduced by antacids

Anti-arrhythmics: for concomitant use of thyroid hormones and amiodarone see p. 110

Antibacterials: metabolism of levothyroxine accelerated by rifampicin (may increase requirements for levothyroxine in hypothyroidism)

• Anticoagulants: thyroid hormones enhance anticoagulant effect of ●coumarins and ●phenindione

Antidepressants: thyroid hormones enhance effects of amitriptyline and imipramine; thyroid hormones possibly enhance effects of tricyclics

Antiepileptics: metabolism of thyroid hormones accelerated by carbamazepine and primidone (may increase requirements for thyroid hormones in hypothyroidism); metabolism of thyroid hormones accelerated by phenytoin (may increase requirements in hypothyroidism), also plasma concentration of phenytoin possibly increased

Barbiturates: metabolism of thyroid hormones accelerated by barbiturates (may increase requirements for thyroid hormones in hypothyroidism)

Beta-blockers: levothyroxine accelerates metabolism of propranolol

Calcium Salts: absorption of levothyroxine reduced by calcium salts

Cytotoxics: plasma concentration of levothyroxine possibly reduced by imatinib

Thyroid Hormones *(continued)*

Iron: absorption of levothyroxine reduced by *oral* iron (give at least 2 hours apart)

Lipid-regulating Drugs: absorption of thyroid hormones reduced by colestipol and colestyramine

Oestrogens: requirements for thyroid hormones in hypothyroidism may be increased by oestrogens

Orlistat: possible increased risk of hypothyroidism when levothyroxine given with orlistat

Polystyrene Sulphonate Resins: absorption of levothyroxine reduced by polystyrene sulphonate resins

Sevelamer: absorption of levothyroxine possibly reduced by sevelamer

Ulcer-healing Drugs: absorption of levothyroxine reduced by cimetidine and sucralfate

Tiagabine

• Antidepressants: anticonvulsant effect of antiepileptics possibly antagonised by MAOIs and ●tricyclic-related antidepressants (convulsive threshold lowered); anticonvulsant effect of antiepileptics antagonised by ●SSRIs and ●tricyclics (convulsive threshold lowered); avoid concomitant use of antiepileptics with ●St John's wort

Antiepileptics: plasma concentration of tiagabine reduced by carbamazepine, phenytoin and primidone

• Antimalarials: possible increased risk of convulsions when antiepileptics given with chloroquine and hydroxychloroquine; anticonvulsant effect of antiepileptics antagonised by ●mefloquine

Barbiturates: plasma concentration of tiagabine reduced by phenobarbital

• Orlistat: possible increased risk of convulsions when antiepileptics given with ●orlistat

Tiaprofenic Acid *see* NSAIDs

Tibolone

Antibacterials: metabolism of tibolone accelerated by rifampicin (reduced plasma concentration)

Antiepileptics: metabolism of tibolone accelerated by carbamazepine and primidone (reduced plasma concentration); metabolism of tibolone accelerated by phenytoin

Barbiturates: metabolism of tibolone accelerated by barbiturates (reduced plasma concentration)

Ticarcillin *see* Penicillins

Tigecycline

Anticoagulants: tigecycline possibly enhances anticoagulant effect of coumarins

Oestrogens: antibacterials that do not induce liver enzymes possibly reduce contraceptive effect of oestrogens (risk probably small, see p. 486)

Vaccines: antibacterials inactivate oral typhoid vaccine–see p. 760

Tiludronic Acid *see* Bisphosphonates

Timolol *see* Beta-blockers

Tinidazole

Alcohol: possibility of disulfiram-like reaction when tinidazole given with alcohol

Oestrogens: antibacterials that do not induce liver enzymes possibly reduce contraceptive effect of oestrogens (risk probably small, see p. 486)

Vaccines: antibacterials inactivate oral typhoid vaccine–see p. 760

Tinzaparin *see* Heparins

Tioguanine

Antiepileptics: cytotoxics possibly reduce absorption of phenytoin

• Antipsychotics: avoid concomitant use of cytotoxics with ●clozapine (increased risk of agranulocytosis)

Cardiac Glycosides: cytotoxics reduce absorption of digoxin tablets

Cytotoxics: increased risk of hepatotoxicity when tioguanine given with busulfan

Tiotropium *see* Antimuscarinics

Tipranavir

Analgesics: plasma concentration of tipranavir possibly reduced by buprenorphine

Antacids: absorption of tipranavir reduced by antacids

• Antibacterials: tipranavir increases plasma concentration of ●clarithromycin (reduce dose of clarithromycin in renal impairment), also plasma concentration of tipranavir increased by clarithromycin; tipranavir increases plasma concentration of ●rifabutin (reduce dose of rifabutin); plasma concentration of tipranavir possibly reduced by ●rifampicin—avoid concomitant use; avoidance of concomitant tipranavir in severe renal and hepatic impairment advised by manufacturer of ●telithromycin

Anticoagulants: avoidance of tipranavir advised by manufacturer of rivaroxaban

• Antidepressants: plasma concentration of tipranavir possibly reduced by ●St John's wort—avoid concomitant use

Antiepileptics: plasma concentration of tipranavir possibly reduced by carbamazepine

Antifungals: plasma concentration of tipranavir increased by fluconazole

Antimalarials: caution with tipranavir advised by manufacturer of artemether/lumefantrine

Antimuscarinics: avoidance of tipranavir advised by manufacturer of darifenacin

• Antivirals: tipranavir reduces plasma concentration of ●abacavir, ●didanosine, ●fosamprenavir, ●lopinavir, ●saquinavir and ●zidovudine; plasma concentration of tipranavir increased by atazanavir (also plasma concentration of atazanavir reduced); tipranavir reduces plasma concentration of ●etravirine, also plasma concentration of tipranavir increased (avoid concomitant use)

• Beta-blockers: manufacturer of tipranavir advises avoid concomitant use with ●metoprolol for heart failure

• Lipid-regulating Drugs: tipranavir possibly increases plasma concentration of ●atorvastatin (consider reducing dose of atorvastatin); tipranavir possibly increases plasma concentration of ●rosuvastatin—manufacturer of rosuvastatin advises avoid concomitant use; tipranavir possibly increases plasma concentration of ●simvastatin—avoid concomitant use

• Ranolazine: tipranavir possibly increases plasma concentration of ●ranolazine—manufacturer of ranolazine advises avoid concomitant use

• Ulcer-healing Drugs: tipranavir reduces plasma concentration of ●esomeprazole and ●omeprazole

Vitamins: increased risk of bleeding when tipranavir given with high doses of vitamin E

Tirofiban

Iloprost: increased risk of bleeding when tirofiban given with iloprost

Tizanidine *see* Muscle Relaxants

Tobacco

Cinacalcet: tobacco smoking increases cinacalcet metabolism (reduced plasma concentration)

Cytotoxics: tobacco smoking reduces plasma concentration of erlotinib

Theophylline: tobacco smoking increases theophylline metabolism (reduced plasma concentration)

Tobramycin *see* Aminoglycosides

Tocilizumab

• Vaccines: avoid concomitant use of tocilizumab with live ●vaccines (see p. 733)

Tolazoline *see* Alpha-blockers

Tolbutamide *see* Antidiabetics

Tolcapone

Antidepressants: avoid concomitant use of tolcapone with MAOIs

Memantine: effects of dopaminergics possibly enhanced by memantine

Tolcapone *(continued)*

Methyldopa: antiparkinsonian effect of dopaminergic antagonised by methyldopa

Tolfenamic Acid *see* NSAIDs

Tolterodine *see* Antimuscarinics

Tolvaptan

Antibacterials: plasma concentration of tolvaptan reduced by rifampicin

Antifungals: plasma concentration of tolvaptan increased by ketoconazole

Cardiac Glycosides: tolvaptan increases plasma concentration of digoxin (increased risk of toxicity)

• Grapefruit Juice: plasma concentration of tolvaptan increased by ●grapefruit juice—avoid concomitant use

Topiramate

• Antidepressants: anticonvulsant effect of antiepileptics possibly antagonised by MAOIs and ●tricyclic-related antidepressants (convulsive threshold lowered); anticonvulsant effect of antiepileptics antagonised by ●SSRIs and ●tricyclics (convulsive threshold lowered); avoid concomitant use of antiepileptics with ●St John's wort

Antidiabetics: topiramate possibly reduces plasma concentration of glibenclamide

• Antiepileptics: plasma concentration of topiramate often reduced by carbamazepine; topiramate increases plasma concentration of ●phenytoin (also plasma concentration of topiramate reduced); CNS toxicity reported when topiramate given with valproate

• Antimalarials: possible increased risk of convulsions when antiepileptics given with chloroquine and hydroxychloroquine; anticonvulsant effect of antiepileptics antagonised by ●mefloquine

Lithium: topiramate possibly affects plasma concentration of lithium

• Oestrogens: topiramate accelerates metabolism of ●oestrogens (reduced contraceptive effect—see p. 486)

• Orlistat: possible increased risk of convulsions when antiepileptics given with ●orlistat

• Progestogens: topiramate accelerates metabolism of ●progestogens (reduced contraceptive effect—see p. 486)

Torasemide *see* Diuretics

Toremifene

• Anticoagulants: toremifene possibly enhances anticoagulant effect of ●coumarins

Antiepileptics: metabolism of toremifene possibly accelerated by carbamazepine (reduced plasma concentration); metabolism of toremifene possibly accelerated by phenytoin; metabolism of toremifene accelerated by primidone (reduced plasma concentration)

Barbiturates: metabolism of toremifene possibly accelerated by barbiturates (reduced plasma concentration)

Diuretics: increased risk of hypercalcaemia when toremifene given with thiazides and related diuretics

Sugammadex: toremifene possibly reduces response to sugammadex

Trabectedin

Antiepileptics: cytotoxics possibly reduce absorption of phenytoin

• Antipsychotics: avoid concomitant use of cytotoxics with ●clozapine (increased risk of agranulocytosis)

Cardiac Glycosides: cytotoxics reduce absorption of digoxin tablets

Tramadol *see* Opioid Analgesics

Trandolapril *see* ACE Inhibitors

Tranylcypromine *see* MAOIs

Trazodone *see* Antidepressants, Tricyclic (related)

Tretinoin *see* Retinoids

Triamcinolone *see* Corticosteroids

Triamterene *see* Diuretics

Triclofos *see* Anxiolytics and Hypnotics

Trientine

Iron: trientine reduces absorption of *oral* iron

Zinc: trientine reduces absorption of zinc, also absorption of trientine reduced by zinc

Trifluoperazine *see* Antipsychotics

Trihexyphenidyl *see* Antimuscarinics

Trilostane

Diuretics: increased risk of hyperkalaemia when trilostane given with potassium-sparing diuretics and aldosterone antagonists

Trimethoprim

• Anti-arrhythmics: increased risk of ventricular arrhythmias when trimethoprim (as co-trimoxazole) given with ●amiodarone—avoid concomitant use of co-trimoxazole

Antibacterials: plasma concentration of trimethoprim possibly reduced by rifampicin; plasma concentration of both drugs may increase when trimethoprim given with dapsone

Anticoagulants: trimethoprim possibly enhances anticoagulant effect of coumarins

Antidiabetics: trimethoprim possibly enhances hypoglycaemic effect of repaglinide—manufacturer advises avoid concomitant use; trimethoprim rarely enhances the effects of sulphonylureas

• Antiepileptics: trimethoprim increases plasma concentration of ●phenytoin (also increased antifolate effect)

• Antimalarials: increased antifolate effect when trimethoprim given with ●pyrimethamine

Antivirals: trimethoprim (as co-trimoxazole) increases plasma concentration of lamivudine—avoid concomitant use of high-dose co-trimoxazole

• Azathioprine: increased risk of haematological toxicity when trimethoprim (also with co-trimoxazole) given with ●azathioprine

Cardiac Glycosides: trimethoprim possibly increases plasma concentration of digoxin

• Ciclosporin: increased risk of nephrotoxicity when trimethoprim given with ●ciclosporin, also plasma concentration of ciclosporin reduced by *intravenous* trimethoprim

• Cytotoxics: increased risk of haematological toxicity when trimethoprim (also with co-trimoxazole) given with ●mercaptopurine or ●methotrexate

Diuretics: increased risk of hyperkalaemia when trimethoprim given with eplerenone

Oestrogens: antibacterials that do not induce liver enzymes possibly reduce contraceptive effect of oestrogens (risk probably small, see p. 486)

Vaccines: antibacterials inactivate oral typhoid vaccine–see p. 760

Trimipramine *see* Antidepressants, Tricyclic

Tripotassium Dicitratobismuthate

Antibacterials: tripotassium dicitratobismuthate reduces absorption of tetracyclines

Tropicamide *see* Antimuscarinics

Trospium *see* Antimuscarinics

Tryptophan

• Antidepressants: possible increased serotonergic effects when tryptophan given with duloxetine; CNS excitation and confusion when tryptophan given with ●MAOIs (reduce dose of tryptophan); agitation and nausea may occur when tryptophan given with ●SSRIs

• Antimalarials: avoidance of antidepressants advised by manufacturer of ●artemether/lumefantrine

Atomoxetine: possible increased risk of convulsions when antidepressants given with atomoxetine

• Sibutramine: increased risk of CNS toxicity when tryptophan given with ●sibutramine (manufacturer of sibutramine advises avoid concomitant use)

Typhoid Vaccine (oral) *see* Vaccines

Typhoid Vaccine (parenteral) *see* Vaccines

Ubidecarenone

Anticoagulants: ubidecarenone may enhance or reduce anticoagulant effect of warfarin

Ulcer-healing Drugs *see* Histamine H$_2$-antagonists, Proton Pump Inhibitors, Sucralfate, and Tripotassium Dicitratobismuthate

Ulipristal

- Antacids: manufacturer of ulipristal advises avoid concomitant use with •antacids (plasma concentration of ulipristal possibly reduced)
- Antibacterials: manufacturer of ulipristal advises avoid concomitant use with •rifampicin (contraceptive effect of ulipristal possibly reduced)
- Antidepressants: manufacturer of ulipristal advises avoid concomitant use with •St John's wort (contraceptive effect of ulipristal possibly reduced)
- Antiepileptics: manufacturer of ulipristal advises avoid concomitant use with •carbamazepine and •phenytoin (contraceptive effect of ulipristal possibly reduced)
- Antivirals: manufacturer of ulipristal advises avoid concomitant use with •ritonavir (contraceptive effect of ulipristal possibly reduced)
- Barbiturates: manufacturer of ulipristal advises avoid concomitant use with •phenobarbital (contraceptive effect of ulipristal possibly reduced)
- Progestogens: ulipristal possibly reduces contraceptive effect of •progestogens
- Ulcer-healing Drugs: manufacturer of ulipristal advises avoid concomitant use with •histamine H$_2$-antagonists and •proton pump inhibitors (plasma concentration of ulipristal possibly reduced)

Ursodeoxycholic Acid

Antacids: absorption of bile acids possibly reduced by antacids

- Ciclosporin: ursodeoxycholic acid increases absorption of •ciclosporin

Lipid-regulating Drugs: absorption of bile acids possibly reduced by colestipol and colestyramine

Oestrogens: elimination of cholesterol in bile increased when bile acids given with oestrogens

Ustekinumab

- Vaccines: avoid concomitant use of ustekinumab with live •vaccines (see p. 733)

Vaccines

Note. For a general warning on live vaccines and high doses of corticosteroids or other immunosuppressive drugs, see p. 733; for advice on live vaccines and immunoglobulins, see under Normal Immunoglobulin, p. 763

- Abatacept: avoid concomitant use of live vaccines with •abatacept (see p. 733)
- Adalimumab: avoid concomitant use of live vaccines with •adalimumab (see p. 733)
- Anakinra: avoid concomitant use of live vaccines with •anakinra (see p. 733)

Antibacterials: oral typhoid vaccine inactivated by antibacterials–see p. 760

Anticoagulants: influenza vaccine possibly enhances anticoagulant effect of warfarin

Antiepileptics: influenza vaccine enhances effects of phenytoin

Antimalarials: oral typhoid vaccine inactivated by antimalarials–see p. 760

- Certolizumab pegol: avoid concomitant use of live vaccines with •certolizumab pegol (see p. 733)
- Corticosteroids: immune response to vaccines impaired by high doses of •corticosteroids, avoid concomitant use with live vaccines (see p. 733)
- Etanercept: avoid concomitant use of live vaccines with •etanercept (see p. 733)
- Infliximab: avoid concomitant use of live vaccines with •infliximab (see p. 733)

Interferons: avoidance of vaccines advised by manufacturer of interferon gamma

- Leflunomide: avoid concomitant use of live vaccines with •leflunomide (see p. 733)

Vaccines *(continued)*

Theophylline: influenza vaccine possibly increases plasma concentration of theophylline

- Tocilizumab: avoid concomitant use of live vaccines with •tocilizumab (see p. 733)
- Ustekinumab: avoid concomitant use of live vaccines with •ustekinumab (see p. 733)

Valaciclovir *see* Aciclovir

Valganciclovir *see* Ganciclovir

Valproate

Analgesics: effects of valproate enhanced by aspirin

- Antibacterials: metabolism of valproate possibly inhibited by erythromycin (increased plasma concentration); plasma concentration of valproate reduced by •carbapenems (possible therapeutic failure of valproate)

Anticoagulants: valproate possibly enhances anticoagulant effect of coumarins

- Antidepressants: anticonvulsant effect of antiepileptics possibly antagonised by MAOIs and •tricyclic-related antidepressants (convulsive threshold lowered); anticonvulsant effect of antiepileptics antagonised by •SSRIs and •tricyclics (convulsive threshold lowered); avoid concomitant use of antiepileptics with •St John's wort
- Antiepileptics: plasma concentration of valproate reduced by carbamazepine, also plasma concentration of active metabolite of carbamazepine increased; valproate possibly increases plasma concentration of ethosuximide; valproate increases plasma concentration of lamotrigine; valproate sometimes reduces plasma concentration of an active metabolite of oxcarbazepine; valproate increases or possibly decreases plasma concentration of phenytoin, also plasma concentration of valproate reduced; valproate possibly increases plasma concentration of •primidone (plasma concentration of active metabolite of primidone increased), also plasma concentration of valproate reduced; valproate possibly increases plasma concentration of rufinamide (reduce dose of rufinamide); CNS toxicity reported when valproate given with topiramate
- Antimalarials: possible increased risk of convulsions when antiepileptics given with chloroquine and hydroxychloroquine; anticonvulsant effect of antiepileptics antagonised by •mefloquine
- Antipsychotics: anticonvulsant effect of valproate antagonised by •antipsychotics (convulsive threshold lowered); increased risk of neutropenia when valproate given with •olanzapine

Antivirals: valproate possibly increases plasma concentration of zidovudine (increased risk of toxicity)

Anxiolytics and Hypnotics: plasma concentration of valproate possibly increased by clobazam; increased risk of side-effects when valproate given with clonazepam; valproate possibly increases plasma concentration of diazepam and lorazepam

Barbiturates: valproate increases plasma concentration of phenobarbital (also plasma concentration of valproate reduced)

Bupropion: valproate inhibits the metabolism of bupropion

Cytotoxics: valproate increases plasma concentration of temozolomide

Lipid-regulating Drugs: absorption of valproate possibly reduced by colestyramine

- Orlistat: possible increased risk of convulsions when antiepileptics given with •orlistat

Sodium Benzoate: valproate possibly reduces effects of sodium benzoate

Sodium Phenylbutyrate: valproate possibly reduces effects of sodium phenylbutyrate

- Ulcer-healing Drugs: metabolism of valproate inhibited by •cimetidine (increased plasma concentration)

Valsartan *see* Angiotensin-II Receptor Antagonists

Vancomycin

Anaesthetics, General: hypersensitivity-like reactions can occur when *intravenous* vancomycin given with general anaesthetics

- Antibacterials: increased risk of nephrotoxicity and ototoxicity when vancomycin given with ●aminoglycosides, capreomycin or colistin; increased risk of nephrotoxicity when vancomycin given with polymyxins

Antifungals: possible increased risk of nephrotoxicity when vancomycin given with amphotericin

- Ciclosporin: increased risk of nephrotoxicity when vancomycin given with ●ciclosporin

Cytotoxics: increased risk of nephrotoxicity and possibly of ototoxicity when vancomycin given with cisplatin

- Diuretics: increased risk of ototoxicity when vancomycin given with ●loop diuretics

Lipid-regulating Drugs: effects of *oral* vancomycin antagonised by colestyramine

- Muscle Relaxants: vancomycin enhances effects of ●suxamethonium

Oestrogens: antibacterials that do not induce liver enzymes possibly reduce contraceptive effect of oestrogens (risk probably small, see p. 486)

Tacrolimus: possible increased risk of nephrotoxicity when vancomycin given with tacrolimus

Vaccines: antibacterials inactivate oral typhoid vaccine–see p. 760

Vardenafil

- Alpha-blockers: enhanced hypotensive effect when vardenafil given with ●alpha-blockers (excludes tamsulosin)—separate doses by 6 hours—see also

Antibacterials: plasma concentration of vardenafil increased by erythromycin (reduce dose of vardenafil)

- Antifungals: plasma concentration of vardenafil increased by ●ketoconazole—avoid concomitant use; plasma concentration of vardenafil possibly increased by ●itraconazole—avoid concomitant use
- Antivirals: plasma concentration of vardenafil possibly increased by fosamprenavir; plasma concentration of vardenafil increased by ●indinavir and ●ritonavir—avoid concomitant use; plasma concentration of vardenafil possibly increased by saquinavir—reduce initial dose of vardenafil

Calcium-channel Blockers: enhanced hypotensive effect when vardenafil given with nifedipine

- Grapefruit Juice: plasma concentration of vardenafil possibly increased by ●grapefruit juice—avoid concomitant use
- Nicorandil: possible increased hypotensive effect when vardenafil given with ●nicorandil—avoid concomitant use
- Nitrates: possible increased hypotensive effect when vardenafil given with ●nitrates—avoid concomitant use

Vasodilator Antihypertensives

ACE Inhibitors: enhanced hypotensive effect when hydralazine, minoxidil or sodium nitroprusside given with ACE inhibitors

Adrenergic Neurone Blockers: enhanced hypotensive effect when hydralazine, minoxidil or sodium nitroprusside given with adrenergic neurone blockers

Alcohol: enhanced hypotensive effect when hydralazine, minoxidil or sodium nitroprusside given with alcohol

Aldesleukin: enhanced hypotensive effect when hydralazine, minoxidil or sodium nitroprusside given with aldesleukin

Alpha-blockers: enhanced hypotensive effect when hydralazine, minoxidil or sodium nitroprusside given with alpha-blockers

Anaesthetics, General: enhanced hypotensive effect when hydralazine, minoxidil or sodium nitroprusside given with general anaesthetics

Vasodilator Antihypertensives (continued)

Analgesics: hypotensive effect of hydralazine, minoxidil and sodium nitroprusside antagonised by NSAIDs

Angiotensin-II Receptor Antagonists: enhanced hypotensive effect when hydralazine, minoxidil or sodium nitroprusside given with angiotensin-II receptor antagonists

Antidepressants: enhanced hypotensive effect when hydralazine, minoxidil or sodium nitroprusside given with MAOIs; enhanced hypotensive effect when hydralazine or sodium nitroprusside given with tricyclic-related antidepressants

Antipsychotics: enhanced hypotensive effect when hydralazine, minoxidil or sodium nitroprusside given with phenothiazines

Anxiolytics and Hypnotics: enhanced hypotensive effect when hydralazine, minoxidil or sodium nitroprusside given with anxiolytics and hypnotics

Beta-blockers: enhanced hypotensive effect when hydralazine, minoxidil or sodium nitroprusside given with beta-blockers

Calcium-channel Blockers: enhanced hypotensive effect when hydralazine, minoxidil or sodium nitroprusside given with calcium-channel blockers

Clonidine: enhanced hypotensive effect when hydralazine, minoxidil or sodium nitroprusside given with clonidine

Corticosteroids: hypotensive effect of hydralazine, minoxidil and sodium nitroprusside antagonised by corticosteroids

Diazoxide: enhanced hypotensive effect when hydralazine, minoxidil or sodium nitroprusside given with diazoxide

Diuretics: enhanced hypotensive effect when hydralazine, minoxidil or sodium nitroprusside given with diuretics

Dopaminergics: enhanced hypotensive effect when hydralazine, minoxidil or sodium nitroprusside given with levodopa

Methyldopa: enhanced hypotensive effect when hydralazine, minoxidil or sodium nitroprusside given with methyldopa

Moxisylyte: enhanced hypotensive effect when hydralazine, minoxidil or sodium nitroprusside given with moxisylyte

Moxonidine: enhanced hypotensive effect when hydralazine, minoxidil or sodium nitroprusside given with moxonidine

Muscle Relaxants: enhanced hypotensive effect when hydralazine, minoxidil or sodium nitroprusside given with baclofen; enhanced hypotensive effect when hydralazine, minoxidil or sodium nitroprusside given with tizanidine

Nicorandil: possible enhanced hypotensive effect when hydralazine, minoxidil or sodium nitroprusside given with nicorandil

Nitrates: enhanced hypotensive effect when hydralazine, minoxidil or sodium nitroprusside given with nitrates

Oestrogens: hypotensive effect of hydralazine, minoxidil and sodium nitroprusside antagonised by oestrogens

Prostaglandins: enhanced hypotensive effect when hydralazine, minoxidil or sodium nitroprusside given with alprostadil

Vasodilator Antihypertensives: enhanced hypotensive effect when hydralazine given with minoxidil or sodium nitroprusside; enhanced hypotensive effect when minoxidil given with sodium nitroprusside

Vecuronium see Muscle Relaxants

Venlafaxine

- Analgesics: increased risk of bleeding when venlafaxine given with ●NSAIDs or ●aspirin; possible increased serotonergic effects when venlafaxine given with tramadol

Venlafaxine *(continued)*
- Anticoagulants: venlafaxine possibly enhances anticoagulant effect of ●warfarin
- Antidepressants: possible increased serotonergic effects when venlafaxine given with St John's wort, duloxetine or mirtazapine; enhanced CNS effects and toxicity when venlafaxine given with ●MAOIs (venlafaxine should not be started until 2 weeks after stopping MAOIs, avoid MAOIs for 1 week after stopping venlafaxine); after stopping SSRI-related antidepressants do not start ●moclobemide for at least 1 week
- Antimalarials: avoidance of antidepressants advised by manufacturer of ●artemether/lumefantrine
- Antipsychotics: venlafaxine increases plasma concentration of ●clozapine and haloperidol

  Atomoxetine: possible increased risk of convulsions when antidepressants given with atomoxetine
- Dopaminergics: caution with venlafaxine advised by manufacturer of entacapone; increased risk of hypertension and CNS excitation when venlafaxine given with ●selegiline (selegiline should not be started until 1 week after stopping venlafaxine, avoid venlafaxine for 2 weeks after stopping selegiline)

  Lithium: possible increased serotonergic effects when venlafaxine given with lithium
- Sibutramine: increased risk of CNS toxicity when SSRI-related antidepressants given with ●sibutramine (manufacturer of sibutramine advises avoid concomitant use)

Verapamil *see* Calcium-channel Blockers

Vigabatrin
- Antidepressants: anticonvulsant effect of antiepileptics possibly antagonised by MAOIs and ●tricyclic-related antidepressants (convulsive threshold lowered); anticonvulsant effect of antiepileptics antagonised by ●SSRIs and tricyclics (convulsive threshold lowered); avoid concomitant use of antiepileptics with ●St John's wort

  Antiepileptics: vigabatrin reduces plasma concentration of phenytoin; vigabatrin possibly reduces plasma concentration of primidone
- Antimalarials: possible increased risk of convulsions when antiepileptics given with chloroquine and hydroxychloroquine; anticonvulsant effect of antiepileptics antagonised by ●mefloquine

  Barbiturates: vigabatrin possibly reduces plasma concentration of phenobarbital
- Orlistat: possible increased risk of convulsions when antiepileptics given with ●orlistat

Vildagliptin *see* Antidiabetics

Vinblastine
- Aldesleukin: avoidance of vinblastine advised by manufacturer of ●aldesleukin
- Antibacterials: toxicity of vinblastine increased by ●erythromycin—avoid concomitant use

  Antiepileptics: cytotoxics possibly reduce absorption of phenytoin
- Antifungals: metabolism of vinblastine possibly inhibited by ●posaconazole (increased risk of neurotoxicity)
- Antipsychotics: avoid concomitant use of cytotoxics with ●clozapine (increased risk of agranulocytosis)

  Antivirals: plasma concentration of vinblastine possibly increased by ritonavir

  Cardiac Glycosides: cytotoxics reduce absorption of digoxin tablets

Vincristine
  Antiepileptics: cytotoxics possibly reduce absorption of phenytoin
- Antifungals: metabolism of vincristine possibly inhibited by ●itraconazole and ●posaconazole (increased risk of neurotoxicity)
- Antipsychotics: avoid concomitant use of cytotoxics with ●clozapine (increased risk of agranulocytosis)

Vincristine *(continued)*
  Calcium-channel Blockers: metabolism of vincristine possibly inhibited by nifedipine

  Cardiac Glycosides: cytotoxics reduce absorption of digoxin tablets

Vinorelbine
- Antibacterials: possible increased risk of neutropenia when vinorelbine given with ●clarithromycin

  Antiepileptics: cytotoxics possibly reduce absorption of phenytoin
- Antifungals: metabolism of vinorelbine possibly inhibited by ●itraconazole (increased risk of neurotoxicity)
- Antipsychotics: avoid concomitant use of cytotoxics with ●clozapine (increased risk of agranulocytosis)

  Cardiac Glycosides: cytotoxics reduce absorption of digoxin tablets

Vitamin A *see* Vitamins
Vitamin D *see* Vitamins
Vitamin E *see* Vitamins
Vitamin K (Phytomenadione) *see* Vitamins
Vitamins
  Antibacterials: absorption of vitamin A possibly reduced by neomycin
- Anticoagulants: vitamin E possibly enhances anticoagulant effect of ●coumarins; vitamin K antagonises anticoagulant effect of ●coumarins and ●phenindione

  Antiepileptics: vitamin D requirements possibly increased when given with carbamazepine, phenytoin or primidone

  Antifungals: plasma concentration of paricalcitol possibly increased by ketoconazole

  Antivirals: increased risk of bleeding when high doses of vitamin E given with tipranavir

  Barbiturates: vitamin D requirements possibly increased when given with barbiturates

  Ciclosporin: vitamin E possibly affects plasma concentration of ciclosporin

  Diuretics: increased risk of hypercalcaemia when vitamin D given with thiazides and related diuretics

  Dopaminergics: pyridoxine reduces effects of levodopa when given without dopa-decarboxylase inhibitor

  Retinoids: risk of hypervitaminosis A when vitamin A given with retinoids

  Selenium: ascorbic acid possibly reduces absorption of selenium (give at least 4 hours apart)

Voriconazole *see* Antifungals, Triazole
Warfarin *see* Coumarins
Xipamide *see* Diuretics
Xylometazoline *see* Sympathomimetics
Zafirlukast *see* Leukotriene Receptor Antagonists
Zaleplon *see* Anxiolytics and Hypnotics
Zidovudine
  Note. Increased risk of toxicity with nephrotoxic and myelosuppressive drugs—for further details consult product literature

  Analgesics: increased risk of haematological toxicity when zidovudine given with NSAIDs; plasma concentration of zidovudine possibly increased by methadone

  Antibacterials: absorption of zidovudine reduced by clarithromycin tablets (give at least 2 hours apart); manufacturer of zidovudine advises avoid concomitant use with rifampicin

  Antiepileptics: zidovudine increases or decreases plasma concentration of phenytoin; plasma concentration of zidovudine possibly increased by valproate (increased risk of toxicity)
- Antifungals: plasma concentration of zidovudine increased by ●fluconazole (increased risk of toxicity)

  Antimalarials: increased antifolate effect when zidovudine given with pyrimethamine
- Antivirals: profound myelosuppression when zidovudine given with ●ganciclovir (if possible avoid concomitant administration, particularly during initial ganciclovir therapy); increased risk of anaemia

Zidovudine

- Antivirals *(continued)*

    when zidovudine given with ●ribavirin—avoid concomitant use; zidovudine possibly inhibits effects of ●stavudine (manufacturers advise avoid concomitant use); plasma concentration of zidovudine reduced by ●tipranavir

    Atovaquone: metabolism of zidovudine possibly inhibited by atovaquone (increased plasma concentration)

- Probenecid: excretion of zidovudine reduced by ●probenecid (increased plasma concentration and risk of toxicity)

Zinc

    Antibacterials: zinc reduces absorption of ciprofloxacin, levofloxacin, moxifloxacin, norfloxacin and ofloxacin; zinc reduces absorption of tetracyclines, also absorption of zinc reduced by tetracyclines

    Calcium Salts: absorption of zinc reduced by calcium salts

    Iron: absorption of zinc reduced by *oral* iron, also absorption of *oral* iron reduced by zinc

    Penicillamine: absorption of zinc reduced by penicillamine, also absorption of penicillamine reduced by zinc

    Trientine: absorption of zinc reduced by trientine, also absorption of trientine reduced by zinc

Zoledronic Acid *see* Bisphosphonates

Zolmitriptan *see* 5HT$_1$ Agonists

Zolpidem *see* Anxiolytics and Hypnotics

Zonisamide

- Antidepressants: anticonvulsant effect of antiepileptics possibly antagonised by MAOIs and ●tricyclic-related antidepressants (convulsive threshold lowered); anticonvulsant effect of antiepileptics antagonised by ●SSRIs and ●tricyclics (convulsive threshold lowered); avoid concomitant use of antiepileptics with ●St John's wort

    Antiepileptics: plasma concentration of zonisamide reduced by carbamazepine and phenytoin

- Antimalarials: possible increased risk of convulsions when antiepileptics given with chloroquine and hydroxychloroquine; anticonvulsant effect of antiepileptics antagonised by ●mefloquine

    Barbiturates: plasma concentration of zonisamide reduced by phenobarbital

- Orlistat: possible increased risk of convulsions when antiepileptics given with ●orlistat

Zopiclone *see* Anxiolytics and Hypnotics

Zotepine *see* Antipsychotics

Zuclopenthixol *see* Antipsychotics

A2 Borderline substances

In certain conditions some foods (and toilet preparations) have characteristics of drugs and the Advisory Committee on Borderline Substances (ACBS) advises as to the circumstances in which such substances may be regarded as drugs. Prescriptions issued in accordance with the Committee's advice and endorsed 'ACBS' will normally not be investigated.

> General Practitioners are reminded that the ACBS recommends products on the basis that they may be regarded as drugs for the management of specified conditions. Doctors should satisfy themselves that the products can safely be prescribed, that patients are adequately monitored and that, where necessary, expert hospital supervision is available.

Foods which may be prescribed on FP10, GP10 (Scotland), or WP10 (Wales) All the food products listed in this appendix have ACBS approval. The clinical condition for which the product has been approved is included with each entry. **Note** Foods included in this appendix may contain cariogenic sugars and appropriate oral hygiene measures should be taken.

Enteral feeds and nutritional supplements For most enteral feeds and nutritional supplements, the main source of **carbohydrate** is either maltodextrin or glucose syrup; other carbohydrate sources are listed in the relevant table, below. Feeds containing residual lactose (less than 1 g lactose/100 mL formula) are described as 'clinically lactose-free' or 'lactose-free' by some manufacturers. The presence of lactose (including residual lactose) in feeds is indicated in the relevant table, below. The primary sources of **protein** or **amino acids** are included with each product entry. The **fat** or **oil** content is derived from a variety of sources such as vegetables, soya bean, corn, palm nuts, and seeds; where the fat content is derived from animal or fish sources, this information is included in the relevant table, below. The presence of medium chain triglycerides (MCT) is also noted where the quantity exceeds 30% of the fat content.

Enteral feeds and nutritional supplements can contain varying amounts of **vitamins**, **minerals**, and **trace elements**—the manufacturer's product literature should be consulted for more detailed information. For further information on enteral nutrition, see section 9.4.2. Feeds containing vitamin K may affect the INR in children receiving warfarin; see **interactions**: Appendix 1 (vitamins).

The suitability of food products for patients requiring a vegan, kosher, halal, or other compliant diet should be confirmed with individual manufacturers.

Note Feeds containing more than 6 g/100 mL protein or 2 g/100 mL fibre should be avoided in children unless recommended by an appropriate specialist or dietician.

> **Standard ACBS indications:** Disease-related malnutrition, intractable malabsorption, pre-operative preparation of malnourished patients, dysphagia, proven inflammatory bowel disease, following total gastrectomy, short-bowel syndrome, bowel fistula
>
> **Paediatric ACBS indications:** Disease-related malnutrition, intractable malabsorption, growth failure, pre-operative preparation of malnourished patients, dysphagia, short-bowel syndrome, bowel fistula

Appendix 2: Borderline substances

Appendix 2: Borderline substances

A2.1 Enteral feeds (non-disease specific)

A2.1.1 Enteral feeds (non-disease specific): less than 5 g protein/100 mL
For further information on composition of feeds, see p.895

A2.1.1.1 Enteral feeds: 1 kcal/mL and less than 5 g protein/100 mL
Not suitable for use in child under 1 year; not recommended for child 1–6 years unless otherwise stated

Product	Formulation	Energy	Protein	Carbohydrate	Fat	Fibre	Special Characteristics	ACBS Indications	Presentation & Flavour
Fresubin® Original (Fresenius Kabi)	Liquid (sip or tube feed) **per 100 mL**	420 kJ (100 kcal)	3.8 g cows' milk soya	13.8 g (sugars 3.5 g[1])	3.4 g	Nil	Gluten-free. Residual lactose. Contains fish gelatin. Feed in flexible pack contains fish oil and fish gelatin	Standard, p.895	Bottle: 200 mL = £1.74. Black currant, chocolate, mocha, nut, peach, vanilla. Flexible pack: 500 mL = £3.36, 1000 mL = £6.63, 1500 mL = £9.97
Fresubin® Original Fibre (Fresenius Kabi)	Liquid (tube feed) **per 100 mL**	420 kJ (100 kcal)	3.8 g cows' milk soya	13.8 g (sugars 1 g)	3.4 g	2 g	Gluten-free. Residual lactose. Contains fish oil and fish gelatin	Standard, p.895 except bowel fistula. Not suitable for child under 2 years	Flexible pack: 500 mL = £3.80, 1000 mL = £7.59, 1500 mL = £10.69
Isosource® Fibre (Nestlé)	Liquid (tube feed) **per 100 mL**	422 kJ (100 kcal)	3.8 g cows' milk	13.6 g	3.4 g	1.4 g	Gluten-free. Residual lactose	Standard, p.895. Not suitable for child under 2 years	Flexible pack: 500 mL = £3.58, 1000 mL = £7.16
Isosource® Standard (Nestlé)	Liquid (tube feed) **per 100 mL**	420 kJ (100 kcal)	4 g cows' milk	13.6 g	3.3 g	Nil	Gluten-free. Residual lactose	Standard, p.895	Flexible pack: 500 mL = £3.15, 1000 mL = £6.30
Jevity® (Abbott)	Liquid (tube feed) **per 100 mL**	441 kJ (106 kcal)	4 g caseinates	14.1 g (sugars 470 mg)	3.47 g	1.76 g	Gluten-free. Residual lactose	Standard, p.895 except bowel fistula. Not suitable for child under 2 years	Flexible pack: 500 mL = £4.04, 1000 mL = £7.59, 1500 mL = £11.40
Novasource® GI Control (Nestlé)	Liquid (tube feed) **per 100 mL**	444 kJ (106 kcal)	4.1 g cows' milk	14.4 g (sugars 500 mg)	3.5 g (MCT 40%)	2.2 g	Gluten-free. Residual lactose	Standard, p.895	Flexible pack: 500 mL = £4.78
Nutrison® (Nutricia Clinical)	Liquid (tube feed) **per 100 mL**	420 kJ (100 kcal)	4 g cows' milk	12.3 g (sugars 1 g)	3.9 g	Nil	Gluten-free. Residual lactose	Standard, p.895	Bottle: 500 mL = £3.76. Flexible pack: 500 mL = £4.17, 1000 mL = £7.32, 1500 mL = £10.97

1. Sugar content varies with flavour

Preparation	Formulation	Energy	Protein	Carbohydrate	Fat	Fibre	Special characteristics	Indications	Presentation
Nutrison® Multi Fibre (Nutricia Clinical)	Liquid (tube feed) **per 100 mL**	420 kJ (100 kcal)	4 g cows' milk	12.3 g (sugars 1 g)	3.9 g	1.5 g	Gluten-free; Residual lactose	Standard, p.895 except bowel fistula	Bottle: 500 mL = £4.09; Flexible pack: 500 mL = £4.51; 1000 mL = £8.16; 1500 mL = £12.25
Osmolite® (Abbott)	Liquid (tube feed) **per 100 mL**	424 kJ (100 kcal)	4 g caseinates soy isolate	13.6 g (sugars 630 mg)	3.4 g	Nil	Gluten-free; Residual lactose	Standard, p.895	Can: 250 mL = £1.83; Bottle: 500 mL = £3.47; 1000 mL = £6.62; 1500 mL = £9.93

◼ Soya protein formula (see also section A2.3.1)

Preparation	Formulation	Energy	Protein	Carbohydrate	Fat	Fibre	Special characteristics	Indications	Presentation
Fresubin® Soya Fibre (Fresenius Kabi)	Liquid (tube feed) **per 100 mL**	420 kJ (100 kcal)	3.8 g soya protein	13.3 g (sugars 4.1 g)	3.6 g	2 g	Gluten-free; Lactose-free; Contains fish oil	Standard, p.895; *also* cows' milk protein intolerance, lactose intolerance	Flexible pack: 500 mL = £3.93
Nutrison® Soya (Nutricia Clinical)	Liquid (tube feed) **per 100 mL**	420 kJ (100 kcal)	4 g soy isolate	12.3 g (sugars 1 g)	3.9 g	Nil	Gluten-free; Residual lactose; Milk protein-free	Standard, p.895; *also* cows' milk protein and lactose intolerance	Bottle: 500 mL = £4.34; Flexible pack: 1000 mL = £8.69
Nutrison® Soya Multi Fibre (Nutricia Clinical)	Liquid (tube feed) **per 100 mL**	420 kJ (100 kcal)	4 g soy isolate	12.3 g (sugars 700 mg)	3.9 g	1.5 g	Gluten-free; Residual lactose; Milk protein-free	Standard, p.895 except bowel fistula; *also* cows' milk protein and lactose intolerance	Flexible pack: 1500 mL = £14.46

◼ Peptide-based formula

Preparation	Formulation	Energy	Protein	Carbohydrate	Fat	Fibre	Special characteristics	Indications	Presentation
Peptamen® (Nestlé)	Liquid (sip or tube feed) **per 100 mL**	420 kJ (100 kcal)	4 g whey peptides	12.7 g (sugars 480 mg¹)	3.7 g (MCT 70%)	Nil	Gluten-free; Residual lactose	Short bowel syndrome, intractable malabsorption, proven inflammatory bowel disease, bowel fistula	Cup (vanilla flavour): 200 mL = £2.83; Flexible pack: 500 mL = £5.86; 1000 mL = £11.00
Peptisorb® (Nutricia Clinical)	Liquid (tube feed) **per 100 mL**	425 kJ (100 kcal)	4 g whey protein hydrolysate	17.6 g (sugars 1.7 g)	1.7 g (MCT 47%)	Nil	Gluten-free; Residual lactose	Short bowel syndrome, intractable malabsorption, proven inflammatory bowel disease, bowel fistula	Bottle: 500 mL = £5.76; Flexible pack: 500 mL = £6.31; 1000 mL = £11.41
Survimed® OPD (Fresenius Kabi)	Liquid (tube feed) **per 100 mL**	420 kJ (100 kcal)	4.5 g lactalbumin hydrolysate	15 g (sugars 300 mg)	2.4 g (MCT 54%)	Nil	Gluten-free; Residual lactose; Contains fish oil and fish gelatin	Standard, p.895; *also* growth failure	Flexible pack: 500 mL = £5.60

1. Sugar content varies with flavour

Appendix 2: Borderline substances

Appendix 2: Borderline substances

A2.1.1.2 Enteral feeds: Less than 1 kcal/mL and less than 5 g protein/100 mL

Not suitable for use in child under 1 year; not recommended for child 1–6 years unless otherwise stated

Amino acid formula (essential and non-essential amino acids)

Product	Formulation	Energy	Protein	Carbohydrate	Fat	Fibre	Special Characteristics	ACBS Indications	Presentation & Flavour
Elemental 028® Extra (SHS)	Liquid (sip or tube feed) **per 100 mL**	360 kJ (86 kcal)	2.5 g (protein equivalent)	11 g (sugars 4.7 g)	3.5 g (MCT 35%)	Nil		Short bowel syndrome, intractable malabsorption, proven inflammatory bowel disease, bowel fistula	Carton: 250 mL = £2.95 Grapefruit, orange and pineapple, summer fruits
	Standard dilution (20%) of powder (sip or tube feed) **per 100 mL**	374 kJ (89 kcal)[1]	2.5 g (protein equivalent)	11.8 g (sugars 1.8 g)	3.5 g (MCT 35%)	Nil			Sachet: 100 g = £5.73 Banana, citrus, orange, unflavoured[2]

Powder provides protein equivalent 12.5 g, carbohydrate 59 g, fat 17.45 g, energy 1871 kJ (443 kcal)/100 g

1. Nutritional values vary with flavour—consult product literature
2. Flavouring: see *Modjul*® Flavour System, p. 925

A2.1.2 Enteral feeds (non-disease specific): 5 g (or more) protein/100 mL

For further information on composition of feeds, see p. 895

A2.1.2.1 Enteral feeds: 1.5 kcal/mL and 5 g (or more) protein/100 mL

Not suitable for use in child under 1 year; not recommended for child 1–6 years unless otherwise stated

Product	Formulation	Energy	Protein	Carbohydrate	Fat	Fibre	Special Characteristics	ACBS Indications	Presentation & Flavour
Fresubin® 2250 Complete (Fresenius Kabi)	Liquid (tube feed) **per 100 mL**	630 kJ (150 kcal)	5.6 g cows' milk	18.8 g (sugars 1.5 g)	5.8 g	2 g	Gluten-free Residual lactose Contains fish oil and fish gelatin	Standard, p. 895	Flexible pack: 1500 mL = £11.94
Fresubin® Energy (Fresenius Kabi)	Liquid (sip feed) **per 100 mL**	630 kJ (150 kcal)	5.6 g cows' milk	18.8 g (sugars[1])	5.8 g	Nil	Gluten-free[2] Residual lactose Contains fish gelatin	Standard, p. 895	Bottle: 200 mL = £1.74 Banana, black current, cappuccino, chocolate, lemon, neutral, strawberry, tropical fruits, vanilla
	Liquid (tube feed) **per 100 mL**	630 kJ (150 kcal)	5.6 g cows' milk	18.8 g (sugars 1.4 g)	5.8 g	Nil	Gluten-free Residual lactose Contains fish oil and fish gelatin	Standard, p. 895	Flexible pack: 500 mL = £4.10 1000 mL = £8.07 1500 mL = £10.82

1. Sugar content varies with flavour
2. Strawberry flavour may contain traces of wheat starch and egg

Product	Form	Energy	Protein source	Carbohydrate	Fat	Special characteristics	Standard	Presentation and flavour
Fresubin® Energy Fibre (Fresenius Kabi)	Liquid (sip feed) **per 100 mL**	630 kJ (150 kcal)	5.6 g cows' milk	18.8 g (sugars[1])	2 g	Gluten-free Residual lactose Contains fish gelatin	Standard, p. 895	Bottle: 200 mL = £1.82 Banana, caramel, cherry, chocolate, strawberry, vanilla
	Liquid (tube feed) **per 100 mL**	630 kJ (150 kcal)	5.6 g cows' milk	18.8 g (sugars 1.5 g)	2 g	Gluten-free Residual lactose Contains fish oil and fish gelatin	Standard, p. 895	Flexible pack: 500 mL = £4.51 1000 mL = £8.59
Fresubin® HP Energy (Fresenius Kabi)	Liquid (tube feed) **per 100 mL**	630 kJ (150 kcal)	7.5 g cows' milk	17 g (sugars 1 g)	5.8 g (MCT 57 %)	Nil	Gluten-free Residual lactose Contains fish oil and fish gelatin	Standard, p. 895; *also* CAPD and haemodialysis	Flexible pack: 500 mL = £4.18 1000 mL = £8.38
Isosource® Energy Fibre (Nestlé)	Liquid (tube feed) **per 100 mL**	630 kJ (150 kcal)	4.9 g cows' milk	20.2 g	5.5 g	1.5 g	Gluten-free Residual lactose	Standard, p. 895 except bowel fistula	Flexible pack: 500 mL = £4.19 1000 mL = £8.39
Jevity® 1.5 kcal (Abbott)	Liquid (tube feed) **per 100 mL**	640 kJ (152 kcal)	6.38 g caseinates and soy isolate	20.1 g (sugars 1.47 g)	4.9 g	2.2 g	Gluten-free Residual lactose	Standard, p. 895 Not suitable for child under 2 years; not recommended for child 2–10 years	Flexible pack: 500 mL = £4.78 1000 mL = £9.14 1500 mL = £14.26
Novasource® GI Forte (Nestlé)	Liquid (tube feed) **per 100 mL**	631 kJ (150 kcal)	6 g cows' milk	18.3 g (sugars 1.8 g)	5.9 g	2.2 g	Gluten-free Residual lactose	Standard, p. 895	Flexible pack: 500 mL = £4.75 1000 mL = £9.50
Nutrison® Energy (Nutricia Clinical)	Liquid (tube feed) **per 100 mL**	630 kJ (150 kcal)	6 g cows' milk	18.5 g (sugars 1.5 g)	5.8 g	Nil	Gluten-free Residual lactose	Standard, p. 895	Bottle: 500 mL = £4.38 Flexible pack: 500 mL = £4.86 1000 mL = £8.81 1500 mL = £13.18
Nutrison® Energy Multi Fibre (Nutricia Clinical)	Liquid (tube feed) **per 100 mL**	630 kJ (150 kcal)	6 g cows' milk	18.5 g (sugars 1.5 g)	5.8 g	1.5 g	Gluten-free Residual lactose	Standard, p. 895	Bottle: 500 mL = £4.90 Flexible pack: 500 mL = £5.39 1000 mL = £9.77 1500 mL = £15.66
Osmolite® 1.5 kcal (Abbott)	Liquid (tube feed) **per 100 mL**	632 kJ (150 kcal)	6.25 g cows' milk soya protein isolate	20 g (sugars 4.9 g)	5 g	Nil	Gluten-free Residual lactose	Standard, p. 895	Flexible pack: 500 mL = £4.15 1000 mL = £8.10 1500 mL = £12.13
Resource® Energy (Nestlé)	Liquid (sip feed) **per 100 mL**	630 kJ (150 kcal)	5.6 g cows' milk	21 g (sugars 5.2 g[1])	5 g	less than 500 mg	Gluten-free Residual lactose	Standard, p. 895 Not suitable for use in child under 3 years	Bottle: 4 × 200 mL = £6.97 Apricot, banana, chocolate, coffee, strawberry-raspberry, vanilla

Formerly *Clinutren®* 1.5

1. Sugar content varies with flavour

Appendix 2: Borderline substances

A2.1.2.2 Enteral feeds: Less than 1.5 kcal/mL and 5 g (or more) protein/100 mL

Not suitable for use in child under 1 year; not recommended for child 1–6 years unless otherwise stated

Product	Formulation	Energy	Protein	Carbohydrate	Fat	Fibre	Special Characteristics	ACBS Indications	Presentation & Flavour
Fresubin® 1000 Complete (Fresenius Kabi)	Liquid (tube feed) **per 100 mL**	420 kJ (100 kcal)	5.5 g cows' milk	12.5 g (sugars 1.1 g)	3.1 g	2 g	Gluten-free Residual lactose Contains fish oil	Standard, p. 895	Flexible pack: 1000 mL = £8.59
Fresubin® 1200 Complete (Fresenius Kabi)	Liquid (tube feed) **per 100 mL**	500 kJ (120 kcal)	6 g cows' milk	15 g (sugars 1.22 g)	4.1 g	2 g	Gluten-free Residual lactose Contains fish oil	Standard, p. 895	Flexible pack: 1000 mL = £11.12
Fresubin® 1800 Complete (Fresenius Kabi)	Liquid (tube feed) **per 100 mL**	500 kJ (120 kcal)	6 g cows' milk	15 g (sugars 1.22 g)	4.1 g	2 g	Gluten-free Residual lactose Contains fish oil	Standard, p. 895	Flexible pack: 1500 mL = £10.95
Jevity® Plus (Abbott)	Liquid (tube feed) **per 100 mL**	504 kJ (120 kcal)	5.5 g caseinates soy isolates	15.1 g (sugars 890 mg)	3.93 g	2.2 g	Gluten-free Residual lactose	Standard, p. 895 Not suitable for child under 2 years; not recommended for child 2–10 years	Flexible pack: 500 mL = £4.35 1000 mL = £8.90 1500 mL = £13.36
Jevity® Plus HP (Abbott)	Liquid (tube feed) **per 100 mL**	547 kJ (130 kcal)	8.13 g cows' milk soy isolates	14.2 g (sugars 950 mg)	4.33 g	1.5 g	Gluten-free Residual lactose	Standard, p. 895; *also* CAPD, haemodialysis Not suitable for child under 2 years; not recommended for child 2–10 years	Flexible pack: 500 mL = £4.57
Jevity® Promote (Abbott)	Liquid (tube feed) **per 100 mL**	427 kJ (101 kcal)	5.55 g caseinates soy isolates	12 g (sugars 670 mg)	3.32 g	1.7 g	Gluten-free Residual lactose	Standard, p. 895 Not suitable for child under 2 years; not recommended for child 2–10 years	Flexible pack: 1000 mL = £8.70
Nutrison® MCT (Nutricia Clinical)	Liquid (tube feed) **per 100 mL**	420 kJ (100 kcal)	5 g cows' milk	12.6 g (sugars 1 g)	3.3 g (MCT 61%)	Nil	Gluten-free Residual lactose	Standard, p. 895	Flexible pack: 1000 mL = £8.15
Nutrison® Protein Plus (Nutricia Clinical)	Liquid (tube feed) **per 100 mL**	525 kJ (125 kcal)	6.3 g cows' milk	14.2 g (sugars 1.1 g)	4.9 g	Nil	Gluten-free Residual lactose	Standard, p. 895	Flexible pack: 1000 mL = £8.39
Nutrison® Protein Plus Multi Fibre (Nutricia Clinical)	Liquid (tube feed) **per 100 mL**	525 kJ (125 kcal)	6.3 g cow's milk	14.1 g (sugars 1.1 g)	4.9 g	1.5 g	Gluten-free Residual lactose	Disease related malnutrition	Flexible pack: 1000 mL = £9.34
Nutrison® 1000 Complete Multi Fibre (Nutricia Clinical)	Liquid (tube feed) **per 100 mL**	420 kJ (100 kcal)	5.5 g cows' milk	11.3 g (sugars 700 mg)	3.7 g	2 g	Gluten-free Residual lactose	Disease related malnutrition in patients with low energy and/or low fluid requirements	Flexible pack: 1000 mL = £9.06

Product	Formulation	Energy	Protein	Carbohydrate	Fat	Fibre	Special Characteristics	ACBS Indications	Presentation & Flavour
Nutrison® 1200 Complete Multi Fibre (Nutricia Clinical)	Liquid (tube feed) **per 100 mL**	505 kJ (120 kcal)	5.5 g cows' milk	15 g (sugars 1.2 g)	4.3 g	2 g	Gluten-free Residual lactose	Standard, p. 895 except bowel fistula	Bottle: 500 mL = £4.80 Flexible pack: 1000 mL = £9.59 1500 mL = £14.41
Osmolite® Plus (Abbott)	Liquid (tube feed) **per 100 mL**	508 kJ (121 kcal)	5.55 g caseinates	15.8 g (sugars 730 mg)	3.93 g	Nil	Gluten-free Residual lactose	Standard, p. 895 Not suitable for child 1–10 years	Flexible pack: 500 mL = £4.06 1000 mL = £7.83 1500 mL = £11.73
Peptamen® HN (Nestlé)	Liquid (tube feed) **per 100 mL**	556 kJ (133 kcal)	6.6 g whey protein hydrolysates	15.6 g (sugars 1.4 g)	4.9 g (MCT 70%)	Nil	Gluten-free Residual lactose Hydrolysed with pork trypsin	Short bowel syndrome, intractable malabsorption, proven inflammatory bowel disease, bowel fistula Not suitable for child under 3 years	Flexible pack: 500 mL = £6.32
Perative® (Abbott)	Liquid (sip or tube feed) **per 100 mL**	552 kJ (131 kcal)	6.7 g caseinate whey protein hydrolysates	17.7 g (sugars 660 mg)	3.7 g (MCT 42%)	Nil	Gluten-free Residual lactose	Standard, p. 895 Not suitable for child under 5 years	Flexible pack: 500 mL = £5.66 1000 mL = £11.32

A2.1.2.3 Enteral feeds: More than 1.5 kcal/mL and 5 g (or more) protein/100 mL

Not suitable for use in child under 1 year; not recommended for child 1–6 years unless otherwise stated

Product	Formulation	Energy	Protein	Carbohydrate	Fat	Fibre	Special Characteristics	ACBS Indications	Presentation & Flavour
Ensure® Twocal (Abbott)	Liquid (sip or tube feed) **per 100 mL**	838 kJ (200 kcal)	8.4 g cows' milk	21 g (sugars 4.5 g)	8.9 g	1 g	Gluten-free Residual lactose	Standard, p. 895; *also* haemodialysis and CAPD	Bottle or carton: 200 mL = £2.08 Banana, neutral, strawberry, vanilla
Isosource® Energy (Nestlé)	Liquid (tube feed) **per 100 mL**	670 kJ (160 kcal)	5.7 g cows' milk	20 g	6.2 g	Nil	Gluten-free Residual lactose	Standard, p. 895	Flexible pack: 500 mL = £3.87 1000 mL = £7.73

A2.1.3 Enteral feeds (non-disease specific): Child under 12 years

For further information on composition of feeds, see p. 895

A2.1.3.1 Enteral feeds, Child: Less than 1 kcal/mL and less than 4 g protein/100 mL

Product	Formulation	Energy	Protein	Carbohydrate	Fat	Fibre	Special Characteristics	ACBS Indications	Presentation & Flavour
Nutrini® Low Energy Multi Fibre (Nutricia Clinical)	Liquid (tube feed) **per 100 mL**	315 kJ (75 kcal)	2.1 g whey protein and caseinate	9.3 g (sugars 600 mg)	3.3 g	800 mg	Gluten-free Residual lactose Contains fish oil	Paediatric, p. 895 except bowel fistula, in child 1–6 years, body-weight 8–20 kg	Bottle: 200 mL = £2.11 Flexible pack: 500 mL = £5.34
Nutriprem® 1 (Cow & Gate)	Liquid (sip feed) **per 100 mL**	335 kJ (80 kcal)	2.5 g whey protein and casein	7.6 g (lactose 6.3 g)	4.4 g	800 mg	Gluten-free Residual lactose Contains soya, fish oil and egg lipid	Low birth-weight formula	Bottle: 60 mL Hospital supply only

Appendix 2: Borderline substances

Appendix 2: Borderline substances

A2.1.3.1 Enteral feeds, Child: Less than 1 kcal/mL and less than 4 g protein/100 mL *(product list continued)*

Product	Formulation	Energy	Protein	Carbohydrate	Fat	Fibre	Special Characteristics	ACBS Indications	Presentation & Flavour
Nutriprem® 2 (Cow & Gate)	Liquid (sip feed) **per 100 mL**	310 kJ (75 kcal)	2 g whey protein and casein	7.4 g (lactose 5.8 g)	4.1 g	800 mg	Contains soya, fish oil and egg lipid	Catch-up growth in pre-term infants (less than 35 weeks at birth) and small for gestational-age infants up to 6 months corrected age	Carton: 200 mL = £1.54 (Bottle: 100 mL Hospital supply only) Can: 900 g = £10.28 (5.1-g measuring scoop provided)
	Standard dilution (15.4%) of powder (sip feed) **per 100 mL**	315 kJ (75 kcal)	2 g whey protein and casein	7.4 g (lactose 5.8 g)	4.1 g (including MCT oil)	800 mg			
Powder provides: protein 13 g, carbohydrate 48.3 g, fat 26.7 g, fibre 5.2 g, energy 2030 kJ (485 kcal)/100 g									
SMA® Gold Prem 1 (SMA Nutrition)	Liquid (sip feed) **per 100 mL**	343 kJ (82 kcal)	2.2 g cows' milk	8.4 g (sugars 4.5 g)	4.4 g	Nil	Contains lactose		Bottle: 100 mL Hospital supply only
SMA® Gold Prem 2 (SMA Nutrition)	Standard dilution (14%) of powder (sip feed) **per 100 mL**	305 kJ (73 kcal)	1.9 g cows' milk	7.5 g sugars 6.4 g	3.9 g	Nil	Contains lactose	Catch-up growth in preterm and small for gestational age infants on discharge from hospital, up to 6 months corrected age	Can: 400 g = £4.57 (4.7-g measuring scoop provided)
Powder provides: protein 14 g, carbohydrate 54 g, fat 28 g, energy 2180 kJ (524 kcal)/100 g									
SMA® High Energy (SMA Nutrition)	Liquid (sip feed) **per 100 mL**	382 kJ (91 kcal)	2 g whey protein and casein	9.8 g lactose	4.9 g	Nil	Contains lactose	Disease related malnutrition and malabsorption, and growth failure in child from birth to 18 months	Carton: 250 mL = £1.80

■ Amino acid formula (essential and non-essential amino acids)

Product	Formulation	Energy	Protein	Carbohydrate	Fat	Fibre	Special Characteristics	ACBS Indications	Presentation & Flavour
Emsogen® (SHS)	Standard dilution (20%) of powder (sip or tube feed) **per 100 mL**	368 kJ (88 kcal)[1]	2.5 g protein equivalent (essential and non-essential amino acids)	12 g (sugars 1.6 g)	3.3 g[2] (MCT 83%)	Nil	Lactose-free	Short-bowel syndrome, intractable malabsorption, proven inflammatory bowel disease, bowel fistula Not suitable for child under 1 year or as sole source of nutrition in child 1–5 years	Sachet: 100 g = £5.90 Orange, unflavoured[3]
Powder provides: protein equivalent 12.5 g, carbohydrate 60 g, fat 16.4 g, energy 1839 kJ (438 kcal)/100 g									

1. Nutritional values vary with flavour—consult product literature
2. Additional source of alpha linolenic acid needed if used as sole source of nutrition
3. Flavouring: see *Modjul®* Flavour System, p. 925

A2.1.3.2 Enteral feeds (Child: 1 kcal/mL and less than 4 g protein/100 mL)

Not suitable for child under 1 year unless otherwise stated

Product	Formulation	Energy	Protein	Carbohydrate	Fat	Fibre	Special Characteristics	ACBS Indications	Presentation & Flavour
Clinutren® Junior (Nestlé)	Standard dilution (22%) of powder (sip or tube feed) **per 100 mL**	420 kJ (100 kcal)	2.97 g whey protein and caseinate	13.3 g	3.9 g	Nil	Gluten-free Residual lactose	Standard, p.895; *also* growth failure in child 1–10 years	Can: 400 g = £10.57 Vanilla (7.85-g measuring scoop provided)
Powder provides: protein 13.9 g, carbohydrate 62.2 g, fat 18.3 g, energy 1950 kJ (467 kcal)/100 g									
Frebini® Original (Fresenius Kabi)	Liquid (tube feed) **per 100 mL**	420 kJ (100 kcal)	2.5 g cows' milk	12.5 g (sugars 700 mg)	4.4 g	Nil	Gluten-free Residual lactose Contains fish oils and fish gelatin	Standard, p.895; *also* growth failure in child 1–10 years, body-weight 8–30 kg	Flexible pack: 500 mL = £4.96
Frebini® Original Fibre (Fresenius Kabi)	Liquid (tube feed) **per 100 mL**	420 kJ (100 kcal)	2.5 g cows' milk	12.5 g (sugars 700 mg)	4.4 g	750 mg	Gluten-free Residual lactose Contains fish oils and fish gelatin	Standard, p.895; *also* growth failure in child 1–10 years, body-weight 8–30 kg	Flexible pack: 500 mL = £5.50
Infatrini® (Nutricia Clinical)	Liquid (sip or tube feed) **per 100 mL**	415 kJ (100 kcal)	2.6 g cows' milk	10.3 g (lactose 5.2 g)	5.4 g	800 mg	Gluten-free Contains fish oil	Failure to thrive, disease-related malnutrition and malabsorption, in child from birth up to body-weight 8 kg	Bottle: 100 mL = £1.08 200 mL = £2.07 Flexible pack: 500 mL = £5.25
Nutrini® (Nutricia Clinical)	Liquid (tube feed) **per 100 mL**	420 kJ (100 kcal)	2.8 g cows' milk	12.3 g (sugars 1 g)	4.4 g	Nil	Gluten-free Residual lactose	Standard, p.895; *also* growth failure in child 1–6 years, body-weight 8–20 kg	Bottle: 200 mL = £2.58 Flexible pack: 500 mL = £5.80
Nutrini® Multi Fibre (Nutricia Clinical)	Liquid (tube feed) **per 100 mL**	420 kJ (100 kcal)	2.8 g whey protein and caseinate	12.3 g (sugars 800 mg)	4.4 g	800 mg	Gluten-free Residual lactose Contains fish oil	Standard, p.895; *also* growth failure in child 1–6 years, body-weight 8–20 kg	Bottle: 200 mL = £2.58 Flexible pack: 500 mL = £6.45
Paediasure® (Abbott)	Liquid (sip or tube feed) **per 100 mL**	422 kJ (100 kcal)[1]	2.8 g cows' milk	11.2 g (sugars 3.92 g)	4.98 g	Nil	Gluten-free Residual lactose	Paediatric, p.895 in child 1–10 years, body-weight 8–30 kg	Bottle: 200 mL = £2.04 Banana, chocolate, strawberry, vanilla Can: 250 mL = £2.54 Vanilla Flexible pack: 500 mL = £5.09 Vanilla
Paediasure® Fibre (Abbott)	Liquid (sip or tube feed) **per 100 mL**	420 kJ (100 kcal)[1]	2.8 g caseinates and whey protein	10.9 g (sugars 3.84 g)	4.98 g	730 mg	Gluten-free Residual lactose	Paediatric, p.895 in child 1–10 years, body-weight 8–30 kg	Bottle: 200 mL = £2.24 Banana, strawberry, vanilla Flexible pack: 500 mL = £5.66 Vanilla

1. Nutritional values vary with flavour—consult product literature

Appendix 2: Borderline substances

Appendix 2: Borderline substances

A2.1.3.2 Enteral feeds, Child: 1 kcal/mL and less than 4 g protein/100 mL (product list continued)

Not suitable for child under 1 year unless otherwise stated

Product	Formulation	Energy	Protein	Carbohydrate	Fat	Fibre	Special Characteristics	ACBS Indications	Presentation & Flavour
Tentrini® (Nutricia Clinical)	Liquid (tube feed) per 100 mL	420 kJ (100 kcal)	3.3 g whey protein and caseinate	12.3 g (sugars 800 mg)	4.2 g	Nil	Gluten-free Residual lactose Contains fish oil	Standard, p. 895; also growth failure in child 7–12 years, body-weight 21–45 kg	Bottle or Flexible pack: 500 mL = £4.80
Tentrini® Multi Fibre (Nutricia Clinical)	Liquid (tube feed) per 100 mL	420 kJ (100 kcal)	3.3 g whey protein and caseinate	12.3 g (sugars 800 mg)	4.2 g	1.1 g	Gluten-free Residual lactose Contains fish oil	Standard, p. 895 except bowel fistula; also growth failure in child 7–12 years body-weight 21–45 kg	Bottle or Flexible pack: 500 mL = £5.27

Hydrolysate Formula See also Infant Formula (Hydrolysate), section 2.3.1

Product	Formulation	Energy	Protein	Carbohydrate	Fat	Fibre	Special Characteristics	ACBS Indications	Presentation & Flavour
Nutrini® Peptisorb (Nutricia Clinical)	Liquid (tube feed) per 100 mL	420 kJ (100 kcal)	2.8 g whey protein hydrolysate	13.7 g (sugars 800 mg)	3.9 g (MCT 46 %)	Nil	Gluten-free Residual lactose	Standard, p. 895; also growth failure in child 1–6 years, body-weight 8–20 kg	Flexible pack: 500 mL = £8.51
Peptamen® Junior (Nestlé)	Liquid (tube feed) per 100 mL	420 kJ (100 kcal)	3 g whey protein hydrolysate	13.2 g	4 g (MCT 60 %)	Nil	Gluten-free Residual lactose Hydrolysed with pork trypsin	Short bowel syndrome, intractable malabsorption, proven inflammatory bowel disease, bowel fistula, in child 1–10 years	Flexible pack: 500 mL = £5.71
	Standard dilution (22%) of powder (sip or tube feed) per 100 mL	420 kJ (100 kcal)	3 g whey protein hydrolysate	13.8 g	3.85 g (MCT 60 %)	Nil	Gluten-free Residual lactose Hydrolysed with bacterial trypsin		Can: 400 g = £15.36 Vanilla (7.86-g measuring scoop provided)

Powder provides: protein 13.7 g, carbohydrate 62.9 g, fat 17.5 g, energy 1910 kJ (457 kcal)/100 g

A2.1.3.3 Enteral feeds, Child: More than 1 kcal/mL and less than 4 g protein/100 mL

Not suitable for child under 1 year unless otherwise stated

Product	Formulation	Energy	Protein	Carbohydrate	Fat	Fibre	Special Characteristics	ACBS Indications	Presentation & Flavour
Fortini® (Nutricia Clinical)	Liquid (sip feed) per 100 mL	630 kJ (150 kcal)	3.4 g cows' milk	18.8 g (sugars 7.4 g)	6.8 g	Nil	Gluten-free Residual lactose	Disease-related malnutrition and growth failure in child 1–6 years, body-weight 8–20 kg	Bottle: 200 mL = £2.77 Strawberry, vanilla
Fortini® Multifibre (Nutricia Clinical)	Liquid (sip feed) per 100 mL	630 kJ (150 kcal)	3.4 g cows' milk	18.8 g (sugars 7.4 g)	6.8 g	1.5 g	Gluten-free Residual lactose	Disease-related malnutrition and growth failure in child 1–6 years, body-weight 8–20 kg	Bottle: 200 mL = £2.91 Banana, chocolate, strawberry, vanilla, and unflavoured

Product	Formulation	Energy	Protein	Carbohydrate	Fat	Fibre	Special Characteristics	ACBS Indications	Presentation & Flavour
Frebini® Energy Drink (Fresenius Kabi)	Liquid (sip feed) per 100 mL	630 kJ (150 kcal)	3.8 g cows' milk	18.7 g (sugars 4.5 g)	6.7 g	Nil	Gluten-free Residual lactose	Disease-related malnutrition and growth failure in child 1–10 years, body-weight 8–30 kg	Bottle: 200 mL = £2.36 Banana, strawberry
Frebini® Energy (Fresenius Kabi)	Liquid (tube feed) per 100 mL	630 kJ (150 kcal)	3.75 g cows' milk	18.75 g (sugars 830 mg)	6.7 g	Nil	Gluten-free Residual lactose Contains fish oil and fish gelatin	Standard, p.895; *also* growth failure in child 1–10 years, body-weight 8–30 kg	Flexible pack: 500 mL = £6.21
Frebini® Energy Fibre Drink (Fresenius Kabi)	Liquid (sip feed) per 100 mL	630 kJ (150 kcal)	3.8 g cows' milk	18.75 g (sugars 4.5 g[1])	6.7 g	1.1 g	Gluten-free Residual lactose	Disease-related malnutrition and growth failure in child 1–10 years, body-weight 8–30 kg	Bottle: 200 mL = £2.41 Chocolate, vanilla
Frebini® Energy Fibre (Fresenius Kabi)	Liquid (tube feed) per 100 mL	630 kJ (150 kcal)	3.75 g cows' milk	18.75 g (sugars 830 mg)	6.7 g	1.13 g	Gluten-free Residual lactose Contains fish oils and fish gelatin	Standard, p.895; *also* growth failure in child 1–10 years, body-weight 8–30 kg	Flexible pack: 500 mL = £6.64
Isosource® Junior (Nestlé)	Liquid (tube feed) per 100 mL	512 kJ (122 kcal)	2.7 g cows' milk	17 g	4.7 g	Nil	Gluten-free Residual lactose	Standard, p.895; *also* growth failure in child 1–6 years, body-weight 8–20 kg	Flexible pack: 500 mL = £4.99
Resource® Junior (Nestlé)	Liquid (sip feed) per 100 mL	630 kJ (150 kcal)[2]	3 g cows' milk	20.6 g (sugars 4.9 g)	6.2 g	Nil	Gluten-free Residual lactose	Standard, p.895 in child 1–10 years	Carton: 200 mL = £1.79 Chocolate, strawberry, vanilla

1. Sugar content varies with flavour
2. Nutritional values vary with flavour—consult product literature

A2.1.3.4 Enteral feeds, Child: 1.5 kcal/mL and more than 4 g protein/100 mL

Not suitable for child under 1 year unless otherwise stated

Product	Formulation	Energy	Protein	Carbohydrate	Fat	Fibre	Special Characteristics	ACBS Indications	Presentation & Flavour
Nutrini® Energy (Nutricia Clinical)	Liquid (tube feed) per 100 mL	630 kJ (150 kcal)	4.1 g caseinate whey protein	18.5 g (sugars 1.1 g)	6.7 g	Nil	Gluten-free Residual lactose Contains fish oil	Standard, p.895; *also* growth failure in child 1–6 years, body-weight 8–20 kg	Bottle: 200 mL = £2.84 Flexible pack: 500 mL = £7.28
Nutrini® Energy Multi Fibre (Nutricia Clinical)	Liquid (tube feed) per 100 mL	630 kJ (150 kcal)	4.1 g caseinate whey protein	18.5 g (sugars 1.1 g)	6.7 g	800 mg	Gluten-free Residual lactose Contains fish oil	Paediatric, p.895 except bowel fistula; *also* total gastrectomy, in child 1–6 years, body-weight 8–20 kg	Bottle: 200 mL = £3.01 Flexible pack: 500 mL = £7.50
Paediasure® Plus (Abbott)	Liquid (sip or tube feed) per 100 mL	632 kJ (151 kcal)	4.2 g caseinates whey protein	16.7 g[1]	7.47 g	Nil	Gluten-free Residual lactose	Paediatric, p.895 in child 1–10 years, body-weight 8–30 kg	Bottle: 200 mL = £2.49 Banana, strawberry, vanilla Flexible pack: 500 mL = £6.39 Vanilla

1. Sugar content varies with presentation

Appendix 2: Borderline substances

Appendix 2: Borderline substances

A2.1.3.4 Enteral feeds, Child: 1.5 kcal/mL and more than 4 g protein/100 mL (product list continued)

Not suitable for child under 1 year unless otherwise stated

Product	Formulation	Energy	Protein	Carbohydrate	Fat	Fibre	Special Characteristics	ACBS Indications	Presentation & Flavour
Paediasure® Plus Fibre (Abbott)	Liquid (sip or tube feed) **per 100 mL**	626 kJ (150 kcal)	4.2 g caseinates whey protein	16.4 g[1]	7.47 g	1.1 g	Gluten-free Residual lactose	Paediatric, p. 895 in child 1–10 years, body-weight 8–30 kg	Bottle: 200 mL = £2.71 Vanilla Flexible pack: 500 mL = £6.80 Vanilla
Tentrini® Energy (Nutricia Clinical)	Liquid (tube feed) **per 100 mL**	630 kJ (150 kcal)	4.9 g whey protein and caseinate	18.5 g (sugars 1.1 g)	6.3 g	Nil	Gluten-free Residual lactose Contains fish oil	Standard, p. 895; *also growth failure, in child 7–12 years, body-weight 21–45 kg*	Bottle or Flexible pack: 500 mL = £5.93
Tentrini® Energy Multi Fibre (Nutricia Clinical)	Liquid (tube feed) **per 100 mL**	630 kJ (150 kcal)	4.9 g whey protein and caseinate	18.5 g (sugars 1.1 g)	6.3 g	1.1 g	Gluten-free Residual lactose Contains fish oil	Paediatric, p. 895; *also proven inflammatory bowel disease, in child 7–12 years, body-weight 21–45 kg*	Bottle or Flexible pack: 500 mL = £6.54

1. Sugar content varies with presentation

A2.2 Nutritional supplements (non-disease specific)

A2.2.1 Nutritional supplements: less than 5 g protein/100 mL

For further information on composition of feeds, see p. 895

A2.2.1.1 Nutritional supplements: 1 kcal/mL and less than 5 g protein/100 mL

Not suitable for use in child under 1 year; use with caution in child 1–5 years unless otherwise stated

Product	Formulation	Energy	Protein	Carbohydrate	Fat	Fibre	Special Characteristics	ACBS Indications	Presentation & Flavour
Ensure® (Abbott)	Liquid (sip or tube feed) **per 100 mL**	423 kJ (100 kcal)[1]	4 g caseinates soy isolate	13.6 g (sugars 3.93 g)	3.36 g	Nil	Gluten-free Residual lactose	Standard, p. 895	Can: 250 mL = £2.01 Chocolate, vanilla

1. Nutritional values vary with flavour—consult product literature

A2.2.1.2 Nutritional supplements: More than 1 kcal/mL and less than 5 g protein/100 mL

Not suitable for use in child under 1 year; use with caution in child 1–5 years unless otherwise stated

Product	Formulation	Energy	Protein	Carbohydrate	Fat	Fibre	Special Characteristics	ACBS Indications	Presentation & Flavour
Ensure® Plus Juce (Abbott)	Liquid (sip feed) **per 100 mL**	638 kJ (150 kcal)	4.8 g whey protein isolate	32.7 g (sugars 9.4 g[1])	Nil	Nil	Gluten-free Residual lactose Non-milk taste	Standard, p. 895	Bottle: 220 mL = £1.75 Apple, fruit punch, grapefruit, lemon-lime, orange, peach, pine-apple, strawberry
Fortijuce® (Nutricia Clinical)	Liquid (sip feed) **per 100 mL**	640 kJ (150 kcal)	4.0 g cows' milk	33.5 g (sugars 13.1 g[1])	Nil	Nil	Gluten-free Residual lactose Non-milk taste	Standard, p. 895 Not suitable for child under 3 years	Bottle: 200 mL = £1.85 Apple, black currant, forest fruits, lemon, orange, strawberry, tropical Starter pack (mixed) 4 × 200 mL = £7.40
Paediasure® Plus Juce (Abbott)	Liquid (sip feed) **per 100 mL**	638 kJ (150 kcal)[2]	4.2 g cows' milk	33.3 g (sugars 9.4 g)	Nil	Nil	Gluten-free Residual lactose Non-milk taste	Nutritional supplement for use in children body-weight 8–30kg with disease-related malnutrition and, or growth failure	Bottle: 200 mL = £2.77 Apple, very berry
Provide® Xtra Juice Drink (Fresenius Kabi)	Liquid (sip feed) **per 100 mL**	525 kJ (125 kcal)	3.75 g pea and soya protein hydrolysates	27.5 g[1]	Nil	Nil[3]	Gluten-free Lactose-free Non-milk taste Sweet-flavoured products contain fish gelatin	Standard, p. 895	Carton: 200 mL = £1.71 Apple, black currant, carrot-apple, cherry, citrus-cola, lemon-lime, melon, orange-pineapple, tomato
Resource® Dessert Energy (Nestlé)	Semi-solid **per 100 g**	671 kJ (160 kcal)	4.8 g cows' milk	21.2 g (sugars 9.9 g[1])	6.2 g	Nil	Gluten-free Contains lactose	Standard, p. 895; also CAPD, haemodialysis	Cup: 125 g = £1.43 Caramel, chocolate, vanilla
Resource® Fruit (Nestlé)	Liquid (sip feed) **per 100 mL**	520 kJ (125 kcal)	4 g whey protein hydrolysate	27 g (sugars 9.5 g[1])	less than 200 mg	less than 200 mg[3]	Gluten-free Residual lactose Non-milk taste	Standard, p. 895 Not suitable for child under 3 years	Bottle: 4 × 200 mL = £7.02 Apple, orange, pear-cherry, rasp-berry-black currant

Formerly Clinutren® Fruit
1. Sugar content varies with flavour
2. Nutritional values vary with flavour—consult product literature
3. Fibre content varies with flavour

Appendix 2: Borderline substances

Appendix 2: Borderline substances

A2.2.2 Nutritional supplements: 5 g (or more) protein/100 mL
For further information on composition of feeds, see p.895

A2.2.2.1 Nutritional supplements: 1.5 kcal/mL and 5 g (or more) protein/100 mL
Not suitable for use in child under 1 year; use with caution in child 1–5 years unless otherwise stated

Product	Formulation	Energy	Protein	Carbohydrate	Fat	Fibre	Special Characteristics	ACBS Indications	Presentation & Flavour
Ensure® Plus Fibre (Abbott)	Liquid (sip or tube feed) **per 100 mL**	642 kJ (153 kcal)[1]	6.25 g cows' milk soya protein isolate	20.2 g (sugars 5.5 g)	4.92 g	2.5 g	Gluten-free Residual lactose	Standard, p.895; *also* CAPD, haemodialysis	Bottle: 200 mL = £1.80 Banana, chocolate, fruits of the forest, raspberry, strawberry, vanilla
Ensure® Plus Milkshake style (Abbott)	Liquid (sip or tube feed) **per 100 mL**	632 kJ (150 kcal)[1]	6.25 g cows' milk soya protein isolate	20.2 g (sugars 5.6 g incl. sucrose)	4.92 g	Nil	Gluten-free Residual lactose	Standard, p.895; *also* CAPD, haemodialysis	Can: 250 mL = £2.28 (vanilla) 250 mL = £2.28 (chicken or mushroom) Bottle: 220 mL = £1.80 Banana, black currant, caramel, chocolate, coffee, fruits of the forest, orange, peach, raspberry, strawberry, vanilla, neutral
Ensure® Plus Yoghurt style (Abbott)	Liquid (sip feed) **per 100 mL**	632 kJ (150 kcal)[1]	6.25 g cows' milk	20.2 g (sugars 11.7 g)	4.92 g	Nil	Gluten-free Residual lactose	Standard, p.895; *also* CAPD, haemodialysis	Bottle: 220 mL = £1.80 Orange, peach, pineapple, strawberry
Ensure® Plus Commence (Abbott)	Starter pack (5–10 day's supply), contains: Ensure® Plus Milkshake Style (various flavours), 1 pack (10 × 220-mL) = £18.00.								
Fortisip® Bottle (Nutricia Clinical)	Liquid (sip feed) **per 100 mL**	630 kJ (150 kcal)	6 g cows' milk	18.4 g[2]	5.8 g	Nil	Gluten-free Residual lactose	Standard, p.895 Not suitable for child under 3 years	Bottle: 200 mL = £1.85 Banana, chocolate, neutral, orange, strawberry, toffee, tropical fruits, vanilla
Fortisip® Multi Fibre (Nutricia Clinical)	Liquid (sip feed) **per 100 mL**	630 kJ (150 kcal)	6 g cows' milk	18.4 g (sugars 7.0 g)	5.8 g	2.3 g	Gluten-free Residual lactose	Standard, p.895 Not suitable for child under 3 years	Bottle: 200 mL = £1.91 Banana, chocolate, orange, strawberry, vanilla
Fortisip® Yoghurt Style (Nutricia Clinical)	Liquid (sip feed) **per 100 mL**	630 kJ (150 kcal)	6 g cows' milk	18.7 g (sugars 10.8 g)	5.8 g	200 mg	Gluten-free Contains lactose	Standard, p.895 Not suitable for child under 3 years	Bottle: 200 mL = £1.85 Peach-orange, raspberry, vanilla-lemon
Fortisip® Range (Nutricia Clinical)	Starter pack contains 4 × Fortisip® Bottle, 4 × Fortijuce®, 2 × Fortisip® Yogurt Style, 1 pack (10 × 200 mL) = £18.50.								

1. Nutritional values vary with flavour—consult product literature
2. Sugar content varies with flavour

Product	Formulation	Energy	Protein	Carbohydrate	Fat	Fibre	Special Characteristics	ACBS Indications	Presentation & Flavour
Fresubin® Protein Energy Drink (Fresenius Kabi)	Liquid (sip feed) per 100 mL	630 kJ (150 kcal)	10 g cows' milk	12.4 g (sugars 6.4 g[1])	6.7 g	Nil[2]	Gluten-free, Residual lactose, Contains fish gelatin	Standard, p.895; also CAPD, haemodialysis	Bottle: 200 mL = £1.77 Cappuccino, chocolate, strawberry, tropical fruits, vanilla

1. Sugar content varies with flavour
2. Fibre content varies with flavour

A2.2.2.2 Nutritional supplements: Less than 1.5 kcal/mL and 5 g (or more) protein/100 mL

Not suitable for use in child under 1 year; use with caution in child 1–5 years unless otherwise stated

Product	Formulation	Energy	Protein	Carbohydrate	Fat	Fibre	Special Characteristics	ACBS Indications	Presentation & Flavour
Clinutren® Dessert (Nestlé)	Semi-solid per 100 g	520 kJ (125 kcal)	9.5 g cows' milk	15.5 g (sugars 14 g[1])	2.6 g	500 mg[2]	Gluten-free, Contains lactose	Standard, p.895; also CAPD, haemodialysis; Not suitable for child under 3 years	Pot: 4 × 125 g = £5.73 Caramel, chocolate, peach, vanilla
Ensure® Plus Crème (Abbott)	Semi-solid per 100 g	574 kJ (137 kcal)[3]	5.68 g[5] cows' milk and soy protein isolate	18.4 g (sugars 12.4 g)	4.47 g	Nil	Gluten-free, Residual lactose, Contains soya	Standard, p.895; also CAPD, haemodialysis; Not suitable for child under 3 years	Pot: 125 g = £1.67 Banana, chocolate, neutral, vanilla
Fortimel® Regular (Nutricia Clinical)	Liquid (sip feed) per 100 mL	420 kJ (100 kcal)	10 g cows' milk	10.3 g (sugars 8.1 g[1])	2.1 g	Nil	Gluten-free, Contains lactose	Standard, p.895; Not suitable for child under 3 years	Bottle: 200 mL = £1.57 Chocolate, forest fruits, strawberry, vanilla
Fortisip® Fruit Dessert (Nutricia Clinical)	Semi-Solid per 100 g	560 kJ (133 kcal)	7 g whey isolate	16.7 g (sugars 11.3 g)	4 g	2.6 g	Residual lactose	Standard, p.895 except bowel fistula; also CAPD, haemodialysis; Not suitable for child under 3 years	Pot: 3 × 150 g = £6.49 Apple, strawberry
Oral Impact® (Nestlé)	Standard dilution of powder (74 g in 250 mL water) (sip feed) per 100 mL	425 kJ (101 kcal)[3]	5.6 g cows' milk	13.4 g (sugars 7.4 g)	2.8 g	1 g	Residual lactose, Contains fish oil	Pre-operative nutritional supplement for malnourished patients or patients at risk of malnourishment; Not suitable for child under 3 years	Sachet: 5 × 74 g = £15.41 Citrus, coffee, tropical

Powder provides: protein 16.8 g, carbohydrate 40.1 g, fat 8.3 g, fibre 3 g, energy 1276 kJ (303 kcal)/74 g

Product	Formulation	Energy	Protein	Carbohydrate	Fat	Fibre	Special Characteristics	ACBS Indications	Presentation & Flavour
Resource® Protein (Nestlé)	Liquid (sip feed) per 100 mL	530 kJ (125 kcal)[3]	9.4 g cows' milk	14 g (sugars 4.5 g)	3.5 g	Nil	Gluten-free, Contains lactose	Standard, p.895; Not suitable for child under 3 years	Bottle: 200 mL = £1.41 Apricot, chocolate, forest fruits, strawberry, vanilla

1. Sugar content varies with flavour
2. Fibre content varies with flavour
3. Nutritional values vary with flavour—consult product literature

Appendix 2: Borderline substances

Appendix 2: Borderline substances

A2.2.2.3 Nutritional supplements: More than 1.5 kcal/mL and 5 g (or more) protein/100 mL

Not suitable for use in child under 1 year; use with caution in child 1–5 years unless otherwise stated

Product	Formulation	Energy	Protein	Carbohydrate	Fat	Fibre	Special Characteristics	ACBS Indications	Presentation & Flavour
Complan® Shake (Complan Foods)	Powder **per 57 g**	1057 kJ (251 kcal)[1]	8.8 g cows' milk	35.2 g (sugars 22.7 g)	8.4 g	Trace	Gluten-free Contains lactose	Standard, p.895	Sachet: 4 × 57 g = £3.44 Banana, chocolate, original, strawberry, vanilla; Starter pack: 5 × 57 g = £5.07
Powder 57 g reconstituted with 200 mL whole milk provides: protein 15.6 g, carbohydrate 44.5 g, fat 16.4 g, energy 1621 kJ (387 kcal)									
Foodlink® Complete (Foodlink)	Powder **per 100 g**	1838 kJ (437 kcal)[1]	21.9 g cows' milk	57.3 g	13.3 g	Nil	Contains lactose	Standard, p.895	Carton: 450 g = £3.29 Banana, chocolate, neutral, strawberry
Recommended serving = 3 heaped tablespoonfuls in 250 mL water provides: protein 12.5 g, carbohydrate 32.7 g, fat 7.6 g, energy 1048 kJ (249 kcal)[1]									
Foodlink® Complete with Fibre (Foodlink)	Powder **per 100 g**	1804 kJ (428 kcal)[1]	19.5 g cows' milk	57.1 g (sugars 36.8 g)	12.3 g	8 g	Contains lactose	Standard, p.895	Sachet: 10 × 63 g = £6.67 Vanilla + fibre
Recommended serving = 4 heaped tablespoonfuls in 250 mL water provides: protein 12.3 g, carbohydrate 38 g, fat 7.5 g, fibre 5 g, energy 1137 kJ (270 kcal)[1]									
Forticreme® Complete (Nutricia Clinical)	Semi-solid **per 100 g**	675 kJ (160 kcal)	9.5 g cows' milk	19.2 g (sugars 10.6 g)	5 g	100 mg[2]	Gluten-free Residual lactose	Standard, p.895; *also* CAPD, haemodialysis Not suitable for child under 3 years	Pot: 4 × 125 g = £7.20 Banana, chocolate, forest fruits, vanilla
Fortisip® Compact (Nutricia Clinical)	Liquid (sip feed) **per 100 mL**	1010 kJ (240 kcal)	9.6 g cows' milk	29.7 g (sugars 15 g)	9.3 g	Nil	Residual lactose	Standard, p.895 Not suitable for child under 3 years	Bottle: 125 mL = £1.85 Banana, mocha, strawberry, vanilla; Starter pack: 4 × 125 mL = £7.40
Fortisip® Extra (Nutricia Clinical)	Liquid (sip feed) **per 100 mL**	675 kJ (160 kcal)	10 g cows' milk	18.1 g (sugars 9 g)	5.3 g	Nil[2]	Gluten-free Contains lactose	Standard, p.895 Not suitable for child under 3 years	Bottle: 200 mL = £1.85 Chocolate, forest fruits, mocha, strawberry, vanilla; Starter pack 4 × 200 mL = £7.40
Fresubin® 2 kcal (Fresenius Kabi)	Liquid (sip feed) **per 100 mL**	840 kJ (200 kcal)	10 g cows' milk	22.5 g (sugars 5.8 g)	7.8 g	Nil	Gluten-free Contains lactose	Standard, p.895; *also* CAPD, haemodialysis	Bottle: 200 mL = £1.69 Apricot-peach, cappuccino, fruits of the forest, toffee, vanilla
Fresubin® 2 kcal Fibre (Fresenius Kabi)	Liquid (sip feed) **per 100 mL**	840 kJ (200 kcal)	10 g cows' milk	22.5 g (sugars 5.8 g)	7.8 g	1.6 g	Gluten-free Contains lactose	Standard, p.895; *also* CAPD, haemodialysis	Bottle: 200 mL = £1.69 Cappuccino, chocolate, lemon, vanilla
Fresubin® Crème (Fresenius Kabi)	Semi-solid **per 100 g**	756 kJ (180 kcal)	10 g cows' milk	19 g (sugars 14.4 g)	7.2 g	2 g	Gluten-free Residual lactose	Standard, p.895; *also* CAPD, haemodialysis Not suitable for child under 3 years	Pot: 4 × 125 g = £6.92 Cappuccino, strawberry, vanilla
Renilon® 7.5 (Nutricia Clinical)	Liquid (sip feed) **per 100 mL**	840 kJ (200 kcal)	7.5 g cows' milk	20 g (sugars 4.8 g)	10 g	Nil	Gluten-free Residual lactose	Standard, p.895 Not suitable for child under 3 years	Carton: 125 mL = £1.85 Apricot, caramel

1. Nutritional values vary with flavour—consult product literature
2. Fibre content varies with flavour

Product	Formulation	Energy	Protein	Carbohydrate	Fat	Fibre	Special Characteristics	ACBS Indications	Presentation & Flavour
Resource® 2.0 Fibre (Nestlé)	Liquid (sip feed) **per 100 mL**	836 kJ (200 kcal)[1]	9 g cows' milk	21.4 g (sugars 5.5 g)	8.7 g	2.5 g	Gluten-free Residual lactose	Standard, p.895 Not suitable for child under 6 years; caution in child 6–10 years	Carton: 200 mL = £1.75 Apricot, coffee, neutral, strawberry, summer fruits, vanilla
Resource® Dessert Fruit (Nestlé)	Semi-solid **per 100 g**	678 kJ (160 kcal)[1]	5 g cows' milk	24 g (sugars 16.4 g)	5 g	1.4 g	Gluten-free Residual lactose	Standard, p.895; also CAPD, haemodialysis	Cup: 3 × 125 g = £4.30 Apple, apple-peach, apple-strawberry[2]
Vegenat-med® Balanced Protein (Vegenat)	Powder **per 110 g serving**	1924 kJ (458 kcal)[1]	18 g cows' milk	62 g	15.35 g	5.8 g	Gluten-free Residual lactose	Standard, p.895 except bowel fistula Not suitable for child under 14 years	Sachet: 12 × 110 g = £35.58 Apple, chocolate, honey, orange
Vegenat-med® High Protein (Vegenat)	Powder **per 110 g serving**	1940 kJ (463 kcal)[1]	23.3 g cows' milk	57.2 g	15.6 g	6 g	Gluten-free Residual lactose	Standard, p.895 except bowel fistula Not suitable for child under 14 years	Sachet: 12 × 110 g = £49.81 Chicken, chickpea, fish, fish-vegetable, ham, lentil, veal, vegetable, winter vegetable 12 × 110 g = £48.04 Curry chicken 12 × 110 g = £47.32 Lemon, rice with lemon 24 × 55 g = £45.63 Rice with apple

1. Nutritional values vary with flavour—consult product literature
2. Flavour not suitable for child under 3 years

A2.3 Specialised formulas
For further information on composition of feeds, see p.895

A2.3.1 Specialised formulas: Infant and child
Specialised formulas are suitable for infants from birth unless otherwise indicated (see also A2.1.3.1 Enteral feeds (non-disease specific); Child under 12 years)

■ Specialised formulas: Infant and child: Amino acid-based formula
ACBS Indications: Proven whole protein intolerance, short bowel syndrome, intractable malabsorption, or other gastro-intestinal disorders where an elemental diet is indicated

Product	Formulation	Energy	Protein	Carbohydrate	Fat	Fibre	Special Characteristics	ACBS Indications	Presentation & Flavour
Neocate® Active (SHS)	Standard dilution (21%) of powder **per 300 mL serving (63-g sachet made up to 300 mL with water)**	1255 kJ (300 kcal)	8.3 g protein equivalent (essential and non-essential amino acids)	34 g (sugars 3.1 g[1])	14.5 g	Nil	Milk protein-free	See above Nutritional supplement only Not suitable for child under 1 year	Sachet: 15 × 63 g = £56.04 Black currant, unflavoured[2]

Powder provides: protein equivalent 13.1 g, carbohydrate 54 g, fat 23 g, energy 1992 kJ (475 kcal)/100 g

1. Sugar content varies with flavour
2. Flavouring: see Modjul® Flavour System, p.925

Appendix 2: Borderline substances

Appendix 2: Borderline substances

A2.3.1 Specialised formulas: Infant and child (product list continued)

Specialised formulas are suitable for infants from birth unless otherwise indicated (see also A2.1.3.1 Enteral feeds (non-disease specific); Child under 12 years)

Product	Formulation	Energy	Protein	Carbohydrate	Fat	Fibre	Special Characteristics	ACBS Indications	Presentation & Flavour
Neocate® Advance (SHS)	Standard dilution (25%) of powder **per 100 mL**	420 kJ (100 kcal)	2.5 g protein equivalent (essential and non-essential amino acids)	14.6 g (sugars 1.3 g[1])	3.5 g (MCT 35%)	Nil	Milk protein-free	See above Not suitable for child under 1 year	Sachet: 100 g = £4.82 Unflavoured[2] 15 × 50 g = £38.99 Banana-vanilla
Powder provides: protein equivalent 10 g, carbohydrate 58.5 g, fat 14 g, energy 1683 kJ (400 kcal)/100 g									
Neocate® LCP (SHS)	Standard dilution (14.7%) of powder **per 100 mL**	293 kJ (70 kcal)	1.9 g protein equivalent (essential and non-essential amino acids)	7.9 g (sugars 720 mg)	3.4 g	Nil	Milk protein-free	Cows' milk allergy, multiple food protein intolerance, and conditions requiring an elemental diet	Can: 400 g = £23.83 (4.9-g measuring scoop provided)
Powder provides: protein equivalent 13 g, carbohydrate 54 g, fat 23 g, energy 1990 kJ (475 kcal)/100 g									
Neocate® Nutra (SHS)	Powder for paste (spoon feed) **per 100 g**	1981 kJ (472 kcal)	8.2 g protein equivalent (essential and non-essential amino acids)	67.4 g (sugars 12.3 g)	18.8 g	Nil	Gluten free Milk protein-free	Nutritional supplement for dietary management of cows' milk allergy, multiple food protein intolerance, and other conditions requiring an amino-acid based food, in children over 6 months	Can: 400 g = £23.83 (measuring scoop provided)
Powder 37 g (8 scoopfuls) provides: protein equivalent 3 g, carbohydrate 24.9 g, fat 7 g, energy 733 kJ (175 kcal)									
Nutramigen® AA (Mead Johnson)	Standard dilution (13.6 %) of powder **per 100 mL**	286 kJ (68 kcal)	1.89 g essential and non-essential amino acids	7 g	3.6 g	Nil	Gluten-free Lactose-free	Severe cows' milk protein intolerance, or multiple food intolerance, and other gastro-intestinal disorders where an elemental diet is specifically indicated	Can: 400 g = £22.05 (4.5-g measuring scoop provided)
Powder provides: protein 13.9 g, carbohydrate 51 g, fat 26 g, energy 2092 kJ (498 kcal)/100 g									

1. Sugar content varies with flavour
2. Flavouring: see Modjul® Flavour System, p.925

Specialised formulas: Infant and child: Hydrolysate formula

Product	Standard dilution (per 100 mL)	Energy	Protein	Carbohydrate	Fat		Notes	Description	Price
Aptamil® Pepti® (Milupa) Formerly Cow & Gate Pepti®	Standard dilution (13.6%) of powder per 100 mL	275 kJ (66 kcal)	1.6 g whey hydrolysed	7.1 g (sugars 6.4 g)	3.5 g	800 mg	Contains lactose and fish oil	Established cows' milk protein intolerance, with or without secondary lactose intolerance	Can: 400 g = £8.62 900 g = £19.39 (4.5-g measuring scoop provided)
Powder provides: protein 11.6 g, carbohydrate 52 g, fat 25.6 g, energy 2025 kJ (484 kcal)/100 g									
Cow & Gate Pepti-Junior® (Cow & Gate)	Standard dilution (12.8%) of powder per 100 mL	275 kJ (66 kcal)	1.8 g whey hydrolysed	6.8 g (sugars 1.1 g)	3.5 g	Nil	Residual lactose Contains fish oil	Disaccharide and/or whole protein intolerance, or where amino acids and peptides are indicated in conjunction with medium chain triglycerides	Can: 450 g = £10.68 (4.3-g measuring scoop provided)
Powder provides: protein 14 g, carbohydrate 53.4 g, fat 27.3 g, energy 2155 kJ (515 kcal)/100 g									
Nutramigen® 1 (Mead Johnson)	Standard dilution (13.5%) of powder per 100 mL	280 kJ (68 kcal)	1.9 g casein hydrolysed	7.5 g	3.4 g	Nil	Gluten-free Lactose-free	Disaccharide and/or whole protein intolerance where additional medium chain triglycerides are not included	Can: 400 g = £8.95 (4.5-g measuring scoop provided)
Powder provides: protein 14 g, carbohydrate 55 g, fat 25 g, energy 2100 kJ (500 kcal)/100 g									
Nutramigen® 2 (Mead Johnson)	Standard dilution (14.6%) of powder per 100 mL	285 kJ (68 kcal)	1.7 g casein hydrolysed	8.6 g	2.9 g	Nil	Gluten-free Lactose-free	Established disaccharide and/or whole protein intolerance (where additional chain triglycerides are not indicated) Not suitable for child under 6 months	Can: 400 g = £8.95 (4.9-g measuring scoop provided)
Powder provides: protein 11.6 g, carbohydrate 59 g, fat 20 g, energy 1950 kJ (466 kcal)/100 g									
Pepdite® (SHS)	Standard dilution (15%) of powder per 100 mL	297 kJ (71 kcal)	2.1 g protein equivalent (non-milk hydrolysate)	7.8 g (sugars 700 mg)	3.5 g	Nil	Lactose-free Contains meat (pork) and soya derivatives	Disaccharide and/or whole protein intolerance	Can: 400 g = £15.05 (5-g measuring scoop provided)
Powder provides: protein equivalent 13.8 g, carbohydrate 52 g, fat 23.2 g, energy 1977 kJ (472 kcal)/100 g									
Pepdite® 1+ (SHS)	Standard dilution (22.8%) of powder per 100 mL	423 kJ (100 kcal)	3.1 g protein equivalent (non-milk hydrolysate, essential amino acids)	13 g (sugars 1.2 g)	3.9 g (MCT 35%)	Nil	Lactose-free Contains meat (pork) and soya derivatives	Disaccharide and/or whole protein intolerance, or where amino acids or peptides are indicated in conjunction with medium chain triglycerides Not suitable for child under 1 year	Can: 400 g = £15.81 Unflavoured[1]
Powder provides: protein equivalent 13.8 g, carbohydrate 57 g, fat 17.3 g, energy 1844 kJ (439 kcal)/100 g									

1. Flavouring: see *Modjul®* Flavour System, p. 925

Appendix 2: Borderline substances

A2.3.1 Specialised formulas: Infant and child (product list continued)

Specialised formulas are suitable for infants from birth unless otherwise indicated (see also A2.1.3.1 Enteral feeds (non-disease specific); Child under 12 years)

Product	Formulation	Energy	Protein	Carbohydrate	Fat	Fibre	Special Characteristics	ACBS Indications	Presentation & Flavour
Pregestimil® (Mead Johnson)	Standard dilution (13.5 %) of powder **per 100 mL**	280 kJ (68 kcal)	1.89 g casein hydrolysed	6.9 g	3.8 g (MCT 54 %)	Nil	Gluten-free Lactose-free	Disaccharide and/or whole protein intolerance, or where amino acids or peptides are indicated in conjunction with medium chain triglycerides	Can: 400 g = £9.81 (4.5-g measuring scoop provided)

Powder provides: protein 14 g, carbohydrate 51 g, fat 28 g, energy 2100 kJ (500 kcal)/100 g

◼ Specialised formulas: Infant and child: Residual lactose formula

Product	Formulation	Energy	Protein	Carbohydrate	Fat	Fibre	Special Characteristics	ACBS Indications	Presentation & Flavour
Enfamil® O-Lac (Mead Johnson)	Standard dilution (13 %) of powder **per 100 mL**	280 kJ (68 kcal)	1.42 g cows' milk	7.2 g	3.7 g	Nil	Gluten-free Residual lactose	Proven lactose intolerance	Can: 400 g = £4.01 (4.3-g measuring scoop provided)

Powder provides: protein 10.9 g, carbohydrate 55 g, fat 28 g, energy 2200 kJ (524 kcal)/100 g

| Galactomin 17® (SHS) | Standard dilution (13.6 %) of powder **per 100 mL** | 295 kJ (70 kcal) | 1.7 g protein equivalent (cows' milk) | 7.5 g (sugars 1.4 g) | 3.7 g | Nil | Residual lactose | Proven lactose intolerance in pre-school children, galactosaemia, and galactokinase deficiency | Can: 400 g = £13.48 Unflavoured[1] (4.3-g measuring scoop provided) |

Powder provides: protein equivalent 12.3 g, carbohydrate 55.3 g, fat 27.2 g, energy 2155 kJ (515 kcal)/100 g

| SMA® LF (SMA Nutrition) | Standard dilution (13 %) of powder **per 100 mL** | 281 kJ (67 kcal) | 1.5 g casein, whey | 7.2 g (sugars 2.6 g) | 3.6 g | Nil | Residual lactose | Proven lactose intolerance | Can: 430 g = £3.97 |

Powder provides: protein equivalent 12 g, carbohydrate 55.6 g, fat 28 g, energy 2185 kJ (522 kcal)/100 g

◼ Specialised formulas: Infant and child: MCT-enhanced formula

Product	Formulation	Energy	Protein	Carbohydrate	Fat	Fibre	Special Characteristics	ACBS Indications	Presentation & Flavour
Caprilon® (SHS)	Standard dilution (12.7 %) of powder **per 100 mL**	277 kJ (66 kcal)	1.5 g cows' milk	7 g (sugars 1.3 g)	3.6 g (MCT 75 %)	Nil	Contains lactose	Disorders in which a high intake of MCT is beneficial	Can: 420 g = £14.62 (4.2-g measuring scoop provided)

Powder provides: protein 11.8 g, carbohydrate 55.1 g, fat 28.3 g, energy 2184 kJ (522 kcal)/100 g

| MCT Pepdite® (SHS) | Standard dilution (15 %) of powder **per 100 mL** | 286 kJ (68 kcal) | 2 g protein equivalent (non-milk peptides, essential amino acids) | 8.8 g (sugars 1.2 g) | 2.7 g (MCT 75 %) | Nil | Gluten-free Lactose-free Contains meat (pork) and soya derivatives | Disorders in which a high intake of MCT is beneficial | Can: 400 g = £16.39 (5-g measuring scoop provided) |

Powder provides: protein equivalent 13.8 g, carbohydrate 59 g, fat 18 g, energy 1903 kJ (453 kcal)/100 g

1. Flavouring: see Modjul® Flavour System, p. 925

Product	Standard dilution / per 100 mL	Protein	Carbohydrate	Fat		Special characteristics	Indication	Presentation
MCT Pepdite® +1 (SHS)	Standard dilution (20 %) of powder **per 100 mL** — 381 kJ (91 kcal)	2.8 g protein equivalent (non-milk peptides, essential amino acids)	11.8 g (sugars 1.6 g)	3.6 g (MCT 75 %)	Nil	Gluten-free. Lactose-free. Contains meat (pork) and soya derivatives	Disorders in which a high intake of MCT is beneficial. Not suitable for child under 1 year	Can: 400 g = £16.39 Unflavoured[1]

Powder provides: protein equivalent 13.8 g, carbohydrate 59 g, fat 18 g, energy 1903 kJ (453 kcal)/100 g

Monogen® (SHS)	Standard dilution (17.5 %) of powder **per 100 mL** — 313 kJ (74 kcal)	2 g protein equivalent (whey)	12 g (sugars 1.2 g)	2.1 g (MCT 90 %)	Nil	Residual lactose. Supplementation with essential fatty acids may be needed	Long-chain acyl-CoA dehydrogenase deficiency (LCAD), carnitine palmitoyl transferase deficiency (CPTD), primary and secondary lipoprotein lipase deficiency	Can: 400 g = £16.29 Unflavoured[1] (5-g measuring scoop provided)

Powder provides: protein equivalent 11.4 g, carbohydrate 68 g, fat 11.8 g, energy 1786 kJ (424 kcal)/100 g

■ Specialised formulas: Infant and child: Soya-based formula

InfaSoy® (Cow & Gate)	Standard dilution (12.8 %) of powder **per 100 mL** — 275 kJ (66 kcal)	1.6 g soya	7 g (sugars 1 g)	3.5 g	Nil	Lactose-free	Proven lactose and associated sucrose intolerance in pre-school children, galactokinase deficiency, galactosaemia, and proven whole cows' milk sensitivity	Can: 900 g = £7.47 (4.3-g measuring scoop provided)

Powder provides: protein 12.8 g, carbohydrate 54.5 g, fat 27.3 g, energy 2150 kJ (514 kcal)/100 g

Wysoy® (Wyeth)	Standard dilution (13.2 %) of powder **per 100 mL** — 280 kJ (67 kcal)	1.8 g soya protein isolate	6.9 g (sugars 2.5 g)	3.6 g	Nil	Lactose-free	Proven lactose and associated sucrose intolerance in pre-school children, galactokinase deficiency, galactosaemia, and proven whole cows' milk sensitivity	Can: 430 g = £3.89, 860 g = £7.37

Powder provides: protein equivalent 14 g, carbohydrate 54 g, fat 27 g, energy 2155 kJ (515 kcal)/100 g

■ Specialised formulas: Infant and child: Low calcium formula

Locasol® (SHS)	Standard dilution (13.1 %) of powder **per 100 mL** — 278 kJ (66 kcal)	1.9 g cows' milk	7 g (sugars 6.9 g)	3.4 g	Nil	Contains lactose. Calcium less than 7 mg/100 mL. No added vitamin D	Conditions of calcium intolerance requiring restriction of calcium and vitamin D intake	Can: 400 g = £18.37 (4.4-g measuring scoop provided)

Powder provides: protein 14.6 g, carbohydrate 53.7 g, fat 26.1 g, energy 2125 kJ (508 kcal)/100 g

■ Specialised formulas: Infant and child: Fructose-based formula

Galactomin 19® (SHS)	Standard dilution (12.9 %) of powder **per 100 mL** — 288 kJ (69 kcal)	1.9 g protein equivalent (cows' milk)	6.4 g (fructose 6.3 g)	4 g	Nil	Residual lactose, galactose and glucose	Conditions of glucose plus galactose intolerance	Can: 400 g = £35.48

Powder provides: protein equivalent 14.6 g, carbohydrate 49.7 g, fat 30.8 g, energy 2233 kJ (534 kcal)/100 g

1. Flavouring: see Modjul® Flavour System, p. 925

Appendix 2: Borderline substances

Appendix 2: Borderline substances

A2.3.1 Specialised formulas: Infant and child (product list continued)

Specialised formulas are suitable for infants from birth unless otherwise indicated (see also A2.1.3.1 Enteral feeds (non-disease specific); Child under 12 years)

■ Specialised formulas: Infant and child: Pre-thickened infant feeds

Note Not to be used for a period of more than 6 months; not to be used in conjunction with any other feed thickener or antacid products

Product	Formulation	Energy	Protein	Carbohydrate	Fat	Fibre	Special Characteristics	ACBS Indications	Presentation & Flavour
Enfamil® AR (Mead Johnson)	Standard dilution (13.5%) of powder **per 100 mL**	285 kJ (68 kcal)	1.7 g cows' milk	7.6 g (lactose 4.6 g)	3.5 g	Nil	Contains lactose, pregelatinised rice starch	Significant gastro-oesophageal reflux	Can: 400 g = £3.01 (4.5-g measuring scoop provided)

Powder provides: protein 12.5 g, carbohydrate 56 g, fat 26 g, energy 2093 kJ (500 kcal)/100 g

| SMA® Staydown (SMA Nutrition) | Standard dilution (12.9%) of powder **per 100 mL** | 279 kJ (67 kcal) | 1.6 g casein, whey | 7 g (lactose 5 g) | 3.6 g | Nil | Contains lactose, pre-cooked corn starch | Significant gastro-oesophageal reflux | Can: 900 g = £5.64 |

Powder provides: protein 12.4 g, carbohydrate 54.3 g, fat 28 g, energy 2166 kJ (518 kcal)/100 g

A2.3.2 Specialised formulas for specific clinical conditions

For further information on composition of feeds, see p. 895

Product	Formulation	Energy	Protein	Carbohydrate	Fat	Fibre	Special Characteristics	ACBS Indications	Presentation & Flavour
Alicalm® (SHS)	Standard dilution (30%) of powder **per 100 mL**	567 kJ (135 kcal)	4.5 g caseinate whey	17.4 g (sugars 3.2 g)	5.3 g	Nil	Residual lactose	Crohn's disease Not suitable for child under 1 year; use as nutritional supplement only in children 1–6 years.	Powder: 400 g = £17.25 Vanilla

Powder provides: protein 15 g, carbohydrate 58 g, fat 17.5 g, energy 1889 kJ (450 kcal)/100 g

| Forticare® (Nutricia Clinical) | Liquid (sip feed) **per 100 mL** | 675 kJ (160 kcal) | 9 g cows' milk | 19.1 g (sugars 13.6 g) | 5.3 g | 2.1 g | Gluten-free Residual lactose Contains fish oil | Nutritional supplement in patients with lung cancer undergoing chemotherapy, or with pancreatic cancer Not suitable in child under 3 years | Carton: 125 mL = £1.98 Cappuccino, orange-lemon, peach-ginger |
| Generaid® (SHS) | Powder **per 100 g** | 1586 kJ (374 kcal) | 76 g protein equivalent (whey protein, plus branched chain amino acids) | 5 g (sugars 5 g) | 5.5 g | Nil | Electrolytes/100 g: Na⁺ 6.1 mmol K⁺ 10.8 mmol Ca²⁺ 6.5 mmol P³⁻ 6.45 mmol | Nutritional supplement for use in chronic liver disease and/or porto-hepatic encephalopathy | Tub: 200 g = £24.55 Unflavoured[1] |

1. Flavouring: see Modjul® Flavour System, p. 925

Product	Energy / dilution	Protein	Carbohydrate	Fat		Electrolytes	Indication	Presentation
Generaid® Plus (SHS)	Standard dilution (22%) of powder **per 100 mL** — 428 kJ (102 kcal)	2.4 g protein equivalent (whey protein, branched chain amino acids)	13.6 g (sugars 1.4 g)	4.2 g (MCT 32%)	Nil	Electrolytes/100 mL: Na⁺ 0.7 mmol, K⁺ 2.7 mmol, Ca²⁺ 1.72 mmol, P* 1.67 mmol	Enteral feed or nutritional supplement in children over 1 year with hepatic disorders	Can: 400 g = £17.56 Unflavoured[1] (5-g measuring scoop provided)

Powder provides: protein equivalent 11 g, carbohydrate 62 g, fat 19 g, energy 1944 kJ (463 kcal)/100 g

Product	Energy / dilution	Protein	Carbohydrate	Fat		Electrolytes	Indication	Presentation
Heparon® Junior (SHS)	Standard dilution (18%) of powder **per 100 mL** — 363 kJ (86 kcal)	2 g cows' milk	3.6 g (sugars 2.9 g)	3.6 g	Nil	Contains lactose. Electrolytes/100 mL: Na⁺ 0.56 mmol, K⁺ 1.9 mmol, Ca²⁺ 2.3 mmol, P* 1.6 mmol	Enteral feed or nutritional supplement for children with acute or chronic liver failure	Can: 400 g = £18.20 (4.5-g measuring scoop provided)

Powder provides: protein 11.1 g, carbohydrate 64.2 g, fat 19.9 g, energy 2016 kJ (480 kcal)/100 g

Product	Energy / dilution	Protein	Carbohydrate	Fat		Electrolytes	Indication	Presentation
KetoCal® (SHS)	Standard dilution (20%) of powder **per 100 mL** — 602 kJ (146 kcal)	3.1 g cows' milk with additional amino acids	600 mg (sugars 120 mg)	14.6 g (LCT 100%)	Nil	Electrolytes/100 mL: Na⁺ 4.3 mmol, K⁺ 4.1 mmol, Ca²⁺ 2.15 mmol, P* 2.77 mmol	Enteral feed or nutritional supplement as part of ketogenic diet in management of epilepsy resistant to drug therapy, in children over 1 year, only on the advice of secondary care physician with experience of ketogenic diet	Can: 300 g = £24.44 Vanilla, Unflavoured

Powder provides: protein 15.25 g, carbohydrate 3 g, fat 73 g, energy 3011 kJ (730 kcal)/100 g

Product	Energy / dilution	Protein	Carbohydrate	Fat		Electrolytes	Indication	Presentation
Kindergen® (SHS)	Standard dilution (20%) of powder **per 100 mL** — 421 kJ (101 kcal)	1.5 g whey protein	11.8 mg (sugars 1.2 g)	5.3 g (LCT 93%)	Nil	Electrolytes/100 mL: Na⁺ 2 mmol, K⁺ 0.6 mmol, Ca²⁺ 2.8 mmol, P* 3 mmol, Low Vitamin A	Enteral feed or nutritional supplement for children with chronic renal failure receiving peritoneal rapid overnight dialysis	Tub: 400 g = £23.32 (5-g measuring scoop provided)

Powder provides: protein 7.5 g, carbohydrate 59 g, fat 26.3 g, energy 2104 kJ (504 kcal)/100 g

Product	Energy / dilution	Protein	Carbohydrate	Fat		Electrolytes	Indication	Presentation
Modulen IBD® (Nestlé)	Standard dilution (20%) of powder **per 100 mL** (sip or tube feed) — 420 kJ (100 kcal)	3.6 g casein	11 g (sugars 3.98 g)	4.7 g	Nil	Gluten-free. Residual lactose	Crohn's disease active phase, and in remission if malnourished	Can: 400 g = £14.38 Unflavoured[2] (8.3-g measuring scoop provided)

Powder provides: protein 18 g, carbohydrate 54 g, fat 23 g, energy 2070 kJ (500 kcal)/100 g

1. Flavouring: see *Modjul®* Flavour System, p. 925
2. Flavouring: see *Flavour Mix®*, p. 925

Appendix 2: Borderline substances

Appendix 2: Borderline substances

A2.3.2 Specialised formulas for specific clinical conditions (product list continued)

For further information on composition of feeds, see p. 895

Product	Formulation	Energy	Protein	Carbohydrate	Fat	Fibre	Special Characteristics	ACBS Indications	Presentation & Flavour
Nepro® (Abbott)	Liquid (sip or tube feed) **per 100 mL**	838 kJ (200 kcal)[1]	7 g cows' milk	20.6 g (sugars 3.26 g)	9.6 g	1.56 g	Gluten-free Residual lactose Electrolytes/100 mL: Na$^+$ 3.67 mmol K$^+$ 2.72 mmol Ca^{2+} 3.43 mmol P$^+$ 2.23 mmol	Enteral feed or nutritional supplement in patients with chronic renal failure who are on haemodialysis or CAPD, or with cirrhosis, or other conditions requiring a high energy, low fluid, low electrolyte diet. Not suitable for child under 1 year; use with caution in child 1–5 years	Carton: 200 mL = £2.34 Strawberry, vanilla Flexible pack: 500 mL = £5.07 Vanilla
ProSure® (Abbott)	Liquid (sip or tube feed) **per 100 mL**	529 kJ (125 kcal)[1]	6.65 g cows' milk	18.3 g (sugars 2.95 g)	2.56 g	2.07 g	Gluten-free Residual lactose Contains fish oil	Nutritional supplement for patients with pancreatic cancer Not suitable for child under 1 year; use with caution in child 1–4 years	Carton: 240 mL = £2.77 Vanilla
Renamil® (KoRa)	Powder (sip or tube feed when reconstituted) **per 100 g**	2003 kJ (477 kcal)	4.6 g cows' milk	70.8 g	19.3 g	Nil	Contains lactose Gluten-free Electrolytes/100 g: Na$^+$ 1.04 mmol K$^+$ 0.13 mmol Ca^{2+} 10.22 mmol P$^+$ 1.06 mmol Contains no vitamin A or vitamin D	Enteral feed or nutritional supplement for adults and children over 1 year with chronic renal failure	Sachet: 10 × 100 g = £25.40
Renapro® (KoRa)	Powder **per 100 g**	1580 kJ (372 kcal)	90 g whey protein	800 mg	1 g	Nil	Gluten-free Residual lactose Electrolytes/100 g: Na$^+$ 23 mmol K$^+$ 2 mmol P$^+$ 4.84 mmol	Nutritional supplement for biochemically proven hypoproteinaemia and patients undergoing dialysis Not suitable for child under 1 year	Sachet: 30 × 20 g = £69.60

Powder provides: protein 18 g, energy 316 kJ (74 kcal)/20-g sachet

Product	Formulation	Energy	Protein	Carbohydrate	Fat	Fibre	Special Characteristics	ACBS Indications	Presentation & Flavour
Renastart® (Vitaflo)	Standard dilution (20%) of powder **per 100 mL**	411 kJ (98 kcal)	1.5 g cows' milk soya	12.6 g (sugars 1.2 g)	4.6 g	Nil	Contains lactose Electrolytes/100 mL: Na$^+$ 2.1 mmol K$^+$ 0.6 mmol Ca^{2+} 0.58 mmol P$^+$ 0.58 mmol	Dietary management of renal failure in child from birth to 10 years	Powder: 10 × 100 g = £56.93 Unflavoured (7-g measuring scoop provided)

Powder provides: protein 7.5 g, carbohydrate 63 g, fat 23.2 g, energy 2053 kJ (491 kcal)/100 g

1. Nutritional values vary with flavour—consult product literature

| | | | | | | | Gluten-free Residual lactose Electrolytes/100 mL: Na⁺ 3.39 mmol K⁺ 2.87 mmol Ca²⁺ 3.48 mmol P* 2.39 mmol | Enteral feed or nutritional supplement in patients with chronic or acute renal failure who are not undergoing dialysis, or with chronic or acute liver disease with fluid restriction; other conditions requiring high energy, low protein, low electrolyte, low volume enteral feed Not suitable for child under 1 year; use with caution in child 1–5 years | Can: 237 mL = £2.40 Vanilla |

Suplena® (Abbott) — Liquid (sip or tube feed) per 100 mL | 840 kJ (200 kcal) | 3 g caseinates | 25.5 g (sugars 2.7 g) | 9.6 g | Nil | Na^+ 3.39 mmol, K^+ 2.87 mmol, Ca^{2+} 3.48 mmol, P^* 2.39 mmol

A2.4 Feed supplements

A2.4.1 High-energy supplements
For further information on composition of feeds, see p.895

A2.4.1.1 High-energy supplements: carbohydrate
Flavoured carbohydrate supplements are not suitable for child under 1 year; liquid supplements should be diluted before use in child under 5 years

ACBS Indications: disease-related malnutrition, malabsorption states, or other conditions requiring fortification with a high or readily available carbohydrate supplement

Product	Formulation	Energy	Protein	Carbohydrate	Fat	Fibre	Special Characteristics	ACBS Indications	Presentation & Flavour
Caloreen® (Nestlé)	Powder per 100 g	1640 kJ (390 kcal)	Nil	96 g Maltodextrin	Nil	Nil	Gluten-free Lactose-free	See above Not suitable for child under 3 years	Powder: 500 g = £3.52 Unflavoured (10-g measuring scoop provided)
Maxijul® Super Soluble (SHS)	Powder per 100 g	1615 kJ (380 kcal)	Nil	95 g Glucose polymer (sugars 8.6 g)	Nil	Nil	Gluten-free Lactose-free	See above	Sachets: 4 × 132 g = £5.17 Can: 200 g = £1.96 2.5 kg = £18.37 25 kg = £124.77 Unflavoured
Maxijul® Liquid (SHS)	Liquid per 100 mL	850 kJ (200 kcal)	Nil	50 g Glucose polymer (sugars 4.5 g[1])	Nil	Nil	Gluten-free Lactose-free	See above	Carton: 200 mL = £1.31 Orange, unflavoured

1. Sugar content varies with flavour

Appendix 2: Borderline substances

A2.4.1.1 High-energy supplements: carbohydrate (product list continued)

Flavoured carbohydrate supplements are not suitable for use in child under 1 year; liquid supplements should be diluted before use in child under 5 years

ACBS Indications: disease-related malnutrition, malabsorption states, or other conditions requiring fortification with a high or readily available carbohydrate supplement

Product	Formulation	Energy	Protein	Carbohydrate	Fat	Fibre	Special Characteristics	ACBS Indications	Presentation & Flavour
Polycal® (Nutricia Clinical)	Powder per 100 g	1630 kJ (384 kcal)	Nil	96 g Maltodextrin (sugars 6 g)	Nil	Nil	Gluten-free Lactose-free	See above	Can: 400 g = £3.66 Neutral (5-g measuring scoop provided)
	Liquid per 100 mL	1050 kJ (247 kcal)	Nil	61.9 g Maltodextrin (sugars 12.2 g)	Nil	Nil		Liquid not suitable for child under 3 years	Bottle: 200 mL = £1.46 Neutral, orange
S.O.S.® (Vitaflo)	Powder per 100 g	1590 kJ (380 kcal)	Nil	95 g (sugars 9 g)	Nil	Nil		For use as an emergency regimen in the dietary management of inborn errors of metabolism in adults and children from birth	Sachets: 30 × 21 g (S.O.S. 10) = £6.30; 30 × 31 g (S.O.S. 15) = £9.30; 30 × 42 g (S.O.S. 20) = £12.60; 30 × 52 g (S.O.S. 25) = £15.60

Contents of each sachet should be reconstituted with water to a total volume of 200 mL

Product	Formulation	Energy	Protein	Carbohydrate	Fat	Fibre	Special Characteristics	ACBS Indications	Presentation & Flavour
Vitajoule® (Vitaflo)	Powder per 100 g	1610 kJ (380 kcal)	Nil	96 g Dried glucose syrup	Nil	Nil	Gluten-free Lactose-free	See above	Can: 500 g = £3.58 2.5 kg = £17.65 25 kg = £105.03 (10-g measuring scoop provided)

A2.4.1.2 High-energy supplements: fat

Liquid supplements should be diluted before use in child under 5 years

ACBS Indications: disease-related malnutrition, malabsorption states, or other conditions requiring fortification with a high fat (or fat and carbohydrate) supplement

Product	Formulation	Energy	Protein	Carbohydrate	Fat	Fibre	Special Characteristics	ACBS Indications	Presentation & Flavour
Calogen® (Nutricia Clinical)	Liquid (emulsion) per 100 mL	1850 kJ (450 kcal)[1]	Nil	100 mg	50 g (LCT 100 %)	Nil	Gluten-free Lactose-free	See above	Bottle: 200 mL = £3.91 500 mL = £9.60 Banana², neutral, strawberry²
Liquigen® (SHS)	Liquid (emulsion) per 100 mL	1850 kJ (450 kcal)	Nil	Nil	50 g (MCT 97 %) Fractionated coconut oil	Nil	Gluten-free Lactose-free	Steatorrhoea associated with cystic fibrosis of the pancreas, intestinal lymphangiectasia, intestinal surgery, chronic liver disease, liver cirrhosis, other proven malabsorption syndromes, ketogenic diet in epilepsy, and in type 1 lipoproteinaemia Not suitable for child under 1 year	Bottle: 250 mL = £7.43

1. Nutritional values vary with flavour—consult product literature
2. Flavour not suitable for child under 3 years

		Energy	Protein	Carbohydrate	Fat	Special characteristics	Presentation
Medium-chain Triglyceride (MCT) Oil (SHS)	Liquid **per 100 mL**	3515 kJ (855 kcal)	Nil	Nil	MCT 100 %	Nil	Nutritional supplement for steatorrhoea associated with cystic fibrosis of the pancreas, intestinal lymphangiectasia, intestinal surgery, chronic liver disease and liver cirrhosis, other proven malabsorption syndromes, ketogenic diet in management of epilepsy, type 1 hyperlipoproteinaemia	Bottle: 500 mL = £11.78

■ Fat and Carbohydrate

		Energy	Protein	Carbohydrate	Fat	Special characteristics	Presentation
Duobar® (SHS)	Bar **per 45 g**	1211 kJ (292 kcal)	Less than 20 mg	22.5 g (sucrose)	22.5 g	Contains phenylalanine 180 micrograms/45-g bar Gluten-free Lactose-free	See above	Bar: 45 g = £1.58 Neutral, strawberry, toffee
Duocal® (SHS)	Liquid **per 100 mL**	695 kJ (166 kcal)	Nil	23.7 g (sugars 2.1 g)	7.9 g (MCT 30 %)	Contains vitamin E	See above	Bottle: 250 mL = £3.22
Duocal® Super Soluble (SHS)	Powder **per 100 g**	2061 kJ (492 kcal)	Nil	72.7 g (sugars 6.5 g)	22.3 g (MCT 35 %)	Gluten-free Lactose-free	See above	Can: 400 g = £14.50 (5-g measuring scoop provided)
Energivit® (SHS)	Standard dilution (15%) of powder **per 100 mL**	309 kJ (74 kcal)	Nil	10 g (sugars 900 mg)	3.75 g	Lactose-free With vitamins, minerals, and trace elements	For children requiring additional energy, vitamins, minerals, and trace elements following a protein-restricted diet	Can: 400 g = £17.64 (5-g measuring scoop provided)
	Powder provides: carbohydrate 66.7 g, fat 25 g, energy 2059 kJ (492 kcal)/100 g							
MCT Duocal® (SHS)	Powder **per 100 g**	2082 kJ (497 kcal)	Nil	72 g (sugars 10.1 g)	23.2 g (MCT 83 %)		See above	Can: 400 g = £17.24

Appendix 2: Borderline substances

Appendix 2: Borderline substances

A2.4.1.3 High-energy supplements: protein

ACBS indications: disease-related malnutrition, malabsorption states, or other conditions requiring fortification with a high fat or carbohydrate (with protein) supplement

Product	Formulation	Energy	Protein	Carbohydrate	Fat	Fibre	Special Characteristics	ACBS Indications	Presentation & Flavour
Casilan 90® (Heinz)	Powder **per 100 g**	1572 kJ (370 kcal)	90 g cows' milk	300 mg	1 g	Nil	Gluten-free Electrolytes/100 g: Na⁺ 1.3 mmol K⁺ 8.7 mmol Ca²⁺ 35 mmol P⁺ 22.6 mmol	Nutritional supplement for use in biochemically proven hypoprotein-aemia	Can: 250 g = £6.49
Protifar® (Nutricia Clinical)	Powder **per 100 g**	1580 kJ (373 kcal)	88.5 g cows' milk	less than 1.5 g	1.6 g	Nil	Gluten-free Residual lactose Electrolytes/100 mL: Na⁺ 1.3 mmol K⁺ 1.28 mmol Ca²⁺ 33.75 mmol P⁺ 22.58 mmol	Nutritional supplement for use in biochemically proven hypoprotein-aemia	Can: 225 g = £7.44 Unflavoured (2.5-g measuring scoop provided)

Powder provides: protein 2.2 g per 2.5 g.

Product	Formulation	Energy	Protein	Carbohydrate	Fat	Fibre	Special Characteristics	ACBS Indications	Presentation & Flavour
Vitapro® (Vitaflo)	Powder **per 100 g**	1506 kJ (360 kcal)	75 g whey protein isolate	9 g	6 g	Nil	Contains lactose	Biochemically proven hypoprotein-aemia	Tub: 250 g = £7.31 2 kg = £57.40 (5-g measuring scoop provided)

▣ Protein and carbohydrate

Product	Formulation	Energy	Protein	Carbohydrate	Fat	Fibre	Special Characteristics	ACBS Indications	Presentation & Flavour
Dialamine® (SHS)	Standard dilution (20%) of powder **per 100 mL**	264 kJ (62 kcal)	4.3 g protein equivalent (essential and non-essential amino acids)	11.2 g (sugars 10.2 g)	Nil	Nil	Contains vitamin C	Hypoproteinaemia, chronic renal failure, wound fistula leakage with excessive protein loss, conditions requiring a controlled nitrogen intake, and haemodialysis Not suitable for child under 6 months	Can: 400 g = £58.91 Orange

Powder provides: protein equivalent 25 g, carbohydrate 65 g, vitamin C 125 mg, energy 1530 kJ (360 kcal)/100 g

Product	Formulation	Energy	Protein	Carbohydrate	Fat	Fibre	Special Characteristics	ACBS Indications	Presentation & Flavour
ProSource® (Nutrinovo)	Liquid **per 30 mL**	420 kJ (100 kcal)	10 g collagen protein whey protein isolate	15 g (sugars 7 g)	Nil	Nil	Gluten-free Lactose-free May contain porcine derivatives	Biochemically proven hypoprotein-aemia Not recommended for child under 3 years	Sachet: 100 × 30 mL = £80.00 Neutral

Protein, fat, and carbohydrate

Product	Form	Energy	Protein	Carbohydrate	Fat	Fibre	Special characteristics	Suitability	Presentation and flavour
Calogen® Extra (Nutricia Clinical)	Liquid per 100 mL	1650 kJ (400 kcal)	5 g cows' milk	4.5 g (sugars 3.5 g)	40.3 g	Nil	Residual lactose; Contains vitamins, minerals, and trace elements	See above; Not suitable for child under 3 years; may require dilution for child 3–5 years	Bottle: 200 mL = £4.56; Neutral, strawberry
Calshake® (Fresenius Kabi)	Powder per 87 g	1841 kJ (439 kcal)[1]	4.1 g cows' milk	56.4 g (sugars 20 g)	22 g	Nil	Contains lactose; Gluten-free	See above; Not suitable for child under 1 year	Sachet: 87 g = £1.96 Banana, neutral, strawberry, vanilla; 90 g = £1.96 Chocolate
Powder: one sachet reconstituted with 240 mL whole milk provides approx. 2 kcal/mL and protein 12 g									
Enshake® (Abbott)	Powder per 100 g	1893 kJ (450 kcal)[1]	8.4 g cows' milk, soy protein isolate	69 g (sugars 14.5 g)	15.6 g	Nil	Residual lactose; Contains vitamins and minerals	See above; Not suitable for child under 1 year; use with caution in child 1–6 years	Sachet: 96.5 g = £1.92 Banana, chocolate, strawberry, vanilla
Powder: 96.5 g reconstituted with 240 mL whole milk provides approx. 2 kcal/mL and protein 16 g									
Pro-Cal® (Vitaflo)	Powder per 100 g	2788 kJ (667 kcal)	13.5 g cows' milk	27 g	56 g	Nil	Contains lactose	See above; Not suitable for child under 1 year	Sachets: 25 × 15 g = £13.21; Tub: 510 g = £12.24; 1.5 kg = £24.94; 12.5 kg = £177.29; 25 kg = £273.21 (15 g measuring scoop provided)
Powder 15 g provides: protein 2 g, carbohydrate 4 g, fat 8.4 g, energy 418 kJ (100 kcal)									
Pro-Cal® Shot (Vitaflo)	Liquid per 100 mL	1393 kJ (334 kcal)	6.7 g cows' milk	13.4 g	28.2 g	Nil	Contains lactose	See above; Not suitable for child under 1 year	Bottle: 6 × 250 mL = £26.22 Banana, neutral, strawberry[2]
QuickCal® (Vitaflo)	Powder per 100 g	3263 kJ (780 kcal)	4.6 g cows' milk	17 g	77 g	Nil	Contains lactose	See above; Not suitable for child under 1 year	Sachets: 25 × 13 g = £11.89
Powder 13 g provides: protein 600 mg, carbohydrate 2.2 g, fat 10 g, energy 418 kJ (100 kcal)									
Scandishake® Mix (Nutricia Clinical)	Powder per 100 g	2099 kJ (500 kcal)[1]	4.7 g cows' milk	65 g (sugars 14.3 g)	24.7 g	Nil	Gluten-free; Contains lactose	See above; Not suitable for child under 3 years	Sachet: 85 g = £2.08 Banana, caramel, chocolate, strawberry, vanilla, unflavoured
Powder: 85 g reconstituted with 240 mL whole milk provides: protein 11.7 g, carbohydrate 66.8 g, fat 30.4 g, energy 2457 kJ (588 kcal)									
Vitasavoury® (Vitaflo)	Powder per 100 g	2590 kJ (619 kcal)[1]	12.7 g cows' milk	23.5 g (sugars 1.5 g)	52.3 g	6.2 g	Contains lactose	See above; Not suitable for child under 3 years	Cup (200 kcal): 24 × 33 g = £26.53; Sachet (300 kcal); 10 × 50 g = £15.99 Chicken, leek and potato, mushroom, vegetable

1. Nutritional values vary with flavour—consult product literature
2. Flavour not suitable for child under 3 years

Appendix 2: Borderline substances

Appendix 2: Borderline substances

A2.4.2 Fibre, vitamin, and mineral supplements

Product	Formulation	Energy	Protein	Carbohydrate	Fat	Fibre	Special Characteristics	ACBS Indications	Presentation & Flavour
High-fibre supplements									
Resource® Optifibre® (Nestlé) Formerly *Resource® Benefiber®*	Powder **per 100 g**	323 kJ (76 kcal)	Nil	19 g guar gum, partially hydrolysed	Nil	78 g	Gluten-free Lactose-free	Standard, p. 895 except dysphagia Not suitable for child under 5 years	Sachet: 16 x 10 g = £7.52 Can: 250 g = £9.26 (5-g measuring scoop provided)
Vitamin and Mineral supplements									
Metabolic Mineral Mixture® (SHS)	Powder **per 100 g**	729 kJ (175 kcal)	Nil	Nil	Nil	Nil	Contains trace elements Electrolytes/100 g: Na⁺ 172 mmol K⁺ 212 mmol Ca²⁺ 205 mmol P⁺ 192 mmol Energy source: Calcium lactate	Mineral supplement for synthetic diets Suitable for infants (but may require further dilution)	Tub: 100 g = £10.18
Paediatric Seravit® (SHS)	Powder **per 100 g**	1275 kJ (300 kcal)	Nil	75 g (sugars 6.75 g¹)	Nil	Nil		Vitamin and mineral supplement in infants and children with restrictive therapeutic diets	Tub: 200 g = £14.37 Unflavoured² 200 g = £15.30 Pineapple³ (5-g measuring scoop provided)

1. Sugar content varies with flavour
2. Flavouring: see *Modjul*® Flavour System, p. 925
3. Flavour not suitable for child under 6 months

A2.5 Feed additives

A2.5.1 Special additives for conditions of intolerance

Colief® (Britannia)
Liquid, lactase 50 000 units/g, net price 7-mL dropper bottle = £8.40
For the relief of symptoms associated with lactose intolerance in infants, provided that lactose intolerance is confirmed by the presence of reducing substances and/or excessive acid in stools, a low concentration of the corresponding disaccharide enzyme on intestinal biopsy or by breath hydrogen test or lactose intolerance test. For dosage and administration details, consult product literature

Fructose
(Laevulose)
For proven glucose/galactose intolerance

A2.5.2 Feed thickeners and pre-thickened foods

Carobel, Instant® (Cow & Gate)
Powder, carob seed flour. Net price 135 g = £2.92.
For thickening feeds in the treatment of vomiting

Nutilis® (Nutricia Clinical)
Powder, modified maize starch, gluten- and lactose-free, net price 20 × 9-g sachets = £5.88, 225 g = £4.51.
For thickening of foods in dysphagia. Not suitable for children under 3 years

Resource® Thickened Drink (Nestlé)
Liquid, carbohydrate 22 g, energy: orange 382 kJ (90 kcal); apple 376 kJ (89 kcal)/100 mL. Flavours; apple or orange, syrup or custard consistencies. Gluten- and lactose-free, net price 12 × 114-mL cups = £7.32.
For dysphagia. Not suitable for children under 1 year

Resource® ThickenUp® (Nestlé)
Powder, modified maize starch. Gluten- and lactose-free, net price 227 g = £4.35; 74 × 4.5-g sachet = £16.66.
For thickening of foods in dysphagia. Not suitable for children under 1 year

SLO Drinks® (SLO Drinks)
Powder, carbohydrate content varies with flavour and chosen consistency (3 consistencies available), see product literature. Flavours: black currant, lemon, orange; hot drinks: chocolate, white coffee, net price 25 × 115 mL = £7.50
Nutritional supplement for patient hydration in the dietary management of dysphagia. Not suitable for children under 3 years

Thick and Easy® (Fresenius Kabi)
Powder. Modified maize starch, net price 225-g can = £4.35; 100 × 9-g sachets = £26.35; 4.54 kg = £70.53.
Thickened Juices, liquid, modified food starch. Flavours: apple or orange, net price 118-mL pot = 57p; apple, black currant, cranberry, kiwi-strawberry, orange, 1.42-litre bottle = £3.61.
For thickening of foods in dysphagia. Not suitable for children under 1 year except in cases of failure to thrive

Thixo-D® (Sutherland)
Powder, modified maize starch, gluten-free. Net price 375-g tub = £6.75.
For thickening of foods in dysphagia. Not suitable for children under 1 year except in cases of failure to thrive

Vitaquick® (Vitaflo)
Powder. Modified maize starch. Net price 300 g = £6.59; 2 kg = £33.57; 6 kg = £85.90.
For thickening of foods in dysphagia. Not suitable for children under 1 year except in cases of failure to thrive

A2.5.3 Flavouring preparations

Flavour Mix® (Nestlé)
Powder, flavours: banana, chocolate, coffee, lemon-lime, or strawberry, net price 60 g = £6.67

FlavourPac® (Vitaflo)
Powder, flavours: black currant, lemon, orange, tropical or raspberry, net price 30 × 4-g sachets = £11.29
For use with Vitaflo's range of unflavoured protein substitutes for metabolic diseases

Modjul® Flavour System (SHS)
Powder, carbohydrate-based flavours, black currant, orange, pineapple, 100 g = £9.77; cherry-vanilla, grapefruit, lemon-lime, 20 × 5-g sachets = £9.77
For use with unflavoured SHS products based on peptides or amino acids; not suitable for child under 6 months

Appendix 2: Borderline substances

A2.6 Foods for special diets

A2.6.1 Gluten-free foods

ACBS indications: established gluten-sensitive enteropathies including steatorrhoea due to gluten sensitivity, coeliac disease, and dermatitis herpetiformis.

Bread

◢ Loaves

Barkat® (Gluten Free Foods Ltd)
Gluten-free. Loaf, multigrain 500 g = £4.44. Loaf, sliced, wholemeal 500 g = £3.36. Loaf, sliced, part-baked, country-style 250 g = £3.36. Loaf, sliced, part-baked, white 300 g = £2.70. Rice bread, brown 500 g = £4.44; white 500 g = £4.44

Dietary Specials® (Nutrition Point)
Gluten-free. Loaf, sliced, multigrain, brown 400 g = £2.94; white 400 g = £2.94.

Ener-G® (General Dietary)
Gluten-free. Loaf, sliced Seattle brown 600 g = £5.05. Rice bread, sliced, brown 474 g = £4.39; white 456 g = £4.39. Rice loaf, sliced 612 g = £4.39. Tapioca bread, sliced 480 g = £4.39

Glutafin® (Nutrition Point)
Gluten-free. Loaf, sliced, fibre 400 g = £3.41; white 400 g = £3.41

Glutafin® Select (Nutrition Point)
Gluten-free. Loaf, sliced, fresh, brown 400 g = £3.17; white 400 g = £3.17. Loaf, sliced, fibre 400 g = £3.04; white 400 g = £3.04. Loaf, seeded 400 g = £3.31. Loaf, part-baked, white 400 g = £3.41

Juvela® (Juvela)
Gluten-free. Loaf, sliced, fresh, fibre 400 g = £3.05; white 400 g = £3.17. Loaf, sliced, white 400 g = £3.05; fibre 400 g = £3.05. Loaf, white 400 g = £3.05; fibre 400 g = £3.05. Loaf, part-baked, fibre 400 g = £3.27; white 400 g = £3.27

Lifestyle® (Ultrapharm)
Gluten-free. Loaf, sliced, brown 400 g = £2.82; high fibre 400 g = £2.82; white 400 g = £2.82. Loaf, brown 400 g = £2.82; high fibre 400 g = £2.82; white 400 g = £2.82

Livwell® (Livwell)
Gluten-free. Loaf, sliced, brown (seeded) 200 g = £2.25; white 200 g = £2.25

Pastically® (GFF Trade)
Gluten-free. Loaf, sandwich 260 g = £3.29; rustic 260 g = £3.29.

Proceli® (Sigma)
Gluten-free. Loaf, sliced, white 165 g = £2.19; sandwich 155 g = £2.06. Rice bread, brown 220 g = £2.19; sandwich 220 g = £2.19.

Schar® (Nutrition Point)
Gluten-free. Loaf, sliced, white 2 x 200 g = £3.05. Loaf, ertha, brown 400 g = £3.34

Sunnyvale® (Everfresh)
Gluten-free. Loaf, mixed grain, sour dough 400 g = £1.91

Ultra® (Ultrapharm)
Gluten-free. Loaf, part-baked, white 400 g = £2.46; high fibre 500 g = £3.35

Valpiform® (Ultrapharm)
Gluten-free. Loaf, country 400 g = £3.75

Wellfoods® (Wellfoods)
Gluten-free. Loaf, sliced 600 g = £4.95; unsliced 600 g = £4.85

◢ Baguettes, buns and rolls

Barkat® (Gluten Free Foods Ltd)
Gluten-free. Baguette, part-baked 200 g = £3.36. Rolls, part-baked 2 x 100 g = £3.30; 6 x 50 g = £3.69

Ener-G® (General Dietary)
Gluten-free. Rolls, dinner × 6 = £2.97; white, long 4 × 55 g = £2.39; round 4 × 55 g = £2.39

Glutafin® (Nutrition Point)
Gluten-free. Baguette 2 × 175 g = £3.20. Rolls, fibre 4 × 50 g = £3.41; white 4 × 50 g = £3.41

Glutafin® Select (Nutrition Point)
Gluten-free. Rolls, fibre 4 × 65 g = £3.17; white 4 × 65 g = £3.17. Rolls, part-baked, white 4 × 50 g = £3.41; long 2 × 75 g = £3.41

Juvela® (Juvela)
Gluten-free. Rolls, fibre 5 × 85 g = £4.11; white 5 × 85 g = £4.11. Rolls, part-baked, fibre 5 × 75 g = £4.25; white 5 × 75 g = £4.25

Lifestyle® (Ultrapharm)
Gluten-free. Rolls, brown 5 × 80 g = £2.82; high fibre 5 × 80 g = £2.82; white 5 × 80 g = £2.82

Livwell® (Livwell)
Gluten-free. Baguette, white 250 g = £2.50. Buns, toasting 4 × 50 g = £2.50. Rolls, white 4 = £2.25. Rolls, part-baked, circle (bagel) 2 × 90 g = £2.50; dinner (square) 2 × 80 g = £2.09

Pastically® (GFF Trade)
Gluten-free. Baguette 160 g = £1.99. Rolls, part-baked, white 2 × 80 g = 2.39; rustic, part-baked, white 2 × 105 g = £2.39

Proceli® (Sigma)
Gluten-free. Baguette, part-baked 2 × 125 g = £2.90. Buns 4 × 50 g = £3.26. Lunch rolls, white 8 × 34 g = £3.11. Rolls, part-baked, white, dinner 4 × 35 g = £1.86; hotdog 3 × 35 g = £1.96; long 3 × 83 g = £2.74.

Schar® (Nutrition Point)
Gluten-free. Rolls 2 × 75 g = £1.91

Ultra® (Ultrapharm)
Gluten-free. Baguette, part-baked 2 × 200 g = £2.46. Rolls, part-baked 4 × 70 g = £2.46

Wellfoods® (Wellfoods)
Gluten-free. Burger buns 4 × 75 g = £3.95. Rolls 4 × 70 g = £3.65

◢ Speciality breads

Livwell® (Livwell)
Gluten-free. Flat bread (pitta) 4 = £3.00. Tear-drop shape (naan) 2 × 90 g = £3.00

Proceli® (Sigma)
Gluten-free. Flat bread (pitta), part-baked 3 × 40 g = £4.04

Cookies and biscuits

Barkat® (Gluten Free Foods Ltd)
Gluten-free. Biscuits, coffee-style 200 g = £ 1.68; digestive 175 g = £2.20

Dietary Specials® (Nutrition Point)
Gluten-free. Biscuits, tea (hoops) 220 g = £2.10

Ener-G® (General Dietary)
Gluten-free. Cookies, vanilla 435 g = £5.00

Glutafin® (Nutrition Point)
Gluten-free. Biscuits, plain 200 g = £3.68; digestive 150 g = £1.89; savoury 125 g = £1.89; savoury shorts 150 g =

£2.59; shortbread 100 g = £1.56; sweet (without chocolate or sultanas) 150 g = £1.89; tea 150 g = £1.89

Juvela® (Juvela)
Gluten-free. Biscuits, digestive 150 g = £2.62; savoury 150 g = £3.29; sweet 150 g = £2.48, tea 150 g = £2.62

Schar® (Nutrition Point)
Gluten-free. Biscuits, savoy 150 g = £2.57

Ultra® (Ultrapharm)
Gluten-free. Biscuits, sweet 250 g = £2.93

Crackers, crispbreads, and breadsticks

Barkat® (Gluten Free Foods Ltd)
Gluten-free. Crackers, round (matzo) 200 g = £2.52

Dietary Specials® (Nutrition Point)
Gluten-free. Cracker bread 150 g = £1.89

Glutafin® (Nutrition Point)
Gluten-free. Crackers, high fibre 200 g = £2.58; plain 200 g = £3.08; mini 175 g = £2.70.

Juvela® (Juvela)
Gluten-free. Crispbread, plain 200 g = £4.06

Schar® (Nutrition Point)
Gluten-free. Breadsticks, grissini 150 g = £2.05. Crackers, plain 200 g = £2.68. Crispbread, plain 250 g = £3.68

Ultra® (Ultrapharm)
Gluten-free. Crackerbread 200 g = £1.77

Valpiform® (Ultrapharm)
Gluten-free. Crac'form toast 250 g = £3.52

Flour mixes and xanthan gum

◀**Flour mixes**
Aproten® (Ultrapharm)
Gluten-free. Flour mix, plain 500 g = £4.99

Barkat® (Gluten Free Foods Ltd)
Gluten-free. Flour mix, bread 500 g = £5.74. Plain 750 g = £5.35

Dietary Specials® (Nutrition Point)
Gluten-free. Flour mix, bread, white 500 g = £5.20. Cake, white 750 g = £5.20. Plain, white 500 g = £5.20

Glutafin® (Nutrition Point)
Gluten-free. Flour mix, fibre 500 g = £5.91; white 500 g = £5.91

Glutafin Select® (Nutrition Point)
Gluten-free. Flour mix, bread, fibre 500 g = £5.91; white 500 g = £5.91. Cake 500 g = £5.91. Fibre 500 g = £5.91; white 500 g = £5.91. Pastry 500 g = £5.91

Heron Foods® (Gluten Free Foods Ltd)
Gluten-free. Flour mix, organic, bread, standard 500 g = £6.33; high fibre 500 g = £6.33

Il Pane di Anna® (GFF Trade)
Gluten-free. Flour mix, bread, white 500 g = £5.25. Cake, white 500 g = £5.25. Pizza base 500 g = £5.25

Juvela® (Juvela)
Gluten-free. Flour mix, fibre 500 g = £6.33; plain 500 g = £6.33; harvest 500 g = £6.33

Orgran® (Community)
Gluten-free. Flour mix, bread 450 g = £3.10. Self-raising 500 g = £2.89. Pastry and pizza 375 g = £3.52

Proceli® (Sigma)
Gluten-free. Flour mix, white 1 kg = £5.14

Pure® (Innovative)
Gluten-free. Flour mix, blended 1 kg = £3.75. Potato starch 500 g = £1.49. Rice, brown 500 g = £1.40; white 500 g = £1.50. Tapioca starch 500 g = £1.99. Teff, brown 1 kg = £4.20; white 1 kg = £4.20

Schar® (Nutrition Point)
Gluten-free. Flour mix, bread 1 kg = £4.99. Cake 500 g = £4.99. Plain 1 kg = £4.99

Tobia® (Tobia Teff)
Gluten-free. Flour mix, teff, brown 1 kg = £2.95; white 1 kg = £2.95

Tritamyl® (Gluten Free Foods Ltd)
Gluten-free. Flour mix, bread, brown 1 kg = £6.60; white 2 kg = £13.20. Plain 2 kg = £13.20

Valpiform® (Ultrapharm)
Gluten-free. Flour mix, bread 1 kg = £6.73. Pastry 1 kg = £6.73

Wellfoods® (Wellfoods)
Gluten-free. Flour mix, plain 1 kg = £7.65

◀**Xanthan gum**
Ener-G® (General Dietary)
Gluten-free. Xanthan gum 170 g = £6.93

Pure® (Innovative)
Gluten-free. Xanthan gum 100 g = £5.75

Pasta

Barkat® (Gluten Free Foods Ltd)
Gluten-free. Pasta, animal shapes 500 g = £4.95; macaroni 500 g = £4.95; spaghetti 500 g = £4.95; spirals 500 g = £4.95; tagliatelle 500 g = £4.95. Buckwheat, penne 250 g = £2.03; spirals 250 g = £2.03

Bi-Aglut® (Ultrapharm)
Gluten-free. Pasta, fusilli 500 g = £5.23; macaroni 500 g = £5.23; penne 500 g = £5.23; spaghetti 500 g = £5.23

BiAlimenta® (Drossa)
Gluten-free. Pasta, potato-based, gnocchi 500 g = £5.59; perle di gnocchi 500 g = £5.60. Tubetti 500 g = £5.90

Dietary Specials® (Nutrition Point)
Gluten-free. Pasta, fusilli 500 g = £3.36; penne 500 g = £3.36; spaghetti 500 g = £3.36

Ener-G® (General Dietary)
Gluten-free. Pasta, rice-based, lasagne 454 g = £4.08; macaroni 454 g = £4.08; shells, small 454 g = £4.08; spaghetti 454 g = £4.08; vermicelli 300 g = £4.08

Glutafin® (Nutrition Point)
Gluten-free. Pasta, lasagne 250 g = £3.13; macaroni penne 500 g = £5.97; shells 500 g = £5.97; spirals 500 g = £5.97; spaghetti, long 500 g = £5.97; tagliatelle 250 g = £3.13

Juvela® (Juvela)
Gluten-free. Pasta, fusilli 500 g = £6.20; lasagne 250 g = £3.16; macaroni 500 g = £6.20; spaghetti 500 g = £6.20; tagliatelle 250 g = £2.99. Fibre, linguine 500 g = £6.20; penne 500 g = £6.20

Orgran® (Community)
Gluten-free. Pasta, rice and corn, lasagne 200 g = £3.03; macaroni 250 g = £2.35; spaghetti 375 g = £2.35. Spirals, buckwheat 250 g = £2.35; corn 250 g = £2.35; brown rice

250 g = £2.60; rice and corn 250 g = £2.35; rice and millet 250 g = £2.35

Pasticely® (GFF Trade)
Gluten-free. Pasta, macaroni 500 g = £2.99; elbow 500 g = £2.99; spaghetti 500 g = £2.99.

Proceli® (Sigma)
Gluten-free. Pasta, macaroni penne 250 g = £2.59; puntini 2 × 250 g = £5.17; spaghetti, short 2 × 250 g = £5.17; spirals 250 g = £2.59

Rizopia® (PGR Health Foods)
Gluten-free. Pasta, brown rice, fusilli 500 g = £2.50; lasagne 375 g = £2.50; penne 500 g = £2.50; spaghetti 500 g = £2.50

Ultra® (Ultrapharm)
Gluten-free. Pasta, fusilli 250 g = £2.95; penne 250 g = £2.95; spaghetti 250 g = £2.95

Pizza bases

Barkat® (Gluten Free Foods Ltd)
Gluten-free. Pizza crust, rice, brown 150 g = £3.83; white 150 g = £3.83

Dietary Specials® (Nutrition Point)
Gluten-free. Pizza base 2 × 150 g = £5.15

Glutafin® (Nutrition Point)
Gluten-free. Pizza base 2 × 150 g = £5.83

Juvela® (Juvela)
Gluten-free. Pizza base 2 × 180 g = £7.56

Pasticely® (GFF Trade)
Gluten-free. Pizza base 165 g = £2.99

Proceli® (Sigma)
Gluten-free. Pizza base 3 × 125 g = £5.18

Ultra® (Ultrapharm)
Gluten-free. Pizza base 2 × 200 g = £2.65

Wellfoods® (Wellfoods)
Gluten-free. Pizza base 2 × 300 g = £8.95

A2.6.1.1 Gluten- and wheat-free foods

> **ACBS indications:** established gluten-sensitive enteropathies with coexisting established wheat sensitivity only.

Ener-G® (General Dietary)
Gluten-free, wheat-free. Bread loaf, six flour 576 g = £3.60. Rolls, Seattle brown, round (hamburger) 4 × 119 g = £3.00; long (hot dog) 4 × 119 g = £3.00. Pizza base, 3 × 124 g = £3.75

Glutafin® (Nutrition Point)
Gluten-free, wheat-free. Flour mix, bread 500 g = £5.63; fibre 500 g = £5.63. Cake mix 500 g = £5.63. Crispbread 150 g = £3.82

Heron Foods® (Gluten Free Foods Ltd)
Gluten-free, wheat-free. Flour mix, organic, bread, fibre 500 g = £6.33. Bread and cake mix 500 g = £6.33

A2.6.2 Low-protein foods

> **ACBS indications:** inherited metabolic disorders, renal or liver failure, requiring a low-protein diet

Bread

Ener-G® (General Dietary)
Low protein, Rice bread, 600 g = £4.39

Juvela® (SHS)
Low protein. Loaf, sliced 400 g = £3.19. Rolls 5 × 70 g = £3.96

Loprofin® (SHS)
Low protein. Loaf, sliced 400 g = £3.19. Rolls, white 4 × 65 g = £2.98; part-baked 4 × 65 g = £3.36

PK Foods® (Gluten Free Foods Ltd)
Low protein. Loaf, white, sliced 550 g = £4.00

Ultra PKU® (Ultrapharm)
Low-protein. Loaf 400 g = £2.65

Cake, biscuits, and crackers

Aproten® (Ultrapharm)
Low protein. Biscuits 180 g = £2.88. Crispbread 260 g = £4.06

Harifen® (Ultrapharm)
Low protein. Cracker toast, 200 g = £2.75

Juvela® (SHS)
Low-protein. Cookies, cinnamon 125 g = £6.67; chocolate chip 125 g = £6.67; orange 125 g = £6.51

Loprofin® (SHS)
Low-protein. Cookies, chocolate chip 100 g = £5.64. Cream-filled biscuits, chocolate 125 g = £2.13. Crunch bar 8 × 41 g = £11.36. Sweet biscuits 150 g = £2.13. Wafers, chocolate 100 g = £2.07; orange 100 g = £2.07; vanilla 100 g = £2.07. Crackers 150 g = £2.91, herb 150 g = £2.91

PK Foods® (Gluten Free Foods Ltd)
Low-protein. *Aminex®* biscuits 200 g = £4.67; cookies 150 g = £4.67. Cookies, chocolate chip 150 g = £4.25; cinnamon 150 g = £4.25; orange 150 g = £4.25. Rusks 200 g = £4.25. Cripsbread 75 g = £2.00

Taranis® (Firstplay Dietary)
Low-protein. Cake bars, lemon 6 × 40 g = £5.10

Ultra PKU® (Ultrapharm)
Low-protein. Biscuits 200 g = £2.21; savoy 150 g = £2.06

Valpiform® (Ultrapharm)
Low-protein. Biscuits, shortbread 120 g = £4.06

Vita Bite® (Vitaflo)
Low protein. Bar, protein 30 mg (less than 2.5 mg phenylalanine), carbohydrate 15.35 g, fat 8.4 g, energy 572 kJ (137 kcal)/25 g. Chocolate flavoured, 25 g = 99p.
Not recommended for any child under 1 year

Cereals

Loprofin® (SHS)
Low-protein. Breakfast cereal flakes, apple 375 g = £6.39; chocolate 375 g = £6.39; strawberry 375 g = £6.39. Cereal loops 375 g = £6.64

Promin® (Firstplay Dietary)
Low-protein. Hot breakfast (powder sachets), apple and cinnamon 6 × 57 g = £7.14, banana 6 × 57 g = £7.14, chocolate 6 × 57 g = £7.14; original 6 × 56 g = £7.14

Desserts

Loprofin® (SHS)
Low-protein. Powder, chocolate 150 g = £3.91; strawberry 150 g = £3.91; vanilla 150 g = £3.91

PK Foods® (Gluten Free Foods Ltd)
Low-protein. Jelly, orange 4 × 80 g = £6.76, cherry 4 × 80 g = £6.76

Promin® (Firstplay Dietary)
Low-protein. Dessert mix, caramel 6 × 36.5 g = £5.60; custard 6 × 36.5 g = £5.60; chocolate and banana 6 × 36.5 g = £5.60; strawberry and vanilla 6 × 36.5 g = £5.60. Rice pudding imitation, apple 4 × 69 g = £5.60; banana 4 × 69 g = £5.60; original 4 × 69 g = £5.60; strawberry 4 × 69 g = £5.60

Flour mixes and egg substitutes

Ener-G® (General Dietary)
Low-protein. Egg replacer 454 g = £4.05

Fate® (Fate)
Low protein. All purpose mix 500 g = £6.39. Cake mix, 2 × 250 g = £6.39; chocolate-flavour 2 × 250 g = £6.39

Juvela® (SHS)
Low-protein. Mix 500 g = £6.82

Loprofin® (SHS)
Low-protein. Mix, plain 500 g = £6.77; chocolate 500 g = £7.16; lemon 500 g = £7.16. Egg replacer 2 × 250 g = £12.43. Egg-white replacer 100 g = £8.00

PK Foods® (Gluten Free Foods Ltd)
Low-protein. Flour mix 750 g = £9.60. Egg replacer 350 g = £4.25

Pasta

Aproten® (Ultrapharm)
Low-protein. Pasta, ditalini 500 g = £4.06; rigatini 500 g = £4.06; spaghetti 500 g = £4.06; tagliatelle 250 g = £2.16

Loprofin® (SHS)
Low-protein. Pasta, animal shapes 500 g = £6.80; conchigle 500 g = £6.82; spirals 500 g = £7.08; gnoccetti sardi 500 g = £6.82; lasagne 250 g = £3.44; macaroni elbows 250 g = £3.40; penne 500 g = £7.08; spaghetti 500 g =

£7.08; tagliatelle 250 g = £3.40; vermicelli 250 g = £3.52. Rice, imitation 500 g = £6.87

Promin® (Firstplay Dietary)
Low-protein. Pasta, alphabet shapes 500 g = £6.35; lasagne sheets 200 g = £2.70; macaroni 500 g = £6.35; shells 500 g = £6.35; spaghetti, short-cut 500 g = £6.35; spirals 500 g = £6.35. Rice, imitation 500 g = £6.35. Tricolour pasta, alphabet shapes 500 g = £6.35; shells 500 g = £6.35; spirals 500 g = £6.35.

Pizza bases

Juvela® (SHS)
Low-protein. Pizza base 2 × 180 g = £7.55

Ultra PKU® (Ultrapharm)
Low-protein. Pizza base 5 × 80 g = £2.45

Savoury meals and mixes

Loprofin® (SHS)
Low-protein. Snack pot, curry 47 g = £3.76; tomato and basil 47 g = £3.76

Promin® (Firstplay Dietary)
Low-protein. Burger mix 2 × 62 g = £5.60; lamb & mint 2 × 62 g = £5.77. Couscous 500 g = £6.35. Pasta elbows in

cheese and broccoli sauce 4 × 66 g = £7.32. Pasta meal 500 g = £6.35. Pasta shells in tomato, pepper, and herb sauce 4 × 72 g = £7.32. Pasta spirals in Moroccan sauce 4 × 72 g = £7.32. Sausage mix, apple & sage 4 × 30 g = £6.30; original 4 × 30 g = £6.30; tomato & basil 4 × 30 g = £6.30

Spreads

Promin® (Firstplay Dietary)
Low-protein. Spread, chocolate and hazelnut 230 g = £6.80

Appendix 2: Borderline substances

A2.7 Nutritional supplements for metabolic diseases

Glutaric aciduria (type 1)

GA1 Anamix® Infant (SHS)

Powder, protein equivalent (essential and non-essential amino acids except lysine, and low tryptophan) 13.1 g, carbohydrate 49.5 g, fat 23 g, fibre 5.3 g, energy 1915 kJ (457 kcal)/100 g, with vitamins, minerals, and trace elements; *standard dilution* (15%) provides protein equivalent 2 g, carbohydrate 7.4 g, fat 3.5 g, fibre 800 mg, energy 287 kJ (69 kcal)/100 mL. Unflavoured, net price 400 g = £31.20 (5-g measuring scoop provided)

Nutritional supplement for the dietary management of proven glutaric aciduria (type 1) in children from birth to 3 years

GA Gel® (Vitaflo)

Gel, protein equivalent (essential and non-essential amino acids except lysine, and low tryptophan) 8.4 g, carbohydrate 8.6 g. fat trace, energy 286 kJ (68 kcal)/20 g, with vitamins, minerals, and trace elements. Unflavoured (flavouring: see *FlavourPac®*, p. 925), net price 30 × 20-g sachets = £145.76

Nutritional supplement for dietary management of type 1 glutaric aciduria in children 1–10 years

[1]XLYS, Low TRY, Maxamaid (SHS)

Powder, protein equivalent (essential and non-essential amino acids except lysine, and low tryptophan) 25 g, carbohydrate 51 g, fat less than 500 mg, energy 1311 kJ (309 kcal)/100 g, with vitamins, minerals, and trace elements. Unflavoured, (flavouring: see *Modjul®* Flavour System, p. 925), net price 500 g = £76.94.

Nutritional supplement for dietary management of type 1 glutaric aciduria

XLYS, TRY, Glutaridon (SHS)

Powder, protein equivalent (essential and non-essential amino acids except lysine and tryptophan) 79 g, carbohydrate 4 g, energy 1411 kJ (332 kcal)/100 g, Lactose-free. Unflavoured, (flavouring: see *Modjul®* Flavour System, p. 925), net price 2 × 500 g = £298.46

Nutritional supplement for type 1 glutaric aciduria in children and adults; requires additional source of vitamins, minerals and trace elements

Glucogen storage disease

Corn flour and corn starch

For hypoglycaemia associated with glycogen-storage disease

Glucose
(Dextrose monohydrate)

Net price 500 g = £1.14.

For glycogen storage disease and sucrose/isomaltose intolerance

Glycosade® (Vitaflo)

Powder, protein 200 mg, carbohydrate (maize starch) 47.6 g, fat nil, fibre less than 600 mg, energy 803 kJ (192 kcal)/60 g, net price 30 × 60-g sachets = £90.00

A nutritional supplement for use in the dietary management of glycogen storage disease and other metabolic conditions where a constant supply of glucose is essential. Not suitable for use in children under 2 years

Homocystinuria or hypermethionimaemia

HCU Anamix® Infant (SHS)

Powder, protein equivalent (essential and non-essential amino acids except methionine) 13.1 g, carbohydrate 49.5 g, fat 23 g, fibre 5.3 g, energy 1915 kJ (457 kcal)/100 g, with vitamins, minerals, and trace elements; *standard dilution* (15%) provides protein equivalent 2 g, carbohydrate 7.4 g, fat 3,5 g, fibre 800 mg, energy 287 kJ (69 kcal)/100 mL. Unflavoured, net price 400 g = £31.20 (5-g measuring scoop provided)

Nutritional supplement for the dietary management of proven vitamin B_6 non-responsive homocystinuria or hypermethioninaemia in children from birth to 3 years

HCU cooler® (Vitaflo)

Liquid, protein (essential and non-essential amino acids except methionine) 15 g, carbohydrate 7.8 g, fat trace, energy 386 kJ (92 kcal)/130 mL, with vitamins, minerals and trace elements. Orange flavour, net price 30 × 130-mL pouch = £271.20

A methionine-free protein substitute for use as a nutritional supplement in children over 3 years with homocystinuria

HCU Express® (Vitaflo)

Powder, protein (essential and non-essential amino acids except methionine) 15 g, carbohydrate 3.8 g, fat 30 mg, energy 315 kJ (75.3 kcal)/25 g with vitamins, minerals and trace elements. Unflavoured, (flavouring: see *Flavour Pac®*, p. 925), net price 30 × 25- g sachets = £265.90

A methionine-free protein substitute for use as a nutritional supplement in children over 8 years with homocystinuria

HCU gel® (Vitaflo)

Powder, protein (essential and non-essential amino acids except methionine) 8.4 g, carbohydrate 8.6 g, fat 30 mg, energy 286 kJ (68 kcal)/20 g with vitamins, minerals and trace elements. Unflavoured, (flavouring: see *Flavour Pac®*, p. 925), net price 30 × 20- g sachets = £148.59

A methionine-free protein substitute for use as a nutritional supplement for the dietary management of children 1–10 years with homocystinuria

HCU LV® (SHS)

Powder, protein (essential and non-essential amino acids except methionine) 20 g, carbohydrate 2.5 g, fat 190 mg, energy 390 kJ (92 kcal)/27.8-g sachet, with vitamins, minerals, and trace elements. Unflavoured (flavouring: see *Modjul®* Flavour System, p. 925), or tropical flavour (formulation varies slightly), net price 30 × 27.8-g sachets = £395.44

Nutritional supplement for the dietary management of hypermethioninaemia or vitamin B_6 non-responsive homocystinuria in children over 8 years

XMET Homidon (SHS)

Powder, protein equivalent (essential and non-essential amino acids except methionine) 77 g, carbohydrate 4.5 g, fat nil, energy 1386 kJ (326 kcal)/100 g. Unflavoured, (flavouring: see *Modjul®* Flavour System, p. 925), net price 500 g = £149.26.

Nutritional supplement for the dietary management of hypermethioninaemia or homocystinuria in children

---

1. Maxamaid products are generally intended for use in children 1–8 years

¹XMET Maxamaid (SHS)

Powder, protein equivalent (essential and non-essential amino acids except methionine) 25 g, carbohydrate 51 g, fat less than 500 mg, energy 1311 kJ (309 kcal)/100 g, with vitamins, minerals, and trace elements. Unflavoured (flavouring: see *Modjul*® Flavour System, p. 925), net price 500 g = £78.79

Nutritional supplement for the dietary management of hypermethioninaemia or homocystinuria

²XMET Maxamum® (SHS)

Powder, protein equivalent (essential and non-essential amino acids except methionine) 39 g, carbohydrate 34 g, fat less than 500 mg, energy 1260 kJ (297 kcal)/100 g, with vitamins, minerals, and trace elements. Unflavoured, (flavouring: see *Modjul*® Flavour System, p. 925), net price 500 g = £126.30.

Nutritional supplement for the dietary management of hypermethioninaemi or homocystinuria

Hyperlysinaemia

HYPER LYS Anamix® Infant (SHS)

Powder, protein equivalent (essential and non-essential amino acids except lysine) 13.1 g, carbohydrate 49.5 g, fat 23 g, fibre 5.3 g, energy 1915 kJ (457 kcal)/100 g, with vitamins, minerals, and trace elements; *standard dilution* (15%) provides protein equivalent 2 g, carbohydrate 7.4 g, fat 3.5 g, fibre 800 mg, energy 287 kJ (69 kcal)/100 mL. Unflavoured, net price 400 g = £31.20 (5-g measuring scoop provided)

Nutritional supplement for the dietary management of proven hyperlysinaemia in children from birth to 3 years

¹XLYS Maxamaid (SHS)

Powder, protein equivalent (essential and non-essential amino acids except lysine) 25 g, carbohydrate 51 g, fat less than 500 mg, energy 1311 kJ (309 kcal)/100 g with vitamins, minerals, and trace elements. Unflavoured, (flavouring: see *Modjul*® Flavour System, p. 925), net price 500 g = £78.79.

Nutritional supplement for the dietary management of hyperlysinaemia

Isovaleric acidaemia

IVA Anamix® Infant (SHS)

Powder, protein equivalent (essential and non-essential amino acids except leucine) 13.1 g, carbohydrate 49.5 g, fat 23 g, fibre 5.3 g, energy 1915 kJ (457 kcal)/100 g, with vitamins, minerals, and trace elements; *standard dilution* (15%) provides protein equivalent 2 g, carbohydrate 7.4 g, fat 3.5 g, fibre 800 mg, energy 287 kJ (69 kcal)/100 mL. Unflavoured, net price 400 g = £31.20 (5-g measuring scoop provided)

Nutritional supplement for the dietary management of proven isovaleric acidaemia or other proven disorders of leucine metabolism in children from birth to 3 years

XLEU Faladon (SHS)

Powder, protein equivalent (essential and non-essential amino acids except leucine) 77 g, carbohydrate 4.5 g, fat

nil, energy 1386 kJ (326 kcal)/100 g. Unflavoured, (flavouring: see *Modjul*® Flavour System, p. 925), net price 200 g = £59.69.

Nutritional supplement for the dietary management of isovaleric acidaemia in children

¹XLEU Maxamaid (SHS)

Powder, protein equivalent (essential and non-essential amino acids except leucine) 25 g, carbohydrate 51 g, fat less than 500 mg, energy 1311 kJ (309 kcal)/100 g with vitamins, minerals, and trace elements. Unflavoured, (flavouring: see *Modjul*® Flavour System, p. 925), net price 500 g = £78.79.

Nutritional supplement for the dietary management of isovaleric acidaemia

Maple syrup urine disease

Isoleucine Amino Acid Supplement (Vitaflo)

Powder, isoleucine 50 mg, carbohydrate 4 g, fat nil, energy 64 kJ (15 kcal)/4 g, net price 30 × 4-g sachets = £43.50

Nutritional supplement for use in the dietary management of maple syrup urine disease and other inborn errors of amino acid metabolism in children over 1 year and adults

MSUD Aid III® (SHS)

Powder, protein equivalent (essential and non-essential amino acids except isoleucine, leucine, and valine) 77 g, carbohydrate 4.5 g, fat nil, energy 1386 kJ (326 kcal)/100 g. Unflavoured, (flavouring: see *Modjul*® Flavour System, p. 925), net price 500 g = £149.26.

Nutritional supplement for the dietary management of maple syrup urine disease and related conditions in children and adults where it is necessary to limit the intake of branched chain amino acids

MSUD Anamix® Infant (SHS)

Powder, protein equivalent (essential and non-essential amino acids except isoleucine, leucine, and valine) 13.1 g, carbohydrate 49.5 g, fat 23 g, fibre 5.3 g, energy 1915 kJ (457 kcal)/100 g, with vitamins, minerals, and trace elements; *standard dilution* (15%) provides protein equivalent 2 g, carbohydrate 7.4 g, fat 3.5 g, fibre 800 mg, energy 287 kJ (69 kcal)/100 mL. Unflavoured, net price 400 g = £31.20 (5-g measuring scoop provided)

Nutritional supplement for the dietary management of proven maple syrup urine disease in children from birth to 3 years

MSUD Anamix® Junior (SHS)

Powder, protein equivalent (essential and non-essential amino acids except isoleucine, leucine, and valine) 8.4 g, carbohydrate 11 g, fat 3.9 g, energy 474 kJ (113 kcal)/29-g sachet, with vitamins, minerals, and trace elements. Unflavoured, (flavouring: see *Modjul*® Flavour System, p. 925), net price 30 × 29-g sachets = £166.73.

Nutritional supplement for the dietary management of maple syrup urine disease in children 1–10 years

MSUD Anamix® Junior LQ (SHS)

Liquid, protein equivalent (essential and non-essential amino acids except isoleucine, leucine, and valine) 10 g, carbohydrate 8.8 g, fat 4.8 g, fibre 310 mg, energy 497 kJ (118 kcal)/125 mL, with vitamins, minerals, and trace elements. Lactose-free. Orange flavour, net price 125-mL carton = £7.58

Nutritional supplement for the dietary management of maple syrup urine disease in children 1–10 years

MSUD express® (Vitaflo)

Powder, protein equivalent (essential and non-essential amino acids except isoleucine, leucine, and valine) 15 g, carbohydrate 3.8 g, fat less than 100 mg, energy 315 kJ (75 kcal)/25 g, with vitamins, minerals, and trace elements. Unflavoured, (flavouring: see *Flavour Pac*®, p. 925), net price 30 × 25-g sachets = £265.90.

Nutritional supplement for the dietary management of maple syrup urine disease in children over 8 years and adults

Appendix 2: Borderline substances

1. Maxamaid products are generally intended for use in children 1–8 years
2. Maxamum products are generally intended for use in children over 8 years

MSUD express cooler® (Vitaflo)
Liquid, protein equivalent (essential and non-essential amino acids except leucine, isoleucine, and valine) 15 g, carbohydrate 7.8 g, fat trace, energy 386 kJ (92 kcal)/130-mL pouch, with vitamins, minerals, and trace elements. Orange flavour, net price 30 × 130-mL = £271.20.
Nutritional supplement for the dietary management of maple syrup urine disease in children over 3 years and adults

MSUD Gel® (Vitaflo)
Powder, protein equivalent (essential and non-essential amino acids except leucine, isoleucine, and valine) 8.4 g, carbohydrate 8.6 g, fat less than 100 mg, energy 286 kJ (68 kcal)/20 g, with vitamins, minerals, and trace elements. Unflavoured, (flavouring: see *Flavour Pac®*, p. 925), net price 30 × 20-g sachets = £148.59.
Nutritional supplement for the dietary management of maple syrup urine disease in children 1–10 years

¹MSUD Maxamaid® (SHS)
Powder, protein equivalent (essential and non-essential amino acids except isoleucine, leucine, and valine) 25 g, carbohydrate 51 g, fat less than 500 mg, energy 1311 kJ

(309 kcal)/100 g, with vitamins, minerals, and trace elements. Unflavoured, (flavouring: see *Modjul®* Flavour System, p. 925), net price 500 g = £78.79.
Nutritional supplement for the dietary management of maple syrup urine disease

²MSUD Maxamum® (SHS)
Powder, protein equivalent (essential and non-essential amino acids except isoleucine, leucine, and valine) 39 g, carbohydrate 34 g, fat less than 500 mg, energy 1260 kJ (297 kcal)/100 g, with vitamins, minerals, and trace elements. Orange flavour or unflavoured, (flavouring: see *Modjul®* Flavour System, p. 925), net price 500 g = £126.30.
Nutritional supplement for the dietary management of maple syrup urine disease

Valine Amino Acid Supplement (Vitaflo)
Powder, valine 50 mg, carbohydrate 4 g, fat nil, energy 64 kJ (15 kcal)/4 g, net price 30 × 4-g sachets = £43.50
Nutritional supplement for the dietary management of maple syrup urine disease and other inborn errors of amino acid metabolism in children over 1 year

Methylmalonic propionic acidaemia

MMA/PA Anamix® Infant (SHS)
Powder, protein equivalent (essential and non-essential amino acids except methionine, threonine, and valine, and low isoleucine) 13.1 g, carbohydrate 49.5 g, fibre 5.3 g, energy 1915 kJ (457 kcal)/100 g, with vitamins, minerals, and trace elements; *standard dilution* (15%) provides protein equivalent 2 g, carbohydrate 7.4 g, fat 3.5 g, fibre 800 mg, energy 287 kJ (69 kcal)/100 mL. Unflavoured, net price 400 g = £31.20 (5-g measuring scoop provided)
Nutritional supplement for the dietary management of proven methylmalonic acidaemia or propionic acidaemia in children from birth to 3 years

XMTVI Asadon (SHS)
Powder, protein equivalent (essential and non-essential amino acids except methionine, threonine, and valine, and low isoleucine) 77 g, carbohydrate 4.5 g, fat nil, energy 1386 kJ (326 kcal)/100 g. Unflavoured, (flavouring: see *Modjul®* Flavour System, p. 925), net price 200 g = £59.69.
Nutritional supplement for the dietary management of methylmalonic acidaemia or propionic acidaemia in children and adults

¹XMTVI Maxamaid (SHS)
Powder, protein equivalent (essential and non-essential amino acids except methionine, threonine, and valine, and low isoleucine) 25 g, carbohydrate 51 g, fat less than 500 mg, energy 1311 kJ (309 kcal)/100 g, with vitamins, minerals, and trace elements. Unflavoured, (flavouring: see *Modjul®* Flavour System, p. 925), net price 500 g = £78.79.
Nutritional supplement for the dietary management of methylmalonic acidaemia or propionic acidaemia

²XMTVI Maxamum (SHS)
Powder, protein equivalent (essential and non-essential amino acids except methionine, threonine, and valine, and low isoleucine) 39 g, carbohydrate 34 g, fat less than 500 mg, energy 1260 kJ (297 kcal)/100 g, with vitamins, minerals, and trace elements. Unflavoured, (flavouring: see *Modjul®* Flavour System, p. 925), net price 500 g = £126.30.
Nutritional supplement for the dietary management of methylmalonic acidaemia or propionic acidaemia

Other inborn errors of metabolism

Cystine Amino Acid Supplement (Vitaflo)
Powder, cystine 500 mg, carbohydrate 3.4 g, fat nil, energy 63 kJ (15 kcal)/4 g, net price 30 × 4-g sachets = £43.50
Nutritional supplement for the dietary management of inborn errors of amino acid metabolism in children over 1 year

DocOmega® (Vitaflo)
Powder, protein (cows' milk, soya) 100 mg, carbohydrate 3.2 g, fat 500 mg (of which docosahexaenoic acid 200 mg), fibre nil, energy 74 kJ (18 kcal)/4 g, with minerals, net price 30 × 4-g sachets = £32.20
Nutritional supplement for the dietary management of inborn errors of metabolism for adults and children from birth

EAA® Supplement (Vitaflo)
Powder, protein equivalent (essential amino acids) 5 g, carbohydrate 4 g, fat nil, energy 151 kJ (36 kcal)/12.5 g,

with vitamins, minerals, and trace elements. Tropical flavour, net price 50 × 12.5-g sachets = £170.64
Nutritional supplement for the dietary management of disorders of protein metabolism including urea cycle disorders in children over 3 years

KeyOmega® (Vitaflo)
Powder, protein (cows' milk, soya) 170 mg, carbohydrate 2.8 g, fat 800 mg (of which arachidonic acid 200 mg, docosahexaenoic acid 100 mg), energy 80 kJ (19 kcal)/4 g, net price 30 × 4-g sachet = £32.30
Nutritional supplement for the dietary management of inborn errors of metabolism

Leucine Amino Acid Supplement (Vitaflo)
Powder, leucine 100 mg, carbohydrate 4 g, fat nil, energy 64 kJ (15 kcal)/4 g, net price 30 × 4-g sachets = £43.50
Nutritional supplement for the dietary management of inborn errors of amino acid metabolism in children over 1 year

1. Maxamaid products are generally intended for use in children 1–8 years
2. Maxamum products are generally intended for use in children over 8 years

Low protein drink (Milupa)

Powder, protein (cows' milk) 4.5 g (phenylalanine 100 mg), carbohydrate 59.5 g, fat 29.9 g, fibre nil, energy 2194 kJ (528 kcal)/100 g, with vitamins, minerals, and trace elements. Contains lactose. Net price 400 g = £7.23 (5-g measuring scoop provided).

Nutritional supplement for the dietary management of inborn errors of amino acid metabolism in adults and children over 1 year

Note Termed *Milupa® lp-drink* by manufacturer

Phenylalanine Amino Acid Supplement (Vitaflo)

Powder, phenylalanine 50 mg, carbohydrate 3.8 g, energy 64 kJ (15 kcal)/4 g, net price 30 × 4-g sachets = £42.23

Nutritional supplement for use in the dietary management of inborn errors of metabolism only

ProZero® (Vitaflo)

Liquid, carbohydrate 8.1 g (of which sugars 3.5 g), fat 3.8 g, energy 278 kJ (66 kcal)/100 mL. Contains lactose. Net price 18 × 250 mL = £22.50; 6 × 1 litre = £30.00

A protein-free nutritional supplement for the dietary management of inborn errors of metabolism in children over 6 months and adults

Phenylketonuria

Add-Ins® (SHS)

Powder, protein equivalent (containing essential and non-essential amino acids except phenylalanine) 10 g, carbohydrate nil, fat 5.1 g, energy 359 kJ (86 kcal)/18.2-g sachet, with vitamins, minerals, and trace elements. Unflavoured, net price 60 × 18.2-g sachets = £301.06.

Nutritional supplement for the dietary management of proven phenylketonuria in children over 4 years

Easiphen® (SHS)

Liquid, protein equivalent (containing essential and non-essential amino acids except phenylalanine) 6.7 g, carbohydrate 5.1 g, fat 2 g, energy 275 kJ (65 kcal)/100 mL with vitamins, minerals, and trace elements. Forest berries flavour, net price 250-mL carton = £7.56.

Nutritional supplement for the dietary management of proven phenylketonuria in children over 8 years

Lophlex® (SHS)

Powder, protein equivalent (essential and non-essential amino acids except phenylalanine) 20 g, carbohydrate 2.5 g, fat 60 mg, fibre 220 mg, energy 385 kJ (91 kcal)/27.8-g sachet, with vitamins, minerals, and trace elements. Flavours: berry, orange, or unflavoured, net price 30 x 27.8-g sachets = £232.31.

Nutritional supplement for the dietary management of proven phenylketonuria in children over 8 years and adults including pregnant women

Loprofin® PKU Drink (SHS)

Liquid, protein (cows' milk) 400 mg (phenylalanine 10 mg), lactose 9.4 g, fat 2 g, energy 165 kJ (40 kcal)/100 mL. Net price 200-mL carton = 61p.

Nutritional supplement for the dietary management of phenylketonuria in children over 1 year

Milupa PKU 2-prima® (Milupa)

Powder, protein equivalent (essential and non-essential amino acids except phenylalanine) 60 g, carbohydrate 10 g, fat nil, energy 1190 kJ (280 kcal)/100 g, with vitamins, minerals, and trace elements. Vanilla flavour, net price 500 g = £125.64

Nutritional supplement for the dietary management of phenylketonuria in children 1–8 years

Milupa PKU 2-secunda® (Milupa)

Powder, protein equivalent (essential and non-essential amino acids except phenylalanine) 70 g, carbohydrate 6.8 g, fat nil, energy 1306 kJ (307 kcal)/100 g, with vitamins, minerals, and trace elements. Vanilla flavour, net price 500 g = £146.59

Nutritional supplement for the dietary management of phenylketonuria in children 9–15 years

Milupa PKU 3-advanta® (Milupa)

Powder, protein equivalent (essential and non-essential amino acids except phenylalanine) 70 g, carbohydrate 4.7 g, fat nil, energy 1270 kJ (299 kcal)/100 g, with vitamins, minerals, and trace elements. Vanilla flavour, net price 500 g = £146.59

Nutritional supplement for the dietary management of phenylketonuria in children over 15 years

Phlexy-10® Exchange System (SHS)

Capsules, protein equivalent (essential and non-essential amino acids except phenylalanine) 416.5 mg/capsule. Net price 200-cap pack = £34.13

Tablets, protein equivalent (essential and non-essential amino acids except phenylalanine) 833 mg tablet. Net price 75-tab pack = £22.11

Drink Mix, powder, protein equivalent (essential and non-essential amino acids except phenylalanine) 8.33 g, carbohydrate 8.8 g/20-g sachet. Apple-black currant, citrus, or tropical flavour. Net price 30 × 20-g sachet = £102.92

Nutritional supplement for the dietary management of phenylketonuria

Phlexy-Vits® (SHS)

Powder, vitamins, minerals, and trace elements, net price 30 × 7-g sachets = £57.43.

Tablets, vitamins, minerals, and trace elements, net price 180-tab pack = £65.13.

For use as a vitamin and mineral component of restricted therapeutic diets in children over 11 years and adults with phenylketonuria and similar amino acid abnormalities

PK Aid 4® (SHS)

Powder, protein equivalent (essential and non-essential amino acids except phenylalanine) 79 g, carbohydrate 4.5 g, fat nil, energy 1420 kJ (334 kcal)/100 g. Unflavoured, (flavouring: see *Modjul* Flavour System, p. 925), net price 500 g = £114.73 (5-g measuring scoop provided).

Nutritional supplement for the dietary management of phenylketonuria in children and adults

PKU Anamix® Infant (SHS)

Powder, protein equivalent (essential and non-essential amino acids except phenylalanine) 13.1 g, carbohydrate 49.5 g, fat 23 g, fibre 5.3 g, energy 1915 kJ (457 kcal)/100 g, with vitamins, minerals, and trace elements; *standard dilution* (15%) provides protein equivalent 2 g, carbohydrate 7.4 g, fat 3.5 g, fibre 800 mg, energy 287 kJ (69 kcal)/100 mL. Unflavoured, net price 400 g = £28.36 (5-g measuring scoop provided)

Nutritional supplement for the dietary management of proven phenylketonuria in children from birth to 3 years

PKU Anamix® Junior (SHS)

Powder, protein equivalent (essential and non-essential amino acids except phenylalanine) 8.4 g, carbohydrate 9.9 g, fat 3.9 g, energy 455 kJ (108 kcal)/29-g sachet, with vitamins, minerals, and trace elements. Flavours: chocolate, pineapple-vanilla, or unflavoured (carbohydrate 11 g, energy 474 kJ (113 kcal)/29-g sachet), net price 30 × 29-g sachets = £101.29.

Nutritional supplement for the dietary management of phenylketonuria in children 1–10 years

PKU Anamix Junior LQ® (SHS)

Liquid, protein equivalent (essential and non-essential amino acids except phenylalanine) 10 g, carbohydrate 8.8 g, fat 4.8 g, fibre 310 mg, energy 497 kJ (118 kcal)/125 mL, with vitamins, minerals, and trace elements. Lactose-free. Flavours: Berry, orange, or unflavoured, net price 125-mL carton = £4.50

Nutritional supplement for the dietary supplement of phenylketonuria in children 1–10 years

Appendix 2: Borderline substances

Appendix 2: Borderline substances

PKU cooler10® (Vitaflo)
Liquid, protein equivalent (essential and non-essential amino acids except phenylalanine) 10 g, carbohydrate 5.1 g, energy 258 kJ (62 kcal)/87-mL pouch, with vitamins, minerals, and trace elements. Unflavoured (white) or flavoured (orange, purple, or red), net price 30 × 87-mL = £110.40.
Nutritional supplement for the dietary management of phenylketonuria in children over 3 years

PKU cooler15® (Vitaflo)
Liquid, protein equivalent (essential and non-essential amino acids except phenylalanine) 15 g, carbohydrate 7.8 g, energy 386 kJ (92 kcal)/130-mL pouch, with vitamins, minerals, and trace elements. Unflavoured (white) or flavoured (orange, purple, or red), net price 30 x 130 mL = £164.40.
Nutritional supplement for the dietary management of phenylketonuria in children over 3 years

PKU cooler20® (Vitaflo)
Liquid, protein equivalent (essential and non-essential amino acids except phenylalanine) 20 g, carbohydrate 10.2 g, energy 517 kJ (124 kcal)/174-mL pouch, with vitamins, minerals, and trace elements. Unflavoured (white) or flavoured (orange, purple, or red), net price 30 × 174 mL = £220.50.
Nutritional supplement for the dietary management of phenylketonuria in children over 3 years

PKU express® (Vitaflo)
Powder, protein equivalent (essential and non-essential amino acids except phenylalanine) 15 g, carbohydrate 3.8 g, energy 315 kJ (76 kcal)/25 g, with vitamins, minerals, and trace elements. Orange, lemon, orange, tropical, or unflavoured, net price 30 x 25-g sachets = £161.21.
Nutritional supplement for the dietary management of phenylketonuria in children over 8 years

PKU gel® (Vitaflo)
Powder, protein equivalent (essential and non-essential amino acids except phenylalanine) 8.4 g, carbohydrate 8.6 g, fat less than 100 mg, energy 286 kJ (68 kcal)/20 g, with vitamins, minerals and trace elements. Orange, raspberry, or unflavoured (flavouring: see *Flavour Pac®*, p. 925), net price 30 × 20-g sachets = £92.94.
For use as part of the low-protein dietary management of phenylketonuria in children 1–10 years

PKU Lophlex® LQ 10 (SHS)
Liquid, protein equivalent (essential and non-essential amino acids except phenylalanine) 10 g, carbohydrate 4.4 g, fibre 170 mg, energy 245 kJ (58 kcal)/62.5 mL, with vitamins, minerals, and trace elements. Flavours: berry, citrus, orange, or tropical, net price 60 × 62.5 mL = £243.00.
Nutritional supplement for the dietary management of phenylketonuria in children over 4 years and adults including pregnant women

PKU Lophlex® LQ 20 (SHS)
Liquid, protein equivalent (essential and non-essential amino acids except phenylalanine) 20 g, carbohydrate 8.8 g, fibre 340 mg, energy 490 kJ (115 kcal)/125 mL, with vitamins, minerals, and trace elements. Flavours: berry, citrus, orange, or tropical, net price 3 × 125 mL = £24.27.
Nutritional supplement for the dietary management of phenylketonuria in children over 4 years and adults including pregnant women

PKU Start® (Vitaflo)
Liquid, protein equivalent (essential and non-essential amino acids except phenylalanine) 2 g, carbohydrate 8.3 g, fat 2.9 g, energy 286 kJ (68 kcal)/100 mL with vitamins, minerals, and trace elements. Contains lactose and fish oil. Net price 500-mL bottle = £5.46
For the dietary management of phenylketonuria in children under 12 months

Sno-Pro® (SHS)
Liquid, protein (cows' milk) 220 mg (phenylalanine 12.5 mg), carbohydrate 8 g, fat 3.8 g, energy 273 kJ (65 kcal)/100 mL. Contains lactose. Net price 200 mL = 98p
Nutritional supplement for the dietary management of phenylketonuria, chronic renal failure and other inborn errors of amino acid metabolism

L-Tyrosine (SHS)
Powder, net price 100 g = £12.53.
Nutritional supplement for the dietary management of phenylketonuria in pregnant women with low plasma tyrosine concentrations

Tyrosine Amino Acid Supplement (Vitaflo)
Powder, tyrosine 1 g, carbohydrate 2.9 g, energy 62 kJ (15 kcal)/4-g sachet, net price 30 × 4-g sachets = £37.80.
Nutritional supplement for the dietary management of phenylketonuria and other inborn errors of amino acid metabolism

[1]XP Maxamaid (SHS)
Powder, protein equivalent (essential and non-essential amino acids except phenylalanine) 25 g, carbohydrate 51 g, fat less than 500 mg, energy 1311 kJ (309 kcal)/100 g, with vitamins, minerals, and trace elements. Orange flavour, or unflavoured (flavouring: see *Modjul®* Flavour System, p. 925), net price 500 g = £46.61.
Nutritional supplement for the dietary management of phenylketonuria in children 1– 8 years

[2]XP Maxamum® (SHS)
Powder, protein equivalent (essential and non-essential amino acids except phenylalanine) 39 g, carbohydrate 34 g, fat less than 500 mg, energy 1260 kJ (297 kcal)/100 g, with vitamins, minerals, and trace elements. Orange, or unflavoured (flavouring: see *Modjul®* Flavour System, p. 925), net price 30 × 50-g sachets = £216.21, 500 g = £72.08.
Nutritional supplement for the dietary management of phenylketonuria in children over 8 years

Tyrosinaemia

Methionine-free TYR Anamix® Infant (SHS)
Powder, protein equivalent (essential and non-essential amino acids except methionine, phenylalanine, and tyrosine) 13.1 g, carbohydrate 49.5 g, fat 23 g, fibre 5.3 g, energy 1915 kJ (457 kcal)/100 g, with vitamins, minerals, and trace elements; *standard dilution* (15%) provides protein equivalent 2 g, carbohydrate 7.4 g, fat 3.5 g, fibre 800 mg, energy 287 kJ (69 kcal)/100 mL. Unflavoured, net price 400 g = £31.20 (5-g measuring scoop provided)
Nutritional supplement for the dietary management of proven tyrosinaemia type 1 in children from birth to 3 years

TYR Anamix® Infant (SHS)
Powder, protein equivalent (essential and non-essential amino acids except phenylalanine and tyrosine) 13.1 g, carbohydrate 49.5 g, fat 23 g, fibre 5.3 g, energy 1915 kJ (457 kcal)/100 g, with vitamins, minerals, and trace elements; *standard dilution* (15%) provides protein equivalent 2 g, carbohydrate 7.4 g, fat 3.5 g, fibre 800 mg, energy 287 kJ (69 kcal)/100 mL. Unflavoured, net price 400 g = £31.20 (5-g measuring scoop provided)
Nutritional supplement for the dietary management of proven tyrosinaemia where plasma-methionine concentrations are normal in children from birth to 3 years

1. Maxamaid products are generally intended for use in children 1–8 years
2. Maxamum products are generally intended for use in children over 8 years

TYR Anamix® Junior (SHS)

Powder, protein equivalent (essential and non-essential amino acids except phenylalanine and tyrosine) 8.4 g, carbohydrate 11 g, fat 3.9 g, energy 475 kJ (113 kcal)/29-g sachet, with vitamins, minerals, and trace elements. Unflavoured, net price 30 x 29-g sachets = £165.38

Nutritional supplement for the dietary management of proven tyrosinaemia in children 1–10 years

TYR cooler® (Vitaflo)

Liquid, protein equivalent (essential and non-essential amino acids except tyrosine and phenylalanine) 15 g, carbohydrate 7.8 g, fat nil, energy 386 kJ (92 kcal)/130 mL, with vitamins, minerals, and trace elements. Orange flavour, net price 30 × 130-mL pouch = £271.20.

Nutritional supplement for the dietary management of tyrosinaemia in children over 8 years

TYR express® (Vitaflo)

Powder, protein equivalent (essential and non-essential amino acids except tyrosine and phenylalanine) 15 g, carbohydrate 3.8 g, fat less than 100 mg, energy 315 kJ (76 kcal)/25 g, with vitamins, minerals, and trace elements. Unflavoured (flavouring: see *Flavour Pac®*, p. 925), net price 30 × 25-g sachets = £265.90

Nutritional supplement for the dietary management of tyrosinaemia in children over 8 years

TYR Gel® (Vitaflo)

Gel, protein equivalent (essential and non-essential amino acids except tyrosine and phenylalanine) 8.4 g, carbohydrate 8.6 g, fat less than 100 mg, energy 286 kJ (68 kcal)/20 g, with vitamins, minerals and trace elements. Unflavoured (flavouring: see *Flavour Pac®*, p. 925), net price 30 × 20-g sachets = £148.59

Nutritional supplement for the dietary management of tyrosinaemia in children 1–10 years

¹XPHEN TYR Maxamaid (SHS)

Powder, protein equivalent (essential and non-essential amino acids except phenylalanine and tyrosine) 25 g, carbohydrate 51 g, fat less than 500 mg, energy 1311 kJ (309 kcal)/100 g, with vitamins, minerals, and trace elements. Unflavoured (flavouring: see *Modjul®* Flavour System, p. 925), net price 500 g = £78.79.

Nutritional supplement for the dietary management of tyrosinaemia in children 1–8 years

XPHEN TYR Tyrosidon (SHS)

Powder, protein equivalent (essential and non-essential amino acids except phenylalanine and tyrosine) 77 g, carbohydrate 4.5 g, fat nil, energy 1386 kJ (326 kcal)/100 g. Unflavoured (flavouring: see *Modjul®* Flavour System, p. 925), net price 500 g = £149.26

Nutritional supplement for the management of tyrosinaemia in children and adults where plasma-methionine concentrations are normal

XPTM Tyrosidon (SHS)

Powder, protein equivalent (essential and non-essential amino acids except methionine, phenylalanine, and tyrosine) 77 g, carbohydrate 4.5 g, fat nil, energy 1386 kJ (326 kcal)/100 g. Unflavoured (flavouring: see *Modjul®* Flavour System, p. 925), net price 500 g = £149.26.

Nutritional supplement for the dietary management of tyrosinaemia type I in children and adults where plasma-methionine concentrations are above normal

Urea cycle disorders (other than arginase deficiency)

L-Arginine (SHS)

Powder, net price 100 g = £11.70.

For use as a supplement in urea cycle disorders other than arginase deficiency, such as hyperammonaemia types I and II, citrullaemia, arginosuccinic aciduria, and deficiency of N-acetyl glutamate synthetase

Conditions for which ACBS products can be prescribed

Note This is a list of clinical conditions for which the ACBS has approved toilet preparations. For details of the preparations see Chapter 13.

Birthmarks

See Disfiguring skin lesions, below

Dermatitis

Aveeno® Bath Oil; *Aveeno®* Cream; *Aveeno®* Colloidal; *E45®* Emollient Bath Oil; *E45®* Emollient Wash Cream; *E45®* Lotion

Dermatitis herpetiformis

See also Gluten-sensitive enteropathies, p. 926

Disfiguring skin lesions (birthmarks, mutilating lesions, scars, vitiligo)

Covermark® classic foundation and finishing powder; *Dermacolor®* Camouflage cream and fixing powder; *Keromask®* masking cream and finishing powder; *Veil®* Cover cream and Finishing Powder. (Cleansing Creams, Cleansing Milks, and Cleansing Lotions are excluded)

Disinfectants (antiseptics)

May be prescribed on an FP10 only when ordered in such quantities and with such directions as are appropriate for the treatment of patients, but not for general hygenic purposes.

Dry mouth (xerostomia)

For patients suffering from dry mouth as a result of having (or having undergone) radiotherapy, or sicca syndrome.

AS Saliva Orthana®; *Biotène Oralbalance®*; *BioXtra®*; *Glandosane®*; *Saliveze®*; *Salivix®*.

For details of preparations see section 12.3.5, p. 670

Eczema

See Dermatitis, above

Photodermatoses (skin protection in)

Delph® Sun Lotion SPF 30; *Spectraban®* Ultra; *Sunsense Ultra®*; *Uvistat®* Lipscreen SPF 50, *Uvistat®* Suncream SPF 30 and 50.

Pruritus

See Dermatitis, above

Appendix 2: Borderline substances

---

1. Maxamaid products are generally intended for use in children 1–8 years

A3 Cautionary and advisory labels for dispensed medicines

Preparations in the *BNF for Children* include code numbers of the cautionary labels that pharmacists are recommended to add when dispensing. It is also expected that, when necessary, pharmacists will counsel children or their carers.

Counselling needs to be related to the age, experience, background, and understanding of the child or carer. The pharmacist should ensure understanding of how to take or use the medicine and how to follow the correct dosage schedule. Any effects of the medicine on co-ordination, performance of skilled tasks, any foods or medicines to be avoided, and what to do if a dose is missed should also be explained. Other matters, such as the possibility of staining of the clothes or skin, or discoloration of urine or stools by a medicine should also be mentioned.

For some preparations there is a special need for counselling, such as an unusual method or time of administration or a potential interaction with a common food or domestic remedy, and this should be mentioned where necessary.

Original packs Most preparations are now dispensed in unbroken original packs (see Patient Packs, p. xiv) that include further advice for the patient in the form of patient information leaflets. The advice in patient information leaflets may be less appropriate when the medicine is for a child, particularly for unlicensed medicines or indications. Pharmacists should explain discrepancies to carers, if necessary. The patient information leaflet should only be withheld in exceptional circumstances because it contains other information that should be provided. Label 10 may be of value where appropriate. More general leaflets advising on the administration of preparations such as eye drops, eye ointments, inhalers, and suppositories are also available.

Scope of labels In general, no label recommendations are provided for injections on the assumption that they will be administered by a healthcare professional or a well-instructed child or carer. The labelling is not exhaustive and pharmacists are recommended to use their professional discretion in labelling new preparations and those for which no labels are shown.

Individual labelling advice is not given on the administration of the large variety of antacids. In the absence of instructions from the prescriber, and if on enquiry the patient has had no verbal instructions, the directions given under 'Dose' should be used on the label.

It is recognised that there may be occasions when pharmacists will use their knowledge and professional discretion and decide to omit one or more of the recommended labels for a particular child. In this case counselling is of the utmost importance. There may also be an occasion when a prescriber does not wish additional cautionary labels to be used, in which case the prescription should be endorsed 'NCL' (no cautionary labels). The exact wording that is required instead should then be specified on the prescription.

Pharmacists label medicines with various wordings in addition to those directions specified on the prescription. Such labels include 'Shake the bottle', 'For external use only', and 'Store in a cool place', as well as 'Discard . . . . days after opening' and 'Do not use after . . . .', which apply particularly to antibiotic mixtures, diluted liquid and topical preparations, and to eye-drops. Although not listed in the *BNF for Children* these labels should continue to be used when appropriate; indeed, 'For external use only' is a legal requirement on external liquid preparations, while 'Keep out of the reach of children' is a legal requirement on all dispensed medicines. Care should be taken not to obscure other relevant information with adhesive labelling.

It is the usual practice for patients to take standard tablets with water or other liquid and for this reason no separate label has been recommended.

The label wordings recommended by the *BNF for Children* apply to medicines dispensed against a prescription. Children and carers should be made aware that a dispensed medicine should never be taken by, or shared with, anyone other than for whom the prescriber intended it. Therefore, the *BNF for Children* does not include warnings against the use of a dispensed medicine by persons other than for whom it was specifically prescribed.

The label or labels for each preparation are recommended after careful consideration of the information available. However, it is recognised that in some cases this information may be either incomplete or open to a different interpretation. The BNF will therefore be grateful to receive any constructive comments on the labelling suggested for any preparation.

Recommended label wordings

Wordings which can be given as separate warnings are labels 1–19 and labels 29–33. Wordings which can be incorporated in an appropriate position in the directions for dosage or administration are labels 21–28. A label has been omitted for number 20.

If separate labels are used it is recommended that the wordings be used without modification. If changes are made to suit computer requirements, care should be taken to retain the sense of the original.

1   Warning. May cause drowsiness
To be used on *preparations for children* containing antihistamines, or other preparations given to children where the warnings of label 2 on driving or alcohol would not be appropriate.

2   Warning. May cause drowsiness. If affected do not drive or operate machinery. Avoid alcoholic drink
To be used on *preparations for adults that can cause drowsiness*, thereby affecting coordination and the ability to drive and operate hazardous machinery; label 1 is more appropriate for children. *It is an offence to drive while under the influence of drink or drugs.* It should be remembered that children and adolescents do, on occasion, consume alcohol and should be made aware of potential problems.
Some of these preparations only cause drowsiness in the first few days of treatment and some only cause drowsiness in higher doses.
In such cases the patient should be told that the advice applies until the effects have worn off. However many of these preparations can produce a slowing of reaction time and a loss of mental concentration that can have the same effects as drowsiness.
Avoidance of alcoholic drink is recommended because the effects of CNS depressants are enhanced by alcohol. Strict prohibition however could lead to some patients not taking the medicine. Pharmacists should therefore explain the risk and encourage compliance, particularly in patients who may think they already tolerate the effects of alcohol (see also label 3).
Queries from patients with epilepsy regarding fitness to drive should be referred back to the patient's doctor.
Side-effects unrelated to drowsiness that may affect a patient's ability to drive or operate machinery safely include *blurred vision, dizziness, or nausea.* In general, no label has been recommended to cover these cases, but the patient should be suitably counselled.

3   Warning. May cause drowsiness. If affected do not drive or operate machinery
To be used on *preparations containing monoamine-oxidase inhibitors*; the warning to avoid alcohol and dealcoholised (low alcohol) drink is covered by the patient information leaflet.
Also to be used as for label 2 but where alcohol is not an issue.

4   Warning. Avoid alcoholic drink
To be used on *preparations where a reaction such as flushing may occur if alcohol is taken* (e.g. metronidazole). Alcohol may also enhance the hypoglycaemia produced by some oral antidiabetic drugs but

routine application of a warning label is not considered necessary.

5   Do not take indigestion remedies at the same time of day as this medicine
To be used with label 25 on *preparations coated to resist gastric acid* (e.g. enteric-coated tablets). This is to avoid the possibility of premature dissolution of the coating in the presence of an alkaline pH.
Label 5 also applies to drugs such as ketoconazole *where the absorption is significantly affected by antacids*; the usual period of avoidance recommended is 2 to 4 hours.

6   Do not take indigestion remedies or medicines containing iron or zinc at the same time of day as this medicine
To be used on *preparations containing ofloxacin and some other quinolones, doxycycline, lymecycline, minocycline, and penicillamine.* These drugs chelate calcium, iron and zinc and are less well absorbed when taken with calcium-containing antacids or preparations containing iron or zinc. These incompatible preparations should be taken 2–3 hours apart.

7   Do not take milk, indigestion remedies, or medicines containing iron or zinc at the same time of day as this medicine
To be used on *preparations containing ciprofloxacin, norfloxacin or tetracyclines that chelate calcium, iron, magnesium, and zinc,* and are thus less available for absorption; these incompatible preparations should be taken 2–3 hours apart. Doxycycline, lymecycline and minocycline are less liable to form chelates and therefore only require label 6 (see above).

8   Do not stop taking this medicine except on your doctor's advice
To be used on *preparations that contain a drug which is required to be taken over long periods without the patient necessarily perceiving any benefit* (e.g. anti-tuberculous drugs).
Also to be used on *preparations that contain a drug whose withdrawal is likely to be a particular hazard* (e.g. clonidine for hypertension). Label 10 (see below) is more appropriate for corticosteroids.

9   Take at regular intervals. Complete the prescribed course unless otherwise directed
To be used on *preparations where a course of treatment should be completed* to reduce the incidence of relapse or failure of treatment.
The preparations are antimicrobial drugs given by mouth. Very occasionally, some may have severe side-effects (e.g. diarrhoea in patients receiving clindamycin) and in such cases the patient may need

to be advised of reasons for stopping treatment quickly and returning to the doctor.

10 Warning. Follow the printed instructions you have been given with this medicine
To be used particularly on *preparations containing anticoagulants, lithium and oral corticosteroids*. The appropriate treatment card should be given to the patient and any necessary explanations given.
This label may also be used on other preparations to remind the patient of the instructions that have been given.

11 Avoid exposure of skin to direct sunlight or sun lamps
To be used on *preparations that may cause phototoxic or photoallergic reactions* if the patient is exposed to ultraviolet radiation. Many drugs other than those listed (e.g. phenothiazines and sulphonamides) may, on rare occasions, cause reactions in susceptible patients. Exposure to high intensity ultraviolet radiation from sunray lamps and sunbeds is particularly likely to cause reactions.

12 Do not take anything containing aspirin while taking this medicine
To be used on *preparations containing probenecid and sulfinpyrazone* whose activity is reduced by aspirin.
Label 12 should not be used for anticoagulants since label 10 is more appropriate.

13 Dissolve or *mix with water* before taking
To be used on *preparations that are intended to be dissolved in water* (e.g. soluble tablets) or *mixed with water* (e.g. powders, granules) before use. In a few cases other liquids such as fruit juice or milk may be used.

14 This medicine may colour the urine
To be used on *preparations that may cause the patient's urine to turn an unusual colour*. These include phenolphthalein (alkaline urine pink), triamterene (blue under some lights), levodopa (dark reddish), and rifampicin (red).

15 Caution flammable: keep away from fire or flames
To be used on *preparations containing sufficient flammable solvent to render them flammable if exposed to a naked flame.*

16 Allow to dissolve under the tongue. Do not transfer from this container. Keep tightly closed. Discard eight weeks after opening
To be used on *glyceryl trinitrate tablets* to remind the patient not to transfer the tablets to plastic or less suitable containers.

17 Do not take more than . . . in 24 hours
To be used on *preparations for the treatment of acute migraine* except those containing ergotamine, for which label 18 is used. The dose form should be specified, e.g. tablets or capsules.
It may also be used on preparations for which no dose has been specified by the prescriber.

18 Do not take more than . . . in 24 hours or . . . in any one week
To be used on preparations containing ergotamine. The dose form should be specified, e.g. tablets or suppositories.

19 Warning. Causes drowsiness which may continue the next day. If affected do not drive or operate machinery. Avoid alcoholic drink
To be used on *preparations containing hypnotics (or some other drugs with sedative effects) prescribed to be taken at night.* On the rare occasions (e.g. nitrazepam in epilepsy) when hypnotics are prescribed for daytime administration this label would clearly not be appropriate. Also to be used as an *alternative to the label 2 wording* (the choice being at the discretion of the pharmacist) *for anxiolytics prescribed to be taken at night.*

It is hoped that this wording will convey adequately the problem of residual morning sedation after taking 'sleeping tablets'.

21 . . . with or after food
To be used on *preparations that are liable to cause gastric irritation, or those that are better absorbed with food.*
Patients should be advised that a *small amount of food is sufficient.*

22 . . . half to one hour before food
To be used on some preparations *whose absorption is thereby improved.*
Most oral antibacterials require label 23 instead (see below).

23 . . . an hour before food or on an empty stomach
To be used on *oral preparations whose absorption may be reduced by the presence of food and acid in the stomach.*

24 . . . sucked or chewed
To be used on *preparations that should be sucked or chewed.*
The pharmacist should use discretion as to which of these words is appropriate.

25 . . . swallowed whole, not chewed
To be used on *preparations that are enteric-coated or designed for modified-release.*
Also to be used on *preparations that taste very unpleasant or may damage the mouth* if not swallowed whole.

26 . . . dissolved under the tongue
To be used on *preparations designed for sublingual use.* Patients should be advised to hold under the tongue and avoid swallowing until dissolved. The buccal mucosa between the gum and cheek is occasionally specified by the prescriber.

27 . . . with plenty of water
To be used on *preparations that should be well diluted* (e.g. chloral hydrate), *where a high fluid intake is required* (e.g. sulphonamides), or *where water is required to aid the action* (e.g. methylcellulose). The patient should be advised that 'plenty' means at least 150 mL (about a tumblerful). In most cases fruit juice, tea, or coffee may be used.

28 To be spread thinly . . .
To be used on *external preparations* that should be applied sparingly (e.g. corticosteroids, dithranol).

29 Do not take more than 2 at any one time. Do not take more than 8 in 24 hours
To be used on containers of dispensed *solid dose preparations containing paracetamol for adults when the instruction on the label indicates that the dose can be taken on an 'as required' basis.* The dose form should be specified, e.g. tablets or capsules.
This label has been introduced because of the serious consequences of overdosage with paracetamol.

30 Do not take with any other paracetamol products
To be used on all containers of dispensed *preparations containing paracetamol.*

31 Contains aspirin and paracetamol. Do not take with any other paracetamol products
To be used on all containers of dispensed *preparations containing aspirin and paracetamol.*

32 Contains aspirin
To be used on containers of dispensed *preparations containing aspirin when the name on the label does not include the word 'aspirin'.*

33 Contains an aspirin-like medicine
To be used on containers of dispensed *preparations containing aspirin derivatives.*

A4 Intravenous infusions for neonatal intensive care

Intravenous policy   A local policy on the dilution of drugs with intravenous fluids should be drawn up by a multi-disciplinary team and issued as a document to the members of staff concerned.

Centralised additive services are provided in a number of hospital pharmacy departments and should be used in preference to making additions on wards.

The information that follows should be read in conjunction with local policy documents.

Guidelines

1. Drugs should only be diluted with infusion fluid when constant plasma concentrations are needed or when the administration of a more concentrated solution would be harmful.
2. In general, only one drug should be mixed with an infusion fluid in a syringe and the components should be compatible. Ready-prepared solutions should be used whenever possible. Drugs should not normally be added to blood products, mannitol, or sodium bicarbonate. Only specially formulated additives should be used with fat emulsions or amino-acid solutions (section 9.3).
3. Solutions should be thoroughly mixed by shaking and checked for absence of particulate matter before use.
4. Strict asepsis should be maintained throughout and in general the giving set should not be used for more than 24 hours (for drug admixtures).
5. The infusion syringe should be labelled with the neonate's name and hospital number, the name and quantity of drug, the infusion fluid, and the expiry date and time. If a problem occurs during administration, containers should be retained for a period after use in case they are needed for investigation.
6. Administration using a suitable motorised syringe driver is advocated for preparations where strict control over administration is required.
7. It is good practice to examine intravenous infusions from time to time while they are running. If cloudiness, crystallisation, change of colour, or any other sign of interaction or contamination is observed the infusion should be discontinued.

Problems

Microbial contamination   The accidental entry and subsequent growth of micro-organisms converts the infusion fluid pathway into a potential vehicle for infection with micro-organisms, particularly species of Candida, Enterobacter, and Klebsiella. Ready-prepared infusions containing the additional drugs, or infusions prepared by an additive service (when available) should therefore be used in preference to making extemporaneous additions to infusion containers on wards etc. However, when this is necessary strict aseptic procedure should be followed.

Incompatibility   Physical and chemical incompatibilities may occur with loss of potency, increase in toxicity, or other adverse effect. The solutions may become opalescent or precipitation may occur, but in many instances there is no visual indication of incompatibility. Interaction may take place at any point in the infusion fluid pathway, and the potential for incompatibility is increased when more than one substance is added to the infusion fluid.

Common incompatibilities   Precipitation reactions are numerous and varied and may occur as a result of pH, concentration changes, 'salting-out' effects, complexation or other chemical changes. Precipitation or other particle formation must be avoided since, apart from lack of control of dosage on administration, it may initiate or exacerbate adverse effects. This is particularly important in the case of drugs which have been implicated in either thrombophlebitis (e.g. diazepam) or in skin sloughing or necrosis caused by extravasation (e.g. sodium bicarbonate and parenteral nutrition). It is also especially important to effect solution of colloidal drugs and to prevent their subsequent precipitation in order to avoid a pyrogenic reaction (e.g. amphotericin).

It is considered undesirable to mix beta-lactam antibiotics, such as semi-synthetic penicillins and cephalosporins, with proteinaceous materials on the grounds that immunogenic and allergenic conjugates could be formed.

A number of preparations undergo significant loss of potency when added singly or in combination to large volume infusions. Examples include ampicillin in infusions that contain glucose or lactates.

Blood Because of the large number of incompatibilities, drugs should not be added to blood and blood products for infusion purposes. Examples of incompatibility with blood include hypertonic mannitol solutions (irreversible crenation of red cells), dextrans (rouleaux formation and interference with cross-matching), glucose (clumping of red cells), and oxytocin (inactivated).

If the giving set is not changed after the administration of blood, but used for other infusion fluids, a fibrin clot may form which, apart from blocking the set, increases the likelihood of microbial growth.

Intravenous fat emulsions These may break down with coalescence of fat globules and separation of phases when additions such as antibacterials or electrolytes are made, thus increasing the possibility of embolism. Only specially formulated products such as *Vitlipid N*® (section 9.3) may be added to appropriate intravenous fat emulsions.

Other infusions Infusions that frequently give rise to incompatibility include amino acids, mannitol, and sodium bicarbonate.

Method

Ready-prepared infusions should be used whenever available. When dilution of drugs is required to be made extemporaneously, any product reconstitution instructions such as those relating to concentration, vehicle, mixing, and handling precautions should be strictly followed using an aseptic technique throughout. Once the product has been reconstituted, further dilution with the infusion fluid should be made immediately in order to minimise microbial contamination and, with certain products, to prevent degradation or other formulation change which may occur; e.g. reconstituted ampicillin injection degrades rapidly on standing, and also may form polymers which could cause sensitivity reactions.

It is also important in certain instances that an infusion fluid of specific pH be used (e.g. **furosemide** injection requires dilution in infusions of pH greater than 5.5).

When drug dilutions are made it is important to mix thoroughly; additions should not be made to an infusion container that has been connected to a giving set, as mixing is hampered. If the solutions are not thoroughly mixed, a concentrated layer of the drug may form owing to differences in density. **Potassium chloride** is particularly prone to this 'layering' effect when added without adequate mixing to infusions; if such a mixture is administered it may have a serious effect on the heart.

A time limit between dilution and completion of administration must be imposed for certain admixtures to guarantee satisfactory drug potency and compatibility. For admixtures in which degradation occurs without the formation of toxic substances, an acceptable limit is the time taken for 10% decomposition of the drug. When toxic substances are produced stricter limits may be imposed. Because of the risk of microbial contamination a maximum time limit of 24 hours may be appropriate for additions made elsewhere than in hospital pharmacies offering central additive service.

Certain injections must be protected from light during continuous infusion to minimise oxidation, e.g. amphotericin and sodium nitroprusside.

Table of drugs given by continuous intravenous infusion to neonates

The table lists key drugs given by continuous intravenous infusion to neonates.

> Covers dilution with *Glucose intravenous infusion* 5% and 10% and *Sodium chloride intravenous infusion* 0.9%. Compatibility with glucose 5% and with sodium chloride 0.9% indicates compatibility with *Sodium chloride and glucose intravenous infusion*. Infusion of a large volume of hypotonic solution should be avoided, therefore care should be taken if water for injections is used.

Adrenaline/Epinephrine (p. 146)

Dilute 3 mg/kg body-weight to a final volume of 50 mL with Glucose 5% or Sodium Chloride 0.9%; an intravenous infusion rate of 0.1 mL/hour provides a dose of 100 nanograms/kg/minute; infuse through a central venous catheter. Incompatible with bicarbonate and alkaline solutions.

Note Usually made up with adrenaline 1 in 1000 (1 mg/mL) solution; this concentration of adrenaline is not licensed for intravenous administration

Alprostadil (*Prostin VR*®) (p. 168)

Dilute 150 micrograms/kg body-weight to a final volume of 50 mL with Glucose 5% or Sodium Chloride 0.9%; an intravenous infusion rate of 0.1 mL/hour provides a dose of 5 nanograms/kg/minute. Undiluted solution must not come into contact with the barrel of the plastic syringe; add the required volume of alprostadil to a volume of infusion fluid in the syringe, and then make up to final volume

Atracurium besilate (p. 790)

Dilute 60 mg/kg body-weight to a final volume of 50 mL with Glucose 5% or Sodium Chloride 0.9%; an intravenous infusion rate of 0.1 mL/hour provides a dose of 120 micrograms/kg/hour; minimum concentration of 500 micrograms/mL, max. concentration of 5 mg/mL.

Dobutamine (as hydrochloride) (p. 143)

Dilute 30 mg/kg body-weight to a final volume of 50 mL with Glucose 5% or Sodium Chloride 0.9%; an intravenous infusion rate of 0.5 mL/hour provides a dose of 5 micrograms/kg/minute; max. concentration of 5 mg/mL; infuse higher concentration solutions through central venous catheter only. Incompatible with bicarbonate and other strong alkaline solutions

Dopamine hydrochloride (p. 144)

Dilute 30 mg/kg body-weight to a final volume of 50 mL with Glucose 5% or Sodium Chloride 0.9%; an intravenous infusion rate of 0.3 mL/hour provides a dose of 3 micrograms/kg/minute; max. concentration of 3.2 mg/mL; infuse higher concentration solutions through central venous catheter. Incompatible with bicarbonate and other alkaline solutions

Epoprostenol (*Flolan*®) (p. 125)

Reconstitute the 500 microgram vial using the glycine buffer diluent provided to make a 10 micrograms/mL concentrate (pH 10.5); filter the concentrate using the filter provided; the concentrate can be administered via a central venous catheter, or it may be diluted further.

Neonate body-weight under 2 kg, using the concentrate, dilute 150 micrograms/kg body-weight to a final volume of 50 mL with Sodium Chloride 0.9%; an intravenous infusion rate of 0.1 mL/hour provides a dose of 5 nanograms/kg/minute.

Neonate body-weight over 2 kg, using the concentrate, dilute 60 micrograms/kg body-weight to a final volume of 50 mL with Sodium Chloride 0.9%; an intravenous infusion rate of 0.1 mL/hour provides a dose of 2 nanograms/kg/minute.

Note Diluted solution stable for 12 hours at room temperature, although some units use for 24 hours and allow for loss of potency. Minimum concentration of 1.43 micrograms/mL

> Intravenous infusion information for neonatal intensive care *only*; for information in other children, see individual drug monographs.

Glyceryl trinitrate (p. 135)

Dilute 3 mg/kg body-weight to a final volume of 50 mL with Glucose 5% or Sodium Chloride 0.9%; an intravenous infusion rate of 1 mL/hour provides a dose of 1 microgram/kg/minute; max. concentration of 400 micrograms/mL (but concentration of 1 mg/mL has been used via a central venous catheter).

Note Glass or polyethylene apparatus is preferable; loss of potency will occur if PVC is used

Heparin (as sodium) (p. 148)

Maintenance of umbilical arterial catheter, dilute 50 units to a final volume of 50 mL with Sodium Chloride 0.45% or use ready-made bag containing 500 units in 500 mL Sodium Chloride 0.9%; infuse at 0.5 mL/hour.

Treatment of thrombosis, dilute 1250 units/kg body-weight to a final volume of 50 mL with Glucose 5% or Sodium Chloride 0.9%; an intravenous infusion rate of 1 mL/hour provides a dose of 25 units/kg/hour

Insulin (soluble) (p. 429)

Dilute 5 units to a final volume of 50 mL with Sodium Chloride 0.9% and mix thoroughly; an intravenous infusion rate of 0.1 mL/kg/hour provides a dose of 0.01 units/kg/hour.

Note Insulin may be absorbed by plastics, flush giving set with 5 mL of infusion fluid containing insulin

Midazolam (p. 293 and p. 784)

Dilute 15 mg/kg body-weight to a final volume of 50 mL with Glucose 5% *or* Sodium Chloride 0.9%; an intravenous infusion rate of 0.1 mL/hour provides a dose of 30 micrograms/kg/hour

> Intravenous infusion information for neonatal intensive care *only*; for information in other children, see individual drug monographs.

Morphine sulphate (p. 262)

Dilute 2.5 mg/kg body-weight to a final volume of 50 mL with Glucose 5% *or* 10% *or* Sodium Chloride 0.9%; an intravenous infusion rate of 0.1 mL/hour provides a dose of 5 micrograms/kg/hour

Noradrenaline/Norepinephrine (p. 145)

Dilute 600 micrograms (base)/kg body-weight to a final volume of 50 mL with Glucose 5% *or* Sodium Chloride and Glucose; an intravenous infusion rate of 0.1 mL/hour provides a dose of 20 nanograms (base)/kg/minute; infuse through central venous catheter; max. concentration of noradrenaline (base) 40 micrograms/mL (higher concentrations can be used if fluid restricted). Discard if discoloured. Incompatible with bicarbonate or alkaline solutions.

Note 1 mg of noradrenaline acid tartrate is equivalent to 500 micrograms of the base. Dose expressed as the base

Vecuronium (p. 792)

Reconstitute each vial with 5 mL Water for Injections to give a 2 mg/mL solution. Dilute 5 mg/kg body-weight to a final volume of 50 mL with Glucose 5% or Sodium Chloride 0.9%; an intravenous infusion rate of 0.5 mL/hour provides a dose of 50 micrograms/kg/hour; minimum concentration of 40 micrograms/mL

Dental Practitioners' Formulary

List of Dental Preparations

The following list has been approved by the appropriate Secretaries of State, and the preparations therein may be prescribed by dental practitioners on form FP10D (GP14 in Scotland, WP10D in Wales).

Sugar-free versions, where available, are preferred.

Aciclovir Cream, BP
Aciclovir Oral Suspension, BP, 200 mg/5 mL
Aciclovir Tablets, BP, 200 mg
Aciclovir Tablets, BP, 800 mg
Amoxicillin Capsules, BP
Amoxicillin Oral Powder, DPF
Amoxicillin Oral Suspension, BP
Amphotericin Lozenges, BP[1]
Ampicillin Capsules, BP
Ampicillin Oral Suspension, BP
Artificial Saliva Liquid, DPF
Artificial Saliva Oral Spray, DPF
Artificial Saliva Substitutes as listed below (to be prescribed only for indications approved by ACBS[2]):
    AS Saliva Orthana®
    Glandosane®
    Biotene Oralbalance®
    BioXtra®
    Saliveze®
    Salivix®
Aspirin Tablets, Dispersible, BP[3]
Azithromycin Oral Suspension, 200 mg/5 mL, DPF
Beclometasone Pressurised Inhalation, BP, 50 micrograms/metered inhalation, CFC-free, as:
    Clenil Modulite®
Benzydamine Mouthwash, BP 0.15%
Benzydamine Oromucosal Spray, BP 0.15%
Betamethasone Soluble Tablets, 500 micrograms, DPF
Carbamazepine Tablets, BP
Carmellose Gelatin Paste, DPF
Cefalexin Capsules, BP
Cefalexin Oral Suspension, BP
Cefalexin Tablets, BP
Cefradine Capsules, BP
Cefradine Oral Solution, DPF[1]
Cetirizine Hydrochloride Tablets, 10 mg, DPF
Chlorhexidine Gluconate Gel, BP
Chlorhexidine Mouthwash, BP
Chlorhexidine Oral Spray, DPF
Chlorhexidine Oromucosal Solution, Alcohol-free, 0.2%, DPF
Chlorphenamine Oral Solution, BP
Chlorphenamine Tablets, BP
Choline Salicylate Dental Gel, BP

Clindamycin Capsules, BP
Co-amoxiclav Tablets, BP, 250/125 (amoxicillin 250 mg as trihydrate, clavulanic acid 125 mg as potassium salt)
Co-amoxiclav Oral Suspension, 125/31 (amoxicillin 125 mg as trihydrate, clavulanic acid 31.25 mg as potassium salt)/5 mL, DPF
Co-amoxiclav Oral Suspension, 250/62 (amoxicillin 250 mg as trihydrate, clavulanic acid 62.5 mg as potassium salt)/5 mL, DPF
Diazepam Oral Solution, BP, 2 mg/5 mL
Diazepam Tablets, BP
Diclofenac Sodium Tablets, BP
Dihydrocodeine Tablets, BP, 30 mg
Doxycycline Capsules, BP, 100 mg
Doxycycline Tablets, 20 mg, DPF
Ephedrine Nasal Drops, BP
Erythromycin Ethyl Succinate Oral Suspension, BP
Erythromycin Ethyl Succinate Tablets, BP
Erythromycin Stearate Tablets, BP
Erythromycin Tablets, BP
Fluconazole Capsules, 50 mg, DPF
Fluconazole Oral Suspension, 50 mg/5 mL, DPF
Hydrocortisone Cream, BP, 1%
Hydrocortisone Oromucosal Tablets, BP
Hydrogen Peroxide Mouthwash, BP
Ibuprofen Oral Suspension, BP, sugar-free
Ibuprofen Tablets, BP
Lansoprazole Capsules, DPF
Lidocaine 5% Ointment, DPF
Lidocaine Spray 10%, DPF
Loratadine Tablets, 10 mg, DPF
Menthol and Eucalyptus Inhalation, BP 1980[4]
Metronidazole Oral Suspension, BP
Metronidazole Tablets, BP
Miconazole Cream, BP
Miconazole Oromucosal Gel, BP
Miconazole and Hydrocortisone Cream, BP
Miconazole and Hydrocortisone Ointment, BP
Mouthwash Solution-tablets, DPF
Nitrazepam Tablets, BP
Nystatin Oral Suspension, BP
Gastro-resistant Omeprazole Capsules, BP
Oxytetracycline Tablets, BP
Paracetamol Oral Suspension, BP[5]
Paracetamol Tablets, BP

---

1. May be difficult to obtain
2. Indications approved by the ACBS are: patients suffering from dry mouth as a result of having (or having undergone) radiotherapy or sicca syndrome
3. The BP directs that when soluble aspirin tablets are prescribed, dispersible aspirin tablets should be dispensed
4. This preparation does not appear in subsequent editions of the BP
5. The BP directs that when Paediatric Paracetamol Oral Suspension or Paediatric Paracetamol Mixture is prescribed and no strength stated Paracetamol Oral Suspension 120 mg/5 mL should be dispensed

Paracetamol Tablets, Soluble, BP
Penciclovir Cream, DPF
Phenoxymethylpenicillin Oral Solution, BP
Phenoxymethylpenicillin Tablets, BP
Promethazine Hydrochloride Tablets, BP
Promethazine Oral Solution, BP
Saliva Stimulating Tablets, DPF
Sodium Chloride Mouthwash, Compound, BP
Sodium Fluoride Mouthwash, BP
Sodium Fluoride Oral Drops, BP

Sodium Fluoride Tablets, BP
Sodium Fluoride Toothpaste 0.619%, DPF
Sodium Fluoride Toothpaste 1.1%, DPF
Sodium Fusidate Ointment, BP
Temazepam Oral Solution, BP
Temazepam Tablets, BP
Tetracycline Tablets, BP

Nurse Prescribers' Formulary

Nurse Prescribers' Formulary for Community Practitioners

Nurse Prescribers' Formulary Appendix (Appendix NPF). List of preparations approved by the Secretary of State which may be prescribed on form FP10P (form HS21(N) in Northern Ireland, form GP10(N) in Scotland, forms FP10(CN) and FP10(PN) in Wales or, when available, WP10CN and WP10PN in Wales) by Nurses for National Health Service patients.

Community practitioners who have completed the necessary training may only prescribe items appearing in the nurse prescribers' list set out below. Community Practitioner Nurse Prescribers are recommended to prescribe generically, except where this would not be clinically appropriate or where there is no approved generic name.

Medicinal Preparations

Almond Oil Ear Drops, BP
Arachis Oil Enema, NPF
¹Aspirin Tablets, Dispersible, 300 mg, BP
Bisacodyl Suppositories, BP (includes 5-mg and 10-mg strengths)
Bisacodyl Tablets, BP
Catheter Maintenance Solution, Chlorhexidine, NPF
Catheter Maintenance Solution, Sodium Chloride, NPF
Catheter Maintenance Solution, 'Solution G', NPF
Catheter Maintenance Solution, 'Solution R', NPF
Chlorhexidine Gluconate Alcoholic Solutions containing at least 0.05%
Chlorhexidine Gluconate Aqueous Solutions containing at least 0.05%
Choline Salicylate Dental Gel, BP
Clotrimazole Cream 1%, BP
Co-danthramer Capsules, NPF
Co-danthramer Capsules, Strong, NPF
Co-danthramer Oral Suspension, NPF
Co-danthramer Oral Suspension, Strong, NPF
Co-danthrusate Capsules, BP
Co-danthrusate Oral Suspension, NPF
Crotamiton Cream, BP
Crotamiton Lotion, BP
Dimeticone barrier creams containing at least 10%
Dimeticone Lotion, NPF
Docusate Capsules, BP
Docusate Enema, NPF
Docusate Oral Solution, BP
Docusate Oral Solution, Paediatric, BP
Econazole Cream 1%, BP
Emollients as listed below:
  Aquadrate® 10% w/w Cream
  Aqueous Cream, BP
  Arachis Oil, BP
  Balneum® Plus Cream
  Cetraben® Emollient Cream
  Dermamist®

Diprobase® Cream
Diprobase® Ointment
Doublebase®
E45® Cream
E45® Itch Relief Cream
Emulsifying Ointment, BP
Eucerin® Intensive 10% w/w Urea Treatment Cream
Eucerin® Intensive 10% w/w Urea Treatment Lotion
Hydromol® Cream
Hydromol® Ointment
Hydrous Ointment, BP
Linola® Gamma Cream
Lipobase®
Liquid and White Soft Paraffin Ointment, NPF
Neutrogena® Norwegian Formula Dermatological Cream
Nutraplus® Cream
Oilatum® Cream
Oilatum® Junior Cream
Paraffin, White Soft, BP
Paraffin, Yellow Soft, BP
QV® Cream
QV® Lotion
QV® Wash
Ultrabase®
Unguentum M®
Zerobase® Cream
Emollient Bath Additives as listed below:
  ²Balneum®
  Cetraben® Emollient Bath Additive
  Dermalo® Bath Emollient
  Diprobath®
  Doublebase® Emollient Bath Additive
  Doublebase® Emollient Shower Gel
  Doublebase® Emollient Wash Gel
  Hydromol® Bath and Shower Emollient
  Oilatum® Emollient
  Oilatum® Junior Emollient Bath Additive
  Oilatum® Gel
  QV® Bath Oil

1. Max. 96 tablets; max. pack size 32 tablets
2. Except pack sizes that are not to be prescribed under the NHS (see Part XVIIIA of the Drug Tariff, Part XI of the Northern Ireland Drug Tariff)

Nurse Prescribers' Formulary

Folic Acid 400 micrograms/5 mL Oral Solution, NPF
Folic Acid Tablets 400 micrograms, BP
Glycerol Suppositories, BP
[1]Ibuprofen Oral Suspension, BP
[1]Ibuprofen Tablets, BP
Ispaghula Husk Granules, BP
Ispaghula Husk Granules, Effervescent, BP
Ispaghula Husk Oral Powder, BP
Lactulose Solution, BP
Lidocaine Ointment, BP
Lidocaine and Chlorhexidine Gel, BP
Macrogol Oral Powder, Compound, NPF
Macrogol Oral Powder, Compound, Half-strength, NPF
Magnesium Hydroxide Mixture, BP
Magnesium Sulphate Paste, BP
Malathion aqueous lotions containing at least 0.5%
Mebendazole Oral Suspension, NPF
Mebendazole Tablets, NPF
Methylcellulose Tablets, BP
Miconazole Cream 2%, BP
Miconazole Oromucosal Gel, BP
Mouthwash Solution-tablets, NPF
Nicotine Inhalation Cartridge for Oromucosal Use, NPF
Nicotine Lozenge, NPF
Nicotine Medicated Chewing Gum, NPF
Nicotine Nasal Spray, NPF
Nicotine Sublingual Tablets, NPF
Nicotine Transdermal Patches, NPF
Nystatin Oral Suspension, BP
Olive Oil Ear Drops, BP

Paracetamol Oral Suspension, BP (includes 120 mg/5 mL and 250 mg/5 mL strengths—both of which are available as sugar-free formulations)
[2]Paracetamol Tablets, BP
[2]Paracetamol Tablets, Soluble, BP (includes 120-mg and 500-mg tablets)
Permethrin Cream, NPF
Phosphates Enema, BP
Phosphate suppositories, NPF
Piperazine and Senna Powder, NPF
Povidone–Iodine Solution, BP
Senna Oral Solution, NPF
Senna Tablets, BP
Senna and Ispaghula Granules, NPF
Sodium Chloride Solution, Sterile, BP
Sodium Citrate Compound Enema, NPF
Sodium Picosulfate Capsules, NPF
Sodium Picosulfate Elixir, NPF
Spermicidal contraceptives as listed below:
  Gygel® Contraceptive Jelly
Sterculia Granules, NPF
Sterculia and Frangula Granules, NPF
Titanium Ointment, BP
Water for Injections, BP
Zinc and Castor Oil Ointment, BP
Zinc Cream, BP
Zinc Ointment, BP
Zinc Oxide and Dimeticone Spray, NPF
Zinc Oxide Impregnated Medicated Bandage, NPF
Zinc Oxide Impregnated Medicated Stocking, NPF
Zinc Paste Bandage, BP 1993
Zinc Paste and Ichthammol Bandage, BP 1993

Appliances and Reagents (including Wound Management Products)

Community Practitioner Nurse Prescribers in England, Wales and Northern Ireland can prescribe any appliance or reagent in the relevant Drug Tariff. In the Scottish Drug Tariff, Appliances and Reagents which may **not** be prescribed by Nurses are annotated **Nx**.

Appliances (including Contraceptive Devices[3]) as listed in Part IXA of the Drug Tariff (Part III of the Northern Ireland Drug Tariff, Part 3 (Appliances) and Part 2 (Dressings) of the Scottish Drug Tariff)

Incontinence Appliances as listed in Part IXB of the Drug Tariff (Part III of the Northern Ireland Drug Tariff, Part 5 of the Scottish Drug Tariff)

Stoma Appliances and Associated Products as listed in Part IXC of the Drug Tariff (Part III of the Northern Ireland Drug Tariff, Part 6 of the Scottish Drug Tariff)

Chemical Reagents as listed in Part IXR of the Drug Tariff (Part II of the Northern Ireland Drug Tariff, Part 9 of the Scottish Drug Tariff)

> The Drug Tariffs can be accessed online at:
>
> National Health Service Drug Tariff for England and Wales: www.ppa.org.uk/ppa/edt_intro.htm
>
> Health and Personal Social Services for Northern Ireland Drug Tariff: www.centralservicesagency.com/display/ni_drug_tariff
>
> Scottish Drug Tariff: www.isdscotland.org/isd/2245.html

1. Except for indications and doses that are [PoM]
2. Max. 96 tablets; max. pack size 32 tablets
3. Nurse Prescribers in Family Planning Clinics—where it is not appropriate for nurse prescribers in family planning clinics to prescribe contraceptive devices using form FP10(P) (forms FP10(CN) and FP10(PN), or when available WP10CN and WP10PN, in Wales), they may prescribe using the same system as doctors in the clinic

Nurse Independent Prescribing

Nurse Independent Prescribers (formerly known as Extended Formulary Nurse Prescribers) are able to prescribe any medicine for any medical condition, including some Controlled Drugs (see BNF).

Nurse Independent Prescribers must work within their own level of professional competence and expertise. They are recommended to prescribe generically, except where this would not be clinically appropriate or where there is no approved non-proprietary name.

Up-to-date information and guidance on nurse independent prescribing is available on the Department of Health website at
www.dh.gov.uk/nonmedicalprescribing

Non-medical prescribing

A range of non-medical healthcare professionals can prescribe medicines for patients as either Independent or Supplementary Prescribers.

Independent prescribers are practitioners responsible and accountable for the assessment of patients with previously undiagnosed or diagnosed conditions and for decisions about the clinical management required, including prescribing. They are recommended to prescribe generically, except where this would not be clinically appropriate or where there is no approved non-proprietary name.

Supplementary prescribing is a partnership between an independent prescriber (a doctor or a dentist) and a supplementary prescriber to implement an agreed Clinical Management Plan for an individual patient with that patient's agreement.

Independent and Supplementary Prescribers are identified by an annotation next to their name in the relevant professional register.

Up-to-date information and guidance on non-medical prescribing is available on the Department of Health website at www.dh.gov.uk/nonmedicalprescribing.

For information on the supply and administration of medicines to groups of patients using Patient Group Directions, see, p. 4.

Nurses

For further information on Nurse Independent Prescribing, see Nurse Prescribers' Formulary, p. 947.

Optometrists

Optometrist Independent Prescribers can prescribe any licensed medicine for ocular conditions affecting the eye and the tissues surrounding the eye, except Controlled Drugs or medicines for parenteral administration. Optometrist Independent Prescribers must work within their own level of professional competence and expertise.

Pharmacists

Pharmacist Independent Prescribers can prescribe any medicine, except Controlled Drugs, for any medical condition. Pharmacist Independent Prescribers must work within their own level of professional competence and expertise.

Index of manufacturers

The following is an alphabetical list of manufacturers and their medicines information contact details. For information on 'special-order' manufacturers and specialist importing companies see p. 957.

3M
3M Health Care Ltd
tel: (01509) 611611

A&H
Allen & Hanburys Ltd
See GSK

A1 Pharmaceuticals
A1 Pharmaceuticals Plc
tel: (01708) 528 900
sales@a1plc.co.uk

Abbey
Abbey Pharmaceuticals Ltd
tel: (01628) 771 036

Abbott
Abbott Laboratories Ltd
tel: (01628) 773 355
ukmedinfo@abbott.com

Abraxis
Abraxis BioScience Ltd
tel: 0207 081 0850
abraxismedical@idispharma.com

ABT Healthcare
ABT Healthcare UK Ltd
tel: (01565) 757783

Acorus
Acorus Therapeutics Ltd
tel: (01244) 625 152
enquiries@acorus-therapeutics.com

Actavis
Actavis UK Ltd
tel: (01271) 311 257
medinfo@actavis.co.uk

Actelion
Actelion Pharmaceuticals UK Ltd
tel: (020) 8987 3333

Activa
Activa Healthcare
tel: (0845) 060 6707
advice@activahealthcare.co.uk

ADI Medical
ADI Medical Ltd
tel: 01494 882 666
info@adimedical.co.uk

Advancis
Advancis Medical Ltd
tel: (01623) 751 500
info@advancis.co.uk

Agepha
Agepha GmbH
tel: (0203) 239 6241
uk@agepha.com

Aguettant
Aguettant Ltd
tel: (01934) 835 694
info@aguettant.co.uk

Air Products
Air Products plc
tel: (0800) 373 580

Alan Pharmaceuticals
Alan Pharmaceuticals
tel: (020) 8346 4311

Alcon
Alcon Laboratories (UK) Ltd
tel: (01442) 341 234

Alexion
Alexion Pharma UK Ltd
tel: (01932) 359 220
alexion.uk@alxn.com

ALK-Abelló
ALK-Abelló (UK) Ltd
tel: (01488) 686 016
info@uk.alk-abello.com

Allergan
Allergan Ltd
tel: (01628) 494 026

Allergy
Allergy Therapeutics Ltd
tel: (01903) 844 702
infoservices@allergytherapeutics.com

Alliance
Alliance Pharmaceuticals Ltd
tel: (01249) 705 145
medinfo@alliancepharma.co.uk

Almirall
Almirall Ltd
tel: (0800) 0087399
almirall@professionalinformation.co.uk

Alphashow
Alphashow Ltd
tel: (0870) 240 2775
info@alphashow.co.uk

Altacor
Altacor Ltd
tel: (01223) 421 411
info@altacor-pharma.com

Amdipharm
Amdipharm plc
tel: (0870) 777 7675
medinfo@amdipharm.com

Amgen
Amgen Ltd
tel: (01223) 420 305
infoline@uk.amgen.com

Anpharm
See Goldshield

Archimedes
Archimedes Pharma UK Ltd
tel: (0118) 931 5060
medicalinformation@archimedespharma.com

Ardana
Ardana Bioscience Ltd
tel: (0131) 226 8550
info@ardana.co.uk

Ardern
Ardern Healthcare Ltd
tel: (01584) 781 777
info@ardernhealthcare.com

Ark Therapeutics
Ark Therapeutics Group Plc
tel: (020) 7388 7722
info@arktherapeutics.com

Aspen
Aspen Europe GmbH
tel: 0049 (4531) 8940 2301

AS Pharma
AS Pharma Ltd
tel: (08700) 664 117
info@aspharma.co.uk

Astellas
Astellas Pharma Ltd
tel: (01784) 419 615

AstraZeneca
AstraZeneca UK Ltd
tel: 0800 7830 033
medical.informationuk@astrazeneca.com

Auden Mckenzie
Auden Mckenzie (Pharma Division) Ltd
tel: (020) 8900 2122

Aurum
Aurum Pharmaceuticals Ltd
tel: (01277) 266600
info@martindalepharma.co.uk

Axcan
Axcan Pharma SA
tel: (0033) 130 461900

Ayrton Saunders
Ayrton Saunders Ltd
tel: (0151) 709 2074
info@ayrtons.com

Bard
Bard Ltd
tel: (01293) 527 888

Basilea
Basilea Pharmaceuticals Ltd
tel: (01483) 790 023
ukmedinfo@basilea.com

Bausch & Lomb
Bausch & Lomb UK Ltd
tel: (01748) 828 864
medicalinformationUK@bausch.com

Baxter
Baxter Healthcare Ltd
tel: (01635) 206 345
surecall@baxter.com

Bayer Consumer Care
See Bayer Schering

Bayer Diabetes Care
See Bayer Schering

Bayer Diagnostics
See Bayer Schering

Bayer Schering
Bayer Schering Pharma
tel: (01635) 563 116
medical.information@bayer.co.uk

BBI Healthcare
BBI Healthcare
tel: (01792) 229 333
info@bbihealthcare.com

Beacon
Beacon Pharmaceuticals Ltd
tel: (01892) 600 930
info@beaconpharma.co.uk

Beiersdorf
Beiersdorf UK Ltd
tel: (0121) 329 8800

BHR
BHR Pharmaceuticals Ltd
tel: (024) 7635 3742
info@bhr.co.uk

Bioenvision
Bioenvision Ltd
tel: (0131) 248 3555
info@bioenvision.com

Biogen
Biogen Idec Ltd
tel: (0800) 008 7401

Biolitec
Biolitec Pharma Ltd
tel: (00353) 14637415
medical.info@biolitec.com

BioMarin
tel: (020) 7420 0800

Biotest UK
Biotest (UK) Ltd
tel: (0121) 733 3393
MedicinesInformation@biotestuk.
com

Biovitrum
Biovitrum AB
tel: (0046) 8697 2000
medical.info@biovitrum.com

Blackwell
Blackwell Supplies Ltd
tel: (01634) 877 620

BOC
BOC Medical
tel: 0800 111 333

Boehringer Ingelheim
Boehringer Ingelheim Ltd
tel: (01344) 424 600
medinfo@bra.boehringer-ingelheim.
com

Boots
Boots The Chemists
tel: (0115) 959 5165

BPC 100
The Bolton Pharmaceutical 100 Ltd
tel: (0845) 602 3907
info@bpc100.com

BPL
Bio Products Laboratory
tel: (020) 8258 2200

Braun
B Braun (Medical) Ltd
tel: (0114) 225 9000
info.bbmuk@bbraun.com

Bray
Bray Health & Leisure
tel: (01367) 240 736
info@bray.co.uk

Bristol-Myers Squibb
Bristol-Myers Squibb
Pharmaceuticals Ltd
tel: (01895) 523 000
medical.information@bms.com

Britannia
Britannia Pharmaceuticals
tel: (0870) 851 0207
enquiries@medinformation.co.uk

BSN Medical
BSN Medical Ltd
tel: (0845) 1223 600

Cambridge
Cambridge Laboratories
tel: (0191) 296 9300
customer.services@camb-labs.com

Cardinal
Cardinal Health Martindale Products
tel: (01277) 266 600
info@martindalepharma.co.uk

C D Medical
C D Medical Ltd
tel: (01629) 733 860

Celgene
Celgene Ltd
tel: (08448) 010 045
medinfo.uk.ire@celgene.com

Centrapharm
See Derma UK

Cephalon
Cephalon Ltd
tel: 0800 783 4869
ukmedinfo@cephalon.com

Chattem UK
Chattem UK Ltd
tel: (01256) 844 144

Chefaro UK
Chefaro UK Ltd
tel: (01480) 421 800

Chemidex
Chemidex Pharma Ltd
tel: (01784) 477 167
info@chemidex.co.uk

Chiesi
Chiesi Ltd
tel: (0161) 488 5555
medinfo@chiesi.uk.com

CHS
Cambridge Healthcare Supplies Ltd
tel: (01603) 735 200
customerservices@typharm.com

Chugai
Chugai Pharma UK Ltd
tel: (020) 8987 5680

Clement Clarke
Clement Clarke International Ltd
tel: (01279) 414 969
resp@clement-clarke.com

CliniMed
CliniMed Ltd
tel: (01628) 535 250
enquires@clinimed.co.uk

Clinisupplies
Clinisupplies Ltd
tel: (020) 8863 4168
info@clinisupplies.co.uk

Colgate-Palmolive
Colgate-Palmolive Ltd
tel: (01483) 302 222

Coloplast
Coloplast Ltd
tel: (01733) 392 000
gbcareteam@coloplast.com

Community
Community Foods Ltd
tel: (020) 8450 9411
email@communityfoods.co.uk

Complan Foods
Complan Foods Ltd
tel: (020) 7395 7565

ConvaTec
ConvaTec Ltd
tel: (01895) 628 400

Co-Pharma
Co-Pharma Ltd
tel: (0870) 851 0207
copharma@medicalinformation.co.
uk

Covidien
Covidien UK Commercial Ltd
tel: (01329) 224 226
medicalcustomerservices@covidien.
com

Cow & Gate
Cow & Gate
tel: (08457) 623 624
careline@inpractice.co.uk

CP
See Wockhardt

Cranage
Cranage Healthcare Ltd
tel: (01477) 549 392
db@cranagehealth.com

Crawford
Crawford Pharmaceuticals
tel: (01477) 537 596

Crucell
Crucell (UK) Ltd
tel: (0127) 462 3172
medicalinformation@crucell.co.uk

CSL Behring
CSL Behring UK Ltd
tel: (01444) 447 400
medinfo@cslbehring.com

Daiichi Sankyo
Daiichi Sankyo UK Ltd
tel: (01753) 482 771
medinfo@daiichi-sankyo.co.uk

Dallas Burston Ashbourne
Dallas Burston Ashbourne Ltd
tel: (01858) 525 643

Danetre
Danetre Health Products Ltd
tel: (01327) 310 909
enquiries@danetrehealthproducts.
com

DDD
DDD Ltd
tel: (01923) 229 251

Dee
Dee Pharmaceuticals Ltd
tel: (01978) 661993
enquiries@deepharmaceuticalsltd.
co.uk

Dental Health
Dental Health Products Ltd
tel: (01622) 749 222

Dentsply
Dentsply Ltd
tel: (01932) 837 279

Dermal
Dermal Laboratories Ltd
tel: (01462) 458 866

Derma UK
Derma UK Ltd
tel: (01462) 733 500
info@dermauk.co.uk

De Vilbiss
De Vilbiss Healthcare UK Ltd
tel: (01384) 446 688

De Witt
E C De Witt & Co Ltd
tel: (01928) 756 800
info@ecdewitt.com

Dexcel
Dexcel-Pharma Ltd
tel: (01327) 312 266
office@dexcelpharma.co.uk

DHP Healthcare
DHP Healthcare Ltd
tel: (01622) 749 222
sales@dhphealthcare.co.uk

Diatos
Diatos SA
tel: (00800) 3286 6966

Dimethaid
Dimethaid International
tel: (01491) 825 016
medinfo@dimethaid.com

Dr Falk
Dr Falk Pharma UK Ltd
tel: (01628) 536 600

Drossa
Drossa Ltd
tel: (020) 7431 9382
sales@drossa.co.uk

Durbin
Durbin plc
tel: (020) 8869 6500
info@durbin.co.uk

Eakin
T G Eakin
tel: (028) 9187 1000
mail@eakin.co.uk

Easigrip
Easigrip Ltd
tel: (01926) 497 108
enquiry@easigrip.co.uk

Ecolab
Ecolab UK
tel: (0113) 232 0066
info.healthcare@ecolab.co.uk

Egis
Egis Pharmaceuticals UK Ltd
tel: (020) 7266 2669
enquiries@medimpexuk.com

Eisai
Eisai Ltd
tel: (020) 8600 1400
lmedinfo@eisai.net

Encysive
Encysive (UK) Ltd
tel: (01895) 876 168
enquiries@encysive.co.uk

Enturia
Enturia Ltd
tel: (0800) 043 7546
enquiries@enturia.co.uk

Espere
Espere Healthcare Ltd
tel: (01234) 834 614
info@esperehealth.co.uk

Ethicon
Ethicon Ltd
tel: (01506) 594 500

Eumedica
Eumedica S.A.
tel: (0208) 444 3377
enquiries@eumedica.com

EUSA Pharma
EUSA Pharma (Europe) Ltd
tel: (01438) 740 720
medinfo-uk@eusapharma.com

Everfresh
Everfresh Natural Foods
tel: (01296) 425 333

Exelgyn
Exelgyn Laboratories
tel: (01491) 642 137

Fabre
Pierre Fabre Ltd
tel: (01962) 874 435
medicalinformation@pierre-fabre.co.
uk

Fate
Fate Special Foods
tel: (01215) 224 433

Fenton
Fenton Pharmaceuticals Ltd
tel: (020) 7224 1388
mail@Fent-Pharm.co.uk

Ferndale
Ferndale Pharmaceuticals Ltd
tel: (01937) 541 122
info@ferndalepharma.co.uk

Ferring
Ferring Pharmaceuticals (UK)
tel: (01753) 214 800

Firstplay Dietary
Firstplay Dietary Foods Ltd
tel: (0161) 474 7576

Flynn
Flynn Pharma Ltd
tel: (01438) 727 822
medinfo@flynnpharma.com

Foodlink
Foodlink (UK) Ltd
tel: (01752) 344 544
info@foodlinkltd.co.uk

Ford
Ford Medical Associates Ltd
tel: (01233) 633 224
enquiries@fordmedical.co.uk

Forest
Forest Laboratories UK Ltd
tel: (01322) 550 550
medinfo@forest-labs.co.uk

Forum
Forum Health Products Ltd
tel: (01737) 773711
health@forumgroup.co.uk

Fox
C. H. Fox Ltd
tel: (020) 7240 3111

Freebake
Freebake Ltd
tel: (0845) 603 9230
info@freebake.co.uk

Fresenius Kabi
Fresenius Kabi Ltd
tel: (01928) 533 575
med.info-uk@fresenius-kabi.com

Fresenius Medical Care
Fresenius Medical Care UK Ltd
tel: (01623) 445 139
medinfo-uk@fmc-ag.com

Kestrel
Kestrel Ltd
tel: (01530) 562 301
kestrel@ventiv.co.uk

Kestrel Ophthalmics
Kestrel Ophthalmics Ltd
tel: (01202) 658 444
info@kestrelophthalmics.co.uk

King
King Pharmaceuticals Ltd
tel: (01438) 356 924

KoRa
KoRa Healthcare Ltd
tel: (01142) 994 979
info@kora.ie

Kyowa Hakko
Kyowa Hakko UK Ltd
tel: (01753) 566 020

Labopharm
Labopharm Europe Ltd
tel: (0800) 678 3765 (UK only) or
(01908) 542 374
labopharm.uk@canreginc.com

Lantor
Lantor UK Ltd
tel: (01204) 855 000
help@lantor.co.uk

Lederle
See Wyeth

LEO
LEO Pharma
tel: (01844) 347 333
medical-info.uk@leo-pharma.com

LifeScan
LifeScan
tel: (01494) 658 750

Lilly
Eli Lilly & Co Ltd
tel: (01256) 315 000
ukmedinfo@lilly.com

Lincoln Medical
Lincoln Medical Ltd
tel: (01748) 828 785
info@lincolnmedical.co.uk

Linderma
Linderma Ltd
tel: (01942) 816 184
linderma@virgin.net

Link
See Archimedes

Lipomed
Lipomed GmbH
tel: (0049) 776 155 9222
lipomed@lipomed.com

Livwell
Livwell Ltd
tel: (0845) 120 0038
info@livwell.eu

Lornamead
Lornamead UK Ltd
tel: (01276) 674000
lornamead@dhl.com

LPC
LPC Pharmaceuticals Ltd
tel: (01582) 560 393
info@lpcpharma.com

Lundbeck
Lundbeck Ltd
tel: (01908) 638 972
ukmedicalinformation@lundbeck.com

M & A Pharmachem
M & A Pharmachem Ltd
tel: (01942) 816184
buy@mapharmachem.co.uk

Manx
Manx Healthcare
tel: (01926) 482 511
info@manxhealthcare.com

Marlborough
Marlborough Pharmaceuticals
tel: (01672) 514 187
info@marlborough-pharma.co.uk

Martindale
See Cardinal

MASTA
MASTA
tel: (0113) 238 7500
medical@masta.org

McNeil
McNeil Products Ltd
tel: (01628) 822 222

MDE
Medical Diagnostics Europe Ltd
tel: (08453) 708 077
info@mdediagnostic.co.uk

Mead Johnson
Mead Johnson Nutritionals
tel: (01895) 523 764

Meadow
Meadow Laboratories Ltd
tel: (020) 8597 1203
enquiries@meadowlabs.fsnet.co.uk

Meda
Meda Pharmaceuticals Ltd
tel: (01748) 828 810
meda@professionalinformation.co.uk

Medac
Medac (UK)
tel: (01786) 458 086
info@medac-uk.co.uk

Medical House
The Medical House plc
tel: (0114) 261 9011
info@themedicalhouse.com

Medicare
Medicare Plus International Ltd
tel: (020) 8799 7891
info@medicare-plus.com

Medihoney
Medihoney (Europe) Ltd
tel: (0800) 071 3912

Medlock
Medlock Medical Ltd
tel: (0161) 621 2100
medical.information@medlockmedical.com

MedLogic
MedLogic Global Ltd
tel: (01752) 209 955
enquiries@mlgl.co.uk

Menarini
A. Menarini Pharma UK SRL
tel: (01628) 856 400

Menarini Diagnostics
A. Menarini Diagnostics
tel: (0118) 944 4100

Merck Serono
Merck Serono Ltd
tel: (020) 8818 7373
medinfo.uk@merckserono.net

Merz
Merz Pharma UK Ltd
tel: (020) 8236 0000
info@merzpharma.co.uk

Micro Medical
Micro Medical Ltd
tel: (01634) 893 500
sales@micromedical.co.uk

Milupa
Milupa Aptamil
tel: (0845) 762 3676
careline@aptamil4hcps.co.uk

Mölnlycke
Mölnlycke Health Care Ltd
tel: (0161) 777 2628
info.uk@molnlycke.net

Morningside
Morningside Healthcare Ltd
tel: (0116) 204 5950

Movianto
Movianto UK
tel: (01234) 248 500
movianto.uk@movianto.com

MSD
Merck Sharp & Dohme Ltd
tel: (01992) 467 272

Nagor
Nagor Ltd
tel: (01624) 625 556
enquiries@nagor.com

Napp
Napp Pharmaceuticals Ltd
tel: (01223) 424 444

Neolab
Neolab Ltd
tel: (01256) 704 110
info@neolab.co.uk

Neomedic
Neomedic Ltd
tel: (01923) 836 379
marketing@neomedic.co.uk

Nestlé
Nestlé Nutrition
tel: (020) 8667 5130
nutrition@uk.nestle.com

Nordic
Nordic Pharma UK Ltd
tel: (0118) 929 8233
info@nordicpharma.co.uk

Norgine
Norgine Pharmaceuticals Ltd
tel: (01895) 826 600

Novartis
Novartis Pharmaceuticals UK Ltd
tel: (01276) 692 255

Novartis Consumer Health
Novartis Consumer Health
tel: (01403) 210 211
medicalaffairs.uk@novartis.com

Novartis Vaccines
Novartis Vaccines Ltd
tel: (08457) 451 500
service.uk@novartis.com

Novo Nordisk
Novo Nordisk Ltd
tel: (01293) 613 555
customercareuk@novonordisk.com

nSPIRE Health
nSPIRE Health Ltd
tel: (01992) 526 300
info@nspirehealth.com

Nutricia Clinical
Nutricia Clinical Care
tel: (01225) 711 688
resourcecentre@nutricia.com

Nutrinovo
Nutrinovo Ltd
tel: (01304) 829 068
info@nutrinovo.com

Nutrition Point
Nutrition Point Ltd
tel: (07041) 544 044
info@nutritionpoint.co.uk

Nycomed
Nycomed UK Ltd
tel: (0800) 633 5797
medinfo@nycomed.com

OakMed
OakMed Ltd
tel: (0800) 592 786
orders@oakmed.co.uk

Octapharma
Octapharma Ltd
tel: (0161) 837 3770
octapharma@octapharma.co.uk

Omron
Omron Healthcare (UK) Ltd
tel: (0870) 750 2771
info.omronhealthcare.uk@eu.omron.
com

Organon
Organon Laboratories Ltd
tel: (01223) 432 700
medrequest@organon.co.uk

Orion
Orion Pharma (UK) Ltd
tel: (01635) 520 300
medicalinformation@orionpharma.
com

Orphan Europe
Orphan Europe (UK) Ltd
tel: (01491) 414 333
infouk@orphan-europe.com

Otsuka
Otsuka Pharmaceutical (UK) Ltd
tel: (020) 8742 4300
medinfo@otsuka.co.uk

Ovation
Ovation Healthcare International Ltd
tel: (00353) 161 39 707

Owen Mumford
Owen Mumford Ltd
tel: (01993) 812 021
customerservices@owenmumford.
co.uk

Oxford Nutrition
Oxford Nutrition Ltd
tel: (01626) 832 067
info@nutrinox.com

Paines & Byrne
Paines & Byrne Ltd
tel: (01784) 419 620

Pari
PARI Medical Ltd
tel: (01932) 341 122
infouk@pari.de

Parkside
Parkside Healthcare
tel: (0161) 795 2792

Peckforton
Peckforton Pharmaceuticals Ltd
tel: (01270) 582 255
info@peckforton.com

Penn
Penn Pharmaceuticals Services Ltd
tel: (01495) 711 222
penn@pennpharm.co.uk

Pfizer
Pfizer Ltd
tel: (01304) 616 161

PGR Health Foods
PGR Health Foods Ltd
tel: (01992) 581715
info@pgrhealthfoods.co.uk

Pharmacia
See Pfizer

Pharma-Global
Pharma-Global Ltd
tel: (00353) 1280 1104
eyecare@pharmaglobal.ie

Pharma Mar
See IDIS

Pharma Nord
Pharma Nord (UK) Ltd
tel: (01670) 519989
info@pharmanord.co.uk

Pharmasure
Pharmasure Ltd
tel: (01923) 233 466
info@pharmasure.co.uk

Pinewood
Pinewood Healthcare
tel: (00353) 523 6253
info@pinewood.ie

Potters
Potters Herbal Medicines
tel: (01942) 219 960
info@pottersherbals.co.uk

Procter & Gamble
Procter & Gamble UK
tel: (01932) 896 000

Procter & Gamble Pharm.
Procter & Gamble Technical Centres
tel: (01784) 474 900

Profile
Profile Pharma Ltd
tel: (0800) 1300 855
info@profilepharma.com

ProStrakan
ProStrakan Ltd
tel: (01896) 664 000
medinfo@prostrakan.com

Protex
Protex Healthcare (UK) Ltd
tel: (08700) 114 112
orders@protexhealthcare.co.uk

Ranbaxy
Ranbaxy UK Ltd
tel: (020) 8280 1986
medinfoeurope@ranbaxy.com

Ransom
Ransom Consumer Healthcare
tel: (01462) 437 615
info@williamransom.com

Ratiopharm UK
Ratiopharm UK Ltd
tel: (02392) 313 587
info@ratiopharmdirect.co.uk

Reckitt Benckiser
Reckitt Benckiser Healthcare
tel: (01482) 326 151
info.MIU@reckittbenckiser.com

Recordati
Recordati Pharmaceuticals Ltd
tel: (01491) 576 336
medinfo@recordati.co.uk

ReSource Medical
ReSource Medical UK Ltd
tel: (01484) 531 489
info@resource-medical.co.uk

Respironics
Philips Respironics (UK) Ltd
tel: (0800) 1300 840
rukmarketing@respironics.com

Richardson
Richardson Healthcare Ltd
tel: (08700) 111 126
info@richardsonhealthcare.com

Riemser
Riemser Arzneimittel AG
tel: (0049) 38351 76 679
info@RIEMSER.de

RIS Products
RIS Products Ltd
tel: (01438) 840 135
info@risproducts.co.uk

Robinsons
Robinson Healthcare Ltd
tel: (01909) 735 001
enquiries@robinsoncare.com

Roche
Roche Products Ltd
tel: (0800) 328 1629
medinfo.uk@roche.com

Roche Diagnostics
Roche Diagnostics Ltd
tel: (01444) 256 000
burgesshill.accu-chek@roche.com

Rosemont
Rosemont Pharmaceuticals Ltd
tel: (0800) 919 312
infodesk@rosemontpharma.com

Rowa
Rowa Pharmaceuticals Ltd
tel: (00 353 27) 50077
rowa@rowa-pharma.ie

S&N Hlth.
Smith & Nephew Healthcare Ltd
tel: (01482) 222 200
advice@smith-nephew.com

Sallis
Sallis Healthcare Ltd
tel: (0115) 978 7841

Sandoz
Sandoz Ltd
tel: (01420) 478 301
uk.drugsafety@sandoz.com

Sanochemia
Sanochemia Diagnostics UK Ltd
tel: (0117) 906 3562

Sanofi-Aventis
Sanofi-Aventis Ltd
tel: (01483) 505 515
uk-medicalinformation@
sanofi-aventis.com

Sanofi Pasteur
Sanofi Pasteur MSD Ltd
tel: (01628) 785 291

Schering-Plough
Schering-Plough Ltd
tel: (01707) 363 636
medical.info@spcorp.com

Schuco
Schuco International Ltd
tel: (020) 8368 1642
sales@schuco.co.uk

Schülke
Schülke UK
tel: (0114) 254 3500
mail.uk@schuelke.com

Scope Ophthalmics
Scope Ophthamics Ltd
tel: (0161) 266 1011
info@scopeophthalmics.com

Servier
Servier Laboratories Ltd
tel: (01753) 666 409
medical.information@uk.netgrs.com

Seven Seas
Seven Seas Ltd
tel: (01482) 375 234

Shermond
Shermond
tel: (0870) 242 7701
sales@shermond.com

Shire
Shire Pharmaceuticals Ltd
tel: (0800) 055 6614
medinfoglobal@shire.com

SHS
SHS International Ltd
tel: (0151) 228 8161
nutrition@shsint.co.uk

Siemens
Siemens Healthcare Diagnostics Ltd
tel: (0845) 600 1966
dx-diag_sales-uk.med@siemens.com

Sigma
Sigma Pharmaceuticals plc
tel: (01923) 444 999
info@sigpharm.co.uk

Sigma-Tau
Sigma-Tau Pharma Ltd (UK)
tel: (0800) 043 1268
medical.information@sigma-tau.co.
uk

Skin Camouflage Co.
The Skin Camouflage Company Ltd
tel: (01507) 343 091
smjcovermark@aol.com

Skinnies
Skinnies UK
tel: (01562) 546 123
info@skinniesuk.com

SLO Drinks
SLO Drinks Ltd
tel: (08452) 22 22 05
info@slodrinks.com

SMA Nutrition
See Wyeth

SNBTS
Scottish National Blood Transfusion
Service
tel: (0131) 536 5700
Contact.pfc@snbts.csa.scot.nhs.uk

Solvay
Solvay Healthcare Ltd
tel: (023) 8046 7000
medinfo.shl@solvay.com

Sovereign
See Amdipharm

Speciality European
Speciality European Pharma Ltd
tel: (0207) 421 7400
info@SpePharma.com

Spectrum
Spectrum Thea Pharmaceuticals
tel: (0845) 521 1290

SpePharm
SpePharm UK Ltd
tel: (0844) 800 7579
medinfo.uk@spepharm.com

Squibb
See Bristol-Myers Squibb

SSL
SSL International plc
tel: (08701) 222 690
medical.information@
ssl-international.com

STD Pharmaceutical
STD Pharmaceutical Products Ltd
tel: (01432) 373 555
enquiries@stdpharm.co.uk

Steraid
Steraid (Gainsborough) Ltd
tel: (01427) 677 659

Stiefel
Stiefel Laboratories (UK) Ltd
tel: (01628) 612 000
general@stiefel.co.uk

Stragen
Stragen UK Ltd
tel: (0870) 351 8744
info@stragenuk.com

Su-Med
Su-Med International UK Ltd
tel: (01457) 890 980
sales@sumed.co.uk

Sutherland
Sutherland Health Ltd
tel: (01635) 874 488

Swedish Orphan
Swedish Orphan International Ltd
tel: (01638) 722 380

Synergy Healthcare
Synergy Healthcare (UK) Ltd
tel: (0161) 624 5641
healthcaresolutions@
synergyhealthplc.com

Syner-Med
Syner-Med (Pharmaceutical
Products) Ltd
tel: (0845) 634 2100
mail@syner-med.com

Systagenix
Systagenix Wound Management
tel: (01344) 871 000

Takeda
Takeda UK Ltd
tel: (01628) 537 900

Talley
Talley Group Ltd
tel: (01794) 503 500

Taro
Taro Pharmaceuticals (UK) Ltd
tel: (08707) 369 544
customerservice@taropharma.co.uk

Teofarma
Teofarma S.r.l.
tel: (01748) 828 857
teofarma@professionalinformation.
co.uk

Teva
Teva Pharmaceuticals Ltd
med.info@tevapharma.co.uk

TEVA UK
TEVA UK Ltd
tel: (08705) 020 304
medinfo@tevauk.com

The Medicines Company
The Medicines Company
tel: (00) 800 8436 3326
GCHS.MI@Quintiles.com

Therabel
Therabel Pharma UK Ltd
tel: (0800) 066 5446
info@dyloject.co.uk

Thomas Blake
Thomas Blake Cosmetic Creams Ltd
tel: (01207) 279 432
sales@veilcover.com

Thornton & Ross
Thornton & Ross Ltd
tel: (01484) 842 217
mail@thorntonross.com

Tillomed
Tillomed Laboratories Ltd
tel: (01480) 402 400
info@tillomed.co.uk

Tobia Teff
Tobia Teff UK Ltd
tel: (0207) 328 2045
info@tobiateff.co.uk

TopoTarget
TopoTarget A/S
tel: (00 45 39) 178 392

Torbet
Torbet Laboratories Ltd
tel: (01603) 735 200
torbet@typharm.com

Transdermal
Transdermal Ltd
tel: (020) 8654 2251
transdermal@transdermal.co.uk

TRB Chemedica
TRB Chemedica (UK) Ltd
tel: (0845) 330 7556

Typharm
Typharm Ltd
tel: (01603) 735 200
customerservices@typharm.com

UCB Pharma
UCB Pharma Ltd
tel: (01753) 534 655
medicalinformationuk@ucb.com

Ultrapharm
Ultrapharm Ltd
tel: (01491) 578 016
orders@glutenfree.co.uk

Univar
Univar Ltd
tel: (01908) 362 200
trientine@univareurope.com

Unomedical
Unomedical Ltd
tel: (01527) 587 700

Urgo
Urgo Ltd
tel: (01509) 502 051
medical@parema.com

Valeant
Valeant Pharmaceuticals Ltd
tel: (01256) 707 744
valeantuk@valeant.com

Vegenat
c/o Archaelis Ltd
tel: (0870) 803 2484
info@vegenat.co.uk

ViiV
ViiV Healthcare UK Ltd
See GSK

Viridian
Viridian Pharma Ltd
tel: (01633) 400 335
info@viridianpharma.co.uk

Vitaflo
Vitaflo International Ltd
tel: (0151) 709 9020
vitaflo@vitaflo.co.uk

Vitaline
Vitaline Pharmaceuticals UK Ltd
tel: (01844) 269 007
vitalineinfo@aol.com

Vitalograph
Vitalograph Ltd
tel: (01280) 827 110
sales@vitalograph.co.uk

Wallace Cameron
Wallace Cameron Ltd
tel: (01698) 354 600
sales@wallacecameron.com

Wallace Mfg
Wallace Manufacturing Chemists Ltd
tel: (01235) 538 700
info@alinter.co.uk

WaveSense
WaveSense Europe Ltd
tel: (01235) 838 639
enquiries@wavesense.co.uk

Wellfoods
Wellfoods Ltd
tel: (01226) 381 712
wellfoods@talk21.com

Williams
Williams Medical Supplies Ltd
tel: (01685) 844 739

Winthrop
Winthrop Pharmaceuticals UK Ltd
tel: (01483) 554 101
winthrop@professionalinformation.
co.uk

Wockhardt
Wockhardt UK Ltd
tel: (01978) 661 261

Wyeth
Wyeth Pharmaceuticals
tel: (01628) 604 377
ukmedinfo@wyeth.com

Wynlit
Wynlit Laboratories
tel: (07903) 370 130

Wyvern
Wyvern Medical Ltd
tel: (01531) 631 105

Zeroderma
Zeroderma Ltd
tel: (01858) 525 643
info@ixlpharma.com

ZooBiotic
ZooBiotic Ltd
tel: (0845) 230 1810
maggots@smtl.co.uk

Special-order Manufacturers

Unlicensed medicines are available from 'special order' manufacturers and specialist importing companies; the MHRA maintains a register of these companies at http://tinyurl.com/cdslke.

Licensed **hospital manufacturing units** also manufacture 'special-order' products as unlicensed medicines, the principal NHS units are listed below. A database (*Pro-File*; www.pro-file.nhs.uk) provides information on all medicines manufactured in the NHS; access is restricted to NHS pharmacy staff.

The Association of Commercial Specials Manufacturers may also be able to provide further information about commercial companies (www.acsm.uk.com).

The characteristics of unlicensed formulations may vary, see also Unlicensed Medicines (p. 7) and Extemporaneous Preparations (p. 8).

> The MHRA recommends that an unlicensed medicine should only be used when a patient has special requirements that cannot be met by use of a licensed medicine

England

London

Barts and the London NHS Trust
Mr J. Singh
Production Manager
Barts and the London NHS Trust
Pathology and Pharmacy Building
Royal London Hospital
80 Newark St
Whitechapel
London, E1 2ES.
tel: (020) 3246 0399
jasdeep.singh@bartsandthelondon.nhs.uk

Guy's and St. Thomas' NHS Foundation Trust
Mr P. Forsey
Associate Chief Pharmacist
Guy's and St. Thomas' NHS Foundation Trust
Pharmacy Department
Guy's Hospital
Great Maze Pond
London, SE1 9RT.
tel: (020) 7188 5003
fax: (020) 7188 5013
paul.forsey@gstt.nhs.uk

Moorfields Pharmaceuticals
Mr N. Precious
Technical Director
Moorfields Pharmaceuticals
25 Provost St
London, N1 7NH.
tel: (020) 7684 8574
fax: (020) 7502 2332
Nick.Precious@moorfields.nhs.uk

North West London Hospitals NHS Trust
Dr K. Middleton
North West London Hospitals NHS Trust
Northwick Park Hospital
Watford Rd
Harrow
Middlesex, HA1 3UJ.
tel: (020) 8869 2204/2223
keith.middleton@nwlh.nhs.uk

Royal Free Hampstead NHS Trust
Ms C. Trehane
Production Manager
Royal Free
Pond St
London, NW3 2QG.
tel: (020) 7830 2282
fax: (020) 7794 1875
christine.trehane@royalfree.nhs.uk

St George's Healthcare NHS Trust
Mr V. Kumar
Assistant Chief Pharmacist
Technical Services
St George's Hospital
Blackshaw Rd
Tooting
London, SW17 0QT.
tel: (020) 8725 1770/1768
fax: (020) 8725 3947
Vinodh.kumar@stgeorges.nhs.uk

University College Hospital NHS Foundation Trust
Mr T. Murphy
Production Manager
University College Hospital
235 Euston Rd
London, NW1 2BU.
tel: (020) 7380 9472
fax: (020) 7380 9726
Tony.murphy@uclh.nhs.uk

Midlands and Eastern

Burton Hospitals NHS Trust
Mr P. Williams
Pharmacy Technical and Support Services Manager
Pharmacy Manufacturing Unit
Queens Hospital
Burton Hospitals NHS Trust
Belvedere Rd
Burton-on-Trent, DE13 0RB.
tel: (01283) 511 511 (or 566 333) ext: 5138
fax: (01283) 593 036
Paul.Williams@burtonh-tr.wmids.nhs.uk

Colchester Hospital University NHS Foundation Trust
Dr R. Needle
Chief Pharmacist
Colchester Hospital University NHS Foundation Trust
Tuner Rd
Colchester, C04 5JL.
tel: (01206) 742 433
fax: (01206) 841 249
richard.needle@colchesterhospital.nhs.uk

Ipswich Hospital NHS Trust
Dr J. Harwood
Production Manager
Pharmacy Manufacturing Unit
Ipswich Hospital NHS Trust
Heath Rd
Ipswich, IP4 5PD.
tel: (01473) 703 603
fax: (01473) 703 609
john.harwood@ipswichhospital.nhs.uk

Nottingham University Hospitals NHS Trust
Ms J. Kendall
Assistant Head of Pharmacy, Technical, and Logistical Services
Pharmacy Production Units
Nottingham University Hospitals
NHS Trust
Queens Medical Centre Campus
Nottingham, NG7 2UH.
tel: (0115) 924 9924 ext: 64177
fax: (0115) 970 9780
Jeanette.Kendall@nuh.nhs.uk

University Hospital of North Staffordshire NHS Trust
Ms K. Ferguson
Chief Technician
Pharmacy Technical Services
University Hospital of North Staffordshire NHS Trust
City General Site
Stoke-on-Trent, ST4 6QG.
tel: (01782) 552 290
fax: (01782) 552 916
Caroline.ferguson@uhns.nhs.uk

North East

The Newcastle upon Tyne Hospitals NHS Foundation Trust
Mr Y. Hunter-Blair
Production Manager
Newcastle Specials
Pharmacy Production Unit
Royal Victoria Infirmary
Queen Victoria Rd
Newcastle-upon-Tyne, NE1 4LP.
tel: (0191) 282 0389
fax: (0191) 282 0469
yan.hunter-blair@nuth.nhs.uk

North West

Preston Pharmaceuticals
Mr A. Cole
Preston Pharmaceuticals
Royal Preston Hospital
Fulwood
Preston, PR2 9HT.
tel: (01772) 522 316
fax: (01772) 523 645
alan.cole@lthtr.nhs.uk

Stockport Pharmaceuticals
Mr M. Booth
Principal Pharmacist/Deputy Chief Pharmacist
Stockport Pharmaceuticals
Pharmacy Department
Stepping Hill Hospital
Stockport
Cheshire, SK2 7JE.
tel: (0161) 419 5657
fax: (0161) 419 5426
mike.booth@stockport.nhs.uk

South East

East Sussex Hospitals NHS Trust
Mr J. Sullivan
Pharmacy Manufacturing Unit Services Manager
Eastbourne DGH Pharmaceuticals
Eastbourne District General Hospital
East Sussex Hospitals NHS Trust
Kings Drive, Eastbourne
East Sussex, BN21 2UD.
tel: (01323) 417 400 ext: 3076
fax: (01323) 414 931
John.Sullivan@esht.nhs.uk

South West

Torbay PMU
Mr P. Bendell
Pharmacy Manufacturing Services Manager
Torbay PMU
South Devon Healthcare
Kemmings Close, Long Rd
Paignton
Devon, TQ4 7TW.
tel: (01803) 664 707
fax: (01803) 664 354
phil.bendell@nhs.net

Yorkshire

Calderdale and Huddersfield NHS Foundation Trust
Dr S. Langford
Pharmacy Production Director
Pharmacy Manufacturing Unit
Huddersfield Royal Infirmary
Gate 2-Acre Mills, School St
Lindley
Huddersfield, HD3 3ET.
tel: (01484) 355 371
fax: (01484) 355 377
stephen.langford@cht.nhs.uk

Northern Ireland

Victoria Pharmaceuticals
Ms C. McBride
Victoria Pharmaceuticals
Belfast Health and Social Care Trust
77 Boucher Crescent
Belfast, BT12 6HU.
tel: (02890) 553 407
fax: (02890) 328 972 (sterile)
fax: (02890) 553 498 (non-sterile)
colettemcbride@belfasttrust.hscni.net

Scotland

NHS Greater Glasgow and Clyde
Mr G. Conkie
Pharmacy Manager
Western Infirmary
Dumbarton Rd
Glasgow, G11 6NT.
tel: (0141) 211 2882
fax: (0141) 211 1967
graham.conkie@ggc.scot.nhs.uk

Tayside Pharmaceuticals
Dr B.W. Millar
General Manager
Tayside Pharmaceuticals
Ninewells Hospital
Dundee, DD1 9SY.
tel: (01382) 632 183
fax: (01382) 632 060
baxter.millar@nhs.net

Wales

Cardiff and Vale University Health Board
Mr P. Spark
Principal Pharmacist (Production)
Cardiff and Vale University Health Board
20 Fieldway
Cardiff, CF14 4HY.
tel: (02920) 748 120
fax: (02920) 748 130
paul.spark@wales.nhs.uk

Index

Index

Index

Index

Index

Index

Index

Yellowcard

In Confidence

COMMISSION ON HUMAN MEDICINES

SUSPECTED ADVERSE DRUG REACTIONS

MHRA

If you suspect that an adverse reaction may be related to a drug, or a combination of drugs, you should complete this Yellow Card or complete a report on the website at www.yellowcard.gov.uk. For *intensively monitored medicines* (identified by ▼) report **all** suspected reactions (including any considered not to be serious). For *established drugs* and *herbal remedies* report **all serious** adverse reactions in adults; report **all serious and minor** adverse reactions in **children** (under 18 years). You do not have to be certain about causality: if in doubt, please report. Do not be put off reporting just because some details are not known. See BNFC (page 15) or the MHRA website (www.yellowcard.gov.uk) for additional advice.

PATIENT DETAILS Patient Initials: _____ Sex: M / F Weight if known (kg): _____

Age (at time of reaction): _____ Identification (Your Practice / Hospital Ref.)*: _____

SUSPECTED DRUG(S)

Give brand name of drug and batch number if known	Route	Dosage	Date started	Date stopped	Prescribed for

---

SUSPECTED REACTION(S)

Please describe the reaction(s) and any treatment given:

Outcome

☐ Recovered
☐ Recovering
☐ Continuing
☐ Other

Date reaction(s) started: _____ Date reaction(s) stopped: _____

Do you consider the reaction to be serious? Yes / No

If *yes*, please indicate why the reaction is considered to be serious (please tick all that apply):

☐ Patient died due to reaction ☐ Involved or prolonged inpatient hospitalisation
☐ Life threatening ☐ Involved persistent or significant disability or incapacity
☐ Congenital abnormality ☐ Medically significant; please give details:

---

* This is to enable you to identify the patient in any future correspondence concerning this report

Please attach additional pages if necessary

Please list other drugs taken in the last 3 months prior to the reaction (including self-medication & herbal remedies)

Was the patient on any other medication? Yes / No If *yes*, please give the following information if known:

Drug (Brand, if known)	Route	Dosage	Date started	Date stopped	Prescribed for

Additional relevant information e.g. medical history, test results, known allergies, rechallenge (if performed), suspected drug interactions. For congenital abnormalities please state all other drugs taken during pregnancy and the date of the last menstrual period.

REPORTER DETAILS Name and Professional Address:	**CLINICIAN (if not the reporter)** Name and Professional Address:
Post code:	Post code:
Speciality: _____ Tel No:	Tel No: _____ Speciality:
Signature:	If you would like information about other adverse reactions
Date:	associated with the suspected drug, please tick this box ☐

If you report from an area served by a Yellow Card Centre (YCC), MHRA may ask the Centre to communicate with you, on its behalf, about your report. See BNFC (page 15) for further details on YCCs. If you want only MHRA to contact you, please tick this box. ☐

Send to **Medicines and Healthcare products Regulatory Agency, CHM FREEPOST SW2991, LONDON SW8 5BR**

Yellowcard®

COMMISSION ON HUMAN MEDICINES

In Confidence

MHRA

SUSPECTED ADVERSE DRUG REACTIONS

If you suspect that an adverse reaction may be related to a drug, or a combination of drugs, you should complete this Yellow Card or complete a report on the website at www.yellowcard.gov.uk. For *intensively monitored medicines* (identified by ▼) report **all** suspected reactions (including any considered not to be serious). For *established drugs* and *herbal remedies* report **all serious** adverse reactions in adults; report **all serious and minor** adverse reactions in **children** (under 18 years). You do not have to be certain about causality: if in doubt, please report. Do not be put off reporting just because some details are not known. See BNFC (page 15) or the MHRA website (www.yellowcard.gov.uk) for additional advice.

PATIENT DETAILS   Patient Initials: _____   Sex: M / F   Weight if known (kg): _____

Age (at time of reaction): _____   Identification (Your Practice / Hospital Ref.)*: _____

SUSPECTED DRUG(S)
Give brand name of drug
and batch number if known

Route	Dosage	Date started	Date stopped	Prescribed for

SUSPECTED REACTION(S)
Please describe the reaction(s) and any treatment given:

Outcome

☐ Recovered
☐ Recovering
☐ Continuing
☐ Other

Date reaction(s) started: _____   Date reaction(s) stopped: _____

Do you consider the reaction to be serious? Yes / No

If *yes*, please indicate why the reaction is considered to be serious (please tick all that apply):

☐ Patient died due to reaction   ☐ Involved or prolonged inpatient hospitalisation
☐ Life threatening   ☐ Involved persistent or significant disability or incapacity
☐ Congenital abnormality   ☐ Medically significant; please give details:

* This is to enable you to identify the patient in any future correspondence concerning this report

Please attach additional pages if necessary

Please list other drugs taken in the last 3 months prior to the reaction (including self-medication & herbal remedies)

Was the patient on any other medication?   Yes / No   If *yes*, please give the following information if known:

Drug (Brand, if known)	Route	Dosage	Date started	Date stopped	Prescribed for

Additional relevant information e.g. medical history, test results, known allergies, rechallenge (if performed), suspected drug interactions. For congenital abnormalities please state all other drugs taken during pregnancy and the date of the last menstrual period.

REPORTER DETAILS	**CLINICIAN (if not the reporter)**
Name and Professional Address:	Name and Professional Address:
Post code: _____	Post code: _____
Speciality: _____ Tel No: _____	Speciality: _____ Tel No: _____
Signature: _____ Date: _____	
	If you would like information about other adverse reactions associated with the suspected drug, please tick this box ☐

If you report from an area served by a Yellow Card Centre (YCC), MHRA may ask the Centre to communicate with you, on its behalf, about your report. See BNFC (page 15) for further details on YCCs. If you want only MHRA to contact you, please tick this box. ☐

Send to **Medicines and Healthcare products Regulatory Agency, CHM FREEPOST SW2991, LONDON SW8 5BR**

Yellowcard

COMMISSION ON HUMAN MEDICINES

In Confidence

SUSPECTED ADVERSE DRUG REACTIONS

MHRA

If you suspect that an adverse reaction may be related to a drug, or a combination of drugs, you should complete this Yellow Card or complete a report on the website at www.yellowcard.gov.uk. For *intensively monitored medicines* (identified by ▼) report **all** suspected reactions (including any considered not to be serious). For *established drugs* and *herbal remedies* report **all serious** adverse reactions in adults; report **all serious and minor** adverse reactions in **children** (under 18 years). You do not have to be certain about causality: if in doubt, please report. Do not be put off reporting just because some details are not known. See BNFC (page 15) or the MHRA website (www.yellowcard.gov.uk) for additional advice.

PATIENT DETAILS	Patient Initials:		Sex: M / F	Weight if known (kg):
Age (at time of reaction):		Identification (Your Practice / Hospital Ref.)*:		

SUSPECTED DRUG(S) Give brand name of drug and batch number if known	Route	Dosage	Date started	Date stopped	Prescribed for

SUSPECTED REACTION(S)
Please describe the reaction(s) and any treatment given:

Outcome

Recovered ☐
Recovering ☐
Continuing ☐
Other ☐

Date reaction(s) started: _____ Date reaction(s) stopped: _____

Do you consider the reaction to be serious? Yes / No

If *yes*, please indicate why the reaction is considered to be serious (please tick all that apply):

Involved or prolonged inpatient hospitalisation ☐
Patient died due to reaction ☐ Involved persistent or significant disability or incapacity ☐
Life threatening ☐ Medically significant; please give details:
Congenital abnormality ☐

* This is to enable you to identify the patient in any future correspondence concerning this report

Please attach additional pages if necessary

Please list other drugs taken in the last 3 months prior to the reaction (including self-medication & herbal remedies)

Was the patient on any other medication?   Yes / No   If yes, please give the following information if known:

Drug (Brand, if known)	Route	Dosage	Date started	Date stopped	Prescribed for

Additional relevant information e.g. medical history, test results, known allergies, rechallenge (if performed), suspected drug interactions. For congenital abnormalities please state all other drugs taken during pregnancy and the date of the last menstrual period.

REPORTER DETAILS
Name and Professional Address:

CLINICIAN (if not the reporter)
Name and Professional Address:

Post code: _____   Tel No: _____
Post code: _____   Tel No: _____
Speciality: _____
Speciality: _____
Signature: _____
Date: _____

If you would like information about other adverse reactions associated with the suspected drug, please tick this box ☐

If you report from an area served by a Yellow Card Centre (YCC), MHRA may ask the Centre to communicate with you, on its behalf, about your report. See BNFC (page 15) for further details on YCCs. If you want only MHRA to contact you, please tick this box. ☐

Send to **Medicines and Healthcare products Regulatory Agency, CHM FREEPOST SW2991, LONDON SW8 5BR**

Yellowcard°

COMMISSION ON
HUMAN MEDICINES

In Confidence

MHRA

SUSPECTED ADVERSE DRUG REACTIONS

If you suspect that an adverse reaction may be related to a drug, or a combination of drugs, you should complete this Yellow Card or complete a report on the website at www.yellowcard.gov.uk. For *intensively monitored medicines* (identified by ▼) report **all** suspected reactions (including any considered not to be serious). For *established drugs* and *herbal remedies* report **all serious** adverse reactions in adults; report **all serious and minor** adverse reactions in **children** (under 18 years). You do not have to be certain about causality: if in doubt, please report. Do not be put off reporting just because some details are not known. See BNFC (page 15) or the MHRA website (www.yellowcard.gov.uk) for additional advice.

| **PATIENT DETAILS**   Patient Initials: _____   Sex: M / F   Weight if known (kg): _____ |
| Age (at time of reaction): _____   Identification (Your Practice / Hospital Ref.)*: _____ |

SUSPECTED DRUG(S)

Give brand name of drug and batch number if known	Route	Dosage	Date started	Date stopped	Prescribed for

SUSPECTED REACTION(S)
Please describe the reaction(s) and any treatment given:

Date reaction(s) started: _____   Date reaction(s) stopped: _____

Do you consider the reaction to be serious? Yes / No

If *yes*, please indicate why the reaction is considered to be serious (please tick all that apply):

Patient died due to reaction ☐

Life threatening ☐

Congenital abnormality ☐

Involved or prolonged inpatient hospitalisation ☐

Involved persistent or significant disability or incapacity ☐

Medically significant; please give details: ☐

Outcome

Recovered ☐

Recovering ☐

Continuing ☐

Other ☐

* This is to enable you to identify the patient in any future correspondence concerning this report

Please attach additional pages if necessary

Please list other drugs taken in the last 3 months prior to the reaction (including self-medication & herbal remedies)

Was the patient on any other medication? Yes / No If yes, please give the following information if known:

Drug (Brand, if known)	Route	Dosage	Date started	Date stopped	Prescribed for

Additional relevant information e.g. medical history, test results, known allergies, rechallenge (if performed), suspected drug interactions. For congenital abnormalities please state all other drugs taken during pregnancy and the date of the last menstrual period.

REPORTER DETAILS	**CLINICIAN (if not the reporter)**
Name and Professional Address:	Name and Professional Address:
Post code: _____ Tel No: _____	Tel No: _____ Post code: _____
Speciality: _____	Speciality: _____
Signature: _____ Date: _____	If you would like information about other adverse reactions associated with the suspected drug, please tick this box ☐
If you report from an area served by a Yellow Card Centre (YCC), MHRA may ask the Centre to communicate with you, on its behalf, about your report. See BNFC (page 15) for further details on YCCs. If you want only MHRA to contact you, please tick this box. ☐	

Send to **Medicines and Healthcare products Regulatory Agency, CHM FREEPOST SW2991, LONDON SW8 5BR**

NEWBORN LIFE SUPPORT

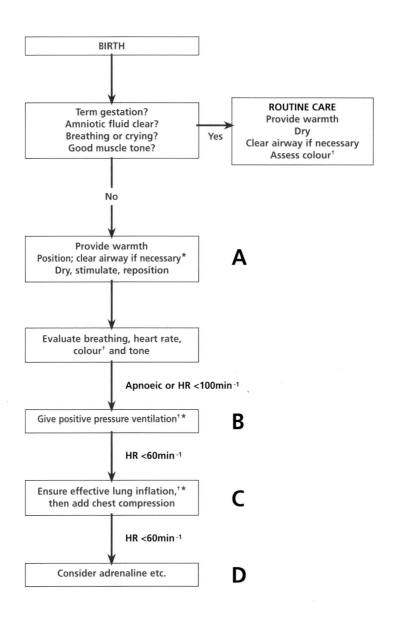

BIRTH

↓

Term gestation?
Amniotic fluid clear?
Breathing or crying?
Good muscle tone?

→ Yes →

ROUTINE CARE
Provide warmth
Dry
Clear airway if necessary
Assess colour†

↓ No

Provide warmth
Position; clear airway if necessary*
Dry, stimulate, reposition

A

↓

Evaluate breathing, heart rate, colour† and tone

↓ **Apnoeic or HR <100min⁻¹**

Give positive pressure ventilation† *   **B**

↓ **HR <60min⁻¹**

Ensure effective lung inflation,† * then add chest compression   **C**

↓ **HR <60min⁻¹**

Consider adrenaline etc.   **D**

*Tracheal intubation may be considered at several steps
†Consider supplemental oxygen at any stage if cyanosis persists

European Resuscitation Council

Resuscitation Council (UK)

PAEDIATRIC BASIC LIFE SUPPORT
(Healthcare professionals with a duty to respond)

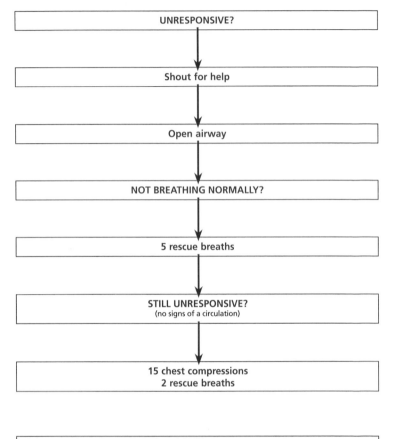

UNRESPONSIVE?

↓

Shout for help

↓

Open airway

↓

NOT BREATHING NORMALLY?

↓

5 rescue breaths

↓

STILL UNRESPONSIVE?
(no signs of a circulation)

↓

15 chest compressions
2 rescue breaths

After 1 minute call resuscitation team then continue CPR

European Resuscitation Council

Resuscitation Council (UK)

PAEDIATRIC ADVANCED LIFE SUPPORT

Unresponsive?

↓

Commence BLS
Oxygenate/ventilate

→ Call Resuscitation Team

CPR 15:2
Until defibrillator/monitor attached

↓

Assess rhythm

Shockable
(VF/pulseless VT)

Non-shockable
(PEA/Asystole)

1 Shock
4 J/kg or AED
(attenuated as appropriate)

Immediately
resume
**CPR 15:2
for 2 min**

During CPR

- Correct reversible causes*
- Check electrode position and contact
- Attempt/verify: IV/IO access, airway and oxygen
- Give uninterrupted compressions when trachea intubated
- Give adrenaline every 3-5 min
- Consider: amiodarone, atropine, magnesium

Immediately
resume
**CPR 15:2
for 2 min**

***Reversible causes**

Hypoxia	Tension pneumothorax
Hypovolaemia	Tamponade, cardiac
Hypo/hyperkalaemia/metabolic	Toxins
Hypothermia	Thromboembolism

European Resuscitation Council

Resuscitation Council (UK)

Reprinted from *Resuscitation*, 67(Suppl. 1): S97–S133, © 2005, with permission from the European Resuscitation Council and Elsevier Ireland Ltd

BODY SURFACE AREA IN CHILDREN

Body-weight under 40kg

Body-weight (kg)	Surface area (m²)	Body-weight (kg)	Surface area (m²)
1	0.10	17	0.71
1.5	0.13	18	0.74
2	0.16	19	0.77
2.5	0.19	20	0.79
3	0.21	21	0.82
3.5	0.24	22	0.85
4	0.26	23	0.87
4.5	0.28	24	0.90
5	0.30	25	0.92
5.5	0.32	26	0.95
6	0.34	27	0.97
6.5	0.36	28	1.0
7	0.38	29	1.0
7.5	0.40	30	1.1
8	0.42	31	1.1
8.5	0.44	32	1.1
9	0.46	33	1.1
9.5	0.47	34	1.1
10	0.49	35	1.2
11	0.53	36	1.2
12	0.56	37	1.2
13	0.59	38	1.2
14	0.62	39	1.3
15	0.65	40	1.3
16	0.68		

Values are calculated using the Boyd equation

Note Height is not required to estimate body surface area using these tables

Adapted by permission from Macmillan Publishers Ltd: Sharkey I et al, *British Journal of Cancer* 2001; **85** (1): 23–28, © 2001

BODY SURFACE AREA IN CHILDREN
Body-weight over 40kg

Body-weight (kg)	Surface area (m²)	Body-weight (kg)	Surface area (m²)
41	1.3	66	1.8
42	1.3	67	1.8
43	1.3	68	1.8
44	1.4	69	1.8
45	1.4	70	1.9
46	1.4	71	1.9
47	1.4	72	1.9
48	1.4	73	1.9
49	1.5	74	1.9
50	1.5	75	1.9
51	1.5	76	2.0
52	1.5	77	2.0
53	1.5	78	2.0
54	1.6	79	2.0
55	1.6	80	2.0
56	1.6	81	2.0
57	1.6	82	2.1
58	1.6	83	2.1
59	1.7	84	2.1
60	1.7	85	2.1
61	1.7	86	2.1
62	1.7	87	2.1
63	1.7	88	2.2
64	1.7	89	2.2
65	1.8	90	2.2

Values are calculated using the Boyd equation

Note Height is not required to estimate body surface area using these tables

Adapted by permission from Macmillan Publishers Ltd: Sharkey I et al, *British Journal of Cancer* 2001; **85** (1): 23–28, © 2001

Approximate conversions and units

lb	kg	stones	kg	mL	fl oz
1	0.45	1	6.35	50	1.8
2	0.91	2	12.70	100	3.5
3	1.36	3	19.05	150	5.3
4	1.81	4	25.40	200	7.0
5	2.27	5	31.75	500	17.6
6	2.72	6	38.10	1000	35.2
7	3.18	7	44.45		
8	3.63	8	50.80		
9	4.08	9	57.15		
10	4.54	10	63.50		
11	4.99	11	69.85		
12	5.44	12	76.20		
13	5.90	13	82.55		
14	6.35	14	88.90		
		15	95.25		

Length

1 metre (m)		= 1000 millimetres (mm)
1 centimetre (cm)		= 10 mm
1 inch (in)		= 25.4 mm
1 foot (ft)	= 12 inches	= 304.8 mm

Mass

1 kilogram (kg)	= 1000 grams (g)
1 gram (g)	= 1000 milligrams (mg)
1 miiligram (mg)	= 1000 micrograms
1 microgram	= 1000 nanograms
1 nanogram	= 1000 picograms

Volume

1 litre	= 1000 millilitres (mL)
1 millilitre (1 mL)	= 1000 microlitres
1 pint	≈ 568 mL

Other units

1 kilocalorie (kcal)	= 4186.8 joules (J)
1000 kilocalories (kcal)	= 4.1868 megajoules (MJ)
1 megajoule (MJ)	= 238.8 kilocalories (kcal)
1 millimetre of mercury (mmHg)	= 133.3 pascals (Pa)
1 kilopascal (kPa)	= 7.5 mmHg (pressure)

> **Plasma-drug concentrations** in *BNF for Children* are expressed in mass units per litre (e.g. mg/litre). The approximate equivalent in terms of amount of substance units (e.g. micromol/litre) is given in brackets.

Prescribing for children
Weight, height, and gender

The table below shows the **mean values** for weight, height and gender by age; these values have been derived from the UK-WHO growth charts 2009 and UK1990 standard centile charts, by extrapolating the 50th centile, and may be used to calculate doses in the absence of actual measurements. However, the child's actual weight and height might vary considerably from the values in the table and it is important to see the child to ensure that the value chosen is appropriate. In most cases the child's actual measurement should be obtained as soon as possible and the dose re-calculated.

Age	Weight kg	Height cm
Full term neonate	3.5	51
1 month	4.3	55
2 months	5.4	58
3 months	6.1	61
4 months	6.7	63
6 months	7.6	67
1 year	9	75
3 years	14	96
5 years	18	109
7 years	23	122
10 years	32	138
12 years	39	149
14 year-old boy	49	163
14 year-old girl	50	159
Adult male	68	176
Adult female	58	164

Recommended wording of cautionary and advisory labels

For details see Appendix 3

1. Warning. May cause drowsiness

2. Warning. May cause drowsiness. If affected do not drive or operate machinery. Avoid alcoholic drink

3. Warning. May cause drowsiness. If affected do not drive or operate machinery

4. Warning. Avoid alcoholic drink

5. Do not take indigestion remedies at the same time of day as this medicine

6. Do not take indigestion remedies or medicines containing iron or zinc at the same time of day as this medicine

7. Do not take milk, indigestion remedies, or medicines containing iron or zinc at the same time of day as this medicine

8. Do not stop taking this medicine except on your doctor's advice

9. Take at regular intervals. Complete the prescribed course unless otherwise directed

10. Warning. Follow the printed instructions you have been given with this medicine

11. Avoid exposure of skin to direct sunlight or sun lamps

12. Do not take anything containing aspirin while taking this medicine

13. Dissolve or mix with water before taking

14. This medicine may colour the urine

15. Caution flammable: keep away from fire or flames

16. Allow to dissolve under the tongue. Do not transfer from this container. Keep tightly closed. Discard 8 weeks after opening

17. Do not take more than... in 24 hours

18. Do not take more than... in 24 hours or... in any one week

19. Warning. Causes drowsiness which may continue the next day. If affected do not drive or operate machinery. Avoid alcoholic drink

21. ... with or after food

22. ... half to one hour before food

23. ... an hour before food or on an empty stomach

24. ... sucked or chewed

25. ... swallowed whole, not chewed

26. ... dissolved under the tongue

27. ... with plenty of water

28. To be spread thinly...

29. Do not take more than 2 at any one time. Do not take more than 8 in 24 hours

30. Do not take with any other paracetamol products

31. Contains aspirin and paracetamol. Do not take with any other paracetamol products

32. Contains aspirin

33. Contains an aspirin-like medicine